G000268736

PSYCHOTROPIC
DRUG
DIRECTORY
2012

THE PROFESSIONALS' POCKET
HANDBOOK AND AIDE MEMOIRE

Dedicated to the memory of:

Paul Woods, June 1948–July 2011
John Maher, July 1938–July 2011
Tubby Reynolds, January 1925–July 2011

The world really would have been a far duller place
without you. Thanks for everything.

The author has made every effort to ensure the
accuracy of drug dosage and other information
contained in this book. However, this does not
diminish the requirement to exercise clinical
judgement, and the author and publisher cannot
accept responsibility for the use of the information
in clinical practice.

The views expressed in this book reflect the
experience of the author and are not necessarily
those of Lundbeck Ltd. Any products referred
to by the author should only be used as
recommended in the manufacturers' Summary of
Product Characteristics.

PSYCHOTROPIC
DRUG
DIRECTORY
2012

THE PROFESSIONALS' POCKET
HANDBOOK AND AIDE MEMOIRE

STEPHEN BAZIRE

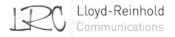

Lloyd-Reinhold
Communications

Lloyd-Reinhold Communications LLP

British Library Cataloguing-in-Publication Data
A catalogue record is available for this book

© Stephen Bazire 2012

ISBN-13 978-0-9569156-0-3

All rights reserved. No part of this publication may be reproduced, stored
in a retrieval system or transmitted in any form or by any means, electronic,
mechanical, photocopying, recording or otherwise, without prior permission from
the publishers

Printed in Malta by Gutenberg Press Limited, Tarxien, Malta

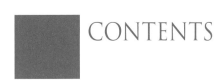

CONTENTS

CHAPTER 4: DRUG INTERACTIONS   297

CHAPTER 5: DRUG-INDUCED PSYCHIATRIC DISORDERS   405

CHAPTER 6: MANAGEMENT OF SIDE-EFFECTS 465

CHAPTER 7: PSYCHOTROPIC DRUGS 515

INDEX AND ABBREVIATIONS 529

INTRODUCTION

Why the *Psychotropic Drug Directory (PDD) 2012*? Well, the title tries to describe the contents, and how you should use them. The 'directory' part is because the book contains general principles, lists, issues, advice and references to help you make decisions but then directs you where to go to get the further information you might need, since it would be virtually impossible to convey all the subtleties of a research paper, case report or review in a couple of lines. I have, for instance, added well over 1500 new references to the text in this edition. If I spent a couple of hours thoroughly reading and analysing each and every paper, I'd never be able to finish the book and would have to give up the day job, before it gives up on me. So, you really should check papers before making important decisions. I would be hugely grateful for any advice or tips about papers that I may have taken at face value and inadvertently missed the errors, hidden bias or multiple publication.

It may be worth pointing out that this book is an entirely independent publication. There is no commercial sponsorship, support or influence on the content, which remains entirely my own work.

How to use the book...

The *PDD 2012* is arranged in a problem-solving way to aid optimum medication use:

- *Chapter 1*: select a mental health problem needing medication management and consider the pharmacological options from the BNF, combination and unlicensed lists.
- *Chapter 2* aids choosing a drug and dose, where a choice exists or is necessary.
- *Chapter 3* aids drug choice in a compromised patient.
- *Chapter 4* allows checking for drug–drug interactions.
- *Chapter 5* is an important check that the mental health problem is not drug-induced.
- *Chapter 6* helps to guide you where a drug works, but side-effects limit effectiveness.
- *Chapter 7* has got historical and other information I couldn't think where else to put.

A minimum level of knowledge is assumed and information given should be followed up in the appropriate sources when time allows. References, where quoted, are either of good recent review articles or of specific information.

Further information can be obtained by referring to the main paper or papers cited and also to the reference sections of those main papers. Lists and references are as comprehensive as viable but could never claim to be fully complete, nor could this book ever be as comprehensive as a MedLine search on a chosen topic. **The listing of a drug use in this book does not in any way imply that it is licensed in your country or safe for this use,** and all information is presented in good faith. Throughout, I have tried to be as objective as possible. It must be up to the reader to make up his or her own mind on a topic, but I hope that the statements and references will have pointed you in the right direction and the time saved in looking papers up will allow more thought. It is inevitable that some papers are from specialist journals but, where possible, I have always quoted more accessible journals in preference. If the only paper published on the use of a drug is from an obscure or ancient source this may well indicate the status of the paper.

Changes to this edition

Updates have been made to all chapters (all marked with a *), with about 1500 new references. To aid navigation we have added chapter tabs and chapter contents at the beginning of each chapter, but you have probably noticed that already. *Chapter 1* has lost epilepsy but gained postpartum depression, antipsychotics in BPSD and a great clozapine plasma level interpretation table, as well as many license changes especially in bipolar mood disorders. *Chapter 3* now has a section on sleep apnea; there is not a lot to say about it but it is a common question my service gets asked. *Chapter 5* has a new cannabis and psychosis summary.

Acknowledgements

Writing and continually updating a book such as this is a tremendous challenge and drain on my stamina and enthusiasm. Subsequently, the continued help, encouragement, constructive criticism and advice I have received from colleagues and correspondents throughout the world has, as ever, been utterly invaluable, not to mention very rewarding. It is wonderful to know that the book has helped improve the pharmaceutical care of many people with mental health needs. I would thus like to thank all the people I have thanked in previous editions, the many members of the College of Mental Health Pharmacy (CMHP) who have conveyed continued enthusiasm, encouragement and support, and all those people I have met at conferences and talks or who have written to me. Thanks as ever must go to my pharmacy staff and colleagues in the trust for continuing to tolerate and humour me, and special thanks to the University of East Anglia's fab School of Pharmacy for the honour. I also wish to thank the many people who have fed back on the book's contents and/or spotted ambiguities in the quarter of a million words, e.g. Laura Regan (for keeping the clozapine section up-to-date), Elaine Linderman, Stephen Bleakley, Alison Marshall, Melinda Cuthbert, Utpal Goswami, Jackie Stark, Dennis Liew, Chris Bazire for helping with my PC (he can solve anything; contact me for details), Sam Illaiee, Bob Flanagan, and special thanks to Richard Owen for his very useful critique and the extra hours it took me to do the developments. And a big hello to Anthony Dimech over in Malta. Thanks also to John Tams and Virgin Radio (especially Geoff and Ben) for the company; to Ossi at Evim (01603-927459) on Prince of Wales Road, Norwich for the great veggie pizzas (especially on a Monday night); and of course, Binkie, for being so amazing to work with; my parents and my Godmother Kate Baxter for continuing to show interest; and Jill, Rosie and Chris for putting up with me.

Stephen Bazire *BPharm, FRPharmS, DipPsychPharm, FCMHP, MBE*
Chief Pharmacist, Norfolk and Waveney Mental Health NHS Foundation Trust,
Hellesdon Hospital, Norwich NR6 5BE
Honorary Professor, School of Pharmacy,
University of East Anglia, Norwich NR4 7TJ
England
E-mail: steve.bazire@nwmhp.nhs.uk or steve.bazire@choiceandmedication.org.uk
CMHP website: www.cmhp.org.uk
Website to aid service user choice of medication: www.choiceandmedication.org

August, 2011

To order a copy of the *Psychotropic Drug Directory 2012*, go online to: www.psychotropicdrugdirectory.com

1 DRUG TREATMENT OPTIONS IN PSYCHIATRIC ILLNESS

Contents

This chapter lists medicines which are indicated for, or have been used in, the conditions listed and the author would welcome suggestions for further inclusions. References should be consulted for fuller details of non-approved uses. In some cases, drugs not available in the UK have been included as possible options if available, and for non-UK readers.

Drugs are classified as follows:

BNF listed

BNF listed drugs are listed in the *British National Formulary* and licensed in the UK for that condition, although there are a few drugs listed in the BNF for which no full licence has been granted. See the appropriate section in the BNF for a review of a drug's role in therapy and its prescribing details. Much information provided here is in addition to that in the standard texts.

+ Combinations

The combinations section includes some combinations that have been used, but carry the risks of additive side-effects and interactions.

● Unlicensed/some efficacy

This section includes drugs of some clinical efficacy (e.g. RCTs) or are strategies which can be used, but where no product licence exists.

■ Unlicensed/possible efficacy

This section includes drugs of minor or un-proven importance or efficacy. No product licence exists.

✹ Case reports

This section includes single cases or small case series. These will await further publications to confirm an early signal, or will move to the 'Others' section if they turn out to be isolated events.

◆ Others

This section includes drugs tried, but where no significant data exists since the original reports.

The lack of positive follow-up data suggests a lack of efficacy although, if you know otherwise, the author would like to hear.

☐ No efficacy

Drugs in this section are not thought to be of clinical use.

Information in these last four categories is given to provide help once all recognised and evidence-based treatments have been tried. These classifications are to some extent arbitrary, and the information is based on data presently available.

It is the prescriber's responsibility to ensure that all precautions are taken when prescribing a drug for an unlicensed use.

1.1 ACUTE PSYCHIATRIC EMERGENCY (APE) including RAPID TRANQUILLISATION

see Aggression (*1.2*), Mania and hypomania (*1.10.2*) and Psychosis and schizophrenia (*1.21*)

Violent patients (usually either schizophrenic, manic or substance abusers) present a risk to themselves and others. Swift, safe and effective treatment is often needed. Rapid tranquillisation (RT) is the term used to describe the procedure of giving varying amounts of antipsychotic medication, usually with benzodiazepines, over brief intervals of time to control agitated, threatening and potentially destructive patients.

Routes: The IM route should generally be the preferred choice except in exceptional circumstances. IV administration may generally be quicker-acting than IM (which is often little quicker than oral drugs, especially if concentrated liquids or melt-in-the-mouth tablets are used) and allows physical restraint to be removed more quickly but IV carries additional dangers. Parenteral (IV/IM) doses generally have a higher potency than oral doses, so 'when required' or regular doses prescribed as 'IM/PO' are entirely inappropriate. All 'PRN' doses should be checked daily to ensure maximum doses are not being exceeded in any 24 hours. Antipsychotics can be fatal in moderate doses in drug-naïve people.

Doses: The need for high doses of antipsychotics is unnecessary, as violent patients respond to standard doses and higher doses may, in fact, be less effective, e.g. inducing akathisia. Use of concomitant benzodiazepines is safer and more effective than using high doses of antipsychotics as monotherapy.

Conditions: Manic patients may respond well to benzodiazepines, with antipsychotics as adjuncts. Schizophrenic patients usually respond best to antipsychotics, with benzodiazepines as adjuncts. In substance misuse, benzodiazepines and antipsychotics may be effective, but more studies are needed.

General principles of the management of acute psychiatric emergency (APE)

1. Obtain a drug history and carry out a physical examination if possible. Unless known previous exposure to psychotropics, use doses at the lower end of the ranges.
2. Antipsychotics in combination with benzodiazepines are preferred.
3. Parenteral administration is generally the quickest and most reliable route, but should be reserved **only** for when the patient cannot be persuaded to take drugs orally.
4. No anticholinergics should be used as this may confuse the clinical picture.
5. Switch to oral doses as soon as possible.
6. Check bp, pulse and temperature frequently.
7. Although APE can be carried out in the community, great care is needed and it is not recommended.

Potential complications of (particularly first generation) antipsychotics in APE:

1. Cardiovascular complications and sudden death — drugs causing QTc prolongation are contraindicated in patients with pre-existing cardiac problems, and care is needed in adrenaline-driven excited patients.
2. Respiratory depression.
3. Extrapyramidal symptoms, especially acute dystonia (may occur in 10–30% of patients within the first 24 hours and later in up to 50% of young males). Akathisia should be considered if agitation occurs, worsens or recurs after antipsychotics have achieved adequate behavioural control, as it may be drug-induced and exacerbate the disturbed behaviour (see *Chapter 6.7*).
4. Seizures, especially in non-compliant epileptics.
5. .Neuroleptic malignant syndrome — see *Chapter 6.8* for risk factors. Close

observation of temperature should be carried out, especially in early stages. Check CPK.

6. Local bruising, pain or extravasations (common, in up to 30% patients).
7. A depot given inadvertently into a vein may be rapidly fatal.
8. Disinhibition may occur with benzodiazepines, especially in people with poor impulse control or impulsivity, high-potency drugs, young or older age, developmental disabilities and/or pre-existing CNS damage. This remains controversial and probably over-rated (controlled study showing no effect: Rothschild *et al, J Clin Psychopharmacol* 2000;**20**:7–11; review by Paton, *Psychiatr Bull* 2002;**26**:460–2 noting the actual incidence may be lower than 1%).
9. In patients already taking antipsychotics, additional acute doses may reach toxic levels.
10. Acute hypotension (minimised if the patient can lie down) can occur, especially with phenothiazines and in the elderly.
11. Mega-colon (rare), heatstroke, aspiration.

Reviews: Use of BDZs and antipsychotics in emergency departments (Rund *et al, J Emerg Med* 2006;**31**:317–24), reappraisal of current options (concludes that parenteral BDZs should now be the mainstay of treatment: McAllister-Williams and Ferrier, *Br J Psychiatry* 2002;**180**:485–9).

BNF listed

Drugs in this section are licensed for emergency, short-term or adjunct therapy of, e.g. acute psychosis, mania, anxiety or exacerbations of chronic psychosis, violent or impulsive behaviour, psychomotor agitation and excitement, or violent or dangerously impulsive behaviour. IM SGAs have a lower incidence of EPSE than IM haloperidol, unless the latter is combined with promethazine (n = 3425, Satterthwaite *et al, J Clin Psychiatry* 2008;**69**:1869–79).

ANTIPSYCHOTICS *

Olanzapine IM, olanzapine orodispersible, risperidone syrup and haloperidol IM appear equally effective in APE, and olanzapine is more effective initially than haloperidol (n = 42, RCT, Hsu *et al, J Clin Psychopharmacol* 2010;**30**:230–4).

Aripiprazole

Aripiprazole is licensed for rapid control of agitation and disturbed behaviour in people with schizophrenia. The initial IM dose is 9.75 mg (range 5.25–15 mg). A second injection can be given after two hours, with no more than three doses in any 24 hours (maximum daily dose 30 mg, including all formulations). In acute psychotic agitation, aripiprazole (15–30 mg/d, n = 298) is as effective as olanzapine (20 mg/d, n = 306) (n = 604, RCT, d/b, 5/7, Kinon et al, J Clin Psychopharmacol 2008;**28**:601–7; MS, Lilly) and haloperidol (n = 448, RCT, d/b, p/c, Andrezina et al, Psychopharmacol [Berl] 2006;**188**:281–92). Aripiprazole IM may have a specific anti-agitation effect rather than just non-specific sedation (s = 3, Currier et al, J Psychiatr Pract 2007;**13**:159–69). Benzodiazepines can be given concomitantly but the patient must be monitored for excessive sedation and postural hypotension.

Chlorpromazine *

Chlorpromazine is licensed for adjunctive short-term treatment of anxiety, agitation, violence or dangerously impulsive behaviour. The injection should be given by deep IM injection only, at 25–50 mg every 6–8 hours, with a lower dose (up to 25 mg eight-hourly) in the elderly. The IM injection is 2–4 times as potent, on a mg for mg basis, as oral chlorpromazine, and so prescriptions for '100 mg po/im' are entirely inappropriate and potentially dangerous. Cochrane concludes that chlorpromazine is as effective as haloperidol, but causes serious postural hypotension and so should be avoided (s = 1, n = 30, Ahmed et al, Cochrane Database Syst Rev 2010;**4**:CD007445).

Haloperidol (see also combinations) *

Haloperidol is licensed for adjunctive short-term treatment of moderate to severe agitation, violence or dangerously impulsive behaviour. It can be used at BNF doses, e.g. up to 30 mg/d orally or 18 mg/d by IM injection only. Due to concerns about QTc prolongation (n = 596, open, Reilly et al, Lancet 2000;**355**:1048–52), especially with IV injection and reports of torsades de pointes, the SmPC now recommends cardiac assessment and an ECG before starting treatment. Akathisia may exacerbate disturbed behaviour.

Olanzapine *

A number of studies have shown olanzapine IM 10 mg to be at least as effective as haloperidol 7.5 mg IM in acute agitation in schizophrenia, with a possibly slightly quicker onset of action (e.g. at 30 minutes), no QT prolongation and significantly fewer EPS, including dystonia and akathisia (n = 311, RCT, p/c, Wright et al, Can J Psychiatry 2003;**48**:716–21, MS; review by Smith, EBMH 2003;**6**:27, noting that the response is in line with what would be expected from other antipsychotics). Other studies show olanzapine IM (n = 1294) to be more effective in APE after the first injection than zuclopenthixol IM or haloperidol IM (n = 2011, 7/7, Castle et al, World J Biol Psychiatry 2009;**10**:43–53), and orodispersible olanzapine was as effective as risperidone orodispersible in acute agitated psychosis, although olanzapine caused less tachycardia (n = 87, open, Hatta et al, Gen Hosp Psychiatry 2008;**30**:367–71). The following are the main recommendations:

- Olanzapine IM can be used to rapidly control agitation and disturbed behaviours in patients with schizophrenia or manic episodes when oral is inappropriate.
- The maximum combined daily dose of oral and IM olanzapine is 20 mg.
- The initial dose of olanzapine IM should be 10 mg as a single injection (use lower doses in elderly patients and those with renal or hepatic impairment).
- A maximum of three injections of olanzapine IM may be administered in any 24 hours, and a minimum of two hours should elapse between each injection.
- Olanzapine IM is intended for short-term use, maximum of three consecutive days.
- Olanzapine 'Velotabs' produce a plasma level profile similar to oral tablets. IM peak plasma levels are five times higher than oral, peaking after a few minutes. Aggressive oral dosing strategies (e.g. up to 40 mg/d) appear reasonably well-tolerated and effective in controlling acutely agitated people with a variety of diagnoses (n = 148, RCT, p/c, 4/7, Baker et al, J Clin Psychopharmacol 2003;**23**:342–8, MS; comment by Citrome, EBMH 2004;**7**:12).
- IM benzodiazepines should not be given concomitantly (or within an hour) of

olanzapine IM. Of 160 cases of ADRs reported to Lilly in USA there were 29 fatalities, of which 66% had concomitant BDZs and 76% had concomitant other antipsychotics (Marder et al, J Clin Psychiatry 2010;**71**:433–41).

- Patients with significant alcohol before olanzapine IM had decreased oxygen saturation after injection, and the effect is more marked in people who also then had BDZs at same time (n = 25, Wilson et al, J Emerg Med 2011; in press).
- Olanzapine pamoate should not be used for acute agitation or severe psychosis in people with schizophrenia (SmPC).

Cochrane is critical of the supporting literature, noting the manufacturer's involvement, poor and incomplete reporting and the borderline ethical nature of the trials (s = 4, n = 769, Belgamwar and Fenton, Cochrane Database Syst Rev 2005; **2**:CD003729).

Reviews: * use in acute agitation (Wagstaff et al, CNS Drugs 2005; **19**:147–64), general (n = 1945, Perrin et al, Eur Psychiatry 2011; in press).

Quetiapine

Quetiapine is licensed for the treatment of acute manic episodes, and 100–200 mg stat may have some efficacy as a sedative in emergency settings, but with no clear dose-response pattern (n = 20, s/b, Currier et al, J Psychiatr Pract 2006; **12**:223–8).

Risperidone *

Risperidone is licensed for acute mania (see combinations). An open prospective study concluded that in acute psychotic agitation risperidone orodispersible was as effective and tolerable as IM haloperidol (n = 124, RCT, open, Lim et al, Neuropsychobiology 2010; **62**:81–6).

Trifluoperazine

Trifluoperazine is licensed as an adjunct therapy for acute anxiety and agitated states.

Zuclopenthixol acetate (Clopixol Acuphase®)

Clopixol Acuphase® (Lundbeck) can be given at a dose of 50–150 mg stat, then repeated after 2–3 days (maximum every 1–2 days) after the first injection. The maximum cumulative dose is 400 mg per 'course', i.e. four injections or over two weeks, whichever comes first. The onset of action is at about eight hours (peaking at about 36 hours; see psychosis 1.21), and so should only be used when initial control has been established with other agents. The maximum single dose in the elderly is 100 mg. While zuclopenthixol acetate appears as effective as haloperidol in APE, sedation at four hours may be greater and there is an advantage of the need for fewer injections. Several reviews have suggested that more data is needed to prove an advantage over standard therapies (Gibson et al, Cochrane Database Syst Rev 2004; **3**:CD000525). Care is needed with Acuphase® to avoid it being given into a vein of a struggling or over-active patient.

BENZODIAZEPINES
(see also combinations)

Diazepam (see also combinations)

The recommended dose of diazepam is 10 mg IV or IM, repeated after not less than four hours. IV infusion is possible, albeit difficult. IV diazepam is much more consistently absorbed than IM which, in turn, is little faster than oral and slower than the rectal route. If the IV route is used, it is strongly recommended to be into the large vein of the antecubital fossa with the patient, if possible, in a supine position to minimise the incidence of hypotension. The maximum IV dose is 5 mg per minute. Mechanical ventilation and flumazenil should be available in case of respiratory depression, as hypoxic drive can be affected. Diazepam has a long half-life and active metabolites, and so accumulation and toxic delirium (especially in the elderly or hepatic impairment) must be avoided by use of decreased doses later on. A wide safety margin makes diazepam and lorazepam the drugs of choice.

Lorazepam (see also combinations)

Lorazepam IM absorption is as slow as oral administration, but more rapid in an active patient and IM carries less risk than IV. IM lorazepam alone was as effective as lorazepam IM plus either risperidone or haloperidol (both oral) in acute agitation and/or psychosis, although the combination therapy was numerically superior (n = 30, RCT, d/b, d/b, Veser et al, J Psychiatr Pract 2006;**12**:103–8). Lorazepam injection may be diluted 50:50 with water or normal saline pre-injection. The dose in acute anxiety is 0.025–0.05 mg/kg (1.75–3.5 mg for a 70 kg person), repeated six-hourly. Some services use 0.5–2 mg PO/IM every 1–2 hours until symptoms are controlled, omitting doses when excessive sedation occurs. This can be a highly effective therapy. Caution is needed in renal and hepatic impairment and in the elderly, where lower doses may be needed. Lorazepam does not accumulate with repeated doses or in hepatic impairment; distinct advantages over diazepam.

+ Combinations

Combinations of antipsychotics and benzo-diazepines are effective and allow lower doses of both to be used. Patients receiving monotherapy in APE at first are more likely to need second injections. A review concluded that combinations of a newer antipsychotic and a BDZ are optimal due to the lower incidence of EPS (s = 11, n = 701, Yildiz et al, Emerg Med J 2003;**20**:339–46).

Antipsychotic + benzodiazepine (see also separate drugs)

This combination is widely and strongly recommended, as the drugs act synergistically, reducing the amount of each drug (particularly the antipsychotic) required. The effect of the combination is rapid and predictable and the patient is less likely to require a second injection. **Lorazepam** is the most widely used benzodiazepine, with 2 mg IM plus haloperidol IM 5 mg being significantly better than lorazepam alone after 60–180 minutes (n = 98, RCT, Battaglia et al, Am J Emerg Med 1997;**15**:335–40). **Diazepam** 10 mg IM/IV is a suitable alternative. In acute psychotic agitation, oral risperidone 2 mg plus lorazepam 2 mg was as effective and as well tolerated as haloperidol 5 mg IM plus lorazepam 2 mg IM over two hours (n = 83 + 79, RCT, s/b, Currier et al, J Clin Psychiatry 2004;**65**:386–94). The orodispersible risperidone tablets may be useful to ensure administration, and as the peak plasma level occurs at 1.4–1.8 hours (the same as plain tablets) it can be as effective as an alternative

to IM antipsychotics (n = 191, open, Normann et al, Pharmacopsychiatry 2006;**39**:209–12). Risperidone liquid 2 mg plus oral lorazepam 2 mg was shown to be as effective in psychotic agitation as haloperidol 5 mg IM plus lorazepam 2 mg IM, but with less complications (n = 30, Currier and Simpson, J Clin Psychiatry 2001;**62**:153–7). In another trial, where patients were given a choice of oral risperidone (2 mg) plus oral lorazepam (2–2.5 mg) or standard IM antipsychotics, with or without lorazepam, most chose oral, which was more successful at two hours and significantly non-inferior with fewer side-effects (n = 226, open, Lejeune et al, Int Clin Psychopharmacol 2004;**19**:259–69). Risperidone 2–6 mg/d was superior to oral zuclopenthixol (20–50 mg/d) when combined with lorazepam in acute psychosis (n = 75, open, 14/7, Hovens et al, J Psychopharmacol 2005;**19**:51–7).
Review: general (Wilhelm et al, BMC Psychiatry 2008;**8**:61)

Haloperidol + promethazine (HAL-PRO)

Three large trials have shown IM promethazine to be an effective adjunct to haloperidol, e.g. promethazine 25–50 mg plus haloperidol 10 mg IM was as effective as lorazepam IM 4 mg and 96% patients in each group were 'tranquil or asleep' after four hours, but 76% were asleep with the HAL-PRO combination, compared with only 45% with lorazepam IM monotherapy (n = 200, RCT, Alexander et al, Br J Psychiatry 2004;**185**:63–9; favourable comment by McAllister-Williams, EBMH 2005; **8**:7; see also n = 316 [c = 311], open, Huf et al, Br Med J 2007;**335**:839). Haloperidol IM plus promethazine IM was as effective as olanzapine IM alone in agitated and violent people with mental health problems. However, the combination required fewer additional medical interventions at four hours (n = 300 [c = 298], RCT, open, 2/52, Raveendran et al, Br Med J 2007;**335**:865).
Cochrane concludes that:
- 1% people given any haloperidol treatment experience a seizure.
- After 20 minutes, HAL-PRO is more tranquillising than haloperidol alone.
- After 15 minutes olanzapine is as tranquillising as HAL-PRO but does

not have an enduring effect and more people need additional treatment at four hours (s = 4, n = 1117, Huf et al, Cochrane Database Syst Rev 2009;**3**:CD005146; see also s = 4, Huf et al, Rev Bras Psiquiatr 2009;**31**:265–70).

● **Unlicensed/some efficacy**

Clonazepam

Clonazepam is licensed only for status epilepticus but can be used as an alternative to diazepam and lorazepam, albeit slower-acting. The dose is 1 mg (1 ml) by slow (1 mg per 30 seconds) IV injection, which is strongly recommended to be into the large vein of the antecubital fossa with the patient in a supine position, if possible, to minimise the incidence of hypotension. Care is needed in the elderly and caution in chronic pulmonary insufficiency.

Midazolam *

Midazolam may be useful for short-term sedation, with a quick onset and offset. IM can be used but IV is too dangerous in non-specialist mental health settings due to the potential for acute respiratory depression. Midazolam 2.5–10 mg IM/IV may be rapidly effective (6–20 minutes) in controlling acute agitation, repeated every 20 minutes up to 20 mg per sedation event and monitored for at least four hours after the last dose. In a pragmatic real-world trial, with a simple end-point and only 1% drop-outs, IM midazolam was superior to haloperidol plus promethazine at 20 and 40 minutes in aggressive or agitated emergency room patients, with few side-effects (n = 301, RCT, TREC-CG, BMJ 2003;**317**:708–13; comment by Waraich, EBMH 2004;**7**:42). Midazolam IM 5 mg was also as effective as (and much quicker acting than) lorazepam IM 2 mg or haloperidol IM 5 mg in acute agitation, but the effects were shorter-lived (82 minutes vs 217 minutes vs 126 minutes respectively; n = 111, RCT, d/b, Nobay et al, Acad Emerg Med 2004;**11**:744–9). Buccal midazolam, when used as an alternative to IM lorazepam, had an onset of action of 15 minutes, peaking at 30 minutes and lasting for at least an hour, with no serious adverse reactions or over-

sedation in a naturalistic study (n = 25, 115 doses, open, Taylor et al, Int J Psychiatr Clin Pract 2008;**12**:309–11). With concentrated intranasal midazolam solution, effective plasma levels are reached within 10 minutes (n = 8, Haschke et al, Br J Clin Pharmacol 2010;**69**:607–16).

■ **Unlicensed/possible efficacy**

Topiramate

A retrospective study suggested topiramate might have some efficacy for the control of aggression in psychosis (n = 45, Gobbi et al, J Clin Psychopharmacol 2006;**26**:467–73).

Valproate

While valproate loading may have an antimanic effect over 48–72 hours, it has no detectable effect when given IV over 120 minutes (n = 7, open, Phroloiv et al, J Clin Psychiatry 2004;**65**:68–70). See entry under mania (1.10.2).

Ziprasidone IM (not UK)

Ziprasidone IM is effective in doses of 10 mg IM every two hours or 20 mg IM every four hours. The maximum dose is 40 mg/day (n = 79, RCT, d/b, Daniel et al, Psychopharmacol 2001;**155**:128–34). Although lorazepam may be given at the same time, the two must not be mixed in the same syringe due to compatibility issues.

1.2 AGGRESSION

see also Acute psychiatric emergency (1.1), Borderline personality disorder (1.11) and Self-injurious behaviour (1.25)

Aggression is defined as behaviour accompanied by verbal or physical threats which, if carried out, would cause harm to others, self or property. It can include situational (provoked), non-situational (unprovoked), passive, physical or interictal (especially in temporal lobe epilepsy). Aggression is not a diagnosis in itself, but as well as being potentially drug-induced (through either intoxication or withdrawal), can be a symptom of many conditions, including dementia, personality disorders, PTSD, PMS, trauma, etc, or as an expression of a variety of emotional or behavioural motivations. Low

GABA and serotonin levels in various parts of the brain are associated with aggressive behaviour, and enhanced norepinephrine and dopamine levels in the brain are associated with increased aggression.

Role of drugs

Drugs may be useful in helping control some cases where suppression of aggression is considered important on safety grounds.

Reviews: * pharmacotherapy (Goedhard et al, J Clin Psychiatry 2006;**67**:1013–24; in brain injury, Fleminger et al, Cochrane Database Syst Rev 2006;**4**:CD003299), general (Volavka et al, Actas Esp Psiquiatr 2006;**34**:123–35), AEDs for aggression and impulsivity (s = 14, n = 672, Huband et al, Cochrane Database Syst Rev 2010;**2**:CD003499), neurobiology (Siever, Am J Psychiatry 2008;**165**:429–42), in children (Parikh et al, J Child Adolesc Psychopharmacol 2008;**18**:157–78).

BNF listed

Lithium

Most studies with lithium have involved aggression in people with learning disabilities and a two-month trial at 0.6–1.0 mmol/L may be justified in patients unmanageable by environmental factors. Lithium has been shown to reduce aggression and the frequency of episodes in learning disabilities (e.g. Langee, Am J Ment Retard 1990;**94**:448–52), reducing impulsive aggression with organic brain damage (n = 2, two years, Bellus et al, Brain Inj 1996;**10**:849–60) and in children with aggression or conduct disorder, albeit poorly tolerated (e.g. n = 86, RCT, d/b, p/c, Malone et al, Arch Gen Psychiatry 2000;**57**:649–54). Lithium may exert an effect via several mechanisms, e.g. enhancement of serotonin, but the potential adverse consequences of sudden discontinuation (accidental or deliberate) should be considered.

■ Unlicensed/some efficacy

Antipsychotics

Raised dopamine levels may be associated with aggression, and so dopamine-blocking drugs may have some rationale. Use of higher doses of antipsychotics are generally considered to be effective only via a chemical strait-jacket or sedating effect. Indeed, in a trial in aggressive challenging behaviour in learning disabilities, aggression decreased substantially over 4/52 with haloperidol, risperidone and placebo, with no differences between the groups. The placebo group at no point showed a worse response than the antipsychotics and the authors concluded that antipsychotics should no longer be accepted routine therapy for aggressive behaviour in learning disabilities (n = 86, RCT, d/b, p/c, 26/52, Tyrer et al, Lancet 2008;**371**:57–63).

However, they may still have a role if used carefully. An analysis of 19 studies suggested that **risperidone** is useful for treating aggression in a range of behavioural disorders, agitation and dementia (s = 19, De Deyn and Buitelaar, Eur Psychiatry 2006;**21**:21–8), especially at lower dose, e.g. for severe, primary aggressive behaviour in adolescents with disruptive behaviours compounded by sub-average cognitive abilities (n = 38, RCT, p/c, 6/52, Buitelaar et al, J Clin Psychiatry 2001;**62**:239–48; review by Young, EBMH 2002;**5**:11). **Clozapine** is not easy to use but reduced seclusion and restraint rates in aggressive, psychotic inpatients over 12 months have been shown, the effect not related to sedation (n = 137, Chengappa et al, Schizophr Res 2002;**53**:1–6). **Quetiapine** may help at 25–300 mg/d for aggression due to traumatic brain injury (n = 7, open, 6/52, Kim and Bijlani, J Neuropsychiatry Clin Neurosci 2006;**18**:547–9). In aggression and SIB in learning disabilities, 80% improved on all measures with **zuclopenthixol** and discontinuation reversed the effect (n = 39, RCT, d/b, p/c, Hässler et al, Pharmacopsychiatry 2008;**41**:232–9), so it either works and/or there is a rebound aggression on withdrawal (n = 49 [c = 39], RCT, d/b, p/c, 6/52, Haessler et al, Br J Psychiatry 2007;**190**:447–8).

Benzodiazepines

Benzodiazepines are reported to be effective in episodic behavioural disorders by aborting aggression in the prodromal stage. **Lorazepam** has been used in resistant aggression in dementia. Use should normally be limited to only a few weeks to minimise the incidence of disinhibition or paradoxical reactions (review by Paton, *Psychiatr Bull* 2002;**26**:460–2, although the actual incidence may be lower than 1%).

Valproate

Valproate may exert an effect by correcting any abnormally low GABA levels. Several small studies have shown a rapid effect, e.g. compared to quetiapine (n = 33, RCT, d/b, 28/7, Barzman et al, *J Child Adolesc Psychopharmacol* 2006;**16**:665–70) and oxcarbazepine (n = 31, MacMillan et al, *J Psychiatr Pract* 2006;**12**:214–22), although earlier studies were less than encouraging (s = 17, n = 164, Lindenmayer and Kotsaftis, *J Clin Psychiatry* 2000;**61**:123–8).

■ Unlicensed/possible efficacy

Aromatherapy

Lavender reduced agitation in Chinese patients with dementia (n = 70, RCT, c/o, 3 + 3/52, Lin et al, *Int J Geriatr Psychiatry* 2007;**22**:405–10).

Beta-blockers

Beta-blockers have been reported to help control aggression in learning disabilities, autism, schizophrenia and in intermittent explosive disorders but have potential effects on bp and heart-rate (review by Haspel, *Harv Rev Psychiatry* 1995;**2**:274–81).

Buspirone

A three-month trial at 30 mg/d seems necessary, and a transient worsening may occur initially (n = 20, 3/12, Stanislav et al, *J Clin Psychopharmacol* 1994;**14**:126–30). Buspirone 90 mg/d has been successful for reducing aggressive behaviour in an autistic woman with profound learning disabilities (n = 1, Brahm et al, *Ann Pharmacother* 2008;**42**:131–7).

Carbamazepine

Evidence for carbamazepine in aggression is largely anecdotal, based on the proposed association between aggression and TLE or other EEG abnormalities. CBZ 600 mg/d may reduce aggressive behaviour in schizophrenia and has also been used in paroxysmal behaviour disorder and the elderly demented (n = 51, RCT, 6/52, Tariot et al, *Am J Psychiatry* 1998; **155**:54–61), 200 mg/d has been successful for BDZ-resistant impulsive aggression (n = 1, Nagata et

al, *Psychiatry Clin Neurosci* 2007;**61**:695–7; n = 1, Pae, *Psychiatry Clin Neurosci* 2008;**62**:483). Beware of an interaction with antipsychotics.

Clonidine

Clonidine 150–400 mcg/d may reduce aggressiveness in destructive children (n = 17, open, Kemph et al, *J Am Acad Child Adolesc Psychiatry* 1993;**32**:577–81), possibly via increased CSF GABA levels.

Estrogens (estrogens)

See dementia (*1.13*).

Gabapentin

Gabapentin has been used in episodic agitation in severely mentally ill patients (n = 11, 6/12, Megna et al, *Ann Pharmacother* 2002;**36**:12–6). See also dementia (*1.13*).

Lamotrigine

See dementia (*1.13*).

Oxcarbazepine

Oxcarbazepine has improved a variety of measures of impulsive aggressiveness (n = 48 [c = 45], RCT, d/b, p/c, 4–10/52, Mattes, *J Clin Psychopharmacol* 2005;**25**:575–9).

Phenytoin

Phenytoin 300 mg/d may reduce impulsive aggressive acts but not premeditated attacks in prisoners (n = 60, d/b, p/c, Barratt et al, *J Clin Psychopharmacol* 1997;**17**:341–9).

SSRIs

The use of SSRIs may be rational if low serotonin levels associated with aggression can be corrected. Aggression in learning disabilities may also be associated with unrecognised mood disorders, e.g. depression. **Citalopram** 20–60 mg/d has significantly reduced aggressive incidents with no deterioration or significant side-effects (e.g. n = 12, open, 6/52, Armentos and Lewis, *J Am Acad Child Adolesc Psychiatry* 2002;**41**:522–9; n = 25, open, 8/52, Reist et al, *J Clin Psychiatry* 2003;**64**:81–5). A similar effect has been suggested with **sertraline** 50–200 mg/d (open, Kavoussi et al, *J Clin Psychiatry* 1994;**55**:137–41). **Fluoxetine** seems to have a clear anti-aggressive effect in IED (intermittent explosive disorder), although less than 50% achieve a full or partial remission (n = 100, RCT, d/b, p/c, Coccaro et al, J Clin Psychiatry 2009;**70**:653–62) and 20–60 mg/d was ineffective in reducing abuse and aggression by men against intimate-partners (n = 26, RCT, p/c, Lee et al, Int Clin Psychopharmacol 2008;**23**:337–41).

Vitamins

Nutritional supplements (containing vitamins, minerals and fatty acids) caused dramatic reductions in antisocial behaviour and violent incidents of young offenders within just two weeks (n = 231, RCT, p/c, Gesch et al, Br J Psychiatry 2002;**181**:22–8; complimentary comment by Benton, EBMH 2003;**6**:41).

◆ Others

Other drugs tried include **cyproterone** 200 mg/d (e.g. n = 1, Byrne et al, Br J Psychiatry 1992;**160**:282–3) and **trazodone** (e.g. n = 1, Mashiko et al, Psychiatry Clin Neurosci 1996; **50**:133–6).

☐ No efficacy

Levetiracetam

Levetiracetam was of no efficacy for impulsive aggression in one study (n = 40 [c = 34], RCT, d/b, p/c, 10/52, Mattes, J Clin Psychiatry 2008;**69**:310–5).

1.3 AGORAPHOBIA
see also Anxiety disorder (1.6), Panic disorder (1.19) and Social anxiety (1.25)

Agoraphobia is an overwhelming and disabling anxiety provoked by being alone or in places where escape might be difficult or embarrassing and so these situations are avoided. Panic attacks may accompany the phobia and depression may be present in up to a half of patients. A link with serotonin deficiency has been shown.

Role of drugs
Drug treatment may be effective in many patients, with psychotherapy being an essential component of the treatment package for many. A meta-analysis of published studies has shown

that symptoms are improved by tricyclics and high potency benzodiazepines and, although there may be a short-term deterioration, this usually turns to a longer-term improvement (s = 43, n = 2367, Bakker et al, Acta Psychiatr Scand 2002;**106**:163–7). The best long-term benefit is from exposure therapy, particularly combined with antidepressants. There is a weak but significant placebo response in drug trials. Adding a CBT package to SSRIs for panic (with or without agoraphobia) seems of little additional benefit, with SSRIs more effective than CBT alone (n = 150, 9/12, van Apeldoorn et al, Acta Psychiatr Scand 2008;**117**:260–70). **Reviews:** general (Perugi et al, CNS Drugs 2007; **21**:741–64), epidemiology (Goodwin et al, Eur Neuropsychopharmacol 2005;**15**:435–43).

BNF listed

Citalopram
Citalopram is licensed for the symptoms of panic disorder, with or without agoraphobia (see also 1.19). The dose is 10 mg/d for a week, increasing to 20–30 mg/d, with a maximum of 60 mg/d. The maximal effect may take three months to develop.

Escitalopram
Escitalopram is licensed for the symptoms of panic disorder, with or without agoraphobia (see also 1.19). The dose is 5 mg/d for the first week, then 10 mg/d (maximum 20 mg/d). The maximal effect may take three months to develop.

Paroxetine
Paroxetine is licensed for the symptoms and prevention of relapse of panic disorder, with or without agoraphobia. See panic disorder (1.19).

● Unlicensed/some efficacy

Benzodiazepines
Alprazolam (n = 69, 3.5 years, Kilic et al, Psychother Psychosom 1997;**66**:175–8) and **diazepam** have been used and shown to help, particularly with anxiety symptoms. **Clonazepam** 1–2 mg/d has also shown significant efficacy (n = 24, RCT, p/c, 6/52, Valenca et al, Arq Neuropsiquiatr 2000;**58**:1025–9).

Review: general (Bruce et al, Am J Psychiatry 2003;**160**:1432–8).

Tricyclics

While SSRIs are now first choice, up to 70% may respond to tricyclics, but with 30% dropping out due to side-effects. 20% may worsen, with an increase in panic attacks. **Clomipramine**, at doses up to 300mg/d, has been shown to be effective (n = 108, d/b, p/c, 8/52, Johnson et al, Arch Gen Psychiatry 1988;**45**:453–9), with a continuous improvement shown over many weeks. See also panic (1.19).

■ Unlicensed/possible efficacy

Buspirone

Buspirone has been shown to be well-tolerated and enhance the effect of CBT in panic disorder with agoraphobia (n = 41, d/b, 68/52, Cottraux et al, Br J Psychiatry 1995;**167**:635–41), although a subsequent naturalistic study was unable to replicate this long-term effect (open, p/c, Bouvard et al, Psychother Psychosom 1997;**66**:27–32).

✴ Case reports

- Tranylcypromine * (n = 1, Boerner and Lühring, Psychiatr Prax 2010;**37**:350–2)

1.4 ALCOHOL DEPENDENCE AND ABUSE

see also Alcohol withdrawal syndrome (1.5)

Symptoms

The main diagnostic symptoms of alcohol dependence are a primacy of drinking over other activities, increased tolerance of alcohol, symptoms of repeated withdrawal, stereotyped pattern of drinking, compulsion to drink and relief drinking.

Risk factors

Some risk factors for alcohol abuse or being an alcohol-dependent drinker include:

1. Occupation, e.g. brewers, reps, doctors.
2. Genetics (up to 30–40% influence).
3. Marital/social problems, e.g. work.
4. Personality, e.g. high anxiety levels.
5. Psychopaths and criminals, e.g. taking alcohol

before criminal events.
6. Psychiatric illness, e.g. depression, phobia, etc.
7. Use for hypnotic or analgesic purposes.
8. Adverse childhood or adolescent experiences, including prenatal alcohol exposure (n = 433, Baer et al, Arch Gen Psychiatry 2003;**60**: 377–85).
9. Parental misuse of alcohol (n = 2427, Lieb et al, Psychol Med 2002;**32**:63–78).
10. Sweet taste preference (n = 122, Kranzler et al, Am J Psychiatry 2001;**158**:813–5).
11. Celebrating Norwich City promotions.

The body metabolises approximately one unit of alcohol per hour (varies between individuals but is the same regardless of the inital quantity), and peak levels occur one hour after the drink is consumed (absorption is more rapid with low volume drinks, e.g. spirits and slower with higher volumes, e.g. beer, small amounts). One unit gives a man an alcohol blood level of about 15mg/100ml and a woman about 20mg/100ml. Alcohol consumption of 7.7–12.9 units per week is associated with the lowest mortality in men (White, J Clin Epidemiol 1999;**52**:967–75, review by Caan, EBMH 2000;**3**:61), a finding often quoted in bars throughout the world.

Role of drugs *

Pharmacological treatment can play its part in an overall plan. Any vitamin deficiency needs correcting (see AWS, 1.5). Other drugs may be useful to treat associated psychiatric morbidity, such as withdrawal, affective disorders, suicidal thoughts and hallucinations. The COMBINE study compared naltrexone, acamprosate and Combined Behavioural Intervention (CBI) and concluded that acamprosate is ineffective but that naltrexone, CBI or both performed best (n = 1383, RCT, p/c, 16/52 and follow-up, Anton et al, JAMA 2006;**295**:2003–17). Other findings from COMBINE include that there is a significant placebo effect in large trial from pills, AA and seeing a healthcare professional (n = 1383 Weiss et al, J Stud Alcohol Drugs 2008;**69**:878–84), and CBI had little practical effect (Zweben et al, Alcohol Clin Exp Res 2008;**32**:1661–9).

In the longer term, disulfiram, naltrexone and acamprosate have roles to play. Despite COMBINE, **acamprosate** has a reasonable evidence base, is superior to placebo and is more effective in preventing a lapse, whereas naltrexone is better at preventing a lapse becoming a relapse (Rösner et al, J Psychopharmacol 2008;**22**:11–23; see also s = 42, Snyder and Bowers, Am J Drug Alcohol Abuse 2008;**34**:449–61), and so may be more useful for programmes aimed at controlled consumption. **Disulfiram** probably has limited efficacy, but, when given as thrice-weekly supervised consumption, may be superior to acamprosate daily unsupervised, which may be logical but I suppose it needed testing (n = 353, retrospective, Diehl et al, Alcohol Alcohol 2010;**45**:271–7). **SSRIs** and/or **lithium** may be useful but the evidence base is not robust due to the difficulty of carrying out these types of study, e.g. high drop-out rates.

Reviews: * pharmacotherapy (Johnson, Am J Psychiatry 2010;**167**:630–9, Garbutt, J Subst Abuse Treat 2009;**36**:S15–23), serotonergic drugs (Kenna, Curr Pharm Des 2010;**16**:2126–35), genetics (Kranzler and Edenberg, Curr Pharm Des 2010;**16**:2141–8; Stacey et al, Curr Psychiatry Rep 2009;**11**:364–9), non-benzodiazepine GABAergic medicines (Leggio et al, Prog Neuropsychopharmacol Biol Psychiatry 2008;**32**:1106–17), opioid antagonists (Soyka and Rösner, Curr Drug Abuse Rev 2008;**1**:280–91), management of Korsakoff's (Kopelman et al, Alcohol Alcohol 2009;**44**:148–54).

BNF listed

Acamprosate *

Acamprosate is licensed in some countries for abstinence maintenance therapy for up to one year in motivated alcohol-dependent patients. It is a GABA analogue and may act to reduce the severity and frequency of relapse by enhancing GABA inhibitory neurotransmission and antagonising glutamate excitation by antagonising mGluR5 receptors, reduces reward, and craving (n = 29, p/c, 6/52, Weinstein et al, Addict Biol 2003;**8**:229–32). It takes about seven days to reach therapeutic levels and so can be started soon after detoxification, although this may have no particular advantage (n = 40, RCT, d/b, p/c, 2/52 plus 10/52, Kampman et al, Addict Behav 2009;**34**:581–6). Continued alcohol consumption negates the therapeutic effect, but occasional lapses do not necessarily do this. Many RCTs have shown clinical effect

and a large meta-analysis concluded that acamprosate has a significant beneficial effect in enhancing abstinence in recently detoxified alcohol-dependent individuals (s = 20, n = 4087, Mann et al, Alcohol Clin Exp Res 2004;**28**:51–63) and as part of a therapeutic approach targeted at achieving abstinence (s = 33, Carmen et al, Addiction 2004;**99**:811–28), although COMBINE was not too encouraging. There appear to be no predictors of the likelihood of efficacy (s = 7, n = 1485, RCT, p/c, Verheul et al, Psychopharmacol [Berl] 2005;**178**:167–73), but may have no effect when craving is high (n = 169, RCT, d/b, p/c, 12/52, Richardson et al, Addiction 2008;**103**:953–9). Its efficacy may be enhanced in combination with disulfiram, and may be effective as an adjunct to psychosocial and behavioural therapies including counselling (see combinations) for the maintenance of abstinence in detoxified patients. It should be combined with continued counselling. Cochrane concludes that acamprosate is effective and safe albeit with a rather moderate effect size, and an NNT of 9 (s = 24, n = 6915, RCT, d/b, Rösner et al, Cochrane Database Syst Rev 2010;**9**:CD004332).

Reviews: * general (Kennedy et al, Expert Opin Drug Metab Toxicol 2010;**6**:363–80; Mann et al, Alcohol Clin Exp Res 2008;**32**:1105–10), mode of action (Mason and Heyser, Expert Opin Drug Saf 2010;**9**:177–88; Mason and Heyser, CNS Neurol Disord Drug Targets 2010;**9**:23–32).

Disulfiram *

Disulfiram acts as a negative reinforcer for abstinence via the potential for the disulfiram-alcohol interaction, i.e. an adversive/conditioning and maintenance therapy in alcoholics. It irreversibly inhibits ALDH (hepatic Aldehyde-NAD reductase) leading to accumulation of acetaldehyde from incomplete alcohol metabolism (Petersen, Acta Psychiatr Scand 1992;**369**[Suppl]:S7–S13, see also 4.7.1). Some published advice tends to underestimate doses needed, e.g. <250mg/d has only a minor interaction with alcohol (Malcolm et al, Expert Opin Drug Saf 2008;**7**:459–72), so it is suggested to start with a loading dose of 400mg/d, with 365mg/d the average dose used (n = 33, retrospective, Mueser et al, Am

J Addict 2003;**12**:242–52). A recent review has concluded that short-term supervised use is effective, but unproven in the long-term (s=11, n=1527, RCT, Jørgensen et al, Alcohol Clin Exp Res 2011; in press). Disulfiram seems superior to naltrexone in relapse prevention (n=100[c=97], RCT, open, one year, De Sousa and De Sousa, Alcohol Alcohol 2004;**39**:528–31). 'Antabuse®' (Alpharma) tablets are dispersible and so can be given as a liquid in a supervised setting. It can also be given as a twice-a-week dose (i.e. daily dose x 7 divided by 2), as the enzyme inhibition is irreversible and the clinical effect lasts about 7–10 days.

Review: * thorough and positive (Krampe and Ehrenreich, Curr Pharm Des 2010;**16**:2076–90).

Vitamin B$_1$ (thiamine)

Vitamin deficiency occurs after chronic alcohol abuse, and is due to inadequate diet, impaired absorption, increased metabolic demand and impaired utilisation. Thiamine (B$_1$) maintenance may be necessary to help reverse the mental confusion secondary to thiamine deficiency where 250mg IM for 3–5 days will minimise the risk of Wernicke's encephalopathy (Thompson and Marshall, Alcohol Alcohol 2006; **41**:159–67), but possibly only about 4.5mg is absorbed from each oral dose, via a saturable mechanism. Cochrane concludes that data to guide dose, frequency, route or duration is lacking (Day et al, Cochrane Database Syst Rev 2004;**1**:CD004033). See AWS 1.5.

Reviews: general (Jackson and Teece, Emerg Med J 2004;**21**:501–2; Meier and Daeppen, Rev Med Suisse 2005;**1**:1740–4), thiamine utilisation (Singleton and Martin, Curr Mol Med 2001; **1**:197–207).

+ Combinations

The COMBINE study provides some guidance but combining drugs with different modes of action may be useful.

Review: general (Mattson and Litten, J Stud Alcohol Suppl 2005;**15**:8–16).

Acamprosate + disulfiram

In one study, alcoholics were randomised over one year to placebo or acamprosate, and could request additional disulfiram. Disulfiram improved the effectiveness of acamprosate, but a high drop-out did not allow full analysis (n=118, RCT, p/c, Besson et al, Alcohol Clin Exp Res 1998;**22**:573–9).

Acamprosate + naltrexone

Combined naltrexone and acamprosate were slightly superior to monotherapy and significantly superior to placebo for time to first drink and time to relapse (n=160, RCT, d/b, p/c, 12/52, Kiefer et al, Arch Gen Psychiatry 2003;**60**:92–9).

Review: Mason, J Stud Alcohol Suppl 2005;**15**: 148–56).

Naltrexone + disulfiram

In a four-arm study, active medication produced lower craving and improved abstinence, but combining naltrexone and disulfiram had no advantage over either agent individually

---

Disulfiram test dose

A test dose is now considered dangerous due to the risks involved and because the mode of action is via a conditioning process. If considered necessary, wait five days after starting treatment for full enzyme block to occur.

1. Give 10–15ml of 95% alcohol (or 15–25ml spirits).
2. Reaction should start in 5–15 minutes.
3. Repeat in 30 minutes if no reaction. Reaction shows as flushed face, tachycardia, nausea, vomiting, fall in blood pressure. (Have crash box plus personnel available.)

Usual cause of no reaction is too low a dose of disulfiram. Bronchospasm has also been reported (Beri et al, Br Med J 1993;**306**:396). Noradrenaline has been effective in severe life-threatening hypotension with the disulfiram-alcohol reaction, when volume resuscitation and dopamine infusion failed (n=1, Ho et al, Am J Med Sci 2007;**333**:53–5).

(n = 254, RCT, p/c, 12/52, Petrakis et al, Biol Psychiatry 2005;**57**:1128–37).

Naltrexone + ondansetron

Augmentation of naltrexone 50 mg/d by ondansetron 0.5 mg/d can decrease alcohol craving (n = 90, RCT, d/b, p/c, 7/7, Myrick et al, Arch Gen Psychiatry 2007;**64**:466–75; n = 20, RCT, d/b, 8/52, Ait-Daoud et al, Alcohol Clin Exp Res 2001;**25**:847–9).

Naltrexone + sertraline *

In comorbid depression and alcohol dependence, sertraline 200 mg/d plus naltrexone 100 mg/d was superior to either drug separately or placebo (n = 170, RCT, d/b, p/c, 14/52, Pettinati et al, Am J Psychiatry 2010; **167**:668–75).

● Unlicensed/some efficacy

Aripiprazole

Aripiprazole 5–15 mg/d was equivalent in efficacy to naltrexone 50mg/d (n = 57 [c = 43], RCT, d/b, 16/52, Martinotti et al, J Psychopharmacol 2009;**23**:123–9) and may reduce the reward and euphoria from alcohol and increase sedation (n = 18, RCT, 3/7, p/c, c/o, Kranzler et al, Alcohol Clin Exp Res 2008;**32**:573–9).

Baclofen *

There is growing evidence for the use of baclofen. In alcohol-dependent people with cirrhosis of the liver, baclofen 10 mg/d TDS produces a well-tolerated and highly significantly reduction in abstinence (71% vs 29% for placebo; n = 84, RCT, d/b, p/c, 12/52, Addolorato et al, Lancet 2007;**370**:1915–22), although 20mg TDS seemed more effective, suggesting a dose-response in alcohol dependence (n = 42, RCT, d/b, p/c, 12/52, Addolorato et al, Alcohol Alcohol 2011;**46**:312–7). It doubles cumulative abstinence duration (n = 148 [c = 129], RCT, p/c, 12/52, Gache and Hadengue, J Hepatol 2008; **49**:1083–5) and reduces craving, consumption and other measures of alcohol dependence (n = 39, RCT, d/b, p/c, 30/7, Addolorato et al, Alcohol Alcohol 2002;**37**:504–8). In case reports, baclofen 140 mg/d produced dramatic reductions in craving and preoccupation

with alcohol (n = 1, Bucknam, Alcohol Alcohol 2007;**42**:158–60), and 270 mg/d (reduced to 120mg/d) allowed one person to become 'effortlessly' alcohol-free (n = 1, 9/12, Ameisen, Alcohol Alcohol 2005;**40**:147–50). However, a US study was unable to show baclofen was superior to placebo in alcohol dependence, albeit well-tolerated (n = 80 [c = 61], RCT, d/b, p/c, 12/52, Garbutt et al, Alcohol Clin Exp Res 2010;**34**:1849–57).
Reviews: * general (Addolorato and Leggio, Curr Pharm Des 2010;**16**:2113–7; Leggio et al, CNS Neurol Disord Drug Targets 2010;**9**:33–44).

Gabapentin

Gabapentin 600 mg/d monotherapy post-detox significantly reduced alcohol consumption and craving, improving outcomes, and was very well tolerated and safe (n = 60, RCT, d/b, p/c, 4/52, Furieri et al, J Clin Psychiatry 2007;**68**:1691–1700). Gabapentin may have some use at night for reducing heavy drinking and improving insomnia (n = 21, RCT, d/b, p/c, 8/52, Brower et al, Alcohol Clin Exp Res 2008; **32**:1429–38).

Naltrexone *

A systematic analysis has concluded that naltrexone reduces the risk of heavy drinking to 83%, decreased drinking days by 4%, with mainly GI and sedative ADRs (s = 50, n = 7793, RCT, d/b, Rösner et al, Cochrane Database Syst Rev 2010;**12**:CD001867). Sweet taste preference has a strong correlation with response to naltrexone (n = 78, p/c, 32/52, Laaksonen et al, Alcohol Alcohol 2011;**46**:308–11). Another extensive review concluded that the majority of double-blind trials support that naltrexone reduces heavy alcohol drinking (s = 29, n = 5997, Pettinati et al, J Clin Psychopharmacol 2006;**26**:610–25). This may be through blocking the pleasure (or 'high') caused by alcohol and reducing alcohol-seeking behaviour or reducing craving (n = 43, O'Malley et al, Am J Psychiatry 1996;**153**:281–3). The efficacy may be enhanced by limited psychosocial interventions (n = 111, RCT, p/c, 12/52, Morris et al, Addiction 2001;**96**:1565–73), CBT (n = 131, RCT, Anton et al, Am J Psychiatry 1999;**156**:1758–64; reviewed by Chick, EBMH 2000;**3**:75), short interventions (n = 107, RCT, d/b, p/c, 12/52,

Latt *et al*, *Med J Aust* 2002;**176**:530–4), prescribing with an antidepressants (n = 627, Krystal *et al*, *Alcohol Clin Exp Res* 2008;**32**:85–91), or by targetted naltrexone, i.e. prior to situations that might have a high risk of heavy drinking (n = 153, RCT, p/c, 8/52, Kranzler *et al*, *J Clin Psychopharmacol* 2003;**23**:294–304). One trial came to the reassuring conclusion that, while naltrexone is only moderately effective in reducing alcohol intake, its efficacy is far greater in people who actually take it (n = 97, p/c, Volpicelli *et al*, *Arch Gen Psychiatry* 1997;**54**:737–42).

Reviews: * general (Garbutt, *Curr Pharm Des* 2010;**16**:2091–7; Ray *et al*, *CNS Neurol Disord Drug Targets* 2010;**9**:13–22), depot injection (Mannelli *et al*, *Expert Rev Neurother* 2007;**7**:1265–77; Roozen *et al*, *Eur Addict Res* 2007;**13**:201–6; Comer *et al*, *Expert Opin Investig Drugs* 2007;**16**:1285–94).

Naltrexone depot injection
(UK license delayed) *

A long-acting naltrexone injection (Vivitrex®, Alkermes; n = 315, RCT, p/c, DASNDSG, *Alcohol Clin Exp Res* 2004;**28**:1051–9) may help, e.g. 380 mg monthly significantly reduced heavy drinking days (n = 627 [c = 401], RCT, d/b, p/c, 6/12, Garbutt *et al*, *JAMA* 2005;**293**:1617–25; comment by Killeen, *EBMH* 2005;**8**:100). The monthly injection may be effective within two days and have a sustained action over at least 6/12 (n = 624, RCT, d/b, p/c, 24/52, Ciraulo *et al*, *J Clin Psychiatry* 2008;**69**:190–5).

Reviews: * general (Gastfriend, *Ann N Y Acad Sci* 2011;**1216**:144–66), systematic review (Lobmaier *et al*, *CNS Neurosci Ther* 2010; in press).

Ondansetron *(see also combinations)*
Ondansetron, a 5-HT3 antagonist, at 8 mcg/kg/d was superior to placebo in increasing drink-free days, especially for early-onset (pre-25 years) alcoholism (n = 271, RCT, Johnson *et al*, *JAMA* 2000;**284**:963–71).

Topiramate *
Data is accumulating that topiramate may be a promising treatment, e.g. topiramate (around 300 mg/d) is superior to placebo for reducing the percentage of heavy drinking days and the number of abstinent days (s = 3, p/c, Arbaizar *et al*, *Actas Esp Psiquiatr* 2010;**38**:8–12) and at least as effective as naltrexone for reducing drinking (n = 102, RCT, 6/12, Flórez *et al*, *Alcohol Clin Exp Res* 2008;**32**:1251–9; n = 155, RCT, d/b, p/c, 12/52, Baltieri *et al*, *Addiction* 2008;**103**:2035–44), superior to naltrexone 50 mg/d for reducing alcohol intake and cravings (n = 182, RCT, open, 6/12, Flórez *et al*, *Eur Addict Res* 2011;**17**:29–36), and in reducing heavy drinking days and all other drinking outcomes (n = 371, RCT, d/b, p/c, 14/52, Johnson *et al*, *JAMA* 2007;**298**:1641–51). It may also reduce relapse (n = 155, RCT, d/b, p/c, 12/52, Baltieri *et al*, *Addiction* 2008;**103**:2035–44).

Reviews: * general (De Sousa, *CNS Neurol Disord Drug Targets* 2010;**9**:45–9; Olmsted and Kockler, *Ann Pharmacother* 2008;**42**:1475–80).

Valproate
Valproate augmentation of TAU has decreased heavy drinking in people with bipolar I with comorbid alcohol dependence, an important finding (n = 59, RCT, d/b, p/c, 24/52, Salloum *et al*, *Arch Gen Psychiatry* 2005;**62**:37–45; enthusiastic review by Le Fauve, *EBMH* 2005;**8**:79), e.g. valproate 3 g/d has been used successfully to treat alcoholic hallucinosis (n = 40, RCT, d/b, 10/7, Aliyev and Aliyev, *Alcohol Alcohol* 2008;**43**:456–9).

■ Unlicensed/possible efficacy

Benzodiazepines
Although not recommended in alcoholics for the very real fear of addiction, benzodiazepines have been advocated if they are able to reduce alcohol dependence (as a 'lesser of two evils' strategy). Any use should be well-documented in the patient's notes.

Buspirone
Two trials in anxious alcoholics have shown reduced anxiety, alcohol consumption and drinking days (n = 61, 12/52, Kranzer *et al*, *Arch Gen Psychiatry* 1994;**51**:720–31), and a significant reduction in alcohol craving and consumption in motivated patients (n = 50, d/b, p/c, Bruno, *Psychopathology* 1989;**22**[Suppl 1]:S49–S59), but no effect on drinking or anxiety has been noted in two other studies

(e.g. n = 156, RCT, Fawcett et al, Alcohol Clin Exp Res 2000;**24**:666–74). It may need four weeks at full therapeutic dose to achieve the effect and so a proper trial is necessary.

Carbamazepine

A significant long-term effect has been shown on time to first drink and survival rates (n = 29, RCT, 12/12, Mueller et al, Alcohol Clin Exp Res 1997;**21**:86–92).

Levetiracetam

In two pilot studies, levetiracetam 3 g/d reduced anxiety and alcohol consumption (n = 3, open, 8/52, Mariani and Levin, Am J Drug Alcohol Abuse 2008;**34**:683–91), and 2 g/d reduced alcohol consumption by 65% (n = 20, open, Sarid-Segal et al, Am J Drug Alcohol Abuse 2008;**34**:441–7).

Memantine

There are two main conflicting studies. Memantine 20–40 mg/d produced a dose-dependent attenuation of alcohol cue-induced craving (n = 38, RCT, 3/7, Krupitsky et al, Am J Psychiatry 2007;**164**:519–23) but up to 40 mg/d had no effect on any measures of alcohol use in treatment-seeking alcoholic-dependent patients (n = 34 [c = 27], d/b, p/c, 16/52, Evans et al, Alcohol Clin Exp Res 2007;**31**:775–82). Also, memantine 20 mg/d was as effective as escitalopram 20 mg/d for reducing drinking in depressed alcoholics, although it was more effective if abstinent at the start and the study had placebo arm (n = 80, d/b, 26/52, Muhonen et al, Subst Abuse Treat Prev Policy 2008;**3**:20).

Oxcarbazepine

In a pilot study, oxcarbazepine was as effective as acamprosate in preventing alcohol relapse and as well tolerated (n = 30, RCT, open, 24/52, Croissant et al, Alcohol Clin Exp Res 2006;**30**:630–5; review by Martinotti et al, Am J Addict 2007;**16**:247–8).

Oxybate, gamma-hydroxybutyrate (GHB) *

Oxybate is the approved name for pharmaceutical quality and marketed GHB, whereas GHB is the chemical name, generally used to describe illicit formulations (of highly variable quality and concentrations) for non-medical

uses (review by Carter et al, Drug Alcohol Dependence 2009;**104**:1–10). It is approved in some countries for alcohol and opiate withdrawal. The doses used for alcohol dependence are 50–100/kg/d (usually a 1.75 g vial 3–4 times a day). For alcohol dependence, Cochrane concludes that GHB is as effective as naltrexone and disulfiram for preventing relapse over 3/12, but has the risks of abuse, misuse and dependence, especially in polydrug abusers (s = 13, Leone et al, Cochrane Database Syst Rev 2010;**2**:CD006266; e.g. n = 55, RCT, 3/12, Caputo et al, Eur Neuropsychopharmacol 2007;**17**:781–9).

Pregabalin *

Pregabalin 150–450 mg/d was as effective as naltrexone for drinking indices and craving scores, but its effect may be more related to management of comorbid psychiatric symptoms (n = 71 [c = 48], RCT, d/b, 16/52, Martinotti et al, J Psychopharmacol 2010; **24**:1367–74), although it may help prevent relapse (n = 20 [c = 15], open, 16/52, Martinotti et al, Adv Ther 2008;**25**:608–18).

Review: * general (Oulis and Konstantako-poulos, CNS Neurosci Ther 2010;**16**:45–50).

Quetiapine *

Quetiapine as monotherapy in dual diagnosis (alcohol dependence and bipolar) markedly reduced alcohol consumption, craving and symptoms (n = 28, open, 16/52, Martinotti et al, Hum Psychopharmacol 2008;**23**:417–24; review by Ray et al, Drug Alcohol Rev 2010; **29**:568–75). However, 25–200 mg/d had no additional effect as an adjunct to naltrexone (n = 62 [c = 47], RCT, d/b, p/c, 12/52, Guardia et al, Addict Behav 2011;**36**:265–9).

SSRIs (see also SSRIs, no efficacy)

Citalopram has produced a modest (16–17%) but significant reduction in alcoholic drink intake and increase in drink-free days in studies of alcoholics, possibly by decreasing desire or reducing the reward (see also n = 62, d/b, p/c, Tiihonen et al, Pharmacopsychiatry 1996;**29**:27–9). **Fluoxetine** at 20–60 mg/d can reduce alcoholic and total drink intake compared to placebo (n = 51, RCT, d/b, p/c, 12/52, Cornelius et al, Arch Gen Psychiatry

1997;**54**:700–5; review by Haslam, *EBMH* 1998;**1**:41), but a larger study failed to reproduce these findings (n = 101, RCT, p/c, 6/12, Kranzler *et al*, *Am J Psychiatry* 1995; **152**:391–7).
Review: (Naranjo and Knoke, *J Clin Psychiatry* 2001;**62**[Suppl 20]:S18–S25).

Tiagabine *
Adjunctive tiagabine (mean 17 mg/d) showed improved craving, global functioning and psychopathology, and lower relapse (7% vs 14%) than placebo (n = 120, open, RCT, 6/12, Paparrigopoulos *et al*, *J Psychopharmacol* 2010;**24**:1375–80), although it does not attenuate alcohol-induced activation of the human reward system (n = 20, Fehr *et al*, *Psychopharmacol [Berl]* 2007;**191**:975–83).

Zonisamide *
Two pilot studies showed <300mg/d well-tolerated and improved craving and alcohol intake (n = 22, open, 12/52, Rubio *et al*, *Clin Neuropharmacol* 2010;**33**:250–3) and a reduced urge to drink in risky drinkers (n = 10, open, d/b, p/c, 13/52, Sarid-Segal *et al*, *Am J Drug Alcohol Abuse* 2010;**36**:102–5).

✷ Case reports

- **Mirtazapine** (n = 1, Crockford and White, *J Clin Psychiatry* 2005;**66**:540).

◆ Others

Other drugs tried include **imipramine** (n = 60, Nunnes *et al*, *Am J Psychiatry* 1993;**150**:963–5), and **trazodone** (open, n = 25, Janiri *et al*, *Alcohol Alcoholism* 1998;**33**:362–5).

☐ No efficacy

Amisulpride
Low dose amisulpride 50 mg/d is ineffective in preventing relapse in primary alcohol dependence (n = 71, RCT, d/b, p/c, 6/12, Marra *et al*, *Alcohol Clin Exp Res* 2002;**26**:1545–52).

Donepezil
While donepezil was ineffective in reversing Wernicke-Korsakoff's disease memory changes (n = 7, s/b, p/c, c/o, 30/7, Sahin *et al*, *Clin Neuropharmacol* 2002;**25**:16–20), high dose donepezil may help the memory deficits from Korsakoff's psychosis (n = 2, Codina *et al*, *Rev Neurol* 2002; **35**:341–5).

Flupentixol decanoate
After detoxification, flupentixol decanoate 10 mg 2/52 actually increased relapses compared to placebo (85% vs 65% for placebo), and so appears to have no role (n = 281, RCT, d/b, 12/12, Weisbeck *et al*, *Alcohol Alcohol* 2001;**36**:329–34).

Lithium
Three trials have shown no advantage over placebo (e.g. n = 156, RCT, 6/12, Fawcett *et al*, *Alcohol Clin Exp Res* 2000;**24**:666–74).

Olanzapine
Olanzapine was well tolerated but ineffective in reducing drinking outcomes (n = 60, RCT, b/d, 12/52, Guardia *et al*, *Alcohol Clin Exp Res* 2004;**28**:736–45).

SSRIs (see also SSRIs, possible efficacy)
Fluvoxamine was worse than placebo on measures of abstinence and relapse (n = 493, RCT, d/b, p/c, 12/12, Chick *et al*, *Drug Alcohol Depend* 2004;**74**:61–70), and **sertraline** was ineffective on measures of drinking when used as an adjunct to naltrexone (n = 113, RCT, d/b, p/c, 10/52, Farren *et al*, *Drug Alcohol Depend* 2009;**99**:317–21).

1.5 ALCOHOL WITHDRAWAL SYNDROME (AWS)
see also Alcohol dependence and abuse (*1.4*)

Symptoms
The presentation of AWS includes psychological symptoms (e.g. anxiety, insomnia and restlessness), psychotic symptoms (e.g. hallucinations), tremor, sweating, tachycardia, gastrointestinal symptoms, GTC seizures, hallucinations and illusions, clouding of consciousness, delirium tremens (DT) and Wernicke's encephalopathy (WE). WE is the acute phase, lasting for about 48 hours after the last drink, and results from thiamine (B1) deficiency. If untreated it can lead on to the chronic form (Korsakoff psychosis, KP)

characterised by severe short-term memory loss. Fits may first occur within 6–8 hours after cessation of alcohol use and peak at 12–24 hours (chronic alcohol consumption causes adaptation and downregulation of GABA receptors and upregulation of NMDA, so sudden withdrawal leads to hyperexcitability and hence seizures). In DT, seizures may occur (either primary or secondary to hypoglycaemia, hypomagnesaemia or hyponatraemia) as may suicidal ideation, gross disorientation, delusions, violence and marked tremor. DT peaks on the third or fourth day, and physical complications are common, e.g. pulmonary infection and hepatic encephalopathy. Risk factors for alcohol withdrawal delirium include concurrent infection, tachycardia, symptoms of withdrawal with blood levels above 1 g/L, and a history of epileptic seizures or delirious episodes (n = 334, Palmstierna et al, *Psychiatr Serv* 2001;**52**:820–3).

Role of drugs *

Seizures and psychiatric disturbances are serious problems and treatment of severe AWS is essential. Withdrawal symptoms in hospital may be underestimated and this may lead to undertreatment. Cochrane concludes that benzodiazepines are protective against seizures and other outcomes but the data was inconclusive, and there is insufficient evidence for the use of anticonvulsants, baclofen and GHB (s = 114, n = 7333, Amato et al, *Cochrane Database Syst Rev* 2011;**6**:CD008537). NICE recommends (June 2010):

For alcohol withdrawal syndrome:
1. First-line therapy is benzodiazepines (diazepam and CDZ are licensed) or carbamazepine — dosage should be individualised according to withdrawal severity, comorbidity and history of withdrawal seizures.
2. Clomethiazole is an alternative, in in-patient settings.
3. Do not offer phenytoin for AWS.

For delirium tremens:
1. Use lorazepam orally (unlicensed), then if refused or it fails try lorazepam injection, haloperidol or olanzapine (all unlicensed).

For prevention of Wernicke's encephalopathy:
1. Offer prophylactic thiamine at top end of BNF range, orally or parenterally.

2. If Wernicke's encephalopathy is suspected, offer parenteral thiamine for minimum of five days then maintenance oral thiamine.

Reviews: * practice guideline (Chang and Steinberg, *Med Clin North Am* 2001;**85**:1191–212), general (McKeon et al, *J Neurol Neurosurg Psychiatry* 2008;**79**:854–62), seizures (Hughes, *Epilepsy Behav* 2009;**15**:92–7), anticonvulsants in AWS (s = 56, n = 4076, Minozzi et al, *Cochrane Database Syst Rev* 2010;**3**:CD005064).

BNF listed

Benzodiazepines

Benzodiazepines are the drugs of choice for treating acute AWS (meta-analysis of 11 RCTs, n = 1286, Holbrook et al, *Can Med Ass J* 1999;**160**:649–55). Chlordiazepoxide (and diazepam) are the established treatments in the UK. Lorazepam (n = 186, p/c, D'Onofrio et al, *N Engl J Med* 1999;**340**:915–9; reviewed in *EBMH* 1999;**2**:107) has also been used, as it has an intermediate half-life and no active metabolites, e.g. lorazepam starting at 8 mg/d was as effective as chlordiazepoxide 80 mg/d (both reducing over eight days) in alcohol withdrawal, and may be a suitable option at lower doses in people with impaired liver function (n = 100, RCT, d/b, 12/7, Kumar et al, *J Stud Alcohol Drugs* 2009;**70**:457–74). Doses may be adjusted in a symptom-triggered way, with adequate monitoring of symptoms in patients with particular needs (e.g. chlordiazepoxide n = 108, Wiseman et al, *J Clin Psychiatry* 1998;**59**:289–93; and oxazepam, n = 117, RCT, Daeppen et al, *Arch Intern Med* 2002;**162**:1117–21). Higher doses of benzodiazepines may reduce the need for mechanical ventilation in acute DTs (n = 54, Gold et al, *Crit Care Med* 2007;**35**:724–30). Beware of an extended metabolism in liver damage (see 3.6), and of respiratory depression.

Reviews: * BDZs in AWS (s = 64, n = 4309, Amato et al, *Cochrane Database Syst Rev* 2010;**3**:CD00506), chlordiazepoxide withdrawal regimens (Chick, *Adv Psychiatr Treat* 1996;**2**:249–57), chlordiazepoxide vs clomethiazole (Duncan and Taylor, *Psychiatr Bull* 1996: **20**:601–3).

Clomethiazole (chlormethiazole)

Clomethiazole is regarded as a safe and effective treatment of AWS at up to 16 capsules/d, reducing over five to nine days. It has a low addictive potential, although dependence (mainly psychological) can be seen in some patients on longer-term therapy (Hession et al, Lancet 1979;**1**:953–4). Clomethiazole was as effective as carbamazepine for alcohol withdrawal, and was associated with less risk of premature discharge (n = 168, Hillemacher et al, Pharmacopsychiatry 2008;**41**:134–7). Clomethiazole may markedly suppress REM sleep in AWS (n = 20, RCT, p/c, d/b, 13/7, Gann et al, Pharmacopsychiatry 2004;**37**:228–35).
Reviews: Clomethiazole home detoxification schedules, and discussion that clomethiazole may not be as toxic as reputed (Sowerby and Hunter, J Substance Misuse 1997;**2**:62–3; 114–7), general (Duncan and Taylor, Psychiatr Bull 1996;**20**:6013).

Vitamin B supplementation

Classic signs of vitamin deficiency may only occur in extreme depletion and so are easily missed, being interpreted as intoxication. B vitamins act as co-enzymes for essential carbohydrate metabolism. Deficiency of nicotinamide, riboflavine (B_2) and pyridoxine (B_6) can cause neuropathies. Thiamine (B_1) supplementation must be primary and priority treatment to reverse the mental confusion secondary to thiamine deficiency (Wernicke's encephalopathy). Oral thiamine has a saturable absorption mechanism which allows only about 4.5 mg of a single dose to be absorbed. Thiamine 100 mg TDS allows about 13.5 mg to be absorbed, adequate only for mild deficiency. In chronic alcohol misusers, oral absorption can be reduced by 70%. Large oral doses are thus futile and adequate parenteral therapy should be routine, and is essential to treat or prevent KP (review, Thompson, Alcohol Alcohol 2000;**35**[Suppl 1]:S2–S7). Indeed, only 16% patients with WE recovered when given low parenteral thiamine doses (50–100 mg/d) and 20% died (see Thompson et al, Alcohol Alcohol 2002;**37**:513–21). The parenteral dose necessary is about 500–1000 mg for three to five days (Thompson and Marshall, Alcohol Alcohol 2006;**41**:159–67). Although anaphylaxis

has been reported with 'Parentrovite®' (Link), the incidence is about one report for every 5,000,000 IM ampoules used. It may be necessary to administer glucose after thiamine when administering thiamine to prevent Wernicke's encephalopathy (Chataway and Hardman, Postgrad Med J 1995;**71**:249–53).
Reviews: Thompson et al, Alcohol Alcohol 2002;**37**:513–21; McIntosh et al, Psychiatr Bull 2005;**29**:94–7.

+ Combinations

Carbamazepine + tiapride

This combination was more effective than either drug separately for alcohol withdrawal (n = 56, RCT, open, Croissant et al, Pharmacopsychiatry 2009;**42**:175–81).

● Unlicensed/some efficacy

Baclofen *

Baclofen (30 mg/d, n = 15) was as effective as diazepam (n = 19) in uncomplicated AWS (n = 37, RCT, 10/7, Addolorato et al, Am J Med 2006;**119**:13–8; n = 42, Stallings and Schrader, J Okla State Med Assoc 2007;**100**:354–60). Cochrane concludes that the evidence for baclofen is currently insufficient to recommend use (s = 1, n = 37, RCT, p/c, Amato et al, Cochrane Database Syst Rev 2011;**6**:CD008537).

Carbamazepine *

A review of CBZ for AWS showed it was safe, tolerable and effective for moderate-to-severe AWS in in-patient settings, but was unproven for seizures and DTs compared to BDZs (s = 7, n = 612, Barrons and Roberts, J Clin Pharm Ther 2010;**35**:153–67). Carbamazepine is probably active via an anti-kindling effect. It is non-addictive and its metabolism is generally little affected by liver dysfunction but may be inhibited by higher doses of alcohol. It has also been used for outpatient detoxifications due to its safety and lack of abuse potential (n = 76 [c = 60], open, Collins et al, Br J Psychiatry 1990;**156**:871–4).
Review: general (suggests limited evidence of efficacy and cannot be recommended; s = 6, RCT, Prince and Turpin, Am J Health Syst Pharm 2008;**65**:1039–47).

Oxcarbazepine

A pilot study suggested that oxcarbazepine was more effective than carbamazepine in AWS, with less craving (n = 29, RCT, s/b, Schik et al, Addict Biol 2005;10:283–8).

■ Unlicensed/possible efficacy

Alcohol IV

In an acute setting, IV alcohol had no advantage over diazepam for acute AWS and the previously reported advantages were not evident (n = 50, RCT, 4/7, Weinberg et al, J Trauma 2008;64:99–104).

Antipsychotics

Decreased dopamine activity may occur in DT so care is needed with anti-dopaminergic drugs, as these may aggravate symptoms and lower the seizure threshold. NMS may also occur and not be recognised. Temperature regulation and liver function pose further difficulties.

Beta-blockers

Beta-blockers, such as atenolol and propranolol, have been used in treating some symptoms of mild-to-moderate AWS, e.g. tachycardia and tremor, and to reduce craving, but are generally not recommended (Neff and McQueen, Drug Intell Clin Pharm 1991;25:31–2). The variable kinetics of propranolol in cirrhosis and portal hypertension must be considered (Cales et al, Br J Clin Pharmacol 1989;27:763–70; comparison with diazepam, Worner, Am J Drug Alcohol Abuse 1994;20:115–24).

Gabapentin *

Gabapentin (1200 mg/d tapering down) may be as effective as lorazepam for AWS and more effective at reducing post-withdrawal drinking (n = 100, RCT, d/b, 12/7, Myrick et al, Alcohol Clin Exp Res 2009;33:1582–8). Gabapentin orally (loaded up to 3200mg in the first 24 hours) may be helpful in less severe and uncomplicated AWS but probably not for more severe AWS (n = 37, open, Bonnet et al, Alcohol Alcohol 2010;45:143–5). A review of previous papers suggested no evidence of efficacy and that it should not be used (s = 2, Prince and Turpin, Am J Health Syst Pharm 2008; 65:1039–47). Augmentation of clomethiazole

is well tolerated but ineffective (n = 61, RCT, d/b, 7/7, Bonnet et al, J Clin Psycho-pharmacol 2003;23:514–19).

Lofexidine

Several studies have shown lofexidine (e.g. 0.4 mg qds for 2–3 days) to be superior to placebo in controlling AWS (e.g. n = 23, Cushman and Sowers, Alcohol Clin Exp Res 1989;13:361–4), but it appeared ineffective as an adjunct to chlordiazepoxide, with more withdrawal, hypotension, adverse effects and poorer retention with the combination compared to chlordiazepoxide alone (n = 72, RCT, Keaney et al, Alcohol Alcohol 2001;36:426–30).

Mirtazapine

Adjunctive mirtazapine 30–60 mg/d reduced anxiety and depressive symptoms during the detox process (n = 68, 4/52, Liappas et al, J Psychopharmacol 2004;18:88–93).

Oxybate, gamma-hydroxybutyrate (GHB) *

GHB 50 mg is effective for AWS and may be available in UK under a special license as Alcover®. Alcohol stimulates GABA-A and increases sedation, whereas stopping alcohol leads to increased CNS excitability, and oxybate counteracts this. GHB can be started before the blood alcohol level would have reached zero, as the onset is 20 minutes after the first dose. Although oxybate has anticonvulsant activity, this is unquantified so during withdrawal it is appropriate to use BDZs for about five days. It has relatively short half-life (4 hours; 8-hour action), so in people who have continued craving, it may be needed 4–6 times a day initially. There are no long-term studies but a duration of 7–10 days is recommended for alcohol withdrawal, with longer for dependence (see 1.5). For AWS it has been shown to be superior to diazepam (n = 42, RCT, open, 3/52, Nava et al, Am J Drug Alcohol Abuse 2007;33:379–92) and flunitrazepam, albeit with more hallucinations and other ADRs (n = 42, RCT, Lenzenhuber et al, Anaesthetist 1999;48:89–96) and as effective as clomethiazole (n = 98 [c = 65], RCT, d/b, p/c, 8/7, Nimmerrichter et al, Alcohol Alcoholism 2002; 37:67–73). The main ADR is slight 'subjective dizziness' in most people after first dose, which resolves in 15–30 minutes and does not occur with subsequent administrations. GHB risks abuse and dependence in polysubstance misuse, so it should not be offered to them.

Reviews: * general (Addolorato et al Expert Opin Investig Drugs 2009;**18**:675-86), mode of action (Ameisen, Alcohol and Alcoholism 2007; **42**:506-7).

Phenobarbital *

Phenobarbital IV (mean 509 mg/d) has been as effective as lorazepam oral (mean 4.2 mg/d) for mild-to-moderate AWS at 48 hours (n = 44, RCT, Hendey et al, Am J Emerg Med 2011;**29**:382–5), and a retrospective study suggested that phenobarbital was a safer alternative to diazepam in DTs (n = 194, Hjermø et al, Dan Med Bull 2010;**57**:A4169). In a more extreme case, phenobarbital IV 65 mg with 130 mg 15 minutes later was effective for BDZ-resistant DTs (n = 1, Hayner et al, Pharmacotherapy 2009; **29**:875–8). For those academically minded, the seizures had failed to respond to lorazepam at over 40 mg/ hr IV, so that indisputably classifies as BDZ-resistant.

Pregabalin *

Pregabalin up to 450 mg/d was as effective as lorazepam and superior to tiapride in uncomplicated AWS, and is a potentially useful treatment (n = 111, RCT, s/b, 14/7, Martinotti et al, Addiction 2010;**105**:288–99) and 200–450 mg/d might be a suitable alternative out-patient detoxification agent for AWS (n = 40, open, Di Nicola et al, Hum Psychopharmacol 2010;**25**:268–75).

Propofol

Benzodiazepine refractory AWS has been successfully treated with propofol infusion (n = 4, McCowan and Marik, Critical Care Med 2000;**28**:1781–4; n = 1, Takeshita, J Clin Psychiatry 2004;**65**:134–5).

Tiapride

A retrospective and then open prospective study concluded that tiapride has potential efficacy (n = 60 + 80, Franz et al, Eur Arch Psychiatry Clin Neurosci 2001;**251**:185–92).

Valproate

A review has concluded that only two of the six available studies show a significant effect for valproate and that it should not become a standard treatment (s = 6, Lum et al, Ann Pharmacother 2006;**40**:441–8), although it may be a suitable alternative to BDZs due to its lack of abuse potential (n = 16, RCT, 6/52, Longo et al, J Addict Dis 2002;**21**:55–64).

Zonisamide *

Zonisamide <600 mg/d (reducing to 100–300 mg/d) was superior to diazepam <130 mg/d (reducing to 5–15 mg/d) for AWS (n = 40, RCT, 3/52, Rubio et al, Pharmacopsychiatry 2010;**43**:257–62).

✱ Case reports

- **Trazodone** 600 mg/d (n = 1, Borras et al, Pharmacopsychiatry 2006;**39**:232).

◆ Others

Other drugs tried include **buprenorphine** (for abrupt withdrawal; Fudala et al, Clin Pharmacol Ther 1990;**47**:525–34), **dexamethasone** (as 4 mg injections; n = 110, Arch Int Med 1991;**114**:705–6), **flumazenil** (for AWS; n = 20, RCT, s/b, Gerra et al, Curr Ther Res 1991;**50**:62–6), **magnesium sulphate** (Ann Pharmacother 1992;**26**:650–2) and **nitrous oxide** (rapid relief of AWS; n = 104, Br J Psychiatry 1991;**159**:672–5), although its use is not recommended (s = 6, Prince and Turpin, Am J Health Syst Pharm 2008;**65**:1039–47).

☐ No efficacy

Fluvoxamine

A trial of fluvoxamine in alcoholic Korsakoff syndrome showed no therapeutic role and included two apparently fluvoxamine-induced episodes of depression (n = 8, O'Carroll et al, Psychopharmacol 1994;**116**:85–8).

Levetiracetam *

A prospective study showed no apparent efficacy or difference in diazepam rescue medication compared with placebo (n = 106, RCT, d/b, p/c, 6/7, Richter et al, J Clin Psychopharmacol 2010; **30**:72–5).

Nitrous oxide

Although rapid relief of AWS has been reported (n = 104, Gillman and Lichtigfeld, *Br J Psychiatry* 1991;**159**:672–5), its use is not recommended (s = 6, Prince and Turpin, *Am J Health Syst Pharm* 2008;**65**:1039–47).

ALZHEIMER'S DISEASE
see Dementia (*1.13*)

ANOREXIA AND BULIMIA NERVOSA
see Eating disorders (*1.15*)

1.6 ANXIETY DISORDER
(generalised) — Generalised Anxiety disorder (GAD) includes also Panic disorder (*1.19*) with or without Agoraphobia (*1.3*), OCD (*1.18*) and Social phobia (*1.25*)

Symptoms
There are numerous symptoms of generalised anxiety disorder (although anxiety can in itself be a symptom of many conditions), but they can be classified into two main groups:

- Psychological symptoms include fearful apprehension, irritability, poor concentration, restlessness, being easily fatigued, sensitivity to noise, disturbed sleep (lying awake worrying, waking intermittently, unpleasant dreams, but not usually early morning waking) and poor memory (due to poor concentration).
- Physical symptoms are mainly due to overactivity of the sympathetic system or increased muscle tension, e.g. gastrointestinal (dry mouth, difficulty swallowing, wind, loose motions, etc), CNS (tinnitus, blurred vision, dizziness), respiratory (constricted chest, difficulty inhaling, overbreathing), cardiovascular (palpitations, heart pain, missed or ectopic beats, neck throbbing), genitourinary (increased micturition, lack of libido and impotence), muscular tension (tension headache, tremor) and panic attacks (sudden episodes of extreme anxiety or apprehension).

Anxiety must be differentiated from depression, early schizophrenia, dementia, drugs/alcohol abuse including withdrawal and physical illness, e.g. thyroid dysfunction (n = 169, Simon *et al*, *J Affect Disord* 2002;**69**:209–17). The lifetime prevalence of anxiety disorders is about 17% in USA (Grant *et al*, *Can J Psychiatry* 2006;**51**:100–3; comment by Starcevic, *EBMH* 2006;**9**:115). GAD has a 90% lifetime comorbidity and only about 25% of GAD cases present without any comorbidity (Maier *et al*, *Acta Psychiatr Scand* 2000;**101**:29–36).

Role of drugs *
Anxiolytics such as benzodiazepines used as a 'first-line' measure are quite appropriate, but it is difficult to assess the longer-term effectiveness of these drugs, as anxiety tends to fluctuate for reasons other than pharmacotherapy. The decision for longer-term treatment must be considered on an individual basis, with the risk:benefit analysis varying with the disability caused by the symptoms and the age of the person. Choice of therapy is not easy but an independent and thorough analysis concluded that the effect sizes were:

- 0.5 pregabalin
- 0.45 antihistamines (hydroxyzine)
- 0.42 SNRI (venlafaxine)
- 0.38 benzodiazepines
- 0.36 SSRIs
- 0.17 buspirone
- -0.31 complementary and alternative medicines (Kava kava and homeopathy).

Children and adolescents responded better to medication and Kava kava was worse than placebo, with significant ADRs (s = 21, d/b, p/c, Hidalgo *et al*, *J Psychopharmacol* 2007;**21**: 864–72), although another systematic review concluded that of the herbal remedies there was only sound evidence for Kava kava for anxiety and it is not free from risks (Ernst, *Adv Psych Treat* 2007;**13**:312–6). The most recent systematic review and meta-analysis concluded that the top ranking drugs in mixed states were fluoxetine (response and remission) and sertraline (tolerability); and for pure GAD, the top drugs were duloxetine (response), escitalopram (remission), pregabalin (tolerability), with venlafaxine and paroxetine lower ranked (s = 27, RCT, Baldwin *et al*, *BMJ* 2011;**342**:1199).

The SSRIs and venlafaxine are effective across the range of anxiety disorders and are generally considered first-line treatment. Initial worsening and rare suicidal ideation can occur, so specific monitoring is needed early in treatment. BDZs are effective but use is not recommended by

NICE and should only be used in the short-term unless anxiety is treatment-resistant. Low-dose trifluoperazine has been shown to be superior to placebo for GAD, but is about the only antipsychotic that has (review by Gao et al, J Clin Psychiatry 2006;**67**:1327–40).TCAs and anticonvulsants can be tried in resistant cases but need an individual risk-benefit assessment. The role of pregabalin is yet to be established. Efficacy should be assessed at 12 weeks and, if successful, continued for six months. Psychological interventions include explanations, reassurance, support and, in more persistent conditions, cognitive and behavioural therapy.

Reviews: * evidence-base for drugs, review (Baldwin et al, J Psychopharmacol 2005;**19**:567–96; Baldwin and Polkinghorn, Int J Neuropsychopharmacol 2005;**8**:293–302), strategies for refractory GAD (Samuel et al, Int Clin Psychopharmacol 2011;**26**:63–8) in primary care (Davidson et al, Prim Care Companion J Clin Psychiatry 2010;**12**:PCC.09r00772), neurobiology (Stein, J Clin Psychiatry 2009;**70**(Suppl 2):15–9), pharmacotherapy (Davidson, J Clin Psychiatry 2009;**70** Suppl 2:25–31), general (Thuile et al, Curr Opin Psychiatry 2009:**22**:84–9, Gale and Davidson, Br Med J 2007;**334**:579–81).

BNF listed

BENZODIAZEPINES *

Benzodiazepines may be extremely useful for chronic anxiety and should not be overlooked, remembering that while indiscriminate benzodiazepine prescribing is inappropriate, they have a distinct role as safe and effective treatments, and that long-term use will not inevitably lead to dose escalation or other problems. A systematic review and meta-analysis of benzodiazepines showed robust evidence for efficacy if later, more rigorous, trials are favoured (s = 23, RCT, p/c, Martin et al, J Psychopharmacol 2007;**21**:774–82). Use of benzodiazepines can be restricted to short-term (up to four weeks) or intermittent courses.

Risks:

- All benzodiazepines are capable of being fatal in overdose (especially combined with alcohol) and should not be prescribed for patients at high risk of overdose.

There may be some difference between different drugs, e.g. temazepam (with rapid absorption and high sedative effect), alprazolam (n = 2063, Isbister et al, Br J Clin Pharmacol 2004;**58**:88–95) and possibly flurazepam may have a greater toxicity in overdose than other benzodiazepines (303 overdose study by Buckley et al, Br Med J 1995;**310**:219–21).

- BDZ users are significantly more likely to have road accidents, possibly as a result of greater difficulty in maintaining road position (s = 27, Rapoport et al, J Clin Psychiatry 2009; **70**:663–73).

- A retrospective review of hip fractures indicated that doses of > 3 mg/d diazepam (or equivalent) increased the risk of hip fractures by 50%, especially after initiation and after more than a month of treatment. Shorter half-life drugs did not appear to reduce this risk (n = 1 222 + 4 888, Wang et al, Am J Psychiatry 2001;**158**:892–8).

Reviews: * general (Cloos and Ferreira, Curr Opin Psychiatry 2009;**22**:90–5), withdrawing BDZs (Lader et al, CNS Drugs 2009;**23**:19–34).

Alprazolam
Alprazolam (review, Verster and Volkerts, CNS Drug Rev 2004;**10**:45–76) is a widely-used (except UK) BDZ.

Chlordiazepoxide
Chlordiazepoxide has a slower onset of action and many active metabolites.

Clobazam
Clobazam is licensed for the short-term (two to four weeks) treatment of anxiety.

Benzodiazepines are indicated for short-term relief of severe anxiety. Other treatment methods should then be started, e.g. relaxation, psychotherapy, treating any underlying depression, etc. Caution is advised for the use of benzodiazepines, e.g. use for short-term use, and avoid in depression and personality disorder.

Diazepam

Diazepam is the standard longer-acting benzo-diazepine, with sedative, anxiolytic and muscle relaxant properties (among others). It has a long half-life and many active metabolites.

Lorazepam

Lorazepam is a shorter-acting benzodiazepine with potent receptor-binding properties. Despite previous media interest in alleged dependence it remains widely used.

Oxazepam

A shorter-acting benzodiazepine (the ultimate metabolite of diazepam and some other benzodiazepines) with no active metabolites.

Non-benzodiazepines

Beta-blockers

Propranolol at 20–60 mg/d may be useful for somatic anxiety symptoms such as tachycardia, sweating and tremor (n = 120, open, c/o, Milanov, *Electromyogr Clin Neuophysiol* 2007;**47**:3–9). The best response appears to be in doses sufficient to reduce resting pulse by 7 bpm (Hallström *et al*, *Br J Psychiatry* 1981;**139**:417–21), and in patients presenting with autonomic complaints, e.g. palpitations, shortness of breath, sweating, rapid ventilation, etc.

Buspirone

Buspirone is a non-benzodiazepine anxiolytic with negligible sedative, cognitive (n = 60, RCT, d/b, Chamberlain *et al*, *J Psychopharmacol* 2007; **21**:210–5), hypnotic, anticonvulsant and muscle relaxant properties. In general, it is considered as effective as the benzodiazepines in GAD, with a better side-effect profile, although it has been noted that early efficacy studies were not performed in patients diagnosed with GAD using current criteria. It has a slow onset of action and may be underused, as it needs four weeks at 10 mg TDS for optimum efficacy. Buspirone possibly acts on 5-HT$_{1A}$ receptors and has no effect on withdrawal in benzodiazepine-dependent persons. Indeed, patients with GAD who have recently discontinued BDZs may suffer more ADRs and respond slower to buspirone than those who have neither had BDZs nor discontinued more

than a month before (n = 735, DeMartinis *et al*, *J Clin Psychiatry* 2000;**61**:91–4). Buspirone does not significantly reduce anxiety symptoms in opioid-dependent individuals (n = 36, RCT, p/c, McRae *et al*, *Am J Addict* 2004;**13**:53–63), although it has a non-existent abuse potential and abrupt discontinuation has not been shown to produce withdrawal symptoms. Cochrane concludes that buspirone is superior to placebo but less effective than BDZs (s = 36, n = 5908, Chessick *et al*, *Cochrane Database Syst Rev* 2006;**3**:CD006115).

Reviews: general (Apter and Allen, *J Clin Psychopharmacol* 1999;**19**:86–93), pharmaco-kinetics (Salazar *et al*, *J Clin Pharmacol* 2001; **41**:1351–8).

Duloxetine *

Duloxetine is licensed for GAD, with a starting dose of 30 mg/d, increasing to 60 mg/d if ineffective and with a maximum dose of 120 mg/d. Data from three independent trials showed duloxetine 60–120 mg/d to consistently improve functioning in GAD (s = 3, n = 1163, RCT, d/b, p/c, 9–10/52, Endicott *et al*, *J Clin Psychiatry* 2007;**68**:518–24) and 120 mg/d is non-inferior to venlafaxine 75–225 mg/d (56–58% response cf 40% with placebo) in adults with GAD (s = 2, n=984, RCT, d/b, p/c, 10/52, Allgulander *et al*, *J Psychopharmacol* 2008;**22**:417–25). In non-responders to duloxetine, 60 mg/d 6/52 there was some benefit from a further 6/12, but not from increasing the dose to 120 mg/d (n = 39 [c = 22], RCT, d/b, p/c, 24/52, Simon *et al*, *CNS Spectr* 2010;**15**:367–73). In responders from an open active treatment phase, relapse with duloxetine 60–120 mg/d was 14% vs 42% with placebo (n = 405, RCT, d/b, p/c, 26/52, Davidson *et al*, *Eur Neuropsychopharmacol* 2008;**18**:673–81).

Reviews: * general (s = 4, d/b, p/c, 9–10/52, Kornstein *et al*, *Expert Rev Neurother* 2009; **9**:155–65 Khan and Macaluso, *Neuropsychiatr Dis Treat* 2009;**5**:23–31), comprehensive review in GAD (Carter and McCormack, *CNS Drugs* 2009;**23**:523–41), use in comorbid depression (Mancini *et al*, *Expert Opin Pharmacother* 2010; **11**:1167–81, MS).

Escitalopram *

Escitalopram is licensed for generalised anxiety

disorder, with a 10mg/d starting dose and a 20mg/d maximum. There may be a significant improvement in GAD symptoms as early as the first week and the majority of patients respond by week eight with a significant improvement in functioning (n = 315, RCT, d/b, p/c, 8/52, Davidson et al, Depress Anxiety 2004;**19**:234–40). However, a trial should last at least four weeks before further intervention is considered (s = 40, Baldwin et al, Hum Psychopharmacol 2009;**24**:269–75). Several large studies have shown that escitalopram 10mg/d and 20mg/d are equally effective for GAD and superior to paroxetine (suggesting that perhaps not all SSRIs are the same in GAD) and placebo (n = 681, RCT, d/b, 12/52, Baldwin et al, Br J Psychiatry 2006;**189**:264–72; comment by Gale, EBMH 2007;**10**:45; n = 121, d/b, 24/52, Bielski et al, Ann Clin Psychiatry 2005;**17**:65–9; s = 3, RCT, p/c, Stein et al, Ann Clin Psychiatry 2005;**17**:71–5). It also seems effective in the long-term with relapse on escitalopram (20%) less than placebo (50%) (s = 4, RCT, d/b, 24/52, Bech et al, J Clin Psychiatry 2010;**71**:121–9). In older (>60) people with GAD, escitalopram is superior to placebo, but not significantly so (n = 177, RCT, d/b, p/c, 12/52, Lenze et al, JAMA 2009;**301**:295–303).

Hydroxyzine *

Hydroxyzine is an antihistamine related to the phenothiazines, which may be mildly useful in some cases. Cochrane is scathing about the available studies and does not think it possible to recommend hydroxyzine as a reliable anxiolytic in GAD (s = 5, n = 884, Guaiana et al, Cochrane Database Syst Rev 2011;**12**:CD006815).

Paroxetine

Paroxetine is licensed for GAD and a number of RCTs have shown 20–50mg/d to be rapidly effective (e.g. n = 324, RCT, p/c, Pollack et al, J Clin Psychiatry 2001;**62**:350–7). Paroxetine 20mg/d may be adequate (e.g. n = 278, RCT, d/b, p/c, 12/52, Baldwin et al, Br J Psychiatry 2006;**189**:264–72) and 40mg/d may be only slightly more effective than 20mg/d (n = 566, RCT, p/c, d/b, 8/52, Rickels et al, Am J Psychiatry 2003;**160**:749–56). Paroxetine may also be effective and well tolerated for long-term management of GAD and reduces relapse

(n = 652, d/b, p/c extension, 32/52, Stocchi et al, J Clin Psychiatry 2003;**64**:250–8; MS).
Reviews: overview of studies (s = 4, n = 1800, RCT, d/b, p/c, Rickels et al, J Clin Psychiatry 2006;**67**:41–7), use in anxiety (Snyderman et al, Expert Opin Pharmacother 2004;**5**:1799–806).

Pregabalin *

Pregabalin is licensed for GAD and one review concluded that 200–450mg/d is the optimal dose range, with 600mg/d being no more effective (s = 4, Bech, Pharmacopsychiatry 2007;**40**:163–8). Pregabalin 300mg/d appears reasonably well tolerated, significantly superior to placebo, and equivalent to alprazolam (n = 454, RCT, d/b, p/c, 4/52, Rickels et al, Arch Gen Psychiatry 2005;**62**:1022–30) and to venlafaxine (n = 21, RCT, d/b, p/c, 6/52, Montgomery et al, J Clin Psychiatry 2006;**67**:771–82; MS). It may also be a quick-acting anxiolytic and a dental anxiety scenario suggests pregabalin's effect may start after 3–4 hours (n = 89, RCT, d/b, p/c, 1/7, Nutt et al, J Psychopharmacol 2009;**23**:867–73). In responders, continuation therapy reduces relapse compared to placebo (42% vs 65%) and is reasonably well tolerated (n = 624, open, 8/52; then n = 338, RCT, p/c, d/b, 6/12, Feltner et al, Int Clin Psychopharmacol 2008;**23**:18–28, MS).
Reviews: * general (Anon, DTB 2010;**48**:19–22; Bendelow et al, Expert Rev Neurother 2007;**7**:769–81; Frampton and Foster, CNS Drugs 2006;**20**:685–95), kinetics (Bockbrader et al, J Clin Pharmacol 2010;**50**:941–50).

Venlafaxine XL

Venlafaxine is licensed for GAD, with 75mg/d considered the optimum dose, 150mg/d also effective but 37.5mg ineffective (n = 541, p/c, d/b, 24/52, Allgulander et al, Br J Psychiatry 2001;**179**:15–22, MS). Venlafaxine 75mg/d and pregabalin (400–600mg/d) may be equipotent and superior to placebo for GAD, but venlafaxine was less well tolerated and pregabalin possibly had an earlier onset (n = 426, RCT, d/b, 6/52, Montgomery et al, J Clin Psychiatry 2006;**67**:771–82; comment by Stein, EBMH 2007;**10**:23). It is also effective for depression with anxiety, e.g. 75–225mg/d was slightly more effective than fluoxetine (20–60mg/d) in 92 patients with comorbid

GAD and MDD (n = 368, 12/52, Silverstone and Salinas, J Clin Psychiatry 2001;**62**:523–9). Higher doses are not routinely recommended but can be used, e.g. venlafaxine up to 225mg/day was superior to placebo in non-depressed outpatients with generalised anxiety disorder (n = 251, RCT, 6/52, Gelenberg et al, JAMA 2000;**283**:3082–8). In a pooled analysis, venlafaxine was found to be as well tolerated and effective in older adults for anxiety as in younger adults (s = 5, n = 1839, RCT, Katz et al, J Am Geriatr Soc 2002;**50**:18–25).

Review: general (Thase, Expert Rev Neurother 2006;**6**:269–82).

> ● **Unlicensed/some efficacy**

Agomelatine *

Agomelatine 25–50mg/d has been shown to be effective and well tolerated for pure GAD (n = 121, RCT, d/b, p/c, 12/52, Stein et al, J Clin Psychopharmacol 2008;**28**:561–6; enthusiastic comment by Baldwin and Lopes, EBMH 2009;**12**:54; review by Baldwin and Lopes, Br J Hosp Med (Lond) 2010;**71**:153–6).

Antipsychotics *

Antipsychotics have little proven efficacy in GAD and have marked side-effects. **Quetiapine** is not licensed for GAD (and the license application suspended in 2010), but 150mg/d seems the optimum dose, and as effective as paroxetine (n = 873, RCT, d/b, 8/52, Bandelow et al, Int J Neuropsychopharmacol 2009;**20**:1–16), e.g. quetiapine 50–150mg/d is effective for GAD at 8 weeks, but 300mg/d was not superior to placebo at all points (n = 951, RCT, d/b, p/c, 10/52, Khan et al, J Clin Psychopharmacol 2011;**31**:418–28). A mean dose of 386mg/d may have some efficacy in resistant GAD as an adjunct to standard treatments (n = 40, open, 12/52, Katzman et al, J Anxiety Disord 2008; **22**:1480–6). Recurrence was lower on quetiapine than placebo (39% to 10%) (n = 432, RCT, d/b, p/c, up to 1 year, Katzman et al, Int Clin Psychopharmacol 2011:**26**:11–24). In a discontinuation maintenance study, 59% responded to open quetiapine; 51% entered the relapse prevention phase; and 10% relapsed on quetiapine vs 54% placebo after 6/12 (n = 268, RCT, d/b, p/c, 6/12 + 6/12, Rickels

et al, Arch Gen Psychiatry 2010;**67**:1274–81). **Trifluoperazine** 2–6mg/d may be superior to placebo (n = 415, d/b, p/c, 4/52, Mendels et al, J Clin Psychiatry 1986;**47**:170–4). Some newer antipsychotics have been used but the evidence for this currently makes it a costly strategy and PRN antipsychotics makes assessment of the underlying causes of agitation more difficult, especially as akathisia can be a side-effect. Antipsychotics should be used carefully and only for infrequent, sustained agitation. A pilot study suggested **aripiprazole** may be useful as an adjunct in resistant GAD (n = 13, open, 8/52, Hoge et al, CNS Spectr 2008;**13**:522–7; review by Katzman, J Aff Disord 2011;**128**[Suppl 1]:S11–20). Adjunctive low-dose **risperidone** (0.5–1.5 mg/d) was superior (but not statistically) to placebo as add-on to existing anxiolytics (n = 40, RCT, d/b, p/c, 5/52, Brawman-Mintzer et al, J Clin Psychiatry 2005;**66**:1321–5), and up to 3mg/d may be useful in refractory anxiety disorders (n = 30[c = 21], open, 8/52, Simon et al, J Clin Psychiatry 2006;**67**:381–5), but was ineffective for anxiety comorbid within bipolar disorder (n = 111, RCT, d/b, p/c, 8/52, Sheehan et al, J Affect Disord 2009:**115**:376–85) and even low doses up to 2mg/d risk hyperprolactinaemia (n = 12, Kopecek et al, Neuro Endocrinol Lett 2006;**27**:803–6). **Ziprasidone** was ineffective as monotherapy for GAD but might have some activity as an adjunct (n = 62[c = 47], RCT, d/b, p/c, 8/52, Lohoff et al, J Clin Psychopharmacol 2010;**30**:185–9). Cochrane concludes that the evidence for olanzapine and risperidone is too limited but that quetiapine monotherapy seems effective but with a lower tolerability (s = 11, n = 4144, Depping et al, Cochrane Database Syst Rev 2010;**12**:CD008120).

Reviews: * general (Gao et al, Expert Rev Neurother 2009;**9**:1147–58; Nemeroff, J Clin Psychiatry 2005;**66** Suppl 8:13–21), antipsychotics as adjuncts (Lorenz et al, Pharmacotherapy 2010; **30**:942–51).

Mirtazapine

Mirtazapine (15–45mg/d) may be effective within a week for the symptoms of GAD with comorbid depression and 30mg produced response in 78% and remission in 36% in a pilot study (n = 44, open, 12/52, Gambi et al, J Psychopharmacol 2006;**20**:483–7).

SSRIs
(see also paroxetine and escitalopram)

SSRIs have some efficacy in anxiety, with paroxetine and escitalopram licensed. Lower doses may be needed initially, as SSRIs may exacerbate symptoms over the first 1–2 weeks of treatment. **Citalopram** has been shown to be effective in 85% patients with GAD, including some who had failed with other SSRIs (n = 13, 12/52, Varia and Rauscher, *Int Clin Psychopharmacol* 2002;**17**:103–7). **Fluvoxamine** CR was superior to placebo for anxiety in adults, with few sexual side-effects (n = 300, RCT, d/b, p/c, 12/52, Westenberg *et al*, *J Clin Psychopharmacol* 2004;**24**:49–55) and it may be mildly effective for anxiety in children and adolescents (review by Irons, *Neuropsychiatr Dis Treat* 2005;**1**:289–99). **Sertraline** 50–150 mg/d was more effective than placebo for GAD (n = 370, RCT, d/b, p/c, 12/52, Allgulander *et al*, *Am J Psychiatry* 2004;**161**:1642–9), including acute treatment (n = 326, RCT, d/b, p/c, 10/52, Brawman-Mintzer *et al*, *J Clin Psychiatry* 2006;**67**:874–81).

Tricyclic antidepressants

Although not recommended by NICE, tricyclics may be useful for persistent or disabling anxiety. They may take several weeks to act but may be effective, e.g. imipramine may be at least as effective as diazepam and trazodone (see also trazodone) (n = 230, d/b, p/c, 8/52, Rickels *et al*, *Arch Gen Psychiatry* 1993;**50**:884–95).

■ Unlicensed/possible efficacy

Acamprosate *

Acamprosate 1998 mg/d had a 62% remission rate when used as an adjunct to SSRIs/SNRIs (n = 13, open, 8/52, Schwartz *et al*, *Ann Pharmacother* 2010;**44**:1930–2).

Gabapentin

In patients with a history of alcohol dependency or abuse, gabapentin 100–900 mg/d may produce sustained clinical improvement in symptoms of anxiety (n = 4, Pollack *et al*, *Am J Psychiatry* 1998;**155**:992–3; review by Norton and Quarles, *Hosp Pharm* 2001;**36**:843–5). Gabapentin 800 mg has reduced public-speaking provoked anxiety (n = 32, d/b, p/c, de-Paris *et al*, *J Psychopharmacol* 2003;**17**:184–8).

Galphimia glauca

Galphimia glauca is a traditional Mexican herbal medicine and was as effective and better tolerated than lorazepam 1 mg/d in GAD (n = 152, RCT, d/b, 4/52, Herrera-Arellano *et al*, *Planta Med* 2007;**73**:713–7).

Kava kava

Kava kava has been reported to be as effective as sub-therapeutic buspirone and a drug I've never heard of (opipramol), with a 75% response rate for all treatment arms which must say something about the illness severity in the trial (n = 129, RCT, 8/52, d/b, Boerner *et al*, *Phytomedicine* 2003;**10**[Suppl 4]:S38–S49). A meta-analysis showed it less than useful (see introduction).

Levetiracetam *

Levetiracetam up to 3000 mg/d appears to have no efficacy in moderate-to-severe GAD, although it was well tolerated (n = 217, RCT, d/b, p/c, 12/52, Stein *et al*, *J Clin Psychiatry* 2010;**71**:627–31), but a mean dose of 2 g/d may have some efficacy for resistant GAD (n = 40, open, 9/52, Kinrys *et al*, *J Clin Psychiatry* 2007;**68**:1010–3).

Omega-3 fatty acids *

There is a review of its possible role, but no clear evidence as yet (Ross, *Prostaglandins Leukot Essent Fatty Acids* 2009;**81**:309-12).

Passionflower (*Passiflora*)

Passionflower may have an anxiolytic effect, with a low incidence of drowsiness compared to oxazepam (n = 36, RCT, d/b, p/c, 4/52, Akhondzadeh *et al*, *J Clin Pharm Ther* 2001; **26**:363–7), although Cochrane concludes that the data is too sparse to draw any conclusions (s = 2, n = 198, Miyasaka *et al*, *Cochrane Database Syst Rev* 2007:**1**:CD004518).

Riluzole

Riluzole 100 mg/d was rapidly effective in 80%, producing remission in 53% over 2–3 weeks (n = 18 [c = 15], open, 8/52, Mathew *et al*, *Am J Psychiatry* 2005;**162**:2379–81).

Tiagabine

An analysis of the three trials showed no significant advantage over placebo in adults with GAD (s = 3, RCT, p/c, d/b, 10/52, Pollack *et al, J Clin Psychopharmacol* 2008;**28**:308–16), although the two less robust studies suggested some efficacy at 8–20 mg/d (e.g. n = 40, open, RCT, 10/52, Rosenthal, *J Clin Psychiatry* 2003;**64**:1245–9; n = 18 [c = 17], open, 8/52, Schwartz et al, *Ann Clin Psychiatry* 2005;**17**:167–72).

Review: in anxiety (Schwartz and Nihalani, *Expert Opin Pharmacother* 2006; **7**:1977–87).

Trazodone

Trazodone has been claimed to be equipotent with some benzodiazepines, e.g. at least as effective as diazepam and imipramine in GAD, although the antidepressants had more side-effects (n = 230, d/b, p/c, 8/52, Rickels et al, *Arch Gen Psychiatry* 1993;**50**:884–95).

❋ Case reports

- **Testosterone** injections (n = 1, Cooper and Ritchie, *Am J Psychiatry* 2000; **157**:1884).

◆ Others

Other drugs tried include **barbiturates** (such as amylobarbital), **mianserin** (n = 106, d/b, 6/52, Bjertnaes et al, *Acta Psychiatr Scand* 1982;**66**:199–207), **nabilone** (n = 8, RCT, Glass et al, *J Clin Pharmacol* 1981;**21**[Suppl 8–9]:S383–S96) and **St John's wort** (n = 100, d/b, 2/52, Panijel, *Therapiewoche* 1985;**41**:4659–68).

☐ No efficacy

Caffeine

Caffeine consumption should be calculated in GAD (*see Caffeinism 1.28*), as higher intakes can cause nervousness, anxiety, restlessness, irritability and palpitations, probably by an abnormal sensitivity to caffeine (n = 36, p/c, Bruce et al, *Arch Gen Psychiatry* 1992;**49**:867–9). One study, however, of chronic schizophrenic in-patients showed no change in anxiety when caffeine was removed from the diet (n = 26, Mayo et al, *Br J Psychiatry* 1993;**162**:543–5).

Review: anxiogenic effects of caffeine (Broderick and Benjamin, *J Okla State Med Assoc* 2004;**97**:538–42).

Homeopathy

Classical homeopathy was no different in one study to placebo, although both groups had high response rates (n = 44, RCT, d/b, p/c, 10/52, Bonne et al, *J Clin Psychiatry* 2003;**64**:282–7).

Ondansetron

One study showed 4 mg/d to be no better than placebo, although placebo response was high (n = 97, RCT, Romach et al, *J Clin Psychopharmacol* 1998;**18**:121–31).

Yohimbine

Yohimbine increases self-rated anxiety in anxiety-prone children (n = 32, Sallee et al, *Am J Psychiatry* 2000;**157**:1236–42).

1.7 ATTENTION DEFICIT HYPER-ACTIVITY DISORDER (ADHD), including HYPERKINETIC DISORDER

1.7.1 ADHD IN CHILDREN AND ADOLESCENTS

Symptoms: *

Attention deficit hyperactivity disorder (ADHD) is characterised by a developmentally inappropriate degree of gross motor activity, impulsivity, inattention to detail and temper outbursts. Children with ADHD have extreme and persistent restlessness, sustained and prolonged motor activity and difficulty in organising and maintaining attention to work or play. They are also easily distracted, fidget, careless, reckless, impulsive, reward seeking, prone to accidents, have learning difficulties (partly due to poor concentration), sleep problems (n = 466, Gau and Chiang, *Sleep* 2009;**32**:671–9), and often have antisocial behaviour and a fluctuating mood. Onset is before seven years of age. Symptoms can fade by puberty but inattention and antisocial behaviour may persist into adult life and may, but not always, lead to poor achievement (see *1.7.2*). ADHD is the most inheritable of all mental health conditions (up to 85%) and so there is a major genetic component. Studies implicate dysregulation of frontal-subcortical-cerebellar catecholamine circuits, including abnormal dopamine transport and impaired neurotransmission (e.g. Kuntsi et al, Neuromolecular Med 2006;**8**:461–84), especially in the nucleus accumbens and midbrain, areas that regulate reward and motivation (n = 97, Volkow et al, JAMA 2009;**302**:1084–91) and lead to a permanent state of dopamine deficiency.

Role of drugs

Pharmacotherapy is an essential component for the treatment package for ADHD. Careful medication management is effective in reducing core ADHD symptoms and superior to behavioural therapy. Stimulants have an immediate effect compared to a delayed effect from noradrenergic agents, e.g. atomoxetine (Wilens et al, J Atten Disord 2002;**5**:189–202). Methylphenidate is clearly the first-line stimulant (s = 62, n = 2897, RCT, Schachter et al, CMAJ 2001;**165**:1475–88; review by Connor, EBMH 2002;**5**:50). There is a natural reluctance by many prescribers to use stimulants in younger children and so mild symptoms should be managed with environmental changes, but moderate-to-severe symptoms may require drug therapy. A meta-analysis of methylphenidate and psychosocial treatments alone or together in adolescent ADHD showed that both were effective, but methylphenidate alone or in combination was superior to psychosocial treatments alone (s = 26, RCTs, Van der Oord et al, Clin Psychol Rev 2008;**28**:783–800; comment by Jensen, EBMH 2009;**12**:18).

Reviews: * general (Newcorn, J Clin Psychiatry 2011; **72**:12; Dopheide and Pliszka, Pharmacotherapy 2009;**29**:656–79), newer treatments (May and Kratochvil, Drugs 2010;**70**:15–40) treatment of comorbid ADHD and autism (Hazell, J Paediatr Child Health 2007;**43**:19–24), non-stimulant medications (Mohammadi and Akhondzadeh, Expert Rev Neurother 2007;**7**:195–201).

NB: Drug trials need to be interpreted carefully as different diagnostic criteria have been used in different studies.

BNF listed *

There are some comparisons between stimulants and atomoxetine. The most robust two show that atomoxetine is non-inferior to methylphenidate, and equally well tolerated, although atomoxetine

had more TEAEs (n = 330, RCT, d/b, 8/52, Wang et al, Aust N Z J Psychiatry 2007;**41**:222–30). The other showed that methylphenidate was superior to atomoxetine and both were superior to placebo, but that in non-responders to one, 42% then responded when switched to the other one (n=516, RCT, d/b, p/c, 6/52, Newcorn et al, Am J Psychiatry 2008;**165**:721–30).

- Although there is still some concern about prescribing stimulants in adolescents, a long-term follow-up of methylphenidate in male children (6–12 years of age) with ADHD showed that an early age of initiation does not increase the risk for negative outcomes (e.g. substance misuse) and probably has the opposite effect (n = 354, Mannuzza et al, Am J Psychiatry 2008;**165**:604–9).
- There is no statistically significant association between stimulant treatment between six and 17 years, and increased or decreased alcohol, drug or nicotine use in adult life (n = 140 [c = 112], 10-year follow-up, Biederman et al, Am J Psychiatry 2008;**165**:597–603)
- There is no evidence for increased risk of sudden death with stimulants in ADHD (n = 18637, McCarthy et al, Drug Saf 2009; **32**:1089–96).
- There is no evidence that ADHD is associated with changes in trajectories of height over time cf controls, or that stimulants have any effect on growth (n = 261, 10–11 years, Biederman et al, J Pediatrics 2010;**157**:635–40). For switching, see Chapter 2.

Review: atomoxetine vs stimulants (s = 5, Gibson et al, Ann Pharmacother 2006;**40**:1134–42).

Atomoxetine *

Atomoxetine is a noradrenaline reuptake inhibitor (NARI) with minimal effects on other transmitters. It is non-stimulant, with minimal abuse potential and no discontinuation syndrome. A meta-analysis of data has shown efficacy, although the authors thought it heterogenous and inconsistent (s = 9, RCT, p/c, Cheng et al, Psychopharmacology 2007;**194**:197–209). The usual dose is 0.5 mg/kg up to 40 mg/d for the first week, increased up to 100 mg/d. Higher doses have been shown to have no advantages over standard doses (s = 2, n = 247, RCT, d/b, Kratochvil et al, J Am Acad Child Adolesc

Psychiatry 2007;**46**:1128–37). In adolescents, higher doses may be more effective than lower doses (1.4 vs 0.8 mg/kg/d; n = 267, RCT, 40/52, Wietecha et al, J Child Adolesc Psychopharmacol 2009;**19**:719–30; MS). Atomoxetine takes 3–4 weeks to work, so if switching from a stimulant continue the stimulant for several weeks while the atomoxetine kicks in. Once-daily dosing of atomoxetine seems equally effective and as well tolerated as twice a day (e.g. n = 218, RCT, d/b, Adler et al, Ann Clin Psychiatry 2006;**18**:107–13), and may be effective throughout the day, including the next morning, unlike methylphenidate (n = 197, RCT, d/b, p/c, 8/52, Kelsey et al, Pediatrics 2004;**114**:1–8, MS). Long-term treatment seems effective (e.g. n = 125, 4 years, Adler et al, J Atten Disord 2008;**12**:248–53) and well-tolerated (s=13, n=714, open, 3-4yrs, Donnelly et al, J Am Acad Child Adolesc Psychiatry 2009;**48**:176-85). A meta-analysis of long-term follow-up data, showed atomoxetine had only a minor effect on height, with none on those with the lowest height (n = 412, >2 years, Spencer et al, Pediatrics 2005;**116**:74–80). While atomoxetine is effective for ADHD, it has no apparent efficacy for comorbid MDD (n = 142, d/b, 9/52, Atomoxetine ADHD-MDD study group, J Child Adolesc Psychopharmacol 2007;**17**:407–20, MS). In 2006, the UK MHRA issued guidance that people on atomoxetine should be monitored for signs of depression, suicidal thoughts or suicidal behaviour and referred for appropriate treatment if necessary, as increased suicidal thoughts or behaviour have been in association with atomoxetine (s = 12, n = 1357), although the incidence was only 0.4% and with no completed suicides.

Reviews:* general (Garnock-Jones and Keating, CNS Drugs 2010;**24**:85-8, Hammerness et al, Neuropsychiatr Dis Treat 2009;**5**:215–26; Vaughan et al, Expert Opin Pharmacother 2009;**10**:669–76).

Dexamfetamine

Amfetamine is clearly superior to placebo on a variety of key measures, remaining effective over 15 months (n = 62, RCT, 15/12, Gillberg et al, Arch Gen Psychiatry 1997;**54**:857–64; review by Hall, EBMH 1998;**1**:86). Exacerbation of chronic tic disorder by methylphenidate

or dexamfetamine has not been shown (n = 19, d/b, p/c, 1 year, Nolan et al, Pediatrics 1999;**103**:730–7).

Methylphenidate

At appropriate doses of methylphenidate (10–80 mg/d), a large proportion of children with ADHD obtain remission of symptoms. Methylphenidate's mode of action may be blockade of central dopamine transporters (Volkow et al, Am J Psychiatry 1998;**155**:1325–31), and may enhance the motivation to complete a task by increasing dopamine (n = 16, Volkow et al, Am J Psychiatry 2004;**161**:1173–80). Predictors of a positive response include demonstrable inattention, normal or near normal IQ, low anxiety (Buitelaar et al, J Am Acad Child Adolesc Psychiatry 1995; **34**:1025–32), high levels of hyperactivity at school and relatively low age (n = 36, RCT, Zeiner et al, Acta Pediatr 1999;**88**:298–303). However, a recent meta-analysis concluded that while methylphenidate is clearly superior to placebo, the effect size is smaller than would be expected (s = 16, Koesters et al, J Psychopharmacol 2009;**23**:733–44). The new SR preparations (eg. Concerta® XL, Janssen, Equasym®, UCB Pharma, Medikinet®, Flynn) have made dosing much easier. The response to methylphenidate in ADHD does not appear to be moderated by comorbid anxiety (n = 91, RCT, 4/12, Diamond et al, J Am Acad Chold Adolesc Psychiatry 1999;**38**:402–9; reviewed in EBMH 1999;**2**:108).

Reviews: pharmacokinetics and efficacy (Kimko et al, Clin Pharmacokinet 1999;**37**:457–70, 75 refs), side-effects (review, Rappaport and Moffitt, Clin Psychol Rev 2002;**22**:1107–31).

+ Combinations

Review: general (Adler et al, Curr Psychiatry Rep 2006;**8**:409–15).

Antipsychotics (e.g. risperidone) + stimulants

See unlicensed/some efficacy.

Atomoxetine + methylphenidate

Adding methylphenidate to atomoxetine

non-responders in previous stimulant non-responders seems a pointless exercise (n = 25, RCT, p/c, d/b, Carlson et al, Child Adolesc Psychiatry Mental Health 2007;**1**:10), although there is a case of successful use in a 10-year-old boy (n = 1, J Child Adolesc Psychopharmacol 2006;**16**:365–70).

● Unlicensed/some efficacy

Amantadine *

A pilot study showed that amantadine 100-150mg/d had efficacy equivalent to methylphenidate 20-30mg/d (n=40, RCT, d/b, 6/52, Mohammadi et al, Hum Psychopharmacol 2010; in press).

Antipsychotics

The 2008 NICE guidelines do not recommend use of antipsychotics in ADHD as, although they have been used for uncontrollable and explosive behaviour, their side-effect profile makes them unsatisfactory. This potential for long-term side-effects and worsening cognitive learning function usually outweighs their potential advantages. However, **risperidone** may be at least as effective as methylphenidate for ADHD in children and adolescents with moderate learning disabilities (n = 45, s/b, 4/52, Filho et al, J Am Acad Child Adolesc Psychiatry 2005;**44**:748–55), and risperidone (mean 1mg/d) was very useful for treating aggression in ADHD (n = 25, RCT, p/c, 4/52, Armenteros et al, J Am Acad

Methylphenidate formulations: plasma profiles

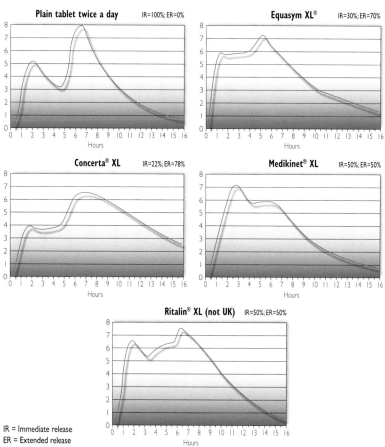

Plain tablet twice a day IR=100%; ER=0%

Equasym XL® IR=30%; ER=70%

Concerta® XL IR=22%; ER=78%

Medikinet® XL IR=50%; ER=50%

Ritalin® XL (not UK) IR=50%; ER=50%

IR = Immediate release
ER = Extended release

Child Adolesc Psychiatry 2007;**46**:558–65). In methylphenidate-resistant ADHD, addition of **quetiapine** produced significant improvement in 47% and was well tolerated (n = 30, open, 3 + 9/52, Kronenberger et al, J Child Adolesc Psychopharmacol 2007;**17**:334–47). **Aripiprazole** (mean 6.7 mg/d), reduced ADHD symptoms and improved overall functioning (n = 23, open, 6/52, Findling et al, J Child Adolesc Psychopharmacol 2008;**18**:347–54).

Bupropion

There is a growing body of evidence supporting the use of bupropion in ADHD. Bupropion XL up to 450 mg/d may be effective (53% vs 31% for placebo) providing well tolerated and sustained benefit throughout the day (n = 162, RCT, d/b, p/c, 8/52, Wilens et al, Biol Psychiatry 2005;**57**:793–801). Bupropion (mean 3.3 mg/kg/d) and methylphenidate (mean 0.7 mg/kg/d) were equipotent in children with ADHD in one trial (n = 15, RCT, 6/52, Barrickman et al, J Am Acad Child Adolesc Psychiatry 1995;**34**:649–57) and provides another pharmacological alternative to stimulants in ADHD.

Clonidine *

Clonidine (an alpha-2 agonist) has been widely used for treatment-resistant ADHD. and an SR version (Kapvay®) is now licensed in USA as add-on or monotherapy for ADHD in 6–17-year-olds. 0.1–0.3 mg/d may be effective (but less so than methylphenidate) in ADHD (n = 122, RCT, d/b, p/c, 16/52, Palumbo et al, J Am Acad Child Adolesc Psychiatry 2008;**47**:180–8; see also s = 11, n = 150, Connor et al, J Am Acad Child Adolesc Psychiatry 1999;**38**:1551–9; reviewed by Greenhill, EBMH 2000;**3**:74). It may be useful as a well tolerated (Daviss et al, J Am Acad Child Adolesc Psychiatry 2008;**47**:189–98) and cheaper alternative to methylphenidate (n = 50, RCT, d/b, Nair and Mahadevan, J Trop Pediatr 2009;**55**:116–21). Clonidine augmentation of stimulants can be used to improve conduct, (e.g. n = 198, RCT, d/b, p/c, Kollins et al, Pediatrics 2011;**127**:1406–13) and may help reduce stimulant adverse effects (n = 67, RCT, p/c, 6/52, Hazell and Stuart, J Am Acad Child Adolesc Psychiatry 2003;**42**:886–94).

Review: * clonidine and alpha-2 adrenergic

agonists (Sallee, Postgrad Med 2010;**122**:78–87)

Modafinil

Modafinil appears to be promising in ADHD, e.g. once-daily modafinil (170–425 mg/d) was well tolerated and effective in children and adolescents on all rating systems and 200–300 mg/d was superior to placebo for ADHD (n = 46, RCT, d/b, p/c, 6/52, Kahbazi et al, Psychiatry Res 2009;**168**:237–7). The most recent review concludes that modafinil improves ADHD symptoms and behaviours compared to placebo (s = 3, n = 638, d/b, p/c, < 9/52, Biederman and Pliszka, J Pediatr 2008;**152**:394–9), with no withdrawal symptoms on abrupt withdrawal (n = 190, RCT, d/b, p/c, 9/52, Swanson et al, J Clin Psychiatry 2006;**67**:137–47). Once-daily dosing is better tolerated than divided doses (n = 248 [c = 223], RCT, d/b, p/c, 4/52, Biederman et al, J Clin Psychiatry 2006;**67**:727–35).

Reboxetine

Reboxetine is a NARI, like atomoxetine, and so logically it could be useful in ADHD. Reboxetine 4–6 mg/d was as effective as methylphenidate 20–50 mg/d (n = 33, d/b, 6/52, Arabgol et al, Eur Child Adolesc Psychiatry 2008; **18**:53–9), and 2–8 mg/d almost as effective as methylphenidate 10–20 mg/d (n = 27, open, 8/52, Cohen-Yavin et al, Clin Neuropharmacol 2009;**32**:179–82). It may have some efficacy in stimulant-resistant ADHD (n = 31, RCT, open, 6/52, Ratner et al, J Am Acad Child Adolesc Psychiatry 2005;**44**:428–33).

Selegiline

In an active comparison, selegiline and methylphenidate were equally effective for child and adolescent ADHD (n = 40, RCT, 60/7, Mohammadi et al, J Child Adolesc Psychopharmacol 2004;**14**:418–25).

Tricyclics

Tricyclics are considered useful in patients non-responsive or intolerant of stimulants. Imipramine, clomipramine, nortriptyline and desipramine have been used in doses of 10–150 mg/d (mean 80 mg). In a retrospective, naturalistic study, tricyclics were shown to be effective at antidepressant doses (n = 37,

Wilens et al, J Nerv Ment Dis 1995; **183**:48–9), although other authors have suggested that lower doses (e.g. 25–50 mg/d) are effective. Sudden death, including cardiac arrest, has been reported with relatively low plasma levels (Riddle et al, J Am Acad Child Adolesc Psychiatry 1991; **30**:104–8) and so close monitoring is warranted.

Venlafaxine *

Venlafaxine 50–75 mg/d was equivalent to methylphenidate in a pilot study, with tolerable side-effects (n = 38, RCT, d/b, Zarinara et al, Hum Psychopharmacol 2010; **25**:530–5).

■ Unlicensed/possible efficacy

Buspirone *

Buspirone (0.5 mg/kg/d) was equivalent to methylphenidate for symptoms of ADHD except inattention (MHP better than buspirone) (n = 34, RCT, d/b, 6/52, Davari-Ashtiani et al, Child Psychiatry Hum Dev 2010; **41**:641–8).

Ginkgo biloba

GB has been shown to be less effective than methylphenidate in ADHD, but we do not know if it is better than placebo (n = 50, RCT, d/b, 6/52, Salehi et al, Prog Neuropsychopharmacol Biol Psychiatry 2010; **34**:76–80; see also n = 6, Niederhofer, Phytother Res 2010; **24**:26–7).

MAOIs

MAOIs are not considered as effective as stimulants but may help some non-responders, e.g. tranylcypromine has been considered as effective as stimulants but the dietary restrictions proved too difficult to manage.

Melatonin *

Although melatonin advances circadian rhythms and enhances sleep time (review by Bendz and Scates, Ann Pharmacother 2010; **44**:185–91), there appears no effect on behaviour, cognition or QoL in ADHD (n = 105, RCT, d/b, p/c, 4/52, Van der Heijden et al, J Am Acad Child Adolesc Psychiatry 2007; **46**:233–41).

Memantine

A pilot study suggested a dose-dependent improvement in ADHD-IV and CGI-S with memantine 10–20 mg/d (n = 16, open, 8/52, Findling et al, J Acad Adolesc Psychopharmacol 2007; **17**:19–33).

Nicotine

Daily transdermal nicotine reduced hyper-activity and learning problems in a pilot study, but was poorly tolerated and so other methods of nicotinic receptor modulation may be worth investigating (n = 10, RCT, d/b, p/c, 2/52, Shytle et al, World J Biol Psychiatry 2002; **3**:150–5).

SSRIs

Serotonin function may be abnormal in ADHD (Fargason and Ford, South Med J 1994; **87**:302–9) and fluoxetine 20–60 mg/d may produce some statistical improvements in some rating scales (n = 22, open, Barrickman et al, J Am Acad Child Adolesc Psychiatry 1991; **30**:762–7).

Valproate *

In stimulant-resistant aggression in ADHD, 57% remitted on valproate compared with only 15% with placebo (n = 27, RCT, d/b, p/c, 8/52, Blader et al, Am J Psychiatry 2009; **166**:1392–401).

Zinc *

Zinc seemed to have some efficacy, but only at doses of 15 mg twice a day, not once a day (n = 52, RCT, d/b, p/c, 13/52, Arnold et al, J Child Adolesc Psychopharmacol 2011; **21**:1–19).

✱ Case reports

- **Duloxetine** * (n = 1, Niederhofer, Eur Psychiatry 2010; **25**:214–5).
- **Gabapentin** (n = 1, Ryback and Ryback, Am J Psychiatry 1995; **152**:1399; n = 1, Hamrin and Bailey, J Child Adolesc Psychopharmacol 2001; **11**:301–9).

◆ Others

Other drugs tried include **thyroid** (n = 1, N Engl J Med 1993; **328**:997–1001).

☐ No efficacy

Barbiturates

These have been tried but excitation and agitation may be counter-productive.

Benzodiazepines

As for barbiturates.

Caffeine

Caffeine is ineffective as a minor stimulant (Dulcan, *Pediatr Ann* 1985;**14**:383–400) as tolerance develops too rapidly.

Donepezil

Adjunctive donepezil seems poorly tolerated and ineffectual for residual ADHD and cognitive symptoms (n = 13 [c = 7], open, 12/52, Wilens *et al*, *J Child Adolesc Psychopharmacol* 2005;**15**:947–55).

Homeopathy

There is no evidence for any efficacy for homeopathy in ADHD (s = 4, n = 168, Coulter and Dean, *Cochrane Database Syst Rev* 2007; **4**:CD005648).

Omega-3 fatty acids *

Recent trials of omega-3/6 only show limited response in a small sub-group of inattentive ADHD adolescents (n = 75, RCT, p/c, c/o, 6/12, Johnson *et al*, *J Atten Disord* 2009;**12**:394–401; n = 37 [c = 26], RCT, d/b, p/c, c/o, 16/52, Bélanger *et al*, *Paediatr Child Health* 2009;**14**:89–98), and a systematic review concluded that EFA supplements do not have an evidence base for routine use (Raz and Gabis, *Dev Med Child Neurol* 2009;**51**:580–92; see also Aben and Danckaerts, *Tijdschr Psychiatr* 2010;**52**:89–97).

Selegiline

Selegiline may be mildly useful for the in-attentive ADHD sub-type, but has little effect on impulsivity (n = 11, RCT, d/b, p/c, c/o, Rubenstein *et al*, *J Child Adolesc Psychopharmacol* 2006;**16**:404–15).

St John's wort

SJW was ineffective in improving symptoms of ADHD (n = 54, RCT, d/b, p/c, 8/52, Weber *et al*, *JAMA* 2008;**299**:2633–41).

1.7.2 ADHD IN ADULTS

Incidence and importance

Adult ADHD is widely under-recognised. Up to 65% adolescents with ADHD will have enduring symptoms, with around 3–4% adults affected, remarkably similar in different countries (n = 11422, Fayyad *et al*, *Br J Psychiatry* 2007;**190**:402–9; comment by Thome, *EBMH* 2008;**11**:31: n = 966, Faraone and Biederman, *J Atten Disord* 2005;**9**:384–91). Comorbidity is common (review by Barkley and Brown, *CNS Spectr* 2008;**13**:977–84), e.g. anxiety (n = 349, Karam *et al*, *J Psychiatr Res* 2009;**43**:697–701), BPD, SUD (Bukstein, *Medscape J Med* 2008;**10**:24), depression (McIntosh *et al*, *Neuropsychiatr Dis Treat* 2009;**5**:137–50), bipolar disorder (n = 159, Tamam *et al*, *Eur Arch Psychiatry Clin Neurosci* 2008;**258**:385–93), conduct disorders (Dowson, *Acta Psychiatr Scand* 2008;**117**:299–305), eating disorders (Nazar *et al*, *Rev Bras Psiquiatr* 2008;**30**:384–9), thus making diagnosis tricky. Indeed, around 20% adults with SUD have ADHD (11–35%, Kalbag and Levin, *Subst Use Misuse* 2005;**40**:1955–81;2043–8; review Wilens, *J Clin Psychiatry* 2007;**68**[Suppl 11]:4–8). Adults with ADHD may have lower educational achievement levels, but not because of low IQ (n = 117, Antshel *et al*, *Psychol Med* 2009;**39**:1325–35). There is an 85% genetic link (adult ADHD having a greater inheritability), with some association with the D4 gene (Faraone, *Psychiatr Clin North Am* 2004;**27**:303–21).

Symptoms *

Adult ADHD (Hesslinger *et al*, *Psychiatry Res* 2003;**119**:217–23) may present as:

- Continuation of symptoms from adolescence
- Re-presentation after a treatment gap by young adults now realising they cannot cope
- First diagnosis, never diagnosed as children but with a history of symptoms
- Late-onset (as opposed to late diagnosis), which is controversial and relatively rare.

Over 90% adults with ADHD suffer from poor attention as the main symptoms (n = 107, Wilens *et al*, *J Clin Psychiatry* 2009;**70**:1557–62) with work, family and social activities also affected, although hyperactivity diminishes and impulsivity is less. Driving is a particular problem, as they get fatigued quickly and are more likely to have accidents on motorways or open roads when attention lapses (Reimer *et al*, *Traffic Inj Prev* 2007;**8**:290–9), and have more tickets and offences, often as result of impulsivity (n = 355, Thompson *et al*, *J Pediatr Psychol* 2007;**32**:745–

59). They are likely to have a lifetime history of sleep problems (n=2284, Gau et al, Sleep 2007;**30**:195–201).

Role of drugs

Prescribing of ADHD treatments drops significantly from age 15–21, but at a greater rate than age-reported lessening of symptoms, suggesting premature stopping in some people who need treatment (McCarthy et al, Br J Psychiatry 2009;**194**:273–7). Stimulants are as effective in adults as in younger people, albeit currently unlicensed. Pharmacotherapy for ADHD is not compromised by psychiatric co-morbidity (Babock and Ornstein, Postgrad Med 2009;**121**:73–82). A systematic review and meta-analysis has concluded that the main evidence in adults is for immediate release methylphenidate, rather than the SR preparations (s=22, n=2203, Peterson et al, Psychopharmacology (Berl) 2008; **197**:1–11). Compliance is often good, and self-reported compliance correlates well with actual compliance (Safren et al, J Atten Disord 2007;**10**:257–60). Many will self-medicate, e.g. with amphetamines if sub-optimally treated. Although diversion is possible (reportedly 16–29%), it is less likely with SR preps (s=21, n=113,104, Wilens et al, J Am Acad Child Adolesc Psychiatry 2008;**47**:21–31). CBT in addition to medications can improve response (Rostain, Postgrad Med 2008;**120**:27–38).

Reviews: * general (Rösler et al, World J Biol Psychiatry 2010;**11**:684–98; Simon et al, Br J Psychiatry 2009;**194**:204–11, comment by Asher-son, EBMH 2009;**12**:128; Feifel and MacDonald, Postgrad Med 2008;**120**:39–47; Tcheremissine and Salazar, Expert Opin Pharmacother 2008;**9**:1299–310. Rostain, Postgrad Med 2008; **120**:27–38; Thomsen and Damm, Igeskr Laeger 2008;**170**:3395–9), pharmacotherapy (Adler, J Clin Psychiatry 2009;**70**:e12; Mészáros et al, Int J Neuropsychopharmacol 2009;**12**:1137–47; Kolar et al, Neuropsychiatr Dis Treat 2008;**4**:107–21; non-stimulants, Newcorn, CNS Spectr 2008;**13**(9 Suppl 13):12–6; stimulants, Stein, CNS Spectr 2008;**13**(9 Suppl 13):8–11), antidepressants in adult ADHD (s=8, Verbeeck et al, Adv Ther 2009;**26**:170–84), managing adult ADHD and SUD (Upadhyaya, J Clin Psychiatry 2007;**68**[Suppl 11]:23–30), clinical guidelines (Gibbins and Weiss, Curr Psychiatry Rep 2007;**9**:420–6), BAP guidelines for adolescents

in transition to adult services and in adults (Nutt et al, J Psychopharmacol 2007;**21**:10–41), neurobiological and genetics (Spencer, CNS Spectr 2008;**13**(9 Suppl 13):5–7).

Unlicensed (but BNF listed for adolescents)

Atomoxetine *

Atomoxetine is not licensed for adult ADHD in UK (but is in e.g. USA). It has advantages in that the risk of diversion is minimal and it is not a controlled drug. A two-trial analysis showed discontinuations at under 10% in adult ADHD (s=2, n=536, RCT, d/b, p/c, 10/52, Michelson et al, Biol Psychiatry 2003;**53**:112–20). Atomoxetine 1.2 mg/kg/d has been shown to improve simulated driving performance (n=18, p/c, c/o, 3/52, Barkley et al, J Atten Disord 2007;**10**:306–16) and can help with comorbid social anxiety (n=442, RCT, d/b, p/c, 16/52, Adler et al, Depress Anxiety 2009;**26**:212–21). Analysis of four studies shows no discontinuation symptoms or rebound, and tapering is not required when stopped (s=4, 9–10/52, Wernicke et al, J Clin Psychopharmacol 2004;**24**:30–5, MS). Atomoxetine can be given once-daily in adults, with an effect lasting into the evening, and for at least 6/12 (n=501, RCT, d/b, p/c, 6/12, Adler et al, J Clin Psychopharmacol 2009;**29**:44–50), and effective (68% vs 42% response) over the longer-term (n=502, RCT, d/b, p/c, 24/52, Young et al, Clin Neuropharmacol 2011;**34**:51-60).

Reviews: general (Vaughan et al, Expert Opin Pharmacother 2009;**10**:669–76; Durell et al, J Atten Disord 2010;**13**:401–6; SM).

Dexamfetamine

Dexamfetamine has been shown to be superior to placebo in adult ADHD (n=68 [c=67], RCT, d/b, p/c. Paterson et al, Aust N Z J Psychiatry 1999;**33**:494–502).

Methylphenidate *

Methylphenidate is not yet licensed for adult ADHD in the UK but has recently been approved in USA, and Medikinet® is licensed for adults in Germany. A recent study showed a statistical and clear efficacy, with a 50% response at 8/52 (cf. 18% in placebo group) and no difference in bp at any visit, albeit with a transient heart rate increase (n = 162, RCT, d/b, p/c, 8/52, Retz et al, World J Biol Psychiatry 2011; in press), although a modest rise in blood pressure and heart rate can occur (s = 26, n = 811, Godfrey, J Psychopharmacol 2009;**23**:194–205). There remains some controversy about dosing. Large studies have suggested that 'robust' dosing (mean 1 mg/kg/d) may be highly effective (response 76% vs 19% placebo) compared to more traditional dosing (e.g. n = 146, RCT, d/b, p/c, 6/52, Spencer et al, Biol Psychiatry 2005;**57**:456–63). A meta-regression analysis concludes that methylphenidate improves adult ADHD in a dose-dependent fashion, but the efficacy is reduced with comorbid SUD (s = 18, Castells et al, CNS Drugs 2011;**25**:157–69). There is a lower risk for diversion with SR preparations (n = 50[c = 39], RCT, d/b, p/c, c/o, 2×5/52, Jain et al, J Clin Psychiatry 2007;**68**:268–77). Methylphenidate improves simulated driving performance in adult ADHD (e.g. n = 19 [c = 18], RCT, d/b, p/c, c/o, 11/7, Verster et al, J Psychopharmacol 2008;**22**:230–7).

Review: general (Nair and Moss, Neuropsychiatr Dis Treat 2009;**5**:421–32).

● Unlicensed/some efficacy

Bupropion

Bupropion has been investigated and it seems effective in adult ADHD, with a more rapid response than the significant placebo effect (n = 162, RCT, p/c, d/b, 8/52, Wilens et al, Biol Psychiatry 2005;**57**:793–801). Bupropion was equivalent to methylphenidate and superior (but not statistically) to placebo in adult ADHD (n = 30, RCT, d/b, p/c, 7/52, Kuperman et al, Ann Clin Psychiatry 2001;**13**:129–34) and up to 400 mg/d has been shown to be significantly superior to placebo (76% vs 37% improved) and, although the exclusion criteria were unclear, further trials are warranted (n = 40[c = 38], RCT, d/b, 6/52, Wilens et al, Am J Psychiatry 2001;**158**:282–8; reviewed by Ferre and Nutt, EBMH 2001;**4**:92). Bupropion up to 400 mg/d may be effective in ADHD with comorbid SUD (n = 14[c = 13], open, 6/12, Solhkhah et al, J Child Adolesc Psychopharmacol 2005;**15**:777–86). Usefully, in comorbid ADHD and bipolar, bupropion may be effective for ADHD without

precipitating mania (n = 36 [c = 30], open, 6/52, Wilens et al, Biol Psychiatry 2003;**54**:9–16).

Clonidine

A license application for a CR product for adult ADHD has been submitted in USA.

■ Unlicensed/possible efficacy

Duloxetine *

There are cases of duloxetine 30 mg/d having some efficacy (n = 2, p/c, c/o, 8/52, Niederhofer, Prim Care Companion J Clin Psychiatry 2010; **12**:PCC.09l00807), including in a 53-year-old male (n = 1, Tourjman and Bilodeau, J Atten Disord 2009;**13**:95–6).

Fish oils

High dose fish oil was better than flax oil or olive oil for correcting low serum phospholipid fatty acid levels in adults with ADHD (n = 30, RCT, 12/52, Young et al, Reprod Nutr Dev 2005; **45**:549–58).

Guanfacine

This alpha-2 noradrenergic agonist (similar to clonidine) may have some potential (n = 17, d/b, p/c, c/o, Taylor and Russo, J Clin Psychopharmacol 2001;**21**:223–8).

Lithium

Lithium (up to 1200 mg/d) was equivalent to methylphenidate (up to 40 mg/d) on most outcome measures in one study (RCT, d/b, c/o, 2×8/52, Dorrego et al, J Neuropsychiatry Clin Neurosci 2002;**14**:289–95).

Modafinil

Modafinil was comparable to dexamfetamine and superior to placebo in adult ADHD (n = 22[c = 21], RCT, p/c, c/o, 3×3/52, Taylor and Russo, J Child Adolesc Psychopharmacol 2000;**10**:311–20).

Nicotine

This indirect dopamine agonist (smoked or transdermally) improves concentration in adult ADHD (s = 2, n = 17, d/b, c/o, Conners and Levin, Psychopharmacol Bull 1996;**32**:55–73), and is frequently used as self-medication by adults with ADHD.

Oxcarbazepine

Oxcarbazepine 300–1500 mg/d may be effective in some adults with ADHD (n = 9 [c = 8], open, 8/52, Davids et al, Prog Neuropsychopharmacol Biol Psychiatry 2006;**30**:1033–8).

Tianeptine

Tianeptine may be 'a slightly effective beneficial and useful treatment for adult ADHD' according to a Medline abstract (n = 68, open, Niederhofer, Neuropsychobiology 2004;**49**:130–3).

Venlafaxine

Although 70% completers responded to venlafaxine 50–150 mg/d, it was poorly tolerated (n = 18 [c = 11], Hedges et al, Psychopharmacol Bull 1995;**31**:779–83). There has been one positive trial of 75 mg/d (n = 10 [= 9], open, 8/52, Findling et al, J Clin Psychiatry 1996;**57**:184–9).

✽ Case reports

- **Milnacipran** (n = 1, Kako et al, Prog Neuropsychopharmacol Biol Psychiatry 2007;**31**:772–5).
- **Moclobemide** (n = 1, Vaiva et al, Prog Neuropsychopharmacol Biol Psychiatry 2002;**26**:609–11).
- **Varenicline** (n = 1, 6/52, Cocores and Gold, J Neuropsychiatry Clin Neurosci 2008;**20**:494–5).

☐ No efficacy

Anticholinesterases

A small open study of adjunctive **donepezil** showed it to be poorly tolerated and ineffective in adults (n = 6, open, 12/52, Wilens et al, J Child Adolesc Psychopharmacol 2005;**15**:947–55) and **galantamine** had no detectable effects (n = 36, RCT, d/b, p/c, 12/52, Biederman et al, J Clin Psychopharmacol 2006;**26**:163–6).

Homeopathy

There is no significant treatment effect on ADHD or related symptoms (s = 4, n = 168, Coulter and Dean, Cochrane Database Syst Rev 2007;**17**:CD005648).

Selegiline

Selegiline up to 60 mg/d was no more effective than placebo in adults and had significant ADRs (n = 24, RCT, d/b, p/c, 10/52, Ernst et al, Psychopharmacol Bull 1996;**32**:327–34), although it may have some efficacy in adolescents.

1.8 AUTISTIC SPECTRUM DISORDERS (ASD)

Symptoms

Autistic spectrum disorders (ASD) are neuro-developmental in origin, characterised by an excessive or morbid dislike of others or society, not responding with normal human emotions towards other people, a morbid self-centred attitude and with major impairments or abnormalities in language, communication, reciprocity, social interactions, imagination and behaviour. The main features include 'autistic aloneness', poor speech and language development, an obsessive desire for sameness, bizarre behaviour or mannerisms, a restricted repertoire of activities and interests, rituals and compulsive behaviour. Onset is not later than three years of age, the incidence 0.04%, or up to 0.2% if including associated conditions (Gillberg and Wing, Acta Psychiatr Scand 1999; **99**:399–406). Up to 25% develop seizures in adolescence, 75% have an IQ in the retarded range, and up to 60% need long-term residential care. There is some evidence that dietary gluten could be implicated in ASDs, and that a gluten-free diet may ameliorate symptoms, particularly if implemented at a very early stage (review by Shattock and Whiteley, Pharm J 2001; **267**:17–9), although Cochrane concludes that there is insufficient data (Millward et al, Cochrane Database Syst Rev 2008;**2**:CD003498).

Role of drugs

Drugs may be of limited use in treating some of the more severe behavioural symptoms. Self-injurious behaviour (SIB) is common (see 1.25) and may be helped by low dose antipsychotics, to which autistic individuals seem very sensitive and so lower doses may be needed. Only risperidone and methylphenidate have more than one trial to show efficacy for aggressive symptoms in ASD (s = 21, Parikh et al, J Child Adolesc Psychopharmacol 2008;**18**:157–78). A therapeutic window may exist, and higher doses may be counter-productive. Family support,

1

education, skills training, behavioural therapy and social support can be significant aspects of the overall management.

Reviews: * general (Levy et al, Lancet 2009; **374**:1627–38; Moss and Howlin, J Intellect Disabil Res 2009;**53**:852–73; Wink et al, Curr Treat Options Neurol 2010;**12**:529–38), systematic review of new treatments (Rossignol, Ann Clin Psychiatry 2009;**21**:213–36), sleep in ASD (Miano and Ferri, Paediatr Drugs 2010;**12**:75–84), drug therapy (s = 21, Parikh et al, J Child Adolesc Psychopharmacol 2008;**18**:157–78), genetics (Grigorenko, Future Neurol 2009;**4**:591–99; Kumar and Christian, Curr Neurol Neurosci Rep 2009;**9**:188–97), ADHD in ASD (Hazell, J Paediatr Child Health 2007;**43**:19–24).

● Unlicensed/some efficacy

Antipsychotics *

Low-dose antipsychotics have a role to play. As adverse reactions can be significant, a 'start low and go slow' routine is recommended. **Risperidone** is licensed in US for irritability associated with autistic disorder in children aged 5–16 years. Two reviews have concluded that although risperidone does not effect the core symptoms of ASDs, it has moderate efficacy in helping behavioural aspects, e.g. irritability, aggression, hyperactivity and stereotyping (s = 4, d/b, Canitano and Scandurra, Neuropsychiatr Dis Treat 2008;**4**:723–30), at 0.5–3.5 mg/d. Even Cochrane concludes that there is some evidence for the benefits of risperidone on irritability, repetition and social withdrawal in ASDs (s = 3, Jesner et al, Cochrane Database Syst Rev 2007;1:CD005040). Long-term use seems safe and effective, e.g. for up to three years (n = 35, open, one year, Reyes et al, Eur Child Adolesc Psychiatry 2006;**15**:97–104), and a long-term discontinuation study suggested a significant relapse prevention efficacy, reducing disruptive behaviour in about half the children taking it (n = 36, d/b, 24/52, Troost et al, J Am Acad Child Adolesc Psychiatry 2005;**44**:1137–44), although this may disappear rapidly on discontinuation (n = 32, 6/12, d/b, Autism Network, Am J Psychiatry 2005;**162**:1361–9). It is well tolerated

(n = 101, RCT, d/b, p/c, 8/52, Aman et al, J Child Adolesc Psychopharmacol 2005;**15**:844–5), although raised prolactin and weight gain are risks so monitor carefully (n = 20, 24/52, Gagliano et al, J Child Adolesc Psychopharmacol 2004;**14**:39–47). **Aripiprazole** is also now licensed in USA, for irritability associated with autism in 6–17-year-olds, including aggression, SIB, temper and mood lability. Doses of 5, 10 and 15 mg/d all significantly improved aberrant behaviour and were well tolerated Aripiprazole may improve irritability in ASDs and be reasonably well-tolerated (s = 2, RCT, d/b, p/c, Curran, Paediatr Drugs 2011;**13**:197–204). A review of 19 studies of SGAs concluded that risperidone (n = 133, s = 13) may be effective in reducing hyperactivity, aggression and repetitive behaviour (with low EPS), **olanzapine** (n = 11, s = 3; e.g. see n = 12, RCT, open, 6/52, Malone et al, J Am Acad Child Adolesc Psychiatry 2001;**40**:887–94) and **clozapine** (open, n = 3, Zuddas et al, Am J Psychiatry 1996;**153**:738) may also be effective, but there is little evidence that **amisulpride** (RCT, n = 9) or **quetiapine** (open, n = 6) are useful in this population (s=13, n=133, Barnard et al, J Psychopharmacol 2002;**16**:93–101). **Haloperidol** has been widely used, with 0.5–3 mg/d used to reduce behavioural symptoms (e.g. aggression and SIB) and improve learning (n = 60, 6/12, Perry et al, J Am Acad Child Adolesc Psychiatry 1989;**28**:87–92). **Ziprasidone** may have some promise in treating adolescents with ASDs (n = 12, open, 6/52, Malone et al, J Child Adolesc Psychopharmacol 2007;**17**:779–90).

Reviews: SGAs (McDougle et al, J Clin Psychiatry 2008;**69** (Suppl 4):15–20), general (Posey et al, J Clin Invest 2008;**118**:6–14; Malone and Waheed, Drugs 2009;**69**:535–48).

Methylphenidate

Methylphenidate has considerable negative effects on tantrums and moods but this may sometimes be outweighed by the positive effects on hyperactivity, attention and stereotype behaviour (e.g. n = 13, d/b, p/c, c/o, Handen et al, J Autism Dev Disord 2000;**30**:245–55; n = 72 [c = 66], RCT, RUPPAN, Arch Gen Psychiatry 2005;**62**:1266–74).

■ Unlicensed/possible efficacy

Antidepressants *

Serotonin reuptake inhibitors may have an occasional role to play, particularly in adults with strong behavioural rigidity. Children and adolescents may be more sensitive to SSRIs and so 'start low and go slow' is the advice. **Fluoxetine** liquid (mean 10mg/d) was superior to placebo for repetitive behaviours in ASDs (n=45, RCT, d/b, p/c, c/o, 2×8/52, Hollander et al, Neuropsychopharmacology 2005;**30**:582–9). Low dose **venlafaxine** (18.75 mg/d) may help reduce SIB and ADHD-like symptoms in ASDs (n=3, Carminati et al, Prog Neuropsychopharmacol Biol Psychiatry 2006;**30**:312–5). However, **citalopram** had no effect on repetitive behaviour in ASDs (n=149, RCT, p/c, 12/52, King et al, Arch Gen Psychiatry 2009;**66**:583–90). **Mirtazapine** 15–30 mg/d had some efficacy (50% were very much improved) in reducing inappropriate sexual behaviours in ASDs (n=10, open, 8/52, Coskun et al, J Child Adolesc Psychopharmacol 2009;**19**:203–6), but is only modestly effective in treating other ASD-related symptoms (n=26, open, Posey et al, J Child Adolesc Psychopharmacol 2001;**11**:267–77). Cochrane concludes there is no evidence of a beneficial effect in children and some suggestion of harm, and the evidence in adults is weak (s=7, n=271, Williams et al, Cochrane Database Syst Rev 2010;**8**:CD004677), although some anxiety and global functioning may improve.

Atomoxetine

Atomoxetine has been used successfully for hyperactivity in autism spectrum disorders, so more trials are warranted (n=16, RCT, p/c, c/o, 13/52, Arnold et al, J Am Acad Child Adolesc Psychiatry 2006;**45**:1196–205).

Cicloserin (D-cycloserine)

Cicloserin was well tolerated and improved measures of social withdrawal (n=12, 6/52, Posey et al, Am J Psychiatry 2004;**161**:2115–7).

Cyproheptadine

Cyproheptadine plus haloperidol was superior to haloperidol alone for ABC-C (aberrant behaviour) listed symptoms (RCT, d/b, p/c,

8/52, Akhondzadeh et al, J Clin Pharm Ther 2004;**29**:145–50).

Melatonin *

A systematic review and meta-analysis concludes that melatonin improves sleep duration, onset and wakenings (s=18, inc. s=5, RCT, d/b, p/c, Rossignol and Frye, Dev Med Child Neurol 2011: in press). Melatonin 3–9mg/d may be dramatically effective for severe circadian disturbances in adults with ASDs (n=6, 6/52, Galli-Carminati et al, Swiss Med Wkly 2009;**139**:293–6), although long-term use may be needed as the effect may disappear on discontinuation (n=25, open, 7/12, Giannotti et al, J Autism Dev Disord 2006;**36**:741–52). Melatonin may improved sleep latency (mean 47 minutes) and total sleep (mean 52 minutes), but not the number of night wakenings (n=22 [c=17], RCT, d/b, c/o, 2×3/12, Wright et al, J Autism Dev Disord 2011;**41**:175–84). **Review:** * practical advice on use (Doyen et al, Eur Child Adolesc Psychiatry 2011;**20**:231–9).

Memantine

Memantine significantly improved disruptive behaviour (n=1, Erickson and Chambers, J Clin Psychiatry 2006;**67**:1000), and language and social behaviour and appeared to have no serious side-effects (n=151, open, 21/12, Chez et al, J Child Neurol 2007;**22**:574–9).

Naltrexone

A review concluded that naltrexone was worth a try, especially if SIB occurs and other interventions have failed (s=14, other reports=11, Elchaar et al, Ann Pharmacother 2006;**40**:1086–95).

Oxytocin *

Inhaled oxytocin may improve social behaviour and facial expression recognition (n=16, RCT, d/b, p/c. c/o, Guastella et al, Biol Psychiatry 2010; **67**:692–4).

Pentoxifylline

Pentoxifylline 600mg/d added to risperidone may have some synergistic effects in treating behavioural problems (n=40, RCT, d/b, p/c, 10/52, Akhondzadeh et al, Prog Neuropsychopharmacol Biol Psychiatry 2010; **34**:32–6).

Propranolol

Propranolol may help improve problem-solving in autistic spectrum disorders (see Beversdorf et al, Neurocase 2008;**14**:378–83).

Topiramate *

Topiramate (as an adjunct to risperidone) improved irritability, stereotypy and hyperactivity compared to placebo (n = 40, RCT, d/b, p/c, 8/52, Rezaei et al, Prog Neuropsychopharmacol Biol Psychiatry 2010;**34**:1269–72).

Valproate

There may be some improvement in behavioural symptoms associated with ASDs, e.g. 91% showed sustained improvement in ASD symptoms, e.g. aggression and impulsivity, particularly if an EEG abnormality or seizure history was present (n = 14, open pilot, Hollander et al, J Clin Psychiatry 2001;**62**: 530–4).

✸ Case reports

- **Buspirone** (n = 1, Brahm et al, Ann Pharmacother 2008;**42**:131–7).

◆ Others

Other drugs tried include **carbamazepine** (e.g. Gillberg, J Autism Dev Disord 1991;**21**:61–77), **clonidine** (n = 9, d/b, p/c, Fankhauser et al, J Clin Psychiatry 1992;**53**:77–82) and high dose **pyridoxine** (Findling et al, J Autism Dev Disord 1997;**27**:467–78).

☐ No efficacy

Lamotrigine

Lamotrigine was ineffective on all measures in one study (n = 28, RCT, p/c, 18/52, Belsito et al, J Autism Dev Disord 2001;**31**:175–81).

Levetiracetam

The major study was unable to show an advantage for levetiracetam (mean 860 mg/d) over placebo (n = 20, p/c, d/b, 10/52, Wasserman et al, Int Clin Psychopharmacol 2006;**21**:363–7), although some symptoms may improve (n = 10, open, Rugino and Samsock, J Dev Behav Pediatr 2002;**23**:225–30).

Omega-3 fatty acids *

A systematic review of small studies was unable to show evidence for efficacy in ASDs (s = 6, n = 94, Bent et al, J Autism Dev Disord 2009;**39**:1145–54), and a recent small pilot study found no effect in ASD (n = 27, RCT, open, 12/52, Bent et al, J Autism Dev Disord 2011;**41**:545–54).

Secretin

Despite much interest, a complete lack of significant effect has been shown (Roberts et al, Pediatrics 2001;**107**:E71; reviewed by Levy, EBMH 2002;**5**:22; n = 56, RCT, p/c, 4/52, Owley et al, J Am Acad Child Adolesc Psychiatry 2001;**40**:1293–99).

St. John's wort

SJW was essentially ineffective for measures of autistic behaviour in a small case series (n = 3, Niederhofer, Phytother Res 2009;**23**:1521–3).

1.9 BENZODIAZEPINE DEPENDENCE and WITHDRAWAL

Although short-term benzodiazepine use at standard doses is usually without significant risk of toxicity and dependence, higher dose and longer-term use have potential risks. In BDZ withdrawal, minimal intervention (leaflet or group meeting) and clinician-led systematic discontinuation are both more effective than TAU (s = 29, Voshaar et al, Br J Psychiatry 2006;**189**:213–20; Parr et al, Addiction 2009;**104**:13–24), but psychotherapy during BDZ tapering may actually be detrimental to long-term outcomes (n = 180 [c = 170], RCT, 15/12, Oude Voshaar et al, Br J Psychiatry 2006; **188**:188–9). Predictors of poor long-term abstinence from BDZs includes more severe BDZ-dependence and continued alcohol intake, and this is independent of doses, personality and psychopathology (n = 180 [c = 174], Voshaar et al, Can J Psychiatry 2006;**51**:445–52). Craving is also an independent risk factor for relapse after successful BDZ-discontinuation (n = 124, Mol et al, J Clin Psychiatry 2007;**68**:894–900). The SDS (Severity of Dependence Scale) can be used to accurately assess the potential for BDZ dependence (de la Cuevas et al, Addiction 2000;**95**:245–50; reviewed by Law, EBMH 2000;**3**:119).

Reviews: withdrawing BDZs in primary care (Lader *et al*, *CNS Drugs* 2009;**23**:19–34), treatment (Heberlein *et al*, *Fortschr Neurol Psychiatr* 2009;**77**:7–15), techniques and outcomes of BDZ detoxifications (Ferguson, *Prescriber* 2005;**16**:20–7).

BNF listed

Antidepressants

Antidepressants may be useful for treating any concurrent anxiety and depression. **Mirtazapine** has been useful, particularly for sleep disturbance (n = 1, Chandrasekaran, *Singapore Med J* 2008;**49**:166–7).

Benzodiazepines

Transferring from the current benzodiazepine to diazepam (if necessary) is a common strategy, as diazepam is a longer-acting benzodiazepine and possibly easier from which to withdraw. If withdrawing chronic BDZs from old age in-patients, short-term (one week) substitution with a low-dose BDZ at night to help sleep may be effective (RCT, d/b, p/c, Petrovic *et al*, *Eur J Clin Pharmacol* 2002;**57**:759–64).

● Unlicensed/some efficacy

Buspirone

Caution is advised as buspirone has been reported to aggravate withdrawal symptoms (1.6). However, buspirone (38 mg/d) has been used successfully in stopping long-term BDZs, introduced before a tapered discontinuation

---

Characteristics of benzodiazepine users:

- Elderly maintained symptom-free by low and unchanging doses.
- Chronic physical disorders controlled by BDZs (e.g. epilepsy).
- Where quality of life is so improved by BDZs that long-term use, preferably with intermittent/variable doses, is justified (e.g. chronic or severe anxiety or insomnia and an inadequate personality, people who relapse to alcohol and other more dangerous substances when BDZ-free).

(n = 107, d/b, Rickels *et al*, *Am J Psychiatry* 2000;**157**:1973–9). Buspirone 15 mg/d may relieve lorazepam withdrawal symptoms, with no rebound anxiety on with-drawal (n = 44, RCT, Delle Chiaie *et al*, *J Clin Psychopharmacol* 1995;**15**:12–9).

Carbamazepine

Carbamazepine 600–800 mg/d has been used as an alternative for benzodiazepine withdrawal in several studies (e.g. Kaendler *et*

How to minimise the risks of dependence:

- Carefully select patients (e.g. avoid especially dependence-prone, lower education, multiple drug users, those with a criminal background).
- Keep the dose low.
- Stop where possible, e.g. use shorter courses.
- Use intermittent or variable doses.
- Use antidepressants if depression mixed with anxiety is present.
  (Darke *et al*, *Addiction* 1994;**89**:683–90)

Risk factors for poor withdrawal (need to seek specialist advice):

- Previously severe withdrawal (including history of seizures) or post-withdrawal reaction.
- Elderly or infirm.
- History of abuse of alcohol/other drugs.
- Concomitant severe medical or psychiatric illness (including personality problems).
- High dose/longer-term use (e.g. >30 mg/d diazepam equivalent > 1 year).
- Cluster B personality/Borderline PD (n = 76, Vorma *et al*, *Subst Use Misuse* 2005;**40**:499–510).
- High neuroticism, higher behavioural inhibition and low social support (n = 41, 28/52, O'Connor *et al*, *Addict Behav* 2004;**29**:583–93).

<table>
<tr><td>

Patients where withdrawal should not be attempted:

- *Older medically ill or with spasticity or epilepsy:* Benzodiazepine usually prescribed by a non-psychiatrist. Seldom abused, doses not escalated, effective long-term. Care with subtle cognitive changes can occur.
- *Psychiatric patients with panic or agoraphobic disorders:* Seldom abused, doses not escalated, necessary long-term.
- *Psychiatric patients with recurrent dysphoria:* Long-term indications for use less clear. Abuse of other drugs often occurs.
- *Chronic sleep-disordered problems:* Drug may be active or preventing a rebound syndrome.

</td><td>

Withdrawal symptoms in the dependent patient:

- *Psychological:* Tension (to above pre-treatment levels), restlessness, agitation, panic attacks.
- *Physical:* Dry mouth, sweating, tremor, sleep disturbance, lethargy, headache, nausea, palpitations.
- *Mental:* Impaired memory and concentration, confusion.
- *Moderate:* Perceptual changes (i.e. hypersensitivity to light/sound), dysphoria, flu-like symptoms, anorexia, sore eyes, depersonalisation, depression, abnormal sensations of movement, rebound insomnia.
- *Severe:* (rare) Convulsions, psychoses (e.g. visual hallucinations, paranoia), delusions.

</td></tr>
</table>

al, Nervenarzt 1996; **67**:381–6). It reduces the chance of withdrawal convulsions and other symptoms (especially if withdrawal is abrupt), and reduces the incidence of relapse (n = 40, RCT, 12/52, Schweizer *et al, Arch Gen Psychiatry* 1991;**48**:448–52).

■ Unlicensed/possible efficacy

Antihistamines
These may be useful as non-benzodiazepine hypnotics where insomnia is a problem.

Clonidine
This may be a helpful adjunct in withdrawal, especially at relatively high dose.

Flumazenil
IV flumazenil has been used to reduce BDZ craving, lower relapse rates and improve outcomes (n = 50, RCT, p/c, 6/52, Gerra *et al, Addict Biol* 2002;**7**:385–95). Caution is needed in BDZ dependence.

Melatonin
Controlled-release melatonin has been successfully used to facilitate discontinuation of benzodiazepines (n = 34, d/b, 6/52, Garfinkel *et al, Arch Intern Med* 1999;**159**:2456–60).

Oxcarbazepine
Oxcarbazepine has been reported to facilitate rapid BDZ withdrawal in as little as 11 days (n = 10, Croissant *et al, Am J Drug Alcohol Abuse* 2008;**34**:534–40).

Pregabalin *
A Norwegian pharmacoepidemiological study suggested that 48% people on BDZs were able to reduce their use when starting pregabalin (cf only 14% on gabapentin) (Bramness *et al, Basic Clin Pharmacol Toxicol* 2010;**107**:883–6; see also review by Oulis and Konstantakopoulos, *CNS Neurosci Ther* 2010; **16**:45–50)

Valproate
Valproate 150–1200 mg/d may reduce the intensity of symptoms in protracted withdrawal (eg. n = 4, Apelt and Emrich, *Am J Psychiatry* 1994;**147**:1990), as well as acting as an anticonvulsant.

● Case reports

- **Topiramate** (n = 1, Cheseaux *et al, Hum Psychopharmacol* 2003;**18**:375–7; n = 1, Michopoulos *et al, World J Biol Psychiatry* 2006;**7**:265–7).

◆ Others

Other drugs tried include **propranolol** (*Postgrad Med J* 1988;**64** [Suppl]:40–4).

☐ No efficacy

Antipsychotics
Low dose anxiolytic use may be useful but may make withdrawal symptoms worse (Anon, *Lancet* 1987;i:78–9).

1.10 BIPOLAR MOOD DISORDER

1.10.1 PROPOPHYLAXIS AND MAINTENANCE
1.10.2 MANIA AND HYPOMANIA
1.10.3 BIPOLAR DEPRESSION
1.10.4 RAPID-CYCLING BIPOLAR DISORDER

Introduction
Bipolar mood disorder is a life-long illness with a variety of presentations, phases and sub-divisions. DSM-IV divides the condition into bipolar I (one or more manic or mixed episodes, wide mood swings), bipolar II (the most common form, one or more episodes of depression with at least one hypomanic but no manic episode) and bipolar III (pseudobipolar, often triggered by antidepressants, and which may present as a mixed state). There are many other classifications and sub-categories.

Diagnosis
Bipolar disorders are now more frequently recognised, but misdiagnosis and inadequate treatment is still commonplace. A survey of members of US bipolar association 'Chapters' showed that over 33% sought professional help within a year of the onset of symptoms, but 69% were misdiagnosed (mostly as unipolar depression but also ADHD, anxiety and personality disorders), there was an average of four physicians seen before getting an accurate diagnosis, and over 33% waited over 10 years before getting a diagnosis (n = 600, Hirschfeld et al, *J Clin Psychiatry* 2003;**64**:161–74), a finding stunningly similar to a previous survey (Lish et al, *J Affect Disord* 1994;**31**:281–94). The **average** time from the onset of symptoms to starting maintenance therapy is 8–10 years (e.g. n = 56, Goldberg and Ernst, *J Clin Psychiatry* 2002;**63**: 985–91), and may

be even longer with women (n = 360, Viguera et al, *Bipolar Disord* 2001;**3**:245–52). Sadly, this long delay leads to poorer social functioning, more annual hospitalisations and a higher likelihood of suicide attempts, regardless of the polarity of the first episode (n = 56, Goldberg and Ernst, *J Clin Psychiatry* 2002;**63**:985–91). Those with a more severe illness are more likely to be treated early with better outcomes (n = 147, Baethge et al, *Acta Psychiatr Scand* 2003;**107**:260–7). Excess mortality has been shown in bipolar (n = 15 386) and unipolar (n = 39 182) disorder in Sweden, both in terms of suicides and from natural causes (population study, Osby et al, *Arch Gen Psychiatry* 2001;**58**:844–50); but suicide rates are significantly reduced by long-term medication with an antidepressant, neuroleptic, or lithium, or combinations thereof (n = 406, 22 years, Angst et al, *J Affect Disord* 2002;**68**:167–81).

Reviews: * general (Sie et al, *Clin Pharmacist* 2009;**1**:67–85), systematic (Ceron-Litvoc et al, *Hum Psychopharmacol* 2008;**24**:19–28), meta-analysis of NNTs for bipolar drugs (Popovic et al, *Psychopharmacology (Berl)* 2011;**213**:657–67).

1.10.1 PROPOPHYLAXIS AND MAINTENANCE

Role of drugs *
The optimum outcomes in bipolar occur with appropriate and consistent prescribing and concordance of mood stabilisers, training for the person to cope with stresses and risk factors, and family support. Lithium, valproate, some antipsychotics and carbamazepine are widely used for the prophylaxis of bipolar disorder, although the evidence for carbamazepine is not robust. It is clear that well-being and functioning are inversely proportional to the number of bipolar episodes, and so strategies to reduce relapse must be rigorously followed, especially minimising difficult-to-treat bipolar depression (see *1.10.3*). Inappropriate use of antidepressants in undiagnosed bipolar may lead to cycle worsening in many (n = 85, naturalistic, Ghaemi et al, *J Clin Psychiatry* 2000;**61**:804–8). Regular compliance is important, but be aware that impaired verbal learning and memory in bipolar could passively limit treatment adherence (n = 40, Cavanagh et al, *Br J Psychiatry* 2002; **180**:293–5, 320–6). Rebound relapse on (rapid)

discontinuation may occur with carbamazepine, antipsychotics and valproate (n = 53, Franks et al, J Psychopharmacol 2008;**22**:452–6). The BALANCE study has shown lithium, and valproate plus lithium, to be superior to valproate alone for relapse prevention (n = 330, RCT, open, < 2 years, Geddes et al, Lancet 2010;**375**:385–95).

CBT does not appear to reduce overall episode recurrence in recurrent bipolar disorder (n = 253 [c = 200], RCT, s/b, 18/12, Scott et al, Br J Psychiatry 2006;**188**:313–20; comment by Lam, EBMH 2006;**9**:99), except perhaps in people with fewer episodes.

Reviews: general (Vieta and Sanchez-Moreno, Dialogues Clin Neurosci 2008;**10**:165–79), BAP guidelines on bipolar disorder (Goodwin et al, J Psychopharmacol 2009;**23**:346–88), mood stabilisers and antipsychotics in maintenance bipolar disorder (Smith et al, Bipolar Disord 2007;**9**:394–412), systematic review of relapse prevention (s = 34, Beynon et al, J Psychopharmacol 2009;**23**:574–91), complementary therapies (con-cludes SJW and SAMe [S-adenosyl-l-methionine] are both effective for depression but can cause mania; inconsistent evidence for acupuncture and omega-3-fatty acids; no data on massage, acupuncture, aromatherapy, yoga; Andreescu et al, J Affect Disord 2008;**110**:16–26).

BNF listed

Aripiprazole *

Aripiprazole is recently licensed for prevention of recurrence of manic episodes in bipolar I, in people who have responded acutely. The maintenance dose is the same as the acute dose. In supporting studies, 15–30 mg/d was superior to placebo for reducing relapse in bipolar mania in those responding over 6/52 (e.g. n = 161, RCT, d/b, p/c, 6/12, Keck et al, J Clin Psychiatry 2006;**67**:626–37; two-year extension, n = 161, RCT, d/b, p/c, two years, Keck et al, Am J Psychiatry 2007;**164**:1480–91; see also n = 262, RCT, d/b, p/c, 3/52, Keck et al, Am J Psychiatry 2003;**160**:1651–8).

Reviews: * meta-analysis with NNTs (Fountou-lakis et al, J Affect Disord 2011; in press), maintenance (McIntyre, Clin Ther 2010;**32**(Suppl 1);S32–8).

Carbamazepine

Long-term therapy in affective disorders is licensed as an alternative to lithium. Six studies of maintenance carbamazepine in bipolar disorder have shown equivocal results, e.g. incomplete protection (reviewed by Keck et al, J Clin Psychiatry 1998;**59**[Suppl 6]:S74–S81, 114 refs). One study showed that only 18% of carbamazepine-treated bipolars remained stable for 3–4 years, and another showed a 50% relapse rate (n = 24, open, four years, Post et al, J Clin Psychopharmacol 1990;**10**:318–27). Carbamazepine apparently has a roughly similar efficacy to lithium (s = 10, n = 572, table in Davis et al, Acta Psychiatr Scand 1999;**100**:406–17). It has been suggested that the best thing you can do with carbamazepine in bipolar is to stop it and allow other drugs to reach therapeutic levels.

Lithium *

The use of lithium in bipolar was first published by Cade (Med J Aust 1949;**36**:49–52) and it is now widely used for the treatment and prophylaxis of bipolar illnesses and, with care, can be successful and safe. It is effective in bipolar I and II, by reducing relapses and increasing inter-episodic intervals.

Efficacy: Lithium clearly reduces the risk of relapse in bipolar disorder (61% with placebo, 33% with lithium), particularly for manic episodes (systematic review and meta-analysis, s = 5, n = 770, RCTs, Geddes et al, Am J Psychiatry 2004;**161**:217–22; review by Bauer, EBMH 2004;**7**;72). Bauer's review states it to be the first published, methodologically rigorous meta-analysis of RCT, d/b, p/c trials in relapse prevention, and concludes that lithium reduces the risk of relapse for at least 10 years in affective relapse, especially manic, but that there is less evidence that it prevents depressive relapses.

Prophylaxis: Lithium is most effective if monitored regularly, and the dose and therapy reviewed regularly to minimise side-effects, especially those of weight gain and cognitive dulling. Commencing lithium within the first ten years of illness predicts better preventative outcomes than beginning prophylaxis later, both in major depression, recurrent and bipolar patients (n = 270, Franchini et al, Eur Arch

Psychiatry Clin Neurosci 1999;**249**:227–30).

The main problems appear to be when therapy is given to carelessly selected patients given insufficient support (see compliance), education and supervision, illustrated by naturalistic studies which show a poorer outcome than controlled trials. Goodwin argues strongly that treatment with lithium should be for at least two years (and more probably three years at the minimum), and that up to two years it may have at best no beneficial effect (premature stopping resulting in premature recurrence of mania).

Suicide reduction: * Reduced suicide rate has been strongly associated with lithium, something unique in bipolar, e.g. a systematic review of RCTs showed that people with bipolar disorder taking lithium are less likely to die by suicide (2 vs 11, odds ratio = 0.26), and less likely to self-harm and with lower deaths overall (s = 32, n = 3458, Cipriani et al, Am J Psychiatry 2005;**162**:1805–19; see also Müller-Oerlinghausen et al, Arch Suicide Res 2005;**9**:307–19). In fact, in 18 municipalities in Oita in Japan where lithium is found in tapwater, lithium levels were significantly and negatively associated with SMR averages for 2002–2006, so maybe even very low levels of lithium may reduce the overall risk of suicide (Ohgami et al, B J Psychiatry 2009;**194**:464–5). The effect may be due to reduced dysphoria, anger, aggression and impulsivity (Tondo and Baldessarini, Epidemiol Psichiatr Soc 2009; **18**:179–83; Muller-Oerlinghausen and Lewitzka, Neuropsychobiology 2010;**62**:43–9).

Mode of action: * Lithium may exert its effect via many mechanisms, e.g. inhibiting secondary messenger systems, or Protein Kinase C activity (an action shared with valproate and tamoxifen), neuroprotection, regulating glycogen synthase kinase-3 (GSK-3) gene expression (Moore et al, Lancet 2000;**356**:1241–2), up-regulation of Bcl-2 (major neuroprotective protein, with speculated rebound reduction in Bcl-2 production on withdrawal: Manji et al, J Clin Psychiatry 2000;**61**[Suppl 9]:S82–S96), protection from glutamate apoptosis (programmed cell death) and increased grey matter volume in areas associated with emotional processing (n = 74, Germaná et al, Acta Psychiatr Scand 2010;**122**:481–7).

Dosing: Once-daily lithium reduces side-effects, simplifies dosage requirements and reduces renal damage (review Ljubicic et al, Can J Psychiatry 2008;**53**:323–31). Alternate daily lithium is not recommended (n = 50, d/b, Jensen et al, J Affect Disord 1996;**36**:89–93). There are several methods of predicting lithium dose and levels (e.g. n = 60, Abou-Auda et al, Bipolar Disord 2008;**10**:369–76).

Plasma levels: * Plasma levels of 0.4–0.8 mmol/L are generally considered safe and effective as prophylaxis, but below 0.4–0.6 mEq/L may be less protective against relapse. In the elderly, a third to half less lithium may be needed due to reduced clearance (n = 9, Hardy et al, J Clin Psychopharmacol 1987;**7**:153–8). Lower plasma levels of lithium may be better at preventing relapse of bipolar depression and higher levels better to prevent mania (n = 64, 18/12, Severus et al, J Affect Disord 2009; **115**:466–70). Muslims fast for 12–17 hours a day every year during the month of Ramadan, but a stable mental state and stable lithium levels have no effect on mental state or plasma levels, even in the heat of Pakistan, as long as the dose is taken at the same time every day (n = 62, Farooq et al, Int Clin Psychopharmacol 2010;**25**:323–7).

Monitoring: Plasma monitoring is often poor, with many litigation cases for poor monitoring, and the NPSA in the UK has recently (2009) set targets for adequate monitoring. Local or national databases may be a successful way to achieve this (Holmes and Bazire, Bipolar Disorders 2003;**5**[Suppl 1]:S53; Anderson and Bazire, Bipolar Disorders 2011;**13**(Suppl 1);28).

Compliance or concordance: The main reason for lithium failure is non-compliance (either complete or erratic), and the patient (and any partner or caregiver) should be aware of the long-term commitment needed. Specialised care, e.g. via lithium or mood clinics, may improve patient and professional compliance with lithium use (Guscott and Taylor, Br J Psychiatry 1994;**164**:741–6). For a general review of strategies to improve compliance, see Schou (Acta Psychiatr Scand 1997;**95**:361–3).

Discontinuation: Early (particularly manic) relapse following lithium discontinuation is now well recognised with several important studies showing a significant risk from rapid discontinuation. If stopped in under 14 days, the risk of relapse is much higher (median 50% risk of relapse within four months, 100% over 3.5 years) than with slower (15–30 days) withdrawal, with a significant excess over the first six months (n = 161, Baldessarini et al, J Clin Psychiatry 1996;**57**:441–8; n = 78, Baldessarini et al, Am J Psychiatry 1997; **154**:551–3). At seven-year follow-up, relapse was more common after acute lithium discontinuation, the excess morbidity being attributable to the first episode/relapse after discontinuation (n = 42, seven years, Cavanagh et al, Acta Psychiatr Scand 2004;**109**:91–5). Even controlled lithium discontinuation leads to a high relapse in people who have had a good response for at least five years, so be careful (n = 32, up to nine years, Yazici et al, J Affect Disord 2004;**80**:269–71). Decreasing lithium levels, (either through erratic compliance or major changes in dose) is also a powerful predictor of relapse (n = 94, Perlis et al, Am J Psychiatry 2002;**159**:1155–9; n = 94, RCT, d/b, Gelenberg et al, N Engl J Med 1989;**321**:1489–93).

Lithium refractoriness: Lithium discontinuation in stable patients, despite adequate lithium levels, has been reported to induce a refractory state. However, two studies of lithium maintenance treatment periods (mean four years) were unable to show this (n = 86, Tondo et al, Am J Psychiatry 1997;**154**:548–50; n = 28, Coryell et al, Am J Psychiatry 1998;**155**:895–8), although the latter study might have been underpowered (Maj, Am J Psychiatry 1999;**156**:1130; plus reply). In a longitudinal study of clinic-attending bipolars compliant with lithium for at least a year, and without comorbid substance misuse, retreatment showed a slightly reduced efficacy. There was no tendency for lesser responses later in treatment (n = 360, longitudinal, Tondo et al, Br J Psychiatry 2001;**178**[Suppl 41]:S184–S190).

Reviews: * general (Nivoli et al, Neuropsychobiology 2010;**62**:27–35 ; Grandjean and Aubry, CNS Drugs 2009;**23**:225–40), metabolic adverse effects (Livingstone and Rampes, J Psychopharmacol 2006;**20**:347–55), in renal disease (Smith et al, J Clin Psychiatry 2005;**66**:96–9), intracellular pathways (Pasquali et al, Behav Pharmacol 2010;**21**:473–92; Quiroz et al, Neuropsychobiology 2010;**62**:50–60).

Olanzapine *

Olanzapine is licensed for the prevention of recurrence in patients with bipolar disorder whose manic episode has responded to olanzapine. Two systematic reviews from Cipriani have summarised the data. One concludes that olanzapine helps prevent manic episodes, but only in people who have responded in an acute or mixed episode and have not responded to lithium or valproate, so the actual license is precise and accurate (s = 5, RCT, Cipriani et al, J Psychopharmacol 2010;**24**:1729-38). Cochrane concludes that although the data is limited, olanzapine may prevent relapses in people responding during an index manic or mixed episode and who have previously not responded to lithium or valproate, although the evidence is stronger for lithium as a first-line maintenance treatment of bipolar disorder (s = 5, n = 1165, Cipriani et al, Cochrane Database Syst Rev 2009; **1**:CD004367).

Review: * adolescents with Bipolar I (McCormack, CNS Drugs 2010;**24**:443–52).

Quetiapine *

Quetiapine is now licensed for the prevention of recurrence of mania, mixed states or depressive symptoms that responded to quetiapine in the acute state (review by Popovic et al, Psychopharmacol (Berl) 2011;**213**:657–67).

+ Combinations

There has been an increased use of poly-pharmacy in refractory bipolar disorder over recent decades.

Lithium + antipsychotics

Lithium is frequently used with antipsychotics in maintenance therapy, although the evidence is poor. In patients stabilised on **quetiapine** and lithium, continued treatment reduced the risk of relapse (20% vs 52%) compared to placebo (n = 1953, open, <36/52; then n = 628, RCT, d/b, p/c, <104/52, Suppes et al, Am J Psychiatry 2009;**166**:476–88; see also RCT, d/b, p/c, <2 years, Vieta et al, J Affect Disord 2008;**109**:251–63). See also 'some efficacy' section.

Lithium + calcium-channel blockers

Although there are some reports of efficacy, potential drug interactions make this combination hazardous (reviewed by Freeman and Stoll, *Am J Psychiatry* 1998;**155**:12–21).

Lithium + carbamazepine/oxcarbazepine

Lithium plus carbamazepine has been widely used and can seem safe and effective, especially for rapid-cycling. Some old studies have shown a well tolerated and improved prophylactic effect compared to lithium monotherapy (e.g. n = 33, Small *et al*, *Psychopharmacol Bull* 1995;**31**:265–72), but in a pilot study, oxcarbazepine appeared more effective and better tolerated than carbamazepine as add-on to lithium for residual bipolar I and II symptoms (n = 52 [c = 52], RCT, d/b, 8/52, Juruena *et al*, *Prog Neuropsychopharmacol Biol Psychiatry* 2009;**33**:94–9).

Lithium + lamotrigine *

Lamotrigine was clearly superior to placebo as an adjunct to lithium in bipolar depression, with the effect continued throughout the trial (n = 124, RCT, d/b, p/c, 76/52, van der Loos *et al*, *Bipolar Disord* 2011;**13**:111–7).

Valproate + antipsychotics

In patients stabilised on **quetiapine** and valproate, continued treatment reduced the risk of relapse (20% vs 52%) compared to placebo (n = 1953, open, <36/52; then n = 628, RCT, d/b, p/c, <104/52, Suppes *et al*, *Am J Psychiatry* 2009;**166**:476–88; see also RCT, d/b, p/c, <2 years, Vieta *et al*, *J Affect Disord* 2008;**109**:251–63). There is also some data that valproate may allow reduction in the doses of antipsychotics needed in bipolar disorder with psychosis, or even replace them (Reutens and Castle, *Br J Psychiatry* 1997;**170**:484–5). See also 'some efficacy'.

Valproate + carbamazepine

There have been several reports of efficacy, e.g. 69% responded when valproate was added to carbamazepine non-responders, (n = 29, Schaff *et al*, *J Clin Psychiatry* 1993; **54**:380–4).

Valproate + lamotrigine

An open study has indicated some efficacy (reviewed by Freeman and Stoll, *Am J Psychiatry* 1998;**155**:12–21), although the incidence of rash appears higher and valproate increases lamotrigine levels (see 4.5.5).

1

● Unlicensed/some efficacy

Antidepressants *

See bipolar depression (1.10.3) for use in bipolar disorder, with notes about the risk of inducing a switch to mania in bipolar depression. For long-term antidepressants in bipolar, a meta-analysis concludes that long-term adjunctive AD treatment was not superior to MS-alone, and should further encourage reliance on MSs as the cornerstone of prophylaxis (s = 12, n = 350, RCT, >6/12, Ghaemi *et al*, *Acta Psychiatr Scand* 2008;**118**:347–56; comment by Young and Seim, *EBMH* 2009;**12**:49).

Antipsychotics (see also aripiprazole, olanzapine and quetiapine in BNF listed) *

The main roles of antipsychotics in bipolar disorder are:

1. Adjunctive to mood stabilisers for management of acute mania (see 1.10.2) or psychotic depression.
2. Adjunctive maintenance in treatment-resistance.

There is no compelling evidence that antipsychotics are effective as mood stabilisers as such in bipolar disorder, although some may help prevent relapse of mania. Aripiprazole, quetiapine and olanzapine are licensed for relapse prevention in responders (see BNF section). Many other antipsychotics are licensed for bipolar mania and might thus have some relapse prevention efficacy. **Asenapine** is licensed in some non-EU countries for relapse prevention. **Risperidone** Consta seems to be better at preventing reoccurrence of mania but not depression (n = 303, Quiroz *et al*, *Biol Psychiatry* 2010;**68**:156–62; review by Deeks, *Drugs* 2010;**70**:1001–12). Risperidone RLAI as adjunct to TAU, continuation study in frequent relapsers showed 23% relapses with RLAI + TAU, 46% with placebo injection (n = 12 [c = 64], RCT, d/b, p/c, 1 year, Mac-fadden *et al*, *Bipolar Disord* 2009;**11**:827–39;MS). **Clozapine** may have some significant mood-stabilising effects in treatment-resistant bipolar or schizoaffective patients, e.g. as add-on therapy compared to placebo (n = 38, RCT, p/c, Suppes et al, Am J Psychiatry 1999;**156**:1164–9), and a longer trial showed some efficacy to improve symptoms in bipolar with psychotic features (n = 37, open, two years, Ciapparelli et al, J Clin Psychiatry 2003;**64**:451–8). Ziprasidone is now licensed in US for adjunct to lithium or valproate as maintenance in bipolar I, and a continuation study for relapse prevention showed an NNT = 8 (n = 238, RCT, d/b, p/c, 24/52, Citrome, Expert Rev Neurother 2010;**10**:1031–7).

Reviews: SGAs in bipolar (Derry and Moore, BMC Psychiatry 2007;**7**:40; Gentile, CNS Drugs 2007;**21**:367–87).

Lamotrigine

Lamotrigine is now licensed in UK for the maintenance treatment of bipolar I depression and relapse prevention (see 1.10.3).

Review: use in bipolar (Bhagwagar and Goodwin, Expert Opin Pharmacother 2005;486:1401–8).

Valproate/valproate semisodium/divalproex

Valproate is licensed for mania and relapse prevention (as Depakote and Episenta). The one-year study comparing divalproex, lithium and placebo (2:1:1) just failed to show divalproex to be superior to lithium or placebo in the time to any mood episode, but there was a noticeable trend for divalproex (40/52) over placebo (28/52) and lithium (24/52), and it was superior to placebo on nearly all secondary measures (n = 372, RCT, Bowden et al, Arch Gen Psychiatry 2000;**57**:481–9). Valproate may also reduce depressive symptoms compared to lithium (sub-analysis of Bowden study by Gyulai et al, Neuropsychopharmacol 2003;**28**:1374–82). Reduced suicide in bipolar has not been shown with valproate compared to lithium (n = 20638, Goodwin et al, JAMA 2003;**290**:1467–73). See also entry under mania/hypomania (1.10.2).

■ Unlicensed/possible efficacy

Anticholinesterases

While adjunctive **galantamine** improved some aspects of episodic memory in cognitive dysfunction, it had little overall positive effect (n = 30 [c = 16], RCT, d/b, p/c, 3/12, Ghaemi et al, J Clin Psychopharmacol 2009;**29**:291–5). **Donepezil** 5–10 mg/d was not much use either for ADL or cognitive function in older people with bipolar (n = 12, 3/12, Gildengers et al, Int J Geriatr Psychiatry 2008;**23**:704–11).

Calcium-channel blockers

Verapamil 120–450 mg/d and diltiazem (n = 8, open, 12/12, Silverstone and Birkett, J Psychiatry Neurosci 2000;**25**:276–80) have shown some promise as a mood stabiliser and may have some role as add-on therapy in resistant cases.

Cannabis

One review of cannabinoids in bipolar concluded that there were no published studies of efficacy but much anecdotal evidence (Ashton et al, J Psychopharmacol 2005;**19**:293–300).

Gabapentin

See bipolar depression (1.10.3). Despite lacking efficacy in acute states, gabapentin added to a mood stabiliser (lithium, valproate or carbamazepine) may have some prophylactic effects (n = 25, RCT, d/b, p/c, 12/12, Vieta et al, J Clin Psychiatry 2006;**67**:473–7).

Omega-3 fatty acids

In a not very stringent trial, omega-3 fatty acids produced a significantly longer remission than placebo, and scored higher on most other outcome measures (n = 30, d/b, 4/12, Stoll et al, Arch Gen Psychiatry 1999;**56**:407–12).

Oxcarbazepine (see also combinations)

There are case reports of success in bipolar II with comorbid substance abuse (n = 4, Nasr, Am J Psychiatry 2002;**159**:1793).

Spironolactone *

Adjunctive spironolactone 50–100 mg/d was effective for residual symptoms in some bipolar patients (n = 4, Juruena et al, J Psychopharmacol 2009;**23**:985–7).

Tamoxifen (see also mania)

There is some interest in tamoxifen as a mood stabiliser in that it shares some intra-cellular properties with lithium, e.g. PKC inhibition (see review by Zarate and Manji, *CNS Drugs* 2009; **23**:569–82).

Tiagabine

There are reports of tiagabine 4 mg/d used successfully as adjunctive therapy in multiple drug-resistant bipolar disorder, continuing to be effective over several months (e.g. n = 2, Schaffer and Schaffer, *Am J Psychiatry* 1999; **156**:2014–15), although it was at best only modestly effective in refractory bipolar, with significant ADRs (n = 13, open, Suppes *et al*, *Bipolar Disord* 2002; **4**:283–9).

Topiramate

There is some evidence accumulating from open studies suggesting some efficacy, e.g. mild improvement was seen in 47% and marked-to-moderate in 13% bipolars treated with topiramate (mean 180 mg/d), with a dose-related response and weight loss, as well as significant side-effects (n = 76, open, Ghaemi *et al*, *Ann Clin Psychiatry* 2001; **13**:185–9), as an adjunctive in treatment-resistant bipolar (n = 19, open, 12/52, Vieta *et al*, *World J Biol Psychiatry* 2003; **4**:172–6) and as add-on maintenance in bipolar, with low drop-outs and low relapses (n = 56, open, 12/12, Lykouras and Hatzimanolis, *Curr Med Res Opin* 2004; **20**:843–7).

Vitamins and minerals

A trial of 36 dietary nutrients has produced a 55–66% reduction in bipolar symptoms and a reduction in medication levels, leading to suggestions that bipolar disorder is an inborn error of metabolism, although the mechanism is unknown (n = 11, 6/12, Kaplan *et al*, *J Clin Psychiatry* 2001; **62**:936–44).

1.10.2 MANIA AND HYPOMANIA

Symptoms

Hypomania, the more common and less severe form of mania, includes an abnormal elation of mood, alternating with irritability, great energy, inability to concentrate, flight of ideas (rapid changing of the subject with some connections) and insomnia. Obsessive preoccupation with some idea, activity or desire may occur. The main presenting symptoms are a euphoric and labile mood (irritable, angry, grandiose), bright or untidy appearance, low sleep requirement, increased drive and energy, reduced insight, pressure of speech, flight of ideas, expansive thought and an overactive and intrusive manner.

Risk factors for chronicity of mania:

- Physical illness
- Substance misuse
- Positive family history
- Poor pre-morbid social functioning
- Depressed or mixed cycles
- Rapid-cycling
- Longer episodes and increased episodes (implying effective treatment in acute phases is essential for long-term outcomes).

(review Tyrer, *J Psychopharmacol* 2006; **20**[suppl 2]:4–11).

Role of drugs *

Hypomania or mania is a phase of a bipolar (or rarely a unipolar) illness. Both usually require specific long-term mood-stabiliser treatment for the bipolar component (i.e. lithium, valproate, SGAs, carbamazepine, etc), and non-specific shorter-term treatments (e.g. antipsychotics, benzodiazepines) for the insomnia, agitation and hyperactivity to calm the person and prevent exhaustion and harm. A recent meta-analysis of RCTs in mania (s = 56, n = 10,800, RCT, p/c, Yildiz *et al*, *Neuropsychopharmacology* 2011; **36**:375–89) concluded that:

- Drugs more effective than placebo: aripiprazole, asenapine, carbamazepine, cariprazine, haloperidol, lithium, olanzapine, paliperidone, quetiapine, risperidone, tamoxifen, valproate, and ziprasidone
- Limited data indicated large effect sizes (Hedges' g = 0.51–2.32) for: carbamazepine, cariprazine, haloperidol, risperidone, and tamoxifen.

A night of sleep deprivation is likely to escalate any manic patient to a higher degree of mania and so hypnotic/sedative use should be considered appropriate. Any comorbid substance misuse should be tackled at the same time, as recovery from mania is poorer in people with a history of substance abuse (retrospective review, n = 204, Goldberg *et al*, *J Clin Psychiatry* 1999; **60**:733–40). After recovery from a manic episode with an antipsychotic and a mood stabiliser, many people receive antipsychotics long-term. This may not always be the best thing to do, as one study showed that those continuing antipsychotics long-term had a quicker onset of depression, were more likely to discontinue, and have more EPS and dysphoria — a good collection of detrimental effects (n = 27, RCT, p/c, d/b, 6/12, Zarate and Tohen, *Am J Psychiatry* 2004;**161**:169–71).

Treatment goals for mania should be:

1. Discontinue any agents that may induce symptoms, including antidepressants and substances of misuse (see 5.7 for lists).
2. Stabilise any medical conditions.
3. Start non-specific calming medications, e.g. benzodiazepines, antipsychotics.
4. Start specific mood-stabilisers or relapse prevention agents (see *1.10.1*) preferably when the patient is able to consent to longer-term therapy. For good reasons, in the real world patients presenting with mania are very different to those in clinical trials and inclusions, exclusions and differing assessments of severity (USA tends to rate the same presentation as more severe than UK) may have led to the over-estimating of anti-manic drug efficacy, as only about 16% of acute manic patients presenting in a routine mental hospital would seem to qualify for a standard placebo-controlled RCT (n = 74, Storosum *et al, Eur Neuropsychopharmacol* 2004;**14**:319–23).

See bipolar mood disorder (*1.10.1*) for maintenance strategies.

Reviews: * pharmacological interventions (s = 13, n = 3089, Smith *et al, Bipolar Disord* 2007;**9**:551–60), evidence-based guidelines (Goodwin *et al, J Psychopharmacol* 2009;**23**:346–88), NNTs and response in acute bipolar (Tamayo *et al, Int J Neuropsychopharmacol* 2010;**13**:813–32), general (Pompili *et al, Neuropsychiatr Dis Treat* 2011;**7**:259–65; Chwieduk and Scott, *CNS Drugs* 2011;**25**:251–67).

BNF listed

Aripiprazole *

Aripiprazole is licensed for prevention of recurrence of manic episodes in bipolar I, in people who have responded acutely. The maintenance dose is the same as the acute dose. In the main supporting study, aripiprazole as an adjunct to lithium or valproate was superior to either as monotherapy (n = 337 [c = 192], RCT, d/b, 12/12, Marcus *et al, Bipolar Disord* 2011;**13**:133–44, MS), a study not included in the recent criticism of aripiprazole (Tsai *et al, PLoS Med* 2011;**8**:e1000434). In an open-label extension trial, aripiprazole seemed effective as an adjunct to lithium or valproate in the completers (n = 283 [c = 146], open, 6/12, Vieta *et al, Curr Med Res Opin* 2010;**26**:1485–96). It also seems to be effective for psychotic symptoms in mania and maintenance, even as monotherapy (s = 4, RCT, Fountoulakis *et al, Ann Gen Psychiatry* 2009;**8**:27).

Reviews: * general (McIntyre *et al, Neuropsychiatr Dis Treat.* 2011;**7**:319–23, De Fazio *et al, Clin Drug Investig* 2010;**30**:827–41; Muzina, *Neuropsychiat Dis Treat* 2009;**5**:279–88; Fountoulakis and Vieta, *Ann Gen Psychiatry* 2009;**8**:16), consensus statement on use in mania (Aitchison *et al, J Psychopharmacol* 2009;**23**:231–40).

Asenapine *

Asenapine is licensed for moderate-severe manic episodes associated with bipolar I disorder in adults. It has a high affinity for 5HT1A/ 1B/2A/2B/2C/5/6/7, D1/2/3/4, alpha 1 and 2, H1 and H2 but not cholinergic receptors (Citrome, *Int J Clin Pract* 2009;**63**:1762–84). In manic or mixed episodes, asenapine (mean 18.2 mg/d) was rapidly effective, well tolerated and as effective as olanzapine (n = 488, RCT, d/b, p/c, 3/52, McIntyre *et al, Bipolar Disord* 2009;**11**:673–86), superior to placebo at day 2 and with less weight gain than olanzapine (n = 488, RCT, d/b, p/c, 3/52, McIntyre *et al, J Affect Disord* 2010;**122**:27–38). The main side-effect is somnolence, with some weight gain. It is presented as a sublingual tablet which dissolves in seconds when placed under the tongue. It is 35% bio-available orally, but less than 2% if swallowed, so no drinking or eating for 10 minutes after a dose is recommended (Gerrits *et al, Biopharm Drug Dispos* 2010;**31**:351–7). Food just before a dose decreases absorption by 20% and by 10% up to four hours afterwards.

Reviews: * in bipolar (McIntyre, *CNS Neurosci Ther* 2011; in press; McIntyre, *Expert Rev Neurother* 2010;**10**:645–9), general (Shahid *et al, J Psychopharmacol* 2008;**23**:65–73; Weber and McCormack, *CNS Drugs* 2009;**23**:781–92), in schizophrenia and bipolar mania (Tarazi and Shahid, *Drugs Today (Barc)* 2009;**45**:865–76).

Carbamazepine

Carbamazepine MR up to 1600mg/d was effective in 41% (cf 22% for placebo) as monotherapy in acute bipolar mania (n = 204 [c = 96], RCT, d/b, p/c, 3/52, Weisler et al, *J Clin Psychiatry* 2004;**65**:478–84) and up to 1600mg/d was superior to placebo in acute mania (n = 239 [c = 144], RCT, d/b, p/c, 3/52, Weisler et al, *J Clin Psychiatry* 2005;**66**:323–30; pooled results analysis; n = 443 [c = 240], RCT, Weisler et al, *CNS Drugs* 2006;**20**:219–31). The previous five RCTs of carbamazepine in acute mania showed a response rate equivalent to lithium and chlorpromazine (review by Keck et al, *J Clin Psychiatry* 1998;**59**[Suppl 6]:S74–S81, 114 refs).

Reviews: acute mania (Owen, *Drugs Today [Barc]* 2006;**42**:283–9), CBZ for bipolar and mania (Stoner et al, *Pharmacotherapy* 2007;**27**: 68–88).

Lithium

Lithium is effective in acute mania/hypomania, although the onset of action may be delayed for five to seven days or longer (unless perhaps if loading doses are used). It is difficult to use in mania due to the need to monitor blood levels, problems with stopping later or prematurely, and the need for two to three years minimum treatment duration. Serum levels of 0.9–1.4mmol/L may be necessary in the short-term for a therapeutic effect and should be reduced once mood is normalised. Loading with lithium in mania is surprisingly poorly studied but has been tried with rapid success, many responding within 48 hours. The only recent study available showed that in 15 manic in-patients given 20mg/kg/d for up to 10 days, only five completed the trial (although seven drop-outs improved sufficiently to allow discharge and only two had ADRs). All had levels >0.6mmol/L after the first day, which was generally well tolerated and showed a rapid improvement, although this needs confirming in a full study (n = 15, open, Keck et al, *Bipolar Disord* 2001;**3**:68–72). At least four previous depressive or 10–12 previous manic episodes are associated with reduced antimanic

response to lithium (Swann et al, *Acta Psychiatr Scand* 2000;**101**:444–51; n = 40, RCT, d/b, p/c, 4/52, Kafantaris et al, *J Am Acad Child Adolesc Psychiatry* 2004;**43**:984–93).

Review: efficacy and side-effects in mania (Bowden, *J Clin Psychiatry* 2000;**61**[Suppl 9]: S35–S40).

Olanzapine (see also combinations) *

For olanzapine in acute mania, the starting dose is 15mg/d as monotherapy or 10mg/d in combination. It may be effective in bipolar mania in adolescents (13–17 year-olds) but had a significant side-effect burden (n = 161, RCT, d/b, p/c, 3/52, Tohen et al, *Am J Psychiatry* 2007;**164**:1547–56). Cochrane concludes that olanzapine is effective in mania, possibly more so than valproate, but with more weight gain and somnolence (n = 1422, s = 6, Rendell et al, *Cochrane Database Syst Rev* 2003;**3**:CD004040), although some feel valproate was underdosed (Lu, *EBMH* 2003;**6**:28). Olanzapine 'Velotabs' produce a plasma level profile similar to oral tablets but may be a suitable alternative to injections in some cases by assuring compliance.

Quetiapine (see also combinations) *

Quetiapine is licensed as monotherapy for the short-term treatment of acute manic episodes (and relapse prevention) associated with bipolar I disorder. Two RCTs have shown efficacy, e.g. quetiapine was as effective as haloperidol in acute mania but better tolerated, with a final dose range of 400–800mg/d (n = 302, RCT, d/b, p/c, 12/52, McIntyre et al, *Eur Neuropsychopharmacol* 2005;**15**:573–85), and up to 800mg/d was as effective as lithium and both were superior to placebo in bipolar mania using YMRS (n = 302, RCT, d/b, p/c, 12/52, Bowden et al, *J Clin Psychiatry* 2005;**66**:111–21). Quetiapine was at least as effective as valproate in adolescent mania (n = 50, RCT, d/b, 28/7, DelBello et al, *J Am Acad Child Adolesc Psychiatry* 2006;**45**:305–13). Rapid dose escalation is licensed for the XL formulation as 300mg on day 1, 600mg on day 2 and then up to 800mg/d after that.

Risperidone (see also combinations)

Risperidone is licensed in the UK for

monotherapy in bipolar mania. Two RCTs have shown efficacy, e.g. risperidone was more effective than placebo (42% vs 13% remission) in mania (n=291, RCT, d/b, p/c, 3/52, Gopal *et al, J Clin Psychiatry* 2005;**66**:1016–20, MS; comment by Khanna, *EBMH* 2006;**9**:40) and in acute mania (YMRS >20) risperidone 1–6mg/d produced significant improvement in symptoms (n=290, RCT, d/b, p/c, 3/52, Khanna *et al, Br J Psychiatry* 2005;**187**:229–34, MS). Although there is some controversy about this second study, the mania was severe and with low drop-outs, it shows that risperidone is also effective in very ill patients. Onset can be rapidly effective (within a week) as an adjunctive treatment to mood stabilisers in mania, especially if carbamazepine-treated patients are excluded (n=151, RCT, d/b, p/c, 3/52, Yatham *et al, Br J Psychiatry* 2003;**182**:141–7; see *4.5.1* for reasons) and risperidone can be safely combined with valproate or lithium in acute mania (n=79, 12/52, Yatham *et al, Int Clin Psychopharmacol* 2004;**19**:103–9). Cochrane concludes that risperidone is effective in mania as both monotherapy and adjunctive treatment (s=6, n=1343, Rendell *et al, Cochrane Database Syst Rev* 2006;**1**:CD004043).

Reviews: general (Nguyen and Guthrie, *Ann Pharmacother* 2006;**40**:674–82; Fenton and Scott, *CNS Drugs* 2005;**19**:429–44).

Valproate semisodium (divalproex)

Valproate semisodium (as Depakote®, Sanofi-Aventis, and Episenta®, Beacon) is licensed in the UK as monotherapy for acute mania and now relapse prevention. Several RCTs have shown efficacy, e.g. a robust trial showed valproate to be as effective as lithium in acute mania, independent of a prior responsiveness to lithium (n=174, RCT, p/c, 21/7, Bowden *et al, JAMA* 1994;**271**:918–24) and may be more effective than lithium and as effective as (but better tolerated than) olanzapine (n=348, s=3, RCT, d/b, Hirschfeld *et al, J Clin Psychiatry* 2003;**64**:841–6, MS; n=120, RCT, d/b, 12/52, Zajecka *et al, J Clin Psychiatry* 2003;**63**:1148–55). A realistic study under realistic conditions, including more severely ill patients, suggests that prompt rapid stabilisation with valproate may allow transition to maintenance without antipsychotics (n=136, RCT, d/b, p/c, 21/7,

Müller-Oerlinghausen *et al, J Clin Psychopharmacol* 2000;**20**:195–203; review by Swann, *EBMH* 2000;**3**:113). Cochrane concludes that there is consistent if limited evidence that valproate is effective in acute mania; it may be less effective than olanzapine but with less sedation and weight gain (s=10, Macritchie *et al, Cochrane Database Syst Rev* 2003;**1**:CD004052). There appears to be a linear relationship between valproate serum concentration and response in acute mania, best response being above 94mcg/ml, presumably as trough levels, although this is unclear in the paper (n=374, s=3, RCT, Allen *et al, Am J Psychiatry* 2006;**163**:272–5). Subsequently, oral loading doses of valproate are probably more rapidly effective in mania, e.g. 20mg/kg/d may give a rapid response, often within three days (n=36, RCT, 6/7, McElroy *et al, J Clin Psychiatry* 1996;**57**:142–6). Even more aggressive dosing (30mg/kg/d on days one and two, then 20mg/kg/d days 3–10) may produce more rapid therapeutic levels in acute mania, with no adverse effects (n=59, RCT, Hirschfeld *et al, J Clin Psychiatry* 1999;**60**:815–18). High-dose IV valproate (20mg/kg) over 30 minutes had no effect in acute mania (n=7, Phrolov *et al, J Clin Psychiatry* 2004;**65**:68–70), but IV has been successfully used for adolescent mania (n=5, Thakur *et al, Eur Child Adolesc Psychiatry* 2004;**13**:258–61). The equivalent amount of valproic acid available from Depakote® 500mg (Sanofi-Aventis), Epilim EC® 500mg (Sanofi-Aventis) and Epilim Chrono® 500mg (Sanofi-Aventis) are 500mg, 433mg and 433mg respectively (MI).

Reviews: general (Bowden, *Bipolar Disord* 2003; **5**:189–202), loading dose strategies (Keck *et al, Bipolar Disord* 2000;**2**:42–6).

+ Combinations

In acute mania, combinations are rightfully commonly used. A review of all adjunctive treatment studies in acute mania notes that combinations are more effective than monotherapy and so lower doses can be used and tolerability is higher, improving longer-term retention in therapy (Sachs and Gardner-Schuster, *Acta Psychiatr Scand* Suppl 2007;**434**:27–34). A meta-analysis has concluded that adding an antipsychotic to an established mood stabliser is more effective than a mood stabliser alone (s = 8, n = 1124, RCT, Smith *et al, Acta Psychiatr Scand* 2007;**115**:12–20).

Review: concensus statement on combining antipsychotics with another medicine (Goodwin *et al, Eur Neuropsychopharmacol* 2009;**19**:520–32).

Antipsychotics + benzodiazepines

See individual drugs or groups in this section (see also Acute Psychiatric Emergency *1.1*).

Lithium + allopurinol

Allopurinol 600mg/d was significantly superior to placebo as an adjunct to lithium in mania and may provide an alternative to antipsychotics (n = 120, RCT, d/b, p/c, 4/52, Machado-Vieira *et al, J Clin Psychiatry* 2008;**69**:1237–45).

Lithium + antipsychotics

Olanzapine was superior to placebo as an add-on to valproate in manic and mixed bipolar episodes, although weight gain with olanzapine was significant (n = 344, RCT, d/b, 6/52, Tohen *et al, Arch Gen Psychiatry* 2002;**59**:62–9, MS; comment by Gardner, *EBMH* 2002;**5**:89). Quetiapine was also superior to placebo when added to lithium and well tolerated (n = 191 [c = 105], RCT, 21/7, d/b, p/c, Sachs *et al, Bipolar Disord* 2004;**6**:213–23), and 500mg/d (range 300–700mg/d) was superior to placebo when combined with lithium or divalproex for bipolar mania, and was well tolerated (n = 402, RCT, d/b, p/c, 6/52, Yatham *et al, J Clin Psychopharmacol* 2004;**24**:599–606). Risperidone plus lithium or valproate was as effective as haloperidol plus mood stabiliser and more effective than a mood stabiliser alone in acute mania (n = 156, RCT, d/b, p/c, 3/52, Sachs *et al, Am J Psychiatry* 2002;**159**:1146–54).

Lithium + carbamazepine

Carbamazepine has been used in resistant cases in combination with lithium. See *4.4* for neurotoxicity warning.

Olanzapine + carbamazepine

Olanzapine plus carbamazepine had no advantage (and had more side-effects) compared to carbamazepine alone in mania, (n = 118, RCT, d/b, p/c, 6 + 20/52, Tohen *et al, Br J Psychiatry* 2008;**192**:135–43; MS).

Valproate + antipsychotics

Augmentation of valproate with amisulpride or haloperidol were equally effective but the former had less side-effects and was more tolerable (n = 123, RCT, open, 3/12, Thomas *et al, Neuropsychiatr Dis Treat* 2008;**4**:675–86). Olanzapine was superior to placebo as an add-on to valproate in manic and mixed bipolar episodes, although weight gain with olanzapine was significant (n = 344, RCT, d/b, 6/52, Tohen *et al, Arch Gen Psychiatry* 2002;**59**:62–9, MS; comment by Gardner, *EBMH* 2002;**5**:89). Quetiapine was also superior to placebo when added to valproate semisodium, and well tolerated (n = 191 [c = 105], RCT, 21/7, d/b, p/c, Sachs *et al, Bipolar Disord* 2004;**6**:213–23; n = 402, RCT, d/b, p/c, 6/52, Yatham *et al, J Clin Psychopharmacol* 2004;**24**:599–606). Risperidone plus mood stabiliser (lithium or valproate) was as effective as haloperidol plus mood stabiliser and more effective than a mood stabiliser alone in acute mania (n = 156, RCT, d/b, p/c, 3/52, Sachs *et al, Am J Psychiatry* 2002;**159**:1146–54).

Valproate + folic acid

Folic acid added to valproate was superior to placebo as an adjuvant in acute mania, an astonishing finding (n=88, RCT, d/b, p/c, 3/52, Behzadi *et al, Acta Psychiatr Scand* 2009; **120**:441–5).

Valproate + lithium

Valproate has been used to augment lithium in resistant rapid-cycling mania (e.g. n = 12, open, Reischies *et al, Neuropsychobiol* 2002;**46**[Suppl 1]:S22–S27).

● Unlicensed/some efficacy

Antipsychotics

(see also aripiprazole, asenapine, olanzapine, quetiapine and risperidone in BNF listed)

There is some evidence that hypomania has a hyperdopaminergic component (Cousins *et al, Bipolar Disord* 2009;**11**:787–806). Amisulpride (about 700mg/d) was effective for mania in a pilot study (n = 20 [c = 14], open, 6/52, Vieta *et al, J Clin Psychiatry* 2005;**66**:575–8). Although obviously problematic, clozapine (mean 500mg/d) may be effective in 72%

treatment-resistant manics or schizoaffectives (n = 25, open, Calabrese et al, Am J Psychiatry 1996;**153**:759–64) and compared to TAU in bipolar (n = 38, RCT, one year, Suppes et al, Am J Psychiatry 1999;**156**:1164–9). Haloperidol was superior to placebo at up to 8mg/d (n = 302, RCT, d/b, p/c, 12/52, McIntyre et al, Eur Neuropsychopharmacol 2005;**15**:573–85) and Cochrane concludes that haloperidol is superior to placebo and equivalent to other antimanic antipsychotics (but possibly inferior to aripiprazole), albeit poorly tolerated (s = 15, n = 2022, Cipriani et al, Cochrane Database Syst Rev 2006;**3**:CD004362). Paliperidone 12mg/d (but not 6mg or 3mg) may be superior to placebo for mania (n = 469, RCT, d/b, p/c, 3/52, Berwaerts et al, J Affect Disord 2011; in press), and as effective as quetiapine (n = 493, RCT, d/b, 12/52, Vieta et al, Bipolar Disord 2010;**12**:230–43), although not effective as an adjunct to either lithium or valproate in acute mania (n = 300, RCT, d/b, p/c, 6/52, Berwaerts et al, J Affect Disord 2011;**129**:252–60). Ziprasidone is licensed in the USA for acute mania and 40–80mg BD produced a rapid (within two days) and sustained improvement in acute bipolar symptoms in one study (n = 210, RCT, p/c, d/b, 3/52, Keck et al, Am J Psychiatry 2003;**160**:741–8).

Benzodiazepines

For a group of drugs routinely used in mania, there is remarkably little robust evidence for the efficacy of benzodiazepines, but use is supported by extensive clinical experience. Short-term medium or high doses of benzodiazepines can be used alone or as adjuncts to other therapies in acute phases of hypomania, e.g. diazepam by itself, lorazepam (Salzman et al, Psychosomatics 1986;**27**:17–21), or clonazepam at 4–16mg/d (n = 12, RCT, d/b, c/o, Chouinard et al, Biol Psychiatry 1983;**18**:451–66). For acute symptoms they have a rapid onset, are highly sedative and are well tolerated, with no EPSE side-effect risk, but have little or no long-term role. A meta-analysis concluded that the data supported the safe and effective use of clonazepam in mania, although there was not exactly a lot to meta-analyse (s = 7, n = 206, RCT, Curtin and Schulz, J Affect Disord 2004;**78**:201–8).

Phenytoin

Phenytoin augmentation of haloperidol in acute mania was more effective than haloperidol alone, and may indicate that blockade of voltage-activated sodium channels is a common therapeutic mechanism for anticonvulsants in acute mania (n = 39, RCT, 5/52, Mishory et al, Am J Psychiatry 2000;**157**:463–5).

Tamoxifen *

Tamoxifen (a protein kinase C inhibitor) now has two RCTs confirming that it has significant antimanic activity and is remarkably well tolerated (n = 66 [c=50], RCT, d/b, p/c, 3/52, Yildiz et al, Arch Gen Psychiatry 2007;**64**:255–63), with 80mg/d clearly superior to placebo as an adjunct to lithium (1–1.2mEq/L) in acute mania (n = 40, RCT, d/b, p/c, 6/52, Amrollahi et al, J Affect Disord 2011;**129**:327–31). Tamoxifen 20–140mg/d was also significantly superior (63% response) to placebo (13% response) in bipolar mania, as early as day 5 (n = 16, d/b, p/c, 3/52, Zarate et al, Bipolar Disorders 2007; **9**:561–70).

■ Unlicensed/possible efficacy

Allopurinol

YMRS improved when allopurinol (300mg/d) was added to lithium and haloperidol in acute mania, albeit not quite statistically significant (n = 82, RCT, d/b, p/c, Akhondzadeh et al, Bipolar Disord 2006;**8**:485–9).

Levetiracetam

A pilot trial of adjunctive levetiracetam 500–2000mg/d showed some improvement in most manic patients, but was not wildly encouraging (n = 34, open, 8/52, Post et al, J Clin Psychiatry 2005;**66**:370–4), although there are cases of response to up to 2500mg/d (n = 1, Goldberg and Burdick, Am J Psychiatry 2002;**159**:148), and as an adjunct to haloperidol (n = 10, open, 28/7, Grunze et al, J Clin Psychiatry 2003;**64**:781–4).

Memantine

Memantine may have some efficacy, and appears well tolerated (n = 33, open, Keck et al, Clin Neuropharmacol 2009;**32**:199–204).

Omega-3 fatty acids

Fish oils may have some efficacy (review by

Maidment, *Acta Psychiatr Scand* 2000;**102**: 3–11).

Oxcarbazepine

Oxcarbazepine has been used successfully in acute mania, e.g. 1–2.4g/d was as effective as valproate in acute mania (n = 60, RCT, d/b, 12/52, Kakkar et al, *Eur Psychiatry* 2009;**24**:178–82), and 750–2000mg/d as an add-on to lithium was effective in 60%, and may be helpful long-term in some patients (n = 17, open, 8/52 + 12/12, Benedetti et al, *J Affect Disord* 2004;**79**:273–7). Oxcarbazepine was not significantly superior to placebo in youths (7–18 years) with bipolar mania (n = 116, RCT, d/b, p/c, 7/52, Wagner et al, *Am J Psychiatry* 2006;**163**:1179–86; comment by MacMillan and Heydrich, *EBMH* 2007;**10**:59).

Topiramate

Data on topiramate as an adjunct is mixed. Open trials have suggested modest efficacy in mania but a manufacturer's analysis concluded that there was no evidence to support routine use as monotherapy in mania (s = 4, RCT, Kushner et al, *Bipolar Disord* 2006;**8**:15–27). In the only RCT, topiramate had no effect as an adjunct to lithium or valproate in bipolar I manic or mixed episodes, but at least people lost significant amounts of weight (n = 287, RCT, d/b, p/c, 12/52, Chengappa et al, *J Clin Psychiatry* 2006;**67**:1698–1706; MS). Cochrane has concluded that there was, as yet, insufficient evidence for use as monotherapy or adjunctive for acute mania (Vasudev et al, *Cochrane Database Syst Rev* 2006;**1**:CD003384).

Tryptophan depletion

Acute tryptophan depletion may have an antimanic effect, albeit poorly tolerated (n = 23[c = 17], RCT, d/b, p/c, 7/7, Applebaum et al, *Bipolar Disord* 2007;**9**:884–7).

Verapamil

Verapamil monotherapy appears to have no antimanic activity but may be highly effective in combination with lithium, possibly by enhancing pKC inhibition (n = 45, RCT, open, 9/52, Mallinger et al, *Bipolar Disord* 2008;**10**:856–66; n = 50[c = 50], RCT, d/b, 4/52, Singh, *Int J Psychiatr Clin Pract* 2008;**12**:303–8).

Zonisamide

Adjunctive zonisamide has improved mania and depression in many patients but mood deteriorated in 32% patients, although nearly all lost weight (n = 62[c = 40], open, 8/52, McElroy et al, *J Clin Psychiatry* 2005;**66**:617–24).

✹ Case reports

- **Clonidine** (in antipsychotic-resistant mania; Jouvent et al, *Br J Psychiatry* 1988;**152**:293).
- **Propofol** IV (n = 1, Cluver and Hardesty, *J Clin Psychiatry* 2006; **67**:165–6).
- **Spironolactone** (n = 1, Gillman and Lichtigfeld, *Br Med J* 1986;**292**:661–2).

◆ Others

Other drugs tried include **dexamfetamine** (Clower, *Psychopharmacol Bull* 1988;**24**:168), **methylene blue** (to reduce pathotoxic vanadium ion concentrations; Moody et al, *Biol Psychiatry* 1989; **26**:850–2).

▢ No efficacy

Antidepressants

Antidepressants can either precipitate mania by provoking a mood switch, or exacerbate existing or developing mania (n = 1864, Lim et al, *Bipolar Disord* 2001;**3**:165–73).

Caffeine

A high caffeine intake will risk disturbing sleep patterns and exacerbating mania, e.g. discontinuing heavy use has helped resolve treatment-resistant schizoaffective mania (n = 1, Caykoylu et al, *Prog Neuropsychopharmacol Biol Psychiatry* 2008;**32**:1349–50).

Dipyridamole

Dipyridamole 200mg/d was ineffective as an adjunct to lithium in bipolar mania (n = 120, RCT, d/b, p/c, 4/52, Machado-Vieira et al, *J Clin Psychiatry* 2008;**69**:1237–45; see also allopurinol, another purinergic agent).

Fosphenytoin

IV fosphenytoin appears ineffective in acute mania (n = 7, open, 1 hour; Applebaum et al, *J Clin Psychiatry* 2003;**64**:408–9).

Gabapentin

The only two controlled studies have failed to show any advantage as an adjunct over placebo in mania (e.g. n = 117, d/b, p/c, Pande, Gabapentin study group, *Bipolar Disord* 1999; **1**[Suppl 1]:S17; Pande *et al, J Clin Psychopharmacol* 1999; **19**:341–8), and the trend was towards a negative effect.

Lamotrigine

Lamotrigine has no efficacy in acute mania and only delays the time to manic relapse in pooled data.

Tiagabine

Tiagabine had no detectable anti-manic activity as monotherapy or adjunctive therapy compared to standard treatments (n = 8, open, 14/7, Grunze *et al, J Clin Psychiatry* 1999; **60**:759–62).

1.10.3 BIPOLAR DEPRESSION *

Bipolar depression is longer-lasting than unipolar depression, frequently misdiagnosed (a substantial proportion of antidepressant-refractory depression is probably undiagnosed bipolar; n = 6, Inoue *et al, J Affect Disord* 2006; **95**:61–7) and is more likely to have psychosis, diurnal variation, and hypersomnia during depressive episodes, and a greater number of shorter episodes (e.g. n = 1036, Forty *et al, Br J Psychiatry* 2008; **192**:388–9). It is clear that well-being and functioning are inversely proportional to the number of bipolar episodes and so strategies to reduce relapse must be rigorously followed. Bipolar depression can be potentiated by substance and alcohol misuse and is much more difficult to treat.

A recent analysis of the 10 main studies (on aripiprazole, lamotrigine, quetiapine and olanzapine/fluoxetine) shows that although responding quickly is good news, it appears not to be a particularly good guide to how well someone will do long-term. However, **not** improving at all in the first 14 days does seem to give a good idea that someone is much less likely to respond in the long-term (s = 10, n = 3369, RCT, d/b, p/c, Kemp *et al, J Affect Disord* 2011; **130**:171–9).

The general principles of management include:

1. **Avoid inducing mixed affective states** with antidepressants, particularly in bipolar III, where the risk of self-harm is high.

2. **Use mood stabilisers:** In the largest non-commercial study in acute phase bipolar depression, paroxetine up to 40mg/d or bupropion up to 375mg/d plus a mood stabiliser (lithium, valproate, carbamazepine or a licensed antimanic agent, e.g. olanzapine, risperidone, aripiprazole, quetiapine, ziprasidone) had a slightly poorer response (based on euthymia at 8/52) than people receiving just a mood stabiliser and placebo, indicating that longer-term adjunctive antidepressants have no therapeutic advantage, but at least the antidepressant did not increase the risk of relapse, switch to mania or have greater ADRs (n = 366, RCT, d/b, p/c, 26/52, STEP-BD, Sachs *et al, N Engl J Med* 2007; **356**:1711–22; comment by Rao *et al, EBMH* 2007; **10**:109).

3. **Optimise antidepressants:** Use with a MS and start with lowest switch risk drugs (see 5 below)

4. **Minimise antidepressant exposure** by attempting gradual taper after a continuation phase, provided the patient is genuinely euthymic. Consider, however, that premature discontinuing antidepressants within the first 3–6/12 of an episode (n = 25) has an up to three times higher relapse rate than those (n = 19) continuing for at least 8/12 (n = 44, retrospective, one year, Altshuler *et al, J Clin Psychiatry* 2001; **62**:612–6).

5. **Avoid switching to mania with antidepressants** — in bipolar depression this usually occurs within the first 12 weeks. The risk is highest in bipolar I and bipolar II, lowest with MDD (s = 13 [7 RCTs], Bond *et al, J Clin Psychiatry* 2008; **69**:1589–601), and lower if antidepressants are used with a mood stabiliser (n = 136, Mundo *et al, J Affect Disord* 2006; **92**:227–30). If mania develops, the best plan is to reduce the antidepressant dose immediately and allow the mood to settle for a month or so. The switch rates in trials have been reported to be:
   - placebo 7%
   - sertraline 2%
   - bupropion 4%.

- fluoxetine 0–16%
- venlafaxine 9%
- imipramine 9.5–28%
- tranylcypromine 24%.

Antidepressant-induced switching from depression to mania may be more common in women and with TCAs vs non-TCAs (36% vs 17%), with amitriptyline (42%), imipramine (42%) and clomipramine (35%) being the highest risk (n = 333, Koszewska and Rybakowski, *Neuropsychobiology* 2009; **59**:12–6).

References: n = 174, RCT, 10/52, Post *et al*, *Br J Psychiatry* 2006;**189**:124–31; n = 34, RCT, p/c, d/b, 8/52, Amsterdam and Shults, *J Affect Disord* 2005;**87**:121–30.

6. **Avoid sudden dose changes** or switches.
7. **Offer ECT** for patients at immediate risk of self-harm or unable to tolerate antidepressants (n = 6, Macedo-Soares *et al*, *J ECT* 2005;**21**:31–4) e.g. older people.
8. **Check thyroid function** — poor response in bipolar depression may be related to low FTI and high TSH levels, even if in the alleged therapeutic range (n = 65, Cole *et al*, *Am J Psychiatry* 2002;**159**:116–21).

Reviews: * pharmacotherapy for acute bipolar II depression (s = 21, RCTs, Swartz and Thase, *J Clin Psychiatry* 2011;**72**:356–66), general (s = 19, Vieta *et al*, *J Clin Psychopharmacol* 2010;**30**:579–90; Baldessarini *et al*, *Harv Rev Psychiatry* 2010;**18**:143–57; Azorin and Kaladjian, *Expert Opin Pharmacother* 2009;**10**:161–72; Malhi *et al*, *Bipolar Disorders* 2009;**11**(suppl 2):55–76), Bipolar II postpartum depression (Sharma *et al*, *Am J Psychiatry* 2009; **166**:1217–21), long-term issues (Vieta, *J Clin Psychiatry* 2010;**71**:e07), ECNP consensus (Goodwin *et al*, *Eur Neuropsychopharmacology* 2008;**18**:535–49), BAP guidelines (Goodwin *et al*, *J Psychopharmacol* 2009;**23**:346–88), systematic review of guidelines (Nivoli *et al*, *J Affect Disord* 2011;**129**:14–26), newer antipsychotics (Cruz *et al*, *Int J Neuropsychopharmacol* 2010;**13**:5–14).

BNF listed

Lamotrigine *

Lamotrigine is now licensed in UK for prevention of depressive episodes in people with bipolar I disorder who experience predominantly depressive episodes (but not for acute episodes).

A robust and independent meta-analysis of the five studies (three unpublished) showed a consistently beneficial effect from 50–200 mg/d in bipolar depression, greater in more severe depression (s = 5, n = 1072, RCT, d/b, p/c, Geddes *et al*, *Br J Psychiatry* 2009;**194**:4–9). In patients with bipolar depression unresponsive to a mood stabiliser and at least one antidepressant, response to lamotrigine was 24% (cf. inositol 17% and risperidone 5%; n = 66, RCT, 16/52, open, Nierenberg *et al*, *Am J Psychiatry* 2006; **163**:210–6). Addition of paroxetine helps but not in people who have not responded to lithium and lamotrigine (n = 124, RCT, d/b, p/c, 16/52, van der Loos *et al*, *Acta Psychiatr Scand* 2010;**122**:246–54). Increasing the dose slowly over 6/52 to 200 mg/d minimises the incidence of serious rash, especially with valproate.

Review: general (Thase, *Neuropsychiatr Dis Treat* 2008;**4**:11–21).

Quetiapine *

Quetiapine is now licensed for treatment of severe depressive episodes in bipolar disorder, and for prevention of recurrence if responding acutely. A slower dose increase is recommended: (night-time, day 1 50 mg; day 2 100 mg; day 3 200 mg; day 4 300 mg). Monotherapy efficacy has been shown in two robust RCTs (BOLDER 1 and 2; s = 2, n = 694, RCT, d/b, p/c, 8/52, Weisler *et al*, *J Clin Psychiatry* 2008;**69**:769–82). BOLDER 1 showed response rates in bipolar 1 depression of 58.2% (600 mg/d) and 57.6% (300 mg/d), compared with 36% for placebo (remission was 52.9% vs 28.4%). Treatment for emergent mania was 3–4% for both groups with an NNT = 5 for response and remission of bipolar depression (Cookson *et al*, *Int Clin Psychopharmacol* 2007;**22**:93–100). BOLDER 2 showed quetiapine 300 mg and 600 mg/d monotherapy were equally effective in bipolar 1 and II depression, with less switching than placebo and the effect visible from week 1. These have been replicated in EMBOLDEN 1 (e.g. n = 270, RCT, d/b, p/c, 8/52, Suppes *et al*, *J Affect Disord* 2010;**12**:106–15), and EMBOLDEN II where quetiapine 300–600 mg/d (but not paroxetine) was superior to placebo (n = 740, RCT, d/b, p/c, 8/52, McElroy *et al*, *J Clin Psychiatry* 2010;**71**:163–74). Quetiapine 300 and 600 mg/d were also superior to placebo, whereas lithium was not (n=802, RCT, d/b, p/c, 8/52, Young et al, J Clin Psychiatry 2010;**71**:150–62). In comorbid BD and anxiety (from BOLDER 1 and 2), quetiapine was more effective than placebo (s=2, n=1051, RCT, d/b, p/c, 8/52, Lydiard et al, Prim Care Companion J Clin Psychiatry 2009;**11**:215–25). Its action might be mediated via N-desalkylquetiapine, a norepinephrine reuptake inhibition and partial 5HT1A agonism (Jensen et al, Neuropsychopharmacology 2008;**33**:2303–12).

Reviews: * general (Janicak and Rado, Expert Opin Pharmacother 2011;**12**:1643–51; Thase, Neuropsychiatr Dis Treat 2008;**4**:11–21; s=5, RCT, d/b, p/c, Bogart and Chavez, Ann Pharmacother 2009;**43**:1848–56).

+ Combinations

Lithium + fluoxetine

Fluoxetine-augmentation of lithium in bipolar mood disorder can help prevent breakthrough depression (n=26, open, three-year, Tondo et al, Int J Psychiatry Clin Pract 1997;**1**:203–6).

Lithium + lamotrigine

Significantly more people responded to lamotrigine augmentation of lithium than placebo augmentation in acute bipolar depression (n=124, RCT, d/b, p/c, 8/52, van der Loos et al, J Clin Psychiatry 2009;**70**:223–31).

Olanzapine + fluoxetine (OFC)

The olanzapine-fluoxetine combination (OFC) is licensed for bipolar depression in the US as 'Symbyax' (6/25, 6/50, or 12/50 mg/day), and has been compared to olanzapine (5–20 mg/day), and placebo (n=833, RCT, d/b, p/c, 8/52, Tohen et al, Arch Gen Psychiatry 2003;**60**:1079–88, MS), although there was no fluoxetine arm and so the combination's efficacy might be predominantly from fluoxetine (n=114[c=83], RCT, open, 7+12/52, Tamayo et al, J Clin Psychopharmacol 2009;**29**:358–61). OFC was more effective than lamotrigine 200 mg/d for bipolar I depression but with more side-effects, although relapses were equivalent (n=410, RCT, d/b, 25/52, Brown et al, Int J Neuropsychopharmacol 2009;**12**:773–82, MS; see also n=410, RCT, d/b, 7/52, Brown et al, J Clin Psychiatry 2006;**67**:1025–33: MS;

comment by Nirenberg, EBMH 2007;**10**:12, noting that the 5/52 titration period with lamotrigine would have left only 2/52 at full dose so it is surprising it did so well), and may have some efficacy in relapse prevention (n=560, open, 76/52, Corya et al, J Clin Psychiatry 2003;**64**:1349–56; MS).

Review: general (Deeks and Keating, CNS Drugs 2008;**22**:793–5).

● Unlicensed/some efficacy

Antidepressants *

A meta-analysis of more recent studies concludes that antidepressants are safe in acute bipolar depression, but lack efficacy (s=15, n=2373, Sidor and Macqueen, J Clin Psychiatry 2011;**72**:156–67). A recent review of antidepressants in bipolar depression (Licht et al, Acta Psychiatr Scand 2008;**118**:337–46) concludes:

- switching occurs anyway
- antidepressants seem safe when combined with a mood stabiliser
- antidepressant monotherapy cannot be recommended, especially in bipolar I
- perception of switching may be because antidepressants shorten depressed phases
- if mania develops, stopping or reducing the antidepressant dose is advisable, although no guidance is available
- accelerated episode frequency is unproven but considered likely.

In the STEP-BD study, for bipolars developing a new-onset depressive episode there is no evidence that antidepressants were associated with new-onset suicidality, even in already high-risk populations (n=425, Bauer et al, J Clin Psychiatry 2006;**67**:48–55). One study showed that continuing antidepressants after a depressive episode was **not** associated with an increased risk of manic episodes, but early discontinuation was associated with significantly increased depressive relapse (n=84, one year, naturalistic, Altshuler et al, Am J Psychiatry 2003;**160**:1252–62).

However, antidepressants can be effective in treating bipolar depression, but once mood has lifted there is the risk of inducing a switch to mania or rapid-cycling. In adults with bipolar depression, venlafaxine, bupropion and sertraline all produce similar acute responses (49–53%) and remission (34–41%), but the risk of switching to mania or hypomania is variable (see general principles, point 5). Patients whose bipolar depression remitted with an antidepressant and a mood stabiliser, and then carried on with the antidepressant, had no statistical benefit from ongoing antidepressants, no symptomatic benefit, no enhanced remission, and no relapse prevention, although some mild positive effects were seen (n = 70, 3 years, Ghaemi et al, J Clin Psychiatry 2010;**71**:372–80). **Fluoxetine** may have a low switch rate in bipolar I and II (n = 34, RCT, p/c, d/b, 8/52, Amsterdam and Shults, J Affect Disord 2005;**87**:121–30). **Bupropion** has been used as an adjunct in resistant, bipolar depression (n = 13, open, Erfurth et al, Neuropsychobiology 2001;**45**[Suppl 1]:S33–S36). **Citalopram** has been shown to be effective in bipolar I and II depression, with a robust and sustained response rate and low ADRs (n = 45, open, 8/52, Kupfer et al, Clin Psych 2001;**62**:985–90). Citalopram and lamotrigine may be useful adjunctives in bipolar depression, with response rates rising considerably past the first six weeks (n = 20, RCT, d/b, 12/52, Schaffer et al, J Affect Disord 2006;**96**:95–9). **Escitalopram** may have some efficacy in bipolar depression (n = 20, open, 12/52, Fonseca et al, J Clin Psychiatry 2006;**67**:81–6). **Moclobemide** 450–750 mg/d may be as effective as imipramine (150–250 mg/d) in bipolar depression, with less side-effects and less switches to mania (2 vs 6), indicating a useful potential role (n = 156, RCT, 8/52, Silverstone et al, Acta Psychiatr Scand 2001;**104**:104–9). **Tricyclics** should be avoided unless covered with mood stabilisers (n = 136, Mundo et al, J Affect Disord 2006;**92**:227–30). In lithium non-responders, **venlafaxine** can be effective in bipolar depression, with no switches to mania (n = 17, 12/52, Amsterdam et al, Acta Psychiatr Scand 2010;**121**:210–8), although response can reduce after repeated exposure (n = 83, RCT, open, Amsterdam and Shults, J Aff Disorders 2009;**115**:234–40). **Tranylcypromine** appeared effective (62.5% responded) in refractory bipolar depression in an incomplete study (n = 19, RCT, open, Nolen et al, Acta Psychiatr Scand 2007;**115**:360–5).

Antipsychotics (see also quetiapine & OFC) *

The main roles of antipsychotics in bipolar depression are as adjunctives to mood stabilisers and as adjunctive maintenance in treatment-resistance. The main bipolar maintenance study showed that **aripiprazole** did not delay the time to relapse of depressive symptoms, although it did not increase it either (n = 161 [c = 12], RCT, d/b, p/c, two years, Keck et al, Am J Psychiatry 2007;**164**:1480–91). Low-dose **ziprasidone** (mean 58 mg/d) may have a potential for bipolar depression (n = 30, Liebowitz et al, J Affect Disord 2009;**118**:205–8).

Modafinil *

Modafinil 100–200 mg/d significantly improved depressive symptoms in bipolar depression, with no difference in treatment-emergent mania (n = 85, RCT, p/c, 6/52, Frye et al, Am J Psychiatry 2007;**164**:1242–9). It does not seem to cause switching to mania when used for fatigue and sleepiness in bipolar depression (n = 39, Nasr et al, J Affect Disord 2006;**95**:111–4). Armodafinil 150 mg appears to improve depressive symptoms in bipolar depression, so probably modafinil might do the same (n = 257, RCT, d/b, p/c, 8/52, Calabrese et al, J Clin Psychiatry 2010;**71**:1363–70).

Omega-3 fatty acids

Ethyl-EPA (ethyl-eicopentaenoic acid) was effective in bipolar depression, with 1–2 g/d superior to placebo (n = 75, RCT, d/b, p/c, 12/52, Frangou et al, Br J Psychiatry 2006;**188**:46–50), but in another study EPA 6 g/d had no overall efficacy on any marker in bipolar depression (RCT, p/c, 4/12, Keck et al, Biol Psychiatry 2006;**60**:1020–3) so dose may be important (n = 12 [c = 8], open, 6/12, Osher et al, J Clin Psychiatry 2005; **66**:726–9).

■ Unlicensed/possible efficacy

Gabapentin

While gabapentin has no antimanic activity (see 1.10.2), it may be useful as an adjunct in refractory and comorbid bipolar patients (review, s = 40, Carta et al, J Affect Disord 2003;**75**:83–91). However, in a trial against lamotrigine, gabapentin was no better than placebo (n = 45, RCT, p/c, d/b, c/o, 6/52, Obrocea et al, Biol Psychiatry 2002;**51**:253–60).

Inositol

Inositol may be useful in bipolar (as well as unipolar) depression, e.g. 50% responded to 12 g/d inositol cf. 30% on placebo (n = 24, RCT, 6/52, Chengappa et al, Bipolar Disord 2000;**2**:47–55), and in bipolar depression unresponsive to a mood stabiliser and at least one antidepressant, response to inositol was 17% (cf lamotrigine 24% and risperidone 5%; n = 66, RCT, 16/52, open, Nierenberg et al, Am J Psychiatry 2006;**163**:210–6). However, inositol was numerically, but not statistically or clinically, superior to placebo as augmentation of lithium or valproate (n = 17, RCT, d/b, p/c, 6/52, Eden Evins et al, Bipolar Disord 2006;**8**:168–74).

Ketamine *

Ketamine (an NMDA antagonist) IV infusion (0.5mg/kg) produced a robust, rapid and reliable improvement in depression symptoms (71% vs 6% with placebo), albeit short-lived (n = 18, RCT, d/b, p/c, c/o, 28/7, Diazgranados et al, Arch Gen Psychiatry 2010;**67**:793–802).

Ketoconazole

Ketoconazole, 400 mg/d has been used as add-on therapy in resistant bipolar depression, with no increase in manic symptoms (n = 6, open, Brown et al, Bipolar Disord 2001;**3**:23–9).

Melatonin

Melatonin secretion is altered in bipolar disorder and so melatonin may have some role (review by Srinivasan et al, World J Biol Psychiatry 2006;**7**:138–51).

Methylphenidate

In one study, methylphenidate was effective and tolerable in 78% depressed bipolars (n = 14, open, 12/52, El-Mallakh, Bipolar Disord 2000; **2**:56–9), and a retrospective chart analysis showed that methylphenidate (mean 14/12) could be effective for bipolar depression without apparent major problems, abuse or mood switching (n = 16,

Lydon and El-Mallakh, J Clin Psychopharmacol 2006;**26**:516–8).

Oxcarbazepine

Oxcarbazepine as add-on to lithium in bipolar depression was effective in 60% and may be successful over the longer-term (n = 17, open, 8/52+12/12, Benedetti et al, J Affect Disord 2004;**79**:273–7).

Pramipexole

Pramipexole (a dopamine agonist) was clearly superior (60% response) to placebo (9%) in bipolar depression, when used as an adjunct to either lithium or valproate (n = 21, RCT, d/b, p/c, 6/52, Zarate et al, Biol Psychiatry 2004;**56**:54–60) and a mean 1.7 mg/d added to existing mood stabilisers produced a 67% response (cf 20% with placebo) in bipolar depression (n = 22, RCT, o/p, p/c, 6/52, Goldberg et al, Am J Psychiatry 2004;**161**:564–6).

Review: Whiskey and Taylor, Psychiatr Bull 2004;**28**:438–40).

Triiodothyronine

Triiodothyronine (T3) (mean 90 mg/d) has been successful in treatment-resistant bipolar II (n = 159, retrospective, Kelly and Lieberman, J Affect Disord 2009;**116**:222–6) and low pretreatment thyroid function predicts slower response to antidepressants (n = 65, Cole et al, Am J Psychiatry 2002; **159**:116–21).

Valproate *

A systematic review and meta-analysis has shown some preliminary evidence for some efficacy. Valproate had an NNT of 5.9 (41% response cf 24% response on placebo) (s = 4, n = 142, RCT, d/b, p/c, Smith et al, J Affect Disord 2010;**122**:1–9; bizarrely the same s = 4, n = 142, RCT, d/b, p/c, Bond et al, in the same J Affect Disord 2010;**124**:228–34).

Zonisamide

Adjunctive zonisamide (mean 236 mg/d) may have modest effectiveness in bipolar depression in some patients, with low switching (e.g. Wilson and Findling, Expert Opin Pharmacother 2007;**8**:111–3), but relatively poor tolerability (n = 20 [c = 10], open, 8/ 52, Ghaemi et al, J Clin Psychopharmacol 2006;**26**:385–8), although up to 300 mg/d as add-on had significant effects in 50% of completers (n = 10 [c=8], open, 8/52, Anand et al, J Clin Psychiatry 2005;**66**:195–8).

□ No efficacy

Levetiracetam *

Levetiracetam up to 2500mg/d was ineffective for acute bipolar depression (n = 42, RCT, d/b, p/c, 6/52, Saricicek et al, J Clin Psychiatry 2011; in press).

1.10.4 RAPID-CYCLING BIPOLAR DISORDER

Introduction *

Rapid-cycling bipolar disorder is a variant of bipolar mood disorder, where four or more mood episodes occur in one year. Although it is relatively uncommon (e.g. one in six presenting with bipolar have a rapid-cycling pattern) and often a transient condition (about 80% will resolve in a year), this sub-group accounts for up to 80% of lithium non-responders, that antidepressant therapy of depressive phases can induce or worsen cycling and that rapid-cycling is a risk factor for suicide and suicide attempts (n = 345, mean 13 years, Coryell et al, Arch Gen Psychiatry 2003;**60**:914–20). Rapid-cyclers are more likely (cf non-rapid-cycling) to have a younger age of onset, more enduring symptoms, more severe depression and impairment, more anxiety/mania (n = 54257, Lee et al, Br J Psychiatry 2010;**196**:217–25), be female and bipolar II (n = 1742, STEP-BD, Schneck et al, Am J Psychiatry 2008;**165**:370–7). Risk factors include poor adherence (n = 3640, Perlis et al, J Clin Psychiatry 2010;**71**:296–303), neurological damage, neuroendocrine factors (including hypothyrodism), psychotropic drugs (e.g. alcohol, antidepressants, stimulants), as well as some genetic factors (Sachs, in J Clin Psychiatry 2006;**67**:1140–51).

Role of drugs

There will probably always be a lack of robust data on the pharmacotherapy of rapid-cycling, as research is complicated by the unpredictable and spontaneously remitting nature of the condition.

The initial strategies must be:
1. Reduce or stop any cycle-promoters, e.g. antidepressants.
2. Add/optimise anti-cycling mood stabilisers (start with lithium for treatment-naïve patients).
3. Add other drugs, e.g. lithium, antipsychotics, lamotrigine (especially for bipolar 2), perhaps valproate.
4. If ineffective, levothyroxine and nimodipine may be effective in some patients not responsive to first-line drugs and may be worth a therapeutic trial.
4. Minimise ADRs to enhance compliance.
5. Recognise that the full benefits may not be apparent for several months so do not abandon treatment too early.

References: n = 500, STEP-BD, Schneck et al, J Clin Psychiatry 2006;**67**[Suppl 11]:22–7; Coryell, CNS Drugs 2005;**19**:557–69.

Reviews: general (Bauer et al, Bipolar Disord 2008;**10**:153–62; Mercer, Curr Psychiatr Rep 2007;**9**:53–62; Schneck, J Clin Psychiatry 2006; **67** [Suppl 22]:22–7), BAP evidence-based guidelines (Goodwin et al, J Psychopharmacol 2009;**23**:346–88).

BNF listed

Carbamazepine

The original carbamazepine study (n = 32, Kishimoto et al, Br J Psychiatry 1983;**143**:327–31) showed a particular effect in rapid-cycling and several studies (e.g. n = 18, open, 6/12, Joyce, Int Clin Psychopharmacol 1988;**3**:123–9) have shown a long-term response rate ranging from 20–70%. Doubt has, however, been raised about long-term efficacy as many people seem to lose the therapeutic response over several years (n = 24, open, four years, Post et al, J Clin Psychopharmacol 1990;**10**:318–27).

Lithium

Around 20% of rapid-cyclers are lithium responders, probably by reducing the intensity of relapses rather than the actual number. Lithium response may be better if the sequence of relapse is mania, depression and then remission, rather than depression, then mania and remission (Grof et al, Prog Neuropsychopharmacol Biol Psychiatry 1987; **11**:199–203). Poor compliance with lithium, particularly if intermittent (e.g. frequent abrupt stopping), may complicate treatment by inducing relapse.

Review: Muzina, *Bipolar Disord* 2009;**11**(Suppl 2):84–91.

Lithium + carbamazepine
The combination can be useful in rapid-cyclers non-responsive to the individual drugs (e.g. n = 16, retrospective, Di Costanzo and Schifano, *Acta Psychiatr Scand* 1991;**83**:456–9). See also interactions (4.5.1).

Lithium + valproate
Open studies have included this combination in rapid-cyclers, and reported an additive or potentiating effect (mentioned by Sharma and Persad, *Lithium* 1994;**5**:117–25).

Thyroid + tricyclic
Sub-therapeutic doses of T_3 tri-iodothyronine 25–50 mcg/d or T_4 levothyroxine up to 0.1 mg/d have been used as augmentation to tricyclics and phenelzine (although care is needed with any use of antidepressants in rapid-cycling). See levothyroxine/liothyronine.

Lamotrigine *
In the largest and only prospective placebo-controlled study in rapid-cycling disorder, lamotrigine was well tolerated and appeared useful in some (n = 324, open + n = 182, d/b maintenance phase, Calabrese et al, *J Clin Psychiatry* 2000;**61**:841–50), with survival rates favouring lamotrigine (significantly so in bipolar II patients), and 41% stable without relapse at 6/12 (cf 26% placebo). In a recent trial, lamotrigine seemed potentially useful as an adjunct in non-response to lithium plus valproate (n = 36[c = 16], d/b, p/c, 12/52, Wang et al, *Psychopharmacol Bull* 2010;**43**:5–21). The optimum dose appears to be 50–200 mg/d, although doses as high as 600 mg/d have been used.

Levothyroxine/liothyronine
Levothyroxine has potential efficacy at 0.3–0.5 mg/d (or liothyronine 140–400 mcg/d) for

rapid or 48-hour-cycling mania. Latent thyroid hypofunction may occur, revealed by a lithium challenge (n = 40, Gyulai et al, *Biol Psychiatry* 2003;**53**:899–905). Significant response was seen in a two-year study with high-dose levothyroxine (n = 6, open, Afflelou et al, *Encephale* 1997;**23**:209–17).

Valproate (see also combinations)
Valproate seems as effective as lithium in preventing relapse in recently stabilised rapid-cyclers (n = 60[n = 254 in stabilisation phase], RCT, d/b, 20/12, Calabrese et al, *Am J Psychiatry* 2005;**162**:2152–61). In patients stabilised for 6/12 on lithium plus valproate, the valproate had no additional effect over lithium alone (n = 31, RCT, d/b, 6/12, Kemp et al, *J Clin Psychiatry* 2009;**70**:113–21).

Calcium-channel blockers
There are old reports of response to nimodipine in rapid-cycling with a very marked response in some patients (e.g. n = 12[c=9], RCT, d/b, p/c, Pazzaglia et al, *Psychiatry Res* 1993;**49**:257–72).

Clonazepam
Clonazepam has been used as an adjunct to lithium in lithium-refractory bipolars (n = 5, open, Aronson et al, *Am J Psychiatry* 1989;**146**:77–80).

Clozapine
Clozapine may be effective in treatment-resistant rapid cycling (e.g. Suppes et al, *Biol Psychiatry* 1994;**36**:338–40).

Gabapentin
Some gabapentin studies in mania included some rapid-cycling patients and moderate efficacy was reported (Shelton and Calabrese, *Curr Psychiatry Reports* 2000;**2**:310–15).

Levetiracetam
There are cases of adjunctive treatment improving depression, interrupting rapid cycling (n = 2, Bräunig and Krüger, *J Psycho-pharmacol* 2003;**17**:239–41) and in multiple drug-resistant rapid-cycling (n = 1, Kaufman, *Epilepsy Behav* 2004;**5**:1017–20).

Olanzapine

Ten rapid-cyclers were classified as responding to olanzapine during dysphoric mania (n = 13, open, 4/52, Gonzalez-Pinto et al, J Clin Psychopharmacol 2002;**22**:450–4).

Quetiapine

Quetiapine 300 mg and 600 mg/d were more effective than placebo in treating depressive episodes in rapid-cycling bipolar I and II (n = 108, RCT, d/b, p/c, 8/52, Vieta et al, Bipolar Disorder 2007;**9**:413–25) and it may be more effective than valproate, albeit with more side-effects (n = 17, open, Langosch et al, J Clin Psychopharmacol 2008;**28**:555–60).

❋ Case reports

- **Carbamazepine + valproate** (n = 1 Ketter et al, J Clin Psychopharmacol 1992;**12**:276–81).
- **Clozapine + lamotrigine *** (n = 1, Bastiampillai et al, J Psychopharmacol 2010; **24**:1834–6).
- **Lamotrigine + valproate** (n = 1, Woo et al, Psychiatry Clin Neurosci 2007;**61**:130–1).
- **Lithium + levothyroxine** (n = 1, Bernstein, J Clin Psychopharmacol 1992;**12**:443–4).
- **Topiramate + clozapine** (n = 1, Chen et al, Clin Neuropharmacol 2005;**28**:136–8).

☐ No efficacy

Antidepressants

Antidepressants may induce rapid-cycling, especially in women prior to the first episode and since up to 50% of cases may be antidepressant-induced, discontinuation has to be a first-line treatment. Antidepressants should only be used in rapid-cyclers in low dose and only in acute severe depression.

1.11 BORDERLINE PERSONALITY DISORDER (BPD)
see also Aggression (1.2)

There are a large number of personality disorders, of which borderline personality disorder is but one. Treating personality disorders (and hence personality itself) is obviously somewhat controversial. Research is now often directed towards treating symptom clusters rather than the underlying personality disorder, e.g. anxiety, aggression and impulsiveness.

Symptoms

The main symptoms of BPD are of a deeply ingrained maladaptive pattern of behaviour, recognisable from adolescence and continuing through most of adult life. People with a PD show continued boredom, anger, unstable relationships, impulsive self-harmful behaviour (e.g. gambling, stealing, binge-eating or drinking), feelings of abandonment, variable moods, recurrent suicide threats or behaviour, and uncertainty about their personal identity.

Role of drugs *

People with BPD may account for up to 7.5% of psychiatric admissions, with a raised incidence of psychiatric morbidity and mortality, and use a wide range of medication and services. Pharmacotherapy will not alter ingrained character traits or the effects of abuse, but they may produce modest benefits with the occasional striking result, and be more effective if combined with psychotherapy. Drug therapy, however, is fraught with problems. Side-effects may be grossly exaggerated and patients may be actively antimedication. Several meta-analyses of RCTs have concluded that the beneficial effects are as follows:

	Antipsychotics	Antidepressants	Mood stabilisers
Cognitive-perception	++	?	?
Anger	++/+++	+/++	++
Impulse-behaviour	+	o	++
Anxiety	?	+/++	+++
Depression	o	+	++
Global functioning	+	o	+

+++ Significant effect   + Minor effect
++ Moderate effect   o No effect

Cochrane concludes that the current data for pharmacotherapy in BPD is insufficient to make any recommendations (s = 8, n = 394, Khalifa et al, Cochrane Database Syst Rev 2010;**8**:CD007667; s = 28, n = 1742, Stoffers et al, Cochrane Database Syst Rev 2010;**6**:CD005653; comment by Lieb *et al, Br J Psychiatry* 2010;**196**:4–12).

References: * s=21, Ingenhoven *et al, J Clin Psychiatry* 2010;**17**:14–25; Mercer *et al, J Pers Disord* 2009;**23**:156–74; Dahl, *Curr Opin Psychiatry* 2008;**21**:78–83.

Reviews: * general (Bellion *et al, CNS Drugs* 2008; **22**:671–92; Diaz-Marsa *et al, Actas Esp Psiquiatr* 2008;**36**:39–49; Dahl, *Curr Opin Psychiatry* 2008; **21**:78–83), anticonvulsants (Díaz-Marsá *et al, Actas Esp Psiquiatr* 2008;**36**(Suppl 3):39–45), suicidality (Cardish, *Can J Psychiatry* 2007;**52**[suppl 1]:115S–127S), management of dangerous and severe PDs (Völlm, *Curr Opin Psychiatry* 2009; **22**:501–6).
.

● Unlicensed/some efficacy

Antipsychotics *

It has been generally accepted that people with DSM-IV borderline or schizotypical personality disorders may gain significant benefit from psychotherapy and small doses of antipsychotics. The FGAs **haloperidol** and **trifluoperazine** have been used to improve anger, hostility and behavioural symptoms, but have been largely superseded, especially as two studies showed haloperidol to be no better than placebo (n=108, RCT, d/b, p/c, 6/52, Soloff *et al, Arch Gen Psychiatry* 1993;**150**:377–85) and poorly tolerated. **Aripiprazole** 15mg/d may improve many measures of BPD (n=52, RCT, d/b, p/c, 8/52, Nickel *et al, Am J Psychiatry* 2006;**163**:833–8), including as an adjunct to sertraline (56% responding to 10–15mg/d; n=21[c=16], open, 12/52, Bellion *et al, Psychiatry Res* 2008; **161**:206–12) and a low starting dose may facilitate response (n=3, Mobascher *et al, Pharmacopsychiatry* 2006;**39**:111–2). Two small open trials of **clozapine** (25–100mg/d) in severe BPD produced a general improvement (e.g. n=12, Benedetti *et al, J Clin Psychiatry* 1998;**59**:13–107) and significantly reduced SIB, aggression, seclusion and violence (n=7, Chengappa *et al, J Clin Psychiatry* 1999;**60**:477–84; n=1 Vohra, *Indian J Psychiatry* 2010;**52**:267–9). **Olanzapine** may be effective against a range of symptoms. A recent trial of olanzapine 5–10mg/d showed a modest advantage over placebo for BPD, with predictable side-effects (n=451[c=294], RCT, d/b, p/c, Zanarini *et al, J Clin Psychiatry*

2011; in press), although a previous trial was negative (although placebo did well), with only a modest effect on core traits of BPD, and may only be effective during periods of decompensation (n=314, RCT, d/b, p/c, 12/52, Schulz *et al, Br J Psychiatry* 2008;**193**:485–92; comment by Nosè, *EBMH* 2009;**12**:89). Both olanzapine and haloperidol improved BPD symptoms in women, with no differences between the drugs (n=28, RCT, d/b, 8/52, Shafti and Shahveisi, *J Clin Psychopharmacol* 2010;**30**:44–7). **Quetiapine** (mean 250mg/d, range 175–400mg/d) may be well tolerated and significantly improve impulsivity and other symptoms in severe BPD (n=23, open, 12/52, Villeneuve and Lemelin, *J Clin Psychiatry* 2005;**66**:1298–303) and a mean of 540mg/d may have an effect on hostility, suspiciousness and other rating scales in BPD (n=29[c=23], open, Perrella *et al, Prog Neuropsychopharmacol Biol Psychiatry* 2007; **31**:158–63; n=16[c=9], open, 8/52, Adityananjee *et al, Ann Clin Psychiatry* 2008;**20**:219–26). Low dose **risperidone** may be effective and well tolerated, e.g. risperidone (mean 3.3mg/d) helped as an add-on to existing therapies to improve BPD symptomatology, especially aggression and overall functioning (n=15, open, 8/52, Rocca *et al, J Clin Psychiatry* 2002; **63**:241–4). **Ziprasidone** does not seem to have a significant effect on BPD (n=60, RCT, d/b, p/c, 12/52, Pascual *et al, J Clin Psychiatry* 2008;**69**:603–8).

Review: general (Mobascher *et al, Nervenarzt* 2007;**78**:1003–13).

SSRIs

Some symptoms of BPD are shared with depression, e.g. self-condemnation, emptiness, hopelessness, boredom and somatic complaints, and so the use of antidepressants may have some logic. SSRIs may have a role, e.g. **sertraline** (n=16, 8/52, Kavoussi *et al, J Clin Psychiatry* 1994;**55**:137–41) and **fluoxetine** (n=40, RCT, Coccaro and Kavoussi, *Arch Gen Psychiatry* 1997;**54**:1081–8; review by Hawton, *EBMH* 1998;**1**:79). Combining with IPT may improve outcomes (n=39[c=32], 6/12, Bellino *et al, Can J Psychiatry* 2006;**51**:453-60). **Fluvoxamine** may significantly improve rapid mood shifts in female BPDs, but not impulsivity and aggression (n=38, RCT, d/b, p/c, c/o, 24/52 total, Rinne et al, Am J Psychiatry 2002;**159**:2048–54). Careful dose titration is needed to minimise agitation.

Topiramate

Topiramate may help to reduce anger in men (n = 42, RCT, d/b, p/c, 8/52, Nickel et al, Biol Psychiatry 2005;**57**:495–9) and women (n = 29, RCT, d/b, p/c, 8/52, Nickel et al, J Clin Psychiatry 2004;**65**:1515–9; IS), and up to 200 mg/d reduced stress and some other symptoms, although SIB was not an outcome measure and the exclusion criteria included anyone suicidal or abusing drugs or alcohol, so the cohort was relatively limited (n = 56, RCT, d/b, 10/52, Loew et al, J Clin Psychopharmacol 2006;**26**:61–6; comment by Killaspy, EBMH 2006;**9**:74).

Valproate

Valproate significantly reduced irritability, anger, impulsiveness and relationship tempestuousness in women with comorbid bipolar II and BPD and was well tolerated (n = 20, RCT, p/c, d/b, 6/12, Frankenburg and Zanarini, J Clin Psychiatry 2002;**63**:442–6).

■ Unlicensed/possible efficacy

Carbamazepine

Carbamazepine may be useful for aggression and episodic dyscontrol and, although the latter is not epileptic, there are some common precipitating factors (e.g. prodromal symptoms, severe disturbance and post-episode relief of tension). Carbamazepine has been suggested as superior to placebo for behaviour control (n = 16, d/b, p/c, c/o, 6/52, Cowdry and Gardner, Arch Gen Psychiatry 1988;**45**:111–9) but an RCT failed to show any effects (n = 20, RCT, 30/7, de la Fuente and Lotstra, Eur Neuropsycho-pharmacol 1994; **4**:479–86).

Duloxetine *

A pilot study showed that duloxetine 60 mg/d had a positive effect on somatic and other symptoms in BPD (n = 18 [c = 14], open, 12/52, Bellino et al, J Psychopharmacol 2010;**24**:333–9).

Lamotrigine

Lamotrigine was relatively well tolerated and highly significantly effective for anger in women

with BPD (n = 27, RCT, d/b, p/c, 8/52, Tritt et al, J Psychopharmacol 2005;**9**:287–91).

Lithium

Lithium has been reported to be useful for episodic dyscontrol and aggression, in BPD, emotionally unstable adolescents and in alcoholics with a BPD, although the consequences of erratic compliance would be a significant disadvantage.

Oxcarbazepine

Oxcarbazepine 1.2–1.5 g BD may have a potential role (n = 17, open, Bellino et al, J Clin Psychiatry 2005;**66**:1111–5).

Tricyclics

Generally tricyclics are considered ineffective (or even detrimental) in depression associated with BPD.

✷ Case reports

- **Methylphenidate** (n = 1, Van Reekum and Links, Can J Psychiatry 1994;**39**:186–7).

□ No efficacy

Amfetamines

Dexamfetamine has been used but, with the exception of the occasional patient, has proved ineffective (reviewed by Stein in Br J Psychiatry 1992;**161**:167–84).

Benzodiazepines

Benzodiazepines are considered to be contra-indicated in BPD due to their potential to disinhibit and induce rage reactions and dependence, e.g. **alprazolam** was significantly worse than placebo for behavioural control (n = 16, d/b, p/c, c/o, 6/52, Cowdry and Gardner, Arch Gen Psychiatry 1988;**45**:111–9), in children with anxious or avoidant disorders (n = 30, d/b, p/c, Simeon et al, J Am Acad Child Adolesc Psychiatry 1992;**31**:29–33). The occasional use of rapidly absorbed short-acting drugs (e.g. **lorazepam**) may have some limited use in patients with intermittent explosive disorders.

MAOIs

Two studies have shown phenelzine 60 mg/d to

be no better than placebo (e.g. n = 108, RCT, d/b, p/c, 5/52, Soloff et al, Arch Gen Psychiatry 1993;**150**:377–85).

Phenytoin
Two ancient studies showed an often negative effect (e.g. Rosenblatt et al, Curr Ther Res 1976; **19**:332–6).

Reboxetine
There is a case of worsening symptoms with reboxetine (n = 1, Anghelescu et al, J Neuropsychiatry Clin Neurosci 2005;**17**:559–60).

1.12: CATATONIA
see also Schizophrenia (1.21)

Symptoms
Catatonia is usually a rare and potentially lethal type of schizophrenia, dominated by psychosis, catalepsy, stupor, extreme negativism, resistant rigidity, hyperpyrexia, excitement (purposeless motor activity not influenced by external stimuli), echopraxia, grimacing or posturing. It may be associated with mixed (rather than pure) manic episodes in bipolars, and so may be misdiagnosed (n = 27, Krüger et al, J Affect Disord 2003;**74**:279–85). It may be linked to ASDs (Takaoka and Takata, Psychol Rep 2007;**101**:961–9) or even be a symptom of autism (Dhossche et al, Int Rev Neurobiol 2006;**72**:151–64).

Role of drugs
ECT is generally considered the treatment of choice for various forms of catatonia, e.g. organic, lethal and schizophrenic (n = 50, Hatta et al, J ECT 2007;**23**:233–5). Organic catatonia often responds to treatment of the underlying cause, e.g. withdrawal of the offending drug. Antipsychotic-induced catatonia is also potentially fatal and must be treated symptomatically. A careful history may elicit a drug-symptom association and the potentially offending drug(s) stopped. Antipsychotics are generally unhelpful.
Reviews: * general (Daniels, J Neuropsychiatry Clin Neurosci 2009;**21**:371–80), drug-induced (Duggal and Singh, Drugs Today [Barc] 2005;**41**:599–607), clinical features, diagnosis, management and prognosis (Fink and Taylor, Arch Gen Psychiatry 2009;**66**:1173–7).

+ Combinations

Lorazepam + dexamfetamine
See separate drugs/groups.

Olanzapine + amantadine
Dramatic reduction of symptoms has been reported with olanzapine and amantadine, weak NMDA receptor antagonists (n = 1, Babington and Spiegel, Psychosomatics 2007;**48**:534–6).

● Unlicensed/some efficacy

Amantadine
See memantine.

Benzodiazepines *
There are many case reports of successful benzodiazepine use in catatonia. **Lorazepam** 3–6 mg/d has produced complete response in 32% patients and improvement in 69% (n = 107, Tibrewal et al, Prog Neuropsychopharmacol Biol Psychiatry 2010;**34**:1520–2), and lorazepam IM (or diazepam IV if lorazepam failed) showed a 100% success rate over 24 hours (n = 14, Huang, Psychiatry Clin Neurosci 2005;**59**:52–5; n = 2, Huang and Huang, Chang Gung Med J 2010;**33**:106–9). In an open study comparing lorazepam and ECT, 76% responded to lorazepam (IV and/or oral) within five days; most who failed responded promptly to ECT and a positive response to initial parenteral challenge with lorazepam predicted a positive outcome (n = 28, open, Bush et al, Acta Psychiatr Scand 1996;**93**:137–43). High-dose maintenance lorazepam has been effective long-term (Manjunatha et al, Aust NZ J Psychiatry 2007;**41**:625–7). Lorazepam IM or **diazepam** IV produced 100% resolution within a day in depressed people with catatonic features (n = 7, Hung and Huang, Clin Neuropharmacol 2006;**29**:144–7) and haemodialysis (n = 1, Tsai and Huang, Prog Neuropsychopharmacol Biol Psychiatry 2010;**34**:423–4). **Clonazepam** at 2.5 mg/d orally or 1 mg IV (e.g. n = 1, Kumar, Aust N Z J Psychiatry 2001;**35**:391) and **midazolam** (mentioned in Am J Psychiatry 1991;**148**:809) have also been used. However, Cochrane concludes that the evidence base for use is lacking (s = 0, n = 0, Gibson and Walcott, Cochrane Database Syst Rev 2008;**4**:CD006570).

Memantine and amantadine *

Amantadine and memantine may both have a role in improving symptoms of treatment-resistant catatonia (n = 25, Carroll et al, J Neuropsychiatry Clin Neurosci 2007;**19**:406–12) and there are many case reports of rapid, significant response of catatonic schizophrenia to memantine 10–20mg/d (n = 1, Carpenter et al, Ann Pharmacother 2006;**40**:344–6) and amantadine (e.g. n = 1, Muneoka et al, Pharmacopsychiatry 2010;**43**:151–2).

Zolpidem

There have been a number of reports of dramatic improvement in catatonia with zolpidem (e.g. Mastain et al, Rev Neurol 1995; **151**:52–6), including a dramatic response when due to alcohol withdrawal (n = 1, Cottencin et al, Med Sci Monit 2009;**15**;129–31), to the extent that it has been used as a diagnostic tool for catatonia, e.g. by inducing resolution in people thought to have schizophrenia and allowing interviews to take place (e.g. Thomas et al, Lancet 1997;**349**:702; Zaw and Bates, Lancet 1997;**349**:1914).

■ Unlicensed/possible efficacy

Antipsychotics *

Antipsychotics are generally considered unhelpful but there are cases of catatonic schizophrenia responsive to amisulpride (n = 1, French and Eastwood, Can J Psychiatry 2003;**48**:570; n = 1, Cottencin et al, Prim Care Companion J Clin Psychiatry 2009;**11**:275–6), including a remarkable case of multi-resistant chronic catatonia responding to amisulpride 1200mg/d over six months (n = 1, Srikanth and Baxter, Prog Neurol Psychiatry 2007;**11**:13–6), aripiprazole up to 18mg/d orally (n = 1, Kirino, Clin Schizophr Relat Psychoses 2010;**4**:185–8; n = 3, Vörös and Tényi, Neuropsychopharmacol Hung 2010;**12**:373–6) and IM (n = 3, Vörös et al, Pharmacopsychiatry 2009;**42**:286–7), clozapine (n = 2, Dursun et al, J Psychopharmacol 2005;**19**:432–3; n = 1, Sixt et al, Z Kinder Jugendosychiatr Psychother 2009;**37**:209–14) and risperidone (n = 2, Valevski et al, Clin Neuropharmacol 2001;**24**:228–31), including for periodic catatonia (Duggal and Gandotra, Can J Psychiatry 2005;**50**:241–2).

Olanzapine has been used to successfully treat lethal catatonia (e.g. n = 1, Chang et al, Prog Neuropsychopharmacol Biol Psychiatry 2009;**33**:1559–60) and encephalitis presenting as catatonia (n = 1, Suzuki et al, Rinsho Shinkeigaku 2010;**50**:329–31).

Carbamazepine

Carbamazepine has been used in lorazepam-resistant patients (n = 9, Kritzinger and Jordaan, Int J Neuropsychopharmacol 2001;**4**:251–7).

Valproate

A very short review (entitled 'is there a role for valproic acid in the treatment of catatonia?') discussed the role, so the answer is 'probably not' (Bowers and Ajit, J Neuropsychiatry Clin Neurosci 2007;**19**:197–8), although a prophylactic effect may occur (n = 1, Yoshida et al, J Clin Psychopharmacol 2005;**25**:504–5).

✱ Case reports

- **Methylphenidate** * (n = 1, Prowler et al, Psychosomatics 2010;**51**:74–6).
- **Vitamin B12** (n = 1, Berry et al, Acta Psychiatr Scand 2003;**108**:156–9).

◆ Others

Other drugs tried include **barbiturates** (thiopental and amobarbital; referred to by Masiar, Am J Psychiatry 1992;**149**:144–5), **bromocriptine** (n = 1, Mahmood, Br J Psychiatry 1991;**158**:437–8), IV **dantrolene** (n = 2, Pennati, Am J Psychiatry 1991; **148**:268).

1.13 DEMENTIA including:

1.13.1 Treatment of Alzheimer's disease
1.13.2 BPSD/BPSSD (behavioural and psychological [signs and] symptoms of dementia)
1.13.3 Vascular dementia
1.13.4 Prophylaxis and prevention

Symptoms

Dementia is a progressive and irreversible reduction in the level of previously attained intellectual, memory and personality or emotional functioning. The main clinical features are:
- disturbed behaviour (disorganised, inappropriate, distracted, restless, antisocial)

- lack of insight
- impaired thinking (slow, impoverished, incoherent, rigid)
- poverty of speech and low mood
- poor cognitive function (forgetfulness, poor attention, disorientation in time and place)
- impaired memory.

Symptoms caused by vitamin depletion (e.g. B_{12}, foliate, thiamine), infections (encephalitis, neurosyphilis) or drug toxicity and can be treated.

Alzheimer's disease (AD) is characterised by amyloid plaques and neuro-fibrillary tangles, with reduced levels of acetylcholine and other transmitters in the brain. The amyloid hypothesis is that accumulation of the peptide amyloid beta, a toxic protein, precipitates the development of the sticky plaques that are common in Alzheimer's, although there are other theories. The degree of dementia is associated more with the degree of neurofibrillary pathology than with the amyloid plaque burden. It usually presents with an insidious onset and steady deterioration, forgetfulness, lack of spontaneity, disorientation, depressed mood, decline in self-care, poor sleep (waking disorientated and perplexed) and intellectual impairment (dysphasia, dyspraxia, language decline). The incidence of comorbid cerebrovascular disease may be high, and ranges from 22% (n = 548, Feldman et al, Int J Geriatr Psychiatry 2008;**24**:479–88) to 89% (n = 232, Tabet et al, Int J Clin Pract 2009;**63**:338–45), depending on the threshold for identification.

Lewy body dementia is a variant of Alzheimer's disease and is more common in men. The key features include early onset, persistent and well-formed visual hallucinations, and motor features of Parkinsonism. Patients may be extremely sensitive to antipsychotics and anticholinergics (Gold et al, Front Neurol Neurosci 2009;**24**:107–13), which may result in a sudden onset of EPSEs, profound confusion and deterioration, and can lead to death.

Vascular dementia is a variant of Alzheimer's (see separate section 1.13.3).

Non-pharmacological interventions should include behavioural management, cognitive and multisensory stimulation, environmental design, physical activities, reality orientation and recreational activities.

Role of drugs

Currently there are six main classes of agents for dementia (management and prevention or delay):

- cholinesterase inhibitors
- NMDA receptor blockers (e.g. memantine)
- antioxidants (including gingko biloba)
- anti-inflammatory agents
- neurotrophic factors (including HRT)
- antiamyloid agents (including cholesterol-lowering drugs)
- Tau protein inhibitors
- Mitochondrial dysfunction regulators.

Cholinesterase inhibitors (ChEls) clearly help many people, but the problem seems to be in identifying which ones. Drug trials have many exclusions, and extrapolation of the results to the general population is open to question, but even delaying admission to a nursing home by one month would be cost-effective. Unfortunately, the only extended trial failed to show an effect on time to institutionalisation or any other measure (n = 565, RCT, d/b, three years, Courtney et al, Lancet 2004;**363**:2105–15), concluding that donepezil was not cost-effective (although the trial had shortcomings, see correspondence in Lancet).

However, several independent reviews have concluded that the ChEls are effective. A major systematic review and meta-analysis showed ChEls to have a modest effect on neuropsychiatric and functional outcomes in Alzheimer's, but long-term outcomes, such as quality of life and caregiver burden, are unclear (s = 29, Trinh et al, JAMA 2003;**280**:210–16; comment by Lahiri and Farlow, EBMH 2003;**6**:94). Another review suggested the ChEls result in a modest but significant therapeutic improvement, with an NNT of 7, and an NNH of 12 (s = 16, n = 5159 + 2795 controls, Lanctôt et al, CMAJ 2003;**169**:557–64).

Reviews: * general (Osborn and Saunders, J Am Osteopath Assoc 2010;**110**(9 Suppl 8):S16–26; Gifford and Jones, Prescriber 2009;**20**:45–9), mild-to-moderate dementia (Hogan et al, CMAJ 2008;**179**:1019–26), severe Alzheimer's disease (Herrmann and Gauthier, CMAJ 2008;**179**:1279–

87; Voisin and Vellas, *Drugs Aging* 2009;**26**:135–44; Hsiung and Feldman, *Expert Opin Pharmacother* 2008; **9**:2575–8), vaccines (Foster *et al*, *Mol Psychiatry* 2009; **14**:239–51), medicines for inappropriate sexual behaviours in dementia (Guay, *Am J Geriatr Pharmacother* 2008;**6**:269–88), Alzheimer's and cerebrovascular disease (Gil *et al*, *Clin Drug Investig* 2008;**28**:429–37), genetics (Cacabelos, *Eur Arch Psychiatry Clin Neurosci* 2008;**258**[suppl 1]:28–47; Avramopoulos, *Genome Med* 2009;**27**:34), anticholinesterases and memantine (s = 59, Raina *et al*, *Ann Intern Med* 2008;**148**:379–97).

1.13.1 TREATMENT OF ALZHEIMER'S DISEASE

BNF listed

CHOLINESTERASE INHIBITORS (ChEIs)

Although there is little to clinically separate the three currently available ChEIs, there are slight differences between them. Donepezil inhibits AChE, rivastigmine inhibits AChE and BuChE (which gives more side-effects initially but may have advantages in later illness), and galantamine both inhibits AChE and enhances ACh's action on nicotinic receptors. ChEIs may offer continued benefit for up to two years in moderately-severe AD (n = 994 [c = 575], RCT, d/b, two years, Bullock *et al*, *Curr Med Res Opin* 2005;**21**:1317–27) and in more severe AD (n = 145, RCT, p/c, 24/52, Feldman *et al*, *Int J Geriatr Psychiatry* 2005;**20**:559–69). All ChEIs may improve cognitive functioning in people with Lewy body dementia (s = 3, 12–20/52, Bhasin *et al*, *Int J Ger Psychiatry* 2007;**22**:890–5). Cochrane concludes that all three are effective, there is no evidence that they are **not** cost-effective, and that donepezil may be slightly better tolerated, although careful titration of galantamine and rivastigmine might overcome this (s = 13, RCT, d/b, p/c, Birks, *Cochrane Database Syst Rev* 2006;**1**:CD005593).

Reviews: * general (Musia *et al*, *Curr Med Chem* 2007;**14**:2654–79), systematic review and meta-analysis comparing anticholinesterases (s = 26, Hansen *et al*, *Clin Interv Aging* 2008;**3**:211–25; s = 12, Lockhart *et al*, *Dement Geriatr Cogn Disord* 2009;**8**:389–403).

Donepezil *

Donepezil is licensed for the symptomatic treatment of mild or moderate AD. The dose is 5 mg/d for the first month, increasing to 10 mg/d as tolerated. CYP2D6 ultrarapid metabolisers may have lower steady-state plasma levels than normals, and show no improvement as a consequence, a possible explanation of interindividual variation (n = 42, Varsaldi *et al*, *Eur J Clin Pharmacol* 2006;**62**:721–6). In the early stages of AD, donepezil 10 mg/d may improve daily cognitive functioning (n = 153, RCT, d/b, p/c, 24/52, Seltzer *et al*, *Arch Neurol* 2004;**61**:1852–6) and may help preserve cognitive function in severe AD (n = 343, RCT, d/b, p/c, 24/52, Black *et al*, *Neurology* 2007;**69**:459–69). In moderate AD, a systematic review concluded donepezil was effective for cognitive and global function in AD for up to six months (s = 10, Whitehead *et al*, *Int J Geriatr Psychiatry* 2004;**19**:624–33; comment by Lanctôt, *EBMH* 2005;**8**:15, noting the AD-2000 trial was published too late to be included in the analysis). Donepezil maintains its effectiveness over one year while remaining well tolerated (e.g. n = 286, RCT, p/c, one year, Winblad *et al*, *Neurology* 2001;**57**:489–95), and even perhaps over two years, although the benefits are lost within six weeks of stopping (n = 763, open, two years, Doody *et al*, *Arch Neurol* 2001; **58**:427–33). In severe AD (MMSE 1–10), donepezil improved cognition and preserved function over an extended period (n = 248 [c = 194], RCT, d/b, p/c, 6/12, Winblad *et al*, *Lancet* 2006;**367**:1057–65; enthusiastic comment by Ringman, *EBMH* 2006;**9**:104). Donepezil may be used in Lewy body dementia, but abrupt withdrawal can lead to acute cognitive and behavioural decline (n = 19, 20 + 6/52, Minett *et al*, *Int J Geriatr Psychiatry* 2003;**18**:988–93). In mild cognitive impairment, donepezil 10 mg/d (cf placebo) may slow the progression to AD over the first year, but not over three years (n = 769, three years, RCT, p/c, d/b, Petersen *et al*, *N Engl J Med* 2005;**352**:2379–88). Higher dose donepezil (23 mg/d) may have additional efficacy over 10 mg/d in moderate to severe AD (n = 1371 [c = 988], RCT, d/b, Farlow *et al*, *Clin Ther* 2010;**32**:1234–51). Cochrane concludes that donepezil produces modest improvements in cognitive function, ADL, and behaviour over one year (s = 23, n =5272, Birks et al, Cochrane Database Syst Rev 2006;1:CD001190).

Reviews: general (Tsuno, Expert Rev Neurother 2009;9:591–8; Winblad, Am J Alzheimer's Dis Other Demen 2009;24:185–92).

Galantamine *

Galantamine is a reversible competitive acetyl-cholinesterase inhibitor, but also stimulates pre- and post-synaptic nicotinic receptors and is indicated for mild-to-moderate AD. The sustained-release capsules (Galantamine XL) allow once a day dosing. The optimum dose is 16mg/d for mild Alzheimer's and 24mg/d for moderate Alzheimer's (n = 835, RCT, d/b, p/c, 5/12, Aronson et al, Drugs Aging 2009;26:231–9), with the benefit sustained over 12 months with the 24mg/d dose (e.g. n = 182, RCT, s/b, 12/12, Wilcock et al, Drugs Aging 2003;20:777–89) or even longer (n = 194[c=119], RCT, d/b, p/c, 36/52, Raskind et al, Arch Neurol 2004;61:252–6). In severe Alzheimer's, it seems well tolerated, safe and may improve cognitive function, but not ADL (n = 407 [c = 329], RCT, d/b, p/c, Burns et al, Lancet Neurol 2009;8:39–47; n = 407, RCT, d/b, p/c, 6/12, Burns et al, Lancet Neurology 2009;8:39–47). In Alzheimer's combined with cerebrovascular disease, galantamine showed improved cognitive function (n = 285 [c = 242], RCT, d/b, p/c, 6/12, Erkinjuntti et al, J Psychopharmacol 2008;22:761–8). Cochrane concludes that galantamine is effective at doses of 16–32mg/d, with a consistent effect at 3–6 months (s = 10, n=6805, Loy and Schneider, Cochrane Database Syst Rev 2006;1:CD001747).

Reviews: * general (Prvulovic et al, Expert Opin Drug Metab Toxicol 2010;6:345–54; Razay and Wilcock, Expert Rev Neurother 2008;8:9–17).

Rivastigmine *

Rivastigmine is licensed for the treatment of mild-to-moderately severe AD and for mild-to-moderate dementia in patients with idiopathic Parkinson's disease. Rivastigmine 6–12 mg/d may have a sustained effect in advanced moderate AD (e.g. n = 44, RCT, p/c, 12/12, Karaman et al, Dement Geriatr Cogn Disord 2005;19:51–6).

Rivastigmine may be useful in people with rapidly progressing AD (s = 4, n = 517, 26/52, Farlow et al, Dement Geriatr Cogn Disord 2005;20:192–7) and in Lewy body dementia (n = 49, RCT, d/b, Touchon et al, Curr Med Res Opin 2006;22:49–59). Rivastigmine may also improve dementia in Parkinson's disease but increases nausea, vomiting and tremor (n = 541 [c = 410], RCT, d/b, 24/52, Emre et al, N Engl J Med 2004;351:2509–18; comment by Chow, EBMH 2005;8:41). 3.7% discontinue due to skin reactions, but manufacturer's advice about application should be followed carefully e.g. site rotation (n = 1195, RCT, p/c, 24/52, Cummings et al, Clin Drug Invest 2010;30:41–9). Cochrane concludes that rivastigmine is beneficial at 6–12mg/d in mild-to-moderate AD, with improvements in ADL and reduced rate of decline (s = 9, n = 4775, Birks et al, Cochrane Database Syst Rev 2009;2:CD001191).

Reviews: * general (Cummings et al, Neurology 2007;69 [4 Suppl 1]:S10–3), patches (Grossberg et al, Int J Clin Pract 2010;64:651–60).

NON-ANTICHOLINESTERASES

Memantine *

Memantine (an NMDA antagonist) is licensed in the UK and some European countries for moderate-to-severe dementia (not just mild-to-moderately severe), a unique indication. It replaces the magnesium ion that blocks NMDA receptors, so acts as a voltage-dependent, non-competitive NMDA-antagonist, blocking the effect of excess glutamate release, thought to be responsible for many symptoms and for disease progression. It may also have a neuroprotective action (review, Jann, Expert Opin Investig Drugs 2000;9:1397–406). The dose is 5mg/d, adding 5mg/d each week up to the licensed maintenance dose of 20mg/d once a day (n = 78, RCT, d/b, 12/52, Jones et al, Int J Geriatr Psychiatry 2007;22:258–62). Side-effects seem low compared to placebo (s = 6, n = 2311, d/b, p/c, > 24/52, Farlow et al, Drug Saf 2008;31:577–85), but include hallucinations, confusion, dizziness, headache and tiredness. The NNTs are 3–6 for global outcomes, 7 for cognitive improvement and 3–6 for ADL improvements (s = 2, Livingston and Katona,

Int J Geriatr Psychiatry 2004;**19**:19–25). In mild-to-moderate AD, memantine 20mg/d showed statistically significant improvements at weeks 12 and 18, but not at 24 weeks due to an unexpectedly high placebo response (n=470, RCT, d/b, p/c, 6/12, Bakchine and Loft, J *Alzheimer's Dis* 2007;**11**:471–9), and in another study memantine improved a wide range of cognitive measures without major drop-outs from ADRs (n=403[c=332], RCT, d/b, p/c, 24/52, Peskind *et al, Am J Geriatr Psychiatry* 2006;**14**:704–15). Memantine may decrease agitated and aggressive behaviour and thus reduce psychotropic drug use and nursing home burden (n=31[c=24], open, 3/12, Herrmann *et al, CNS Drugs* 2011;**25**:425–33). Uniquely, memantine has also been shown to reduce deterioration in moderate-to-severe AD (MMSE 3–14, mean 7.9) compared to placebo, based on CIBIC-plus and ADCS-ADLsev, and with low drop-outs (n=252, RCT, p/c, 28/52, Reisberg *et al, N Engl J Med* 2003;**348**:1333–41). A pooled analysis of memantine in moderate-to-severe AD showed memantine was associated with reduced worsening of AD symptoms (s=6, n=1826, RCT, d/b, p/c, 6/12, Wilkinson and Andersen, *Dement Geriatr Cogn Disord* 2007;**24**:138–45; see also n=451[c=412]], 6/12, Clerici *et al, Drugs Aging* 2009;**26**:321–32). Memantine might improve global clinical status and behavioural symptoms in Lewy body dementia (n=199[c=159], RCT, d/b, p/c, 24/52, Emre *et al, Lancet Neurol* 2010;**9**:969–77) and in dementia in Parkinson's disease or Lewy bodies (n=72[c=56], RCT, d/b, p/c, 24/52, Aarsland *et al, Lancet Neurol* 2009;**8**:613–8). Cochrane concludes there is a beneficial effect at six months (McShane *et al, Cochrane Database Syst Rev* 2006; **2**:CD003154).

Reviews: * general (Herrmann and Lanctôt, *Expert Opin Pharmacother* 2011;**12**:787–800; McKeage, *Drugs Aging* 2010;**27**:177–9; Thomas and Grossberg, *Clin Interv Aging* 2009;**4**:367–77; s=7, van Marum, *Neuropsychiatr Dis Treat* 2009;**5**:237–47; McKeage, *CNS Drugs* 2009; **23**:881–97), pharmacodynamics (Rammes *et al, Curr Neuropharmacol* 2008;**6**:55–78), cognitive functions (s=6, n=1826, Emre *et al, J Alzheimer's Dis* 2008;**14**:193–9), in moderate to

severe AD long-term (Puangthong and Hsiung, *Neuropsychiatr Dis Treat* 2009;**5**:553–61).

+ Combinations

Memantine + ChEIs *

Memantine augmentation of **rivastigmine** may improve memory and executive function in mild-to-moderate AD (n=90, open, 12/52, Riepe *et al, Dement Geriatr Cogn Disord* 2007; **23**:301–6) and had a sustained effect on slowing cognitive and functional decline in AD compared to anticholinesterase or no treatment (n=382, 30/12, Atri *et al, Alzheimer Dis Assoc Disord* 2008;**22**:209–21). Rivastigmine and memantine appears tolerable but better with rivastigmine patches rather than capsules (n=117, open, 26/52, Olin *et al, Int J Geriatr Psychiatry* 2010;**25**:419–26), although one trial of memantine as an adjunct to rivastigmine patches did not seem to add much (n=172[c=147], RCT, open, 24.52, Choi *et al, Curr Med Res Opin* 2011;**27**:1375–83). In an observational study of Alzheimer's, those patients taking memantine and an anticholinesterase (15%) had significantly delayed time to nursing home care compared to either as monotherapy (40% and 45% respectively) but made no change to time to death (n=943, open, mean 3 years, Lopez *et al, J Neurol Neurosurg Psychiatry* 2009;**80**:600–7). **Reviews:** memantine and galantamine (Grossberg *et al, J Clin Pharmacol* 2006;**46**[7 suppl 1]:17S–26S), memantine and donepezil (Xiong and Doraiswamy, *Geriatrics* 2005;**60**:13–4).

Sibutramine + ChEIs

Sibutramine had some efficacy in improving cognitive functioning in early and moderate AD when used as an adjunct to donepezil (RCT, p/c, 3/12, Ollat *et al, Encephale* 2007;**33**:211–5).

● Unlicensed/some efficacy

Ginkgo biloba *

Ginkgo biloba (GB) 120mg/d stabilised and in some cases improved cognitive function for 6–12 months in patients with mild-to-moderate AD and multi-infarct dementia (n=155) compared to placebo (n=54), (RCT, Le Bars *et al, JAMA* 1997;**278**:1327–32). It must be given for

at least 1–3 months before the full therapeutic effect is seen. In a trial of mild-to-severe AD, the placebo group showed a significant decline in all measures (ADAS-cog, GERRI and CGI), while the GB group were considered to have at least slightly improved on some scales (n = 309, d/b, p/c, 26/52, Le Bars et al, Dement Geriatr Cogn Disord 2000;11:230–7). GB (special extract EGb 761) has been shown to be equivalent to donepezil and superior to placebo on MMSE (e.g. n = 96, RCT, d/b, 22/52, Yancheva et al, Aging Ment Health 2009;13:183–90). However, GB 120 mg/d had no detectable effect on mild-to-moderate dementia over 6/12 (n = 176, RCT, d/b, p/c, 6/12, McCarney et al, Int J Geriatr Psychiatry 2008;23:1222–30). Cochrane concludes that there is no convincing evidence for its efficacy on cognition in dementia or in healthy adults (s = 9, RCT, d/b, p/c, Geng et al, Cochrane Database Syst Rev 2010;12:CD007769). However, a systematic review concluded that GB is superior to placebo for improving cognitive function in dementia, although the differences were inconsistent (s = 9, n = 2372, 12–52/52, Weinmann et al, BMC Geriatr 2010; 10:14).
Review: Anon, Prescrire Int 2007;16:205–7.

SSRIs (see also sertraline in 'no efficacy') *
Some studies have shown a potential effect, e.g. escitalopram seems to be as effective as risperidone for BPSD (n = 40, RCT, d/b, 6/52, Barak et al, Int Psychogeriatr 2011; in press), and **citalopram** and superior to placebo (favourably with perphenazine) for behavioural disturbances associated with dementia (n = 85, RCT, d/b, 17/7, Pollock et al, Am J Psychiatry 2002;159:460–5).

■ Unlicensed/possible efficacy

Doxycycline and rifampicin
Significantly reduced decline has been shown with doxycycline 200 mg/d and rifampicin 300 mg/d for three months, which was well tolerated (n = 101, RCT, t/b, p/c, 12/12, Loeb et al, J Am Geriatr Soc 2004;52:381–7).

Folic acid
Cochrane concludes that there is no consistent evidence one way or the other for the use of folic acid (with or without B12) to treat or prevent AD (s = 8, RCT, Malouf et al, Cochrane Database Syst Rev 2008;4:CD004514).

Insulin
Elevating insulin levels (with or without hyperglycaemia) improves memory in people with AD (n = 23 + 14 controls, Craft et al, Arch Gen Psychiatry 1999;56:1135–40).

Levodopa
In people with dementia with Lewy bodies, levodopa produced 36% 'responders' for motor symptoms (n = 14 [c = 10], Molloy et al, J Neurol Neurosurg Psychiatry 2005;76:1200–3).

Methylphenidate *
Methylphenidate 10–20 mg/d has been successfully used for chronic apathy in dementia (n = 13, RCT, d/b, p/c, c/o, 5/52, Herrmann et al, J Clin Psychopharmacol 2008;28:296–301; n = 23, open, 12/52, Padala et al, Am J Geriatr Psychiatry 2010;18:371–4).

Masitinib *
Masitinib (a mast cell stabiliser) slowed cognitive decline as an adjunct to an anticholinesterase and/or memantine (n = 34, RCT, p/c, 24/52, Piette et al, Alzheimers Res Ther 2011;3:16).

Naftidrofuryl
This is a cerebral vasodilator with some limited effect on cognitive and global functioning (e.g. n = 84, RCT, Emeriau et al, Clin Ther 2000;22:834–44).

Omega-3 fatty acids
Reduced levels of DHAs have been related to dementia and so supplements may have some efficacy if started early (Cole et al, Prostaglandins Leukot Essent Fatty Acids 2009;81:213–21) and may help cognitive function in very mild AD (n = 204 [c = 174], RCT, d/b, p/c, Freund-Levi et al, Arch Neurol 2006;63:1402–8).

Piracetam
Piracetam stimulates ACh release but Cochrane concludes that the evidence is too weak to prove an effect (Flicker and

Grimley Evans, *Cochrane Database Syst Rev* 2001;**2**:1011).

Raloxifene *

In postmenopausal women (>69 years of age), the oestrogen raloxifen 60mg/d significantly improved verbal memory (n=213, RCT, d/b, p/c, 12/12, Jacobsen *et al, Menopause* 2010; **17**:309–14).

Testosterone

Men with AD receiving weekly testosterone enanthante 100mg performed significantly better in spatial and memory tests, but with no change in aggression or unwanted behaviour (n=32, RCT, p/c, 6/52, Cherrier *et al, Neurology* 2005;**64**:2063–8).

Vinpocetine

Cochrane concludes that vinpocetine is well tolerated but has only a minor effect (s=3, n=583, p/c, Szatmari and Whitehouse, *Cochrane Database Syst Rev* 2003;**1**:CD003119).

✱ Case reports

- **Lamotrigine** 100mg/d (n=1, 6/12, Devarajan *et al, Am J Psychiatry* 2000; **157**:1178).

◆ Others

Other drugs tried include **amantadine** (n=33, Jibiki *et al, Acta Therapeutica* 1993;**19**:389–96) and **naltrexone** and **naloxone** (review in *Ann Pharmacother* 1993;**27**:447–80).

☐ No efficacy

Cannabinoids

Cochrane concludes that there is no evidence yet that cannabinoids are effective for dementia or BPSD (s=1, Krishnan *et al, Cochrane Database Syst Rev* 2009;**2**:CD007204).

Cicloserin (D-cycloserine)

Cicloserin (a partial agonist at NMDA receptors) may enhance implicit memory in Alzheimer's, but Cochrane concludes that it has no place in treatment (Laake and Oeksengaard, *Cochrane Database Syst Rev* 2002;**2**:CD003153).

Melatonin

There is no evidence that melatonin helps cognitive and non-cognitive symptoms of dementia (s=3, Jansen *et al, Cochrane Database Syst Rev* 2006;**1**:CD003802).

Nicotine

There may be reduced nicotinic cholinergic receptors in the frontal cortex in dementia, and nicotine may stimulate the release of acetylcholine in this area. Cochrane concludes that there is no reliable evidence for a beneficial effect (s=1, Lopez-Arrieta *et al, Cochrane Database Syst Rev* 2001; **2**:CD001749).

NSAIDs (see also prevention, *1.13.4*)

Aspirin 75mg e/c had no obvious effect on deterioration in people (median age 75 years) already with diagnosed AD, and produced ADRs (n=310, p/c, open, two years, AD2000 Group, *Lancet Neurology* 2008;**7**:41–9).

Pioglitazone *

Pioglitazone was well tolerated but ineffective in Alzheimer's (n=29[c=25], RCT, d/b, p/c, 18/52, Geldmacher *et al, Arch Neurol* 2011; **68**:45–50).

Prednisone

Prednisone 10–20mg/d has been shown to be ineffective (n=138, RCT, 56/52, Aisen *et al, Neurology* 2000;**54**:588–93).

Procaine

Cochrane concludes that procaine is detrimental in dementia and cognitive impairment (s=2, n=415, Szatmári and Bereczki, *Cochrane Database Syst Rev* 2008; **4**:CD005993).

Selegiline

Selegiline may improve MMSE scores, but with no apparent effect on brain lesions or degenerative changes in brain tissue and Cochrane concludes that the evidence is poor, with no justification for use or any need for further studies (Birks and Flicker, *Cochrane Database Syst Rev* 2003;**1**:CD000442; see also n=1073, Wilcock *et al, Int J Geriatr Psychiatry* 2002;**17**:175–83).

Sertraline *

Sertraline does not seem to do anything for depression in Alzheimer's (e.g. n = 131, RCT, d/b, p/c, 12/52, Rosenberg et al, Am J Geriatr Psychiatry 2010;**18**:136–45; n = 131[c = 117], d/b, 24/52, Weintraub et al, Am J Geriatr Psychiatry 2010;**18**:332–40).

Vitamins

In mild-to-moderate AD in Taiwanese people, addition of multivitamins (e.g. pyridoxine 5 mg, folic acid 1 mg and iron) had no effect on cognition or ADL functions (n = 89, RCT, d/b, p/c, 26/52, Sun et al, Clin Ther 2007;**29**:2204–14). Cochrane concludes that there is no evidence that vitamin E helps cognitive impairment in AD (Isaac et al, Cochrane Database Syst Rev 2008;**3**:CD002854)

1.13.2 BPSD/BPSSD (behavioural and psychological [signs and] symptoms of dementia)

BPSD has a cluster of cognitive and non-cognitive symptoms (Petrovic et al, Acta Clin Belg 2007;**62**:426–32) and occurs in up to 90% of people with dementia (Robert et al, Eur Psychiatry 2005;**20**:490–6). BPSD is likely to be an imbalance in a range of transmitters rather than one neurotransmitter abnormality (Kálmán et al, Neuropsychopharmacol Hung 2008;**10**:233–49). It includes aggression, agitation, anxiety, wandering, hoarding, sexual disinhibition, apathy and disruptive vocal activity.

Role of drugs

Symptoms of BPSD should be monitored for at least a month before treatment is considered, and non-drug approaches (e.g. environment, multisensory stimulation, etc) used first. Anticholinesterases and memantine have modest efficacy, antidepressants help depression (but more data is needed on agitation and aggression), carbamazepine may be effective (but has significant interactions) but use of valproate is not supported by current data (Herrmann and Lanctôt, Can J Psychiatry 2007;**52**:630–46). Antipsychotics may be helpful for severe BPSD symptoms but use low doses, time limit and document fully. They should not be used for mild-to-moderate symptoms.

Reviews: * general (Ballard et al, Curr Opin Psychiatry 2009;**22**:532–40; Restifo et al, Australas Psychiatry 2011;**19**:59–63), symptoms (Chiu et al, J Formos Med Assoc 2006;**105**:556–62), psychopathology (Lanari et al, Mech Ageing Dev 2006;**127**:158–65), anticonvulsants (Pinheiro, Encephale 2008;**34**:409–15; Amann et al, Clin Pract Epidemol Ment Health 2009;**5**:14), and genetics (Borroni et al, Curr Alzheimer Res 2010; **7**:158–64).

BNF listed

Anticholinesterases

Anticholinesterases may help BPSD by slowing disease progression in AD, e.g. **donepezil** may significantly reduce delusions, disinhibition and other BPSD symptoms but not agitation (n = 272, RCT, p/c, 12/52, Howard et al, N Engl J Med 2007;**357**:1382–92; frustrated comment by Pelosi, EBMH 2008;**11**:84). A pooled analysis suggested **galantamine** might improve behavioural symptoms as well (s = 3, n = 2033, RCT, d/b, p/c, 3–6/12, Herrmann et al, Am J Geriatr Psychiatry 2005;**13**:527–34). A meta-analysis of studies of **rivastigmine** 6–12 mg/d shows it may be well tolerated and effective for BPSD (s = 3, p/c, 6/12, Finkel et al, Clin Ther 2004;**26**:980–90). A systematic review of all three anticholinesterases in BPSD concluded the evidence was limited but they were certainly an option (s = 14, median 24/52, Rodda et al, Int Psychogeriatr 2009;**21**:813–24).

Review: general (Miller, Consult Pharm 2007; **22**:754–62).

Memantine

A systematic meta-analysis suggested that memantine decreases NPI (neuropsychiatric inventory) scores and may have a role in managing BPSD, although the effect size is relatively small (s = 5, n = 1750, RCT, d/b, p/c, Maidment et al, Ann Pharmacother 2008;**42**:32–8). In moderately severe to severe Alzheimer's disease, a pooled analysis of three studies showed memantine to have a significant effect on neuropsychiatric symptoms and disease progression (s = 3, RCT, p/c, 6/12, Wilcock et al, J Clin Psychiatry 2008;**69**:341–8).

Risperidone * (see also antipsychotics)

Risperidone is licensed for the short-term treatment (up to 6/52) of persistent aggression in patients with moderate to severe Alzheimer's dementia unresponsive to non-pharmacological approaches and when there is a risk of harm to self or others. A starting dose of 0.25 mg BD is recommended, increased to an optimum of 0.5 mg BD for most patients, although up to 1 mg BD can be used. A mean dose of 1.5 mg/d has been shown to be effective and well tolerated for BPSD, including sleep disturbances (n = 338 [c = 321], open, 12/52, Durán et al, Int Psychogeriatr 2005;**17**:591–604), aggression, agitation and psychosis (n = 337, RCT, p/c, 12/52, Brodaty et al, J Clin Psychiatry 2003;**64**:134–43). Additional care is needed in Lewy body dementia as, although psychotic and behavioural symptoms may respond well to low dose, severe EPSEs (especially rigidity) have occurred at 1 mg/d. Risperidone appears as effective as olanzapine (n = 39, d/b, 14/7, Fontaine et al, J Clin Psychiatry 2003;**64**:726–30), quetiapine (n = 72 [c = 69], RCT, s/b, 8/52, Rainer et al, Eur Psychiatry 2007;**22**:395–403) and superior to haloperidol (n = 114, RCT, d/b, c/o, 18/52, Suh et al, Int J Geriatr Psychiatry 2006;**21**:654–60).

+ Combinations

Memantine + ChEIs

In patients stable on **donepezil**, addition of memantine may significantly improve BPSD in moderate-to-severe AD (n = 404 [c = 322], RCT, d/b, p/c, Tariot et al, JAMA 2004;**291**:317–24; review by McShane, EBMH 2004;**7**:76) and significantly lowered NPI scores by reducing agitation-related stress (d/b, p/c, 24/52, Cummings et al, Neurology 2006;**67**:57–63).

■ Unlicensed/probable efficacy

Antipsychotics (see also risperidone) *

See box overleaf.

The **haloperidol** SmPC now states that elderly patients with dementia-related psychosis treated with antipsychotic drugs are at an increased risk of death (s = 17, p/c), being 1.6–1.7 times higher than placebo-treated patients, most appearing to be either cardiovascular (e.g.

heart failure, sudden death) or infections (e.g. pneumonia) in nature.

Aripiprazole has been suggested as a suitable alternative (Hamuro, Aust N Z J Psychiatry 2007; **41**:556) as 10 mg/d appears safe and effective for psychosis associated with AD, improving psychosis, agitation and CGI (n = 487, RCT, d/b, p/c, 10/52, Mintzer et al, Am J Geriatr Psychiatry 2007;**15**:918–31). Aripiprazole IM was well-tolerated and superior to placebo for BPSD (n = 129, RCT, d/b, p/c, 24 hours, Rappaport et al, J Am Med Dir Assoc 2009;**10**:21–7), but aripiprazole (mean 9 mg/d) was ineffective, albeit well tolerated, for psychotic symptoms in Alzheimer's disease (n = 256, RCT, d/b, p/c, 10/52, Streim et al, Am J Geriatr Psychiatry 2008; **16**:537–50).

Olanzapine at low dose, e.g. 5–10 mg/d (but not 15 mg/d) has been shown to be superior to placebo in treating BPSD and psychosis in patients with AD (n = 206, RCT, d/b, p/c, 6/52, Street et al, Arch Gen Psychiatry 2000;**57**:968–76) and 2.5 mg/d seems a reasonable starting dose (n = 652, RCT, 10/52, d/b, p/c, De Deyn et al, Int J Geriatr Psychiatry 2004;**19**:115–26). It has also been used in Lewy body dementia, e.g. decreased psychotic symptoms but with no exacerbation of EPS (n = 29, RCT, Cummings et al, Dement Geriatr Cogn Disord 2002;**13**:67–73, sub-analysis), albeit not well tolerated (n = 8, open, Walker et al, Int J Geriatr Psychiatry 1999; **14**:459–66).

Quetiapine's UK SmPC has been updated with a warning that it is not approved for dementia-related psychosis due to a three-fold increased risk of CVA seen in RCTs with some SGAs. However, despite lack of safety data, 25–150 mg/d has become standard therapy for BPSD in dementia, e.g. quetiapine (50–400 mg/d) was as effective as risperidone (0.5–2 mg/d) for BPSD with no cognitive impairment (n = 72 [c = 69], RCT, s/b, 8/52, Rainer et al, Eur Psychiatry 2007;**22**:395–403), and 200 mg/d was superior to placebo for BPSD, but 100 mg/d was not superior (n = 333 [c = 63–65%], RCT, d/b, p/c, 10/52, Zhong et al, Curr Alzheimer Res 2007;**4**:61–93). However, quetiapine (mean 200 mg/d) did not improve psychosis or cause cognitive or motor deterioration, but reduced CGI-C scores compared to placebo (n = 40 [c = 27], RCT, d/b,

The use of antipsychotics in elderly people with dementia

Antipsychotics are widely used for symptomatic management of BPSD, but this remains a high-profile and controversial subject. They should not be used as substitutes for poor standards of care, and must be monitored and reviewed regularly.

The EMEA 2008 review concluded that FGAs are associated with excess mortality, compared to SGAs (e.g. n = 37241, 180/7, Schneeweiss et al, CMAJ 2007;**176**:627–32), although no conclusion can be drawn on individual antipsychotics.

The UK CSM recommended in 2004 that risperidone and olanzapine should not be used for BPSD in elderly people with dementia (see SmPCs for restrictions and guidance), as the risk of death with SGAs is 1.6–1.7 times higher than with placebo (4.5% vs 2.6%), mostly cardiovascular (e.g. heart failure, sudden death) or infections (e.g. pneumonia).

Antipsychotic use in elderly people with BPSD

Evidence for safety is sparse:
- A prospective nursing home study did not show any increased mortality with antipsychotics (n = 273, 12/12, Suh et al, Int Psychogeriatr 2005;**17**:429–41).

The actual antipsychotic itself seems to be less important:
- The Medicaid analysis was unable to show that SGAs (including risperidone) were more likely to cause CVEs than haloperidol or benzodiazepines (n = 8 million, Finkel et al, Int Psychogeriatr 2005;**17**;617–29)
- Comparisons of olanzapine, risperidone and quetiapine in BPSD show no significant differences in CVA/TIA events, although dementia appears to be an important risk factor for CVAs? (n = 18236, 26/52, Layton et al, J Psychopharmacol 2006;**20**:473–82), and although olanzapine and risperidone show greater improvement than placebo on anger, aggression and paranoia, none improved functioning, care needs or quality of life (n = 421, RCT, p/c, < 36/52, Sultzer et al, Am J Psychiatry 2008;**165**:844–54).
- Increased mortality can occur with higher doses e.g. > 1 mg/d haloperidol (n = 2217); > 2.5 mg/d olanzapine (n = 3384); and > 1 mg/d risperidone (n = 8249); but not quetiapine (n = 4277); but not at lower doses or for any of the antipsychotics after the first 30/7 (5 years, retrospective, Rossom et al, J Am Geriatr Soc 2010;**58**:1027–34).

The main risks are:
- **Femur fracture**: increased risk (OR = 1.3, n = 7393, Liperoti et al, J Clin Psychiatry 2007;**68**:929–34)
- **Pneumonia**: 60% increased risk (n = 22944, Knol et al, J Am Geriatr Soc 2008;**56**:661–6)
- **Decreased survival and cerebrovascular events**:
  - → Carrying on with antipsychotics had a survival probability of 70% compared to 77% in a switch-to-placebo group at one-year; 46% vs 71% at two years and 30% vs 59% at three years (n = 128, RCT, p/c, Ballard et al, Lancet Neurol 2009;**8**:151–7).
  - → An increased risk of death at 30 days compared to non-users (n = 27,259 pairs, Gill et al, Ann Intern Med 2007;**146**:775–86).
- **Increased risk of stroke**:
  - → The risk of stroke in people > 65 years old prescribed antipsychotics is higher with

The use of antipsychotics in elderly people with dementia *(continued)*

SGAs (47 per 1000 patient years), butyrophenones (47), phenothiazines (72) and benzamides (25) than without (12), but the risk was higher with FGAs than the SGAs (non-users n = 69939 cf n = 4223 on antipsychotics; Sacchetti *et al, J Psychopharmacol* 2008;**22**:39–46).

→ There is an increased risk of stroke in the first four weeks of antipsychotic use, no increase in months 2–3 and a slight increase in months 4–6 (n = 6,180, controls = 128,308 unexposed, Sacchetti *et al, J Psychopharmacol* 2010;**24**:1131–32). Another study suggested the risk of CVAEs is higher from the 1–9th weeks (OR 9.9), but falls to baseline after three months, so chronic use appears not to be associated with CVAEs (n = 26157, Kleijer *et al, J Psychopharmacol* 2009;**23**:909–14).

Conclusion

Use antipsychotics only as a last line of management:

- Nursing staff trained and supported to deliver enhanced psychosocial care can reduce antipsychotic use in nursing homes without an increase in agitation (n = 349, RCT, s/b, 12/12, Fossey *et al, Br Med J* 2006;**332**:756–8; comment by Byrne, *EBMH* 2006;**9**:103).
- ADRs from the SGAs may be the limiting factor and the modest benefits may be outweighed by the risks (n = 421, RCT, d/b, p/c, Schneider *et al, N Engl J Med* 2006;**355**:1525–38; comment by Ballard *et al, EBMH* 2007;**10**:58).
- Cochrane concludes that risperidone and olanzapine reduce aggression in dementia, but the risk of severe CVA and EPSE means that they should not be used routinely unless there is marked distress (s = 16, RCT, p/c, Ballard and Waite, *Cochrane Database Syst Rev* 2006; **1**:CD003476).
- Although they cause harm and the evidence is against them, use may be justified in a palliative care model, reducing stress to the person and relatives where life expectancy is short (Treloar *et al, B J Psychiatry* 2010;**197**:88–90).

Avoid absolutely in possible Lewy body dementia:

- Although psychotic and behavioural symptoms may respond well to low doses, severe EPSEs (especially rigidity) can occur at low doses, resulting in rapid deterioration and death unless discontinued quickly.

Review treatment effects regularly:

- Carry out pre-treatment assessment, repeat every 3–6 months to detect common ADRs such as postural hypotension, anticholinergic effects and EPSE.
- Single daily doses are usually appropriate once stable.
- Review doses regularly, and institute a periodic reduction in dose (e.g. by 10–25% every four weeks), and if no recurrence then continue the reduction every four weeks.

Ensure good fluid intake in the first four weeks:

- The main risk seems to be in the first four weeks (five years, Rossom *et al, J Am Geriatr Soc* 2010;**58**:1027–34) and this may be due to dehydration and poor mobilisation (Ballard and Corbett, *CNS Drugs* 2010;**24**:729–39), rather than a platelet effect. So, ensuring adequate hydration and movement in the first month is essential.

p/c, 6/52, Paleacu *et al, Int J Geriatr Psychiatry* 2008;**23**:393–400). It has, however, been associated with significant cognitive decline (n = 80 [c = 71], RCT, p/c, d/b, 26/52, Ballard *et al, Br Med J* 2005;**330**:874).

IM **ziprasidone** may be safe and effective for the short-term management of BPSD (n = 14, open, 24/24, Rais *et al, Psychiatry (Edgmont)* 2010;**7**:17–24).

Review: general (Liperoti *et al, Curr Neuropharmacol* 2008;**6**:117–24).

Cyproterone *

Cyproterone 100 mg/d showed significantly better efficacy and safety than haloperidol 2 mg/d in controlling mild aggression associated with AD (n = 27, RCT, d/b, 3/12, Huertas *et al, J Clin Psychiatry* 2007;**68**:428–9; n = 1, Bolea-Alamanac *et al, J Psychopharmacol* 2011;**25**:141–5).

Prazosin

Prazosin (mean 6 mg/d) was well tolerated and significantly useful for reducing BPSD (n = 22, RCT, d/b, p/c, 8/52, Wang *et al, Am J Geriatr Psychiatry* 2009;**17**:744–51).

Topiramate *

Topiramate 25–50 mg/d appeared as effective as risperidone 0.5–2 mg/d in BPSD (n = 48 [n = 41], RCT, d/b, 8/52, Mowla and Pani, *J Clin Psychopharmacol* 2010;**30**:40–3).

Yokukansan *

Yokukansan, a traditional Japanese medicine, appears effective and well tolerated (n = 106, RCT, c/o, Mizukami *et al [all 23 of them], Int J Neuropsychopharmacol* 2009;**12**:191–9; n = 61, RCT, open, 4/52, Okahara *et al, Prog Neuropsychopharmacol Biol Psychiatry* 2010; **34**:532–6).

■ Unlicensed/possible efficacy

Antidepressants

Antidepressants may have some use for comorbid depression. **Fluvoxamine** has been reported to be useful for BPSD (n = 3, Kurita *et al, Fukushima J Med Sci* 2006;**52**:143–8). Modest reductions of agitation in AD have been reported with **trazodone** (e.g. n = 149, RCT, 16/52, Teri *et al, Neurology* 2000;**55**:1247–8) and mirtazapine 15–30 mg/d significantly reduced agitation in Alzheimer's, without significant ADRs or cognitive deterioration (n = 16 [c = 13], open, 12/52, Cakir and Kulaksizoglu, *Neuropsychiatr Dis Treat* 2008;**4**:963–6).

Aromatherapy

Melissa, an essential balm oil, may reduce agitation in severe dementia (n = 71, d/b, p/c, Ballard *et al, J Clin Psychiatry* 2002;**63**:553–8) and lavender oil (two hours a day) produced a modest but significant reduction in agitation in dementia in a cunningly placebo-controlled trial (n = 15, p/c, Holmes *et al, Int J Geriatr Psychiatry* 2002;**17**:305–8). However, a review concludes that the evidence is scarce, incomplete, mixed and inconclusive (s = 11, Nguyen and Paton, *Int J Geriatr Psychiatry* 2008;**23**:337–46).

Review: Holmes and Ballard, *Adv Psychiatr Treat* 2004;**10**:296–300.

Carbamazepine

Carbamazepine has proved useful for hostility and aggression in demented patients not responding to antipsychotics (n = 21, RCT, 6/52, Olin *et al, Am J Geriatr Psychiatry* 2001;**9**:400–5), but a literature review was less than enthusiastic about its efficacy (s = 7, Konovalov *et al, Int Psychogeriatr* 2008;**20**:293–308).

Gabapentin

There is limited data in BPSD but gabapentin has been used for BPSD and sexual disinhibition in dementia and in a review of 11 case reports, three case series and one chart review, gabapentin was in most cases well tolerated and effective, but the data is incomplete (Kim *et al, Drugs Aging* 2008;**25**:187–96).

Valproate

Valproate may have some short-term efficacy but has tolerability issues (s = 4, p/c, Porsteinsson, *Drugs Aging* 2006; **23**:877–86). Doses should generally be less than 1000 mg/d (n = 20, RCT, d/b, p/c, Profenno *et al, Curr Alzheimer Res* 2005;**2**:553–8) for decreasing physical agitation and aggression, with 86% response rates reported (n = 46, open, 6/52, Porteinsson *et al, Am J Geriatr Psychiatry* 2003;**11**:434–40). However, other trials showed no benefit in BPSD (e.g. n = 14, RCT, d/b, p/c, c/o, Herrmann et al, Dement Geriatr Cogn Disord 2007;**23**:116–9). Cochrane concludes that valproate is ineffective in treating agitation in dementia, with unacceptable ADRs (s = 3, Lonergan and Luxenberg, Cochrane Database Syst Rev 2009;**3**:CD003945).

Yi-Gan San

Yi-Gan San (a traditional Chinese medicine) improved BPSD and ADL (n = 52 [c = 52], RCT, open, 4/52, Iwasaki et al, J Clin Psychiatry 2005;**66**:248–52; see also n = 5 [c = 5], open, 4/52, Shinno et al, Prog Neuropsychopharmacol Biol Psychiatry 2008;**32**:881–5).

Zolpidem

This has been used for dementia-related insomnia and night-time wandering (Shelton and Hocking, Ann Pharmacother 1997;**31**:319–22).

✱ Case reports

- **Buspirone** (n = 1, Hamner et al, J Clin Psychopharmacol 1996;**16**:261–2).
- **Donepezil + gabapentin** (n = 2, Dallocchio et al, J Clin Psychiatry 2000;**61**:64).
- **Propranolol** (n = 1, Summers, J Alzheimer's Dis 2006;**9**:69–75).

☐ No efficacy

Cannabinoids

Cochrane concludes there is no evidence that cannabinoids improve BPSD or other symptoms of dementia (s = 1, Krishnan et al, Cochrane Database Syst Rev 2009;**2**:CD007204).

Estrogen

Short-term estrogen may increase disturbed and aggressive behaviour in dementia in the elderly (n = 16, RCT, d/b, p/c, 4/52, Kyomen et al, Am J Psychiatry 2002;**159**:1225–7).

Melatonin

Melatonin (1.5-8.5 mg/d) at night had no effect on sleep, circadian rhythms or agitation in Alzheimer's, compared to placebo (n = 41, RCT, p/c, d/b, 10/7, Gehrman et al, Am J Geriatr Psychiatry 2009;**17**:166–9).

Oxcarbazepine

Oxcarbazepine appears to have no significant effect on BPSD in dementia (n = 103, RCT, d/b, p/c, 8/52, Sommer et al, Dement Geriatr Cogn Disord 2009;**27**:155–63).

1.13.3 VASCULAR DEMENTIA

Vascular dementia (VaD) is the second most common cause of dementia, affecting about 1–4% people over 65. It is a non-uniform disease due to a single strategic infarct, and can be comorbid with AD. VaD is characterised by executive dysfunction rather than memory impairment, usually with an acute onset of disorientation. The main symptoms are reading difficulties, loss in insight, apathy, impaired executive function and gait apraxia (n = 219, Chan et al, Dement Geriatr Cogn Disord 2008;**26**:513–21). Neuroimaging shows cerebrovascular lesions (e.g. Murray et al, Panminerva Med 2007;**49**:197–207).

Prevention (i.e. elimination of the main causes) may be the best option:
- hypertension (and lack of use of antihypertensives, probably the main factor)
- diabetes
- atherosclerosis
- cv disease (coronary artery disease, CHF, peripheral vascular disease)
- smoking
- atrial fibrillation
- lipid abnormalities
- hyperhomocystinemia
- sleep apnoea
- chronic infection
- elevation of C-reactive protein.

(McVeigh and Passmore, Clin Interven Aging 2006; **1**:229–35; Román, Cerebrovasc Dis 2005;**20**[suppl 2]:91–100).

Role of drugs

Anticholinesterases and memantine may produce small benefits but more data is needed (s = 8, n = 5183, RCT, 6/12, Kavirajan and Schneider, Lancet Neurol 2007;**6**:782–92), although a recent review concludes that there is insufficient evidence that anticholinesterases or memantine help (Zekry et al, Front Neurol Neurosci 2009;**24**:95–106).

Reviews: general (Rojas-Fernandez and Moorhouse, Ann Pharmacother 2009;**43**:1310–23;

Zekry, *Front Neurol Neurosci* 2009;**24**:95–106 Schneck, *Top Stroke Rehabil* 2008;**15**:22–6; Baskys and Hou, *Clin Interv Aging* 2007;**2**:327–35), symptoms (Stewart, *Am J Geriatr Cardiol* 2007;**16**:165–70), prevention and management (Kirschner,*Curr Neurol Neurosci Rep* 2009;**9**:437–42).

BNF listed

Anticholinesterases *

Two large-scale studies show **donepezil** produces significant improvements in cognition and global functioning in VaD (s = 2, n = 1219, 24/52, Malouf and Birks, *Cochrane Database Syst Rev* 2004;**1**:CD004395), but not global functioning (n = 974, RCT, p/c, 24/52, Román *et al, Stroke* 2010;**41**:1213–21). In an extension study, donepezil appeared to improve cognition (s = 2, n = 885 [c = 707], RCT, 54/52, Wilkinson *et al, Int J Geriatr Psychiatry* 2009;**25**:305–13). **Galantamine** may also be effective for patients with VaD or AD combined with cerebrovascular disease (n = 396 + 196 controls, 6/12, Erkinjuntti *et al, Lancet* 2002;**359**:1283–90; MS). **Rivastigmine** does not provide any consistent response in probable VaD but some improvements may be seen, probably by improving Alzheimer's co-morbidity (n = 710, RCT, d/b, p/c, 24/52, Ballard *et al, Curr Med Res Opin* 2008;**24**:2561–74).

Aripiprazole

Aripiprazole IM was well tolerated and superior to placebo for acute agitation in VaD (n = 129, RCT, d/b, p/c, 24 hours, Rappaport *et al, J Am Med Dir Assoc* 2009;**10**:21–7).

Memantine

In mild-to-moderate VaD, memantine improves cognition and is well tolerated (n = 579, RCT, d/b, p/c, 28/52, Wilcock *et al, Int Clin Psychopharmacol* 2002; **17**:297–305), and memantine 20mg/d has improved ADAS-cog scores compared to placebo (where they declined) in the ITT analysis (n = 321 [c = 288], RCT, p/c, 28/52, Orgogozo *et al, Stroke* 2002;**33**:1834–9). Cochrane, however, concludes that there is a small beneficial effect at six months in AD, but no detectable effect

in VaD (Areosa *et al, Cochrane Database Syst Rev* 2005;**2**:CD003154).

Review: treatment effect sizes in vascular dementia (Smith *et al, Alzheimer Dis Assoc Disord* 2006;**20**:133–7).

■ Unlicensed/possible efficacy

Antihypertensives *

Hypertension is a significant risk factor, and a persistent effect from calcium-channel blockers has been seen (review by Hanes and Weir, *Am J Geriatr Cardiol* 2007;**16**:175–82).

❋ Case reports

- **Finasteride *** (n = 1, Na *et al, J Am Geriatr Soc* 2009;**57**:2161–2).

□ No efficacy

Cyproterone

Cyproterone was effective for aggression and impulsive behaviour but not aberrant motor behaviour in VaD (n = 19, open, Caparros-Lefebvre and Dewailly, *Rev Neurol [Paris]* 2005;**161**:1071–8).

Huperzine A

Cochrane concludes that there is no evidence that Huperzine A (a herbal medicine) has any efficacy in VaD (s = 1, n = 14, Hao *et al, Cochrane Database Syst Rev* 2009;**2**:CD007365).

SSRIs

Citalopram appears to have no efficacy in VaD (n = 98, RCT, d/b, 4/52, Nyth and Gottfries, *Br J Psychiatry* 1990;**157**:894–901).

1.13.4 PROPHYLAXIS AND PREVENTION OF DEMENTIA *

This section may be useful in helping advise patients, carers, friends and relatives about possible strategies for reducing the risk of dementia, especially where a family history exists. The genetic risk only accounts for 7% cases, but new cases could be reduced by:

- Eliminating depression and diabetes and eating more fruit and veg (21% reduction)
- Eliminating depression (10% reduction)

- Increasing education (18% reduction) (n = 1433, 7 years, Ritchie *et al, Br Med J* 2010; **341**:3885).

General measures (see also vascular dementia) include:

- **Alcohol** — light to moderate alcohol consumption in later life is associated with a reduced risk of Alzheimer's and VaD (n = 36746, Anstey *et al, Am J Geriatr Psychiatry* 2009;**17**:542–55).
- **Being overweight** in midlife increases the risk of dementia (n = 1152, 40 years, Hassing *et al, Int J Obes (Lond)* 2009;**33**:893–8). Among women alive at 70, a high mid-life waist-to-hip ratio may increase the odds of dementia (n = 1462, 32 years, Gustafson *et al, Neurology* 2009;**73**:1559–66; n = 6583, mean 36 years, Whitmer *et al, Neurology* 2008; **71**:1057–64; n = 733, Seshadri *et al, Ann Neurol* 2010;**68**:136–44).
- **Physical activity** and exercise modestly improve cognition over two years (n = 170[c = 138], RCT, two years, Lautenschlager *et al, JAMA* 2008;**300**:1027–37).
- **Hypertension** (see antihypertensives); high and low bp is associated with faster cognitive decline in AD patients (s = 11, n = 10625, Sharp *et al, Int J Geriatr Psychiatry* 2011; in press) and in hypertensive men, controlling blood pressure reduces the risk of AD (n = lots and lots, Peila *et al, Stroke* 2006;**37**:1165–70).
- **Lower cholesterol** (see statins).
- **Fruit and vegetables** — the risk of AD is reduced in people taking at least three fruit juices a week, but no effect was seen from vitamins E, C, or beta-carotene (n = 1836, mean eight years, Dai *et al, Am J Med* 2006;**119**:751–9). A diet rich in nuts, fish and vegetables and low in saturated fat and vitamin B12 may have a protective effect (n = 2148, 4 years, Gu *et al, Arch Neurol* 2010; **67**:699–706).
- **Not having diabetes** (slower cognitive decline in AD patients with diabetes; n = 154, Musicco *et al, J Neurol* 2009;**256**:1288–95; n = 103, 4 years, Velayudhan *et al, Br J Psychiatry* 2010;**196**:36–40).
- **Drinking 3–5 cups of tea or coffee a day** in midlife is associated with a 65% reduction

in Alzheimer's. The effect most marked with tea but coffee as well (s = 5, Eskelinen and Kivipelto, *J Alzheimers Dis* 2010;**20**(Suppl 1):167–74).

- **Having depression** is a risk factor for Alzheimer's, not an early sign or an inevitable part as it tends not to get worse or appear at the onset of dementia. The hippocampus creates new nerves and connections, it shrinks in depression, and this might indicate a lack of new cells (n = 357, Wilson *et al, Neurology* 2010;**75**:21–6).
- Not using **anticholinergics** (Jessen *et al, Eur Arch Psychiatry Clin Neurosci* 2010;**260** Suppl 2:S111–5; see also 'No efficacy').

Assessment of risk:

Score	Risk factor
1–2	Older age
2–4	Poor cognitive performance
2	BMI < 18.5
1	> 1 apolipoprotein E epsilon 4 alleles
1	MRI shows white matter disease
1	Ventricular enlargement
1	Carotid artery thickening on ultrasound
1	History of bypass surgery
1	Slow physical performance
1	Lack of alcohol consumption

Range 0–15

Over six years, the percentage of people developing dementia were:

- 4% with low scores
- 23% with moderate scores
- 56% with high scores

(n = 3375, Barnes *et al, Neurology* 2009;**73**:173–9).

Reviews: * general (Gauthier *et al, Int Psychogeriatr* 2010;**22**:346–72 Sano *et al, CNS Drugs* 2008;**22**:887–902; Stephan and Brayne, *Int Rev Psychiatry* 2008;**20**:344–56).

● **Unlicensed/some efficacy**

Anticholinesterases

A systematic review concludes that ChEIs do

not delay the progression to AD or dementia when given to people with mild cognitive impairment (s = 8, RCT, 24/52–3 years, Raschetti et al, PLoS Medicine 2007;**4**:e338), but donepezil may delay the progression in the presence of depression (n = 756, d/b, p/c, three years, Lu et al, Neurology 2009;**72**:2115–21). Previously Cochrane concluded that donepezil does not delay the onset of AD (s = 2, n = 782, RCT, d/b, p/c, Birks and Flicker, Cochrane Database Syst Rev 2006;**3**:CD006104).

NSAIDs

NSAIDs may, or may not, reduce the risk of AD. The case for:

- A pooled analysis showed a significant effect on reducing the risk of AD but with no advantage for SALAs (e.g. diclofenac, flurbiprofen, ibuprofen) over non-SALAs (e.g. celecoxib, etodolac, mefenamic acid, nabu-metone, naproxen) (s = 6, n = 13499, Szekely et al, Neurology 2008;**70**:2291–8).
- Taking NSAIDs for more than five years was protective against AD, with clearest evidence from ibuprofen (e.g. n = 246199, Vlad et al, Neurology 2008;**70**:1672–7).
- They reduce cognitive decline, but only if started in midlife (before 65 years) before cogitive decline starts, for a minimum of two years and if the person happens to have one or more predisposing APOE genotypes (n = 3383, Hayden et al, Neurology 2007;**69**:275–82), e.g. the APOE epsilon 4 allele (n = 3229, Szekely et al, Neurology 2008;**70**:17–24).

The case against:

- A five-year case-control study of post-mortem brain tissue showed no significant differences in the amount of inflammatory glia, plaques, or tangles in either diagnostic group.
- They may not alleviate the progression in people with mild-to-moderate AD (n = 351, RCT, d/b, p/c, one year, Aisen et al, JAMA 2003;**289**:2819–26; comment by Jacoby, EBMH 2003;**6**:110).
- No effect from low-dose aspirin 75 mg/d (n = 310, RCT, open, mean three years, AD2000 Collaborative Group, Lancet Neurol 2008;**7**:41–9), ibuprofen 800 mg/d (n = 132 [c = 97], RCT, d/b, p/c, 12/12,

Pasqualetti et al, Aging Clin Exp Res 2009;**21**:102–10) and from celecoxib and naproxen (n = 2528 [c = 2117], RCT, d/b, p/c, mean two years, ADAPT Group, Arch Neurol 2008;**65**:896–905).

- Prior heavy NSAID users actually had a higher AD incidence than non-users, although this could be because of delayed onset (n = 2736, 10 years, Breitner et al, Neurology 2009;**22**:1899–905).

Review: general (McGeer and McGeer, Neurobiol Aging 2007;**28**:639–47).

■ Unlicensed/possible efficacy

Antihypertensives (see also introduction) *

A recent systematic review concluded that only ACE inhibitors and diuretics significantly reduce the risk for, and progression to, dementia in the majority of studies (s = 12, Shah et al, Am J Geriatr Pharmacother 2009;**7**:250–61). Cochrane concludes that there is no convincing evidence that lowering bp in later life prevents dementia or cognitive impairment in people with no apparent prior cerebrovascular disease, although the data is not robust (s = 4, n = 15936, McGuinness et al, Cochrane Database Syst Rev 2009;**4**: CD004034). However, antihypertensive drug use is associated with a 8% reduction in the risk of dementia per year for people aged <76 (n = 6249, 15 years, Haag et al, Neurology 2009; **72**:1727–34), and a postmortem study showed less Alzheimer's neuropathology in people treated with antihypertensives, even less than non-hypertensive people (n = 291, Hoffman et al, Neurology 2009;**72**:1720–6).

Beer

Beer contains silicone, which may reduce the bioavailability of aluminium (Gonzalez-Munoz et al, Food Chem Toxicol 2008;**46**:49–56). Well, it still seems to be working for my Dad.

Coffee/caffeine/tea (see also introduction)

A pooled analysis shows a protective effect for coffee on developing AD (s = 4, Barranco Quintana et al, Neurol Res 2007;**29**:91–5), and may be from a neuroprotective effect from caffeine (Rosso et al, Am J Alzheimers Dis Other Dement 2008;**23**:417–22). However, coffee drinking did not appear to affect the risk of mild cognitive impairment of dementia in one study (n = 2606, mean follow-up 28 years, Laitala et al, Am J Clin Nutr 2009;**90**:640–6).

Estrogen (oestrogen) *

Estrogen is a potent chemical factor that prevents vascular disease and improves blood flow in diseased vessels in regions of the brain affected by AD. Estrogen also has an important role in the preservation and repair of neurons (n = 143, Manly et al, Neurology 2000;**54**:833–8). Some trials have shown a potential effect in slowing decline or improving cognition, e.g. from long-term HRT in older women (n = 2000, Carlson et al, Neurology 2001;**57**:2210–16), high-dose transdermal 17-beta-estradiol (n = 20, RCT, p/c, 8/52, Asthana et al, Neurology 2001;**57**:605–12) and estrogen HRT, oral or transdermal (n = 184, Maki et al, Am J Psychiatry 2001;**158**:227–33). However, other trials have failed to show a protective effect from, e.g. conjugated estrogens (e.g. n = 120, RCT, 12/12, Mulnard et al, JAMA 2000;**283**:1007–15; review by Hogervorst and McShane, EBMH 2000;**3**:83), from short-term estrogens (n = 42 women, RCT, 16/52, Henderson et al, Neurology 2000;**54**:295–302), or estrogen replacement therapy (ERT) (n = 2859, Alves de Moraes et al, Am J Epidemiol 2001;**154**:733–9). It did not reduce the risk of developing AD (n = 221406, case-control, Seshadri et al, Arch Neurol 2001; **58**:435–40) and actually increased the risk in another study (n = 4000, RCT, d/b, p/c, Shumaker et al, JAMA 2003;**289**:2651–62, 2663–72; comment by Sherwin and McGill, EBMH 2003;**6**:111). It may only help if started before 49 years, and may possibly be detrimental after 60 (review by Craig and Murphy, Ann N Y Acad Sci 2010;**1205**:245–53). Cochrane concludes that HRT and ERT may have some effects but there is insufficient evidence to indicate them for women with cognitive impairment (s = 7, n = 351, RCT, d/b, Hogervorst et al, Cochrane Database Syst Rev 2009;**1**:CD003799).

Reviews: general (Henderson, Semin Reprod Med 2009;**27**:283–93; Pike et al, Front Neuro-endocrinol 2009;**30**:239–58; Zhao and Brinton, BMC Neurosci 2006;**7**:24).

Fish and n-3 fatty acids

People who eat fish at least once a week have 60% lower risk of developing AD compared with people who never, or seldom eat fish (n = 815, Morris et al, Arch Neurol 2003;**60**: 940–6). See also omega-3 fatty acids.

Folate

Cochrane concludes that there is no consistent evidence one way or the other for the use of folic acid (with or without B12) to treat or prevent AD (s = 8, RCT, Malouf et al, Cochrane Database Syst Rev 2008;**4**:CD004514), although some studies were positive (e.g. (n = 965, mean six years, open, Luchsinger et al, Arch Neurol 2007;**64**:86–92).

Lithium *

Lithium may reduce dementia rates by producing a sustained increase in gray matter volume within 10–12 weeks (n = 36, Lyoo et al, Neuropsychopharmacology 2010;**35**:1743–50).

The case for: There is some evidence that lithium could have a preventative role in AD, possibly by blocking accumulation of amyloid-beta peptides. Those with bipolar disorder have an increased risk of dementia compared to the general population (19% vs 7%), but reduced in non-lithium takers (n = 1423, Terao et al, Prog Neuropsychopharmacol Biol Psychiatry 2006; **30**:1125–8; n = 114, Nunes et al, Br J Psychiatry 2007;**190**:359–60; comment by Terao, Br J Psychiatry 2007;**190**:361–2). In bipolar patients, two or more prescriptions for lithium are associated with a significant decrease in the rate dementia cf one prescription, but no association with any other drug group (n = 4856, Kessing et al, Bipolar Disord 2010;**12**:87–94).

The case against: A case-control study failed to show that lithium protects against the onset of dementia (Dunn et al, Alzheimer Dis Assoc Disord 2005;**19**:20–2). A short-term study showed no effect on GSK-3, which regulates the tau protein (n = 71, 10/52, Hampel et al, J Clin Psychiatry 2009;**70**:922–31), and lithium had no effect on MMSE in mild-to-moderate Alzheimer's disease (n = 22 [c = 8], open, < 12/12, Int J Geriatr Psychiatry 2008;**23**:704–11).

Reviews: * use in AD (Zhong and Lee, Expert Opin Drug Saf 2007;**6**:375–83), possible mechanisms (Yeh and Tsai, Med Hypotheses

2008;**71**:948–51), neuroprotection (Caraci *et al, CNS Neurosci Ther* 2011; in press).

Melatonin

Melatonin and its analogues have been proposed as potentially having some value (Srinivasan *et al, Behav Brain Funct* 2006;**2**:15).

Memantine

A pilot study has suggested that memantine may improve cognitive function in some populations of postmenopausal women at risk of dementia (n = 22, open, 6/12, Wroolie *et al, Acta Neurol Scand* 2008;**119**:172–9).

Raloxifene

Raloxifene, a selective estrogen receptor modulator for osteoporosis, at 120 mg/d (but not 60 mg/d) may produce a 33% reduced risk of cognitive impairment in postmenopausal women (n = 5386, three years, Yaffe *et al, Am J Psychiatry* 2005;**62**:683–90).

Red wine *

Moderate consumption could help reduce or slow AD due to the phenolic content (Anon, *Duke Med Health News* 2007;**13**:7–8). I thought you'd like to know.

Statins *

Even moderately raised midlife serum total cholesterol is associated with an increased risk of AD (n = 9844, 43 years, Solomon *et al, Dement Geriatr Cogn Disord* 2009;**28**:75–80), but it is unclear if statins help reverse this.

The case for: statins, e.g. lovastatin, pravastatin and atorvastatin 80 mg/d (n = 67 [c = 63], RCT, p/c, 3/12, Sparks *et al, Arch Neurol* 2005; **62**:753–7), have been reported to substantially lower the risk of developing dementias (n = 1364, Jick *et al, Lancet* 2000;**356**:1627–31; n = 60,000, Josefson, *Br Med J* 2000;**321**:1040). In cognitively normal people, ongoing statin therapy has been associated at autopsy with reduced neurofibrillary tangle burden, so starting statins before the onset of AD is the important part (n = 110, Li *et al, Neurology* 2007;**69**:878–85). Non-statin cholesterol-lowering drugs do not show this effect (n = 6992, 15 years, Haag *et al, J Neurol Neurosurg Psych* 2009;**80**:13–7). Statins may

also help people with increased risk (n = 57, RCT, d/b, p/c, 4/12, Carlsson *et al, J Alzheimers Dis* 2008;**13**:187–97). Statin users are about half as likely to develop dementia as those not taking them (n = 1674, five years, Cramer *et al, Neurology* 2008;**71**:344–50). In people with AD, use of statins and beta-blockers associated with delay in functional decline (n = 216, three years, Rosenberg *et al, Am J Geriatr Psychiatry* 2008;**16**:883–92).

The case against: statin use over 4–5 years had no association with a lower incidence of dementia (n = 355 from n = 4895, Zandi *et al, Arch Gen Psychiatry* 2005; **62**:217–24; see also n = 2798, Rea *et al, Arch Neurol* 2005;**62**:1047–51) and in mild-to-moderate AD, atorvastatin 80 mg/d as add-on to donepezil had no beneficial effect on cognition or global function (n = 640, RCT, d/b, p/c, 72/52, Feldman *et al, Neurology* 2010;**74**:956–64).

Conclusion: Cochrane concludes that there is insufficient information to recommend statins (s = 3, n = 748, McGuinness *et al, Cochrane Database Syst Rev* 2010;**8**:CD007514; critical comment by Haan, noting that only two major trials were used, and that statins reduced LDL, reduced stroke and have at least an indirect impact, Haan, *EBMH* 2009;**12**:114). A balanced review concludes stains do not really harm anyone, but do not work for preventing progression to AD, although might improve MMSE (s = 2, McGuinness and Passmore, *J Alzheimer's Dis* 2010;**20**:925–33).

Vitamins *

High levels of homocysteine have been shown to raise risk of AD, and B vitamins lower homocysteine and might slow the rate of atrophy in older people with mild cognitive impairment. However, brain shrinkage is not the same as dementia, although there might be some relationship (n = 271 [c = 168], RCT, d/b, p/c, 24/12, Smith *et al, PLoS ONE* 2010; **5**:12244).

The case for: Vitamin E and C supplements may protect against VaD and improve cognitive function in later life in men (n = 3385, Masaki *et al, Neurology* 2000;**54**:1265–72) and twice the risk of AD if B12 or folate deficient (n = 370, Wang *et al, Neurology* 2001;**56**:1188–94). Other studies have shown that high dietary intake of vitamins C and E may lower the risk of AD (n = 5395, six years, Engelhart et al, JAMA 2002; **287**:3223–9), and that vitamin E from food (but not other antioxidants or supplements) may lower the risk of AD (n = 815, Morris et al, JAMA 2002;**287**:3230–7). Also, patients taking combined vitamin E (1000 u/d) and donepezil 5 mg/d declined at a slower rate than expected (n = 130, retrospective, one year; Klatte et al, Alz Dis Assoc Disord 2003; **17**:113–6).

The case against: In mild cognitive impairment, vitamin E 2000 IU (cf placebo) has no effect on impairment and did not slow the progression to AD (n = 769, three years, RCT, p/c, d/b, Petersen et al, N Engl J Med 2005;**352**:2379–88) and B6, B12 and folate supplementation was ineffective in reducing dementia symptoms (n = 409 [c = 340], RCT, d/b, p/c, 18/12, Aisen et al, JAMA 2008;**300**:1174–83; comment by Connelly, EBMH 2009;**12**:86). Cochrane concludes that there is no evidence for efficacy from vitamin E in either prevention or treatment of Alzheimer's disease (s = 2, Isaac et al, Cochrane Database Syst Rev 2008;**3**:CD002854).

☐ No efficacy

Anticholinergics *
People taking a drug with an anticholinergic effect have an increased risk of cognitive decline, dementia (HR = 1.65) (n = 6912, four years, Carrière et al, Arch Intern Med 2009; **169**:1317–24) and death (Fox, Maidment et al, J Am Geriatr Soc 2011; in press) but discontinuing decreases the risk.

Omega-3 fatty acids
Numerous studies have now shown that omega-3 fatty acids do not delay the rate of decline (e.g. n = 402 [c = 295], RCT, d/b, p/c, 18/12, Quinn et al, JAMA 2010;**304**:1903–11), or reduce rates of dementia or Alzheimer's (n = 663, 11 years, Kröger et al, Am J Clin Nutr 2009;**90**:184–92). However, it has been suggested that they may be (more) effective if begun early or if used with an antioxidant (Cole et al, Prostaglandins Leukot Essent Fatty Acids 2009;**81**:213–21).

Reviews: * general (Huang, J Alzheimer's Dis 2010;**21**:673–90; Jicha and Markesbery, Clin Interv Aging 2010;**5**:45–61; Cederholm and Palmblad, Curr Opin Clin Nutr Metab Care 2010;**13**:150–5).

Gingko biloba *
Several trials have now shown GB to have no effect on reducing the rates of dementia (n = 3069, RCT, d/b, p/c, median six years, DeKosky et al, JAMA 2008;**300**:2253–62; comment by Hoerr, EBMH 2009;**12**:85; n = 3069 [c = 2901], RCT, d/b, p/c, mean 6 years, Snitz et al, JAMA 2009;**302**:2663–70).

1.14 DEPRESSION
1.14.1 UNIPOLAR DEPRESSION
see also Postpartum depression (1.14.2), Bipolar depression (1.10.3), Rapid-cycling bipolar disorder (1.10.4), Dysthymia (1.14.3) and Mania and hypomania (1.10.2)

Depression is a common illness, affecting up to 3% of the population per year, but remains underdiagnosed, undertreated (especially in men and in those under 30). The overall cost of depression (e.g. work, family, other illnesses) is high for this eminently treatable condition, although the UK press still seems to have generally archaic views on this, with an apparent strong anti-pharmacotherapy bias. For example, the enormous publicity of the 2008 meta-analysis of short-term 4–8 weeks FDA licensing data for antidepressants pre-1999 (Kirsch et al, PLoS Med 2011;**5**:e45:0050045) concluded that antidepressants had no significant efficacy for anything except severe depression, once unpublished and inconvenient studies were excluded. Re-analysis shows the study results were selective, unjustified and overemphasised, e.g. there were important flaws and errors in the calculations, and exclusion of the significant effects from venlafaxine and paroxetine, making the conclusions invalid (Fountoulakis and Möller, Int J Neuropsychopharmacol 2011;**14**:405–12). What this analysis really shows is that short-term trials are not long enough and that the combination of SSRIs and CBT will, in many people, be the most effective treatment (critique of the evidence, or lack thereof, for psychotherapy; Nutt and Sharpe, J Psychopharmacol 2008;**22**:3–6; comment on Kirsch by McAllister-Williams, EBMH 2008; **11**:66–8). Antidepressants may enhance the effectiveness of psychotherapy (NNT = 7) (s = 16, n = 852, Cuijpers et al, Acta Psychiatr Scand 2010;**121**:415–23), but many CBT trials use waiting list controls, which is actually worse than nothing (n = 368, RCT, p/c, 10/52, Hegerl et al, Int J Neuropsychopharmacol 2010;**13**:31–44).

Symptoms

Depression presents with a mixture of biological symptoms (insomnia or hypersomnia, diurnal variation in mood, low appetite, fatigue or loss of energy, constipation, loss of libido, weight loss or gain) and psychiatric symptoms (depressed mood, loss of interest or pleasure, poor memory, psychomotor agitation or retardation, recurrent thoughts of death or suicide, anxiety, feelings of worthlessness or guilt, including delusions, etc). Depression does not include the normal reaction to the death of a loved one. Atypical depression includes the symptoms of depression, plus two from hypersomnia, hyperphagia, rejection sensitivity and severe lethargy (n = 579, Posternak and Zimmerman, Arch Gen Psychiatry 2002;**59**:70–6).

Causes

Risk factors can include prescribed or OTC drugs, substance misuse, genetic susceptibility, physical illness, menopause (n = 643 [c = 420], Cohen et al, Arch Gen Psychiatry 2006;**63**:385–90; comment by Woods, EBMH 2006;**9**:109), stress (e.g. bereavement, loss of job, birth of child, break-up of relationship, work stress), epilepsy (double risk, n = 130,880, Fuller-Thomson and Brennenstuhl, Epilepsia 2009;**50**:1051–8), poor social background and the time of year.

Role of drugs *

Although most depressions will resolve with time, antidepressants have a major role in hastening this recovery and reducing suffering. Antidepressants are effective, not addictive, and do not generally lose efficacy with prolonged use. Adequate doses are needed for clinical effect, and continuation for an appropriate period will minimise relapse.

Treatment of depression *

The general principles of the medicines treatment of depression (with antidepressants) can be summed up by the six Ds:

- Diagnosis
- Drug-related
- Drug
- Dose
- Duration
- Discontinuation

1. **D**iagnosis: Making, or being able to make, a diagnosis helps. An obvious statement, but diagnosis does start with a D.

2. **D**rug-related causes eliminated: See list in Chapter 5.5, as well as physical (e.g. low folate levels) and environmental causes.

3. **D**rug: All the main antidepressants appear to have broadly similar efficacy, although there may be some differences in efficacy and acceptability (see comparative section). As non-compliance or inadequate dosage are the main causes of drug failure, the choice of drug should consider this.

The unique Cipriani meta-analysis compared bupropion, citalopram, duloxetine, escitalopram, fluoxetine, fluvoxamine, milnacipran, mirtazapine, paroxetine, reboxetine, sertraline, and venlafaxine range for the acute treatment of unipolar major depression in adults. Cipriani concluded that:

- Escitalopram, mirtazapine, venlafaxine and sertraline were significantly more efficacious than duloxetine, fluoxetine, fluvoxamine, paroxetine and reboxetine (the least efficacious antidepressant). .

- Escitalopram and sertraline showed the best profile of acceptability, with significantly fewer discontinuations than duloxetine, fluvoxamine, paroxetine, reboxetine, and venlafaxine.

- Clinically important differences exist, both in efficacy and acceptability, in favour of escitalopram and sertraline. Sertraline might be the best first choice because it has the most favourable balance between benefits, acceptability and acquisition cost, although escitalopram was not far behind. (s = 117, n = 25,928, RCT, Cipriani et al, Lancet 2009;**373**:746–58).

Onset of action: * It is commonly stated that antidepressants take four weeks to work. It is more accurate to say that 'time to substantial remission' (full statistical separation from placebo) may take four weeks in clinical trials (partly because trials are not powered to detect an earlier onset). Onset of action may in fact be much quicker:

- detectable positive effects after three hours (n = 26, RCT, d/b, Murphy et al, Br J Psychiatry 2009;**194**:535–40; n = 21 [c = 16], RCT, c/o, s/b, Bruhl et al, Neuropsychopharmacology 2010;**35**:521–33)
- separation from placebo by day 5 (review by Mitchell, Br J Psychiatry 2006; **188**:105–6),
- symptomatic improvement in a week (s = 28, n = 5872, RCT, Taylor et al, Arch Gen Psychiatry 2006;**63**:1217–23)
- 57% differences apparent by week 2 (s = 47, n = 8500, d/b, p/c, Pasternak and Zimmerman, J Clin Psychiatry 2005; **66**:148–58).

Early improvement (within two weeks) strongly predicts later outcomes, lower anxiety, and higher function (n = 568, 12/52, Kim et al, J Affect Disord 2011;**129**:183–90; s = 41, n = 6562, p/c, 4–8/52, Szegedi et al, J Clin Psychiatry 2009;**70**:344–53) and leads to better long-term compliance, as recovery is associated with starting antidepressants. Telling people they take four weeks to work will of course mean any rapid improvement will be attributed to other reasons. Higher starting doses speed response, but lead to increased drop-outs and ADRs (s = 9, n = 2340, RCT, d/b, p/c, Papakostas et al, World J Biol Psychiatry 2010;**11**:300–7), although spreading out the first doses across a day reduces the ADRs from peak plasma levels and can improve tolerability.

4. **D**ose: The therapeutic range of the newer antidepressants has been established through dose-finding studies but is less clear for the tricyclics (e.g. the need for tricyclic doses of 125–150 mg/d in 95% adults). Once-daily dosing is as effective as multiple daily doses, regardless of drug half-life (s = 22, Yıldyz, and Sachs, J Affect Disord 2001;**66**:199–206; review by Barbui, EBMH 2002;**5**:57).

5. **D**uration:

5a. Acute therapy — SSRIs are the standard first-line therapy, although starting at half the standard dose for a few days improves tolerability. The person must be monitored for akathisia, anxiety, agitation and suicidal ideation early in treatment. If depression remains completely unchanged after four weeks of therapeutic dosing, an alternate drug should be tried, and definitely after eight weeks (n = 840, 12/52, open, Quitkin et al, Am J Psychiatry 2003;**160**:734–40). These times should probably be doubled in the elderly and in chronic

Rankings of the top antidepressants for efficacy and cost-effectiveness (NICE, 2009) *

Efficacy	Cost-effectiveness	
	Moderate depression	Severe depression
1 Mirtazapine	1 Mirtazapine	1 Mirtazapine
2 Escitalopram	2 Sertraline	2 Sertraline
3 Venlafaxine	3 Escitalopram	3 Escitalopram
4 Sertraline	4 Citalopram	4 Citalopram
5 Citalopram	5 Venlafaxine	5 Venlafaxine
6 Paroxetine	6 Paroxetine	6 Paroxetine
7 Fluoxetine	7 Fluoxetine	7 Fluoxetine
8 Duloxetine	8 Fluvoxamine	8 Duloxetine
9 Fluvoxamine	9 Duloxetine	9 Fluvoxamine
10 Reboxetine	10 Reboxetine	10 Reboxetine

depression (review by Gelenberg and Chesen, J Clin Psychiatry 2000;**61**:712–21).

5b. Continuation therapy — proper treatment of depression requires not just acute treatment but continuation while the person remains vulnerable. Inadequate or no treatment for six months post-response in controlled trials has resulted in relapse rates as high as 50% (cf <20% with adequate treatment). If a first episode of depression remits in 12 weeks, continued treatment for six months minimises the risk of relapse, but longer therapy may confer little additional benefit, except in people with additional relapse risk factors (n = 395, RCT, 52/52, Reimherr et al, Am J Psychiatry 1998;**155**:1247–53) such as recurrent depression (s = 31, n = 4410, Geddes et al, Lancet 2003;**361**:653–61; comment by Donoghue, EBMH 2003;**6**:84). Continuation doses should be the **same or close to the therapeutic dose** (RCT, 3 years, Frank et al, J Affect Disord 1993;**27**:139–45).

5c. Maintenance or relapse prevention — relapse prevention has been shown for a number of antidepressants, e.g. imipramine over 3–5 years (n = 128, RCT, d/b, p/c, three years, Frank et al, Arch Gen Psychiatry 1990;**47**:1093–9; Kupfer et al, Arch Gen Psychiatry 1992;**49**:769–73), and venlafaxine, but not sertraline (RCT, d/b, p/c, two years, Wilson et al, Br J Psychiatry 2003;**182**:492–7). Those likely to benefit from maintenance (Kasper and Eder in Winkler et al, Curr Opin Psychiatry 2002;**15**:63–8) include those with chronic depression, three episodes, or two episodes with risk factors (late or early onset, short interval between episodes, rapid onset, dysthymia, positive family history, comorbidity, incomplete response and low work adjustment). In a 10-year prospective study of multiple recurrences of major depression, the risk of recurrence increased by 16% with each successive episode, but the risk of recurrence progressively decreased as duration of recovery increased (n = 318, open, 10 years, Solomon *et al, Am J Psychiatry* 2000;**157**:229–33), so keeping people well pays dividends.

General minimum treatment duration recommendations:

- First episode — six months post-recovery.
- Second episode — 2–3 years.
- Third episode — five years or longer.
- Fourth episode — you should need a very good reason to stop.

Pleasingly, the doubling in antidepressant prescribing in the UK over the last decade is apparently due to longer durations of treatment rather than a rise in depression (n = 189,851, Moore *et al, Br Med J* 2009;**339**:b3999).

Review: relapse prevention (various artists, *J Clin Psychiatry* 2007;**68**:619–30).

6. **D**iscontinuation: * When discontinuing, slowly reduce doses over a minimum of four weeks as stopping antidepressants rapidly (1–7 days) leads to a shorter time to relapse compared to slower (14/7 or more) discontinuation (n = 224, open, Baldessarini *et al, Am J Psychiatry* 2010; **167**:934–41). Discontinuation syndromes have been reported for nearly all antidepressants, but particularly paroxetine and venlafaxine. Discontinuation symptoms usually appear within 1–3 days of stopping treatment and they can improve within a week (although can last much longer), while recurrence of depression begins after three weeks and continues to worsen. See switching antidepressants in *2.2.2* for a further review, e.g. symptoms and management.

Treatment-resistant depression (TRD) *

TRD is defined (after STAR*D) as failure of two treatment trials. Remember also that resistant depression may be undiagnosed bipolar (see *1.10.3*).

Options include:

1. Escalate antidepressant doses for an adequate duration: This is appropriate for drugs with a dose-response curve, e.g. up to 300 mg/d or more of a tricyclic or other drug (e.g. venlafaxine), or to tolerance (monitoring plasma levels carefully),

remembering that a few people have multiple copies of, e.g. CYP2D6 and may rapidly metabolise tricyclics. Push SSRI doses to BNF maximum.

2. Check blood levels: to detect possible 2D6 ultrarapid metabolisers or non-concordance.

3. Switch antidepressants: * The pros and cons (Shelton *et al, CNS Drugs* 2010;**24**:131–61) are:

- **Pros**: avoidance of polypharmacy; lower TEAEs; lower costs
- **Cons**: cannot build on a partial response; evidence is that monotherapy switches after two treatments only have a limited effect.

Ensure all drug classes have been tried optimally, e.g. SSRIs, tricyclics, SNRIs, mirtazapine, agomelatine, moclobemide (at much higher doses e.g. over 600 mg/d) and MAOIs (see *Chapter 2.2.6* for advice on switching antidepressants).

4. Augment or combine: * The pros and cons (Shelton *et al, CNS Drugs* 2010;**24**:131–61) are:

- **Pros**: can build on improvements achieved so far; especially with partial response
- **Con**: results in multiple medicines; higher costs; more ADRs.

Use logical combinations of antidepressants, (see later in this section), e.g. mirtazapine, lithium, carbamazepine (but not with tricyclics, see *4.5.1*), valproate, or lithium/SSRI/tryptophan.

5. Assure compliance: Around 42% people stop antidepressants within the first 30 days (mostly from ADRs), 30% in the next 60 days (mostly due to lack of efficacy), and only 28% carry on beyond three months (n = 829, Olfson *et al, Am J Psychiatry* 2006;**163**:101–8).

6. Manage ADRs: If response occurs but ADRs are limiting, see *Chapter 6* for strategies to manage, e.g. sexual dysfunction, sedation, etc.

7. Check folate levels: See adjunctive therapy.

8. Consider individual CBT: This should be considered in combination with antidepressants and may be effective, but requires a high level of expertise (n = 240, RCT, p/c, 16/52, DeRubeis *et al, Arch Gen Psychiatry* 2005;**62**:409–16).

Review: drug treatments (Papakostas, *J Clin Psychiatry* 2009;**70**[Suppl 6]:16–25).

Bipolar depression

See separate section (*1.10.3*).

Loss of antidepressant efficacy (tachyphylaxis)

Loss of antidepressant efficacy (also termed

'operational tolerance', or more graphically as 'poop-out') has been reported during long-term maintenance treatment. The incidence of relapse in people with a true drug response and continuing treatment is around 7.4%, whereas in the relapse rate in placebo responders is 24%, so relapse in continuation treatment is most likely to be in people who were not true drug responders (s = 4, Zimmerman and Thongy, *J Clin Psychiatry* 2007;**68**:1271–6). Possible mechanisms might include non-compliance, loss of initial placebo response, loss of true drug effect, pharmacological tolerance, accumulation of detrimental metabolites, change in illness pathology, unrecognised rapid-cycling, switching and cycle acceleration in bipolars, antidepressant-induced paradoxical effects and a genuine lack of prophylactic efficacy (review by Fava, *J Clin Psychiatry* 2003;**64**:123–33).

Strategies to overcome loss of efficacy include:
1. **Increase** the dose.
2. **Decrease** the dose (this may work if the dose has exceeded any 'therapeutic window', but is poorly supported by published data).
3. **Addition** of dopamine agonists, e.g. bromocriptine.
4. **Augment** with, e.g. mood stabilisers, anti-convulsants, thyroid, another antidepressant.
5. **Drug holiday** (although this is poorly supported by the literature).
6. **Switch** to a different drug or class.
7. **Ensure compliance**.

Suicidality *

The role of antidepressants in reducing or causing suicide or suicidal ideation remains controversial (see *Chap 5.15, pp. 459–460*). The key conclusion seems to be that there may be an increase in under 25s (probably undiagnosed bipolar depression) but not in older adults.

Reviews: * BAP guidelines updated (Anderson *et al, J Psychopharmacol* 2008;**22**:343–96), pharmacotherapy (Reid and Cameron, *Prescriber* 2009;**20**:18–36; Qaseem *et al, Ann Intern Med* 2008;**149**:725–33; Gartlehner *et al, Ann Intern Med* 2008;**149**:734–50), dopamine agonists (Clausius *et al, Neuropsychiatr* 2009; **23**:15–25), complementary and alternative medicines (s = 185, RCTs, Freeman *et al, J Clin Psychiatry* 2010;**71**:682–8; *ibid* 689–81), TDM

of 15 antidepressants (Reis *et al, Ther Drug Monit* 2009;**31**:42–56), SGAs as augmentation (Shelton and Papakostas, *Acta Psychiatr Scand* 2008;**117**:253–9), role of glutamate (Mitchell and Baker, *Acta Psychiatr Scand* 2010;**122**:192–210), adolescent depression (*Br Med J* 2010; **340**:c209).

SELECTIVE SEROTONIN REUPTAKE INHIBITORS (SSRIs)

The SSRIs are now first choice drugs in depression in most patients due to their safety in overdose and side-effect profile. Although chemically distinct from each other, the SSRIs are essentially more similar than different. All effective antidepressants, but their ADR profiles and potential for interactions may show clinical differences, as well as efficacy and tolerability differences (see choice of drugs).

Citalopram *

Citalopram is an established first-line anti-depressant and a review of 30 RCTs showed citalopram to be superior to placebo, of comparable efficacy to other antidepressants (including escitalopram: n = 240 [c = 203], RCT, d/b, 6/52, Ou *et al, Psychopharmacology (Berl)* 2011;**213**:639–46) and well tolerated from 20–60 mg/d. STAR*D's phase I used an average of 42 mg/d for optimum effect. Relapse prevention has been shown over 15 months in adults (n = 427, RCT, 44–77/52, Hochstrasser *et al, Br J Psychiatry* 2001;**178**:304–10) and in the elderly (n = 121, RCT, 48/52, Klysner *et al, Br J Psychiatry* 2002; **181**:29–35; review by Appelberg, *EBMH* 2003: **6**:24).

Reviews: * safety (Nemeroff, *Psychopharmacol Bull* 2003;**37**: 96–121), in later life depression (Seitz *et al, Int J Geriatr Psychiatry* 2010;**25**:1296–305).

Escitalopram *

Escitalopram is the pharmacologically active enantiomer of citalopram (a mix of R- and S-citalopram) and at least twice as potent on a mg for mg basis as citalopram (eg, n = 380, RCT, d/b, 8/52, Wade *et al, Int Clin Psychopharmacol* 2002;**17**:95–102). R-citalopram seems to antagonise escitalopram at serotonin receptors (e.g. Storustovu *et al, Br J Pharmacol* 2004;**142**:172–80); escitalopram binds to the primary binding site **and** the allosteric site; whereas R-citalopram blocks the allosteric site in a dose-dependent manner, reducing the antidepressant effect on the primary site. Escitalopram has a 30–40 times greater affinity for the serotonin transporter than R-citalopram (Sanchez, *Basic Clin Pharmacol Toxicol* 2006; **99**:91–5). The optimal dose in moderate MDD seems to be 10 mg/d with 20 mg/d the optimum in severe depression (p/c, 8/52, Bech *et al, Pharmacopsychiatry* 2006;**39**:128–34).

Numerous meta-analyses have shown escitalopram superior to other antidepressants, e.g. Cochrane concludes that there is a consistent and significant advantage for escitalopram over other antidepressants for efficacy and acceptability (s = 14, Cipriani *et al, Cochrane Database Syst Rev* 2009; **2**:CD006532), was significantly more effective for response and remission of depression than other SSRIs [NNT = 25] and SNRIs [NNT = 15] (s = 16, n = 4549, Kennedy *et al, Curr Med Res Opin* 2009;**25**:161–75), relapse with escitalopram at 20% far better than the 50% with placebo (s = 4, RCT, d/b, 24/52, Bech *et al, J Clin Psychiatry* 2010;**71**:121–9) and there is an NNT for response of 11.9 and 5.7 for remission, with an odds ratio of 1.44 for response and 1.86 for remission in favour of escitalopram over citalopram, a statistically significant superior efficacy (s = 8, n = 2009, RCT, Montgomery *et al, Int J Neuropsychopharmacol* 2011;**14**:261–8). An independent meta-analysis concluded that escitalopram has superior efficacy to citalopram and all SSRIs combined (s = 12, RCT, Ali and Lam, *Neuropsychiatr Dis Treat* 2011;**7**:39–49). While most antidepressants have greater efficacy with more severe depression, escitalopram appears to be effective across all grades of depression, especially severe (s = 15, n = 4301, Kilts *et al, Expert Opin Pharmacother* 2009;**10**:927–36). A trial should last at least four weeks before further intervention is considered (s = 40, Baldwin *et al, Hum Psychopharmacol* 2009;**24**:269–75). Relapse prevention has been shown (n = 590[c = 437], open, 12/12, Wade *et al, Ann Clin Psychiatry* 2006;**18**:83–9;

n = 139, RCT, d/b, p/c, 52/52, Kornstein *et al, J Clin Psychiatry* 2006;**67**:1767–75; MS).
Reviews: * general (Garnock-Jones and McCormack, CNS *Drugs* 2010;**24**:769–96), enantiomer advantages (Leonard and Taylor, *J Psychopharmacol* 2010;**24**:1143–52).

Switching or discontinuing antidepressants

For a table on switching antidepressants and the gaps needed, or advice on the problems of discontinuing, see *Chapter 2.2.7.*

Fluoxetine

Fluoxetine is licensed across the world for depression, with or without anxiety. Although 20 mg/d (s=3, n = 417, d/b, Beasley *et al, J Clin Psychiatry* 2000;**61**:722–8; MS) is the standard dose, some resistant depressions may respond to 60–80 mg/d. It has been shown to be clearly superior to placebo and slightly superior to tricyclics with significantly fewer drop-outs (rigorous meta-analysis, s = 30, n = 4120, Bech *et al, Br J Psychiatry* 2000;**176**:421–8) with evidence of relapse prevention (n = 140, RCT, 48/52, Gilaberte *et al, J Clin Psychopharmacol* 2001;**21**:417–24, MS). An interesting independent review suggesting inferior efficacy to other antidepressants (s = 131, Cipriani *et al, J Clin Psychiatry* 2006;**67**:850–64), and recently 60–80 mg/d was shown not to be superior to venlafaxine or placebo for MDD with melancholic features (n = 289, RCT, d/b, p/c, 6/52, Sheehan *et al, Int Clin Psychopharmacol* 2009;**24**:61–86). Cochrane calls for better trials with fluoxetine, a somewhat futile hope unless used as a comparator (Cipriani *et al, Cochrane Database Syst Rev* 2005;**4**:CD004185).
Review: safety and side-effects (Wernicke, *Expert Opin Drug Saf* 2004;**3**:495–504, MS).

Fluvoxamine

Fluvoxamine's starting dose should be 100–150 mg/d. Recent meta-analyses conclude there are no significant differences between fluvoxamine and other antidepressants (s = 54, n = 5122, RCT, Omori *et al, Cochrane Database*

Syst Rev 2010;**3**:CD006114), but that it has more GI ADRs.

Paroxetine

Paroxetine is licensed for depression, including that accompanied by anxiety, with 20mg/d the optimum dose, although higher plasma levels are associated with early response in severely depressed patients so dose escalation might be effective (n = 84, 4-18/52, Gex-Fabry et al, Prog Neuropsychopharmacol Biol Psychiatry 2007;**31**:892–900). Relapse prevention has been shown with paroxetine in old age (n = 116, RCT, d/b, p/c, two years, Reynolds et al, N Engl J Med 2006;**354**:1130–8). Paroxetine's half-life increases from 10 to 21 hours on chronic dosing, but reduces when this is stopped, which may in part explain the many reports of discontinuation effects (see 2.2.2).
Reviews: general (Marks et al, Expert Opin Drug Saf 2008;**7**:783–94; Tang and Helmeste, Expert Opin Pharmacother 2008;**9**:787–94).

Sertraline

The pharmacological profile of sertraline is similar to fluoxetine, but with a shorter half-life. The optimum dose may be 75mg (n = 82, Morishita and Kinoshita, Hum Psychopharmacol 2008;**23**:647–51). In recurrent depression (three or more episodes of MDD in four years), sertraline 50mg/d and 100mg/d were superior to placebo in preventing recurrences in people switched to sertraline for continuation treatment (n = 371, RCT, p/c, d/b, 18/12, Lépine et al, Am J Psychiatry 2004;**161**:836–42), but not in the elderly (n = 113[c = 31], RCT, d/b, p/c, two years, Wilson et al, Br J Psychiatry 2003; **182**:492–7; MS). Cochrane concludes that there is a trend for sertraline's superiority over other antidepressants, although critical of the study standards (s = 59, Cipriani et al, Cochrane Database Syst Rev 2010;**4**CD006117).
Review: pharmacokinetic profile (DeVane et al, Clin Pharmacokinet 2002;**41**:1247–66).

TRICYCLICS

Doses of 125–150mg/d of tricyclics are effective in depression and clearly superior to placebo, but, due to cardiotoxicity, overdose toxicity (n = 2503, Shah et al, Psychol Med 2001;**31**:1203–

10), sedation and anticholinergic effects are not recommended first-line, and in the UK, NICE recommends performing an ECG before prescribing tricyclics in depressed people at significant risk of cardiovascular disease. If using tricyclics, a therapeutic dose must be used before assessing the response.
Reviews: toxicity (Nutt, J Psychopharmacol 2005; **19**:123–4; pointing out the relative toxicity and sub-therapeutic dosing), cardiovascular toxicity from tricyclic poisoning (Thanacoody and Thomas, Toxicol Rev 2005;**24**:205–14).

Amitriptyline

Cochrane concludes that amitriptyline is at least as effective as other antidepressants, but with a higher side-effect burden (s = 194, Guaiana et al, Cochrane Database Syst Rev 2007; **2**:CD004186).

Clomipramine

Clomipramine is a predominantly serotonergic tricyclic with an active metabolite, also used for depression with an obsessional component.

Dosulepin (dothiepin)

Dosulepin is toxic in overdose and in the UK NICE recommends that it is not used. Although often prescribed to aid sleep, both dosulepin and fluoxetine disrupt REM sleep and no sleep-promoting effects were seen from dosulepin (n = 12, RCT, 5/52, d/b, p/c, Wilson et al, J Psychopharmacol 2002;**16**:321–31).

Doxepin

Doxepin is a standard tricyclic with moderate sedation, which may have fewer anticholinergic and cardiac effects than older tricyclics.

Imipramine

Imipramine is a standard tricyclic. NICE states that women tolerate imipramine more poorly than men. Stimulant side-effects may be troublesome, as may the anticholinergic effects, especially in the elderly, and it may provoke fragmentation of motor activity during sleep (n = 52, Volkers et al, Eur Neuropsychopharm 2002;**12**:273–8).

Lofepramine

Lofepramine is NICE's tricyclic of choice,

Table 1.1: The rationale and risks for combinations of antidepressants

SS	serotonin syndrome very possible
(SS)	serotonin syndrome possible or rarely reported
SSU	serotonin syndrome unlikely
LR	low rationale
SR	some rationale
HR	high rationale
UR	unknown rationale
LH	relatively low hazard or risk
MH	medium hazard or risk either known or predicted
HH	high hazard or risk of problems known or predicted so specialist monitoring required
UH	unknown or undocumented hazard
SM-LDT	specialist monitoring required and limit dose of tricyclic
VM	consider venlafaxine (>200 mg/d) or mirtazapine instead for combined 5-HT and NA/NE reuptake blockade
CI	see *Chapter 1* for data on positive use of combination
C4/5	see *Chapters 4* or *5* for data on risk of interaction or adverse consequences

	Citalopram/ escitalopram	Fluoxetine	Fluvoxamine	Paroxetine	Sertraline	Tricyclics	MAOIs	Venlafaxine	Mirtazapine	Reboxetine	Trazodone	Duloxetine	Moclobemide	Agomelatine
Fluoxetine	SS LR-HH													
Fluvoxamine	SS LR-HH	SS LR-HH												
Paroxetine	SS LR-HH	SS LR-HH	SS LR-HR											
Sertraline	SS LR-HH	SS-C4/5/5 LR-HH	SS LR-HH	SS LR-HH										
Tricyclics	SS-C4/5 LR-HH-CI	SS-C4/5 LR-HH-CI SM-LDT	SS-C4/5 LR-HH-CI SM-LDT	SS-C4/5 LR-HH-CI SM-LDT	SS-C4/5 LR-HH-CI									
MAOIs	(SS)-C4/5 SR-HH	(SS)-C4/5 SR-HH	(SS)-C4/5 SR-HH	(SS)-C4/5 SR-HH	(SS)-C4/5 SR-HH	(SS) SR-HH-CI								
Venlafaxine	SS LR-HH	SS-C4/5 LR-HH	SS LR-HH	SS MR-HH-CI	SS-C4/5 LR-HH	SS LR-HH	SS-C4/5 SR-HH							
Mirtazapine	SSU LR-UH	(SS) LR-UH	SSU LR-UH	SSU C4/5 LR/LH	SSU C4/5 LR-LH	SSU C4/5 LR-LH	SSU C4/5 SR-MH	SSU HR-LH						
Reboxetine	SSU SR-UH VM	SSU SR-UH VM	SSU SR-UH VM	SSU SR-UH VM	SSU SR-UH VM	SSU C4/5 LR-MH	SSU C4/5 LR-HH	SSU LR-UH	SSU MR-UH					
Trazodone	SS LR-UH	SS-C4/5 LR-MH	SS- C4/5 LR-UH	SS LR-UH	SS LR-UH	(SS) SR-MH	(SS)-C4/5 SR-HH	SS LR-HH	SSU SR-UH	SSU SR-UH VM				
Duloxetine	SS LR-HH	SS LR-MH	SS LR-HH	SS LR-HH	(SS) LR-HH	(SS)-C4 SR-LH	(SS)-C4 SR-HH	SS LR-HH	SSU SR-UH	SSU SR-UH VM	SS LR-HH			
Moclobemide	(SS)-C4/5 SR-MH	(SS)-C4/5 SR-LH	(SS)-C4/5 SR-MH	(SS)-C4/5 SR-MH	(SS) SR-MH	(SS0-C4/5 SR-HH	(SS) LR-HH	(SS)-C4/5 SR-HH	SSU SR-UH	SSU SR-UH	(SS) SR-UH	(SS) SR-UH		
Agomelatine	SSU HR-LH	SSU HR-LH	SSU HR-MH	SSU HR-LH	SSU HR-LH	SSU HR-LH	SSU HR-LH	SSU HR-LH	SSU HR-LH	SSU HR-LH	SSU HR-LH	SSU HR-LH	SSU HR-LH	
Tryptophan	(SS)-C4/5 UR-MH	(SS)-C4/5 UR-MH	(SS)-C4/5 UR-MH	(SS)-C4/5 UR-MH	(SS)-C4/5 UR-MH	(SS)-C4/5 UR-MH	(SS)-C4/5 UR-MH	(SS) UR-MH	SSU UR-LH	SSU UR-LH	(SS) UR-MH	(SS) UR-MH	SSU UR-MH	SSU UR-LH

and may have slightly less ADRs than other tricyclics. It is surprisingly safe in over dose, and blocks the cardiotoxic effects of the main metabolite desipramine (full review: Lancaster and Gonzalez, *Drugs* 1989;**37**:123–40).

Nortriptyline

Nortriptyline is a tricyclic with low cardio-toxic side-effects and suitable for once-daily administration. In treatment-resistant depression (failing 1–5 adequate trials), 40% may respond (12% remission) to nortriptyline, although 35% may not tolerate it (n = 92, open, 6/52, Nierenberg et al, *J Clin Psychiatry* 2003;**64**:35–9; n = 116, RCT, 12/52, Mulsant et al, *Am J Geriatr Psychiatry* 2001;**9**:406–14).

Trimipramine

Structurally related to levomepromazine, trimi-pramine has significant sedative properties. High dose trimipramine (up to 400 mg/d) has been shown to be at least as effective as amitriptyline and haloperidol for delusional depression (n = 94 [c = 57], RCT, d/b, p/c, 6/52, Künzel et al, *J Psychiatr Res* 2009;**43**:702–10).

OTHER ANTIDEPRESSANTS

Agomelatine *

Agomelatine is a 5HT2C and 5HT2B anta-gonist and a melatonin M1 and M2 agonist. In responders, the effective dose in 80% is 25 mg/d and 50 mg/d in the remaining 20% (n = 21, RCT, d/b, p/c, 6/52, Kennedy and Emsley, *Eur Neuropsychopharmacol* 2006;**16**:93–100), although 50 mg/d may not have a significant advantage (RCT, d/b, p/c, 8/52, Stahl et al, *J Clin Psychiatry* 2010;**71**:616–26). At 25–50 mg/d it is as effective as venlafaxine 75–150 mg/d, improving sleep quickly and with lower drop-outs (n = 332, RCT, d/b, 6/52, Lemoine et al, *J Clin Psychiatry* 2007;**68**:1723–32, MS). A pooled analysis shows efficacy also in severe depression (s = 3, n = 357, p/c, Montgomery and Kasper, *Int Clin Psychopharmacol* 2007;**22**:283–91), it is exceptionally well tolerated, appearing to have no sexual side-effects, no tolerability issues (n = 192, RCT, d/b, p/c, 2/52, Montgomery et al, *Int Clin Psychopharmacol* 2004;**19**:271–80), with no early relapse on discontinuation, suggesting no withdrawal or rebound effects

(n = 239, RCT, d/b, p/c, 6/12, Goodwin et al, *J Clin Psychiatry* 2009;**70**:1128–37). Agomelatine 25–50 mg/d improved circadian rest-activity/sleep-wake cycle in depressed patients by the end of week 1 and beyond (n = 303, RCT, d/b, 6/52, Kasper et al, *J Clin Psychiatry* 2010;**71**:109–20). Data is accumulating showing a superior effect to other standard antidepressants, e.g. agomelatine 25–50 mg/d was well tolerated and superior to fluoxetine 20–40 mg/d in severe MDD, although the fluoxetine was given at night (n = 515, RCT, d/b, 8/52, Hale et al, *Int Clin Psychopharmacol* 2010;**25**:305–14). Transient aminotransferase elevations can be seen at the higher dose (n = 511, RCT, d/b, p/c, 8/52, Zajecka et al, *J Clin Psychopharmacol* 2010; **30**:135-44).

Reviews: * general (Dolder et al, *Ann Pharmacother* 2008;**42**:1822–31; San and Arranz, *Eur Psychiatry* 2008;**23**:396–402), effect on sleep (Quera-Salva et al, *Hum Psychopharmacol* 2010; **25**:222–9), melatonergic mechanisms (De Berardis et al *CNS Neurol Disord Drug Targets* 2011;**10**:119–32).

Duloxetine *

Duloxetine is an SNRI that also weakly inhibits dopamine reuptake, but has no histamine, dopamine, cholinergic or adrenergic receptor affinity. The standard dose is 60 mg/d (but starting at a lower dose may improve toler-ability; s = 6, n = 1619, d/b, p/c, Pritchett et al, *J Psychiatr Res* 2007;**41**:311–8), and, although there is no published evidence that 120 mg/d is more effective, some believe that to be the case. Efficacy has been shown in two major studies (e.g. n = 267, RCT, d/b, p/c, 9/52, Detke et al, *J Psychiatr Res* 2002;**36**:383–90; n = 245, RCT, d/b, p/c, 9/52, Detke et al, *J Clin Psychiatry* 2002;**63**:308–15). Duloxetine appears at least as effective as paroxetine (e.g. n = 392, RCT, d/b, p/c, 8/52, Perahia et al, *Eur Psychiatry* 2006;**21**:367–78, MS), and non-inferior to escitalopram in depression (n = 684, RCT, d/b, p/c, 8/52, Nierenberg et al, *Curr Med Res Opin* 2007;**23**:401–16). Follow-on studies show relapse prevention efficacy (e.g. n = 288, RCT, d/b, p/c, < 52/52, Perahia et al, *J Clin Psychiatry* 2009;**70**:706–16; MS). Plasma levels may be worth measuring (n = 45, open, 12/52, Volonteri et al, *J Psychopharmacol* 2010;**24**:1193–9). Meta-analysis of all data (including unpublished or not fully reported) concludes that duloxetine is not a first-line choice in depression (s = 16, n = 5364, RCTs, Schueler et al, *Acta Psychiatr Scand* 2011;**123**:247–65), although some of these were under-dosed and the effect on painful physical symptoms in depression is small and statistically non-significant (s = 5, Spielmans, *Psychother Psychosom* 2008;**77**:12–6).

Reviews: general (Gupta et al, *Ann Clin Psychiatry* 2007; **19**: 125–32; Frampton and Plosker, *CNS Drugs* 2007; **21**:581–609).

Flupentixol

The standard initial dosage is 1 mg as a single morning dose, which can be increased to 2 mg/d (maximum 3 mg/d) if there is inadequate clinical response.

Mianserin

Mianserin is a tetracyclic with prominent $5HT_{2A}$ and $5HT_{2C}$ antagonist properties, a good safety profile in overdose, low cardiotoxicity and marked sedative properties.

Mirtazapine *

Mirtazapine blocks presynaptic alpha-2 adreno-receptors (increasing norepinephrine transmission) and indirectly enhances sero-tonergic transmission, with additional $5-HT_2$ and $5-HT_3$ receptor blockade minimising the incidence of serotoninergic side-effects, e.g. nausea, headache and sexual dysfunction. The optimum starting dose of 30 mg/d is well tolerated. Mirtazapine has been shown to be as effective as reference antidepressants (s = 10, n = 1904, RCT, d/b, Papakostas et al, *J Psychopharmacol* 2008;**22**:843–8) and may also be well tolerated and very effective as an adjunctive in antidepressant-resistant persistent MDD (n = 26, RCT, d/b, p/c, 4/52, Carpenter et al, *Biol Psychiatry* 2002;**51**:183–8). A meta-analysis of mirtazapine vs SSRI studies shows that people taking mirtazapine have a 74% higher likelihood of achieving remission in the first two weeks of therapy (s = 15, n = 2971, RCT, d/b, 6–8/52, Thase et al, *Int Clin Psychopharmacol* 2010;**25**:189–98). Relapse prevention is significantly superior to placebo (n = 156, RCT, d/b, 40/52, Thase et al, *J Clin Psychiatry* 2001;**62**:782–8).

Reviews:* general (Benjamin and Doraiswamy, *Expert Opin Pharmacother* 2011;**12**:1623–32 Croom et al, *CNS Drugs* 2009;**23**:427–52), kinetics (Timmer et al, *Clin Pharmacokinet* 2000;**38**:461–74, 56 refs), ADRs (Watanabe et al, *CNS Drugs* 2010;**24**:35–53).

> **Switching or discontinuing antidepressants**
>
> For a table on switching antidepressants and the gaps needed, or advice on the problems of discontinuing, see *Chapter 2.2.7.*

Moclobemide

Moclobemide (a reversible inhibitor of mono-amine oxidase-A) inhibits only MAO-A and not MAO-B, so an excess of tyramine in the body will displace moclobemide from MAO-A, allowing tyramine metabolism to occur, MAO-B remaining free. This results in a 'cheese-reaction', usually only at amounts above 100–150 mg of tyramine (see *4.3.4*), unlikely under normal conditions. A meta-analysis showed it to be about equipotent with reference antidepressants in agitated-anxious depressive patients, and clearly superior to placebo (s = 38, n = 2416, d/b, Delini-Stula et al, *J Affect Disord* 1995;**35**:21–30). Moclobemide appears to be benign even with massive ingestions (n = 106, Isbister et al, *Br J Clin Pharmacol* 2003;**56**:441–50).

Review: Bonnet, *CNS Drug Rev* 2003;**9**:97–140.

Reboxetine *

Reboxetine is a selective norepinephrine re-uptake inhibitor with no dopamine, histamine, adrenergic or serotonin effects at 8 mg/d. The four published RCTs indicate reboxetine to be significantly more effective than placebo in severe depression (s = 4, RCT, d/b, p/c, 8/52, Montgomery et al, *J Clin Psychopharmacol* 2003;**23**:45–50) but a more recent scathing report suggested that as 74% of patient data was not published, the studies en masse do not show reboxetine to be effective, inferior to SSRIs and possibly harmful cf placebo. While early dose-finding studies are often inconclusive this does lend credence to the clinical impression, i.e. it isn't much cop (s = 13, n = 4098, p/c, Eyding et al, Br Med J 2010;**341**:c4737).

Reviews: general (Hajos et al, CNS Drug Rev 2004;**10**:23–44; Page, CNS Drug Rev 2003;**9**: 327–42).

Trazodone

Trazodone increases NE and 5-HT turnover with low cardiotoxicity and anticholinergic side-effects, but a higher incidence of drowsiness and nausea. Trazodone 300–350 mg/d is more effective than placebo (n = 412, RCT, d/b, p/c, 8/52, Sheehan et al, Psychiatry (Edgmont) 2009;**6**:20–33). It is best taken with food to reduce peak blood levels.

Venlafaxine *

Venlafaxine is an SNRI with 5-HT reuptake inhibition across the dosage range, NE reuptake inhibition becoming significant from 150 mg/d (n = 32, Harvey et al, Arch Gen Psychiatry 2000;**57**:503–9) and dopamine reuptake inhibition above 225 mg/d. A meta-analysis of all data (including unpublished) concludes that venlafaxine is a valid alternative for SSRI/TCA non-responders, rather than a first-line choice (s = 56, n = 13652, RCTs, Schueler et al, Acta Psychiatr Scand 2011;**123**:247–65), and with a greater effect on remission rates in more severe depression (s = 31, n = 6492, Schmitt et al, Eur Arch Psychiatry Clin Neurosci 2009;**259**:329–39). There is evidence for a dose-response relationship, e.g. venlafaxine may be more effective at higher doses than certain SSRIs, with comparable tolerability (e.g. s = 32, Smith et al, Br J Psychiatry 2002;**180**:396–404), especially at higher doses, up to 375 mg/d (n = 96, retrospective, Vanoli et al, J Psychopharmacol 2008;**22**:434–40), but less well tolerated so is best reserved for people not responding to standard dose (n = 232, RCT, open, 12/52, Thase et al, J Clin Psychopharmacol 2006;**26**:250–8; comment by Dodd and Berk, EBMH 2007;**10**:17). Relapse prevention has been shown in prior responders to venlafaxine over two years in the PREVENT studies (n = 258, RCT, d/b, p/c, 12/12, Kocsis et al, J Clin Psychiatry 2007;**68**:1014–23; n = 1096, RCT, d/b, two years, Keller et al, J Clin Psychiatry 2007;**68**:1246–56; review by Kornsten, Expert Rev Neurother 2008;**8**:737–42).

The UK MHRA recommendations on venlafaxine are:

- still to be reserved as 2nd line treatment
- shared care is only required for initiation in severely depressed people, or in hospitalised patients who require doses of 300 mg daily, or above
- it is only contraindicated in people with an identified high risk of a serious cardiac ventricular arrhythmia or with uncontrolled hypertension. No baseline ECG is needed, but regular bp is recommended.

The higher overdose toxicity with venlafaxine may be due to increased use in patients at higher risk factors for suicide (including severity of depression), e.g. venlafaxine (n = 27096) patients were 4–6 times more likely to have been previously hospitalised for depression than fluoxetine (n = 134996) or citalopram (n = 52035) (n = 214127, Mines et al, Pharmacoepidemiol Drug Saf 2005;**14**:367–72, MS). Discontinuation effects may be significant (see 2.2.6). Although the UK SmPCs for XL and plain tablets have different maximum doses, this is just a licensing issue not a difference in absorption or safety.

Reviews: * venlafaxine vs TCAs (van den Broek et al, J Psychopharmacol 2009;**23**:708-13), vs SSRIs (s = 17, Weinmann et al, Psychopharmacology (Berl) 2008;**196**:511–20) and vs duloxetine (s = 54, n = 18180, Schueler et al, Acta Psychiatr Scand 2011;**123**:247–65).

MONOAMINE OXIDASE INHIBITORS (MAOIs) *

MAOIs may be being under-used and use is declining (n = 348, 10 years, Shulman et al, J Clin Psychiatry 2009;**70**:1681–6).

Isocarboxazid

Isocarboxazid is a hydrazine derivative that irreversibly blocks the MAO enzyme (editorial by Shader and Greenblatt, J Clin Psychopharmacol 1999;**19**:105).

Phenelzine

Phenelzine is a hydrazine derivative that irreversibly blocks the MAO enzyme, and is NICE's MAOI of choice, although they recommend that it is only initiated by specialist mental health professionals (including GPs with a special interest in mental health). A comparison of tranylcypromine and phenelzine showed no significant difference between them, with a 52% response rate in severe TRD (n = 77 [c = 67], d/b, 5/52, Birkenhäger et al, J Clin Psychiatry 2004;**65**:1505–10).

Tranylcypromine

Tranylcypromine is a non-hydrazine amfetamine-related MAOI with stimulant effects and a greater incidence of adverse drug interactions. Tranylcypromine did poorly in TRD in the STAR*D study (n = 109, open, McGrath et al, Am J Psychiatry 2006;**163**:1531–41), although the mean dose was only 37mg/d (doses towards 100mg/d or more may be much more effective, e.g. n = 77, d/b, 5/52, Birkenhäger et al, J Clin Psychiatry 2004;**65**:1505–10; mean 52mg/d produced a 59% remission rate in treatment-resistant depression; n = 32, Adli et al, Pharmacopsychiatry 2008;**41**:252–7), more patients were switched because of previous medication intolerance and the 2/52 washout/lead-in would have led to shorter duration of treatment.

OTHER ANTIDEPRESSANTS

Lithium (see also combinations)

Lithium monotherapy in the treatment and prophylaxis of unipolar (as well as bipolar) depression has been well-established and is associated with lower mortality, e.g. a meta-analysis of all available studies in MDD that had reported suicide or suicide attempts showed an 88% lower risk with vs without lithium, suggesting an anti-suicide effect in MDD as well as bipolar (s = 8, n = 329, Guzzetta et al, J Clin Psychiatry 2007;**68**:380–3). However, lithium is most effective as an adjunct to tricyclics and SSRIs (s = 9, n = 234, RCT, Bauer and Dopfmer, J Clin Psychopharmacol 1999;**19**:427–34; review by Lam, EBMH 2000;**3**:44; Bandolier 2000; **7**:4–5), where it may show a rapid effect over 1–2 weeks, although it may be of limited use in people resistant to multiple antidepressants (n = 92, RCT, p/c, 12/52, Nierenberg et al, J Clin Psychopharmacol 2003;**23**:92–5). Some antidepressant response to lithium is probably

mood stabilisation in undiagnosed bipolar depression and so sudden withdrawal of lithium would be outright dangerous (Faedda et al, Am J Psychiatry 2001;**158**:1337–9). Cochrane concludes lithium is effective for relapse-prevention of long-term unipolar depression (s = 8, n = 475, Cipriani et al, Cochrane Database Syst Rev 2006;**4**:CD003492).

Reviews: * lithium augmentation and bipolarity (Inoue et al, J Affect Disord 2011;**129**:64–7), predictors of efficacy (Sugawara et al, J Affect Disord 2010;**125**:165–8), long-term outcomes (Adli et al, Neuropsychobiology 2009;**60**:23–30). See main entry under bipolar mood disorder (1.10) and bipolar depression (1.10.3).

Tryptophan

Tryptophan is a naturally occurring amino acid and precursor to serotonin, and is used in combination with other antidepressants. Tryptophan depletion results in a rapid lowering of mood (review by Bell et al, Br J Psychiatry 2001;**178**:399–405) and acutely reverses antidepressant-induced remission, so tryptophan might help if low tryptophan levels have occurred. Cochrane concludes that the trial data is limited and unreliable but suggests tryptophan may be superior to placebo (s = 2, n = 64, Shaw et al, Cochrane Database Syst Rev 2002;**1**:CD003198). Due to a previous association with eosinophilia-myalgia syndrome (EMS), it is now only licensed in the UK for resistant depression, by hospital specialists, in patients with severe depression continuously for more than two years, after adequate trials of standard drug treatments and as an adjunct to other treatments.

+ Combinations (of antidepressants) *

There is some evidence that combined NE and 5-HT reuptake blocking drugs can produce a quicker antidepressant effect, although it could be that combined drug use produces higher success rates by treating different depressive subgroups. It might even be better to start with combined antidepressants from the start, e.g. remission rates in one trial were fluoxetine 20mg/d (25%), mirtazapine 30mg/d + bupropion 150mg/d (46%), mirtazapine

30 mg/d + fluoxetine 20 mg/d (52%), mirtazapine 30 mg/d + venlafaxine 225 mg/d (58%), (n = 105, RCT, d/b, 6/52, Blier et al, Am J Psychiatry 2010;**167**:281–8).

Review: * strategies for combination and augmentation for depression (Carvalho et al, Curr Opin Psychiatry 2009;**22**:7–12).

Bupropion + SSRIs/SNRIs/MAOIs *

Bupropion 200–300 mg/d may be useful in combination, e.g. 56% of **venlafaxine/ SSRI**-resistant depressed patients responded when bupropion was added (n = 25, Spier et al, Depress Anxiety 1998;**7**:73–5). It may also counteract SSRI/venlafaxine-induced sexual dysfunction (n = 18, open, 8/52, Kennedy et al, J Clin Psychiatry 2002;**63**:181–6). Addition of bupropion 150–300 mg/d in **escitalopram** 20 mg/d non-responders led to a marked response cf bupropion monotherapy (n = 135, open, 18/52, Maron et al, J Clin Psychiatry 2009;**70**:1054–6). **Duloxetine** (mean 60 mg/d) combined with bupropion (mean 175 mg/d) was successful (remission 30%, response 60%) in non-responders to initial monotherapy with either drug (n = 10, open, Papakostas et al, Depress Anxiety 2006;**23**:178–81). Bupropion and **tranylcypromine** have been successful for multi-drug resistant depression (n = 1, Pierre and Gitlin, J Clin Psychiatry 2000; **61**:450–1).

Review: reduced side-effects (Zisook et al, Biol Psychiatry 2005;**59**:203–10).

Lithium + antidepressants *

In people non-responsive to antidepressants, the best evidence is for combinations with lithium e.g. there is an NNT of 5 for response (41% vs 14% for placebo) (s = 30, n > 500, open; s = 10, n = 269, RCT, d/b, p/c, Bauer et al, Neuropsychobiology 2010;**62**:36–42). For SSRI augmentation, there is evidence of a substantial effect, mostly within 1–2 weeks (review by Zullino and Baumann, Pharmacopsychiatry 2001;**34**:119–27), maintained for 6/12 (n = 30, RCT, d/b, p/c, 6/52, open 4/12 extension, Bauer et al, Am J Psychiatry 2000;**157**:1429–35), as well as having an anti-suicidal effect in MDD (n = 167, Lauterbach et al, Acta Psychiatr Scand 2008;**118**:469–79). Adequate lithium levels (0.4 mmol/L or more) seem necessary. Predictors of efficacy include being bipolar, > 3

previous MDDs and a family history of MDD/ bipolar in a first-degree relative (n = 79, 8/52, Sugawara J Affect Disord 2010;**125**:165–8). So, lithium works in bipolar depression, even if it has not been diagnosed.

Review: lithium augmentation in refractory MDD (Bschor and Bauer, Curr Pharm Des 2006; 12:2985–92).

Lithium + tryptophan + antidepressants (eg. clomipramine, SSRI or phenelzine)

Variously known as Triple Therapy or the MRC, Newcastle or London Cocktail, there have been reports of 55% remission rates in severe depression, eg. from:

- clomipramine (to 150 mg/d or to tolerance, e.g. 300–400 mg/d) plus
- tryptophan (2–4 g/d) plus
- lithium (standard levels).

Alternatives to clomipramine include phenelzine and the SSRIs (n = 20, RCT, Barker et al, Int Clin Psychopharmacol 1987;**2**:261–72). Tryptophan enhances the action of clomipramine on 5-HT sites and improves 5-HT absorption. Lithium also affects 5-HT and is an antidepressant in its own right.

Mirtazapine + venlafaxine/SSRIs

In persistent MDD, addition of mirtazapine 30 mg to existing therapy produced a response rate of 64% cf 20% with placebo (n = 26, RCT, d/b, p/c, 4/52, Carpenter et al, Biol Psychiatry 2002;**51**:183–88; short review in Fava, J Clin Psychiatry 2001;**62**[Suppl 18]:S4–S11). Mirtazapine has also been used with high-dose venlafaxine, the rationale being to use mirtazapine to block 5HT2 and 5HT3 receptors, reducing sexual and anxiety side-effects from venlafaxine, and allowing higher doses to be tolerated. The combination might have been under-rated in STAR*D phase 4 because the QIDS score was actually 23.5% vs only 12.1% for tranylcypromine. A retrospective study showed response rates of 50% at 8/52, and 56% at 6/12, with mirtazapine ADRs predominant (n = 32, Hannan et al, J Psychopharmacol 2007;**21**:161–4).

Reboxetine + duloxetine *

In duloxetine-resistant depression, a pilot study showed that addition of reboxetine produced an impressive 70% remission rate (n = 79[c=71], open, 12/52, Seguí et al, J Psychopharmacol 2010;**24**:1201–7).

Reboxetine + mirtazapine

Addition of reboxetine in mirtazapine-resistant depression may be a safe and effective strategy (n = 14, 12/52, Lopez-Munoz et al, Clin Neuropharmacol 2006;**29**:192–6).

Reboxetine + SSRIs

This logical combination has been used successfully, e.g. reboxetine added to SSRI/mirtazapine/venlafaxine partial or non-responders produced a well tolerated improvement (n = 61, open, 6/52, Rubio et al, J Affect Disord 2004;**81**:67–72) and combined escitalopram and reboxetine may provide a rapid response (n = 3, Camarasa et al, Prog Neuropsychopharmacol Biol Psychiatry 2005;**29**:165–8). In SSRI partial responders, addition of reboxetine produced 50% response and 34% remission rates, so RCTs would be useful to confirm this effect (n = 141, open, 12/52, López-Muñoz et al, Pharmacopsychiatry 2007;**40**:14–9). We await them.

SSRIs + SSRIs

Although there are anecdotal reports (e.g. Bondolfi et al, Psychopharmacol [Berl] 1996;**128**:421–5), the combination cannot be recommended and risks serotonin syndrome.

Tricyclics + MAOIs

Although extreme caution is advised, this combination is known to be effective in some resistant depressions, e.g. isocarboxazid plus amitriptyline (n = 25, open, Berlanga and Ortega-Soto, J Affect Disord 1995;**34**:187–92). Tranylcypromine plus clomipramine is known to be dangerous (at least two deaths) but other combinations can be used with care in an inpatient setting. Most problems occur when a tricyclic is added to an MAOI. Fewer adverse events have been reported with the reverse. It is best to take great care, e.g. separate the doses (e.g. MAOI in the morning, tricyclic in the evening), add one to the other in low dose and build up slowly or stop all antidepressants, wait a week, and then start both together at low dose and build up again.

Tricyclics + SSRIs

The only robust prospective study on the combination showed that high dose fluoxetine (60 mg/d) was, in fact, more effective in partial or non-responders to 20 mg/d than a fluoxetine/desipramine combination (n = 41, RCT, d/b, 4/52, Fava et al, Am J Psychiatry 1994;**151**:1372–4). Positive studies have not been robust (see Cowen and Power, Br J Psychiatry 1993; **162**:266–7). The combination should generally be avoided due to the high risk of an adverse interaction (4.3.2) and in potentially suicidal patients. (Cheeta et al, Br J Psychiatry 2004;**184**:41–7).

Venlafaxine + SSRIs

SSRIs have been used successfully to augment venlafaxine (n = 4, Gonul et al, Prog Neuropsychopharmacol Biol Psychiatry 2003; **27**:889–91), but the combination is not recommended.

+ Augmentation (by drugs with no intrinsic antidepressant activity *

Reviews: * NNTs and response rates for adjunctives in MDD (Citrome, Postgrad Med 2010;**122**:39–48), systematic review (s = 32, Fleurence et al, Psychopharmacol Bull 2009;**42**:57–90), SGAs as adjuncts and monotherapy (Chen et al, Curr Opin Psychiatry 2011;**24**:10–7).

Anticholinesterases

Donepezil augmentation of sertraline improved cognition in elderly people with depression and cognitive impairment (n = 23, RCT, d/b, p/c, 8/52, Pelton et al, Int J Geriatr Psychiatry 2008;**23**:670–6), but adding galantamine to venlafaxine or citalopram had no effect in MDD in 'older' (> 50) adults and with increased drop-outs (n = 38, RCT, d/b, p/c, 24/52, Holtzheimer et al, Int J Geriatr Psychiatry 2008;**23**:625–31).

Antipsychotics *

Cochrane concludes that quetiapine monotherapy is more effective than placebo, and that augmentation of antidepressants with aripiprazole and quetiapine was superior to placebo, with olanzapine and risperidone showing some promise (s = 28, n = 8487, RCT, d/b, Komossa et al, Cochrane Database Syst Rev

2010;**12**:CD008121). A major meta-analysis has concluded that SGAs can successfully augment antidepressants in MDD but at increased risk of stopping due to side-effects (s = 16, n = 3480, p/c, Nelson and Papakostas, *Am J Psychiatry* 2009;**166**:980–91).

Aripiprazole (s = 2, Weber *et al, CNS Drugs* 2008;**22**:807–13) has been approved in the US as adjunctive or add-on treatment to antidepressants for adults with MDD, but a monotherapy license would require longer-term studies. In incomplete responders to an SSRI or venlafaxine, adjunctive aripiprazole (2–20 mg/d) improved MADRS scores and was well tolerated (n = 362, RCT, d/b, p/c, 8 + 6/52, Berman *et al, J Clin Psychiatry* 2007; **68**:843–53; critical review by Ciprani and Barbui, *EBMH* 2008;**11**:15), and adjunctive aripiprazole 2–20 mg/d was effective in 37% cf 19% with placebo (n = 349 [c = 297], RCT, d/b, p/c, 8/52, Berman *et al, CNS Spect* 2009;**14**:197–206; MS). A 50% response rate from adjunctive aripiprazole was seen in depression in older people (n = 24 [c = 19], open, 12/52, Sheffrin *et al, J Clin Psychiatry* 2009;**70**:208–13). It has also been useful as an adjunct to bupropion (n = 4, 4/12, Sokolski, *Ann Pharmacother* 2008;**42**:1124–9) and escitalopram (n = 16 [c = 13], open, 7/52, Matthews *et al, J Clin Psychopharmacol* 2009;**29**:73–6). Even in people not responding to at least four antidepressants, aripiprazole (mean 11 mg/d) was moderately successful, although rates of akathisia were high at 25% (n = 381, RCT, d/b, 6/52, Marcus *et al, J Clin Psychopharmacol* 2008;**28**:156–65).

Clozapine has been used in refractory psychotic depression (n = 1, Dassa *et al, Br J Psychiatry* 1993;**163**:822–4).

Olanzapine-fluoxetine (OFC) * is licensed in USA for treatment-resistant unipolar and bipolar depression. A pooled analysis showed OFC superior to fluoxetine or olanzapine individually, and that absence of early improvement is highly predictive of overall response failure (s = 5, Tohen *et al, J Clin Psychiatry* 2010;**71**:451–62). However, OFC was no more effective than either drug alone or nortriptyline monotherapy (n = 500, RCT, d/b, 8/52, Shelton *et al*, *J Clin Psychiatry* 2005;**66**:1289–97, MS; comment by Dodd and Berk, *EBMH* 2006;**9**:42), and olanzapine plus sertraline improved psychotic depression better than olanzapine alone, suggesting that olanzapine monotherapy may not be a potent antidepressant (n = 259, RCT, d/b, p/c, 12/52, Meyers *et al, Arch Gen Psychiatry* 2009;**66**:838–47).

Quetiapine (see also monotherapy under unlicensed) XL is now licensed in USA and Europe for adjunctive treatment in recurrent and resistant MDD (Pae *et al, Prog Neuropsychopharmacol Biol Psychiatry* 2010;**34**: 1165–73), with adjunctive quetiapine 300 mg/d effective at week 6, whereas 150 mg was not statistically superior (n = 446, RCT, d/b, p/c, 6/52, El-Khalili *et al, Int J Neuropsychopharmacol* 2010;**13**:917–32). Adjunctive quetiapine 150–300 mg/d was effective for MDD, with some reduction in symptoms as early as a week (n = 493, RCT, d/b, p/c, 6/52, Bauer *et al, J Clin Psychiatry* 2009;**70**:540–9. In psychotic MDD, quetiapine 600 mg/d plus venlafaxine 375 mg/d was more effective than venlafaxine or imipramine monotherapy (n = 122, RCT, d/b, 7/52, Wijkstra *et al, Acta Psychiatr Scand* 2010; **121**:190–200).

Risperidone 1–2 mg/d augmentation of sub-optimally effective antidepressants has increased response and remission (n = 274, RCT, d/b, p/c, 6/52, Mahmoud *et al, Ann Intern Med* 2007;**147**:593–602; comment by Barbee, *EBMH* 2008;**11**:77). In non-psychotic, unipolar TRD, risperidone 0.5–3 mg/d produced more rapid response and higher remission rates (n = 97, RCT, d/b, p/c, 4/52, Keitner *et al, J Psychiatr Res* 2009;**43**:205–14). **Perphenazine** added to a tricyclic did not improve efficacy in late-life psychotic depression (n = 36, RCT, d/b, 4/52, Mulsant *et al, J Clin Psychiatry* 2001;**62**:597–604), although I personally object to late-life being defined as people aged 50 or older. **Sulpiride** 100 mg/d may accelerate the antidepressant effect of paroxetine 10–40 mg/d (n = 41 [c = 33], RCT, open, 12/52, Uchida *et al, J Clin Psychopharmacol* 2005;**25**:545–51). **Ziprasidone** has been used as augmentation in SSRI-resistance (n = 64, RCT, open, 6/52, Dunner *et al, J Clin Psychiatry* 2007;**68**:1071–7; MS).

Reviews: * OFC/olanzapine + fluoxetine (Bobo and Shelton, *Expert Rev Neurother* 2010; **10**:651–70), OFC in TRD (Croxtall and Scott, *CNS Drugs* 2010;**24**:245–62), aripiprazole as augmentation in MDD (Blier and Blondeau, *J Aff*

Disord 2011;**128**[Suppl 1]:S3–10), general (Selis and Peeters, *Tijdschr Psychiatr* 2008;**50**:213–22), SGAs as augmentation (Shelton and Papakostas, *Acta Psychiatr Scand* 2008;**117**:253–9).

Benzodiazepines

Cochrane concludes that BDZ augmentation, e.g. clonazepam (optimum dose 2.5–6 mg/d, response takes 2–4 weeks; Morishita, *Hum Psychopharmacol* 2009;**24**:191–8), of anti-depressants leads to fewer drop-outs and less depression severity at 1–4 weeks, but the effect disappears at 6–8 weeks. So, short-term use may thus be successful, possibly by minimising initial SSRI side-effects (e.g. anxiety), improving sleep, or a direct action (s = 9, n = 679, Furukawa *et al, Cochrane Database Syst Rev* 2002;**1**:CD001026; comment by Gijsman, *EBMH* 2001;**4**:45). Predictors of response to clonazepam augmentation in protracted unipolar TRD include negative family history of psychiatric illness, and doses 2.5–4 mg/d (n = 120, Morishita and Arita, *Hum Psychopharmacol* 2007;**22**:27–31).

Buspirone

Buspirone shares some pharmacodynamic properties with pindolol and augmentation of SSRIs may produce marked improvement in resistant depression, e.g. adding 20–60 mg/d buspirone to SSRI non-responders produced significant reductions in MADRS scores at the end of week one compared to placebo, but both groups were equivalent at six weeks (n = 102, RCT, p/c, d/b, 6/52, Appelberg *et al, J Clin Psychiatry* 2001;**62**:448–52). Another trial, suggested that buspirone actually slowed the onset of action of fluoxetine (n = 120, RCT, open, 12/52, Onder and Tural, *J Affect Disord* 2003;**76**:223–7), so great care is needed.

Carbamazepine (see also unlicensed)

Carbamazepine augmentation may be useful in SSRI non-responders (n = 6, Steinacher *et al, Eur Neuropsychopharmacol* 2002;**12**:255–60), although beware of potential interactions, e.g. carbamazepine does not augment mirtazapine's onset of action compared to placebo, and reduces mirtazapine plasma levels (n = 46, 5/52, open, Schule *et al, World J Biol Psychiatry* 2008;**25**:1–10).

Celecoxib

Celecoxib (400 mg/d) was more effective than placebo as an adjunct to fluoxetine in MDD (n = 40, RCT, p/c, 6/52, Akhondzadeh *et al, Depress Anxiety* 2009;**26**:607–11).

Estradiol/estrogen (see also unlicensed)

Estrogen supplementation of SSRIs may enhance their effectiveness (n = 5, Westlund *et al, J Affect Disord* 2003;**77**:87–92) in, e.g. postnatal depression (see *1.14.2*) and the menopause (n = 145, Miller *et al, J Am Geriatr Soc* 2002;**50**:1826–30). Low-dose estrogen 0.625 mg/d as augmentation to partially effective SSRIs in perimenopausal depression significantly improved mood, but not memory (n = 17, RCT, d/b, p/c, 6/52, Morgan *et al, J Clin Psychiatry* 2005;**66**:774–80).

Folate *

Folate is a naturally occurring B vitamin necessary for synthesis of norepinephrine, serotonin and dopamine (Fava and Mischoulon, *J Clin Psychiatry* 2009;**70**(Suppl 5):12–7), and low RBC folate levels have been linked to depression, persistent symptoms and a poor response to antidepressants (n = 127, RCT, p/c, 10/52, Coppen and Bailey, *J Affect Disord* 2000;**60**:121–30; comment by Goodwin, *EBMH* 2001;**4**:41), an easily rectified problem (e.g. n = 2948, Morris *et al, Psychother Psychosom* 2003;**72**:80–7). Folate 15 mg/d has significantly improved clinical response and recovery (systematic review and meta-analysis by Taylor *et al, J Psychopharmacol* 2004;**18**:251–6). Leucovorin (metabolised to methylfolate) has a modest effect in SSRI non-response (n = 22, 8/52, Alpert *et al, Ann Clin Psychiatry* 2002;**14**:33–8).

Fludrocortisone *

Fludrocortisone (a mineralocorticoid receptor agonist) did not improve the efficacy of escitalopram but speeded up the response (n = 64, RCT, d/b, p/c, 5/52, Otte *et al, J Psychiatr Res* 2010:**44**:339–46).

Lamotrigine *

Lamotrigine's main role is in bipolar depression (see *1.10.3*) but it may have a role as an adjunct at 200 mg/d for refractory unipolar depression, enhancing the onset of paroxetine (n = 40, p/c, d/b, 9/52, Normann et al, J Clin Psychiatry 2002;**63**:337–44), but 100mg/d was not quite statistically superior to placebo as an adjunct to fluoxetine in MDD and bipolar II (n = 23, RCT, d/b, p/c, 6/52, Barbosa et al, J Clin Psychiatry 2003;**64**:403–7). However, in non-bipolar depression, the evidence is sparce (Thomas et al, J Ment Health 2010;**19**:168–75) and lamotrigine augmentation of anti-depressants was ineffective (n = 34, RCT, d/b, p/c, 8/52, Santos et al, Prim Care Companion J Clin Psychiatry 2008;**10**:187–90). Remember that even missing two days' doses means retitrating.

Levothyroxine (thyroxine, synthetic T4) *

Low TSH and higher T4 levels are associated with current depressive syndrome in young adults (n = 6869, Forman-Hoffman et al, Acta Psychiatr Scand 2006;**114**:132–9). Thyroid supplementation, e.g. levothyroxine 150–300 mcg/d may accelerate the onset of tricyclic response in non-refractory depression (5/6 studies found T3 significantly superior to placebo, especially in women: meta-analysis, Altshuler et al, Am J Psychiatry 2001;**158**:1617–22). The combination of T3+T4 may be no better than T4 monotherapy (n = 40, RCT, d/b, p/c, 15/52, Sawka et al, J Clin Endocrinol Metab 2003;**88**:4551–5).

Liothyronine (L-isomer of triiodothyronine, T3) *

A meta-analysis showed liothyronine augmentation to produce twice as many responses in refractory depression compared to controls, with moderately large improvements (s = 5, RCTs, Cooper-Kazaz and Lerer, Int J Neuropsychopharmacol 2008;**11**:685–99). T3 50mcg/d was effective in 35% treatment-resistant depressives, especially for melancholic MDD (n = 20, open, 4/52, Iosifescu et al, J Clin Psychiatry 2005;**66**:1038–42) and 33% achieved full remission with T3 mean 90mg/d after failing an average of 14 agents (n = 159, retrospective, Kelly and Lieberman, J Affect Disord 2009;**116**:222–6; see also n = 17, Kelly and Lieberman, J Affect Disord 2009;**115**:230–3). Augmentation of sertraline 100mg/d by liothyronine 40–50mcg/d improved ITT

response rates from 57% to 70%, a significant effect (n = 124, RCT, d/b, p/c, 8/52, Cooper-Kazaz et al, Arch Gen Psychiatry 2007;**64**:679–88). This may be effective, particularly in rapid-cycling bipolar disorder (1.10.4).
Reviews: STAR*D (Nierenberg et al, Am J Psychiatry 2006;**163**:1519–30), HUNT study (Panicker et al, Clin Endocrinol (Oxf) 2009; **71**:574–80).

Metyrapone

Metyrapone 1g/d accelerated the response to 'standard' antidepressants (nefazodone or fluvoxamine) in MDD, possibly by counteracting stress hormones' inhibition of 5HT release in the forebrain (n = 63, RCT, p/c, 5/52, Jahn et al, Arch Gen Psychiatry 2004;**61**:1235–44; comment by Young, EBMH 2005;**8**:72).

Methylphenidate

Methylphenidate may be effective as augmentation where incomplete response has occurred with antidepressants, including the elderly, where apathy and withdrawal (but not hopelessness) are prominent features. Augmentation of citalopram may be rapidly successful and well tolerated in elderly depressed patients (e.g. n = 16, RCT, d/b, p/c, 10/52, Lavretsky et al, Am J Geriatr Psychiatry 2006;**14**:181–5). Cochrane concludes that there is reasonable evidence for short-term psychostimulants (methylphenidate, dexam-fetamine, modafinil) to reduce the symptoms of depression (s = 24, RCT, Candy et al, Cochrane Database Syst Rev 2008;**2**:CD006722). Methylphenidate had no effect on depression ratings (MADRS) but improved apathy and fatigue (n = 145, RCT, d/b, p/c, 5/52, Ravindran et al, J Clin Psychiatry 2008;**69**:87–94).

Modafinil

A review concluded that open studies show modafinil helps fatigue associated with depression but that RCTs have not been able to show this (Lam et al, Ann Pharmacother 2007;**41**:1005–12). Adjunctive modafinil may help in patients with fatigue and sleepiness in MDD over the short-term, but the effect wears off over 6/52 (n = 136 [c = 118], RCT, d/b, p/c, 6/52, DeBattista et al, J Clin Psychiatry 2003;**64**:1057–64; n = 245 [c = 194], open, p/c,

12/52, Thase et al, CNS Spectr 2006;**11**:93–102).

Nimodipine

Nimodipine augmentation of fluoxetine has been successful for 'vascular depression' (n = 101, RCT, d/b, p/c, 8/52, Taragano et al, Int Psychogeriatr 2005;**17**:487–98).

Pergolide

The dopamine agonist pergolide had moderate success in open trials as an adjunct (n = 20, open, Bouckoms and Mangini, Psychopharmacol Bull 1993;**29**:207–11; n = 20, open, Izumi et al, J Affect Disord 2000; **61**:127–32).

Pindolol *

Antidepressants, e.g. SSRIs may act by inhibiting the 5-HT reuptake pump, increasing 5-HT but this also enhances 5-HT at 5-HT$_{1A}$ receptors situated on the cell body which operate a feedback loop, thus cancelling each other out. Over a period of weeks, however, the pre-synaptic 5-HT$_{1A}$ receptors become desensitised. Pindolol selectively blocks 5-HT$_{1A}$ receptors, and inhibits this initial feedback loop to increase the speed of onset of action. An eloquent systematic review concluded that pindolol is clearly effective to enhance the onset of action of SSRIs, most clearly up to four weeks (s = 11, Whale et al, J Psychopharmacol 2010;**24**:513–20). In another interesting twist, re-analysis of an old study (n = 11, RCT, Perez et al, Lancet 1997;**349**:1594–7) suggested that pindolol improves response (70% vs 40%) and speed of response (53 days vs 19 days) in first episode depression but not in recurrent patients (Portella et al, Eur Neuropsychopharmacol 2009;**19**:516–9). Another trial and meta-analysis of pindolol as an adjunct to SSRIs concludes a significantly quicker onset of action at 2 weeks, maintained at weeks 4 and 6 (n = 30, RCT, d/b, p/c, 6/52, Portella et al, J Clin Psychiatry 2011; in press).

Riluzole

Riluzole (mean 75 mg/d) is another dopamine agonist and may be useful as an adjunct to standard antidepressants, with a significant effect within the first week (n = 10, open, 12/52, Sanacora et al, Biol Psychiatry 2007;**61**:822–5),

and as monotherapy (mean 170 mg/d, n = 19, open, 6/52, Zarate et al, Am J Psychiatry 2004; **161**:171–4).

Topiramate

Adjunctive topiramate may be beneficial for some obese depressed females (n = 16, open, Carpenter et al, J Affect Disord 2002;**69**:251–5).

Valproate

There are some reports of efficacy in TRD as augmentation of lithium (n = 10, Sharma et al, Lithium 1994; **5**:99–103), and it may help reduce depressive agitation (n = 12 [c = 9], open, 4/52, DeBattista et al, J Clin Psychopharmacol 2005;**25**:476–9).

Vitamin B12 (cyanocobalamin)

Oral B12 1 mg/d supplementation has been recommended in TRD (review by Coppen and Bolander-Gouaille, J Psychopharmacol 2005; **19**:59–65).

> ● **Unlicensed/some efficacy**
> **(see also augmentation)**

Amisulpride *

Amisulpride 50 mg/d monotherapy has been shown to have an antidepressant activity comparable with fluoxetine 20 mg/d, (n = 281, d/b, Smeraldi, J Affect Disord 1998;**48**:47–56), paroxetine 20 mg/d (n = 272, RCT, d/b, 56/7, Cassano et al, Int Clin Psychopharmacol 2002; **17**:27–32) and for psychotic depression in the elderly (n = 11, Politis et al, Prog Neuropsychopharmacol Biol Psychiatry 2008;**32**:1227–30).

Bupropion *

Bupropion, a presynaptic dopamine and noradrenaline reuptake inhibitor, is licensed in the USA and other countries for the treatment of depression, as well as for smoking cessation. A meta-analysis of original data from seven studies comparing bupropion (n = 732) with SSRIs (n = 731) showed equivalent efficacy and tolerability, except bupropion caused no more sexual dysfunction than placebo (s = 7, RCT, d/b, Thase et al, J Clin Psychiatry 2005;**66**:974–81), less nausea, diarrhoea and somnolence, but higher cardiovascular, proconvulsive (at doses up to 450 mg/d: Pesola and Avasarala, *J Emerg Med* 2002;**22**:235–9) and overdose toxicity. Bupropion XR 300 mg/d was as effective and as well tolerated as venlafaxine 150 mg/d, with dry mouth and insomnia the most reported ADRs (n = 571, RCT, d/b, p/c, 8/52, Hewett *et al, J Psychopharmacol* 2009;**23**:531–8; MS), although failed in a second trial (n=591, RCT, d/b, p/c, 8/52, Hewett *et al, J Psychopharmacol* 2010;**24**:1209–16). There is no evidence for differential onset of action from SSRIs overall or escitalopram specifically (s = 7, n = 1672, RCT, d/b, 8/52, Papakostas *et al, J Clin Psychiatry* 2007;**68**:1907–12). Bupropion 300 mg/d (max 450 mg/d) helps MDD with decreased energy, pleasure, interest (n = 274, RCT, d/b, p/c, 8/52, Jefferson *et al, J Clin Psychiatry* 2006;**67**:865–73), sleepiness and fatigue (s = 6, n = 1317, RCT, d/b, Papakostas *et al, Biol Psychiatry* 2006;**60**:1350–5), and anxiety symptoms in comorbid depression (s = 10, n = 2890, RCT, d/b, p/c, Papakostas *et al, J Psychiatr Res* 2008;**42**:134–40). A relapse prevention effect has been shown (n = 423, RCT, d/b, p/c, 44/52, Weihs *et al, Biol Psychiatry* 2002;**51**:753–61). The maximum dosage of 450 mg/d should be adhered to since the risk of seizures is dose related (see *3.4*).

Reviews: general (Glayton, *Expert Opin Pharmacother* 2007;**8**:457–66), clinical profile and pharmacology (Dwoskin *et al, CNS Drug Rev* 2006;**12**:178–207).

Carbamazepine (see also augmentation)

Evidence for use as a pure antidepressant is poor (see augmentation) (e.g. n = 16, open, Cullen *et al, J Clin Psychiatry* 1991;**52**:472–6). See main entry under bipolar mood disorder (*1.10.*).

Estradiol/estrogens (see also combinations) *

Estrogen receptors occur in the CNS and loss of estrogen has been shown to reduce serotonergic and other functioning. It may have a role in PDD (see *1.14.2*). It may improve depressive symptoms in postmenopausal women, albeit not cognition (n = 19, RCT, p/c, c/o, 24/52, Schiff *et al, Psychoneuroendocrinology* 2005;**30**:309–15). Conjugated estrogens 0.625 mg/d have significantly improved mood in perimenopausal women with MDD partially responding to antidepressants (n = 17, RCT, p/c, 6/52, Morgan *et al, J Clin Psychiatry* 2005;**66**:774–80), a progesterone derivative (chlormadinone) plus ethinylestradiol improved mood in women in an observational study (n = 50000, < 12/12, Huber *et al, Clin Drug Invest* 2008;**28**:783–91). However, a larger study showed transdermal estradiol did not improve depressive symptoms in postmenopausal women (n = 57, RCT, d/b, p/c, 8/52, Morrison *et al, Biol Psychiatry* 2004;**55**:406–12), nor did it enhance the effectiveness of sertraline in postmenopausal women with MDD, but it might have speeded the onset of response (n = 22, RCT, p/c, 10/52, Rasgon *et al, J Psychiatr Res* 2007;**41**:338–43).

Reviews: * general (Estrada-Camarena *et al, Behav Pharmacol* 2010;**21**:451–64; Studd and Panay, *Best Pract Res Clin Obstet Gynaecol* 2009;**23**:63–71), mechanisms of action (Osterlund, *Biochim Biophys Acta* 2010;**1800**: 1136–44), transdermal estradiol (Moses-Kolko *et al, Clin Obstet Gynecol* 2009;**52**:516–29).

Methylphenidate (see also augmentation)

Methylphenidate can be used as monotherapy in acute depression as it has the major advantage of a rapid action (often within 48 hours), although the effect tends to be transient and it may worsen anxiety and insomnia. The stimulant action of methylphenidate in the elderly may be grossly attenuated and so may not be appropriate in those reporting age-related cognitive decline (n = 60, RCT, p/c, d/b, Turner *et al, Psychopharmacol [Berl]* 2003;**168**:455–64).

Quetiapine (see also augmentation) *

In MDD, quetiapine 150–300 mg/d monotherapy seems effective, (n = 310, RCT, d/b, p/c, 10/52, Bortnick *et al, J Affect Disord* 2011; **128**:83–94) even from the fourth day (n = 723, RCT, d/b, p/c, 6/52, Weisler *et al, CNS Spectr* 2009;**14**:299–313), and 300mg/d XL was as effective as duloxetine for MDD (n = 612, RCT, d/b, p/c, 6/52, Cutler *et al, J Clin Psychiatry* 2009;**70**:526–39). Maintenance monotherapy reduces relapse of MDD cf placebo by 66% (n = 776, RCT, d/b, p/c, 12/12, Liebowitz *et al, Depress Anxiety* 2010;**27**:964–76).

Selegiline

Transdermal selegiline (20mg/d) is licensed in the USA and may be surprisingly effective and well tolerated in MDD, as the transdermal route allows higher doses than possible orally, with no need for dietary restrictions (n = 177, RCT, p/c, 6/52, Bodkin and Amsterdam, *Am J Psychiatry* 2002;**159**:1869–75; comment by Benedictis, *EBMH* 2003;**6**:44; see also n = 289, d/b, p/c, 8/52, Amsterdam, *J Clin Psychiatry* 2003;**64**:208–14).

St John's wort (SJW) *

SJW is available over-the-counter in most European countries in a variety of preparations. The mode of action is uncertain but may include serotonin and/or norepinephrine reuptake inhibition, MAO-A and B inhibition and sigma receptor activity. A variety of systematic reviews and meta-analyses conclude SJW has modest effects in MDD, but older smaller trials in a variety of depressions have shown a marked effect (e.g. s = 13, Rahimi *et al, Prog Neuropsychopharmacol Biol Psychiatry* 2009;**33**:118–27) and relapse prevention over 6/12 (n = 426, RCT, d/b, p/c, 26/52, Kasper *et al, Eur Neuropsychopharmacol* 2008;**18**:803–13). However, a major rigorous trial failed to show a significant antidepressant or anxiolytic effect in MDD (n = 200, RCT, p/c, 8/52, Shelton *et al, JAMA* 2001;**285**:1978–86; review by Hawley and Dale, *EBMH* 2002;**5**:24) and, in a second trial, neither sertraline nor SJW (generously dosed) were effective in moderately-severe depression (n = 340, RCT, d/b, p/c, 8/52, Davidson *et al, JAMA* 2002;**287**:1807–14; review by Swann, *EBMH* 2002;**5**:111; vigorous discussion by Jonas *et al, JAMA* 2002;**288**:446–9). Most studies are short-term (up to 6/52), and many have high (up to 50%) drop-out rates, indicating that transient mild depression may be common in participants. Care is needed in adjunctive therapy (particularly if purchased OTC — see *4.3.3.9*). Cochrane concludes that SJW is superior to placebo in MDD, equivalent to standard antidepressants and with fewer side-effects, although the source of SJW may be relevant (s = 29, n = 5489, Linde *et al, Cochrane Database Syst Rev* 2008;**4**:CD000448; comment by Ernst, *EBMH* 2009;**12**:78).

Reviews: general (Kelly, *Hosp Med* 2001;**62**:274–6) and ADRs (s = 35, Knüppel and Linde, *J Clin Psychiatry* 2004;**5**:1470–9).

■ Unlicensed/possible efficacy

Botox injections

A small study showed that people with depression improved two months after botox injections (n = 10, Finzi and Wasserman, *Dermatologic Surg* 2006;**32**:645–50).

Buspirone (see also augmentation)

Buspirone may be superior than placebo but less effective than imipramine as monotherapy in MDD in old age (n = 177, RCT, Schweizer *et al, J Clin Psychiatry* 1998;**59**:175–83).

Chromium

Chromium picolinate may be an option in atypical depression, with a potential effect within two weeks (n = 15, 8/52, p/c, Davidson *et al, Biol Psychiatry* 2003;**53**:261–4).

Dexamethasone

This synthetic glucocorticoid can show a rapid and marked improvement given IV (n = 37, 4/7, Arana *et al, Am J Psychiatry* 1995;**152**:265–7) or orally (n = 10, 6/52, Dinan *et al, Acta Psychiatr Scand* 1997;**95**:58–61), although probably only a minority of patients respond (letter by Wolkowitz *et al, Am J Psychiatry* 1996;**153**:1112–3). This interesting effect may be via upregulation of glucocorticoid receptors, an effect shared with the SSRIs.

Reviews: glucocorticoids (Kling *et al, Depress Anxiety* 2009;**26**:641–9; Yu *et al, J Steroid Biochem Mol Biol* 2008;**108**:300–9).

Dexamfetamine

Dexamfetamine may be rapidly effective for depression and fatigue, with one successful trial in men with HIV (n = 23, RCT, 2/52, Wagner and Rabkin, *J Clin Psychiatry* 2000;**61**:436–40).

DHEA (dehydroepiandrosterone)

DHEA (an adrenal androgen and neurosteroid) at 90–450mg/d monotherapy was effective for mid-life depression (n = 18/52, RCT, d/b, p/c, c/o, 18/52, Schmidt *et al, Arch Gen*

Psychiatry 2005;**62**:154–62), and in non-major depression in HIV/AIDS (n = 145 [c = 133], RCT, p/c, d/b, 8/52, Rabkin et al, Am J Psychiatry 2006;**163**:59–66), possibly by reducing the vulnerability to stress.

Donepezil
Donepezil may reduce REM latency in depressed patients (n = 16, c/o, Perlis et al, Biol Psychiatry 2002;**51**:457–62).

Glucocorticoid antagonists
See hydrocortisone, ketoconazole, mifepristone and dexamethasone.

Hydrocortisone
IV hydrocortisone produced a significantly greater and robust improvement in HAM-D scores than ovine CRH or placebo (n = 22, RCT, d/b, p/c, 2/7, DeBattista et al, Am J Psychiatry 2000;**157**:1334–7; comment by Watson and Young, Am J Psychiatry 2001;**158**:1536–7).

Hyoscine
A robust and rapid response occurred to short-term treatment with IV scopolamine in TRD (n = 39 [c = 18], RCT, d/b, p/c, c/o, 5/7, Furey and Drevets, Arch Gen Psychiatry 2006;**63**:1121–9).

Ketamine
There is a case of remarkable antidepressant response to inadvertent ketamine induction 'monotherapy' after seizure-free and hence failed ECT sessions (n = 1, Ostroff et al, Am J Psychiatry 2005;**162**:1385–6).

Ketoconazole
Ketoconazole inhibits cortisol secretion, lowering cortisol levels and may have a slow-onset antidepressant effect, particularly in hypercortisolemic (but not normal) patients (n = 20, RCT, d/b, p/c, 4/52, Wolkowitz et al, Biol Psychiatry 1999;**45**:1070–74), but probably not in TRD (n = 16, RCT, Malison et al, J Clin Psychopharmacol 1999;**19**:466–70).

Magnesium *
There is a view that inadequate dietary magnesium is a main cause of TRD (Eby and Eby, Med Hypotheses 2010;**74**:649–60).

Mifepristone
Mifepristone 600–1200 mg/d (another gluco-corticoid antagonist) may be an option for psychotic MDD, the theory being that 'the psychosis in MDD is caused by excessive activation of the HPA axis' (n = 30, open, 7/7, Belanoff et al, Biol Psychiatry 2002;**52**:386–92). Six days of mifepristone can lead to significant improvement in PMD even in the first week, maintained for four weeks, but probably not to eight weeks (n = 20, open, 8/52, Simpson et al, J Clin Psychiatry 2005;**66**:598–602).

Omega-3 fatty acids (PUFAs) *
Systematic reviews conclude that omega-3 fatty acids are a potential treatment for depression (s = 21, Kraguljac et al, Psychopharmacol Bull 2009;**42**:39–54), but note significant heterogeneity and publication bias (s = 10, n = 329, d/b, p/c, > 4/52, Lin and Su, J Clin Psychiatry 2007;**68**:1056–61). The most recent meta-analysis concludes that PUFAs work better in bipolar depression and MDD, as adjunctive or acute (rather than prophylactic) therapy, and where the EPA (eicosapentaenoic acid) content is 51–100% cf the DHA (docosahexaenoic acid) component (s = 28, RCTs, Martins, J Am Coll Nutr 2009;**28**:525–42).

The case for: Omega-3 supplementation in MDD had only a modest effect in depression without comorbid anxiety (n = 432, RCT, d/b, p/c, 8/52, Lespérance et al, J Clin Psychiatry 2011; in press). Intakes of fish and omega-3 fatty acids may be inversely associated with chronic depression, so supplementation may be helpful in people for whom fish is not an acceptable source (n = 3317, 20 years, Colangelo et al, Nutrition 2009;**25**:1011–9).

The case against: There are many negative studies. EPA-E 1 g/d was numerically but not statistically superior to placebo for MDD, albeit well-tolerated (n = 57 [c = 35], RCT, d/b, p/c, 8/52, Mischoulon et al, J Clin Psychiatry 2009;**70**:1636–44) and adjunctive E-EPA had no effect in depression in diabetics (n = 25, RCT, d/b, p/c, 12/52, Bot et al, J Affect Disord 2010;**126**:282–6). DHA (docosahexaenoic acid, an omega-3 fatty acid) was ineffective as monotherapy in MDD (n = 35, p/c, 6/52, Marangell et al, Am J Psychiatry 2003;**160**:996–8) and in people with CHD, augmentation of sertraline 50 mg/d with omega-3 fatty acids had no effects on depression (n = 122, RCT, d/b, 10/52, Carney et al, JAMA 2009;**302**:1651–7). A Finnish study showed low dietary intake of omega-3 fatty acids is **not** associated with low mood (n = 29 133, Hakkarainen et al, Am J Psychiatry 2004;**161**:567–9) and there has been a small negative study in perinatal depression (n = 26, RCT, d/b, p/c, 6/52, Rees et al, Aust N Z J Psychiatry 2008;**42**:199–205).

Reviews: * general (s = 19, Rocha Araujo et al, Expert Rev Neurother 2010;**10**:1117–29), role (reasonable adjunctive strategy, not yet for monotherapy; Freeman, J Clin Psychiatry 2009; **70** [Suppl 5]:7–11).

Opiates *

Some anecdotal cases suggest that oxycodone or oxymorphone may produce a sustained effect in refractory and chronic depression, as well as reducing psychogenic pain and distress (review by Berrocoso et al, Curr Pharm Des 2009;**15**:1612–22) and buprenorphine may be useful in refractory, unipolar depression (see Callaway, Biol Psychiatry 1996;**39**: 989–90). The potential for abuse limits their use.

Phenytoin

Phenytoin (up to 400 mg/d) was as effective as fluoxetine (up to 21 mg/d) for MDD (n = 33 [c = 28], RCT, d/b, Nemets et al, J Clin Psychiatry 2005;**66**:586–90).

Pramipexole

Pramipexole is a dopamine D2/D3 agonist licensed for Parkinson's disease and has been used with some success (n = 22, case series, Ostow, Am J Psychiatry 2002;**159**:320–1; n = 174, RCT, p/c, 8/52, Corrigan et al, Depress Anxiety 2000;**11**:58–65).

SAM-e (S-adenosyl-L-methionine) *

SAMe (a naturally occurring cellular mole-cule) was effective and well-tolerated as an adjunct to SSRIs in SSRI-non-response (n = 73, RCT, d/b, p/c, 6/52, Papakostas et al, Am J Psychiatry 2010;**167**:942–8), with IM or IV use well supported, but less so for oral use (Papakostas, J Clin Psychiatry 2009;**70** [Suppl 5]:18–22).

Testosterone *

Low free testosterone levels are associated with a higher prevalence of depression, e.g. older men with low total or free testosterone levels are 1.5–2.7 times more likely to have depression (n = 3987, Almeida et al, Arch Gen Psychiatry 2008;**65**:283–9), and so supplementation might help (n = 3987, Almeida et al, Arch Gen Psychiatry 2007; **64**:283–9). Weekly testosterone cypionate 100–200 mg/d may be effective in some men with late-onset depression, but not earlier-onset depression (n = 15, RCT, 6/52, Perry et al, J Clin Psychiatry 2002;**63**:1096–101). In men with metabolic syndrome, low testosterone, ED and depression, depot testosterone undecanoate significantly improved mood, most markedly in men with low baseline total testosterone (n = 184, RCT, d/b, p/c, 30/52, Giltay et al, J Sex Med 2010;**7**:2572–82). Testosterone gel may be a non-parenteral route capable of producing an antidepressant effect in men with refractory depression and low testosterone (n = 22, RCT, p/c, 8/52, Pope et al, Am J Psychiatry 2003;**160**:105–11), although it was ineffective for TRD with plasma testosterone < 350 ng/ml (n = 100, RCT, p/c, d/b, 6/52, Pope et al, J Clin Psychopharmacol 2010;**30**:126–34).

Vardenafil

Vardenafil is effective for erectile dysfunction in milder MDD, and depressive symptoms may improve with treatment of one of the potential symptoms (n = 280, RCT, d/b, p/c, Rosen et al, Am J Psychiatry 2006;**163**:79–87).

Zinc *

An extraordinary study (n = 75, d/b, p/c, 12/52, Siwek et al, J Affect Disord 2010;**126**:447–52), that needs replicating, suggested that:

- Serum zinc is significantly lower (by 22%) in depressed cf non-depressed people
- Zinc levels increase with response to imipramine regardless of zinc supplementation
- People with resistant depression have 14% lower zinc levels than people with non-resistant depression
- Oral zinc increases serum zinc levels
- There is an inverse relationship between serum zinc and response.

✱ Case reports

- **Pregabalin** 150–225 mg/d (n = 1, Showraki, *J Psychopharmacol* 2007; **21**:883–4).
- **Tramadol** (n = 1, Shapira et al, *J Clin Psychiatry* 2001; **62**:205–6).
- **Varenicline** (n = 1, Grosshans et al, *Addiction* 2009; **104**:859–61).

◆ Others

Other drugs tried include **bromocriptine** 10–60 mg/d (McGrath et al, *J Clin Psychopharmacol* 1995; **15**: 289–91), **cyproheptadine** (n = 6, RCT, Greenway et al, *Pharmacotherapy* 1995; **15**:357–60), **tetracyclines** (minocycline; Pae et al, *Biomed Pharmacother* 2008; **62**:308–11; demeclocycline; Levine et al, *Am J Psychiatry* 1996; **153**:582) and **thyrotropin-releasing hormone** (n = 5, Marangell et al, *Arch Gen Psychiatry* 1997; **54**:214–22).

□ No efficacy

Atomoxetine

In SSRI-refractory depression, atomoxetine augmentation is of no benefit (n = 276, RCT, d/b, p/c, 8/52, Michelson et al, *J Clin Psychiatry* 2007; **68**:582–7; MS) and atomoxetine is in fact a failed antidepressant monotherapy (n = 15 [c = 11], open, 8/52, Carpenter et al, *J Clin Psychiatry* 2005; **66**:1234–8).

Benzodiazepines

Benzodiazepines have no antidepressant activity but can help with short-term anxiety and when starting SSRIs. Short-term adjunctive use may have some role.

Caffeine

Some depressed people may have increased sensitivity to caffeine (Lee et al, *Am J Psychiatry* 1988; **145**:632–5).

Inositol

Inositol is a precursor of an intracellular secondary messenger system for numerous neurotransmitters but is ineffective as SSRI augmentation (n = 27, RCT, p/c, Levine et al, *Biol Psychiatry* 1999; **45**:270–3), or in SSRI failures (RCT, d/b, Nemets et al, *J Neural Transm* 1999; **106**:795–8).

Memantine

Memantine 5–20 mg/d was ineffective for MDD (n = 32, RCT, d/b, p/c, Zarate et al, *Am J Psychiatry* 2006; **163**:153–5).

Pyridoxine (vitamin B6)

Low B6 levels have been associated with depression and supplementary B6 might be useful but a review (s = 10 including five RCTs) showed no apparent effect in men, although some minor effect in premenopausal women (*Family Pract* 2005; **2**:532–7).

Spironolactone ✱

Spironolactone (a mineralocorticoid receptor antagonist) did not improve the efficacy of escitalopram, even in responders (n = 64, RCT, d/b, p/c, 5/52, Otte et al, *J Psychiatr Res* 2010: **44**:339–46).

1.14.2 POSTPARTUM DEPRESSION (PPD) ✱

see also Depression (*1.14.1*)

Symptoms:

PPD is defined as MDD with a postpartum onset within one month of childbirth, although it can pre-date birth and occur in the first year. The Edinburgh Postnatal Depression Scale (Cox et al, *Br J Psychiatry* 1987; **150**:782–6) is the most widely used assessment tool. The incidence ranges from 6–14% (e.g. (n = 865, Miyake et al, *J Affect Disord* 2006; **96**:133–8), peaking in the third month, then declining over the year. The recurrence rate may be as high as 25% (Wisner et al, *J Clin Psychiatry* 2001; **62**:82–6).

There is a clear and well-established relationship between maternal depression and impaired childhood development, e.g. poor cognitive function, behavioural inhibition, emotional maladjustment, poor bonding, slowed development, and child neglect (e.g. Carter et al, *J Am Acad Child Adolesc Psychiatry* 2001; **40**:18–26). Thus, there is huge risk in not treating, especially as suicide is also a risk.

Causes:

There are many and dramatic changes in hormones in the postnatal period, and estrogen, progesterone and other hormonal fluctuations have been proposed as the main culprits, although rapid changes in estrogen and progesterone may not be a cause (n = 192, 7/12, Klier et al, J Psychiatr Res 2007;**41**:273–9).

Risk factors for PPD:
- Postpartum blues (Reck et al, J Affect Disord 2009;**113**:77–87)
- MDD or anxiety in pregnancy
- Previous depression (n = 588, McCoy et al, J Reprod Med 2008;**53**:166–70)
- Antidepressants discontinued during pregnancy
- Cigarette smoking (n = 588, McCoy et al, J Reprod Med 2008;**53**:166–70)
- Low partner support
- Epilepsy (e.g. 29% incidence, n = 35, Turner et al, Epilepsy Behav 2006;**9**:293–7; n = 110, Turner et al, Epilepsia 2009;**50**(Suppl1):24–7), especially with polypharmacy and multiparity (n = 56, Galanti et al, Epilepsy Behave 2009;**16**:426–30)
- Low serum zinc (n = 66 [c = 58], 30/7, Wójcik et al, Pharmacol Rep 2006;**58**:571–6).

Not risk factors for PPD:
- Low serum magnesium (n = 66 [c = 58], 30/7, Wójcik et al, Pharmacol Rep 2006;**58**:571–6)
- Low folate, pyridoxine or cobalamin (n = 865, Miyake et al, J Affect Disord 2006;**96**:133–8)
- Medroxyprogesterone acetate depot — if given immediately postpartum does not seem to predispose to PPD (n = 55 + 192 controls, Tsai and Schaffir, Contraception 2010; **82**:174–7).

Role of drugs: *
Antidepressants have some issues regarding infant exposure, but the multiple adverse effects of untreated PPD are outweighed by this risk if drugs and doses are chosen carefully. The potential effects of antidepressants in breast-feeding must be considered (see C3.1; review by Freeman, J Clin Psychiatry 2009;**70**:e35; Fortinguerra et al, Pediatrics 2009;**124**:547–56). Non-pharmacological treatments such as IPT (interpersonal psychotherapy) and CBT have shown modest effect sizes (Cuijpers et al, J Clin Psychol 2008;**64**:103–18), although antidepressants show larger effect sizes (Bledsoe et al, Res Soc Work Pract 2006;**16**:109–20) in more robust trials. ECT may be an option in an emergency (n = 5, Forray and Ostroff, J ECT 2007;**23**:188–93). Adding antidepressants to supportive care in PPD can bring forward response (n = 254, RCT, 18/52, Sharp et al, Health Technol Assess 2010;**14**:1–153). SSRIs can delay secretory activation by around 15 hours immediately postpartum so might delay onset of breast-feeding (n = 431, Marshall et al, J Clin Endocrin Metabol 2010;**95**:837–46).

Prevention: *
A protective effect has been shown by nortriptyline (n = 51, RCT, d/b, p/c, 20/52, Wisner et al, J Clin Psychiatry 2001;**62**:82–6) and sertraline (n = 22, RCT, d/b, p/c, 20/52, Wisner et al, Am J Psychiatry 2004;**161**:1290–2), although the effect seemed to go when stopped at 20/52.

Reviews: * pharmacotherapy (Ng et al, Pharmacotherapy 2010;**30**:928–41), diagnosis and treatment of postnatal bipolar depression (Kelly and Sharma, Expert Rev Neurother 2010;**10**:1045–51), General (Lanza di Scalea and Wisner, Expert Opin Pharmacother 2009;**10**:2593–2607; Friedman and Resnick, Women's Health 2009;**5**:287–95; Pearlstein et al, Am J Obs Gynecol 2009;**400**:357–64), prevention (Chabrol and Callahan, Expert Rev Neurother 2007;**7**:557–76), safety index for antidepressants (Gentile, Drug Saf 2007;**30**:107–21), bipolar PPD (Sharma et al, J Affect Dis 2010;**125**:18–25; Sharma et al, Am J Psychiatry 2009;**166**:1217–21), rating scales (Oppo et al, Arch Women's Ment Health 2009;**12**:239–49), psychoneuroimmunology (Corwin and Pajer, J Women's Health [Larchmt] 2008;**17**:1529–34), bipolar II PPD (Sharma et al, Am J Psychiatry 2009; **166**:1217–21).

BNF listed

No antidepressants are specifically licensed for PPD, so all are technically licensed (see 1.14.1). Specific PPD papers are listed below.

Bupropion *
Bupropion 150–400 mg/d showed 37.5% remitting, plus 37.5% responding, but had no effect on comorbid anxiety (n = 8, open, 8/52, Nonacs et al, Int J Neuropsychopharmacol 2005; **8**:445–9).

Fluoxetine *
In the main study fluoxetine 20 mg/d and CBT both improved depressive symptoms more

than placebo, but the combination had no advantage over monotherapy (n = 87, RCT, d/b, p/c, 12/52, Appleby et al, Br Med J 1997; **314**:932–6).

Fluvoxamine *

Fluvoxamine (mean 150 mg/d) showed 67% remission rate (n = 6, open, 8/52, Suri et al, Am J Psychiatry 2001;**158**:1739–40).

Paroxetine *

Paroxetine (max 40 mg/d) has produced remission in 37% vs placebo (14%) at week 8, but this was not statistically significant (n = 70, RCT, d/b, p/c, 8/52, Yonkers et al, J Clin Psychiatry 2008;**69**:659–65). Paroxetine (max 50 mg/d, 87.5% response) and CBT (79% response) were both effective in another study (n = 35, RCT, 12/52, Misri et al, J Clin Psychiatry 2004; **65**:1236–41).

Sertraline *

Sertraline (max 200 mg/d) was as effective as nortriptyline (max 150 mg/d) (n = 109, RCT, 24/52, Wisner et al, J Clin Psychopharmacol 2004;**65**:353–60).

Venlafaxine *

A small study showed possible efficacy, also perhaps also in comorbid anxiety (n = 15, open, 8/52, Cohen et al, J Clin Psychiatry 2001; **62**:592–6).

● **Unlicensed/some efficacy**

Benzodiazepines *

Benzodiazepines may be useful for short-term anxiety and insomnia, but nothing specific has been published.

Calcium *

Calcium has been mentioned in one review (s = 7, Dennis et al, Can J Psychiatry 2004; **49**:467–75).

Estrogens *

Use of sublingual beta-estradiol produced 100% recovery in severe PPD, although 14/23 were also taking antidepressants (n = 23, 8/52, open, Ahokas et al, J Clin Psychiatry 2001;**62**:332–6). Women on transdermal 17-

beta-estradiol may have a greater remission rate (review by Moses-Kolko et al, Clin Obstet 2009;**52**:516–29). Cochrane concluded that estrogen therapy is associated with greater improvement in severe postpartum depression than placebo, and may be of modest value (s = 2, n = 229, Dennis et al, Cochrane Database Syst Rev 2008;**4**:CD001690).

Riboflavin *

Moderate consumption of riboflavin (vitamin B2) may be protective (n = 865, Miyake et al, J Affect Disord 2006;**96**:133–8).

Selenium *

Prenatal selenium 100 mcg/d significantly reduced postnatal depression scores (EPDS) and might thus have a role in prevention of PPD (n = 166 [c = 85], RCT, d/b, p/c, 8/12, Mokhber et al, J Matern Fetal Neonatal Med 2011;**24**:104–8).

St. John's wort *

St John's wort might be considered by some people as 'natural' and hence safe, but that is unproven. There is no published data on use in PPD (short review by Goldman et al, Can Fam Physician 2003;**49**:29–30).

□ **No efficacy**

Omega-3 fatty acids *

A review of Omega-3 fatty acids concludes that the trials so far are not robust and are inconclusive (s = 7, Borja-Hart and Marino, Pharmacotherapy 2010;**30**:210–6; e.g. n = 59 [c = 51], RCT, p/c, 8/52, Freeman et al, J Affect Disord 2008;**110**:142–8; n = 26, RCT, d/b, p/c, 6/52, Rees et al, Aust NZ J Psychiatry 2008; **42**:199–205). Docosahexanoic acid (DHA), a form of omega-3 fish oils, also showed no effect in PPD, on improving cognitive skills or language development in children if taken from < 21/52 to term, although there were lower rates of pre-term birth in mothers on DHA, and it was definitely safe in pregnancy (n = 2399, RCT, d/b, Makrides et al, JAMA 2010;**304**:1675–83; review by Wojcicki and Heyman, J Matern Fetal Neonatal Med 2010;**24**:680–6).

Review: * general (Levant, Depress Res Treat 2011;2011:in press).

Progesterones *

Cochrane concludes that norethisterone enthanate (a synthetic progestogen) administered within 48 hours of delivery significantly increased the risk of postpartum depression (s = 2, n = 229, Dennis et al, Cochrane Database Syst Rev 2008;**4**:CD001690).

Thyroxine *

Women with high antenatal thyroid antibody levels may be at greater risk of developing PPD (e.g. n = 57, Lambrinoudaki et al, J Affect Disord 2010;**121**:278–82), but this is not corrected by daily thyroxine (n = 446, RCT, d/b, p/c, 5/12, Harris et al, Br J Psychiatry 2002;**180**:327–30).

1.14.3 DYSTHYMIA
see also Depression (1.14)

Symptoms

Dysthymia (literally 'ill-humored') is a low-grade chronic depression (often with anxiety) of insidious onset, chronic course (lasting at least two years with permanent or intermittent symptoms) and a high risk of relapse. It has few of the physical symptoms of depression and is compatible with stable social functioning. Almost all sufferers eventually develop super-imposed major depression (n = 86, three-year follow-up, Klein et al, Am J Psychiatry 2000;**157**:931–9). The life-time prevalence rate may be around 3–6%, and higher in the elderly. It has been considered by some to be similar to depressive personality disorder or anxiety and, by others, as a way of medicalising (and hence ignoring) social problems.

Role of drugs *

It is clear that antidepressants are effective in dysthymia, and indeed a meta-analysis showed antidepressants to actually have a wider margin of efficacy than in MDD, partly due to a lower placebo response rate in dysthymia (s = 17, Levkovitz et al, J Clin Psychiatry 2011;**72**:509–14). There is no proven significant differences between classes but they should form part of an overall treatment strategy including, e.g. psychological therapies. A greater sensitivity to side-effects has been noted in dysthymics. SSRIs and moclobemide appear favoured. Cochrane concludes that drug therapy might as well be chosen on the basis of potential side-effects (s = 14, de Lima and Hotopf, Cochrane Database Syst Rev 2003;**3**:CD004047).

Reviews: * diagnosis and treatment (de Lima and Hotopf, Drug Saf 2003;**26**:55–64), in the elderly (Bellino et al, Drugs Aging 2000;**16**:107–21), in children and adolescents (Nobile et al, CNS Drugs 2003;**17**:927–46), general (Kripke, Am Fam Physician 2004;**70**:1269–70).

● Unlicensed/some efficacy

ALCAR (acetyl-l-carnitine)

ALCAR may be as effective and tolerable as amisulpride (n = 204, RCT, d/b, 12/52, Zanardi and Smeraldi, Eur Neuropsychopharmacol 2006;**16**:281–7).

Antipsychotics

Cochrane concludes that for SGAs in dysthymia, quetiapine monotherapy is more effective than placebo, augmentation with aripiprazole or quetiapine (and possibly olanzapine or risperidone) may be superior to placebo (s = 28, n = 8487, Komossa et al, Cochrane Database Syst Rev 2010;**12**:CD008121). There is some evidence for low-dose amisulpride (e.g. n = 313, RCT, d/b, 12/52, Amore et al, Int Clin Psychopharmacol 2001;**16**:317–24).

Review: substituted benzamides in dysthymia (Pani and Gessa, Mol Psychiatry 2002;**7**:247–53).

Bupropion

Bupropion SR up to 400 mg/d was effective in 71% patients in one trial, with those having a history of substance misuse less likely to respond (n = 21, open, 8/52, Hellerstein et al, J Clin Psychopharmacol 2001;**21**:325–9).

Moclobemide

Moclobemide (mean 675 mg/d) has been shown to be significantly more effective for dysthymia than imipramine (mean 220 mg/d), with fewer side-effects (n = 315, RCT, Versiani et al, Int Clin Psychopharmacol 1997;**12**:183–93).

SSRIs

SSRIs are probably the treatment of choice for dysthymia. **Citalopram** (mean 39 mg/d) appeared effective in 73% of 'pure' dysthymics in one study (n = 21, open, 12/52, Hellerstein

et al, Int Clin Psychopharmacol 2004;**19**:143–8).
Fluoxetine 20mg/d may be more effective than placebo, with 50% of the non-responders at three months improving with a dose increase to 40mg/d (n=140, RCT, Vanelle et al, Br J Psychiatry 1997;**170**:345–50), but may have limited efficacy in elderly patients (n=90[c=71], RCT, d/b, p/c, 12/52, Devanand et al, Am J Geriatr Psychiatry 2005;**13**:59–68). **Paroxetine** was superior to psychotherapy and placebo in older dysthymics (n=415, RCT, 11/52, Williams et al, JAMA 2000;**284**:1519–26). In dysthymia without major depression, **sertraline** up to 200mg/d may be effective over a wide range of efficacy and quality of life measures (n=310, RCT, p/c, 12/52, Ravindran et al, J Clin Psychiatry 2000;**61**:821–7), and may improve behaviour and personality in dysthymia (n=410, RCT, d/b, p/c, Hellerstein et al, Am J Psychiatry 2000;**157**:1436–44).

Tricyclics

Tricyclics at robust doses, e.g. 50–300mg/d imipramine may be effective but with high drop-outs in longstanding dysthymia (n=416, RCT, 12/52, p/c, Kocsis et al, Am J Psychiatry 1997;**154**:390).

■ **Unlicensed/possible efficacy**

Chromium

Chromium (as the picolinate) provided a dramatic and complete resolution of dysthymia in a small trial (n=5, s/b, McLeod et al, J Clin Psychiatry 1999;**60**:237).

Duloxetine

A pilot study has suggested some efficacy for duloxetine in dysthymia (n=24[c=19], open, Koran et al, J Clin Psychiatry 2007;**68**:761–5).

Mirtazapine

Mirtazapine 15–45mg/d was effective in 73% in a small trial (n=15[c=11], open, 10/52, Depress Anxiety 1999;**10**:68–72).

Sildenafil

Sildenafil 25mg/d has produced improvement, not related to erectile function, in middle-aged male depression (n=20, open, 6/52, Orr et al, J Nerv Ment Dis 2008;**196**:496–500).

Testosterone

In hypogonadal older men, testosterone gel may be effective for subsyndromal depression (n=33, RCT, d/b, p/c, 24/52, Shores et al, J Clin Psychiatry 2009;**70**:1009–16) and IM injections for middle-aged late-onset dysthymia in men (n=23, RCT, d/b, p/c, Seidman et al, J Clin Psychopharmacol 2009;**29**:216–21).

Venlafaxine

Several open studies suggest some efficacy, e.g. up to 225mg/d was effective in 71% of completers (n=17[c=14], 9/52, Dunner et al, J Clin Psychiatry 1997;**58**:528–31), and up to 300mg/d may be reasonably effective and generally well tolerated for elderly patients (n=23[c=18], open, 12/52, Devanand et al, J Geriatr Psychiatr Neurol 2004;**17**:219–24).

◆ **Others**

Other drugs tried include **phenelzine** and **tranylcypromine** (review, Anon, Br J Psychiatry 1995;**166**:174–83). and **valproate** (n=1, Kemp, Br J Psychiatry 1992; **160**:121–3).

□ **No efficacy**

St John's wort

People with dysthymia seem unresponsive to SJW, although non-dysthymics may improve (n=150, RCT, d/b, p/c, 6/52, Randlov et al, Phytomedicine 2006; **13**:215–21).

1.15 EATING DISORDERS

1.15.1 Anorexia nervosa
1.15.2 Bulimia nervosa
1.15.3 Binge-eating disorder

DSM-IV includes three eating disorders; anorexia nervosa (AN), bulimia nervosa (BN) and eating disorders not otherwise specified (EDNOS), the latter including binge-eating disorder. Although sociocultural explanations are important and relevant, anorexia, bulimia and obesity may be heterogeneous disorders with a complex aetiology, including genetic factors and the environment.

Reviews: * general (Treasure et al, Lancet 2010;**375**:583–93), anticonvulsants for eating disorders (McElroy et al, CNS Drugs 2009;**23**:139–56), pharmacotherapy (Flament et al, Int J Neuropsychopharmacol 2011; in press; Powers and Bruty, Child Adolesc Psychiatr Clin N Am 2009;**18**:175–87), drug treatment of adolescent eating disorders (Couturier and Lock, J Can Acad Child Adolesc Psychiatry 2007;**16**:173–6).

1.15.1 ANOREXIA NERVOSA (AN)

Symptoms:

The main diagnostic symptoms of anorexia nervosa are:

- Amenorrhoea in females (absence of three consecutive menstrual cycles).
- Refusal to maintain body weight over the minimum normal for age and height.
- Intense fear of gaining weight or becoming fat.
- Disturbance in body perception, e.g. feeling fat even when emaciated.

Anorexia usually starts in the late teens, with distorted body image and relentless dieting. Patients may avoid carbohydrates, induce vomiting, abuse laxatives, take excess exercise, binge eat and suffer depression and social withdrawal. It may occur in up to 8–13 per 100 000 population, and 90% are female. Psychotherapy may be useful but with only a few small trials is unproven (s = 6, Hay et al, Cochrane Database Syst Rev 2003;**4**:CD003909).

Role of drugs

Drug therapy is generally most useful as a supportive measure to treat any concurrent conditions. In severely emaciated patients, enteral feeding or even TPN may be necessary. **Reviews:** * overall management (Herpertz-Dahlmann and Salbach-Andrae, Child Adolesc Psychiatr Clin N Am 2009;**18**:131–45), systematic review (s = 32, Bulik et al, Int J Eat Disord 2007;**40**:310–20), genetics (Bulik et al, Annu Rev Nutr 2007;**27**:263–75), adolescent eating disorders: definitions, symptomatology, epidemiology and comorbidity (Herpertz-Dahlmann, Child Adolesc Psychiatr Clin N Am 2009; **18**:31–47), use of SGAs (McKnight and Park, Eur Eat Disord Rev 2010;**18**:10–21), in adolescents (Herpertz-Dahlmann and Salbach-Andrae, Child Adolesc Psychiatr Clin N Am 2009;**18**:131–45.

● Unlicensed/some efficacy

Nutritional feeding

TPN may be necessary in severely anorexic patients where life-threatening weight loss has occurred, particularly if accompanied by low potassium levels and where conventional therapies have failed. Weight gain can be significant in a relatively short period. TPN, with great care (review by Golden and Meyer, Int J Adolesc Med Health 2004;**16**:131–44) and supervised oral feeding with nutritional supplements can be effective. Osteoporosis (Misra and Klibanski, Rev Endocr Metab Disord 2006; **7**:91–9) and osteopenia can be frequent and severe complications (Golden, Adolesc Med 2003;**14**:97–108). Vitamin D and calcium supplements are essential.

Reviews: * medical complications (Mitchell and Crow, Curr Opin Psychiatry 2006;**19**:438–43), tube feeding and nutrition (Gentile et al, Clin Nutr 2010;**29**:627–32; Rigaud et al, Presse Med 2009;**38**:1739–45).

Treatment of any PMS

This may help any premenstrual exacerbations.

■ Unlicensed/possible efficacy

Antipsychotics *

A review of SGAs in AN has concluded that the data is inconclusive (RCT = 4, open = 5, cases = 26, McKnight and Park, Eur Eat Disord Rev 2010;**18**:10–21).

There are some reports that OCD and AN may respond to **olanzapine** 5 mg/d, with reduced fixed body perceptions and improved insight (e.g. n = 20, open, 10/52, Powers et al, Int J Eat Disord 2002;**32**:146–54; n = 1, Tateno et al, Psychiatry Clin Neurosci 2008;**62**:752), and, although a review concludes that olanzapine 2.5–15 mg/d promotes weight gain and may have benefits on psychological symptoms, there are no RCTs (Dunican and DelDotto, Ann Pharmacother 2007;**41**:111–5). It has been used successfully in combination with psychotherapy for adolescent AN (e.g. n = 1, Dadi-Hero et al, Psychiatr Danub 2009;**21**:122–5). **Risperidone** has been used (Newman-Toker, J Am Acad Child Adolesc Psychiatry 2000;**39**:941–2).

Aripiprazole has been used to treat psychosis in AN where weight gain from antipsychotics has been an issue (e.g. n = 5, Trunko et al, Int J Eat Disord 2011;**44**:269–75; n = 1, Aragona, Eat Weight Disord 2007;**12**:54–7). Low-dose **haloperidol** has been suggested as an adjunct in severe AN (n = 13, open, 6/12, Cassano et al, Int J Eat Disord 2003;**33**:172–7). **Quetiapine** 150–300 mg/d has improved some general psychiatric symptoms in anorexia (n = 19 [c = 14], open, 10/52, Powers et al, Int J Eat Disord 2007;**40**:21–6), and TAU plus quetiapine 100–400 mg/d was superior to TAU for a range of AN key symptoms (n = 33, RCT, open, 12/52–1 year, Court et al, J Psychiatr Res 2010;**44**:1027–34).

Reviews: review (s = 4, Court et al, Eat Disord 2008;**16**:217–23), in children and adolescents (Mehler-Wex et al, Eur Eat Disord Rev 2008; **16**:100–8).

Antidepressants (see also fluoxetine)

There is some evidence that serotonergic control of the anterior pituitary function and impaired adrenal function occurs in AN (n = 12, Mondelli et al, Psychoneuroendocrinology 2006;**31**:1139–48). **Citalopram** 20 mg/d has been used successfully (e.g. n = 52, RCT, Fassino et al, Eur Neuropsychopharmacol 2002; **12**:453–9).

Zinc

Zinc has virtually no side-effects. A four-week trial may help some people (e.g. Acta Psychiatr Scand 1990;**82**:14–7), and 100 mg/d produced an increase in BMI twice that of placebo (n = 35, RCT, Birmingham et al, Int J Eat Disord 1994; **15**:251–5). 14 mg/d for two months has been advocated as routine in all people with AN (Birmingham and Gritzner, Eat Weight Disord 2006;**11**:109–11; review by Su and Birmingham, Eat Weight Disord 2002;**7**:20–2).

✻ Case reports

- **Mirtazapine** * (n = 1, Safer et al, Int J Eat Disord 2011;**44**:178–81; n = 1, Jaafar et al, Aust N Z J Psychiatry 2007;**41**:768–9).
- **Mirtazapine + olanzapine** (n = 1, 6/12, Wang et al, Prog Neuropsychopharmacol Biol Psychiatry 2006;**30**:306–9).

- **Sertraline** 50 mg/d (n = 1, Roberts and Lydiard, Am J Psychiatry 1993; **150**:1753).
- **Tramadol** 225 mg/d (n = 1, Mendelson, Am J Psychiatry 2001;**158**:963–94).

□ No efficacy

Fluoxetine

In an important trial, fluoxetine had no advantage over placebo in anorexia following weight restoration (n = 93, RCT, d/b, p/c, < 1 year, Walsh et al, JAMA 2006;**295**:2605–12).

Topiramate

Topiramate caused relapse of anorexia in a patient when used for epilepsy (n = 1, Rosenow et al, Am J Psychiatry 2002;**159**:2112–3).

1.15.2 BULIMIA NERVOSA (BN)

Symptoms

The main diagnostic symptoms of bulimia nervosa are:

- Recurrent binge eating, including lack of control.
- An urge to overeat (including lack of control of eating during binges).
- Regular self-induced vomiting, laxative abuse, strict dieting or fasting.
- Persistent over-concern with body shape and weight.

There must be a minimum of two binge episodes per week for at least three months. Weight and menses are normal. The prevalence rates are about 1% for young women and 0.1% for young men. Mu-opioid receptor binding in bulimic women is lower than in healthy women in the left insular cortex, the area involved in processing taste, as well as the anticipation and reward of eating (n = 16, Bencherif et al, J Nucl Med 2005;**46**:1349–51).

Role of drugs

Cochrane concludes that all antidepressants appear equally effective compared to placebo, but with a high drop-out rate (Bacaltchuk and Hay, Cochrane Database Syst Rev 2003;**4**:CD003391; review by Morgan, EBMH 2002;**5**:75–6) and do not work as antidepressants. Adequate doses are needed, e.g. at least 150 mg/d equivalent of a tricyclic for adequate duration, e.g. at least four weeks. Side-effects (especially anticholinergic) can be severe and result in non-compliance. Drugs should be part of an individualised programme with nutrition and CBT the most effective interventions, although Cochrane concludes that the evidence for the efficacy of CBT in bulimia is small and of variable quality (s = 48, n = 3054, Hay et al, Cochrane Database Syst Rev 2009;**4**:CD000562).

Reviews: * general (Hay and Claudino, Clin Evid (Online) 2010;**2010**:1009; Shapiro et al, Int J Eat Disord 2007;**40**:321–36).

BNF listed

Fluoxetine *

Fluoxetine 60mg/d has a significant effect on binge-eating and purging, eating attitudes, behaviour and food craving, e.g. it was superior to placebo as maintenance therapy, albeit with a high drop-out rate (eg. n = 150, RCT, 12/12, Romano et al, Am J Psychiatry 2002;**159**:96–102; review by Palmer, EBMH 2002;**120**:120). Fluoxetine may also be effective in adolescent bulimia (n = 10, open, 8/52, Kotler et al, J Child Adolesc Psychopharmacol 2003;**13**:329–35), but may have no benefit over a year once weight has been restored (n = 93, RCT, d/b, p/c, 12/12, Walsh et al, JAMA 2006;**295**:2605–12). Patients who fail to report at least a 60% decrease in binge-eating or vomiting by week 3 are unlikely to respond to fluoxetine (s = 2, n = 785, Sysko et al, Psychol Med 2010;**40**:999–1005). It does not work purely as an antidepressant, as the improvement is independent of depression scores and needs higher doses. Its long half-life may help with missed doses.

● Unlicensed/some efficacy

SSRIs (see also fluoxetine above)

Citalopram may be useful for depressed patients with bulimia (n = 37, RCT, s/b, Leombruni et al, Adv Ther 2006;**23**:481–94). **Fluvoxamine** 200mg/d may reduce binge-eating and purging and may be well tolerated (e.g. n = 12, RCT, p/c, 12/52, Milano et al, Adv Ther 2005;**22**:178–83). **Paroxetine** has been reputed to have no beneficial effect in an unpublished study. **Sertraline** was significantly

superior to placebo in most measures in two short studies (n = 34, RCT, d/b, 6/52, McElroy et al, Am J Psychiatry 2000;**157**:1004–6; n = 18, open, 8/52, Sloan et al, Int J Eat Dis 2004; **36**:48–54).

Topiramate

There is growing interest in topiramate in bulimia. A systematic analysis has suggested topiramate is effective for the short-term treatment of BN but long-term use is unproven (s = 5, Arbaizar et al, Gen Hosp Psych 2008;**30**:471–5). Two RCTs have shown that topiramate (median 100mg/d, range 25–400) may significantly improve binge and purge symptoms of BN (n = 64, RCT, p/c, Hoopes et al, J Clin Psychiatry 2003;**64**:1335–41, ibid 1449–54; MS; n = 60, RCT, d/b, p/c, 10/52, Nickel et al, Int J Eat Disord 2005;**38**:295–300). There has been a case series where topiramate was almost completely successful in stopping binging and purging in three patients with comorbid mood disorders, but was ineffective in two (n = 5, Barbee, Int J Eat Disord 2003;**33**:469–72).

■ Unlicensed/possible efficacy

Buspirone

Buspirone may have similar efficacy to fluoxetine in short-term management of bulimic symptoms (n = 57, open, 12/52, Rajewski and Rybakowski, Psychiatr Pol 2006;**40**:75–82).

Lamotrigine

Lamotrigine has been used to treat bulimia with comorbid bipolar (Rybakowski and Kaminska, Prog Neuropsychopharmacol 2008;**32**:2004–5).

MAOIs

MAOIs can be useful drugs if the dietary restrictions can be overcome.

Ondansetron

Ondansetron was reported to be effective in three small, short-term trials by one group of investigators, and may be an option after failure of conventional therapies (reviews by Fung and Ferrill, Ann Pharmacother 2001;**35**:1270–3; Generali and Cada, Hosp Pharm 2001;**36**:547–52;572). Decreased binge-eating and vomiting has been shown with ondansetron 24 mg/d, possibly due to pharmacological decrease in vagal neuro-transmission (n = 28, RCT, Faris et al, Lancet 2000;**355**:792–7; editorial by Kiss, Lancet 2000;**355**:769–70).

Oxcarbazepine

Oxcarbazepine has been used for self-mutilating bulimic patients (Cordas et al, Int J Neuropsychopharmacol 2006;**9**:769–71).

PMS treatments

Pyridoxine and progesterones may help to minimise the effects of premenstrual relapses.

Reboxetine

Reboxetine 4 mg/d has produced a rapid response (50% decrease in bulimic behaviour) in 60% patients (n = 28, RCT, 3/12, Fassino et al, J Psychopharmacol 2004;**18**:423–8).

Stimulants

In women with comorbid ADHD and bulimia, complete response in binge eating has been reported with psychostimulants (n = 6, Dukarm, J Women's Health [Larchmt] 2005;**14**:345–50).

Tricyclics

Many tricyclics, e.g. amitriptyline have been used but poor relapse rates suggest serious limitations with long-term efficacy (RCT, d/b, p/c, 6/12, Walsh et al, Am J Psychiatry 1991; **148**:1206–12).

❊ Case reports ❊

- **Aripiprazole** ❊ (n = 3 Trunko et al, Int J Eat Disord 2010;**44**:269–75).
- **Duloxetine** 120 mg/d (n = 1, Hazen and Fava, J Psychopharmacol 2006;**20**:723–4; n = 1, Christensen and Averbuch, Psychiatry (Edgmont) 2009;**6**:27–8).
- **Flutamide** 500 mg/d (n = 2, Bergman and Eriksson, Acta Psychiatr Scand 1996;**94**:137–9).
- **Naltrexone** + fluoxetine (n = 1, Neumeister et al, Am J Psychiatry 1999;**156**:797).

◆ Others

Other drugs tried include **naltrexone** (n = 19, RCT, Marrazzi et al, Int Clin Psychopharmacol

1995;**10**:163–72), **trazodone** (n = 42, RCT, Pope et al, J Clin Psychopharmacol 1989;**9**:254–9), val**proate** (Tachibana et al, Jpn J Psychiatry Neurol 1989;**43**:77–84).

□ No efficacy

Carbamazepine

No effect was seen in one study (n = 6, Safai-Kutti and Kutti, Am J Psychiatry 1983;**140**:1225–6).

Clozapine

There is a case of bulimia acutely worsening on clozapine 350 mg/d (Brewerton and Shannon, Am J Psychiatry 1992;**149**:1408).

Cyproheptadine

Cyproheptadine appears to be detrimental in bulimia (n = 72, RCT, d/b, Halmi et al, Arch Gen Psychiatry 1986; **43**:177–81).

Lithium

Despite early enthusiasm, lithium appears no more effective than placebo (n = 91, Hsu et al, J Nerv Mental Dis 1991;**179**:351–5).

Mianserin

No effect was seen at 60 mg/d (n = 50, 8/52, Sabine et al, Br J Clin Pharmacol 1983;**15**:S195–S202).

1.15.3 BINGE-EATING DISORDER (BED)

Symptoms

BED is characterised by binge-eating large amounts of food in discrete time periods, which is not then followed by compensatory behaviours such as purging or vomiting. BED is a chronic condition (mean duration 14 years, n = 888, Pope et al, Am J Psychiatry 2006;**163**:2181–3), with a longer duration than bulimia or anorexia. Many (but not all) patients are obese and may seek treatment for this. CBT is effective for behavioural and psychological features of BED but not for the obesity (n = 108 [c = 86], RCT, 16/52, d/b, p/c, Grilo et al, Biol Psychiatry 2005;**57**:301–9). Higher than expected rates of comorbid psychiatric conditions, especially depression, are seen.

Role of drugs

A meta-analysis of p/c trials concluded that pharmacotherapy had a clinical advantage over placebo for achieving short-term remission and weight-loss from BED, but there was no data for a long-term effect. Combining with psychotherapy does not enhance the effect (s = 33, p/c, Reas and Grilo, *Obesity (Silver Spring)* 2008;**16**:2024–38). Studies on desipramine, fluvoxamine, fluoxetine, sertraline, citalopram, dexfenfluramine, sibutramine and topiramate have shown some efficacy. An open trial of venlafaxine suggested a role.

Reviews: * general (Mathes *et al, Appetite* 2009; **52**:545–53; Yager, *Am J Psychiatry* 2008;**165**:4–6; Araujo *et al, World J Biol Psychiatry* 2010;**11**:199-207), pharmacotherapy (Reas and Grilo, *Obesity (Silver Spring)* 2008;**16**:2024–38; Stafano *et al, Eat Behav* 2008;**9**:129–36).

● Unlicensed/some efficacy

Atomoxetine

Atomoxetine 40–120mg/d was fairly well tolerated and significantly reduced binge-eating ratings (n = 40[c = 36], RCT, d/b, p/c, 10/52, McElroy *et al, J Clin Psychiatry* 2007; **68**:390–8).

SSRIs (see also 'no efficacy')

The SSRIs seem to have some efficacy. **Citalopram** may be effective in reducing binge-eating frequency, weight and severity (n = 38, RCT, d/b, p/c, 6/52, McElroy *et al, J Clin Psychiatry* 2003;**64**:807–13). **Sertraline** 100–200mg/d and fluoxetine 40–80mg/d were equally effective for measures of BED (n = 42, RCT, d/b, 6/12, Leombruni *et al, Prog Neuropsychopharmacol Biol Psychiatry* 2008;**32**:1599–605). **Fluoxetine** (mean dose 71mg/d) was well tolerated and effective in reducing binge-eating frequency, weight and illness severity (n = 60, RCT, d/b, 6/52, Arnold *et al, J Clin Psychiatry* 2002;**63**:1028–33), but had a low impact on BED symptoms compared to individualised CBT (n = 116, > 2 years, Devlin *et al, Obesity [Silver Spring]* 2007; **15**:1702–9).

Lamotrigine

Lamotrigine had a significant effect on all measures of BED in one study, but unfortunately placebo had an exceptionally high placebo response, which may have disguised any effect, or not, as the case may be (n = 51, RCT, d/b, p/c, 16/52, Guerdjikova *et al, Int Clin Psychopharmacol* 2009;**24**:150–8).

Lithium

In comorbid bipolar and BED, lithium has helped augment topiramate (n = 12, open, Kotwal *et al, Hum Psychopharmacol* 2006; **21**:425–31).

Memantine

Memantine 5–20mg/d may reduce binge-eating in BED but has little effect on BMI (n = 19[c = 9], open, 12/52, Brennan *et al, Int J Eat Disord* 2008;**41**:520–6), and the effect may be complete within 24 hours, possibly blocking leptin response (n = 5, Hermanussen and Tresguerres, *Econ Hum Biol* 2005;**3**:329–37).

Reboxetine

Reboxetine 8mg/d has produced a remarkable reduction in binge days per week, decreased BMI and improved other measures (n = 9[c = 5], open, 12/52, Silveira *et al, Eat Weight Disorder* 2005;**10**:93–6).

Sibutramine

Two RCTs have shown sibutramine 15mg/d to reduce binge episodes, weight and mental state (n = 60, RCT, d/b, p/c, 12/52, Appolinario *et al, Arch Gen Psychiatry* 2003;**60**:1109–16) and superior to placebo for reducing measures of BED (binges, weight, psychopathology) but with significant ADRs (n = 304, RCT, d/b, p/c, 24/52, Wilfley *et al, Am J Psychiatry* 2008;**165**:51–8).

Topiramate

A systematic analysis has suggested that topiramate is effective for the short-term treatment of BED but long-term use is unproven (s = 5, Arbaizar *et al, Gen Hosp Psychiatry* 2008;**30**:471–5). Some of these studies included topiramate at up to 600mg/d producing an enduring improvement in some patients with BED, albeit poorly tolerated, with a high drop-out rate (e.g. n = 61, 14 + 42/52, RCT, d/b, p/c, McElroy *et al, J Clin Psychiatry* 2004; **65**:1463–9). Adjunctive topiramate 200mg/d improved the short-term efficacy of CBT (n = 73, RCT, d/b, p/c, 21/52, Claudino *et al, J Clin*

Psychiatry 2007;**68**:1324–32) and topiramate has produced binge-eating remission in 58% (cf 29% on placebo) with 30% drop-out in both groups (n = 394, McElroy et al, Biol Psychiatry 2007;**61**:1039–48).

Reviews: * general (Leombruni et al, Neuropsychiatr Dis Treat 2009;**5**:385–92; Tata and Kockler, Ann Pharmacother 2006;**40**:1993–7).

■ **Unlicensed/possible efficacy**

Acamprosate *
Acamprosate was not statistically different to placebo but all measures improved (n = 40, RCT, d/b, p/c, 10/52, McElroy et al, Int J Eat Disord 2011;**44**:81–90).

Sodium oxybate *
Oxybate (mean 7 g/d) appeared very effective for BED but with a high drop-out rate (n = 12 [c = 5], open, 16/52, McElroy et al, Int J Eat Disord 2011;**44**:262–8).

Zonisamide
Zonisamide 100–600 mg/d may significantly reduce binge-eating frequency and other measures (n = 15 [c = 8], open, 12/52, McElroy et al, J Clin Psychiatry 2004;**65**:50–6).

✱ **Case reports ***

• Duloxetine * 120 mg/d (n = 1, Bernardi and Pallanti, J Psychopharmacol 2010;**24**:1269–72).

□ **No efficacy**

Fluvoxamine (see also SSRIs)
Fluvoxamine was no better than placebo in BED (n = 20, RCT, d/b, p/c, Pearlstein et al, Arch Women Ment Health 2003;**6**:147–51).

GILLES DE LA TOURETTE
see Tourette's syndrome (1.28)

1.16 INSOMNIA

Insomnia, the difficulty in initiating or maintaining sleep, is generally a symptom of a condition, not an illness itself and should always be treated as such. Insomnia can be caused by a variety of external (e.g. environment) and internal stimuli

(e.g. mental health problems, e.g. ADHD, stress, emotional conflict, physical illness and drugs, see 5.15), and can be transient, chronic, initial or with early morning wakening. The causes, where possible, should be determined and treated, as well as placing emphasis on sleep hygiene.

Principles of sleep hygiene:
1. Avoid excessive use of caffeine (particularly within 3–4 hours of going to bed), alcohol or nicotine. A hot milky drink may help.
2. Do not stay in bed for prolonged periods if not asleep. Go to another dimly lit room — watching TV can have an alerting effect.
3. Avoid daytime naps or long periods of inactivity.
4. A warm bath or exercise a few hours before bedtime may promote sleep.
5. Avoid engaging in strenuous exercise or mental activity near bedtime (although sex can aid sleep).
6. Make sure that the bed and bedroom are comfortable and avoid extremes of noise, temperature and humidity.
7. Establish a regular bedtime routine, e.g. going to bed at the same time and rising at the same time every morning, regardless of sleep duration.
8. Diet — carbohydrate (e.g. pasta, etc) helps sleep, but not eating a big meal within about two hours of going to bed. Sugar may inhibit sleep, as may some vitamin supplements.

Role of drugs *
Assuming sleep hygiene is good, any hypnotics should always be used on a PRN basis, as tolerance may develop to the sedative effects within 2–3 weeks, especially with the benzodiazepines. Short-term use for short-term reasons is usually without problem and can be very useful and comforting for the patient. Longer-term use needs the risk:benefit analysis considered carefully. The principles of sleep hygiene should be discussed and any problems corrected before prescribing hypnotics. A meta-analysis has concluded that benzodiazepines and non-benzodiazepines are superior to placebo (s = 105, RCTs, d/b, p/c, Buscemi et al, J Gen Intern Med 2007;**22**:1335-50). Anyone who has ever taken an hypnotic would know the differences between the Z hypnotics and the BDZs, but NICE failed to recognise

this (see fervent rebuffs to NICE by Nutt, *J Psychopharmacol* 2005;**19**:125–7 and Alford and Verster, *J Psychopharmacol* 2005;**19**:129–32). About 30% older people prescribed BDZs or Zs may still be taking them two months later, but since they seem to be effective it may be that effort should go into avoiding long-term use, rather than stopping short-term for treatment of some symptoms of mania, anxiety and depression (n = 129, Simon and Ludman, *Gen Hosp Psychiatry* 2006;**28**:374–8).

Reviews: * BAP Guidelines for treatment of insomnia, parasomnias and circadian rhythm disorders (Wilson *et al, J Psychopharmacol* 2010;**24**:1577–1600), comparison of newer agents (Zammit, *Drug Saf* 2009;**32**:735–48), general (Wilson and Nutt, *Prescriber* 2008;**19**:14–24; Passarella and Duong, *Am J Health Syst Pharm* 2008;**65**:927–34; Bhat *et al, Expert Opin Pharmacother* 2008;**9**:351–62), melatonin agonists (Ferguson *et al, Expert Rev Neurother* 2010;**10**:305–18), circadian rhythms and pharmacological management of insomnia (Richardson *et al, Am J Manag Care* 2007;**13**[5 Suppl]:S125–8), melatonin agonists modes of action (Srinivasan *et al, Int J Neurosci* 2009;**119**:821–46).

BNF listed

BENZODIAZEPINES

Benzodiazepines may be extremely useful in the short-term management of insomnia, helping to facilitate essential high-quality sleep. A meta-analysis indicated benzodiazepines are effective in improving sleep latency and duration but ADRs (e.g. drowsiness and dizziness) are common, although methodologically these studies are flawed. Users of benzodiazepines are at greater risk of road-traffic accidents, especially if combined with alcohol (s = 27, Rapoport *et al, J Clin Psychiatry* 2009;**70**:663-73). Although relatively safe in over-dose, BDZs (especially flunitrazepam and nitrazepam) have been implicated in 39% of drug poisoning suicides in Sweden from 1992–1996, so care is needed (Carlsten *et al, Scand J Public Health* 2003;**31**:224–28). Withdrawal of long-term BDZ hypnotics may improve cognitive functioning in the elderly (n = 104, d/b, one year; Curran *et al, Psychol Med* 2003;**33**:1223–37;

comment by Furukawa, *EBMH* 2004;**7**:46, noting a high drop-out rate).

Flunitrazepam

This longer-acting benzodiazepine may have an abuse potential, including in combination with other drugs, and is probably under-rated in this respect, especially in forensic settings (Daderman and Edman, *Psychiatry Res* 2001; **103**:27–42).

Flurazepam

Flurazepam is a benzodiazepine with a short half-life but with longer-acting metabolites that can cause hangover in older people (n = 25, RCT, d/bb, p/c, c/o, Boyle *et al, Hum Psychopharmacol* 2009;**24**:61–71).

Loprazolam

Loprazolam is an intermediate-acting benzo-diazepine with a half-life of 7–15 hours.

Lormetazepam

Lormetazepam is an intermediate acting benzo-diazepine. Short-term use has no effect on daytime vigilance or motor task performance and it may produce minimal psychomotor impairment in younger adults (n = 18, RCT, d/b, p/c, Fabbrini *et al, Clin Ther* 2005;**27**:78–83).

Predicting hypnotic dependence risk
(Tyrer, *Br Med J* 1993;**306**:706–8)

Factor	Score
Benzodiazepine hypnotic used	3
Dose higher than BNF mean	2
Duration of treatment > 3 months	2
Dependent personality	2
Short elimination half-life drug	2
Tolerance or dose escalation	2
Total	
No dependence, abrupt withdrawal	=0
Some dependence risk, withdraw over two weeks recommended	=1–4
Strong dependence risk, withdraw over 4–12 weeks	=5–8
High risk of dependence, withdraw gradually plus support programme	=8–13

Nitrazepam

Nitrazepam is a longer-acting benzodiazepine similar to diazepam, which has active meta-bolites. Stable plasma levels can be attained in five days, so avoid use in the elderly.

Temazepam

Temazepam is a shorter-acting benzodiazepine, whose abuse potential has been well recognised. 7.5 mg and 15 mg appear equally effective (n = 131, RCT, d/b, Erman et al, Curr Med Res Opin 2004;**20**:441–9).

'Z' HYPNOTICS

The 'Z' hypnotics are now widely used and offer many benefits over the benzodiazepines. NICE in the UK concluded that there was nothing to chose between 'Z' hypnotics and the hypnotic benzodiazepines, a conclusion that has been hotly disputed (see introduction) and not reviewed by NICE. **Zolpidem** is potent and quick-acting (often within 15 minutes) and ideal for initiating sleep and has many fans in the pharmaceutical and medical worlds. **Zopiclone** and the benzodiazepines have a slower onset but longer action. A large review concluded that the incidence of dependence with zopiclone and zolpidem is remarkably lower than hypnotic BDZs, and that they are relatively safe (n = 58, Hajak et al, Addiction 2003;**98**:1371–8).
Reviews: * comparative kinetics and dynamics (Drover, Clin Pharmacokinet 2004;**43**:227–38), comparative tolerability of 'Z' hypnotics (Terzano et al, Drug Saf 2003;**26**:261–82), comprehensive (s = 24, n = 3909, Dundar et al, Hum Psychopharmacol 2004;**19**:305–22).

Zaleplon

Zaleplon is a pyrazolopyrimidine hypnotic, a selective full agonist at the omega-1 benzodiazepine receptor (Noguchi et al, Eur J Pharmacol 2002;**434**:21–8).

Zolpidem

Zolpidem is a imidazopyridine hypnotic which binds preferentially to the omega-1 benzo-diazepine receptor. It decreases time to sleep and increases total sleep time and efficiency, but does not affect sleep architecture. It has a rapid onset of action and a short duration.

It has been shown to be at least as effective as zopiclone, with less rebound on discontinuation and is better tolerated, e.g. no metallic taste (n = 479, d/b, 14/7, Tsutsui et al, J Int Med Res 2001;**29**:163–77). Zolpidem causes minimal cognitive, memory and equilibrium adverse effects and should be the preferred hypnotic in the elderly (n = 48, RCT, d/b, p/c, c/o, Allain et al, Eur J Clin Pharmacol 2003;**59**:179–88). In a fascinating study, zolpidem 10mg taken at night up to 3–5 times a week significantly improved overall sleep, which was sustained, with no evidence of rebound, dose escalation or withdrawal, showing that true PRN hypnotic use may be highly effective and safe (n = 199, RCT, p/c, 12/52, Perlis et al, J Clin Psychiatry 2004;**65**:1128–37). It is so safe that it can even be taken by athletes the night before an event without adversely affecting performance (n = 7, d/b, p/c, c/o, Ito et al, Neurosci Res 2007;**59**:309–13).
Reviews: * general (Dang et al, CNS Neurosci Ther 2011; in press), kinetics (de Haas et al, J Psychopharmacol 2010;**24**:1619–29).

Zopiclone

Zopiclone is an established and safe non-benzodiazepine hypnotic, albeit only licensed in the UK for up to 7.5 mg/d for four weeks. Zopiclone is equivalent, but not superior, to BDZs (n = 2672, meta-analysis, Holbrook et al, CMAJ 2000;**162**:225–33; reviewed by Furukawa, EBMH 2000;**3**:81). Zopiclone may impair memory storage during sleep (n = 8, d/b, p/c, c/o, Silva et al, Neurosci Res 2003;**47**:241–3).
Review: extensive, including abuse potential (Cimolai, Can Fam Physician 2007;**53**:2124–9).

OTHER HYPNOTICS

Antihistamines

Antihistamines may be effective and are often used as OTC sleep aids. Promethazine has a relatively long half-life and a low abuse potential. Diphenhydramine may have an abuse potential and has been strongly linked to cognitive impairment and decline in older hospitalised patients and is best avoided in this patient group (n = 426, Agoustini et al, Arch Intern Med 2001;**161**:2091–7). However, while causing drowsiness they do not actually lead to a quality or refreshing sleep.

Barbiturates

Barbiturates should only be used for severe, intractable insomnia where there are compelling reasons, and only in patients already taking barbiturates. Toxicity in overdose can be high.

Chloral hydrate

Chloral hydrate has properties similar to the barbiturates and is relatively safe in the elderly as the half-life is not significantly lengthened. An abuse potential exists and it can be toxic in overdose.

Clomethiazole (chlormethiazole)

Clomethiazole is a thiamine derivative with sedative-hypnotic and anticonvulsant properties. It has a rapid onset of action and short half-life even in the elderly, although they may be more sensitive to it. Dependence and abuse has been reported, but is not considered too important if the patient is not dependence prone (n = 5, Hession et al, Lancet 1979;ii:953–4). It is unsafe in overdose.

Melatonin CR (Circadin PR®) *

Melatonin is an agonist at M1, M2 and M3 receptors. Circadin® (Lundbeck) is the only melatonin product licensed in the UK, as a monotherapy course up to 13 weeks for primary insomnia in people aged 55 and over (although it also works in under 55s; n = 791 [c = 746], RCT, d/b, p/c, 7/12, Wade et al, Curr Med Res Opin 2011;27:87–98). The dose is 2 mg 1–2 hours before bedtime and after food (which slows absorption). The PR tablets contain a synthetic melatonin, which is released over several hours to match the normal human melatonin profile (increasing after dark, peaking at 2–4.00 AM, then diminishing), as older people with primary insomnia secrete significantly lower levels of melatonin than healthy elderly with good sleep quality. Pineal melatonin is synthesized and secreted in close association with the light/dark cycle (review, Srinivasan et al, Int J Neurosci 2009;119:821–46) and melatonin receptors may in fact only be expressed for a few hours. PR-melatonin 2 mg significantly improves sleep quality, morning alertness, sleep

onset and quality of life in primary insomnia (n = 354 [c = 334], RCT, d/b, p/c, 5/52, Wade et al, Curr Med Res Opin 2007;23:2597–2605), with no withdrawal symptoms on discontinuation (n = 170 [c = 164], RCT, d/b, p/c, 7/52, Lemoine et al, J Sleep Res 2007;16:372–80) and improved perceived quality of sleep (n = 40, RCT, d/b, p/c, 6/52, Luthringer et al, Int Clin Psychopharmacol 2009;24:239–49), including in shift workers (n = 86, RCT, d/b, p/c, c/o, Sadeghniiat-Haghighi et al, J Circadian Rhythms 2008;6:10). Both sleep and depression can improve (n = 33 [c = 31], RCT, d/b, p/c, 4/52, Serfaty et al, Int Clin Psychopharmacol 2010;25:132–42). Adjunctive melatonin can also help older people discontinue conventional hypnotics (n = 22, RCT, d/b, c/o, 4/12, Garzón et al, Aging Clin Exp Res 2009;21:38–42) and significantly improve sleep efficiency in chronic schizophrenics with poor sleep (n = 40, RCT, d/b, p/c, 15/7, Kumar et al, J Clin Psychiatry 2007;68:237–41). Circadin is well tolerated, with low drop-outs in clinical trials, and is not associated with impairment of memory, vigilance, and driving performance as compared with placebo, has no discernible withdrawal symptoms and, in older adults (>55), causes no impaired function or cognitive performance compared to zolpidem (n = 16, RCT, d/b, p/c, c/o, Otmani et al, Hum Psychopharmacol 2008;23:693–705). Any loss in efficacy over time may be due to slower metabolism (1A2) and subsequent accumulation and toxicity, so it would be best to lower the dose (n = 3, Braam et al, J Intellect Disabil Res 2010;54:547–55).

Review: use for insomnia in over 55s (Wade and Downie, Expert Opin Investig Drugs 2008; 17:1567–72).

Triclofos

Triclofos is a chloral-related drug with similar actions to chloral but with less gastric irritation and a more palatable taste. It is only available as a liquid in the UK and indicated for short-term treatment of severe resistant insomnia.

● Unlicensed/some efficacy

Other sedative drugs the patient may already be taking, especially antipsychotics and antidepressants, may be prescribed as a single dose at night. In longer-term therapy most can be given this way. It is also important to avoid the use of 'stimulating' drugs at night, e.g. anticholinergics and MAOIs, although again these are only causing sedation, not aiding quality or refreshing sleep, e.g. they may disrupt REM sleep. If using antidepressants, a review suggests choosing sedating ones over activating ones, low anticholinergic effects, HT2A or 2C blockers over pure histamine blockers and use the lowest dose possible (e.g. doxepin 25 mg, mirtazapine 15 mg, trazodone 50 mg, trimipramine 25 mg; Wiegand, *Drugs* 2008;**68**:2411–7).

Agomelatine *

Agomelatine can help sleep if caused by MDD (reviewed by Quera-Salva et al, *Hum Psychopharmacol* 2010;**25**:222–9.

Doxepin *

Doxepin 1 mg, 3 mg and 6 mg may be superior to placebo for improving objective and subjective sleep measures in primary insomnia, with no apparent ADRs or residual effects (n = 67, RCT, d/b, c/o, Roth et al, *Sleep* 2007;**30**:1555–61). In transient insomnia in healthy adults, doxepin 6 mg has shown significant benefits on sleep onset, maintenance, duration and quality (n = 565, RCT, d/b, p/c, Roth et al, *Sleep Med* 2010;**11**:843–7). In older adults, doxepin 1–3 mg at night significantly improved most sleep parameters with no residual effects the next day (n = 240, RCT, d/b, p/c, 12/52, Krystal et al, *Sleep* 2010;**33**:1553–61).

Reviews: * general (Goforth, *Expert Opin Pharmacother* 2009;**10**:1649–55; Weber et al, *CNS Drugs* 2010;**24**:713–20).

Mirtazapine

Insomnia is reported by 90% depressed patients, but stimulation of 5-HT$_2$ receptors is thought to underlie the insomnia and adverse changes in sleep architecture seen with SSRIs/SNRIs. Mirtazapine blocks 5-HT$_2$ receptors and may improve sleep, e.g. 30 mg increased sleep efficiency and decreased wakenings (and their duration), but with no effect on REM (n = 20, RCT, d/b, p/c, 3/7, Aslan et al, *Sleep* 2002;**25**:677–9). Mirtazapine may in fact help normalise abnormal REM sleep (n = 32, Schittecatte et al, *Psychiatry Res* 2002;**109**:1–8),

unlike SSRIs (n = 19, RCT, d/b, 8/52, Winokur et al, *J Clin Psychiatry* 2003;**64**:1224–9).

Quetiapine

Quetiapine 25–10 mg has been shown to improve sleep, probably at least partly through its antihistaminic effects (n = 14, RCT, d/b, p/c, 17/7, Cohrs et al, *Psychopharmacology* 2004;**174**:421–9; see also RCT, d/b, p/c, 3/52, Tassniyom et al, *J Med Assoc Thai* 2010;**93**:729–34).

Review: use in addictive conditions (Terán et al, *Subst Use Misuse* 2008;**43**:2169–71).

Trazodone

A review of trazodone as an hypnotic concluded that, except perhaps in depressed people, there is little or no data on efficacy or tolerability, and no dose-response data for sleep, so more research is needed before use can be considered of lower risk (Mendelson, *J Clin Psychiatry* 2005;**66**:469–76). More recently, 25–150 mg has been shown to be effective (n = 28, open, 3/12, Wichniak et al, *Pol Merkur Lekarski* 2007;**23**:41–6).

■ Unlicensed/possible efficacy

Alcohol

Alcohol is not recommended for routine use as a hypnotic because, although it causes sedation, it increases slow-wave sleep, reduces and disrupts REM sleep, the diuretic effect may be counter-productive and overdose can have serious consequences. Rebound arousal can occur with higher doses when blood concentrations reach zero, leading to awakening. It is, however, widely used as self-medication and is available in a number of highly palatable formulations, e.g. Farmer's, Chalk Hill and anything sold at the Ivy House, Stradbroke. Interestingly, ageing Scotch whisky upregulates GABA receptors more than younger or blended Scotch (regardless of ethanol concentration), and is better at calming and inducing sleep (Koda et al, *J Agriculture Food Chem* 2003;**51**:5238–44). Reasonable quantities of Spanish beer can also provide sufficient melatonin (and the higher the alcohol content, the more the melatonin) to increase the human body's antioxidant capacity (n = 1, b = 18, Maldonado et al, *Clin Nutr* 2009;**28**:188–91).

Cherry tart juice beverage *

Chronic insomnia in older people can respond to Cherry tart juice beverage, albeit with a modest effect (n = 15, RCT, d/b, p/c, 2×2/52, Pigeon et al, J Med Food 2010;**13**:579–83).

Donepezil

Anticholinesterases have been shown to improve REM sleep in younger adults and also in elderly healthy adults (n = 42, d/b, p/c, Schredl et al, Pharmacopsychiatry 2006;**39**:205–8).

Gabapentin *

In alcoholics with persistent insomnia, gabapentin may improve sleep slightly more than trazodone (n = 55, open, 6/52, Karam-Hage and Brower, Psych Clin Neurosci 2003;**57**:542–4), perhaps by enhancing slow-wave sleep and improving sleep quality (n = 18, open, 4/52, Lo et al, Clin Neuropharmacol 2010;**33**:84–90).

Herbal and OTC preparations

There is an extensive review of oral, non-prescription treatments for insomnia, e.g. herbals and others (Meolie et al, J Clin Sleep Med 2005;**1**:173–87), including passionflower, valerian, Jamaican dogwood, hops, Californian poppy, chamomile, lemon balm, St John's wort, kava kava, wild lettuce, skullcap, Patrina root, first-generation histamine-1-receptor antagonists, alcohol, calcium, vitamin A, nicotinamide, magnesium, vitamin B12, tryptophan, 5-hydroxytryptophan, dietary changes, Natrum muriaticum and Yoku-kan-san-ka-chimpi-hange. It concluded that the studies were small, of inadequate design and lacked statistical analysis. There was insufficient data to recommend any, except preliminary but conflicting data on valerian and H1-antagonists. There are significant potential risks for Jamaican dogwood, kava kava, alcohol and tryptophan.

Nicotine

Low concentrations of nicotine can cause mild sedation and relaxation and so a cigarette could help sleep in an anxious person. Higher levels cause arousal and agitation.

Tiagabine

Although tiagabine 4–6 mg was effective in helping insomnia in the elderly (n = 24, RCT, d/b, p/c, Walsh et al, Sleep 2005;**28**:673–6), a second study failed to show any effect (n = 207, RCT, d/b, p/c, Roth et al, Sleep 2006; **29**:335–41).

□ No efficacy

Caffeine

Caffeine competes with the inhibitory neurotransmitter adenosine, causing cortical arousal and decreased sleep. 150 mg before retiring has a marked effect on sleep latency, reduces sleep efficacy and REM periods. Its half-life of five hours means any ingested near bedtime will effect sleep latency. See caffeinism (1.28).

SSRIs

SSRIs can obviously help insomnia caused by depression by treating the root cause but they should not be taken at night as they disrupt REM sleep.

MANIA AND HYPOMANIA

see Bipolar – Mania and hypomania (1.10.2)

1.17 NARCOLEPSY

Symptoms

Narcolepsy is a rare and often misdiagnosed disabling neurological disorder of excessive daytime sleepiness, sleep paralysis, hypnagogic hallucinations, cataplexy (sudden loss of muscle tone provoked by strong emotions, e.g. laughter) and abnormalities in REM sleep. There is a strong genetic linkage, and normally starts in the 20s or 30s. The incidence ranges from one in 1000 to 10 000. Narcolepsy is probably caused by the loss of a relatively few neurons responsible for producing the neuropeptide hypocretin. Other specific symptoms include catalepsy (an abrupt, bilateral loss of skeletal muscle tone), hypnagogic hallucinations (vivid dreams while falling asleep or waking), sleep paralysis and automatic behaviour (unconscious functioning while asleep).

Role of drugs *

The use of stimulants or modafinil is considered first-line treatment, with some antidepressants useful in some resistant cases. The risks of pharmacotherapy are usually outweighed by the risks to the patient of driving, work-place

and other mishaps. The role of oxybate is as yet unclear. However, there is no robust evidence that antidepressants are effective for narcolepsy or improve quality of life (s = 5, n = 246, Vignatelli et al, Cochrane Database Syst Rev 2008;1: CD003724).
Reviews: * general (Ahmed and Thorpy, Clin Chest Med 2010;**31**:371–81; Didato and Nobili, Expert Rev Neurother 2009;**9**:897–910; Mohsenin, Postgrad Med 2009;**121**:99–104), pharmacotherapy (Zaharna et al, Expert Opin Pharmacother 2010;**11**:1633–45), diagnosis (Hohsenin, Postgrad Med 2009;**121**:99–104), newer treatments (Nishino and Okuro, Expert Opin Emerg Drugs 2010;**15**:139–58).

BNF listed

Dexamfetamine

Dexamfetamine acts by enhancing release of noradrenaline, dopamine and serotonin, but the stimulant effect appears to be mainly via dopamine. Dexamfetamine 5–50 mg/d can be highly effective, although doses of 40–60 mg/d have been shown to be more effective than lower doses. If tolerance develops, drug holidays may be necessary. Although dexamfetamine is not immune from problems of chronic stimulant ingestion, many can take it for decades without apparent adverse consequences.

Methylphenidate (unlicensed but BNF listed)

Methylphenidate 2.5–5 mg BD (up to 60 mg/d) can be used (see also dexamfetamine above). Tolerance can be a problem, with drug holidays helpful. It has been considered as good as dexamfetamine and may have a better side-effect profile (reviewed by Challman and Lipsky, Mayo Clin Proc 2000;**75**:711–21).

Modafinil *

Modafinil is now just licensed in UK for symptomatic relief of excessive sleepiness associated with narcolepsy. Its precise mechanism of action is unknown, but it may activate the hippocampus which receives afferents from the hypothalamus, the centre of the sleep–wake rhythm, promoting wakefulness. It significantly increases daytime sleep latency but does not suppress cataplexy. Modafinil offers advantages because of its lack of rebound phenomena after treatment withdrawal and its

low abuse potential. Modafinil 600 mg/d appears the maximum tolerated dose but splitting the doses, e.g. 200 mg BD may help promote wakefulness throughout a day compared to once-daily (s = 2, n = 56, RCT, d/b, Schwartz et al, J Neuropsychiatry Clin Neurosci 2005;**17**:405–12), with no tolerance or withdrawal in a 40-week follow-on (n = 271, RCT, 9/52, Modafinil study group, Neurology 2000;**54**:1166–75). It may also be useful for improving daytime wakefulness in people unresponsive to stimulants (n = 150, open, 6/52, Schwartz et al, Sleep Med 2003;**4**:43–9). A review and meta-analysis concludes that modafinil is effective for excessive daytime sleepiness but not cataplexy (s = 9, n = 1054, RCTs, Golicki et al, Med Sci Monit 2010;**16**:177–86).
Reviews: general (Myrick et al, Ann Clin Psychiatry 2004;**16**:101–9), mode of action (Ballon and Feifel, J Clin Psychiatry 2006;**67**:554–66), pharmacokinetics (Robertson and Hellriegel, Clin Pharmacokinet 2003;**42**:123–37).

Sodium oxybate *

Sodium oxybate is licensed for cataplexy in adults with narcolepsy. Oxybate probably promotes slow (delta) wave sleep consolidating night-time sleep, increasing stage 3 and 4 sleep, reducing the onset of REM sleep. Nocturnal administration of oxybate shows a dose-related improvement in sleep and functional status in people with narcolepsy (n = 285, RCT, d/b, p/c, 4/52, Weaver and Cuellar, Sleep 2006;**29**:1189–94). The starting dose is 4.5 g/d, titrated slowly every two weeks (or longer) up to 9 g/d as a BD dose (bedtime and 2.5–4 hours later, due to its short half-life). If oxybate is stopped for more than 14 days it should be retitrated, although withdrawal symptoms with therapeutic doses are minimal (n = 55, Anon, J Toxicol Clin Toxicol 2003;**41**:131–5). Doses of 4.5, 6 and 9 g at night produce decreases in cataplexy attacks of 57%, 65% and 85% respectively (n = 228, RCT, d/b, p/c, 8/52, Xyrem ISG, Sleep Med 2005;**6**:415–21), and a discontinuation study suggested a long-term efficacy (n = 55, d/b, mean 21/12, US Xyrem MSG, Sleep Med 2004;**5**:119–23). Oxybate 9 g/d and modafinil 200–600 mg/d were both effective for excessive daytime sleepiness and produced additive effects when used together (n=270, RCT, d/b, p/c, 10/52, Black and Houghton, *Sleep* 2006;**29**:939–46). Due to its abuse potential (it is the sodium salt of gamma-hydroxybutyrate [GHB], prescribing is limited to physicians experienced in the treatment of sleep disorders. GHB can be abused for its euphoric and weight loss effects, and its amnesic effect has led to it being used as a date-rape drug (Camacho *et al*, *Am J Drug Alcohol Abuse* 2005;**31**:601–7; Gonzalez and Nutt, *J Psychopharmacol* 2005;**19**:195–204). It has been alleged that the risk of abuse/misuse may have been over-rated and is actually very low (n=26000, Wang *et al*, *J Clin Sleep Med* 2009;**5**:365–71; MS). When switching to oxybate, gradual withdrawal of antidepressants can lead to a short-term increase in cataplexy, especially with TCAs (n=57, Ristanovic *et al*, *Sleep Med* 2009;**10**:416–21).

Reviews: * general (Ahmed and Thorpy, *Clin Chest Med* 2010;**31**:371–81; Owen, *Drugs Today (Barc)* 2008;**44**:197–204), newer treatments (Nishino and Okuro, *Expert Opin Emerg Drugs* 2010;**15**:139–58).

● Unlicensed/some efficacy

Selegiline

Two trials have shown a potent and dose-related effect, at doses of at least 20 mg/d (e.g. n=30, RCT, d/b, p/c, 4/52, Mayer *et al*, *Clin Neuropharmacol* 1995;**18**:306–19), and may be useful in patients who get disturbing side-effects with stimulants.

■ Unlicensed/possible efficacy

SSRIs

These are generally considered less effective than tricyclics but some positive results have been reported with, e.g. fluoxetine (Langdon *et al*, *Sleep* 1986;**9**:371–2).

Tricyclics

Clomipramine and imipramine have been used for cataplexy and sleep paralysis, particularly in stimulant-resistant or intolerant patients. Tricyclic ADRs can be significant and rebound cataplexy can occur with abrupt withdrawal (n=57, 7/52, Ristanovic *et al*, *Sleep Med* 2009;**10**:416–21).

Venlafaxine

Venlafaxine has been used for narcolepsy with cataplexy at 37.5–112.5 mg/d in children (n=6, Møller and Østergaard, *J Child Adolesc Psychopharmacol* 2009;**19**:197–201).

✱ Case reports ✱

- **Donepezil** 10 mg/d (n=1, 3/12, Niederhofer, *J Clin Sleep Med* 2006;**2**:71–2).
- **Tranylcypromine** (n=1, Gernaat *et al*, *Pharmacopsychiatry* 1995;**28**:98–100).
- **Tranylcypromine + modafinil** (n=1, Clemons *et al*, *Sleep Med* 2004;**5**:509–11).

◆ Others

Other drugs used include **codeine** (n=8, RCT, Fry *et al*, *Sleep* 1986;**9**:269–74), and **propranolol** (n=48, 18/12, Meier-Ewart *et al*, *Sleep* 1985;**8**:95–104).

1.18 OBSESSIVE-COMPULSIVE DISORDER (OCD)

Symptoms

OCD probably has a lifetime prevalence of 2–3%, an early onset (childhood or adolescence), and frequently becomes chronic and disabling if untreated. It is characterised by recurrent and intrusive thoughts of compulsive, stereotyped, repetitive behaviour, e.g. recurrent checking, hand-washing, etc. Functioning is impaired by obsessive thoughts and rituals. Resisting these thoughts causes heightened anxiety.

Role of drugs

There is much evidence for the cause of OCD being related to a dysfunctional serotonin system, and SSRIs and clomipramine have been shown to be effective. The available data (meta-analyses/reviews by Ackerman and Greenland, *J Clin Psychopharmacol* 2002;**22**:309–17; Hollander and Kahn, *EBMH* 2003;**6**:23; s=9, n=278, RCT, b/d, Bloch *et al*, *Mol Psychiatry* 2006;**11**:622–32) concludes that:

1. Drug: Only antidepressants affecting the serotonin system are effective:
   - the SSRIs as a class are similarly effective to clomipramine and both are superior to non-serotonergic drugs

- clomipramine is perhaps slightly more effective than SSRIs
- tricyclics (other than clomipramine) and mirtazapine seem ineffective
- concomitant depression does not seem necessary for improvement in obsessive-compulsive symptoms.

2. Dose: The daily dose usually needs to be high, e.g. 250–300 mg clomipramine, or 60–80 mg fluoxetine or paroxetine which, although less well tolerated, are clearly associated with improved efficacy (s = 9, n = 2268, RCT, d/b, p/c, Bloch et al, Mol Psychiatry 2010;[in press]). In resistant OCD, even higher doses may be needed e.g. citalopram up to 120 mg/d, escitalopram up to 50 mg/d, fluoxetine 100 mg/d, paroxetine up to 80 mg/d, sertraline 250–300 mg/d over at least a year (n = 26, retrospective, Pampaloni et al, J Psychopharmacol 2010;**24**:1439–45).

3. Duration: Response is slow and may not occur for many weeks so continue with the maximum tolerated dose of an SSRI for **three months** (25% respond given adequate dose and duration). A minimum of 1–2 years pharmacotherapy is recommended, as relapse is common on discontinuation and the risks of long-term therapy may be outweighed by the risks of relapse and its consequences.

4. Treatment resistance: Switching from an SSRI (paroxetine) to venlafaxine or vice versa if no response may be an effective strategy (n = 150, RCT, d/b, Denys et al, J Clin Psychiatry 2004;**65**:37–43; review by Bhui, EBMH 2004;**7**:114). Failing that, add an antipychotic (best evidence is for risperidone and haloperidol), although only 30% will show a meaningful response.

5. Discontinuation: Very gradual discontinuation over several months is widely recommended.

In the UK, NICE has produced guidance on OCD and uses a stepped care approach. However, this did not emphasise the need to use higher doses for prolonged periods of time. Drugs may only reduce symptomatology by 30–60%, but many patients consider this a significant benefit. The effects of SSRIs may be enhanced by CBT (e.g. 17 sessions, n = 108, RCT, Simpson et al, Am J Psychiatry 2008;**165**:621–30), especially if the CBT is added immediately after drug response (n = 96 [c = 59], RCT, s/b, 12/52, Tenneij et al, J Clin Psychiatry 2005;**66**:1169–75; comment by Cottraux, EBMH 2006;**9**:53).

Reviews: * general (Marazziti and Consoli, Expert Opin Pharmacother 2010;**11**:331–43; Abramowitz et al, Lancet 2009;**374**:491–9; Ravindran et al, Can J Psychiatry 2009;**54**:331–43), BAP evidence-based guidelines (Baldwin et al, J Psychopharmacol 2005;**19**:567–96), BDNF in OCD (Maina et al, J Affect Disord 2010;**122**:174–8), current trends (Decloedt and Stein, Neuropsychiatr Dis Treat 2010;**6**:233–42), drug treatment (Kellner, Dialogues Clin Neurosci 2010;**12**:187–97), IV routes of treatment (Ravindran et al, J Psychopharmacol 2010; **24**:287–96).

BNF listed

Clomipramine

Clomipramine is superior to placebo and non-serotonergic drugs (e.g. n = 122, RCT, d/b, p/c, 12/52, Foa et al, Am J Psychiatry 2005;**162**:151–61; see also review of meta-analyses in introduction).

Escitalopram

Escitalopram is licensed for the treatment of OCD at a dose of 10–20 mg/d. Escitalopram 10 mg/d was as effective as (and better tolerated than) paroxetine 40 mg/d, and escitalopram 20 mg/d was effective as early as six weeks (n = 466, RCT, d/b, p/c, 24/52, Stein et al, Curr Med Res Opin 2007;**23**:701–11). High-dose escitalopram (up to 50 mg/d, mean 34 mg/d) may be needed and is well tolerated and effective in resistant OCD (n = 67 [c = 64], open, 16/52, Rabinowitz et al, Int Clin Psychopharmacol 2008;**23**:49–53). Relapse prevention is well-established, with an NNT for prevention of relapse of 3.3 (s = 4, RCT, d/b, 24/52, Bech et al, J Clin Psychiatry 2010;**71**:121–9).

Fluoxetine

Fluoxetine has shown a significant clinical effect at 20–60 mg/d, developing over 13 weeks, and continuing to be effective for at least nine months with few side-effects (e.g. n = 130, RCT, p/c, 12/12, Romano et al, J Clin Psychopharmacol

2001;**21**:46–52). It may be more effective in washers and with obsessive thoughts rather than checkers (n = 265, Farnam et al, Arch Iran Med 2008;**11**:522–5).

Fluvoxamine

Fluvoxamine has been shown to be partially or very effective in several trials and it may be equivalent to clomipramine but better tolerated (n = 227, RCT, d/b, 10/52, Mundo et al, Hum Psychopharmacol 2001;**16**:461–8).

Paroxetine

Paroxetine is licensed for the symptoms of OCD and for relapse prevention at doses of 40–60 mg (reviews by Owen, Drugs Today (Barc) 2008;**44**:887–93 and Kamijima and Aoki, Expert Rev Neurother 2006;**6**:945–56). Higher doses are necessary, particularly in acute OCD, as 20 mg/d is not effective (n = 348, RCT, d/b, p/c, 12/52, Hollander et al, J Clin Psychiatry 2003; **64**:1113–21).

Sertraline

Sertraline is licensed for OCD in adults and also in children and adolescents (dose: 6–12 years, 25–50 mg/d; for 13–17 years, use the adult dose but with no dose increases after less than a week, and a lower body weight may require lower doses). Sertraline has been shown to be effective in many studies, e.g. slightly more effective than fluoxetine but as well tolerated (n = 150, RCT, d/b, 6/12, Bergeron et al, J Clin Psychopharmacol 2002;**22**:148–54). Rapid titration to 150 mg/d over five days may give a faster onset of action in acute OCD, with similar tolerability to slower (15 days) titration (n = 32, s/b, 12/52, Bogetto et al, Eur Neuropsychopharm 2002;**12**:181–6). Relapse prevention has been shown, with lack of prominent discontinuation symptoms (n = 649[c=223], RCT, 6/12, Koran et al, Am J Psychiatry 2002;**159**:88–95; review by Soomro, EBMH 2002;**5**:115). High-dose sertraline (up to 400 mg/d) may be effective in refractory OCD (n = 66, RCT, d/b, 12/52, Ninan et al, J Clin Psychiatry 2006;**67**:15–22).

+ Combinations of SSRIs/clomipramine

Review: * rationale and use of adjunctive

dopamine antagonists for TR-OCD (Koo et al, Expert Rev Neurother 2010;**10**:275–90).

Antipsychotics + SSRIs/clomipramine *

Cochrane concludes that the data on olanzapine is too limited to draw a conclusion and that quetiapine and risperidone might help SSRI efficacy (s = 11, n = 396[c = 345], RCTs, <6/12, Komossa et al, Cochrane Database Syst Rev 2010;**12**:CD008141). If successful, they should probably continue for at least several months, as relapse on discontinuation is high. **Risperidone** has been shown to be effective as SSRI augmentation at 3 mg/d (e.g. n = 70, RCT, 12/52, McDougle et al, Arch Gen Psychiatry 2000; **57**:794–801; comment by Ramasubbu, Arch Gen Psychiatry 2002;**59**:472–3), and even at really low-dose, e.g. 0.5 mg/d (n = 45, RCT, d/b, p/c, 6/52, Erzeovesi et al, Eur Neuropsychopharmacol 2005;**15**:69–74). For **olanzapine** the only RCT showed no additional advantage of adding olanzapine in fluoxetine-refractory OCD patients (n = 44, RCT, p/c, 6/52, Shapira et al, Biol Psychiatry 2004; **55**:553–5). **Aripiprazole** augmentation of SSRIs in resistant OCD may be well tolerated and effective in completers (c = 30, RCT, d/b, p/c, 16/52, Muscatello et al, J Clin Psychopharmacol 2011;**31**:174–9). **Quetiapine** up to 400 mg/d has some efficacy as an adjunct to SSRIs in resistant OCD (s = 3, n = 102, RCT, d/b, p/c, Fineberg et al, Int Clin Psychopharmacol 2006; **21**:337–43), and starting quetiapine 300–450 mg/d with an SSRI from the start may significantly enhance the number of responses (n = 76[c = 66], RCT, d/b, p/c, 10/52, Vulink et al, J Clin Psychiatry 2009;**70**:1001–8), although quetiapine 400–600 mg/d was ineffective as an adjunct to an SSRI in resistant OCD (n = 40, RCT, d/b, p/c, 12/52, Kordon et al, J Clin Psychopharmacol 2008;**28**:550–4).

Clomipramine + SSRIs

Citalopram plus clomipramine was markedly more effective than clomipramine in treatment-resistant OCD (n = 16, open, 3/12, Pallanti et al, Eur Psychiatry 1999;**14**:101–6) and around 50% people taking clomipramine (after failing at least two SSRIs previously) responded after addition of citalopram up to 60 mg/d (n = 20, 11/12, Marazziti et al, CNS Spectr 2008;**13**:971–6).

Dexamfetamine and caffeine + SSRIs

In partial response to SNRIs or SSRIs, augmentation with d-amphetamine (30 mg/d) and caffeine (300 mg/d) were equally effective in improving residual symptoms, although this book's author would think there are quite a few people who have 300 mg/d caffeine without any need for an augmentation strategy (n = 24, RCT, d/b, 5/52, Koran et al, J Clin Psychiatry 2009; **70**:1530–5).

Gabapentin + SSRIs

Gabapentin up to 3600 mg/d has been used in patients only partially responsive to fluoxetine 30–100 mg/d (n = 5, open, 6/52, Cora-Locatelli et al, J Clin Psychiatry 1998;**59**:480–1).

Inositol + SSRIs

Inositol 18 g/d may significantly reduce Y-BOCS rating scale scores (n = 13, d/b, c/o, 6/52, Fux et al, Am J Psychiatry 1996;**153**:1219–21; n = 10, open, Seedat and Stein, Int Clin Psychopharmacol 1999;**14**:353–6), but the only RCT has shown no effect on symptoms (n = 10, RCT, d/b, p/c, c/o, 6/52, Fux et al, Int J Neuropsychopharmacol 1999;**2**:193–5).

Lithium + SSRIs

Lithium augmentation of fluvoxamine in OCD appears ineffective (n = 30, d/b, p/c, McDougle et al, J Clin Psychopharmacol 1991;**11**:175–84).

Memantine + SSRIs/clomipramine *

Memantine 20 mg/d has been used as augmentation to SSRI-non-responsive OCD, producing a meaningful improvement in 43% completers (n = 15 [c = 14], 12/52, Aboujaoude et al, J Clin Psychopharmacol 2009;**29**:51–5) and a pilot study suggested that memantine augmentation of SSRIs/clomipramine had beneficial effects in severe OCD (n=44, s/b, Stewart et al, J Clin Psychopharmacol 2010; **30**:34–9).

Mirtazapine + citalopram

Mirtazapine 15–30 mg/d may speed the response to citalopram by four weeks, but with similar response rates from week 8,

which could be significant in severe OCD, although a robust study would be needed to confirm this (n = 49, s/b, 12/52, Pallanti et al, J Clin Psychiatry 2004;**65**:1394–9; comment by Schüle and Laakmann, EBMH 2005;**8**:42). In mirtazapine-responders, discontinuation led to relapse suggesting a prophylactic effect (n = 30, d/b, p/c, 8/52, Koran et al, J Clin Psychiatry 2005;**66**:515–20).

Naltrexone + SSRIs/clomipramine

Naltrexone augmentation in SSRI-resistant OCD was ineffective (n = 10, RCT, d/b, p/c, c/o, 5/52, Amiaz et al, Eur Neuropsychopharmacol 2008;**18**:455–61).

Pindolol + SSRIs

Pindolol 7.5 mg/d may possibly improve the response to paroxetine in multiple SSRI-resistant OCD (n = 14, d/b, p/c, 6/52, Dannon et al, Eur Neuropsychopharmacol 2000;**10**:165–9).

Riluzole + SSRIs

Riluzole 100 mg/d appeared to have some activity as an adjunct in a treatment-resistant OCD (n = 13, open, Coric et al, Biol Psychiatry 2005;**58**:424–8).

Topiramate + SSRIs *

Topiramate augmentation of SSRIs may be useful for compulsions, but not obsessions (n = 36, RCT, d/b, p/c, 12/52, Berlin et al, J Clin Psychiatry 2011;**72**:716–21; see also n = 16, < 13/52, Van Ameringen et al, Depress Anxiety 2006;**23**:1–5).

Tricyclics + clomipramine

Addition of nortriptyline 50 mg/d to clomipramine 150 mg/d produced a more rapid onset of action than clomipramine alone (n = 30, d/b, p/c, RCT, Noorbala et al, J Clin Pharm Ther 1998;**23**:155–9).

● Unlicensed/some efficacy

Citalopram

Citalopram has been shown to be as effective as fluvoxamine and paroxetine and predictors of response include longer duration of more severe illness, no previous SSRI and an adequate dose for adequate duration (RCT, Stein et al,

Int Clin Psychopharmacol 2001;**16**:357–61). Very high dose citalopram (160 mg/d) may be effective in severe, resistant OCD (n = 1, Bejerot and Bodlund, *Acta Psychiatr Scand* 1998; **98**:423–4).

Venlafaxine

Venlafaxine has been shown to be as effective as paroxetine but not superior (n = 150, RCT, d/b, Denys *et al*, *J Clin Psychopharmacol* 2003;**23**:568–75), but almost as effective as clomipramine (n = 47; 150–225 mg/d) and better tolerated (n = 73, RCT, s/b, 12/52, Albert *et al*, *J Clin Psychiatry* 2002;**63**:1004–9). **Reviews:** SNRIs in OCD (Phelps and Cates, *Ann Pharmacother* 2005;**39**:136–40; Dell'Osso *et al*, *J Clin Psychiatry* 2006;**67**:600–10).

■ Unlicensed/possible efficacy

Cycloserine

Cycloserine 100 mg given before behavioural therapy improves OCD and depressive symptoms (n = 23, RCT, d/b, p/c, 5/52, Wilhelm *et al*, *Am J Psychiatry* 2008;**165**:335–41), and when used before exposure therapy (d/b, p/c, Kushner *et al*, *Biol Psychiatry* 2007;**62**:835–8).

Glycine

Glycine 60 g/d appears poorly tolerated but may work well in some people, with some significant sustained responses in a pilot study (n = 24 [c = 14], RCT, d/b, p/c, 12/52, Greenberg *et al*, *J Psychiatr Res* 2009;**43**:664–70).

Mirtazapine

Mirtazapine 60 mg/d showed advantage over placebo (n = 30 [c = 26], open,12/52 followed by d/b, p/c discontinuation, 8/52, Koran *et al*, *J Clin Psychiatry* 2005;**66**:515–20).

Morphine

Rather bizarrely, once-weekly oral morphine was effective in some treatment-resistant OCD patients, unlike lorazepam or placebo (n = 23, RCT, d/b, c/o, p/c, 6/52, Koran *et al*, *J Clin Psychiatry* 2005;**66**:353–9).

Ondansetron *

Ondansetron was significantly superior to placebo for OCD as an add-on to fluoxetine

(n = 42, RCT, d/b, p/c, 8/52, Soltani *et al*, *Hum Psychopharmacol* 2010;**25**:509–13).

Phenelzine

Phenelzine 60 mg/d was shown to be inferior to fluoxetine (80 mg/d) except in patients with asymmetry/other atypical obsession, and no preferential response was detected in patients with high anxiety levels (n = 60, RCT, Jenike *et al*, *Am J Psychiatry* 1997;**154**:1261–4).

Psilocybin

Psilocybin reduced acute OCD symptoms in some patients in a carefully controlled situation (n = 9, Moreno *et al*, *J Clin Psychiatry* 2006; **67**:1735–40).

✱ Case reports ✱

- **Amantadine** * augmentation (n = 1, Pasquini *et al*, *J Clin Psychopharmacol* 2010;**30**:85–6).
- **Buspirone + fluoxetine** (n = 1, Alessi and Bos, *Am J Psychiatry* 1991;**148**:1605).
- **Buspirone + sertraline** (n = 2, Menkes, *Br J Psychiatry* 1995;**167**:823–4).
- **Carbamazepine** * 1200 mg/d (n = 1, Aggarwal *et al*, *Indian J Med Soc* 2009;**63**:368–9).
- **Carbamazepine + clomipramine** (n = 1, Iwata *et al*, *J Clin Psychiatry* 2000;**161**:528–9).
- **Lamotrigine** * 150 mg/d (n = 1, Uzun *et al*, *J Psychopharmacol* 2010;**24**:425–7).
- **Nicotine chewing gum** (n = 1, Pasquini *et al*, *Prog Neuropsychopharmacol Biol Psychiatry* 2005;**29**:157–9).
- **Oxcarbazepine** (n = 1, McMeekin, *J S C Med Assoc* 2002;**98**:316–20).
- **Paliperidone** (n = 1, Angelucci *et al*, *Prog Neuropsychopharmacol Biol Psychiatry* 2009; **33**:1277–8).
- **Pregabalin** as an adjunct sertraline-risperidone (n = 1, Oulis *et al*, *Prim Care Companion J Clin Psychiatry* 2008;**10**:249).
- **Tramadol** 100 mg/d (n = 1, Goldsmith *et al*, *Am J Psychiatry* 1999;**156**:660–1).

◆ Others

Other drugs tried include **diphenhydramine** up to 250 mg/d (n = 28, d/b, c/o, 6/52, Hewlett *et al*, *J Clin Psychopharmacol* 1992;**12**:420–30).

□ No efficacy

Bupropion

Bupropion had no significant effect in OCD (n = 12, open, 8/52, Vulink et al, J Clin Psychiatry 2005;**66**:228–30).

Clonazepam

Clonazepam seems ineffective as mono-therapy in treating OCD, although it may be helpful for specific sub-groups with comorbid anxiety (n = 27, d/b, p/c, 10/52, Hollander et al, World J Biol Psychiatry 2003;**4**:30–4) and as augmentation of sertraline (n = 37, RCT, d/b, p/c, 12/52, Crockett et al, Ann Clin Psychiatry 2004;**16**:127–32).

Clozapine

Clozapine has been used for OCD symptoms in schizophrenia (n = 15, open, Reznik et al, Pharmacopsychiatry 2004;**37**:52–6), but has been shown to be ineffective (n = 10, McDougle et al, Am J Psychiatry 1995;**152**:1812–4) or even detrimental (eg. Baker et al, J Clin Psychiatry 1992;**53**:439–42).

Flutamide

The anti-androgen flutamide was ineffective in one trial (n = 8, Altemus et al, J Clin Psychiatry 1999;**60**:442–5).

Minocycline *

A small trial suggested that minocycline was not effective as an adjunct in OCD, except perhaps in early onset and in hoarders (n = 9, 12/52, open, Rodriguez et al, J Clin Psychiatry 2010;**71**:1247–9).

Naltrexone

Naltrexone appears to have no beneficial effect (n = 10, RCT, d/b, p/c, c/o, 2/12, Amiaz et al, Eur Neuropsychopharmacol 2008;**18**:455–61).

Oxytocin

Initial enthusiasm was not confirmed in a study of intranasal administration (n = 3, Salzberg and Swedo, Am J Psychiatry 1992;**149**:713–4).

Trazodone

A study showed trazodone up to 300mg/d to be equipotent with placebo (n = 21, d/b, c/o, 10/52, Pigott et al, J Clin Psychopharmacol 1992; **12**:156–62).

Tricyclics (except clomipramine)

Imipramine (Volavka et al, Psychiatry Res 1985; **14**:85–93), amitriptyline and nortriptyline have been shown to be ineffective.

1.18.1 BODY DYSMORPHIC DISORDER (BDD)

Symptoms

Body dysmorphic disorder (BDD) is characterised by a disabling preoccupation with an imagined or minor defect in appearance (especially skin, hair and nose), with time-consuming behaviours such as mirror gazing, excessive camouflaging and need for reassurance. The adult incidence is thought to be around 0.5–1% (Bohne et al, Psychosomatics 2002;**43**:486–90), although it may be as high as 2.4% (Koran et al, CNS Spectr 2008;**13**:316–22). It has a fluctuating or episodic course, often life-long, with a higher risk/comorbidity in people with depression, social phobia, SUDs, OCD and eating disorders. There is a high risk of suicide (around a quarter may have attempted suicide sometime during their life, 2.6% per year and 0.3% succeed, Phillips and Menard, Am J Psychiatry 2006;**163**:1280–2), which is 45 times higher than the general population and 2–3 times more than depression and bipolar.

Role of drugs

There are few trials or RCTs in BDD. NICE recommends using either an SSRI or more intensive targeted CBT for moderate BDD. The onset of action of SSRIs (as in OCD) may be delayed for up to 12/52. The best evidence is available for fluoxetine; clomipramine monotherapy is a second line; with buspirone as an adjunct in resistant cases. Treatment duration should be 12 months if effective to prevent relapse and allow further improvement. TCAs (other than clomipramine), SNRIs, MAOIs, anxiolytics (except short-term) or antipsychotic mono-therapy are not recommended. Cochrane concludes that SSRIs/clomipramine are superior to placebo and to desipramine (s = 2, n = 96) and CBT may be effective (s = 3, n = 83), mostly in women (s = 5, n = 179, Ipser et al, Cochrane Syst Database Rev 2009; **1**:CD005332).

Reviews: * general (Bjornsson et al, Dialogues Clin Neurosci 2010;**12**:221–32; Fiori and Giannetti, Neuropsychiatr Dis Treat 2009;**5**:477–81), relationship to eating disorders (Phillips and Kaye, CNS Spectr 2007;**12**:347–58) and OC spectrum (Ravindran et al, Can J Psychiatry 2009; **54**:331–43).

■ Unlicensed/possible efficacy

Buspirone

A small open study showed a 46% response with buspirone as augmentation of SSRIs (n = 13, open, Phillips, Psychopharmacol Bull 1996;**32**:175–80).

Citalopram

An open study showed a 73% response rate in BDD (n = 15, open, 12/52, Phillips and Najjar, J Clin Psychiatry 2003;**64**:715–20).

Clomipramine

Clomipramine was clearly superior to desipramine in BDD even if delusions were prominent (n = 29, RCT, d/b, c/o, 16/52, Hollander et al, Arch Gen Psychiatry 1999;**56**:1033–9).

Escitalopram

A small study showed some well tolerated efficacy (47% were much improved) in BDD (n = 15[c = 11], open, Phillips, Int Clin Psychopharmacol 2006;**21**:177–9).

Fluoxetine

A 53% response rate (cf 18% with placebo) has been seen (NNT = 2.7, n = 67, RCT, d/b, p/c, 12/52, Phillips et al, Arch Gen Psychiatry 2002;**59**:381–8). Fluoxetine appears to have a protective effect against suicide (n = 67, RCT, d/b, p/c, 12/52, Phillips and Kelly, Int Clin Psychopharmacol 2009;**24**:26–8).

Fluvoxamine

In an open study, fluvoxamine had a 63% response rate using BDD-YBOCS (n = 30, open, 16/52, Phillips et al, J Clin Psychiatry 2001; **62**:87–91; n = 1, Khan and Decker, J Child Adoles Psychopharmacol 2001;**11**:105–7; reviewed by Irons, Neuropsychiatr Dis Treat 2005;**1**:289–99).

Levetiracetam

A pilot study suggested that levetiracetam (mean 2000mg/d) can improve many measures of BDD (n = 17, open, 12/52, Phillips and Menard, CNS Spectr 2009;**14**:252–60).

Olanzapine

Olanzapine (up to 15mg/d) augmentation of fluoxetine was effective in 33%, but 67% remained unchanged (n = 6, d/b, p/c, 8/52, Phillips, Am J Psychiatry 2005;**162**:1022–3). It has been used to augment paroxetine (n = 1, Nakaaki et al, Psychiatry Clin Neurosci 2008; **62**:370).

Venlafaxine

Venlafaxine (minimum150mg/d) may improve global severity and specific symptoms (n = 17 [c = 11], open, 12–16/52, Allen et al, CNS Spectr 2008;**13**:138–44).

✱ Case reports ✱

- **Aripiprazole + fluvoxamine** * (n = 1, Uzun and Ozdemir, Clin Drug Investig 2010;**30**: 707–10).
- **Bupropion** (n = 1, Nardi et al, Aust N Z J Psychiatry 2005;**39**:112).
- **Glycine** * (n = 1, Cleveland et al, Neural Plast 2009;2009: in press).

□ No efficacy

Pimozide

Pimozide was ineffective as an adjunct to fluoxetine (n = 28, d/b, p/c, 8/52, Phillips, Am J Psychiatry 2005;**162**:377–9).

1.19 PANIC DISORDER

see also Anxiety disorder (1.6)

Symptoms

Panic disorder is usually characterised by sudden attacks of anxiety, where physical symptoms predominate, peaking within 10 minutes and with an associated fear of serious consequences, e.g. heart attack. These attacks need to include four of the following: palpitations, abdominal distress/nausea, numbness/tingling, inability to breathe or shortness of breath, choking, sweating, chest pains, dizziness, depersonalisation (common), flushes/chills, fear of dying and trembling/shaking. The lifetime prevalence of panic disorder is about 5% in the USA (Grant et al, J Clin Psychiatry 2006;**67**:363–74; comment by Bienvenu, EBMH 2006;**9**:114), with a point prevalence of 1.5% (males) and 2.8% (females). There is frequently a family history and it can be a presenting feature of depression.

Role of drugs *

In general, short-term benefits may be gained with drug therapy. The main principle is to start low and go slow (to minimise initial jitteriness), and accept that response may take some time to occur, e.g. SSRIs are effective long-term with a slow onset of action, initial worsening and some exacerbation may occur on discontinuation. After a standard dose SSRI for 6/52, there is little evidence for the efficacy of increasing the dose (n = 39, Simon et al, J Clin Psychiatry 2009;**70**:1563–70). Benzodiazepines have a quicker onset of action but obvious potential problems, e.g. the dependence potential and tolerance, and NICE concludes that they have a poor long-term outcome. Placebo responders tend to show an early and temporary remission. Combining CBT and antidepressants increases the response compared to either therapy alone (meta-analysis, s = 21, n = 1709, RCTs, Furukawa et al, Br J Psychiatry 2006;**188**:305–12; comment by Mitte, EBMH 2006;**9**:98). Relapse rates at 6–12 months can be as high as 75% and stopping antidepressants suddenly (over 1–7 days) leads to an increased relapse rate, occurring more rapidly (half the time it would take otherwise) than stopping more slowly over 14 days or longer (n = 398, mean 3-year follow-up, Baldessarini et al, Am J Psychiatry 2010;**167**:934–41). Adding a CBT package to SSRIs seems of little additional benefit, with SSRIs more effective than CBT alone (n = 150, 9/12, van Apeldoorn et al, Acta Psychiatr Scand 2008;**117**:260–70). Cochrane concludes that there is no evidence for psychotherapy as an adjunct for BDZs in panic (s = 3, n = 243, Watanabe et al, Cochrane Database Syst Rev 2009;**2**:CD005335).

Reviews: * SSRIs (Mochcovitch and Nardi, Expert Rev Neurother 2010;**10**:1285–93), general (Davies et al, Prescriber 2010;**20**:17–27; Katon, N Engl J Med 2006;**354**:2360–7; Taylor, Br Med J 2006;**332**:951–5; Roy-Byrne et al, Lancet 2006;**368**:1023–32), BAP evidence-based guidelines (Baldwin et al, J Psychopharmacol 2005; **19**:567–96), epidemiology (Batelaan et al, Tijdschr Psychiatr 2006;**48**:195–205).

BNF listed

Benzodiazepines *

Benzodiazepines are rapidly effective and useful in people needing immediate relief (review by Kasper and Resinger, Eur Neuropsychopharmacol 2001;**11**:307–21). Many benzodiazepines have been studied, e.g. **clonazepam** is longer-acting, with 1–2 mg/d the best balance between benefit and tolerability and it may have a sustained effect (n = 67, three years, open, Nardi et al, Psychiatry Res 2005;**137**:61–70). The main problem is discontinuation, where relapse may be more common with shorter-acting benzodiazepines so transferring to an SSRI is advisable. In patients asymptomatic for at least a year, tapering clonazepam at 0.25 mg/week can be successful, without major withdrawal symptoms or relapse (n = 73, open, Nardi et al, J Clin Psychopharmacol 2010;**30**:290–3).

Citalopram

Citalopram is licensed in the UK for panic disorder, with or without agoraphobia. The starting dose in panic disorder is 10 mg/d for one week, increasing to 20–30 mg/d as the optimum dose to a maximum of 60 mg/d and 20–60 mg/d appears to be effective and well tolerated over one year. It may be quicker acting than paroxetine, but equipotent (n = 58, RCT, s/b, 60/7, Perna et al, Pharmacopsychiatry 2001;**34**:85–90).

Escitalopram

Escitalopram is licensed in the UK for panic disorder, with or without agoraphobia. The initial dose is 5 mg/d for the first week, then 10 mg/d, increasing to a maximum of 20 mg/d. Escitalopram and citalopram appear equally effective in panic disorder (n = 366, RCT, d/b, p/c, 10/52, Stahl et al, J Clin Psychiatry 2003;**64**: 1322–7, MS).

Paroxetine

Paroxetine is licensed for panic and agoraphobia.

A 10mg/d starting dose is recommended. Several studies have shown a significant effect, e.g. as effective as citalopram (n = 58, RCT, s/b, 60/7, Perna et al, Pharmacopsychiatry 2001;**34**:85–90). The optimum effective dose is 40mg/d. After 12 months treatment, a further year of paroxetine did not reduce relapse rates compared to discontinuation in panic disorder (with or without agoraphobia) (n = 143, open, three years, Dannon et al, BMC Psychiatry 2004;**11**:16). Combining with CBT is significantly more effective than placebo plus CBT (n = 120, RCT, p/c, 12/52, Oehrberg et al, Br J Psychiatry 1995;**167**:374–9).

Tricyclics

Tricyclics are effective in panic disorder. They may take four weeks to start to work and 12 weeks for maximal effect. Initial jitteriness is a common problem and so it is usually necessary to start at a low dose (10–25 mg/d). **Clomipramine** is as effective as paroxetine in panic disorder, but with a slower onset of action and more side-effects and may have a biphasic response, symptoms worsening over 12 weeks before improving. **Imipramine** is effective (vs placebo) in all studies using doses above 150mg/d and with a substantial prophylactic efficacy (n = 18, RCT, Mavissakalian and Perel, Ann Clin Psychiatry 2001;**13**:63–7). Long-term maintenance is needed for most patients, although early detection of relapse may be a viable alternative to long-term therapy (n = 51, RCT, d/b, 12/12, Mavissakalian and Perel, J Clin Psychopharmacol 2002;**22**:294–9).

+ Combinations

Clonazepam + SSRI

Use of clonazepam, slowly tapered after four weeks, as an initial adjunct to paroxetine facilitates longer-term monotherapy (n = 60, RCT, p/c, 12/52, Pollack et al, J Psychopharmacol 2003;**17**:276–82).

● Unlicensed/some efficacy

Fluoxetine

Fluoxetine is effective when initial doses are kept very low (2.5–5 mg/d) then increased, as higher doses produce side-effects such as anxiety and over-stimulation, possibly due to serotonergic supersensitivity. Fluoxetine 20mg/d is clearly superior to placebo over a range of symptoms in panic disorder. If there is no response by 6/52, it may benefit from an increase up to 60mg/d (n = 180 [c = 153], 12/52, RCT, Michelson et al, Br J Psychiatry 2001;**179**:514–8).

Fluvoxamine

Fluvoxamine has been compared favourably with placebo and cognitive therapy (n = 55, RCT, p/c, 8/52, Black et al, Arch Gen Psychiatry 1993;**50**:44–50), but not all placebo trials have shown efficacy.

Gabapentin

Gabapentin 600–3600 mg/d may have anxiolytic effects in severe panic disorder (n = 103, RCT, d/b, p/c, 8/52, Pande et al, J Clin Psychopharmacol 2000;**20**:467–71).

Mirtazapine

Mirtazapine may be a rapidly effective alternative to SSRIs (n = 28, RCT, open, 12/52, Boshuisen et al, Int Clin Psychopharmacol 2001;**16**:363–8) and of similar efficacy and tolerability to fluoxetine (n = 27, RCT, 8/52, Ribeiro et al, Braz J Med Biol Res 2001;**34**:1303–7).

Sertraline *

Pooled data indicates that sertraline is an effective treatment for panic disorder, even in people with risk factors for poor response (s = 4, n = 664, d/b, Pollack et al, J Clin Psychiatry 2000;**61**:922–7) and prevents relapse (n = 240, RCT, d/b, p/c, 8/52, Kamijima et al, Int Clin Psychopharmacol 2005;**20**:265–73). Early response predicts final remission, a useful aid to decision-making (n = 544, p/c, Pollack et al, J Psychiatr Res 2002;**36**:229–36). Sertraline is enhanced by self-administered CBT (n = 251, RCT, p/c, 12/52, Koszycki et al, Psychol Med 2011;**41**:373–83).

Review: Hobgood and Clayton, Drugs Today (Barc) 2009;**45**:351–61.

■ Unlicensed/possible efficacy

Aripiprazole

A pilot study suggested aripiprazole may be

useful as an adjunct in resistant panic disorder (n = 10, open, 8/52, Hoge et al, CNS Spectr 2008;**13**:522–7; see also n = 1, Harada et al, J Clin Psychopharmacol 2009;**29**:301–2).

Cicloserin (D-cycloserine)

D-cycloserine may have a role in enhancing the response to CBT for panic (n = 31, RCT, d/b, p/c, Otto et al, Biol Psychiatry 2010;**67**:365–70).

Duloxetine

A pilot study suggests duloxetine 60–120mg/d may have some efficacy in panic disorder (n = 15, open, 6/52, Simon et al, CNS Neurosci Ther 2009;**15**:19–23).

Inositol

In one trial, inositol 12g/d improved panic symptoms, whereas lorazepam did not (n = 25, d/b, p/c, c/o, 4/52, Benjamin et al, Am J Psychiatry 1995;**152**:1084–6) and was superior to fluvoxamine 150mg/d in another (n = 20, RCT, c/o, 8/52, Palatnik et al, J Clin Psychopharmacol 2001;**21**:335–9).

Lamotrigine *

Some success has been reported in chronic panic (n = 4, 14/12, Masdrakis et al, Clin Neuropharmacol 2010;**33**:126-8).

Levetiracetam

Levetiracetam was effective in 84% completers in a pilot study (n = 18 [c = 13], open, 12/52, Papp, J Clin Psychiatry 2006;**67**:1573–6).

MAOIs *

Tranylcypromine 60mg/d appears to be effective for comorbid panic and social anxiety, but not 30mg/d, or the panic symptoms alone (n = 36, d/b, 12/52, Nardi et al, Psychiatry Res 2010;**175**:260–5). Phenelzine 45–90mg/d may be effective (n = 1, Buch and Wagner, J Clin Psychiatry 2007;**68**:335–6).

Moclobemide

Moclobemide was ineffective as monotherapy (n = 55, RCT, 8/52, Loerch et al, Br J Psychiatry 1999;**174**:205–12), but comparisons with clomipramine (n = 135, RCT, 8/52, Kruger and Dahl, Eur Arch Psych Clin Neurosci 1999; **249** [Suppl 1]:S7–S10) and fluoxetine (RCT, d/b,

8/52, Tiller et al, Eur Arch Psych Clin Neurosci 1999;**249**[Suppl 1]:S19–S24) show similar efficacy, although the comparator drugs may have been at sub-therapeutic doses.

Olanzapine

Olanzapine (mean 12.3mg/d) was remarkably effective in reducing refractory panic attacks, with 50% even being panic-free at the trial end (n = 10, open, 8/52, Hollifield et al, Depress Anx 2005;**21**:33–40).

Reboxetine

Reboxetine is less effective than citalopram (n = 19, RCT, s/b, c/o, 18/52, Seedat et al, Int Clin Psychopharmacol 2003;**18**:279–84) and paroxetine (n = 68, RCT, s/b, Bertani et al, Pharmacopsychiatry 2004;**37**:206–10).

Valproate

Valproate 300–1500mg/d may be useful for resistant panic disorder (e.g. n = 13 [c = 10], open, 8/52, Baetz and Bowen, Can J Psychiatry 1998;**43**:73–7).

Venlafaxine *

Venlafaxine (75–225mg/d) was superior to placebo for panic disorder, higher doses being most effective (n = 624, RCT, p/c, 12/52, Pollack et al, Psychopharmacol [Berl] 2007;**194**:233–42), although a previous study was negative (n = 361, RCT, d/b, p/c, 10/52, Bradwejn et al, Br J Psychiatry 2005;**187**:352–9). Very low dose is sometimes effective (n = 2, Orenstein and Raskind, J Clin Psychiatry 2010;**71**:89–91).

* Case reports *

- **Bupropion** (n = 1, Gebhardt et al, J Clin Pharm Ther 2008;**33**:575–7).
- **Olanzapine + paroxetine** (n = 1, Chao, Pharmacopsychiatry 2004; **37**:239–40).
- **Oxcarbazepine** (n = 1, Windhaber et al, J Clin Psychiatry 1997;**58**:404–5).
- **Pramipexole + SSRIs** (n = 2, Marazziti et al, Am J Psychiatry 2001;**158**: 498–9).

◆ Others

Other drugs tried include **carbamazepine** (review by Keck et al, J Clin Psychopharmacol

1992;**12**[Suppl]:S36–S41), **clonidine** (review by Puzantian and Hart, *Ann Pharmacother* 1993; **2**:1351–3), **ondansetron** (Schneier et al, *Anxiety* 1996;**2**:199–202) and **pindolol** (see Mathew et al, *Psychopharmacol Bull* 2001;**35**:97–110).

□ No efficacy

Buspirone

Buspirone is not superior to placebo (d/b, c/o, *J Clin Psychiatry* 1988;**49**[8, Suppl]:S30–S36), or in combination with CBT (n = 77, RCT, Bouvard et al, *Psychother Psychosom* 1997;**66**:7–32).

Caffeine

Caffeine is anxiogenic and panic patients seem to be more sensitive to its effects. Challenge doses of 480 mg have been shown to provoke panic attacks (n = 98, RCT, d/b, 1/52, Nardi et al, *Psychiatry Res* 2009;**169**:149–53).

1.20 POST-TRAUMATIC STRESS DISORDER (PTSD)

Symptoms

PTSD is an anxiety disorder resulting from an extreme stressful event, e.g. serious threat to life or involvement of a loved one in a catastrophic event, and where a personal vulnerability exists. The person then re-experiences the event recurrently through dreams and feelings. PTSD may be a quite common yet unrecognised cause of significant morbidity and mortality. The lifetime prevalence may be 1–9%. Only drugs with a significant effect on the serotonin system seem to work.

Role of drugs *

Current data suggests that 'positive' symptoms (e.g. nightmares, etc) respond better to drugs, whereas 'negative' symptoms of avoidance (e.g. social withdrawal, etc) are less responsive. SSRIs (e.g. sertraline and paroxetine) have been shown to be effective in short-term studies (6–12/52), and for relapse prevention over 6–12/12. Higher doses of serotonergic drugs for longer periods (at least five weeks) seem necessary. Extended treatment is needed, as there is a great risk of relapse and symptom recurrence if discontinued (s = 3, RCT, d/b, p/c, < 14/52, Davis

et al, *CNS Drugs* 2006;**20**:465–76). SGAs, non-SSRIs and AEDs may also be effective (s = 9, Davis et al, *CNS Drugs* 2006;**20**:465–76). BDZs are probably ineffective (review by Asnis et al, *Drugs* 2004;**64**:383–404). Cochrane concludes medicines can be effective in reducing core symptoms plus depression and disability (s = 35, n = 4597, Stein et al, *Cochrane Database Syst Rev* 2006;**1**:CD002795), but it is unknown if combining PTs and pharmacotherapy is any better (or worse) than either alone (s = 4, Hetrick et al, *Cochrane Database Syst Rev* 2010; **7**:CD007316).

Reviews: general (Mellman and Lydiard, *J Clin Psychiatry* 2008;**69**:e2; Zohar et al, *Curr Opin Psychiatry* 2008;**21**:74–7), BAP evidence-based guidelines (Baldwin et al, *J Psychopharmacol* 2005; **19**:567–96), pharmacotherapy (Mohamed and Rosenheck, *J Clin Psychiatry* 2008;**69**:959–65), alternatives to antidepressants (Berger et al, *Prog Neuropsychopharmacol Biol Psychiatry* 2009; **33**:169–80), AEDs in PTSD (Berlin, *Curr Psychiatry Rep* 2007;**9**:291–300).

BNF listed

Paroxetine

Paroxetine is licensed for PTSD, with a standard dose of 20 mg/d, increasing gradually to 50 mg/d if needed. Doses of 20–40 mg/d have been shown to be effective and well tolerated in adults (both male and female) with chronic PTSD (n = 551, RCT, p/c, 12/52, Marshall et al, *Am J Psychiatry* 2001;**158**:1982–8), in dissociation in chronic PTSD in adults (n = 52, RCT, d/b, p/c, 10/52, Marshall et al, *Depress Anxiety* 2007;**24**:77–84) and in chronic PTSD (n = 30, open, 6/12, Kucukali et al, *Bosn J Basic Med Sci* 2008;**8**:76–9; n = 52[c = 25], 12/12, open, Kim et al, *Psychiatry Clin Neurosci* 2008;**62**:646–52).

Sertraline *

Sertraline is licensed for PTSD in women, but may not be effective in men. Two RCTs in PTSD have shown sertraline (mean dose 150 mg/d) to be superior to placebo in measures of global and functional outcomes and symptom severity (n = 187, RCT, 12/52, Brady et al, *JAMA* 2000;**283**:1837–44; critical review by Bisson, *EBMH* 2000;**3**:109) and at

50–200 mg/d to produce a 60% response rate cf 38% with placebo (n = 208, RCT, p/c, 12/52, Davidson et al, Arch Gen Psychiatry 2001;**58**:485–92). It was effective in Iranian war veterans n = 70[c = 64], RCT, d/b, p/c, 10/52, Panahi et al, Psychol Med 2011; in press). Sertraline seems particularly effective in treating psychological symptoms of PTSD, e.g. anger, anhedonia, detachment and numbing as opposed to somatic symptoms, e.g. insomnia and exaggerated startle response (n = 400, 12/52, Davidson et al, Psychol Med 2002;**32**:661–70), and for PTSD caused by either interpersonal trauma or childhood abuse (n = 395, RCT, d/b, p/c, 12/52, Stein et al, Ann Clin Psychiatry 2006;**18**:243–9), but was not effective for PTSD in a VA clinic setting (n = 169, RCT, d/b, p/c, 12/52, Friedman et al, J Clin Psychiatry 2007;**68**:711–20; MS). A prophylactic effect has been suggested (n = 96, open, 24/52, Davidson et al, Am J Psychiatry 2001;**158**:1974–81; review by Bisson, EBMH 2002;**5**:110).

Review: Schwartz and Rothbaum, Expert Opin Pharmacother 2002;**3**:1489–99.

● Unlicensed/some efficacy

SSRIs (paroxetine and sertraline licensed)

Fluoxetine (up to 60 mg/d) was shown to be superior to placebo in civilians with PTSD, with a very low placebo response rate (e.g. n = 131, RCT, p/c, d/b, 6/12, Martenyi et al, Br J Psychiatry 2002;**181**:315–20; comment by Butterfield, EBMH 2003;**6**:51; strong criticism by Agell, Br J Psychiatry 2003;**182**:366–7 and defence by Eli Lilly; Br J Psychiatry 2003;**182**:367–8) and for relapse prevention in responders over 6/12 (n = 123[c = 114], open, 6/12, Davidson et al, J Clin Psychopharmacol 2005;**25**:166–9). Care may be needed initially with use in patients with comorbid panic attacks, as fluoxetine may increase panic and anxiety so start low and go slow. **Citalopram** was partly effective in two cases (n = 2, Khouzam et al, Mil Med 2001;**166**:921–3). **Escitalopram** (up to 20 mg/d) was effective in 45% patients (n = 25[c = 24], open, 12/52, Robert et al, J Clin Psychiatry 2006;**67**:1522–6). **Fluvoxamine** 100–300 mg/d (mean 150 mg) appeared

to improve combat-related PTSD but not depressive symptoms (n = 15, open, 14/52, Escalona et al, Depress Anxiety 2002;**15**:29–33).

Topiramate

Topiramate (up to 400 mg/d) has shown a significant effect on re-experiencing symptoms and treatment outcome scales in civilian PTSD (e.g. n = 38, RCT, d/b, p/c, Tucker et al, J Clin Psychiatry 2007;**68**:201–6; n = 43[c = 29], open, 8/52, Alderman et al, Ann Pharmacother 2009;**43**:635–41).

Venlafaxine

Venlafaxine 37.5–300 mg/d (mean 222 mg/d) was significantly more effective than placebo for enduring PTSD (n = 329, RCT, d/b, p/c, 6/12, Davidson et al, Arch Gen Psychiatry 2006; **63**:1158–65; review, Pae et al, Expert Rev Neurosci 2007;**7**:603–15).

■ Unlicensed/possible efficacy

Antipsychotics

A meta-analysis of studies shows that **olanzapine** and **risperidone** were superior to placebo for PTSD symptoms, particularly 'intrusion' symptoms (s = 7, n = 192, RCT, d/b, p/c, Pae et al, Int Clin Psychopharmacol 2008;**23**:1–8). **Aripiprazole** was effective in about 60% of those who tolerated the drug, starting at a low dose, i.e. 5 mg/d rather than 10 mg/d, to aid tolerability (n = 22[c = 14], open, 12/52, Villarreal et al, Psychopharmacol Bull 2007;**40**:6–18; n = 32[c = 23], open, 16/52, Mello et al, Rev Bras Psiquiatr 2008;**30**:358–61) and adjunctive aripiprazole (mean 13 mg/d) produced a 53% response rate with PTSD, with a low starting dose (5 mg) and slower titration to improve tolerability (n = 17[c = 8], open, 12/52, Robert et al, Psychopharmacol Bull 2009;**42**:69–80). **Clozapine** has been used successfully in comorbid psychosis and PTSD (n = 1, Hamner, Am J Psychiatry 1996;**153**:841) and in treatment-resistant, abused adolescents with psychosis and PTSD (n = 6, Wheatley et al, J Clin Psychopharmacol 2004;**24**:167–73). **Levomepromazine** may help reduce sleep problems in PTSD (Aukst-Margetic et al, Eur Psychiatry 2004;**19**:235–6).

Olanzapine augmentation of SSRIs may be useful (e.g. n = 19, d/b, p/c, 8/52, Stein *et al, Am J Psychiatry* 2002;**159**:1777–9). Quetiapine (mean 200–250 mg/d) may also be an option as augmentation of SSRIs and encouraging outcomes were seen in small pilot studies as adjunctive treatment in resistant PTSD (n = 20[c = 18], open, 6/52, Hamner *et al, J Clin Psychopharmacol* 2003;**23**:5–20; n = 15, open, 8/52, Ahearn *et al, Int Clin Psychopharmacol* 2006;**21**:29–33). Adjunctive risperidone in resistant combat PTSD was well tolerated and produced a modest improvement in one study (n = 40, RCT, d/b, p/c, 5/52, Hamner *et al, Int Clin Psychopharmacol* 2003;**18**:1–8) and 2–4 mg/d has helped decrease some psychotic and PTSD symptoms in antidepressant-resistant patients (n = 26, open, 6/52, Kozaric-Kovacic *et al, J Clin Psychiatry* 2005;**66**:922–7). However, in sertraline part-response, addition of risperidone is of limited value (n = 45 [c = 34], Rothbaum *et al, J Clin Psychiatry* 2008;**69**:520–5). Ziprasidone has been used successfully (n = 2, Siddiqui *et al, J Psychiatry Neurosci* 2005;**30**:430–1).

Benzodiazepines

Although generally considered ineffective, potential anti-arousal effects can be useful and beneficial effects have been seen with clonazepam at 4–5 mg/d although it was largely ineffective in improving sleep disturbances and nightmares in combat-related PTSD (n = 6, 2 + 2/52, p/c, c/o, s/b, Cates *et al, Ann Pharmacother* 2004;**38**:1395–9). Care is needed with possible abuse, induction of depression, the potential for the release of impulsive or antisocial behaviour and severe withdrawal reactions.

Beta-blockers

Propranolol may reduce the consolidation of emotional memory and is a potential, albeit controversial treatment for minimisation of PTSD (Henry *et al, Am J Bioeth* 2007;**7**:12–20; Rosenberg, *Am J Bioeth* 2007;**7**:27–8), e.g. pro-pranolol 40 mg TDS (n = 19, open, Vaiva *et al, Biol Psychiatry* 2003;**54**:947–9). However, propranolol was ineffective in preventing PTSD in soldiers experiencing burns in conflict (n = 65, McGee *et al, J Burn Care Res* 2009;**30**:92–7).

DHEA (dehydroepiandrosterone)

7-keto DHEA has been used successfully in treatment-resistant PTSD (n = 5, Sageman and Brown, *J Clin Psychiatry* 2006;**67**:493–6).

Duloxetine *

In men with PTSD, duloxetine 60–120 mg/d showed promise (n = 21 [c = 20], open, 8/52, Walderhaug *et al, Pharmacopsychiatry* 2010; **43**:45–9).

Gabapentin

Successful use has been reported (e.g. n = 30, Hamner *et al, Ann Clin Psychiatry* 2001;**13**:141–6; n = 1, Malek-Ahmadi, *Ann Pharmacother* 2003;**37**:664–6).

Levetiracetam

Levetiracetam (mean 2000 mg/d) may be useful as antidepressant augmentation in refractory PTSD (n = 23, retrospective, mean 10/52, Kinrys *et al, J Clin Psychiatry* 2006;**67**:211–4).

Liothyronine/triiodothyronine

Triiodothyronine 25 mcg/d has been used successfully to augment ineffective SSRI mono-therapy (n = 5, 8/52, Agid *et al, J Clin Psychiatry* 2001;**62**:169–73).

MAOIs

Phenelzine may exert a notable effect on intrusive and avoidance symptoms (n = 60, RCT, d/b, 8/52, Kosten *et al, J Nerv Ment Dis* 1991;**179**:366–70). The strong inhibitory effect on REM sleep may be contributory.

Mirtazapine

A number of studies have suggested an effect in some symptoms at 45 mg/d (64% response vs 20% for placebo; n = 29, RCT, d/b, p/c, 8/52, Davidson *et al, Biol Psychiatry* 2003;**53**:188–91). For PTSD nightmares, mirtazapine may have some significant effects, perhaps by an effect on sleep (n = > 300, open, Lewis, *Am J Psychiatry* 2002;**159**:1948–9). A continuation study showed a modest enduring effect for six months (n = 15 [c = 12], 24/52, Kim *et al,*

Psychiatry Clin Neurosci 2005;**59**:743–7).

Phenytoin

Phenytoin may have some use at anticonvulsant doses and may be associated with changes in brain structure (n = 9, open, 3/12, Bremner *et al, J Clin Psychiatry* 2004;**65**:1559–64; Bremner et al, *J Psychopharmacol* 2005;**19**:159–65).

Prazosin *

Prazosin (mean dose 9.5 mg/d) may reduce nightmares in veterans with chronic PTSD if taken for at least eight weeks. In a retrospective study in nighttime PTSD, prazosin was as effective as quetiapine over the first 6/12, but seemed more effective in the long-term, with less side effects (n = 324 [c = 237], open, > 6/12, Byers et al, *J Clin Psychopharmacol* 2010; **30**:225–9). It is well tolerated and superior to placebo on primary outcome measures in PTSD if taken at night (n = 40 [c = 34], RCT, d/b, p/c, 8/52, Raskind *et al, Biol Psychiatry* 2007;**61**:928–34).

Reviews: general (Taylor *et al, Am J Health Syst Pharm* 2008;**65**:716–22; Miller, *Pharmacother* 2008;**28**:656–66).

Pregabalin

A small pilot study suggested pregabalin may be useful for accident-related PTSD (e.g. n = 9, 6/52, Pae *et al, Int Clin Psychopharmacol* 2009; **24**:29–33).

Quetiapine

Quetiapine 25–400 mg/d monotherapy has reduced psychotic and PTSD symptoms (n = 53, open, 8/52, Kozaric-Kovacic and Pivac, *Int J Neuropsychopharmacol* 2007;**10**:253–61).

Tiagabine

Tiagabine 8 mg/d (range 4–12 mg/d) may be worth investigating in PTSD (n = 7, open, 8/52, Taylor, *J Clin Psychiatry* 2003;**64**:1421–5; UG) and a discontinuation study in responders suggested some relapse prevention efficacy (n = 29 [c = 19], open, 12/52, Connor *et al, Psychopharmacol [Berl]* 2006;**184**:21–5).

Tricyclics

Amitriptyline (n = 46, p/c, 8/52, Davidson *et al, Arch Gen Psychiatry* 1990;**4**:259–69) and imipramine (n = 60, RCT, p/c, 8/52, Kosten et al, *J Nerv Ment Dis* 1991;**179**:366–70) have been shown to produce a modest and clinically meaningful effect. However, doses of 300 mg/d for at least eight weeks may be needed.

Valproate

Intrusion, hyperarousal and depressive symptoms may respond to valproate (n = 16, 8/52, Clark *et al, J Trauma Stress* 1999;**12**:395–401) and in civilians with non-combat-related PTSD (open, Otte *et al, J Clin Psychopharmacol* 2004;**24**:106–8).

❋ Case reports ❋

- **Memantine** (n = 4, 12/52, Battista *et al, Psychiatry* 2007;**70**:167–74).
- **Oxcarbazepine** (n = 1, Berigan, *Can J Psychiatry* 2002; **7**:973–4).

◆ Others

Other drugs tried include **buspirone** (e.g. Hamner *et al, Depress Anxiety* 1997;**5**:137–9), **cyproheptadine** for nightmares (e.g. Brophy, *Mil Med* 1991;**156**:100–1), and **trazodone** (n = 6, open, Hertzberg *et al, J Clin Psychopharmacol* 1996;**1**:294–8).

☐ No efficacy

Bupropion

Bupropion may improve depression but not for PTSD (n = 30, d/b, p/c, 8/52, Becker *et al, J Clin Psychopharmacol* 2007; **27**:193–7).

Flumazenil

Two studies have shown no effects (e.g. Coupland *et al, Biol Psychiatry* 1997;**41**:988–90).

Guanfacine

Guanfacine had no effect on any PTSD symptoms (n = 63, RCT, d/b, p/c, 8/52, Neylan *et al, Am J Psychiatry* 2006;**163**:2186–8).

Naltrexone

Only non-significant improvements were seen in a small, short trial (n = 8, open, 2/52, Lubin *et al, Hum Psychopharmacol* 2002;**17**:181–5).

PSYCHIATRIC EMERGENCY, ACUTE
see Acute psychiatric emergency (1.1)

1.21 PSYCHOSIS AND SCHIZOPHRENIA
1.21.1. Psychosis and schizophrenia
1.21.2. First episode (early intervention)
1.21.3. Cognitive impairment
see also Catatonia (1.12)

Symptoms *
Schizophrenia is an enduring and fluctuating mental health problem with a high chance of relapse. Schneider's 'First rank symptoms' are often used as the main diagnostic features. They include hearing thoughts spoken aloud, 'third person' hallucinations, hallucinations in the form of a commentary, somatic hallucinations, thought withdrawal or insertion, thought broadcasting, delusional perceptions and feelings, or actions experienced as being made or influenced by external agents. The most frequent symptoms are a lack of insight, auditory hallucinations, ideas of reference, suspiciousness, flat affect, voices speaking to them, delusional mood, delusions of persecution and thoughts spoken aloud. Japan has apparently dropped schizophrenia as a term, and suggested it now be called 'salience syndrome', i.e. the person's interpretation of what is happening (van Os, *Acta Psychiatr Scand* 2009;**120**:363–72).

Possible causes of schizophrenia
The dopamine hypothesis, i.e. excess dopamine activity in the mesolimbic remains the most enduring explanation for the main symptoms (Toda and Abi-Dargham, *Curr Psychiatry Rep* 2007; **9**:329–36) but is clearly not the whole story and there are many other theories, e.g. hypofunction of the glutamate systems, particularly at the NMDA sub-type of glutamate receptor (Harrison, *Br J Psychiatry* 2008;**192**:86–7), combined dopamine hyperfunction and glutamate hypofunction (Paz et al, *Eur Neuropsychopharmacol* 2008;**18**:773–86) and 5-HT$_2$ hyperfunction (Di Pietro and Seamans, *Pharmacopsychiatry* 2007;**40**(Suppl 1):S27–33). The balance between D$_2$ and 5-HT$_2$ may be important. Abnormal connections between nerves involving amino acid neurotransmitters may be a consequence of developmentally reduced synaptic connectivity (during perinatal and adolescent periods), rather than loss of neuronal or glial cells. Antipsychotics are thought to exert a significant part of their clinical effect via blockade of mesolimbic D$_2$ receptors (Strange, *Trends Pharmacol Sci* 2008;**29**:314–21).

Role of drugs in schizophrenia
Antipsychotics have a major role in the management of the symptoms of schizophrenia but there is no clear choice of first-line antipsychotic. In nearly all RCTs using haloperidol as the comparator, haloperidol doses were higher than recommended even for severely ill patients, so it is not surprising some of the newer drugs appear better tolerated (s = 49, Hugenholtz et al, *J Clin Psychiatry* 2006; **67**:897–903). The terms 'atypical' and 'typical' have no real meaning but until a better classification title is agreed upon, the abbreviations SGA (second generation antipsychotic) and FGA (first generation antipsychotic) respectively will be used here.

1. Choice of antipsychotic
There have only been two major independent comparisons between antipsychotics.
CATIE (n = 1493, RCT, < 18/12, Lieberman et al, *N Engl J Med* 2005;**353**:1209–23) compared olanzapine (7.5–30 mg/d), risperidone (1.5–6 mg/d), perphenazine (8–32 mg/d), quetiapine (200–800 mg/d) and ziprasidone (40–160 mg/d). Among the many findings were:
- 74% patients discontinued their first antipsychotic within 18 months
- Olanzapine had the lowest drop-out rate (but had its known side-effects)
- Perphenazine was as effective as the SGAs
- Those who did not respond to a SGA, clozapine was more effective than switching to another SGA (n = 99, CATIE, McEvoy et al, *Am J Psychiatry* 2006;**163**:600–10)
- Switching to risperidone or olanzapine was more effective than quetiapine or ziprasidone, based on time to discontinuation (n = 444, RCT, d/b, CATIE, Stroup et al, *Am J Psychiatry* 2006;**163**:611–22).

CUtLASS compared switching to either FGAs or SGAs in people who needed a change and showed striking consistency over all drugs for quality of life scores (n = 227, RCT, open-s/b, 12/12, Jones et al, *Arch Gen Psychiatry* 2006; **63**:1079–87). The choice of antipsychotic in the acute phase thus remains an individual decision. A meta-analysis of SGA vs FGA trials has confirmed that SGAs are not a homogenous class (s = 150, n = 21,533, d/b, Leucht et al, Lancet 2009;**373**:31–41).

2. Early-onset and limitation of progression

Evidence is accumulating that antipsychotics started after the symptoms first appear, or even in a prodromal stage, may prevent or delay the progression of schizophrenia. See section *1.21.2*.

3. Acute phase *

Many antipsychotics have an immediate calming effect (relieving distress in the acute stage) and then reduce the intensity of psychotic symptoms. There is little proven advantage of using higher doses of some drugs, e.g. above about 12–15 mg/d of high-potency antipsychotics (e.g. haloperidol), and higher doses potentially give the recipient an adverse experience. Robust differences have been shown for both haloperidol and olanzapine compared to placebo at two weeks (s = 2, n = 422, RCT, d/b, p/c, 6/52, Kinon et al, J Clin Psychopharmacol 2010; **30**:286–9) and a pooled-data analysis has shown that if there was no improvement after two weeks, the person is unlikely to respond at week 4 and so may benefit from an earlier change (s = 7, n = 1708, RCT, Leucht et al, J Clin Psychiatry 2007;**68**:352–60). Most response is likely within 3–4 weeks, so objective rating scales may be a useful, time-effective and cost-effective tool in decision-making.

4. Relapse prevention *

Relapse of schizophrenia occurs in around 80% of untreated schizophrenics and so maintenance therapy, which reduces relapse rates significantly, is usually an important component of the management. If antipsychotics are stopped, relapse may be delayed for 2–6 months, with the individual often feeling better (due to a reduced side-effect burden) before the relapse.

Year	Life expectancy		Difference
	Schizophrenia	General population	
1996	32.5 years	57.5 years	25 years
2006	37.4 years	59.9 years	22.5 years

Intermittent therapy (prodrome-based or crisis intervention) is generally accepted as ineffective (n = 363, RCT, Gaebel et al, Schizophr Res 2002;**53**:145–59) and risks sudden relapse.

Although long-term antipsychotics are the most important relapse-prevention strategy, it is difficult to motivate people to continue while relatively asymptomatic. While compliance and adherence are terms used, 'concordance' implies an agreement between the prescriber and patient as to the degree of medicine-taking acceptable to both. In patients, this will balance the positive effects of the drug (e.g. symptom suppression) and the negative effects (e.g. side-effects) and finding a good reason not to relapse, e.g. family, friends or job, may aid effective maintenance therapy.

Long-term side-effects, particularly the under-rated akathisia, weight gain and dysphoria, tend to reduce compliance. However, an 11-year follow-up study of mortality in people with schizophrenia concluded that there was no evidence of an increase in deaths and that the gap in life expectancy between people with schizophrenia and the general population is reducing, e.g. there was a lower mortality in people with schizophrenia taking antipsychotics (for 7–11 years during study period) than not, (n = 66881 schizophrenics from national register cf 5.2m in general population, 11 years, Tiihonen et al, Lancet 2009;**374**:620–7; critical appraisal De Hert et al, Schizophr Res 2010;**117**:68-74). In people taking antipsychotics, the highest mortality was with quetiapine (OR 1.41), the lowest with clozapine (OR 0.74).

5. Discontinuation

Many people with schizophrenia are on long-term antipsychotics (depot or oral) at the dose they received when acutely ill. With depression 'the dose that got you well keeps you well' is probably true, but there is abundant evidence that this may not be necessary in schizophrenia as continuous antipsychotic intake is 'topping-up' D2 blockade as significant D2 blockade can persist for 16 weeks after discontinuing depots (Pani et al, Eur Psychiatry 2007;**22**:267–75). Reducing doses from their acute levels may actually improve outcomes and symptoms but (and it is a big but) some people appear to need higher doses long-term. This does not mean you

The use of high dose antipsychotic medication (Thompson, *Br J Psychiatry* 1994;**164**:448–58; revised by Royal College of Psychiatrists, 2006)

The upper end of the dose ranges of older antipsychotics is often not clearly established and usually defined by limits of safety and the SPCs. Doses above these limits should only be used 'with caution and under specialist supervision'. 'Chlorpromazine equivalents' have been used to compare drugs or calculate total doses of multiple drugs, but maximum doses vary between drugs, and dosage equivalents are of only limited use (see *2.2.1*). The evidence and scientific rationale for the effectiveness of high doses is very limited.

Main dangers of high dose antipsychotics:

1. Sudden cardiac-related death, e.g. QT prolongation, torsades de pointes.
2. CNS toxicity, e.g. CNS and respiratory depression, hypoxia, seizures.

Main uses of antipsychotics above BNF limits:

1. **Psychiatric emergency:** see 'Acute psychiatric emergency' (*Chapter 1.1*).
2. **Acute treatment:** i.e. after the emergency, but before the antipsychotic takes full effect. Doses should be reduced as soon as possible once the patient has responded.
3. **Long-term treatment:** e.g. in treatment-resistant schizophrenia where residual symptoms impair living or rehabilitation:
   - **as polypharmacy:** the prescribing of multiple antipsychotics is 'not recommended' as it 'may constitute a hazard' and side-effects are not minimised
   - **poor resources:** inadequate resources/environment often result in the need for more medication at higher doses.

Factors to be considered before prescribing high-dose antipsychotics:

- The diagnosis is fully confirmed and documented.
- Plasma levels are therapeutic and compliance with regimen is assured.
- Treatment duration has been fully adequate.
- Reduced doses for a trial period have been tried to rule out, e.g. akathisia.
- Adverse social and psychological factors have been minimised.
- Alternative antipsychotic therapies tried.

If exceeding standard BNF antipsychotic doses, the following should be routine and documented:

- Multidisciplinary team and patient (or advocate) discussion, obtaining valid consent if possible, making a thorough record of the decision and reasoning, including target signs and symptoms, and outcome evaluation.
- Consideration of any contraindications, e.g. cardiac, age, renal, hepatic, weight, and smoking, and any interactions, e.g. with tricyclics, carbamazepine, etc.
- ECG pre-treatment to exclude QTc prolongation, repeated every 1–3 months, especially with haloperidol.
- Doses increased only slowly.
- Regular checks carried out on pulse, bp temperature and hydration.
- Prescription reviewed regularly and reduced after three months if no improvement.

should not try reducing doses but that care is needed to prevent unnecessary and potentially catastrophic relapses.

Reducing doses or stopping antipsychotics in someone on a high dose long-term

- Check the history carefully to confirm that there is clear evidence of previous illness. If so, proceed only with great caution (especially if any evidence of a forensic potential) and document carefully. A history of non-compliance without relapse is a good sign, but not to be taken as confirmation that antipsychotics are not needed.
- Make only small changes each time.
- Remember that the peak for relapse may be at about 3–6 months post-dose reduction or discontinuation. So, leave for six months to assess the outcome of each change.
- Have a robust system in place for detecting early signs of relapse.
- Have a robust plan for increasing or reintroducing doses if early signs of relapse occur, to restabilise the patient.
- Remember that some people need higher doses and there is much to gain by reducing doses but probably more to lose should the person relapse and not be able to return to their previous levels of functioning.
- Consider the consequences of relapse, damage to the individual and others, and previous events.

Risk factors for relapse

Medication risk factors include:

- Drug used, e.g. rehospitalisation rates for schizophrenics discharged on olanzapine (n = 313) or risperidone (n = 268) were similar (31% and 33% respectively) but considerably lower than those (n = 458) discharged on FGAs (48%) (2 years, Rabinowitz *et al*, *Am J Psychiatry* 2001;**58**:266–9), confirmed by CATIE.
- Doses: there are some ethnic trends in drug responses, and doses may need to be lower in some racial groups (n = 192, 6/52, Emsley *et al*, *J Clin Psychiatry* 2002;**63**:9–14). Higher long-term doses lead to extra ADRs and a higher risk of non-compliance.
- Duration of untreated psychosis (DUP): DUP is a good predictor of outcome.

- Unmanaged substance misuse: this reduces antipsychotic effects in dual diagnosis, with sooner and longer readmissions, especially in those non-compliant (n = 99, four years, Hunt *et al*, *Schizophr Res* 2002; **54**:253–64).
- Non-compliance/concordance.

Reviews: * optimal duration of prophylactic antipsychotics in schizophrenia (Bosveld-van Haandel *et al*, *Acta Psychiatr Scand* 2001; **103**:335–46), general (Chan and Ungvari, *Int J Neuropsychopharmacol* 2002;**5**:277–81).

Suicide prevention

Around 5% of schizophrenics will commit suicide, usually near illness onset (n = 22 598, Palmer *et al*, *Arch Gen Psychiatry* 2005;**62**:247–53). A five-year retrospective study suggested both risperidone and olanzapine gave some protection from suicidality compared to other (excluding clozapine) antipsychotics (n = 756, Barak *et al*, *Psychopharmacol [Berl]* 2004;**175**: 215–9). Clozapine has a clear anti-suicide effect.

Reviews: * systematic review of SGAs in TRS (Melnik *et al*, *Sao Paulo Med J* 2010;**128**:141–66), mode of action (Stone *et al*, *J Psychopharmacol* 2010;**24**:953–64), metabolic side-effects of SGAs in children (Fedorowicz and Fombonne, *J Psychopharmacol* 2006;**20**:533–50), systematic review and meta-analysis of SGAs vs low-potency FGAs (s = 150, n = 21,533, d/b, Leucht *et al*, *Lancet* 2009;**373**:31–41), plasma levels of SGAs (Mauri *et al*, *Clin Pharmacokinet* 2007; **46**:359–88).

1.21.1 PSYCHOSIS AND SCHIZOPHRENIA

BNF listed

FIRST GENERATION (OR TYPICAL) ANTIPSYCHOTICS (FGAs)

PHENOTHIAZINES

Chlorpromazine

Chlorpromazine can be used for a wide range of psychotic conditions but use in the elderly is problematic. Cochrane concludes that chlorpromazine remains a global 'benchmark' for schizophrenia, as a well-established, effective but imperfect treatment (Adams *et al*, *Cochrane Database Syst Rev* 2007;**2**:CD000284) with a relapse prevention efficacy (s = 10, n = 1042, Almerie et al, Cochrane Database Syst Rev 2007; 1:CD006329). Cochrane also concludes that, based on available studies (all 1968–78), the optimum dose of chlorpromazine is in the 400–800 mg/d range, with no advantages for lower or higher doses (s = 4, n = 1012, RCT, Liu and De Haan, Cochrane Syst Database Rev 2009; 2:CD007778). IV use is not recommended unless the injection is diluted and the patient is in a supine position.

Fluphenazine (see also depots)
The oral preparation has been discontinued in the UK. Cochrane concluded that oral fluphenazine was effective 'but imperfect' (s = 7, Mataer and Almerie, Cochrane Database Syst Rev 2007; 1:CD006352).

Levomepromazine (methotrimeprazine) *
Cochrane concludes that there is little information on levomepromazine, but that it causes less EPSE than haloperidol and more hypotension than risperidone, not really a ground-breaking conclusion (s = 4, n = 192, Sivaraman et al, Cochrane Database Syst Rev 2010; 10:CD007779). It has sedative effects.

Pericyazine
Pericyazine is a piperidine phenothiazine, with marked sedative and hypotensive side-effects. Use as a low-dose anxiolytic-sedative has increased with the fall of thioridazine. Little is published about the drug.

Perphenazine
Perphenazine is a piperazine phenothiazine with a relatively short half-life (8–12 hours). Chosen as a 'typical' comparator, the CATIE study has shown perphenazine to be as effective as olanzapine, risperidone, quetiapine and ziprasidone (n = 1493, RCT, < 18/12, Lieberman et al, N Engl J Med 2005; 353:1209–23; see also Rosenheck; Kane et al, J Clin Psychiatry 2007; 68:1812–4).

Prochlorperazine
Prochlorperazine is a piperazine phenothiazine better known for its use as an antiemetic and in Ménières disease, but also licensed for schizophrenia and acute mania.

Promazine
Promazine is similar to chlorpromazine and retains a minor role as a non-dependence-prone hypnotic, although the potential for side-effects should not be ignored.

Trifluoperazine
Trifluoperazine is a piperazine phenothiazine widely used as an antipsychotic and sometimes claimed to have 'activating' effects at low doses. Cochrane concludes that trifluoperazine is of similar efficacy to other antipsychotics (s = 13, n = 1162, Marques et al, Cochrane Database Syst Rev 2004; 1:CD003545).

BUTYROPHENONES

Benperidol
Benperidol is a potent D2 blocker marketed originally as specific for antisocial sexual behaviour. Cochrane concludes that there is insufficient evidence to assess the drug's effectiveness, with a single poor RCT, where it was inferior to perphenazine (Leucht and Hartung, Cochrane Database Syst Rev 2005; 2:CD003083). See 1.24.

Haloperidol (see also depots) *
Haloperidol is the prototype and standard reference butyrophenone used for the treatment of acute and chronic psychosis, both orally and as an injection (aqueous and depot), although in the CUtLASS study few patients remained on haloperidol long-term. The BNF oral limit is 30 mg/d, but there is no additional antipsychotic advantage from doses higher than 12 mg/d in psychosis and acute mania, and 4 mg/d may be as effective as 10 mg/d and 40 mg/d (n = 24, RCT, d/b, 2/52, Stone et al, Am J Psychiatry 1995; 152:1210–2). Even ultra-low doses (1–2 mg/d) may be effective and well tolerated in first-episode psychosis (n = 35, open, Oosthuizen et al, J Psychopharmacol 2001; 15:251–5), although reported to cause as much TD as standard dose FGAs (n = 57, 12/12, Oosthuizen et al, J Clin Psychiatry 2003; 64:1075–80). An observational study showed that improvement in the first two weeks was predictive of response, and that increasing the dose above 6.6 mg/d (+/- 2 mg) in non-responders did not improve response (n = 101,

Giegling et al, J Psychiatr Res 2010;**44**:487–92). So, a moderate dose in the first two weeks either works or it doesn't, so there appears to be little point in pushing it up. The elimination half-life in brain tissue is about 6–8 days, with significant amounts still detectable after two weeks. Thus, residual side-effects may continue for many weeks or months after stopping the drug, due to persistence of active CNS levels (Kornhuber et al, Am J Psychiatry 1999;**156**:885–90). Cochrane concludes that haloperidol is superior to placebo but that its ADRs are such that alternative antipsychotics should be prescribed (Joy et al, Cochrane Database Syst Rev 2006;**4**:CD003082). The UK SmPC now recommends an ECG before treatment due to the risk of a dose-related increase in QT-interval (n = 596, Reilly et al, Lancet 2000;**355**:1048–52), especially if given by the IV, rather than IM route.

Review: Pharmacokinetics (Kudo and Ishizaki, Clin Pharmacokinetics 1999;**37**:435–56).

THIOXANTHENES

Flupentixol (see also depots)
Oral flupentixol is usually used in low dose for anxiety and depression. Flupentixol 5–20 mg/d was as effective as olanzapine 5–20 mg/d with more EPS but less weight gain (n = 28, RCT, d/b, 4/52, Gattaz et al, Pharmacopsychiatry 2004;**37**:279–85), and 4–12 mg/d was as effective as risperidone 2–6 mg/d for negative, affective and cognitive symptoms (n = 144, RCT, d/b, 25/52, Ruhrmann et al, Prog Neuropsychopharmacol Biol Psychiatry 2007; **31**:1012–22).

Zuclopenthixol (see also depots)
Zuclopenthixol is a relatively long-acting oral antipsychotic, and in a trial of oral vs depot zuclopenthixol in people with violence and schizophrenia, violence was inversely proportional to compliance, and much lower in the depot group (n = 46, RCT, s/b, one year, Arango et al, Eur Psychiatry 2006;**21**:34–40). Cochrane concludes that oral zuclopenthixol is a viable option but needs routine anticholinergics (s = 18, n = 1578, Kumar and Strech, Cochrane Database Syst Rev 2005; **4**:CD005474).

DIPHENYLBUTYLPIPERIDINES

Fluspirilene
See depots.

Pimozide
Pimozide is licensed for chronic schizophrenia and other psychoses, especially paranoid and monosymptomatic hypochondriacal psychoses, e.g. parasitosis. It is effective against a wide range of positive symptoms (s = 35, n = 1348, Rathbone and McMonagle, Cochrane Database Syst Rev 2007;**3**:CD001949), but with potential cardiotoxic effects (see 3.2). Any use in delusional disorders is based almost entirely on case reports (Gray, EBMH 2000;**3**:117).

BENZAMIDES, substituted

Review: consensus statement on substituted benzamides in psychiatry (Racagni et al, Neuropsychobiol 2004;**50**:134–43).

Amisulpride *
Low dose amisulpride (related to sulpiride) blocks pre-synaptic D2 and D3 autoreceptors, higher doses blocking post-synaptic receptors, with little effect on other receptors. Amisulpride has been compared with risperidone (n = 309, RCT, d/b, 6/12, Sechter et al, Neuropsychopharmacol 2002;**27**:1071–81) and at 200–800 mg/d is equivalent to olanzapine 5–20 mg/d but with less weight gain (n = 377, RCT, d/b, 6/12, Martin et al, Curr Med Res Opin 2002;**18**:355–62) and dose-dependent hyperprolactinaemia (RCT, d/b, 6/12, Mortimer et al, Int Clin Psychopharmacol 2004;**19**:63–9). A meta-analysis showed some effect at 50–100 mg/d for predominantly negative symptoms and lower use of anticholinergic drugs (s = 18, n = 2214, RCT, Leucht et al, Am J Psychiatry 2002;**159**:180–90; caution expressed by Remington and Kapur, EBMH 2002;**5**:85). Another meta-analysis suggests negative symptoms may respond to low-dose amisulpride at the dose necessary for positive symptom response (when it becomes a D2/D3 blocker), its effect is essentially that of a 'typical' agent (s = 4, Storosum et al, Schizo Bull 2002;**28**:193–201). Cochrane concludes that studies vs SGAs are short but that it is more

effective than ziprasidone with less weight gain than risperidone or olanzapine (s = 10, n = 1549, Komossa et al, Cochrane Database Syst Rev 2010;1:CD006624).

Reviews: * general (Nuss and Tessier, Curr Med Res Opin 2010;**26**:787–801; Mortimer, Neuropsychiatr Dis Treat 2009;**5**:267–77), TDM (Sparshatt et al, Acta Psychiatr Scand 2009; **120**:416–28).

Sulpiride

Sulpiride is a specific dopamine (D2, plus some D3 and D4) receptor blocker, well-established in the UK. Cochrane concludes that sulpiride may be effective but the evidence is extremely limited (s = 2, n = 113, Omori and Wang, Cochrane Database Syst Rev 2009;**2**:CD007811). It was the most commonly chosen FGA in the CUtLASS study (n = 227, RCT, open-s/b, 12/12, Jones et al, Arch Gen Psychiatry 2006;**63**:1079–87).

SECOND GENERATION (OR ATYPICAL) ANTIPSYCHOTICS (SGAs)

'Atypical' has been a widely-used term to describe a diverse group of antipsychotics with specific characteristics, e.g. minimal EPS, lack of sedation or a fast dissociation from D2 receptors. The CATIE and CUtLASS studies have shown similar efficacy but different ADRs. CATIE, CUtLASS and the Leucht meta-analysis (s = 150, n = 21533, d/b, Lancet 2009;**373**:31–41) have shown similar efficacy but different ADRs.

Reviews of SGAs: dosing (Cutler et al, CNS Spectr 2008;**13**[Suppl 9]:1–16), TDM (Hiemke et al, Ther Drug Monit 2004;**26**:156–60), doses (Kinon et al, CNS Drugs 2004;**18**:597–616) and mechanisms of action (Horacek et al, CNS Drugs 2006;**20**:389–409).

Aripiprazole *

Aripiprazole is a dopamine D2 and $5HT_{1A}$ receptor partial agonist, and a $5HT_{2A}$ receptor antagonist. It stimulates dopamine receptors but to a lower level than dopamine, while blocking endogenous dopamine (100% D2 occupancy by aripiprazole reduces dopaminergic activity to about 30%). The starting dose should be 5 mg/d if the patient is switching from another antipsychotic, increasing to 10 mg/d, and then

15 mg/d as tolerated. Time to steady state takes one to two and maybe four weeks so rapid dose escalation may not be advisable (Uzun et al, Psychiatr Danub 2005;**17**:67–75). A thorough analysis has concluded that the optimum dose of aripiprazole is 10 mg/d, with doses above 20 mg/d providing no additional benefit (s = 5, Mace and Taylor, CNS Drugs 2009;**23**:773–80), although higher doses have been used, albeit with variable success (e.g. 35–60 mg/d, n = 4, Crossman and Lindenmayer, J Clin Psychiatry 2006;**67**:1158–9). A rather critical systematic review and meta-analysis has concluded that aripiprazole is superior to placebo with less raised prolactin than other antipsychotics, although study attrition rates were large and poorly reported (s = 10, El-Sayeh et al, Br J Psychiatry 2006;**189**:102–8; biting and justified criticism by Mortimer, EBMH 2007;**10**:14). Long-term efficacy equivalent to olanzapine has been shown in a one-year extension trial to a 6/12 RCT (n = 214, one year, Chrzanowski et al, Psychopharmacology [Berl] 2006;**189**:259–66), where 15 mg/d seems well tolerated and effective (n = 310, RCT, p/c, d/b, 6/12, Pigott et al, J Clin Psychiatry 2003;**64**:1048–56; comment by Mortimer, EBMH 2004;**7**:41 noting placebo level side-effects, no dose titration, simple dosing, that 30% of stable people relapsed over 6/12 when switched, and a lack of symptom reduction in more severely ill patients). In olanzapine or risperidone non-responders, switching to either aripiprazole (15–30 mg/d) or perphenazine (8–64 mg/d), resulting in 27% and 25% respectively responding, with aripiprazole better tolerated and with higher QoL scores (n = 300, RCT, d/b, 6/52, Kane et al, J Clin Psychiatry 2007;**68**:213–23; MS). Aripiprazole 9.75 mg IM is rapidly effective and well tolerated for agitation in schizophrenia (n = 357, RCT, p/c, Tran-Johnson et al, J Clin Psychiatry 2007;**68**:111–9; MS). Cochrane concludes that aripiprazole is effective, with a lower risk of akathisia, raised prolactin and QTc prolongation than other SGAs (s = 15, n = 7110, RCT, El-Sayeh and Morganti, Cochrane Database Syst Rev 2006 2:CD004578), efficacy is similar to typicals but with superior tolerability (s = 9, n = 3122, Bhattacharjee and El-Sayeh, Cochrane Database Syst Rev 2008;**3**:CD006617) but somewhat less effective than olanzapine,

albeit better tolerated for metabolic effects and sedation (s=4, n=1404, Komossa et al, *Cochrane Database Syst Rev* 2009;**4**:CD006569; see also n=703, RCT, d/b, 46/52, Fleischacker et al, *Biol Psychiatry* 2009;**65**:510–7).

Reviews: * extensive (Sparshatt et al, *J Clin Psychiatry* 2010;**71**:1447–56), general (Stip and Tourjman, *Clin Ther* 2010;**32**(Suppl 1);S3–20), consensus statement (Sullivan et al, *Curr Med Res Opin* 2007;**23**:1733–44), safety and tolerability (Pae, *Expert Opin Drug Saf* 2009;**8**:373–86), use in children and adolescents (Greenaway and Elbe, *J Can Acad Child Adolesc Psychiatry* 2009;**18**:250–60), oral vs IM kinetics (Boulton et al, *Clin Pharmacokinet* 2008;**47**:475–85).

Clozapine (see also *Tables 1.2–1.6*) *

Clozapine is indicated for treatment-resistant schizophrenia (TRS) and unresponsive psychotic disorders in Parkinson's disease. Before starting, patients should have a physical examination and any cardiac disease excluded.

Efficacy: Clozapine is probably effective in up to 30–50% of treatment-resistant schizophrenics (n=268, RCT, d/b, p/c, 6/52, Kane et al, *Arch Gen Psychiatry* 1988;**45**:789–96). This may rise to 60% if adequate doses are given for up to 12 months, e.g. a one-year study in TRS showed that 50–76% responded to clozapine, the peak response occurring at 12–24 weeks (n=84, open, 52/52, Lieberman et al, *Am J Psychiatry* 1994;**151**:1744–52). There is probably little clinical gain in prolonging exposure to clozapine beyond eight weeks at any particular dose if no response is seen (n=50, open, Conley et al, *Am J Psychiatry* 1997;**154**:1243–7). Cochrane concludes that clozapine is slightly more effective than other SGAs (s=27, n=3099, RCT, Asenjo Lobos et al, *Cochrane Database Syst Rev* 2010;**11**:CD006633), and in TRS where it is clearly superior and has a differential efficacy (s=42, n=3950, Essali et al, *Cochrane Database Syst Rev* 2009; **1**:CD000059).

Mode of action: Clozapine's mode of action remains unclear, e.g. it has a low occupancy of D_2 receptors (30–60%) and thus may act via D_1, $5\text{-}HT_2$, ACh, $5\text{-}HT_6$ and $5\text{-}HT_7$ receptors and inhibition of pre-synaptic alpha-2 autoreceptors. Some D_2 limbic specificity has been shown. Adjunctive aripiprazole (with potent D2 affinity) does not diminish clozapine's efficacy,

suggesting its efficacy is not predominantly D2 blockade.

Blood levels: * Plasma levels may be useful in optimising therapy if poor response occurs. ADRs can be far higher than spontaneously reported, and plasma level related (n=103, Yusufi et al, *Int Clin Psychopharmacol* 2007; **22**:238–43). See table *1.6*.

Blood dyscrasias: Clozapine can cause a usually reversible neutropenia in 3–4% of patients, which may lead on to agranulocytosis in 0.8% of patients over one year, with a non-dose-related higher risk in older people and those with lower base-line wbc counts (n=11555, Alvir et al, *N Engl J Med* 1993;**329**:162–7). The onset peaks at around 8–10 weeks (range 0.5–24+ weeks), lasts between 12 and 20 days and treatment is thus restricted (see *Table 1.2*), although the incidence after three years is minimal. The UK CPMS database study indicated that agranulocytosis is 2.4-fold higher in Asians compared to Caucasians, and there is an age-related increase in risk of 53% per decade, but no dose-relationship (n=12760, Munro et al, *Br J Psychiatry* 1999;**175**:576–80). Clozapine is also able to induce transient granulocytopenia without the usual rise in granulocyte colony stimulating factor (G-CSF) levels. The use of clozapine in people with a low wbc count due to benign ethnic neutropenia (BEN) may be allowed with haematologist advice. Of 53 patients rechallenged after clozapine-induced leucopenia or neutropenia, 38% had a further dyscrasia and, in most of these, it was more severe, longer-lasting and occurred more quickly than the original episode, but 55% were rechallenged successfully and remained in treatment (n=53, Dunk et al, *Br J Psychiatry* 2006;**188**:255–63). G-CSF or GM-CSF stimulates cell production and shortens the period of clozapine-induced agranulocytosis by about a half, at which point it can be discontinued (e.g. n=1, Schuld et al, *Acta Psychiatr Scand* 2000;**102**:153–5).

Reviews: * general (Mckee et al, *Clin Schizophr Relat Psychoses* 2011;**5**:26–32), restarting clozapine after neutropenia (Whiskey and Taylor, *CNS Drugs* 2007;**21**:25–35), genetics of clozapine-induced agranulocytosis (Opgen-Rhein and Dettling, *Pharmacogenomics* 2008; **9**:1101–11).

Clozapine UK prescribing and monitoring summary

Clozapine is indicated in the UK for treatment-resistant schizophrenia and psychosis in Parkinson's disease, ie. patients 'non-responsive' or 'intolerant' of conventional antipsychotics (*Table 1.2*). It can be dispensed on a weekly, fortnightly or four-weekly basis (*Table 1.3*), but only following a satisfactory blood result (*Table 1.4*).

TABLE 1.2: SUMMARY OF UK CLOZAPINE PRESCRIBING RESTRICTIONS

'Non-responsive'	Lack of satisfactory clinical improvements despite the use of at least two marketed antipsychotics prescribed at adequate dose for an adequate duration
'Intolerant'	The impossibility of achieving clinical benefit with conventional antipsychotics because of severe or untreatable neurological or other adverse reactions, eg. extrapyramidal or tardive dyskinesia
Patient requirements	Hospital-based originally. Normal white blood cell and differential blood counts. Enrolled with clozapine non-rechallenge database (CNRD)
Prescriber and dispensing requirements	Consultant must be registered with CNRD (clozapine non-rechallenge database). Hospital or nominated community pharmacy must be registered with CNRD

TABLE 1.3: SUMMARY OF UK CLOZAPINE MINIMUM BLOOD TEST REQUIREMENTS *

Blood tests	Required frequency	Validity
Pre-treatment	Single blood screen	10 days, if satisfactory (green)
First 18 weeks of treatment First sample at three days	Weekly (usually Monday or Tuesday)	11 days (not including day of sample) if satisfactory (green)
Weeks 19–52	Every two weeks if blood results have been satisfactory	21 days (not including day of sample) if satisfactory (green)
Weeks 53 onwards	Every four weeks, if 'stable haematological profile'	42 days (not including day of sample) if satisfactory (green)
Discontinuation (temporary or permanent)	Weekly (up to 18 weeks), or fortnightly (19 weeks onwards) for four weeks after completely stopping clozapine	In total one month's follow-up is required at previous monitoring frequency e.g. 4x1/52, 2x2/52 or 1x4/52. . If test result has not been, or does not go, red clozapine may be restarted. See *Table 1.5*

TABLE 1.4: SUMMARY OF UK TEST RESULTS

Results	Meaning	Action
Green	Satisfactory	Routine tests
Amber	wbc or neutrophil counts below accepted levels	Repeat test twice a week until either red or green
Red	wbc below 3000/mm^3 and/or absolute neutrophils below 1500/mm^3	Immediate cessation of therapy. Sample blood daily until patient recovered. No further prescribing allowed unless an error has occurred or Consultant takes full responsibility.

TABLE 1.5: SUMMARY OF TEMPORARY BREAKS IN CLOZAPINE THERAPY ADVICE *

1. Dose		
Dose on discontinuation	Break	Dose on restart (contact your supplying pharmacy for advice)
Any	<48 hours	Restart on previous dose
Any	>48 hours	Restart at 12.5–25 mg and build up gradually to previous dose to minimise dose-related side-effects
2. Sampling frequency		
Previous monitoring frequency	Break	Monitoring on restart
Weekly	<1 week	Weekly, no need to restart 18-week period
Weekly	>1 week	Weekly, **must** restart 18-week period
After 18 weeks *		
Fortnightly	3 days	Fortnightly
Fortnightly	≥3 days	Weekly for six weeks, then fortnightly
Four-weekly	≤3 days	Four-weekly
Four-weekly	>3 days	Weekly for six weeks, then four-weekly
Fortnightly or four-weekly	>4 weeks	Requires full re-registration and monitoring again fully as if commencing for the first time.

TABLE 1.6: SUMMARY OF CLOZAPINE PLASMA LEVEL INTERPRETATION *

Trough clozapine	Clinical response	Advice
<0.01 ('not detected')	Any	Clozapine unlikely to have been taken for at least a week pre-sample unless early in initiation phase and with dose < 100 mg/d. Low plasma levels may occur in CYP1A2 ultra-rapid metabolisers (review by Greenwood-Smith et al, J Psychopharmacol 2003;17:234–8) and may account for some non-responders
<0.35 mg/l	Good	Repeat at six months, then annually unless response deteriorates or ADRs become troublesome
	Poor or incomplete	If poor adherence possible, consider psychoeducation or supervised administration. Suspension is available, ensure very well shaken before administering. Repeat assay after adherence intervention. If no improvement, consider cautious dose increase (extra care above 450 mg/d because of the increased risk of ADRs, particularly seizures.) Monitor mental state and side-effects. Review patient again and repeat the assay after at least one week on the new dose. Low plasma levels may occur in CYP1A2 ultra-rapid metabolisers (review by Greenwood-Smith et al, J Psychopharmacol 2003;17:234–8) and may account for some non-responders
0.35–0.60 mg/l	Good	Repeat at six months, then annually unless response deteriorates or ADRs become troublesome. If ADRs persist or are serious, consider cautious dose reduction (e.g. 25 mg/d in week 1, and a further 25 mg/d in week 2, etc.), but bear in mind the possible loss of response
	Poor or incomplete	If clozapine has continued for at least 3–6 months at the current dose, consider psychosocial intervention. Augmentation with other psychoactive drugs can be considered (see separate section). It is important that any such attempts should be carefully considered with respect to side-effects (including the risk of neutropenia) and possible interactions. Clozapine should not be used with drugs known to have a substantial potential for causing agranulocytosis
0.61–0.99 mg/l	Good, with no clinical features of toxicity	Review treatment. Consider a cautious dose reduction (e.g. 25 mg/d in week 1 and a further 25 mg/d in week 2, etc.), but balance this reduction against the risk of diminishing the response to clozapine. Consider using an anticonvulsant (not carbamazepine) as prophylaxis against seizures, if dose reduction thought inadvisable. Monitor the patient's mental state. Repeat assay after at least one week on a new dose, otherwise three-monthly
	Poor, incomplete or reduced and/or with clinical features of toxicity	Consider a cautious dose reduction (see above) to bring plasma clozapine to below 0.6 mg/L. Monitor the patient's mental state. Repeat assay after at least one week on a new dose
1.0–1.9 mg/l	Good — no clinical features of toxicity	Review treatment. Consider cautious dose reduction (as above) to bring plasma level below 1.0 and possibly below 0.6 mg/L, but balance this against risk of reduced response to clozapine. Consider using valproate as prophylaxis against seizures. Monitor the patient's mental state. Repeat the assay after at least one week on a new dose, otherwise three-monthly. Remember that plasma levels may continue to rise in the short term, even after dose reduction reduction
	Poor, incomplete or reduced and/or with clinical features of toxicity	Consider a cautious dose reduction (see above) to bring plasma levels to below 1.0 and possibly below 0.6 mg/L. Monitor the patient's mental state. Repeat the assay after at least one week on a new dose. Remember that plasma levels may continue to rise in the short term, even after dose reduction reduction
>2 mg/l	Good, with no clinical features of toxicity	Review urgently. Consider a cautious dose reduction (see above) to bring plasma level to below 1.0 mg/L, and possibly below 0.6 mg/L. Consider an anticonvulsant (not carbamazepine) as prophylaxis against seizures. Monitor the patient's mental state. Repeat the assay after at least one week on a new dose. Bear in mind that plasma clozapine may continue to rise in the short term, even after the dose has been reduced
	Poor, incomplete or reduced and/or with clinical features of toxicity	Review urgently. If the patient is being treated in the community, consider admitting them for observation. Consider withholding clozapine for 24 hours and re-starting at 75% of the last dose, and thereafter reducing the dose cautiously (see above) to bring plasma clozapine to below 1.0 mg/L, and possibly below 0.6 mg/L. Consider using an anticonvulsant prophylaxis (not carbamazepine) as prophylaxis against seizures. Monitor the patient's mental state. Repeat the assay after at least one week on a new dose. Bare in mind that plasma clozapine may continue to rise in the short term, even after the dose has been reduced
Others		Plasma level ratios: Clozapine:norclozapine ratio >2 suggests clozapine N-demethylation has become saturated (n = 26796, Couchman et al, Ther Drug Monit 2010;32:438–47).

Reference: by kind permission Bob Flanaghan, CMHP Bulletin 2011

Suicide reduction: It is now reasonably well-established that clozapine reduces suicide rates in schizophrenia, which can be as high as 10%, a startling comparison with the risk of one in 50 for reversible agranulocytosis. The InterSePT study (n = 980, RCT, d/b, two years, Meltzer et al, Arch Gen Psychiatry 2003;**60**:82–91; comment by Volavka, EBMH 2003;**6**:93) has shown a 25% reduction in suicide events compared to olanzapine (itself with possible antisuicide effects) which appears to be due to clozapine's intrinsic action (e.g. reducing impulsiveness and aggression, n = 44, open, 6/12, prospective, Spivak et al, J Clin Psychiatry 2003;**64**:755–60) not from concomitant medication (Glick et al, J Clin Psychiatry 2004;**65**:679–85), making a contribution to the risk:benefit analysis of clozapine. However, one study failed to show a reduced completed suicide rate with clozapine (9.2–10.5% in each group over four years), as the reduced death rate was entirely due to reduced respiratory disorders (n = 1514 plus 2830 matched-controls, four years, Sernyak et al, Am J Psychiatry 2001;**158**:931–7; disputed by Ertugrul and Meltzer, Am J Psychiatry 2002; **159**:323–5; comment by Reinstein et al, Clin Drug Investig 2002;**22**:341–6).

Reviews: combination therapies (Mouaffak et al, Clin Neuropharmacol 2006;**29**:28–33), in children (Gogtay and Rapoport, Expert Opin Pharmacother 2008;**9**:459–65), ADRs (Flanagan, Curr Drug Saf 2008;**3**:115–22).

Olanzapine

Olanzapine is licensed for the treatment of schizophrenia and relapse prevention. It blocks a wide variety of receptors, e.g. 5-HT$_{2A/C}$, 5-HT$_3$, 5-HT$_6$, D$_{1-5}$, M$_{1-5}$, alpha-one and H1, with some mesolimbic dopamine selectivity. The starting and main therapeutic dose is 10 mg/d (range 5–20 mg/d, mean 15–18 mg/d). Many studies have shown a clinical effect, e.g. where olanzapine (mean dose 15 mg/d) was more effective than haloperidol (10–20 mg/d) on negative symptoms (n = 335, RCT, d/b, 12/12, Tollefson and Sanger, Am J Psychiatry 1997;**154**:466–74). An independent study in TRS suggested that switching from an SGA/haloperidol to olanzapine may improve cognitive function but improve psychopathology in only

9% (n = 45, Lindenmayer et al, J Clin Psychiatry 2002;**63**:931–5). Olanzapine appeared effective in a relapse prevention study (n = 583, RCT, d/b, one year, Beasley et al, J Clin Psycho- pharmacol 2003;**23**:582–94, MS).

Higher doses: Use of higher doses may be increasing, and there is some evidence for efficacy (Citrome and Kantrowitz, Expert Rev Neurother 2009;**9**:1045–58), although high dose olanzapine (10 mg vs 20 mg vs 40 mg/d) had no advantage over lower doses in TRS (n = 599, RCT, d/b, 8/52, Kinon et al, J Clin Psychopharmacol 2008;**28**:392–400; MS). In a comparison of high-dose olanzapine mean 34 mg/d (vs clozapine mean 564 mg/d) showed similar efficacy in TRS (n = 40, RCT, d/b, 6/12, Meltzer et al, J Clin Psychiatry 2008;**69**:274–85; comment by Roth, J Clin Psychiatry 2008;**69**:176–7). Higher dose olanzapine (30–40 mg/d) has similar kinetics as 20 mg/d but akathisia is more common (n = 37, RCT, d/b, Mitchell et al, Clin Ther 2006;**28**:881–92). Olanzapine levels may be useful to optimise doses and assess the influence of gender, smoking and interactions (n = 194, Skogh et al, Ther Drug Monit 2002;**24**:518–26). Cochrane concludes that olanzapine may be effective but that unfamiliar rating scales make firm conclusions difficult to draw (Duggan et al, Cochrane Database Syst Rev 2005;**2**:CD001359), and that, although it may have a small superiority over other SGAs, it has known metabolic and weight ADRs, and a 49% drop-out rate from trials makes this conclusion 'tentative' (s = 50, n = 9476, Komossa et al, Cochrane Database Syst Rev 2010;**3**:CD006654).

Reviews: * TDM/plasma levels, dosing and interactions (Patel, Flanagan et al, J Clin Psychopharmacol 2011;**31**:[in press]), safety (Kantrowitz and Citrome, Expert Opin Drug Saf 2008;**7**:761–9).

Paliperidone *

Paliperidone, the 9-hydroxy metabolite of risperidone, has a starting and standard dose of 6 mg/d, which has placebo level EPS, and no need for dose titration. The oral form uses the OROS sustained release system giving a once-daily dosage and steady plasma levels. Paliperidone is also an antagonist at alpha-1 and alpha-2 adrenergic receptors and HI histaminergic receptors but no affinity for cholinergic muscarinic or beta-1 or beta-2 adrenergic receptors. It has been shown to be effective at 6–12 mg/d in acute schizophrenia (s = 3, n = 1326, RCT, d/b, p/c, 6/52, Meltzer et al, J Clin Psychiatry 2008;**69**:817–29), quicker-acting and more effective than quetiapine in acute schizophrenia (n = 397 [c = 281], RCT, d/b, p/c, 6/52, Canuso et al, Am J Psychiatry 2009;**166**:691–701, MS) and in relapse prevention studies (s = 3, n = 1083, 52/52, open extension, Emsley et al, Int Clin Psychopharmacol 2008;**23**:343–56). Paliperidone is licensed in the EU for schizoaffective disorder, with 12 mg/d the optimum dose (n = 316, RCT, p/c, 6/52, Canuso et al, J Clin Psychiatry 2010;**71**:587–98). Paliperidone 9 mg/d im-proved sleep architecture and continuity in schizophrenia with concomitant insomnia (n = 36, RCT, d/b, p/c, 2/52, Luthringer et al, Int Clin Psychopharmacol 2007;**22**:299–308). Administration with high fat high caloric meal increases peak concentration 60% and the AUC 54% compared with administration under fasting conditions. Cochrane concludes paliperidone is effective (s = 5, n = 3067, RCT, p/c, Nussbaum and Stroup, Cochrane Database Syst Rev 2008;**2**:CD006369; comment by Dolder, EBMH 2008;**11**:114).

Reviews: * general (Yang, CNS Drugs 2011; **25**:523–38; Chwieduk and Keating, Drugs 2010;**70**:1295–317; Marino and Caballero, Pharmacopsychiatry 2008;**28**:1283–98; Dolder et al, Am J Health Syst Pharm 2008;**65**:403–13), tolerability (Harrington and English, Int Clin Psychopharmacol 2010;**25**:334–41), plasma levels (Nazirizadeh et al, Eur J Clin Pharmacol 2010;**66**:797–803; de Leon et al, Psychosomatics 2010;**51**:80–8).

Quetiapine *

Quetiapine is an established antipsychotic with effects on many receptors, e.g. it shows transiently high D2 occupancy which drops rapidly over 12–14 hours, which may explain the low EPS and low prolactin elevation (s = 20, review by Sparshatt et al, J Clin Psychiatry 2011; in press). The target dose of 600 mg/d (range 150–750 mg/d) is probably the most effective,

with once-daily dosing viable with the new XL preparation, although a few may experience worsening symptoms or orthostatic hypo-tension Quetiapine XL was as effective as plain tablets, but with less ADRs (n = 58, RCT, d/b, c/o, Datto et al, Clin Ther 2009 **31**:492–502). Cochrane concludes that although quetiapine is more effective than placebo, no difference could be detected against traditional antipsychotics, (Srisurapanont et al, Cochrane Database Syst Rev 2004;**2**:CD000967) and also that the drop-out rate from quetiapine is relatively high, with most stopping it within a few weeks (s = 21, n = 4101, RCT, Komossa et al, Cochrane Database Syst Rev 2010;**1**:CD006625). Doses need to be increased gradually over several days, initially to reduce the incidence of postural hypotension. An analysis has shown that the onset of action of quetiapine is significant by the end of week one (SANS and BPRS), sooner than usually expected (s = 3, n = 620, RCT, d/b, Small et al, Curr Med Res Opin 2004;**20**:1017–23). A review of high-dose quetiapine concluded that there is little or no evidence for use of supra-BNF doses (Sparshatt et al, CNS Drugs 2008;**22**:49–72).

Reviews: * general (Miodownik and Lerner, Expert Rev Neurother 2006;**6**:983–92), TDM (Wittman et al, Neuro Endocrinol Lett 2010; **31**:203–7).

Risperidone *

Risperidone is licensed for acute and chronic psychosis and has D_2 and $5-HT_2$ blocking actions.

Dose: An extensive literature analysis con-cluded that risperidone's optimum dose is 4 mg/d, lower doses being consistently less effective and > 6 mg/d having more side-effects, and with less efficacy at >10 mg/d (Ezewuzie and Taylor, J Psychopharmacol 2006;**20**:86–90). Cochrane agrees that generally the optimal dose is 4–6 mg/d, with 2–4 mg/d of value in first episodes and doses above 10 mg/d have no advantage (Li et al, Cochrane Database Syst Rev 2009;**4**:CD007474). Titration to 6 mg/d over three days is standard practice, but a slower titration has been recommended (over weeks rather than days, stabilising on 2–4 mg/d initially before proceeding to higher doses), particularly in drug-naive first-episode schizophrenics and in the elderly, as this markedly reduces the final doses needed, EPS and improves compliance (n = 17, Kontakakis et al, Am J Psychiatry 2000;**157**:1178–9), and may lead to better outcomes. Even very low dose (1–2 mg/d) can produce dramatic improvements in the prodromal phase or first episode schizophrenia (see 1.21.2).

Efficacy: Risperidone has shown efficacy across a wide range of symptoms of psychosis and schizophrenia. Relapse prevention has been shown over one year (n = 397, average follow-up one-year, Csernansky et al, N Engl J Med 2002;**346**:16–22; comment by McIntosh, EBMH 2002;**5**:77) and is probably most effective over one year at least (n = 404, RCT, 1 year, Wang et al, Am J Psychiatry 2010;**167**:676–85). Surprisingly, Cochrane is not impressed with risperidone's efficacy vs placebo (s = 1, n = 599, Rattehalli et al, Cochrane Database Syst Rev 2010;**1**:CD006918).

Reviews: * TDM (therapeutic range of 25–150 microg/L, n = 50, Odou et al, Clin Drug Invest 2000;**19**:283–92; Nazirizadeh et al, Eur J Clin Pharmacol 2010;**66**:797–803), plasma levels (n = 51, Yasui-Furukori et al, J Psychopharmacol 2010;**24**:987–94).

Sertindole *

Sertindole is now available in Australia, and on a named-patient basis in the UK. Cochrane concluded that sertindole is effective and as tolerable as placebo at 20 mg/d (s = 3, n = 1104, Lewis et al, Cochrane Database Syst Rev 2005;**3**:CD001715) but with little evidence of superiority over other SGAs (Komossa et al, Cochrane Database Syst Rev 2009;**2**:CD006752).

Review: * general (Azorin et al, Expert Opin Pharmacother 2010;**11**:3053–64; Muscatello et al, Drug Des Devel Ther 2010;**4**:187–201).

Ziprasidone (not available in the UK) *

Ziprasidone is licensed in the USA and some European countries for schizophrenia, and is effective in the treatment of positive, negative and depressive symptoms of schizophrenia and schizoaffective disorder. Ziprasidone 5–20 mg has been shown to be effective in acute psychosis, and better tolerated than

haloperidol IM (e.g. n = 278, RCT, d/b, p/c, one year, Arato et al, Int Clin Psychopharmacol 2002;**17**:207–15) and effective for relapse prevention (e.g. n = 168, d/b, 196/52, Potkin et al, Int J Neuropsychopharmacol 2009;**12**:1233–48). Ziprasidone has been compared with clozapine in TRS, where it showed efficacy, but with less metabolic ADRs than clozapine (n = 147, RCT, d/b, p/c, 18/52, Sacchetti et al, Schizophr Res 2009;**110**:80–9). Cochrane concludes that ziprasidone is slightly less effective than amisulpride, olanzapine and risperidone but with low weight gain (s = 9, n = 3361, Komossa et al, Cochrane Database Syst Rev 2009;**4**:CD006627).

Review: * general (Fagiolini et al, Expert Opin Pharmacother 2010;**11**:2199–220)

DEPOT AND LONG-ACTING INJECTIONS

The major advantage of depots is assured compliance and steady plasma levels, with associated and proven reduction in relapses, rehospitalisation and severity of relapse. There may also be some reduction in bioavailability problems (some people metabolise antipsychotics extensively via the first-pass effect). Used properly, depots can lead to reduced relapses, stable therapeutic effects and better downward titration of doses to reduce the incidence of side-effects. With CATIE's low retention rates, long-acting injections may help improve retention and reduce relapse, readmissions, brain tissue loss, and deterioration (Nasrallah, Acta Psychiatr Scand 2007;**115**:260–7). The major disadvantages include the impossibility of altering a dose if side-effects develop (e.g. dystonia, NMS), patients seeing depot administration as 'being controlled', having no control over or involvement in their treatment or, worse still, as being a punishment. Many users and carers are insufficiently educated about the pros and cons of depot administration. It is not enough just to prevent relapse with a depot.

Depot injections do, of course, also hurt, the pain declining over 10 days and this has a negative effect on patient attitude towards medication (n = 34, Bloch et al, J Clin Psychiatry 2001;**62**:855–9), although there is some evidence to the contrary (Walburn et al, Br J

Psychiatry 2001;**179**:300–7). There is need for a meticulous (Z-tracking) injection technique (Cocoman and Murray, *J Psychiatr Ment Health Nurs* 2008;**15**:424–34).

Licensed UK depot/long-acting injection sites *

Depot/LAI	Licensed IM routes
Flupentixol decanoate	Gluteal, lateral thigh
Fluphenazine decanoate	Gluteal
Fluspirilene	Gluteal, lateral thigh
Haloperidol decanoate	Gluteal
Olanzapine pamoate	Gluteal
Paliperidone palmitate	Gluteal, deltoid
Pipothiazine palmitate	Gluteal
Risperidone	Gluteal, deltoid
Zuclopentixol decanoate	Gluteal, lateral thigh

Reviews: * general (Cañas and Möller, *Expert Opin Drug Saf* 2010;**9**:683–97; Lindenmayer, *Neuropsychiatr Dis Treat* 2010;**6**:261–7), psycho-pharmacology and ADRs (Taylor, *Br J Psychiatry Suppl* 2009;**52**:S13–9).

Pharmacokinetics

The tables on *pages 152–155* show the plasma levels for each depot as single doses (although these have been difficult to obtain and are not reliable), and as computer-generated profiles for multiple doses (based on single-dose profiles). The half-life is often longer on chronic administration.

Flupentixol decanoate *
(e.g. Depixol®, Lundbeck)

Flupentixol is a dopamine specific thioxanthene antipsychotic (Kuhn *et al*, *Fortschr Neurol Psychiatr* 2000;**68**[Suppl 1]: S38–S41) licensed in people stabilised on oral therapy first (UK SmPC). Cochrane recommends standard doses as there are no trials vs placebo (Quraishi and David, *Cochrane Database Syst Rev* 2000;**2**:CD001470). It is contraindicated in people with circulatory collapse or depressed consciousness due to any cause (e.g. intoxication with alcohol or opiates).

- Duration of action = 3–4 weeks.
- Peak = 7–10 days.
- Rate limiting half-life = eight days (single dose), 17 days (multiple doses).
- Time to steady state = 10–12 weeks.

Fluphenazine decanoate
(e.g. Modecate®, Sanofi-Synthelabo)

Fluphenazine decanoate is a phenothiazine and a four-week interval between injections is possible. The efficacy data is very limited, showing little difference between depots and orals (s = 70, n = 1892, RCT, David *et al*, *Cochrane Database Syst Rev* 2005;**1**:CD000307). Fluphenazine 25mg every two or six weeks produces similar side-effects, efficacy and relapse rates, but with reduced drug exposure using the longer dosage interval (n = 50, RCT, 54/52, Carpenter *et al*, *Am J Psychiatry* 1999;**156**:412–8).

- Duration of action = 1–3 weeks.
- Peak = 6–48 hours.
- Rate-limiting half-life = 6–10 days (single doses), 14–100 days (multiple doses).
- Time to steady state = 6–12 weeks.

Fluspirilene
(e.g. Redeptin®, SmithKline French)

Fluspirilene is only available in the UK as an import, as a water-based weekly micro-crystalline injection. Cochrane concludes that it has no advantage over orals or other depots, albeit with limited data (s = 12, n=525, RCT, Abhijnhan *et al*, *Cochrane Database Syst Rev* 2007;**1**:CD001718).

- Duration of action = 1.5 weeks.
- Peak within two days.
- Rate limiting half-life = 7–9 days.
- Time to steady state = 5–6 weeks.

Haloperidol decanoate
(Haldol Decanoate ®, Janssen)

Haloperidol decanoate is a butyrophenone and a four-week interval between injections is possible. An analysis suggests a maximal effect at 50mg/4 weeks, with no evidence that doses above 100mg/4 weeks have any additional effects (s = 13, Taylor, *Psychiatr Bull* 2005;**29**:104–7), e.g. rates of deterioration with 50–100mg/month were not significantly greater in one study compared to 25mg/month, and ADRs were possibly higher (n = 105, RCT, d/b, Kane *et al*, *Am J Psychiatry* 2002;**4**:554–60; review by Marois and Roy, *EBMH* 2002;**5**:113). It is best reserved for chronic relapsing schizophrenics responsive to haloperidol.

Depot and longer-acting injection pharmacokinetics

These graphs show the known plasma levels of the available longer-acting antipsychotic injections in the UK. The single dose kinetics are reasonably well-established for many of these preparations. The multiple-dose graphs are computer-generated as little or no data exists on long-term kinetics, with downward arrows indicating when injections are given. These graphs will, however, give *some* indication of the time to steady state, and the length of time before plasma levels fall to zero after a depot has been stopped, although half-lives tend to lengthen with chronic use. The 'y' axis units are not established for any of the multiple dose graphs, and there will of course be some inter-individual variation.

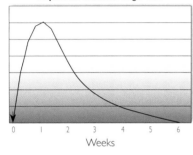

Flupentixol decanoate single dose

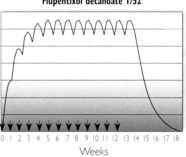

Flupentixol decanoate 1/52

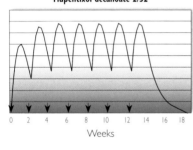

Flupentixol decanoate 2/52

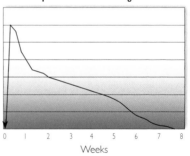

Fluphenazine decanoate single dose

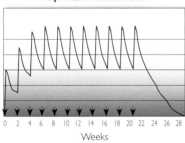

Fluphenazine decanoate 2/52

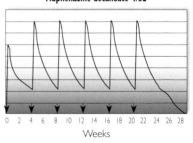

Fluphenazine decanoate 4/52

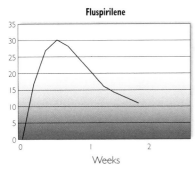

Fluspirilene

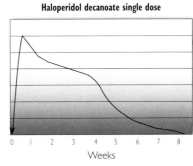

Haloperidol decanoate single dose

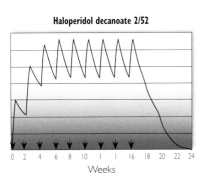

Haloperidol decanoate 2/52

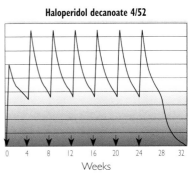

Haloperidol decanoate 4/52

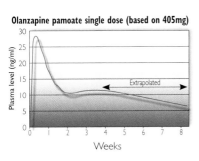

Olanzapine pamoate single dose (based on 405mg)

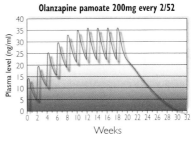

Olanzapine pamoate 200mg every 2/52

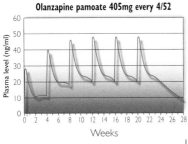

Olanzapine pamoate 405mg every 4/52

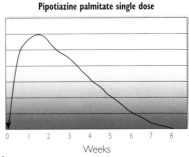

Pipotiazine palmitate single dose

Pipotiazine palmitate 2/52

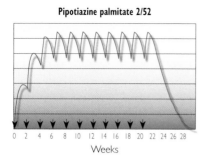

Pipotiazine palmitate 4/52

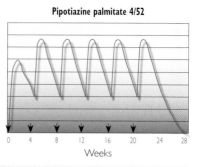

Risperidone Consta single dose

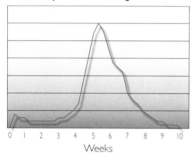

Risperdal Consta 2/52

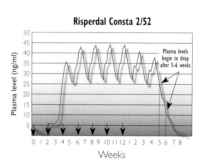

Zuclopenthixol decanoate single dose

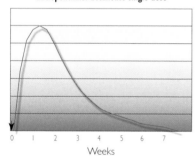

Zuclopenthixol decanoate 1/52

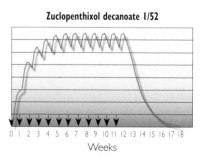

Zuclopenthixol decanoate 2/52

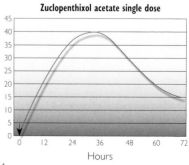

Zuclopenthixol acetate single dose

154

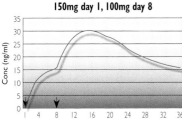

Paliperidone palmitate initiation: 150mg day 1, 100mg day 8

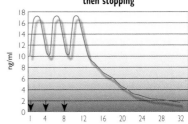

Paliperidone palmitate 50mg monthly then stopping

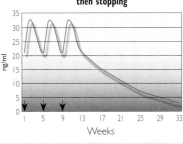

Paliperidone palmitate 100mg monthly then stopping

Weeks

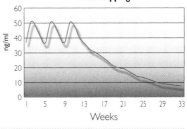

Paliperidone palmitate 150mg monthly then stopping

Weeks

- Duration of action = six weeks.
- Peak = 3–9 days.
- Rate limiting half-life = 18–21 days (single + chronic).
- Time to steady state = 10–12 weeks at monthly dosing.

Olanzapine pamoate
(Zypadhera®, Zyprexa Relprevv®, Lilly) *

Olanzapine pamoate is a long-acting formulation for deep IM gluteal injection in people who have previously received oral doses. Olanzapine pamoate releases olanzapine slowly over approximately 6–8 weeks after each injection, so care is needed after discontinuation. Oral supplementation is not recommended, e.g. in acute TRS, olanzapine pamoate every two or four weeks was more effective than placebo, despite no use of additional oral supplementation (RCT, d/b, p/c, 8/52, Lauriello *et al*, *J Clin Psychiatry* 2008;**69**:790–9). However, if supplementation is used, it should be the equivalent of a maximum of 20mg/d (all preparations) and the 'loading dose' should be reduced after two months (n=9, Mamo *et al*, *Neuropsychopharmacology*

2008;**33**:298–304). A huge study has shown it to be effective and well-tolerated as oral, apart from injection-related adverse events (n=1065, RCT, d/b, 24/52, Kane *et al*, *Am J Psychiatry* 2010;**167**:181–9). Doses should be as per the chart for the first two months, then reduced.

- Duration of action = about six weeks.
- Peak = four days.
- Half-life = 30 days.
- Time to steady state = three months.

Dose conversion:

Oral dose	Starting dose (initial 2/12)	Maintenance dose (after 2/12)
10mg/d	210mg 2/52 or 405mg 4/52	150mg 2/52 or 300mg 4/52
15mg/d	300mg 2/52	210mg 2/52 or 405mg 4/52
20mg/d	300mg 2/52	300mg 2/52

Post-injection syndrome:* There have been reports of unpredictable (0.07% injections, in 1.4% patients; n=2054, injections=45000; Detke *et al*, *BMC Psychiatry* 2010;**10**:43) and idiosyncratic excessive sedation, resembling olanzapine overdose (Citrome, *Int J Clin Pract* 2009;**63**:140–50) 1–6 hours post-injection (usually one hour), with full recovery within 24–72 hours. To avoid adverse consequences, after injection, the patient must be observed in a healthcare facility by appropriately qualified personnel for at least three hours for signs and symptoms of apparent overdose, e.g. sedation (mild to coma), delirium, EPSE, dysarthria, ataxia, aggression and convulsions.

Review: * general (Naber, *Expert Opin Pharmacother* 2011;**12**:627–33; Citrome, *Int J Clin Pract* 2009;**62**:140–50; Frampton, *Drugs* 2010;**70**:2289–313.

Paliperidone palmitate
(Xeplion®, Invega Sustenna,® Janssen) *

Paliperidone palmitate is a long-acting IM injection licensed for maintenance treatment of schizophrenia. It uses a novel nanocrystal technology formulation, allowing an early and sustained release. It is the palmitate ester of paliperidone, the major metabolite of risperidone. Efficacy has been show in a large number of studies in acute schizophrenia (e.g. n = 388, RCT, d/b, p/c, 13/52, Gopal, *Int Clin Psychopharmacol* 2010;**25**:247–56; n = 514, RCT, d/b, p/c, 13/52, Nasrallah *et al*, *Neuropsychopharmacology* 2010;**35**:2072–82; n = 652, RCT, d/b, p/c, 13/52, Pandina *et al*, *J Clin Psychopharmacol* 2010;**30**:235–44; MS), non-inferiority to risperidone LAI (n = 1220, RCT, d/b, 13/52, Pandina *et al*, *Prog Neuropsychopharmacol Biol Psychiatry* 2011; **35**:218–26; MS), where 150 mg separates from placebo after four days in acute exacerbation of schizophrenia (n = 312, RCT, d/b, p/c, 13/52, Alphs *et al*, *Ann Gen Psychiatry* 2011;**11**:12; MS). Relapse prevention (n = 312, RCT, d/b, p/c, 24/52, Hough *et al*, *Schizophr Res* 2010;**116**:107–17; MS) is clear, with an NNT = 2 for prevention of relapse (s = 8, Gopal *et al*, *Neuropsychiatr Dis Treat* 2011;**7**:93–101; MS). It can be started in patients previously responsive to paliperidone or risperidone without prior stabilisation on the oral preparation. Paliperidone palmitate has a specific dose schedule:

- Initial dose 150 mg in the deltoid muscle. No oral supplementation is needed.
- Give 100 mg on day 8 in the deltoid

muscle (if switching directly from risperidone LAI these two starting doses do not have to be in the deltoid).

- Then as per dose equivalent or schedule, and can be in the gluteal or deltoid sites.
- Under exceptional circumstances the day 8 dose can be +/- 2 days, and monthly doses +/- 7 days without a clinically significant effect on plasma concentrations.

Review: * extensive and practical (Gopal *et al*, *Curr Med Res Opin* 2010;**26**:377–87), general (Hoy *et al*, *CNS Drugs* 2010;**24**:227–44; Citrome, *Int J Clin Pract* 2010;**64**:216–39; Bishara, *Neuropsych Dis Treat* 2010;**6**:561–72).

Pipothiazine palmitate
(Piportil®, Sanofi-Aventis)

Pipothiazine is a piperidine phenothiazine marketed in the UK as the palmitate. Cochrane concludes that although better data is needed, pipothiazine is a viable antipsychotic choice (Dinesh *et al*, *Cochrane Database Syst Rev* 2004; **4**:CD001720).

- Duration of action = 4–6 weeks.
- Peak = 9–10 days.
- Rate limiting half-life = 14–21 days.
- Time to steady state = 8–12 weeks.

Risperidone (RLAI)
(Risperdal Consta®, Janssen) *

This novel, long-acting injection uses risperidone molecules in a synthetic and absorbable polymer microsphere base suspended in water. It is licensed for schizophrenic and other psychoses.

Release: The initial dose is 25–37.5 mg fortnightly, with a maximum of 50 mg every two weeks. Plasma levels are stable after 3–4 injections and maintained for 4–5 weeks after the last injection, then decline rapidly. D2 receptor studies show risperidone 25, 50 and 75 mg fortnightly are in the range found in patients effectively treated with 2, 4 and 6 mg/d oral risperidone respectively (n = 13, Gefvert *et al*, *Int J Neuropsychopharmacol* 2005;**8**:27–36; see also Love and Conley, *Am J Health Syst Pharm* 2004; **61**:1792–800), although 75 mg had higher side-effects (n = 400, RCT, d/b, p/c, 12/52, Kane *et al*, *Am J Psychiatry* 2003;**160**:1125–32). Where possible, patients should be pre-treated with risperidone orally for at least a few days before the injection is commenced to rule out any severe EPS, hypotensive or other idiosyncratic reactions. Oral cover may be needed for the first 3–4 weeks, then tapered during weeks 4–5. Steady state occurs about 6–8 weeks after each dose change, some have recommended dose increases only every eight weeks (Knox and Stimmel, *Clin Ther* 2004; **26**:1994–2002). Elimination is complete 7–8 weeks after the last injection. The deltoid and gluteal injection routes have the same release, Cmax and AUC (s = 2, Thyssen *et al*, *J Clin Pharmacol* 2010; **50**:1011–21; MS).

The injection can now be given in the deltoid muscle, with a specific needle for each site.

Efficacy: Risperidone injection 25–50 mg every 2/52 was as effective as olanzapine oral 5–20 mg/d (n = 377, RCT, open, one year; Keks *et al*, *Br J Psychiatry* 2007; **191**:131–9; MS) and more effective than zuclopenthixol depot (n = 115, RCT, open, 6/12, Rubio *et al*, *Can J Psychiatry* 2006; **51**:531–9). Of 65% patients completing one year on Consta, 5% dropped out because of ADRs, and 25% suffered ADRs (n = 615, open, 12/12, Fleischacker *et al*, *J Clin Psychiatry* 2003; **64**:1250–7; see also n = 347 [c = 243], open, 12/12, Rossi *et al*, *Hum Psychopharmacol* 2009; **24**:574–83). In a retrospective case note review, a mirror-image analysis of Consta use showed it resulted in a 58% retention in treatment at one year, and roughly halved readmission rates and stays (n = 67, three years, Niaz and Haddad, *Acta Psychiatr Scand* 2007; **116**:36–46).

Optimum efficacy may take many months, e.g. half of those with a good outcome at 6/12 had not yet improved by 3/12 and oral doses may be needed longer than the first 3/52 (n = 50, naturalistic follow-up, Paton and Okocha, *Psychiatr Bull* 2004; **28**:12–4, IS). There may be a significant effect on negative symptoms when used for a prolonged period of time (n = 842 [c = 631], 6/12, Curtis *et al*, *J Psychopharmacol* 2008; **22**:254–61).

Factors predicting response: RLAI seems to produce more favourable outcomes in previous poor concordance and older people (n = 250, 6/12, Taylor *et al*, *Int J Neuropsychopharmacol* 2006; **9**:685–94), out-patients and those not previously treated with clozapine (n = 211, 6

years, Taylor and Cornelius, *J Psychopharmacol* 2010; **24**:995–9).

Dose and switching: See *C2.2.1.2*.

A careful switching study concluded:
- oral dose < 3 mg/d = Consta 25 mg 2/52
- oral 3–5 mg/d = Consta 37.5 mg 2/52
- oral > 5 mg/d = Consta 50 mg 2/52

(n = 50 [c = 45], RCT, s/b, 48/52, Bai *et al*, *J Clin Psychiatry* 2007; **68**:1218–25).

Reviews: * general (Bobo and Shelton, *Expert Rev Neurother* 2010; **10**:1637–58; Rainer, *Neuropsychiatr Dis Treat* 2008; **4**:919–27).

Zuclopenthixol acetate

(Clopixol Acuphase®, Lundbeck)

Zuclopenthixol acetate is available as 'Clopixol Acuphase' in the UK. 50–150 mg as a single dose provides a reduction in psychotic symptoms over about 78 hours. The maximum cumulative dose is 400 mg over two weeks, with no more than four injections. Cochrane concludes that there is inadequate data on Acuphase and no convincing evidence either way in APE compared to IM haloperidol (Fenton *et al*, *Cochrane Database Syst Rev* 2004; **2**:CD00525). See also *1.1*.

- Duration of action = 2–3 days.
- Peak = 24–40 hours.
- Rate limiting half-life = 32 hours +/- 7.

Zuclopenthixol decanoate

(Clopixol®, Lundbeck)

This is a thioanthene antipsychotic which has also been used in high dose in aggression, particularly in learning disabilities and forensic patients but is not indicated for this.

- Duration of action = 2–4 weeks.
- Peak = 4–9 days.
- Rate limiting half-life = 17–21 days (multiple doses).
- Time to steady state = 10–12 weeks.

+ Combinations

Polypharmacy with antipsychotics falls into three main categories:
- two or more drugs of the same class
- multiclass (two drugs in different classes at full dose)
- adjunctive and augmentation (low dose of one with a standard dose of another).

Appropriate reasons for the use of antipsychotic combinations include:

- Failure to respond to clozapine.
- Poor clozapine tolerance, with a second drug as augmentation of a low clozapine dose.
- As augmentation in clozapine partial response.
- Patients unwilling to stop an existing drug or choosing not to try clozapine.
- During a switch from one antipsychotic to another.
- When discontinuing a depot poses an unacceptable risk, e.g. forensic patients.
- As a temporary measure during an acute exacerbation of illness.

Inappropriate reasons for the use of antipsychotic combinations include:

- Confusing a sedative effect with an antipsychotic effect.
- Not waiting long enough for an antipsychotic to work before making changes.
- As a substitute for failing to plan and communicate a switch, which is then never fully completed.
- Where clinical improvement occurs before a switch is completed, and the clinician 'quits while ahead' rather than risking completing the change.
- Using high doses to make up for in-adequate resources and environment.

Despite widespread use of combinations (with increased ADRs and possibly reduced outcomes; n = 1043, McCue et al, J Clin Psychiatry 2003; **64**:984–9), there are few RCTs of combination antipsychotics in schizophrenia and multiple antipsychotics are associated with a major increase in drug exposure, adverse events and time in hospital, but with no apparent clinical gain compared to monotherapy (n = 70 pairs, Centorrino et al, Am J Psychiatry 2004; **161**:700–6). Combinations should thus only be used once standard monotherapies have been found inadequate, and then with carefully monitored outcomes (clinical and adverse) and discontinued if no clear advantage is seen.
Review: editorial review of the lack of evidence and trials of combinations (Zink et al, Curr Opin Psychiatry 2010;**23**:103–11).

Clozapine combinations & augmentation

A recent meta-analysis was unable to show any short-term benefit from clozapine augmentation over 16 weeks, but longer-term trials are needed (s = 10, n = 522, Taylor and Smith, Acta Psychiatr Scand 2009;**119**:419–25). Similarly Cochrane concludes that there is insufficient data to conclude anything (s = 3, Cipriani et al, Cochrane Database Syst Rev 2009;**3**:CD006324).
Reviews:* general (Mossaheb et al, World J Biol Psychiatry 2010;**11**:502-5; Barbui et al, Schizophr Bull 2008;**35**:458–68), augmentation in TRS insufficiently responsive to clozapine (Sommer et al, Schizophr Bull 2011; in press).

Clozapine + amisulpride (see also sulpiride)

Combining a specific D2-blocker with cloza-pine is a well-known strategy. There are some studies e.g. amisulpride significantly improved response to clozapine without significant additional side-effects (n = 33[c = 28], open, 6/12, Munro et al, Acta Psychiatr Scand 2004;**110**:292–8) and 80% improved with amisulpride 700mg/d (range 520–980mg/d) as adjunctive therapy (n = 56[c = 50], s/b, 8/52, Genç et al, Adv Ther 2007;**24**:1–13).

Clozapine + anticholinesterases

See 1.21.3 for the effect on cognition.

Clozapine + aripiprazole *

Although there have been many case reports and series of aripiprazole combined with clozapine, the only RCT showed aripiprazole augmentation of clozapine slightly to improve negative symptoms but does not lead to a significant improvement in the total symptoms of schizophrenia (n = 62, RCT, d/b, p/c, Chang et al, J Clin Psychiatry 2008;**69**:720-31; comment by Remington, EBMH 2009;**12**:51), but interestingly did not lead to deterioration either. Other open studies include aripiprazole 15mg/d augmentation of clozapine sig-nificantly improving all symptom measures (except PANSS positive) with no increase in ADRs (n = 27[c = 23], open, 16/52, Mitsonis et al, Prog Neuropsychopharmacol Biol Psychiatry 2007;**31**:373–7) and weight loss, reduction in clozapine dosage and improved symptoms (n = 26, Karunakaran et al, J Psychopharmacol 2007;**21**:453–56).

Review: Englisch and Zink, Prog Neuropsycho-pharmacol Biol Psychiatry 2008;**32**:1386–92.

Clonidine + clozapine *

There is a case of clonidine augmentation of clozapine-resistant schizophrenia (n = 1, Dardennes et al, Prog Neuropsychopharmacol Biol Psychiatry 2010;**30**:724–5).

Clozapine + gingko biloba

In TRS, addition of Gingko biloba to clozapine had some beneficial effects on negative symptoms, but not positive or overall symptoms (n = 42, p/c, 12/52, Doruk et al, Int Clin Psychopharmacol 2008;**23**:223–7).

Clozapine + lamotrigine *

A meta-analysis concluded that lamotrigine augmentation of clozapine was superior to placebo with a clinically meaningful benefit (s = 5, n = 161, RCT, p/c, 10–24/52, Tiihonen et al, Schizophr Res 2009;**109**:10–4; concordant comment by Goff, EBMH 2009;**12**:111).

Clozapine + memantine *

Memantine 20 mg/d augmentation of clozapine has been associated with improvement in positive and negative symptoms in TRS (n = 21 [c = 21], RCT, d/b, p/c, 12/52, de Lucena et al, J Clin Psychiatry 2009;**70**:1416–23).

Clozapine + mirtazapine

Mirtazapine augmentation of clozapine has improved negative symptoms (especially apathy and anhedonia) and BPRS scores (n = 24, RCT, d/b, p/c, 8/52, Zoccali et al, Int Clin Psychopharmacol 2004;**19**:71–6).

Clozapine + quetiapine

Although quetiapine has some effect as augmentation of clozapine, it may be less effective than amisulpride (n = 56 [c = 50], s/b, 8/52, Genç et al, Adv Ther 2007;**24**:1–13). Weight loss has been reported when 25% of the clozapine dose was converted to quetiapine (1 mg clozapine:2 mg quetiapine) (n = 65, open, 10/12, Reinstein et al, Clin Drug Invest 1999;**18**:99–104).

Clozapine + risperidone *

An RCT has shown risperidone 4–6 mg/d to improve sub-optimal clozapine response (n = 40, RCT, d/b, p/c, 12/52, Josiassen et al, Am J Psychiatry 2005;**162**:130–6), although a moderate (four-fold) rise in prolactin levels can occur (n = 40, open, Henderson et al, J Clin Psychiatry 2001;**62**:605–8). However, addition of risperidone 3 mg/d (n = 68, RCT, p/c, d/b, 8+18/52, Honer et al, N Engl J Med 2006; **354**:472–82) or 6 mg/d made no difference to psychopathology or quality of life compared to placebo (n = 30, RCT, p/c, d/b, 6/52, Yagcıoglu et al, J Clin Psychiatry 2005;**66**:63–72). A critical review concludes the evidence is encouraging, with the best response with lower risperidone dose and longer duration (s = 15 [2 = RCT], n = 86, Kontaxakis et al, Eur Arch Psychiatry Clin Neurosci 2006;**256**:350–5). In clozapine poor responders (due to non-adherence), addition of risperidone LAI to oral clozapine had a marked effect on reducing relapses and improving social functioning (n = 4, 1 year, Kim et al, J Psychopharmacol 2010;**24**:981–6).

Clozapine + sulpiride *

In the first RCT of combined antipsychotics, clozapine and sulpiride produced a substantially greater improvement than clozapine alone in TRS (n = 24, RCT, Shiloh et al, Br J Psychiatry 1997;**171**:569–73), although the two study groups had some initial differences. Cochrane concludes that sulpiride plus clozapine is probably more effective than clozapine alone (s = 4, n = 221, Wang et al, Cochrane Database Syst Rev 2010;**1**:CD008125).

Clozapine + ziprasidone

In TRS, clozapine augmentation by ziprasidone or risperidone was equally effective and well tolerated, with slight QT prolongation with ziprasidone and prolactin rise with risperidone (n = 24, open, RCT, 6/52, Zink et al, J Psychopharmacol 2009;**23**:305–14).

Other antipsychotic combinations and augmentation

Amisulpride + risperidone or ziprasidone

In a small trial, 80% improved on the combination with amisulpride at a mean dose of 693 mg/d (n = 15, open, Lerner et al, Clin Neuropharmacol 2005;**28**:66–71).

Aripiprazole + quetiapine or risperidone *

In TRS, addition of aripiprazole 2–15mg/d to partially effective risperidone (n = 177) or quetiapine (n = 146) had no effect on symptoms, but helped reduce prolactin levels (n = 323 [c = 225], RCT, d/b, p/c, 16/52, Kane et al, J Clin Psychiatry 2009;**70**:1348–57).

Olanzapine + sulpiride

Sulpiride 600mg/d augmentation of partially effective olanzapine had no effect on PANSS but significantly improved depressive symptoms (n = 17, RCT, 8/52, Kotler et al, Int Clin Psychopharmacol 2004;**19**:23–6).

Risperidone + olanzapine

Risperidone plus olanzapine was successful in TRS resistant to sequential olanzapine, quetiapine and risperidone monotherapy, and was well tolerated albeit with increased side-effects (e.g. n = 17 [c = 17], open, 8/52, Suzuki et al, Hum Psychopharmacol 2008;**23**:455–63).

Quetiapine + amisulpride *

In quetiapine partial response, addition of amisulpride has some beneficial effect but significantly increased weight and prolactin (n = 6, open, 8/52, Englisch et al, Clin Neuropharmacol 2010;**33**:227–9).

● Augmentation (with drugs with no intrinsic antipsychotic activity)

Allopurinol

Allopurinol may increase circulating pools of adenosine (which may make dopamine receptors have a lower affinity for dopamine) and may ultimately have antipsychotic and anxiolytic effects. In the main RCT, 13% improved with adjunctive allopurinol (cf 0% on placebo) so it may have some role (n = 59 [c = 51], RCT, d/b, p/c, 8/52, Dickerson et al, Schizophr Res 2009;**109**:66–9). Haloperidol plus allopurinol was superior to haloperidol (n = 46, RCT, d/b, p/c, 8/52, Akhondzadeh et al, Prog Neuropsychopharmacol Biol Psychiatry 2005;**29**:253–9) and 300–600mg/d may be the effective adjunctive dose in resistant

schizophrenia (n = 35 [c = 22], d/b, p/c, c/o, 12/52, Brunstein et al, J Clin Psychiatry 2005; **66**:213–9).

Review: * general (Buie et al, Ann Pharmacother 2006;**40**:2200–4).

Anticholinesterases

See 1.21.3.

Antidepressants *

A recent systematic review and meta-analysis concluded that antidepressants have modest effects on negative symptoms. This is statistically significant for fluoxetine, trazodone and ritanserin. Other antidepressants (mirtazapine, reboxetine, mianserin, fluvoxamine, sertraline, paroxetine and citalopram) had no apparent beneficial effects, albeit with limited study numbers (s = 23, n = 819, Singh et al, Br J Psychiatry 2010;**197**:174–9).

SSRIs: Citalopram has been successful for depressive/anxiety symptoms of PANSS (RCT, Taiminen et al, Int Clin Psychopharmacol 1997; **12**:31–5) and improving subjective well-being, but addition of citalopram 40mg/d to SGAs had no effect on any clinical or cognition measures (n = 19, RCT, p/c, c/o, 24/52, Friedman et al, J Clin Psychiatry 2005;**25**:237–42). **Escitalopram** is well-tolerated but ineffective for negative symptoms in chronic schizophrenia (n = 40 [c = 34], RCT, d/b, p/c, 10/52, Iancu et al, Psychiatry Res 2010;**179**:19–23). **Fluoxetine** 20 mg/d significantly improved PANSS in open studies of TRS (e.g. n = 9, open, 6/52, Goff et al, Am J Psychiatry 1990;**147**:492–4), but may increase EPS and was ineffective as an adjunct to clozapine (n = 33, open, p/c, 8/52, Buchanan et al, Am J Psychiatry 1996;**153**:1625–7). **Fluvoxamine** was ineffective as augmentation of risperidone-resistant schizophrenia (n = 30, open, 12/52, Takashi et al, Hum Psychopharmacol 2002;**17**:95–8) and must only be used with clozapine with extreme care (see 4.2.4). **Paroxetine** (n = 8, open, 30/12, Jockers-Scherubl et al, J Clin Psychiatry 2001;**62**:573) and **sertraline** (n = 26, d/b, p/c, 8/52, Mulholland et al, J Psychopharmacol 2003;**17**:107–12) may improve negative or depressive symptoms.

Mirtazapine: despite the Singh meta-analysis, mirtazapine appears clearly and robustly superior to placebo on almost all measures of improvement as an adjunct to antipsychotics in TRS (n = 39, RCT, d/b, 6/52, Joffe et al, Schizophr Res 2009;**108**:245–51), and 30 mg/d as an adjunct to risperidone significantly improved negative and PANSS total scores cf placebo (n = 40, RCT, d/b, p/c, 8/52, Abbasi et al, Schizophr Res 2010;**116**:101–6), although it had no efficacy on PANSS scores as an adjunct to SGAs (n = 40, RCT, d/b, p/c, 6/52, Berk et al, Hum Psychopharmacol 2009;**24**:233–8).

Aspirin *

Aspirin 1000 mg/d as an adjunct to regular antipsychotics has a significant effect on PANSS scores, leading to speculation that inflammation may be a new target for treatment (n = 70, RCT, d/b, p/c, 3/12, Laan et al, J Clin Psychiatry 2010;**71**:520–7).

Benzodiazepines

Short-term use may reduce anxiety, tension and insomnia and high doses may have some tranquillising effects. They may also allow lower doses of antipsychotics to be used, as high doses of antipsychotics are often used for their additional sedative properties, e.g. in psychotic agitation. Cochrane concludes that there is little or no evidence that BDZs are useful as monotherapy or even adjunctive therapy in schizophrenia, although widely used to augment antipsychotics in acute states (s = 31, n = 2000, Volz et al, Cochrane Database Syst Rev 2007:**1**:CD006391). See also 'Acute psychiatric emergency' (1.1).

Buspirone *

Buspirone 60 mg/d (as an adjunct to risperidone 6 mg/d) significantly improved PANSS components and was surprisingly well-tolerated (n = 46, RCT, d/b, p/c, 8/52, Ghaleiha et al, J Clin Psychopharmacol 2010;**30**:678–82).

Chinese herbal medicines

A systematic review and meta-analysis suggested that monotherapy was not effective but that adjunctive use might help some outcomes (s = 7, RCTs, Rathbone et al, Br J Psychiatry 2007;**190**:379–84; probably an inappropriate conclusion, comment by Werneke, EBMH 2008;**11**:19).

Cicloserin (D-cycloserine)

Cicloserin is a partial agonist of a glutamate receptor sub-type and addition of 50 mg/d to FGAs, risperidone and olanzapine produced a significant reduction in negative symptoms (n = 24, d/b, p/c, c/o, 6/52, Heresco-Levy et al, Am J Psychiatry 2002;**159**:480–2), supporting the view that glutamate function may be important in schizophrenia.

Cox-2 inhibitors

Celecoxib 400 mg/d added to risperidone in TRS may produce a significant reduction in PANSS compared to risperidone mono-therapy (n = 50, RCT, d/b, p/c, 5/52, Muller et al, Eur Arch Psychiatry Clin Neurosci 2004;**254**:14–22) and reduce EPSEs (n = 60, RCT, d/b, p/c, 8/52, Akhondzadeh et al, Schizophr Res 2007;**90**:179–85).

Cyproheptadine

Adding cyproheptadine 24 mg/d to haloperidol 30 mg/d has significantly reduced negative symptoms (n = 30, RCT, Akhondzadeh et al, J Clin Pharm Ther 1999;**24**:49).

DHEA (dehydroepiandrosterone)

DHEA 100 mg/d produced significant improvements as adjunctive therapy in negative, depressive and anxiety symptoms of schizophrenia, although Cochrane concludes that the available studies are inconclusive and unconvincing (s = 3, n = 126, Elias and Kumar, Cochrane Database Syst Rev 2007; **3**:CD006197).

Dipyridamole

Dipyridamole (75 mg/d) plus haloperidol (16–20 mg/d) was superior to haloperidol alone in schizophrenia, possibly via an effect on the interaction between the adenosine and dopamine systems (n = 30, RCT, Akhondzadeh et al, J Clin Pharm Ther 2000; **25**:131–8).

Folate

Although there have been some reports, a review suggests that the data is inadequate, inconsistent and unconvincing (s = 7, n = 325 + 560, Muntjewerff and Blom, Prog Neuro-psychopharmacol Biol Psychiatry 2005;**29**:1133–9), although low folate levels have been reported in schizophrenia (n = 91, Goff *et al*, *Am J Psychiatry* 2004;**161**:1705–8).

Ginkgo biloba (see also clozapine)

Ginkgo biloba has enhanced the effectiveness of haloperidol and reduced EPS compared to placebo (n = 109, RCT, d/b, p/c, 12/52, Zhang *et al*, *J Clin Psychiatry* 2001;**62**:878–83; comment by Knable, *EBMH* 2002;**5**:90).

Glycine

High-dose glycine (0.8 g/kg/d) as add-on to olanzapine or risperidone significantly reduced negative symptoms by 23% and improved cognitive function (e.g. n = 17, RCT, d/b, p/c, c/o, 6/52, Heresco-Levy *et al*, *Biol Psychiatry* 2004; **15**:165–71), particularly in people with low pre-treatment plasma glycine levels, although some studies are negative (n = 30, d/b, p/c, Evins *et al*, *Am J Psychiatry* 2000;**157**:826–8).

Lamotrigine (see clozapine augmentation) *

Evidence for augmentation (especially of clozapine) is considered reasonable, but monotherapy lacking. In comorbid schizphrenia and OCD, addition of lamotrigine 200 mg/d to existing therapy (olanzapine or quetiapine, plus SSRI or BDZ) gave an 83% response in schizoaffective disorder and a significant effect overall (n = 9, open, 8/52, Poyurovsky *et al*, *J Psychopharmacol* 2010;**24**:861–6).

Reviews: * systematic review (Tiihonen *et al*, *Schizophr Res* 2009;**109**:10–4), mode of action (Large *et al*, *Psychopharmacology [Berl]* 2005; **6**:1–22).

Ondansetron *

Ondansetron 8 mg/d as an adjunct to risperidone significantly improved negative symptoms and general symptoms (n = 30, RCT, d/b, p/c, > 8/52, Akhondzadeh *et al*, *Schizophr Res* 2009;**107**:206–12) and 8 mg/d improved PANSS and reduced EPSE in people with TRS on haloperidol 4–30 mg/d, (n = 121, RCT, d/b, p/c, 12/52, Zhang *et al*, *Schizophr Res* 2006;**88**:102–10). A review concluded that ondansetron may be an effective adjunct, especially for negative symptoms, but that a large RCT is needed (s = 6, Bennett and Vila, *Ann Pharmacother* 2010;**44**:130–6).

Oxcarbazepine

Oxcarbazepine has been used as an adjunctive treatment in acute schizophrenia (n = 6, open, Leweke *et al*, *Am J Psychiatry* 2004;**161**:1130–1).

Pregabalin *

Adjunctive pregabalin may be effective for comorbid anxiety in schizophrenia (n = 11, open, Englisch *et al*, *J Clin Psychopharmacol* 2010;**30**:437–40).

Sarcosine (N-methylglycine) *

Sarcosine was superior to placebo as add-on to TAU for TRS, unlike d-serine, which was not (n = 60, RCT, d/b, p/c, 6/52, Lane *et al*, *Int J Neuropsychopharmacol* 2010;**13**:451–60).

Selegiline

Low-dose oral selegiline as antipsychotic augmentation may improve negative symptoms of schizophrenia (n = 67, d/b, p/c, 12/52, Bodkin *et al*, *Am J Psychiatry* 2005;**162**:388–90).

D-serine (see also sarcosine)

D-serine is a full agonist at glycine NMDA receptors and, when used at 30 mg/kg/d as adjunct to olanzapine or risperidone, significantly improved PANSS, 20% reduction in BRS in 35% of patients, with no detrimental adverse effects (n = 39, RCT, d/b, p/c, c/o, 6/52, Heresco-Levy *et al*, *Biol Psychiatry* 2005;**15**:577–85).

Sildenafil *

Sildenafil 75 mg/d as an adjunct to risperidone 6 mg/d significantly improved negative symptoms of schizophrenia (n = 40, RCT, d/b, p/c, 8/52, Akhondzadeh *et al*, *Psychopharmacol (Berl)* 2011;**213**:809–15).

Topiramate

Topiramate 300 mg/d as an antipsychotic adjunct in TRS has reduced PANSS scores in some (n = 26, RCT, d/b, p/c, c/o, 2×12/52, Tiihonen *et al*, *J Clin Psychiatry* 2005;**66**:1012–5, IS), particularly for negative symptoms and reducing weight gain (n = 32, RCT, d/b, p/c, Afshar *et al*, *J Psychopharmacol* 2009;**23**:157–62). However, topiramate had no effect on BPRS when added to clozapine, risperidone, olanzapine or flupentixol (n = 9, open, Dursun and Deakin, *J Psychopharmacol* 2001;**15**:297–301), and significant deterioration has been reported so it should not be used with clozapine as anticonvulsant cover (e.g. n = 1, Hofer et al, J Clin Psychiatry 2003;**64**:1267–8).

Valproate *

Reviews have concluded that there is no proven advantage for valproate augmentation in schizophrenia. Some studies show inconsistent benefit but that it may be useful in acute management (Basan et al, Schizophr Res 2004;**70**:33–7; Basan and Leucht, Cochrane Database Syst Rev 2004;**1**:CD004028). As an adjunct to risperidone or olanzapine for acute exacerbation of schizophrenia has resulted in an earlier response of psychotic symptoms (n = 249, RCT, d/b, 4/52, Casey et al, Neuropsychopharmacol 2003;**28**:182–92), or as augmentation of SGAs in very severe schizophrenia (n = 28, open, Suzuki et al, Hum Psychopharmacol 2009;**24**:628–38). Cochrane concludes that there is no data to support or refute the use of valproate as monotherapy in schizophrenia (s = 7, n = 519, Schwarz et al, Cochrane Database Syst Rev 2008;**3**:CD004028).

Zotepine *

Zotepine is now discontinued in many countries. Cochrane concludes that there is insufficient evidence to say if it has any advantages over other SGAs (s = 3, n = 289, Subramanian et al, Cochrane Database Syst Rev 2010;**10**:CD006628).

Reviews: * general (Green, Expert Opin Drug Metab Toxicol 2009;**5**:181–6), safety (Riedel et al, Expert Opin Drug Saf 2010;**9**:659–66).

● **Unlicensed/some efficacy**

Asenapine *

Asenapine is licensed in EU for moderate-severe manic episodes associated with bipolar I disorder in adults, but in some non-EU countries also for acute schizophrenia (e.g. US) and relapse prevention. It has a high affinity for 5HT1A/1B/2A/2B/2C/5/6/7, D1/2/3/4, alpha 1 and 2, H1 and H2 but not cholinergic receptors (Citrome, Int J Clin Pract 2009;**63**:1762–84). Asenapine 10mg/d was as effective as risperidone and superior to placebo in acute schizophrenia, and as well tolerated as placebo (n = 174, RCT, p/c, 6/52, Potkin et al, J Clin Psychiatry 2007;**68**:1492–1500;

MS), and 10mg/d was superior to risperidone 6mg/d and placebo in acute schizophrenia (n = 174, RCT, p/c, d/b, 6/52, Potkin et al, J Clin Psychiatry 2007;**68**:1492–1500). Robust long-term relapse prevention efficacy compared to placebo (12% vs 47%) has been shown (n = 386 [c = 207], RCT, d/b, p/c, 26/52, Kane et al, J Clin Psychiatry 2011;**72**:349–55). It is presented as a sublingual tablet which dissolves in seconds when placed under the tongue. It is 35% bioavailable orally, but less than 2% if swallowed, so no drinking or eating for 10 minutes after a dose is recommended. Food just before a dose decreases absorption by 20% and by 10% up to four hours afterwards. The US PI for asenapine recommends gradual discontinuation and minimising overlap with other antipsychotics.

Reviews: * in schizophrenia (Bishara and Taylor, Neuropsychiatr Dis Treat 2009;**5**:483–90), general (Citrome, Neuropsychiatr Dis Treat 2011;**7**:325–39; Shahid et al, J Psychopharmacol 2008;**23**:65–73; Weber and McCormack, CNS Drugs 2009;**23**:781–92).

● **Unlicensed/some efficacy**

Estradiol/estrogen *

Estrogen may have specific antipsychotic-like effects in women with schizophrenia (n = 125, Bergemann et al, Psychol Med 2007;**37**:1427–36), e.g. 100mcg estradiol significantly reduced positive and general psychopathology, suggesting a possible role (n = 102, RCT, p/c, 28/7, Kulkarni et al, Arch Gen Psychiatry 2008; **65**:955–60; generally positive comment by Crespo-Focorro et al, EBMH 2009;**12**:55), e.g. estrogen as an adjunct to haloperidol significantly reduced positive and general symptoms in women (n = 32, RCT, d/b, p/c, 8/52, Akhondzadeh et al, Prog Neuropsychopharmacol Biol Psychiatry 2003;**27**:1007–12). Transdermal estrogen was, however, unable to prevent relapse of postnatal affective psychosis when started within 48 hours of delivery (n = 29, open, 12/7, Kumar et al, J Clin Psychiatry 2003;**64**:112–8).

■ **Unlicensed/possible efficacy**

Bromocriptine

Bromocriptine (n = 6, open, Levi-Minzi et al, Compr Psychiatry 1991;**32**:210–6) may decrease negative symptoms, at least in some patient sub-groups.

Betel nut

Males with schizophrenia chewing large quantities of betel nut (an anti-muscarinic) have significantly milder positive symptoms than low users (n = 65, Sullivan et al, Am J Psychiatry 2007;**164**:670).

Flunarizine

Flunarizine has some dopamine-blocking properties, and has been shown to be as effective as haloperidol and, with a half-life of 2–7 weeks, could have a potential role as a long-acting oral antipsychotic (n = 70, RCT, d/b, 12/52, Bisol et al, J Clin Psychiatry 2008; **69**:1572–9).

Lithium

Lithium-responsive psychosis can occur and may be familial and is perhaps genetically distinct from the bulk of schizophrenias. A meta-analysis has concluded that although a few studies show some efficacy of lithium in schizophrenia, the overall results are inconclusive (n = 611, s = 20, Leucht et al, J Clin Psychiatry 2004;**65**:177–86) and Cochrane agrees that lithium is ineffective as a sole agent, but may potentially be useful in a few patients (n = 611, s = 20, Leucht et al, Cochrane Database Syst Rev 2003;**3**:CD003834; review by Bender and Dittmann-Balcar, EBMH 2004;**7**:104). Lithium augmentation of clozapine may provide additional clinical benefit in schizoaffective but not schizophrenic patients (n = 20, p/c, 4/52, Small et al, J Clin Psychopharmacol 2003; **23**:223–8).

Melatonin

Melatonin 3 mg/d may be useful as a hypnotic in schizophrenia (see insomnia, n = 40, RCT, d/b, p/c, 15/7, Kumar et al, J Clin Psychiatry 2007;**68**:237–41), but not in those with better sleep efficiency (n = 19, RCT, c/o, p/c, Shamir et al, J Clin Psychiatry 2000;**61**:373–7).

Gabapentin *

A pilot study suggested adjunctive gabapentin may have some effect in partially-responsive

schizophrenia (n = 10, 8/52, Gabriel, Neuropsychiatr Dis Treat 2010;**6**:711–7).

L-theanine *

L-theanine is a unique amino acid found virtually only in tea and may have psychoactive properties. A pilot study showed augmentation of antipsychotics in schizophrenia or schizoaffective disorders improved positive, activation and anxiety symptoms, so more studies may be worth it (n = 60 [c = 40], RCT, d/b, p/c, 8/52, Ritsner et al, J Clin Psychiatry 2011;**72**:34–42).

Minocycline *

Minocycline 200 mg/d, which modulates the glutamatergic system, improved negative symptoms and general outcome in first-episode patients as an add-on to SGAs (n = 54, RCT, d/b, p/c, 6/12, Levkovitz et al, J Clin Psychiatry 2010;**71**:138–49). There are cases of acute schizophrenia with predominantly catatonic symptoms responding to minocycline (n = 2, Miyaoka et al, Prog Neuropsychopharmacol Biol Psychiatry 2007;**31**:304–7).

Omega-3 fatty acids *

There is some evidence for abnormal phospholipid metabolism in schizophrenia, and trials with PUVAs have produced inconsistent but usually favourable findings, with 2 g/d the optimum dose (Horrobin, Am J Psychiatry 2003;**160**:188–9). E-EPA (ethyl-eicosapentaenoic acid) may be effective as adjunctive therapy for persistent psychotic symptoms (n = 40, RCT, 12/52, Emsley et al, Am J Psychiatry 2002;**159**:1696–8), e.g. general symptoms may improve by taking a supplement that combines essential poly-unsaturated fatty acids (EPUFAs) with antioxidants (n = 73, 4/12, Arvindaksham et al, Schizophr Res 2003;**62**:195–204). A small open study of adjunctive omega-3 fatty acids and vitamins E and C to haloperidol suggested significantly improved symptoms on all rating scales, particularly on reduced akathisia (n = 17, open, Sivrioglu et al, Prog Neuropsychopharmacol Biol Psychiatry 2007;**31**:1493–9). However, omega-3 fatty acids have been shown to be ineffective in treating residual symptoms of schizophrenia (n = 87, RCT, 16/52, Fenton et al, Am J Psychiatry 2001; **158**:2071–4). Cochrane concludes the evidence is still inconclusive (s = 8, n = 517, Joy et al, Cochrane Database Syst Rev 2006;**3**:CD001257).

Raloxifene *

Raloxifene (an estrogen modulator) 120mg/d produced a significantly quicker recovery cf 60mg/d and placebo, suggesting a potential role in postmenopausal women with schizophrenia (n = 35, p/c, Kulkarni et al, Psychoneuroendocrinology 2010;**35**:1142–7).

Tetrabenazine

Tetrabenazine has been used for the treatment of psychoses and psychoneuroses but the high incidence of side-effects makes this a relatively unsuitable drug.

❋ Case reports *

- **Amisulpride + aripiprazole** worsening psychosis when aripiprazole was added to amisulpride (n = 1, Adan-Manes and Garcia-Parajua, J Clin Pharm Ther 2009;**34**:245–6).
- **Clozapine + olanzapine** (n = 1, Rhoads, J Clin Psychiatry 2000;**61**:678–80).
- **Dronabinol** * (n = 4, Schwarcz and Karajgi, J Clin Psychiatry 2010;**71**:1552–3).
- **Olanzapine + quetiapine** (n = 1, Dunkley and Reveley, J Psychopharmacol 2005;**19**:97–101).
- **Pergolide + amisulpride** (n = 1, Roesch-Ely et al, Pharmacopsychiatry 2006;**39**:115–6).

◆ Others

Other drugs that have been tried include **calcium-channel blockers** (Am J Psychiatry 1992;**149**:1615; Drug Intell Clin Pharm 1990;**24**:838–40), **famotidine** (review by Martinez, Ann Pharmacother 1999;**33**:742–7), **naltrexone/naloxone** (Welch and Thompson, J Clin Pharm Ther 1994;**19**:279–83).

☐ No efficacy

Ayurvedic medicine

Ayurvedic medicine may have some effects, but there is inadequate data to draw any conclusions (s = 3, n = 250, Agarwal et al, Cochrane Database Syst Rev 2007;**4**:CD006867).

Buspirone

Buspirone has various receptor activities, e.g. $5-HT_{1A}$ partial antagonism and dopamine antagonism but exacerbation of psychosis has been reported.

Caffeine

Excess caffeine consumption can present as psychosis, increasing arousal and may have a psychotogenic effect, but moderate use probably has little effect on anxiety, depression and psychosis (e.g. n = 26, RCT, d/b, c/o, Mayo et al, Br J Psychiatry 1993;**162**:543–5).

Cannabidiol

In a small case series in TRS, only one showed mild improvement with cannabidiol, the others showing none (n = 3, 35/7, Zuardi et al, J Psychopharmacol 2006;**20**:683–6).

Cannabis

Cochrane concludes that there is insufficient evidence to support or refute the use of cannabis to treat schizophrenia (s = 1, RCT, Rathbone et al, Cochrane Database Syst Rev 2008;**3**:CD004837).

Carbamazepine *

Cochrane could not recommend carbamazepine for routine use, either as monotherapy, augmentation or maintenance (s = 10, n = 258, RCT, Leucht et al, Cochrane Database Syst Rev 2007;**3**:CD001258). A related systematic review and meta-analysis of carbamazepine augmentation in schizophrenia failed to show any clinically significant positive effect (s = 10, n = 283, Leucht et al, J Clin Psychiatry 2002;**63**:218–24). Remember that carbamazepine will also induce CYP3A4 and reduce the plasma levels of many antipsychotics.

Creatine

Adjunctive creatine 5g/d had no effect on cognitive function or symptoms (n = 12, RCT, d/b, p/c, c/o, 3/12, Kaptsan et al, J Clin Psychiatry 2007;**68**:881–4).

Methylphenidate

Bolus IV methylphenidate has been used to induce an exacerbation of symptoms in an attempt to predict those people most likely to relapse when antipsychotics are discontinued (mentioned in Klein and Wender, *Arch Gen Psychiatry* 1995;**52**:429–33).

Memantine

Memantine 20 mg/d was ineffective on all primary and secondary measures as an adjunct to antipsychotics in schizophrenia (n = 138, RCT, d/b, p/c, 8/52, Lieberman *et al, Neuropsychopharmacology* 2009;**34**:1322–9).

Nifedipine

Adjunctive nifedipine is of little efficacy, although it had a numerical advantage in negative PANSS scores (n = 62, open, 10/52, Dzhuga and Kozlovski, *Zh Nevrol Psikhiatr Im S S Korsakova* 2009;**109**:32–5).

Tricyclics

Tricyclics are at best ineffective for acute psychotic episodes (n = 58, RCT, d/b, p/c, 4/52, Kramer *et al, Arch Gen Psychiatry* 1989; **46**:922–8).

Vitamin B6

No difference in PANSS scores was detectable with B_6 supplementation in stable chronic schizophrenics (n = 15, d/b, p/c, c/o, 9/52, Lerner *et al, J Clin Psychiatry* 2002;**63**:54–8).

1.21.2 FIRST EPISODE (EARLY INTERVENTION)

Early intervention can include both treating a first episode quickly, and treating people at high risk before symptoms actually appear. Social decline, associated with neurocognitive deficits often occurs in the prodromal phase, or in the early course of schizophrenia, thus management is vital.

A longer duration of untreated psychosis (DUP) shows a consistent but modest relationship (s = 26, n = 4490, Marshall *et al, Arch Gen Psychiatry* 2005;**62**:975–83; comment by Perkins, *EBMH* 2006;**9**:36; n = 157, Wunderink *et al, Acta Psychiatr Scand* 2006;**113**:332–9) with:

- worse symptoms, poor social functioning independent of symptoms (n = 98, 1 year, Barnes *et al, Br J Psychiatry* 2008;**193**:203–9; n = 109, White *et al, Psychol Med* 2009; **39**:1447–56)

- less chance of remission, and reduced improvement after one year (n = 49, Fusar-Poli *et al, Br J Psychiatry* 2009;**194**:181–2)
- impaired verbal IQ, verbal learning and working memory (n = 273, Lappin *et al, Schizophr Res* 2007;**95**:103–10).

However, delay in starting antipsychotics in first-episode psychosis is not necessarily neurotoxic for the brain or leads to reduced hippocampal volumes (n = 105, Ho *et al, Am J Psychiatry* 2005;**162**:1527–9). Structured early intervention programmes improve overall functioning and adherence but not necessarily symptoms (n = 144, RCT, 18/12, Garety *et al, Br J Psychiatry* 2006;**188**:37–45; comment by van Meijl, *EBMH* 2006;**9**:69). Substance misuse early in the illness has been linked with increased severity of illness (n = 232, Bühler *et al, Schizophr Res* 2002;**54**:234–51), and so should also be managed. Cochrane concludes that there is insufficient data to draw conclusions for use in children with onset prior to 13 years (Kennedy *et al, Cochrane Database Syst Rev* 2007;**3**:CD004027). Addition of CBT, family therapy and other inputs to optimal pharmacotherapy and case management may improve symptoms and outcomes, although psychotic symptoms and readmissions may be unchanged (n = 50, RCT, two years, Grawe *et al, Acta Psychiatr Scand* 2006;**114**:328–36).

Role of antipsychotics in first episodes: *

- Minimise deterioration (or even perhaps prevent the illness developing, although this remains unproven; s = 18, n = 1808, Marshall and Rathbone, *Cochrane Database Syst Rev* 2011;**6**:CD004718).
- Reduce stigma from symptoms, aiming for complete, not incomplete, remission.
- Increase engagement by minimising adverse experience with medication through use of minimum effective doses.

Antipsychotic therapy is usually considered as essential treatment, and is definitely more effective if taken regularly. Improving concordance (and effectiveness) in a first episode has a number of principles:

1. Optimal antipsychotic initiation:
- Slow titration is needed, both starting and stopping. The mean time to response is nine weeks (n = 118, Robinson *et al, Am J Psychiatry* 1999;**156**:544–9), but may be

longer (n = 522, RCT, median 30/52, Emsley et al, Am J Psychiatry 2006; **163**:743–45).

2. Patient choice considered a high priority: *

- A meta-analysis has concluded that there is no difference in efficacy between SGAs and FGAs in early psychosis, but there is a significant difference in (predictable) ADRs (s = 15, n = 2522, RCT, Crossley et al, Br J Psychiatry 2010;**196**:434–9). So, consider what the patient prefers (weight gain is the most unpopular side-effect and its impact on the user must not be trivialised). Antipsychotic-induced weight gain is 3–4 times more common in younger, first-episode patients compared to older, chronic patients. The increase is consistent by drug but idiosyncratic by individual, with oanzapine, risperidone, haloperidol (s = 51, n = 14769, Alvarez-Jiménez et al, CNS Drugs 2008;**22**:547–62).

- Explain that there is no clear way of treating prodromal symptoms without the high risk of treating 'false positives' (review by Larsen et al, Acta Psychiatr Scand 2001;**103**:323–4).

- Minimise 'obvious' ADRs that might make the person apepar abnormal, e.g. EPSE, and which reduce compliance and engagement (n = 42, Amminger et al, Schizophr Res 2002;**54**:223–30).

3. Adequate duration of treatment: * the relapse rate over five years is high with diagnosed but untreated schizophrenia.

- Long-term treatment retention is low – as few as 12% youths are still on same treatment at 12/12 (n = 54, Findling et al, J Am Acad Child Adolesc Psychiatry 2010;**49**:583–94).

- On discontinuation, up to 78% may experience an exacerbation or relapse within one year, and 96% may do so within two years (n = 53, RCT, open, 18/12, Gitlin et al, Am J Psychiatry 2001;**158**:1835–42).

- Patients should be advised that not taking antipsychotics for several years will almost inevitably lead to relapse and rehospitalisation (n = 104, Robinson et al, Arch Gen Psychiatry 1999;**56**:241–7). The optimum duration of therapy is, as yet, unclear.

4. Optimum long-term dosing

- In a study in remitted first-episode psychosis patients stable for 6/12, maintenance with low-dose antipsychotics was compared

to gradual discontinuation, with an 18/12 follow-up. Twice as many relapses occurred in the discontinuation group compared to maintenance (43% vs 21%), with 30% requiring restarting antipsychotics and only 20% successfully discontinuing. The authors conclude that the risk from low doses appears low compared to the risk of relapse and subsequent potential deterioration (n = 131, RCT, open, 18/12, Wunderink et al, J Clin Psychiatry 2007;**68**:654–61).

- Relatively low doses of risperidone 4 mg/d, olanzapine 15.3 mg/d, haloperidol 5.4 mg/d may be equally effective for first episode psychosis, with haloperidol worst for EPSE and olanzapine worst for weight gain (n = 172, RCT, open, 6/52, Crespo-Facorro et al, J Clin Psychiatry 2006;**67**:1511–21; IS, comment by Barbui et al, EBMH 2007;**10**:54).

5. Treatment is monitored:

- Some antipsychotics have a high incidence of EPS (even with low dose haloperidol; n = 57, 12/12, Oosterhuizen et al, J Clin Psychiatry 2003;**64**:1075–80), raised prolactin and adverse cognitive effects. Others have higher incidence of weight gain (which should be dealt with early) and diabetes, which needs to be screened for, monitored and managed.

Reviews: * the case for early intervention (McGorry, Br Med J 2008;**337**:a695), the case against (Pelosi, Br Med J 2008;**337**:a710), general (Mattai et al, Curr Opin Psychiatry 2010;**23**:304–10; Salimi et al, CNS Drugs 2009;**23**:837–55), efficacy and tolerability (Kumra et al, Schizophrenia Bull 2008;**34**:60–71).

BNF listed

Amisulpride

Amisulpride (mean 250 mg/d) is licensed from age 15 years upwards (n = 14[c = 12], open, 6/52, Murphy et al, Hum Psychopharmacol 2006; **21**:511–7).

Aripiprazole *

Aripiprazole is licensed in the UK for schizophrenia in adolescents aged 15 years or older (US 13–17 years). NICE in UK concludes that aripiprazole is an option for people aged 15–17 who are intolerant or non-responsive to risperidone (NICE TA213, Jan 2011). In first episode patients, aripiprazole had a responder rate of 79% and was well tolerated (n = 45 [c = 42], open, 12/52, Takahashi et al, Clin Neuropharmacol 2009;**32**:149–50; n = 21, open, 8/52, Lee et al, Psychiatry Clin Neurosci 2010; **64**:38–43) and a chart review suggested some efficacy as an adjunct (n = 15, Bachmann et al, Pharmacopsychiatry 2009;**42**:153–7).

Clozapine

Clozapine is licensed from age 16 upwards. Early use of clozapine (after as few as 25 weeks in people failing two other antipsychotics) has been associated with significant and meaningful reductions in symptoms (n = 13, Agid et al, J Clin Psycho-pharmacol 2007;**27**:369–73; see also n = 54, d/b or open, Sporn et al, J Am Acad Child Adolesc Psychiatry 2007;**46**:1349–56), but it has more ADRs and toxicity (n = 25, RCT, d/b, 8/52 + open two-year follow-up, Shaw et al, Arch Gen Psychiatry 2006;**63**:721–30).

Haloperidol

Haloperidol is licensed for childhood behavioural disorders and schizophrenia with no age limit. There is an irony that the only antipsychotic licensed in this age group is probably the one you would not want to use. Haloperidol 2 mg/d is much better tolerated than 8 mg/d and as effective, shown by PANSS scores (n = 40, RCT, d/b, 6/52, Oosthuizen et al, Int J Neuropsychopharmacol 2004;**7**:125–31) and has equivalent efficacy to olanzapine, although drop-out rates were high and this trial excluded more severely ill people (n = 263 [c = 83], RCT, d/b, one year, Strakowski et al, Schizophr Res 2005;**78**:161–9; comment by Awad, EBMH 2006;**9**:47). Unlike olanzapine, haloperidol is associated with reduced grey matter volume in a first episode, either due to haloperidol-induced toxicity or differential olanzapine efficacy (n = 263, RCT, d/b, volunteer controlled, 24/12, Lieberman et al, Arch Gen Psychiatry 2005;**62**:361–70). Haloperidol and risperidone (both 2–4 mg/d) were equally effective in relapse prevention in first-episode schizophrenia, with similar ADRs and drop-outs (n = 151, RCT, d/b, one year, Gaebel et al, J Clin Psychiatry 2007;**68**:1763–74).

Olanzapine *

Olanzapine is only licensed in UK from age 18 years upwards. Low dose olanzapine is preferable to haloperidol in first-episode psychosis, with superior efficacy, lower discontinuations, greater retention in treatment and reduced side-effects (e.g. n = 107, RCT, d/b, p/c, 6/52, Kryzhanovskaya et al, J Am Acad Child Adolesc Psychiatry 2009;**48**:60–70), although weight gain is a significant adverse effect (mean 15.4 kg) in first-episode psychosis (n = 263, open, two years, Zipursky et al, Br J Psychiatry 2005;**187**:537–43; comment by Lambert, EBMH 2006;**9**:72). Olanzapine (2.5–20 mg/d) and risperidone (1–6 mg/d) have been shown to be equipotent in first-episode schizophrenia (e.g. n = 100 [c = 77], RCT, open, 6/12, Cuesta et al, Br J Psychiatry 2009;**194**:439–45) and as effective as quetiapine (n = 50 [c = 32], open, 6/12, Arango et al, Eur Child Adolesc Psychiatry 2009;**18**:418–28), but weight gain was greater with olanzapine and the FDA have warned about the increased risk of weight gain and hyperlipidemia with long-term treatment in the 13–17 age group.
Review: * use in adolescents (McCormack, CNS Drugs 2010;**24**:443–52).

Quetiapine *

Quetiapine is licensed for schizophrenia in adults but not recommended for under 18s due to lack of data. Low EPS, weight gain and prolactin effects make quetiapine a suitable antipsychotic. It seems as effective as olanzapine but with less weight gain (n = 50 [c = 32], open, 6/12, Arango et al, Eur Child Adolesc Psychiatry 2009;**18**:418–28). In people stable after one year of antipsychotics, maintenance with quetiapine for a further year showed relapse of 41% cf 79% placebo (n = 178, RCT, d/b, p/c, 12/12, Chen et al, Br Med J 2010;**341**:c4024). However, a small study failed to show any beneficial effect on cognition in antipsychotic-naïve first episode schizophrenia (n = 48, 6/12, Andersen et al, Psychiatry Res 2011;**187**:49–54).

Risperidone *

Risperidone is licensed from age 15 years upwards and is now the standard first choice. Risperidone needs a low but adequate dose, e.g. 1–3 mg/d seems the optimum dose, and as effective as 4–6mg/d but with less ADRs (n=160, RCT, d/b, p/c, 6/52, Haas et al, J Child Adolesc Psychopharmacol 2009;19:611–21; MS), so it makes little pharmacological sense in escalating doses at an early stage (n=49, d/b, 8/52, Merlo et al, J Clin Psychiatry 2002;63:885–91). In the 75% who initially clinically improve, relapses are delayed longer with risperidone (mean 3.3mg/d; median 466 days) than haloperidol (mean 2.9mg/d; median 205 days) (n=555, RCT, d/b, <5 years, median 30/52, Schooler et al, Am J Psychiatry 2005;162:947–53). Risperidone 1–6mg/d was equipotent with olanzapine (2.5–20mg/d) in first-episode schizophrenia, but patients may be more stable with risperidone (n=112, RCT, open, 4/12, Robinson et al, Am J Psychiatry 2006;163:2096–102; see also n=25, RCT, open, 12/52, Mozes et al, J Child Adolesc Psychopharmacol 2006;16:393–403). Use of RLAI improves compliance and reduces relapse rate (n=50[c=32], open, two years, Emsley et al, Int Clin Psychopharmacol 2008; 23:325–31) in first episode schizophrenia compared to oral risperidone (n=50, Kim et al, Prog Neuropsychopharmacol Biol Psychiatry 2008;32:1231–5) .

Celecoxib *

Adding further weight to the hypothesis of inflammation as a contributor to schizophrenia, amisulpride 200–1000mg/d plus celecoxib 400mg or placebo showed a significantly better outcome in first episodes with celecoxib, including improved negative symptoms (n=49, RCT, d/b, p/c, 6/52, Müller et al, Schizophr Res 2010;121:118–24).

Omega-3 fatty acids (E-EPA) *

In an extraordinary study of young people at ultra-high risk of developing psychotic disorders, a 3/12 course of omega-3 fatty acids 1.2g/d (PUFAs) reduced transition to psychotic disorder from 27.5% (placebo) to 4.9% (PUFA) over one year; an NNT of 4 (n=81[c=76], RCT, d/b, p/c, 12/12, Amminger et al, Arch Gen Psychiatry 2010;67:146–54). Beat that if you can, and it certainly beats the previous negative study (n=69, RCT, d/b, p/c, 12/52, Berger et al, J Clin Psychiatry 2007;68:1867–75).

1.21.3 COGNITIVE IMPAIRMENT

Cognitive impairment is a known complication of schizophrenia and of antipsychotics, and so methods to improve cognitive function are needed. Some antipsychotics may have a better cognitive profile than others, e.g. risperidone over haloperidol (n=533[c=359], RCT, 3/12 follow-up, Harvey et al, Am J Psychiatry 2005;162:1888–95), and olanzapine over haloperidol (n=167, RCT, d/b, 12/52, Keefe et al, Am J Psychiatry 2004;161:985–95). In schizophreniform and first episode psychosis, amisulpride, olanzapine, haloperidol, quetiapine and ziprasidone can all produce a moderate improvement in cognition, with no differences between the drugs, which is weakly related to symptom change (n=498, RCT, open, 6/12, EUFEST, Davidson et al, Am J Psychiatry 2009;166:675–82).

Reviews: * general (Galletly, Psychopharmacol [Berl] 2009;202:259–73), pharmacological treatment of cognition in schizophrenia (Barch, Curr Top Behav Neurosci 2010;4:43–96; Harvey and Cornblatt, Am J Psychiatry 2008;165:163–5).

Anticholinesterases *

A meta-analysis concludes that the three anticholinesterases improve motor speed and executive function (motor speed and attention) as adjuncts, but that more data is needed (s=13, RCT, d/b, Ribeiz et al, CNS Drugs 2010;24:303–17). Of the available drugs, **donepezil** 5–10mg/d appears to have little effect on cognitive deficits in schizophrenia (e.g. n=26, RCT, d/b, p/c, 16/52, Kohler et al, Cognit Neuropsychiatry 2007;12:412–21). However, some mild improvements have been shown (e.g. n=28, open, 12/52, Chung et al World J Biol Psychiatry 2009;10:156–62) and 10mg/d as an adjunct to risperidone significantly improved negative symptoms in chronic schizophrenia with cognitive impairments (n=30, RCT, d/b, p/c, 12/52, Akhondzadeh et al, Prog Neuropsychopharmacol Biol Psychiatry 2008;32:1810–5). Improvement in refractory negative symptoms and cognition has been reported with adjunctive **galantamine**, e.g. improved processing speed, WAIS-III and verbal memory, although it interfered with practice effects in attention tasks (n = 86, RCT, d/b, p/c, 12/52, Buchanan et al, Am J Psychiatry 2008;**165**:82–9), but 24 mg/d had no apparent effect on cognitive function or negative symptoms in stable schizophrenia with low baseline functioning (n = 83 [c = 73], RCT, d/b, p/c, 12/52, Conley et al, Clin Neuropharmacol 2009;**32**:69–74). **Rivastigmine** up to 9 mg/d had no effect on cognitive function in schizophrenics with significant impairment (n = 20, RCT, c/o, 6/12, Chouinard et al, Curr Med Res Opin 2007;**23**:575–83) and adjunctive use had no detectable effect on cognitive function when added to stable antipsychotic therapy in schizophrenia (n = 40 [c = 21], RCT, d/b, p/c, 24/52, Sharma et al, Schizophr Res 2006;**85**:73–83), although up to 16 mg BD has significantly improved quality of life and cognitive functioning with few ADRs (n = 16, 12/12, Lenzi et al, Clin Neuropharmacol 2003; **26**:317–21).

Buspirone

Buspirone augmentation has improved attention in schizophrenia but not statistically (n = 73, RCT, d/b, p/c, 6/12, Sumiyoshi et al, Schizophr Res 2007;**95**:158–68).

Clozapine + risperidone

The combination did not significantly improve cognitive function cf clozapine alone (n = 30, RCT, d/b, p/c, 6/52, Akdede et al, J Clin Psychiatry 2006;**67**:1912–9).

Minocycline *

Minocycline 200 mg/d, which modulates the glutamatergic system, improved cognitive functioning in first-episode patients as an add-on to SGAs (n = 54, RCT, d/b, p/c, 6/12, Levkovitz et al, J Clin Psychiatry 2010;**71**:138–49).

Mirtazapine *

Augmentation of risperidone significantly improved cognitive and negative symptoms, but at the cost of weight gain (n = 21, RCT, d/b, p/c, 8/52, Cho et al, Prog Neuropsychopharmacol Biol Psychiatry 2011;**35**:208–11) and adjunctive mirtazapine was superior to placebo for improving a variety of cognitive functions (n = 37, RCT, d/b, p/c, 6/52, Stenberg et al, Int J Neuropsychopharmacol 2010;**13**:433-41).

Modafinil *

Modafinil 200 mg/d has produced improvements in cognitive functioning in schizophrenia (n = 20, RCT, d/b, p/c, c/o, Turner et al, Neuropsychopharmacol 2004;**29**:1363–73), but had no effect on negative symptoms although some global improvements were seen (n = 20, RCT, d/b, p/c, 8/52, Pierre et al, J Clin Psychiatry 2007;**68**:705–10) and Modafinil 300 mg/d added to clozapine had no effect on impaired cognition (n = 35, RCT, d/b, p/c, 8/52, Freudenreich et al, J Clin Psychiatry 2009; **70**:1674–80).

Pregnenolone *

Adjunctive pregnenolone (a neurosteroid that enhances cognition in rats and modulates NMDA receptors) 30 mg/d was superior to placebo and 200 mg/d for positive symptoms and EPS in schizophrenia (n = 58 [c = 44], RCT, d/b, p/c, 8/52, Ritsner et al, J Clin Psychiatry 2010; **71**:1351–62), supporting a previous pilot study (n = 21 [c = 18], RCT, d/b, p/c, 8/52, Marx et al, Neuropsychopharmacology 2009;**34**:1885–903).

□ No efficacy

Atomoxetine

Adjunctive atomoxetine was ineffective for improving cognitive impairment in schizophrenia (n = 32, RCT, d/b, p/c, 8/52, Kelly et al, J Clin Psychiatry 2009;**70**:518–25).

Cicloserin (D-cycloserine)

In severe negative symptoms and cognitive impairment (without marked positive, depressive or EPSE symptoms) there was no improvement when either glycine or cicloserin were added (n = 157, RCT, d/b, p/c, 12/52, Buchanan et al, Am J Psychiatry 2007;**164**:1593–602).

Dehydroepiandrosterone DHEA *

Adjunctive DHEA 400 mg/d had little effect on positive symptoms and EPS in schizophrenia (n = 58 [c = 44], RCT, d/b, p/c, 8/52, Ritsner et al, J Clin Psychiatry 2010;**71**:1351–62).

Glycine

See cicloserine above.

Reboxetine *

Adjunctive reboxetine 4 mg/d to olanzapine 10 mg/d has no effect on cognitive dysfunction (p/c, d/b, Poyurovsky et al, Isr J Psychiatry Relat Sci 2009;**46**:213–20).

RAPID-CYCLING BIPOLAR DISORDER

see Bipolar disorder, rapid-cycling (1.10.4)

1.22 SEASONAL AFFECTIVE DISORDER (SAD)

see Depression (1.14), Mania and hypomania (1.10.2) and Bipolar mood disorder (1.10)

SAD is a recurrent affective disorder, predominantly major depression, but can include mania or hypomania. It has a characteristic seasonal relationship, usually autumn or winter (s = 20, Magnusson, Acta Psychiatr Scand 2000: **101**:176–84), for at least two or three years, with full remission at a characteristic time of the year and outnumbering any non-seasonal episodes. The incidence may be around 1–10% (e.g. 2.4% in North Wales) and peaks in winter. Atypical depressive features include hypersomnia, increased appetite and weight and carbohydrate cravings. Theories for the cause include excess melatonin secretion, delayed or reduced amplitude circadian rhythms, and serotonergic dysfunction. It is often undiagnosed and half of sufferers are given other depressive diagnoses and antidepressants (n = 1999, Michalak et al, Br J Psychiatry 2001;**179**:31–4). Light therapy is first choice for SAD (n = 96, RCT, Lam et al, Am J Psychiatry 2006;**163**:805–12; comment by Gaynes, EBMH 2007;**10**:26) and, although better tolerated than fluoxetine, it is not without risk, with side-effects including jumpiness (9%), headache (8%), and nausea (16%).

Role of drugs

While phototherapy is well established, drug treatment may also be effective, with bupropion and sertraline appearing as effective. Seasonal major depression can be prevented by starting an antidepressant early in the season while patient is still well (e.g. with bupropion 150–300 mg/d; s = 3, n = 1042, RCT, p/c, Modell et al, Biol Psychiatry 2005;**58**:658–67).

Reviews: general (DTB 2009;**47**:128–32; Westrin

and Lam, Ann Clin Psychiatry 2007;**19**:239–46), long-term treatment (Westrin and Lam, CNS Drugs 2007;**21**:901–9), light therapy (Golden et al, Am J Psychiatry 2005;**162**:656–62; Terman, EBMH 2006;**9**:21).

● Unlicensed/some efficacy

Bupropion

Bupropion XL is licensed in the USA for SAD, using 150–300 mg/d where treatment was started in the autumn while the patients were still well (s = 3, n = 1042, RCT, p/c, d/b, Modell et al, Biol Psychiatry 2005;**58**:658–67).

Sertraline

Sertraline (50–200 mg/d) was significantly superior to placebo in winter pattern SAD in one study (n = 187, RCT, d/b, p/c, O/P, 8/52, Moscovitch et al, Psychopharmacol [Berl] 2004; **171**:390–7).

■ Unlicensed/possible efficacy

Agomelatine

A pilot study suggested that seasonal depression may respond to agomelatine (n = 37, open, 14/52, Pjrek et al, Psychopharmacology [Berl] 2007;**190**:575–9).

Beta-blockers

Propranolol 60 mg/d administered pre-sunrise (5.30–6.00 AM) may produce response in winter depression possibly via short-term, short-acting beta-blocker-induced truncation of nocturnal melatonin secretion early morning but not in the evening (n = 33, d/b, p/c, Schlager, Am J Psychiatry 1994;**151**:1383–5). Atenolol appears less effective (n = 19, d/b, p/c, c/o, Rosenthal et al, Am J Psychiatry 1988;**145**:52–6).

Duloxetine

Duloxetine may be useful for SAD (n = 26, open, 8/52, Pjrek et al, Pharmacopsychiatry 2008;**41**:100–5).

Melatonin

Melatonin secretion is altered in SAD and melatonin may have some role (review by Srinivasan et al, World J Biol Psychiatry 2006; **7**:138–51).

Mirtazapine

A pilot study has shown a rapid and well tolerated effect in SAD (n = 8, open, 4/52, Hesselmann et al, Hum Psychopharmacol Clin Exp 1999;**14**:59–62).

Modafinil

A pilot study suggested modafinil significantly reduces fatigue and sleepiness (n = 13 [c = 9], open, 8/52, Lundt, J Affect Disord 2004; **81**:173–8).

Reboxetine

A pilot study indicated a rapid and significant effect, including atypical symptoms in the first week (n = 16, open, 6/52, Hilger et al, Eur Neuropsychopharmacol 2001;**11**:1–5).

SSRIs (see also sertraline)

Light therapy has an early onset of action and, in responders, **citalopram** significantly reduces relapse in the continuation phase (n = 282, p/c, 15/52, Martiny et al, Acta Psychiatr Scand 2004;**109**:230–4). **Escitalopram** 10–20mg/d appears effective and very well tolerated (n = 20, open, 8/52, Pjrek et al, Pharmacopsychiatry 2007;**40**:20–4) and **fluoxetine** 20mg/d was superior to placebo (59–34%), but was not quite statistically significant (n = 68, p/c, 5/52, Lam et al, Am J Psychiatry 1995;**152**:1765–70).

◆ Others

Other drugs used include **moclobemide** (n = 581, RCT, d/b, 6/52, Partonen and Lonnqvist, J Affect Disord 1996;**41**:93–9), **St John's wort** (s/b, Kasper, Pharmacopsychiatry 1997;**30**[Suppl 2]: S89–S93).

□ No efficacy

Ginkgo biloba

One study was unable to show an effect from 'Bio-Biloba' in preventing winter depression (n = 27, RCT, 10/52, Lingaerde et al, Acta Psychiatr Scand 1999;**100**:62–6).

1.23 SELF-INJURIOUS BEHAVIOUR (SIB)

SIB is a self-destructive behaviour resulting in significant tissue damage, but without lethal intent. It can occur in learning disabilities (e.g. Lesch-Nyhan syndrome), as well as in OCD, sadomasochism, schizophrenia and borderline personality disorder. There seems to be a variety of causes, e.g. relief of dysphoria, poor impulse control and dissociation.

Role of drugs

Opiate antagonists may be useful where a reward mechanism seems to exist. There is some evidence of a serotonergic involvement. Antipsychotics seem to work mainly via a non-specific sedating mechanism.

Reviews: * general (Oliver and Richards, Curr Opin Psychiatry 2010;**23**:412–6), psycho-pharmacology of severe SIB associated with learning disabilities (Clarke, Br J Psychiatry 1998;**172**:389–94).

● Unlicensed/some efficacy

Antipsychotics

Antipsychotics are frequently prescribed but evidence for their efficacy is suggestive rather than conclusive. **Risperidone** was shown to be effective for up to 52 months in 75% of developmentally disabled inpatients (retrospective chart analysis, Brahm et al, Pharmacotherapy 2001;**21**:382). Low-dose **olanzapine** (5mg/d) has been used successfully for SIB (n = 2, Hough, J Clin Psychiatry 2001; **62**:96–7), and **clozapine** 200mg/d has been effective in a few cases (n = 2, Hammock et al, J Autism Dev Disord 2001;**31**:109–13).

Review: Janowsky et al, J Clin Psychopharmacol 2005;**25**:19–25.

Buspirone

In developmentally disabled people with SIB and anxiety, 64% responded to doses of 20–45mg/d with a maximal response seen after three weeks (n = 14, open, Ratey et al, J Clin Psychiatry 1989;**50**:382).

Lithium

Some old studies have suggested that lithium is effective in aggression and SIB, e.g. response was seen in 2–8 weeks with a lithium levels of 0.7–1.0mEq/L (n = 42, d/b, p/c, 4/12, Craft et al, Br J Psychiatry 1987; **150**:685–9).

Naltrexone/naloxone

There is conflicting data about the efficacy of naltrexone in SIB. Some studies show some efficacy when used in adequate dose for adequate duration, e.g. 25–100 mg/d orally (n = 4, Sandman et al, Am J Ment Retard 1990;**95**:93–102), although lower doses (e.g. 10–50 mg/d) may also be effective and it undoubtedly helps some patients (e.g. n = 1, 32/52, Griengl et al, Acta Psychiatr Scand 2001;**103**:234–6; n = 1 plus review, White and Schultz, Am J Psychiatry 2000;**157**:1574–82). Some trials have, however, shown a lack of efficacy (n = 33, d/b, p/c, c/o, Willemsen-Swinkels et al, Arch Gen Psychiatry 1995;**52**:766–73). SIB may get worse over the first few weeks of naltrexone but then improve and so short studies could miss the effect. There is some evidence of raised opioid peptide activity in autism, Fragile-X syndrome and other mental handicaps.

Review: Symons et al, Ment Retard Dev Disabil Res Rev 2004;**10**:193–200.

■ Unlicensed/possible efficacy

Omega-3 fatty acids

Omega-3 fatty acid supplements reduced suicidal markers and improved well-being in recurrent self-harmers, but had no effect on impulsivity, aggression and hostility (n = 49, RCT, d/b, p/c, 12/52, Hallahan et al, Br J Psychiatry 2007;**190**:118–22).

Oxcarbazepine

Oxcarbazepine has been used for self-mutilating bulimic patients (Cordas et al, Int J Neuropsychopharmacol 2006;**9**:769–71).

✱ Case reports ✱

- **Anticholinesterases** (n = 1, Alagiakrishnan et al, J Am Geriatr Soc 2003;**51**:1326).
- **Clozapine + clomipramine** (n = 1, Holzer et al, Am J Psychiatry 1996;**153**:133).
- **Dextromethorphan** (n = 1, Welch and Sovner, Br J Psychiatry 1992;**161**:118–20).
- **Lamotrigine + fluoxetine** (n = 1, Schupak, Prog Neuropsychopharmacol Biol Psychiatry 2007;**31**:1337–8).
- **Topiramate** (n = 1, Cassano et al, Bipolar Disorders 2001;**3**:161).

◆ Others

Other drugs used include **clomipramine** (n = 11, open, Garber et al, J Am Acad Child Adolesc Psych 1992;**31**:1157–60), **fluoxetine** (n = 4, Ricketts et al, J Am Acad Child Adolesc Psychiatry 1993;**32**:865–9).

1.24 SEXUAL DEVIANCY DISORDERS

Sexual deviancy disorders are abnormalities of a basic biological drive and are recognised as psychiatric syndromes. They include exhibitionism, fetishism, sexual masochism or sadism, paedophilia and voyeurism, but not rape (considered a sexual expression of aggression rather than an aggressive expression of sexuality). The main characteristic is of intense, recurrent sexual arousal and fantasies, particularly connected with inanimate objects, children, non-consenting adults or the self.

Role of drugs

Drug therapy is controversial but may sometimes be a useful adjunct to other therapies, due to the chronic nature of the disease and its high and unpredictable relapse rates. One review (Bradford, J Sex Res 2000;**37**:248–57) suggested a treatment hierarchy of CBT, SSRIs, low-dose antiandrogens, higher dose antiandrogens, then very high dose antiandrogens. Deviant sexual behaviour is rare in women and so drug therapy is usually aimed at reducing sexual drive in men. The success of any form of treatment is highly dependent on detailed evaluations and diagnosis. Placebo-controlled studies have huge ethical complications.

Reviews: * drug treatment of paraphilic and non-paraphilic sexual disorders (Codispoti, Psychiatr Clin North Am 2008;**31**:671–9; Guay, Clin Ther 2009;**31**:1–31; Sajith et al, J Intellect Disabil Res 2008;**52**:1078–90), treatment protocols for cyproterone, medroxyprogesterone, etc (Reilly et al, Can J Psychiatry 2000;**45**:559–63).

■ BNF listed

Benperidol

Benperidol is a standard butyrophenone which, although used for the control of deviant antisocial sexual behaviour, has no proven use other than as an antipsychotic. The only double-blind study published showed a slight reduction in sexual thoughts, but not in behaviour (*Drug Ther Bull* 1974;**12**:2).

Cyproterone (acetate)

Cyproterone is available in many countries to treat severe hypersexuality and sexual deviation in men. It has both antiandrogenic and antigonadotropic actions and probably acts by disrupting the receptors' response to androgens. It can reduce sexual interest, drive and arousal, as well as deviant fantasies and behaviour, and significantly reduces some sexual behaviours in paraphilias and paedophilia (n = 19, RCT, d/b, p/c, c/o, Bradford *et al*, *Arch Sex Behav* 1993;**22**:383–402). The onset of action may be delayed for 2–3 weeks and is reversible within 3–6 weeks of stopping. An adequate trial of four months is usually recommended. A depot injection is available on a named patient basis and a syrup can be made.

● Unlicensed/some efficacy

LHRH antagonists

Luteinising hormone-releasing hormone (gonadorelin, LHRH) antagonists can produce complete chemical castration and thus have a potent effect on sexual deviancy. A thorough review concluded that LHRH antagonists offer a treatment option for severe paraphilia, with little or no relapse if the patient remains under treatment (s = 13, n = 118, Briken *et al*, *J Clin Psychiatry* 2003;**64**:890–7). **Nafarelin** has been used and **flutamide**, a pure antiandrogen similar to cyproterone, has been used in conjunction with nafarelin (n = 1, Rousseau *et al*, *Can J Psychiatry* 1990;**35**:338–41). **Leuprolide** acetate is an alternative and a depot leuprolide significantly suppressed self-reported deviant sexual interests and behaviour and was well tolerated, although bone demineralisation occurred in 25% (n = 12, open, Krueger and Kaplan, *Arch Sex Behav* 2001;**30**:409–22). **Triptorelin** has also been used (n = 6, Thibaut *et al*, *Acta Psychiatr Scand* 1993;**87**:445–50), where depot triptorelin palmoate 3.75 mg/month plus psychotherapy was effective for reducing episodes of deviant sexual behaviours over 3–12 months in all men with severe paraphilia

(n = 30, open, Rosler and Witztum, *N Engl J Med* 1998;**338**:416–22).

Medroxyprogesterone (acetate)

Medroxyprogesterone has indirect antiandrogenic activity by preventing testosterone release from the testicles (review by Cooper, *Can J Psychiatry* 1986;**31**:73–9) and increasing the metabolic clearance of testosterone, resulting in suppression of sexual arousal and libido. Adverse effects include weight gain, diabetes and DVTs, although feminisation has not been reported. Few proper trials have been carried out, but there is a case series where it was successful for inappropriate sexual behaviour in elderly men with dementia (n = 5, case series, Light and Holroyd, *J Psychiatry Neurosci* 2006;**31**:132–4).

SSRIs

Reduced daily frequency and duration of paraphilia and related disorders has been shown (n = 26, open case series, Kafka and Hennen, *J Clin Psychiatry* 2000;**61**:664–70; n = 1, Mania *et al*, *Prim Care Companion J Clin Psychiatry* 2006;**8**:106). Citalopram has been used successfully for hypersexuality in early Alzheimer's disease (n = 1, Tosto *et al*, *Neurol Sci* 2008;**29**:269–70). SSRI-induced anorgasmia may be a contributory factor to this effect.

■ Unlicensed/possible efficacy

Imipramine

Some improvements in paraphilic and non-paraphilic sexual addictions and depressive symptoms were noted in 90% of patients treated with imipramine, fluoxetine or lithium (n = 10, Kafka, *J Clin Psychiatry* 1991;**52**:60–5).

Lithium

See imipramine.

Methylphenidate

Methylphenidate may be used cautiously to augment the effect of SSRIs in paraphilias and related disorders (n = 26, Kafka and Hennen, *J Clin Psychiatry* 2000;**61**:664–70).

Mirtazapine

Mirtazapine 15–30 mg/d had some efficacy

(50% were very much improved) in reducing inappropriate sexual behaviours in people with autism (n = 10, open, 8/52, Coskun et al, J Child Adolesc Psychopharmacol 2009;**19**:203–6).

Naltrexone

Compulsive sexual behaviour has been treated with naltrexone and SSRIs (n = 2, Raymond et al, Int Clin Psychopharmacol 2002;**17**:201–5), and naltrexone was reported to have a positive response in 15 adolescent sexual offenders, with a therapeutic window of 50–200mg/d. Of the six non-responders, five responded to leuprolide (n = 21, open, Ryback, J Clin Psychiatry 2004;**65**:982–6).

Valproate

Valproate has been a useful adjunct in bipolar sex offenders, but only for mood, not for paraphilic symptoms (open, retrospective, Nelson et al, J Affect Disord 2001;**64**:249–55).

✷ Case reports ✷

- **Carbamazepine** (n = 1, Freymann et al, Pharmacopsychiatry 2005;**38**:144–5; n = 1, Bach et al, Mov Disord 2009;**24**:1241–2).
- **Gabapentin** (n = 3, Alkhalil et al, Am J Ther 2004;**11**:231–5).
- **Oxcarbazepine** ✷ (n = 1, Corretti and Baldi, Arch Sex Behav 2010;**39**:1025–6).
- **Quetiapine** (n = 1, Prakash et al, Am J Alzheimer's Dis Other Demen 2009;**24**: 136–40).
- **Topiramate** (n = 1, Khazaal and Zullion, BMC Psychiatry 2006;**6**:22).

1.25 SOCIAL ANXIETY DISORDER (SOCIAL PHOBIA DISORDER)

see also Anxiety disorder (1.6)

Social anxiety is the second most common phobia (incidence in USA is 5%; n = 43093, Grant et al, J Clin Psychiatry 2005;**66**:1351–61; comment by Manfro, EBMH 2006;**9**:88) where the sufferers fear public ridicule, scrutiny and negative evaluation, with fear of embarrassment, criticism or making a public mistake. Feared situations include public speaking, social gatherings, writing under supervision or eating and drinking in public. Anticipatory anxiety leads to impaired performance. Two sub-divisions include general and specific social phobia. This is a serious, disabling anxiety disorder associated with reduction in quality of life (s = 3, n = 829, RCTs, p/c, Stein and Kean, Am J Psychiatry 2000;**157**:1606–13) and a high risk of alcohol dependence and abuse, but is underdiagnosed with less than 5% of sufferers receiving a diagnosis (n = 3862, Katzelnick et al, Am J Psychiatry 2001; **158**:1999–2007). Early diagnosis and treatment may be vital (Kahalid-Khan et al, Paediatr Drugs 2007;**9**:227–37).

Role of drugs

Drugs and behavioural approaches are commonly used. Meta-analyses of effect sizes (including all six UK SSRIs) conclude that SSRIs are more effective than placebo, with improvements also in social and occupational functioning (e.g. s = 15, n = 3527, RCT, d/b, p/c, 10–24/52, Hansen et al, Int Clin Psychopharmacol 2008;**23**:170–9). Venlafaxine XL may be second-line, with moclobemide, MAOIs and benzodiazepines third choice. The only predictor of response is length of treatment, which should be at least 12 weeks (Stein et al, J Clin Psychiatry 2002;**63**:152–5). Cochrane concludes that SSRIs have the strongest evidence for short-term and probably the long-term (s = 36, n = 4268, RCT, Stein et al, Cochrane Database Syst Rev 2004;**4**:CD001206). The placebo response may be moderately large (15 p/c studies, Oosterbaan et al, J Psychopharmacol 2001;**15**:199–203). CBT alone is probably more effective than fluoxetine and placebo (n = 60, RCT, d/b, 12/12, Clark et al, J Consult Clin Psychol 2003;**71**:1058–67; review by Taylor, EBMH 2004;**7**:75) but compared to clonazepam alone, combined psychodynamic group therapy (PGT) and clonazepam improved global functioning, but not any secondary measures (n = 57, RCT, 12/52, Knijnik et al, Eur Psychiatry 2008;**23**:567–74).

Reviews: general (Westenberg, CNS Spectr 2009;**14**(2 Suppl 3):24–33; Schneier, N Engl J Med 2006;**355**:1029–36), BAP evidence-based guidelines (Baldwin et al, J Psychopharmacol 2005; **19**:567–96).

BNF listed

Escitalopram ✷

Escitalopram is licensed in the UK with a starting

dose of 10mg/d, increased to a maximum of 20mg/d or reduced to 5mg/d, depending upon the individual's response. Any trial should last at least four weeks before further intervention is considered (s = 40, Baldwin et al, Hum Psychopharmacol 2009;24:269–75). Efficacy has been shown in a number of major trials. Escitalopram 10–20mg/d was superior to placebo (54% vs 39% response) using the LSAS total score (n = 358, RCT, p/c, d/b, 12/52, Kasper et al, Br J Psychiatry 2005;186:222–6; MS). It is effective for relapse prevention (placebo = 50%, escitalopram 20%) with an NNT of 3.3 (s = 4, RCT, d/b, 24/52, Bech et al, J Clin Psychiatry 2010;71:121–9).

Paroxetine

Several studies show paroxetine to be superior to placebo, e.g. at 20–50mg/d reducing symptoms and avoidance, with 40mg/d the optimum dose (n = 384, d/b, 12/52, Liebowitz et al, J Clin Psychiatry 2002;63:66–74). Lack of response at eight weeks does not necessarily predict long-term lack of response and so a minimum of 12 weeks treatment is necessary (review, s = 3, Stein et al, J Clin Psychiatry 2002;63:152–5). It may be effective for relapse prevention (n = 323[c = 257], RCT, p/c, Stein et al, Arch Gen Psychiatry 2002;59:1111–8).

Venlafaxine

Venlafaxine XL is now licensed for moderate-to-severe generalised social anxiety disorder (n = 279[c = 173], RCT, d/b, p/c, 12/52, Liebowitz et al, J Clin Psychiatry 2005;66:238-47). The standard dose of 75mg/d is as effective and well tolerated as paroxetine 20–50mg/d (n = 413[c = 318], RCT, p/c, d/b, 12/52, Liebowitz et al, Arch Gen Psychiatry 2005;62:190–8), although 150–225mg/d has been used (n = 386, d/b, p/c, 6/12, Stein et al, Psychopharmacol [Berl] 2004;177:280–8). Lower doses may be useful in children and adolescents (n = 293, RCT, p/c, 16/52, March et al, Biol Psychiatry 2007;62:1149–54).

Combinations

Paroxetine + clonazepam

Unlike panic disorder, combining a BDZ with paroxetine did not lead to a quicker response

(n = 28[c = 19], d/b, p/c, 10/52, Seedat and Stein, J Clin Psychiatry 2004;65:244–8).

● Unlicensed/some efficacy

Benzodiazepines

Benzodiazepines have a rapid onset, good tolerability and flexible dosing, but cause sedation, lack of coordination and long-term use has some potential risks. **Diazepam** may be ineffective but **clonazepam** has been widely studied (review by Jefferson, J Clin Psychiatry 2001;62[Suppl 1]:S50–S53) and appears safe and effective.

Gabapentin

Gabapentin (900–3600mg/d) was well tolerated and significantly reduced symptoms in one trial (n = 69, RCT, d/b, p/c, 14/52, Pande et al, J Clin Psychopharmacol 1999;19:341–8), and 1800mg/d was as effective as tiagabine for reducing symptoms of social anxiety (n = 8, RCT, d/b, c/o, 2x4/52, Urbano et al, Prim Care Companion J Clin Psychiatry 2009;11:123).

MAOIs *

In a study of CBGT (cognitive behavioural group therapy), response rates were:

Response at	12/52	24/52
Placebo	33%	33%
CBGT	47%	52%
Phenelzine	54%	48%
Both	72%	78%

(n = 128, Blanco et al, Arch Gen Psychiatry 2010;67:286–95). Phenelzine may need robust dosing (e.g. mean dose 66mg/d, n = 7, open, Aarre, Nord J Psychiatry 2003;57:313–5). Tranylcypromine 60mg/d (but not 30mg/d) appears to be effective for comorbid panic and social anxiety (n = 36, d/b, 12/52, Nardi et al, Psychiatry Res 2010;175:260–5).

Moclobemide

In a comparison of moclobemide, CBT and the combination, moclobemide was better for subjective general anxiety, CBT for avoidant behaviour (and best overall) and the combination most rapidly effective (n = 81 [c = 66], RCT, p/c, 6/12 + 24/12, Prasko et al, Neuro Endocrinol Lett 2006;27:473–81).

Pregabalin

Pregabalin 600 mg/d was effective and well tolerated in social anxiety, whereas 150 mg/d and placebo were ineffective (n = 135, RCT, d/b, p/c, 10/52, Pande et al, J Clin Psychopharmacol 2004;**24**:141–9, MS). In a comparative study, it was as effective as lorazepam 6 mg/d (n = 271, RCT, d/b, p/c, 4/52, Feltner et al, J Clin Psychopharmacol 2003;**23**:240–9, MS; see also Pary, EBMH 2004;**7**:17).

SSRIs (paroxetine, escitalopram and venlafaxine are licensed)

Citalopram 40 mg/d appears well tolerated and as effective (75% response) as moclobemide (n = 71, RCT, s/b, 8/52, Atmaca et al, Hum Psychopharmacol 2002;**17**:401–5). Improvement in social anxiety symptoms may lag behind depression resolution, and may need more than 12 weeks for full response (n = 21, open, 12/52, Schneier et al, Depress Anxiety 2003;**17**:191–6). **Fluvoxamine** may have some role, e.g. the CR version was superior to placebo in another (n = 279, RCT, p/c, 12/52, Davidson et al, J Clin Psychopharmacol 2004;**24**:118–25), including for relapse prevention (n = 112, 24/52 extension, Stein et al, Int J Neuropsychopharmacol 2003; **6**:317–23). **Sertraline** is licensed in several countries for social anxiety and at up to 200 mg/d appears more effective than placebo (e.g. n = 204, RCT, 20/52, van Ameringen et al, Am J Psychiatry 2001;**158**:275–81; review by Pieters, EBMH 2001;**4**:91; see also n = 415, RCT, d/b, p/c, 12/52, Liebowitz et al, J Clin Psychiatry 2003;**64**:785–92). Its efficacy may be enhanced by combination with exposure therapy (n = 387, RCT, d/b, 24/52, Blomhoff et al, Br J Psychiatry 2001;**179**:23–30). Sertraline may be effective long-term, but relapse may occur on discontinuation (n = 375, RCT, p/c, d/b, one year, Haug et al, Br J Psychiatry 2003;**182**:312–8). However, a large pilot study failed to show that **fluoxetine** up to 60 mg/d was superior to placebo, although the latter had an unusually high response rate (n = 60, RCT, d/b, 14/52, Kobak et al, J Clin Psychopharmacol 2002; **22**:257–62).

■ Unlicensed/possible efficacy

Botulinum toxin

Severe axillary hyperhydrosis has been treated with botulinum toxin, significantly improving overall disability (n = 40, RCT, p/c, 8/52, Connor et al, J Clin Psychiatry 2006;**67**:30–6).

Quetiapine

One study has shown a slight positive effect as monotherapy (n = 15, RCT, p/c, Vaishnavi et al, Prog Neuropsychopharmacol Biol Psychiatry 2007;**31**:1464–9), but single doses of 25 mg were ineffective for social anxiety, and caused drowsiness (n = 20, RCT, d/b, p/c, c/o, Donahue et al, J Anxiety Disord 2008; **23**:362–8).

◆ Others

Other drugs used include **bupropion** (n = 10, open, 12/52, Emmanuel et al, Depress Anxiety 2000;**12**:111–3) and **tricyclics** (n = 15, open, 8/52, Simpson et al, J Clin Psychopharmacol 1998; **18**:132–5)

□ No efficacy

Atomoxetine *

A small pilot study concluded that atomoxetine was unlikely to be effective for SA (n = 27, RCT, d/b, p/c, 10/52, Ravindran et al, J Clin Psychopharmacol 2009;**29**:561–4).

Beta-blockers

There is no evidence for efficacy, except perhaps in people where management of tremor is essential, e.g. musicians (e.g. nadolol; n = 31, d/b, c/o, s/b, James and Savage, Am Heart J 1984;**108**:1150–5). Pindolol 15 mg/d was no more effective than placebo in augmenting SSRI treatment of generalised social phobia (n = 14, d/b, p/c, c/o, 4/52, Stein et al, Am J Psychiatry 2001;**158**:1725–7). However, illicit self-medication with propranolol (up to 320 mg/d) has been reported (n = 1, Fontanella, Rev Bras Psiquiatr 2003;**25**:228–30), with symptoms manageable with adjunctive paroxetine, so maybe it does work, but at higher doses.

Caffeine

Caffeine induces more severe performance anxiety suggesting a hyperreactivity to caffeine (n = 28 + 26, RCT, d/b, c/o, Nardi et al, Psychiatry Res 2009;**169**:149–53).

Levetiracetam *

Levetiracetam was well-tolerated but slightly inferior to placebo for social anxiety (e.g. n = 217, RCT, d/b, p/c, 12/52, Stein et al, J Clin Psychiatry 2010;**71**:627–31).

Mirtazapine *

Mirtazapine 30–45 mg/d failed to separate from placebo in a major trial (n = 60, RCT, d/b, p/c, 12/52, Schutters et al, Int Clin Psychopharmacol; 2010;**25**:302–4), although it seemed effective and well tolerated in women with social anxiety but not comorbid psychiatric illness (n = 66 [c = 60], RCT, d/b, p/c, 10/52, Muehlbacher et al, J Clin Psychopharmacol 2005;**25**:580–3; comment by Mörtberg, EBMH 2006;**9**:75)

St John's wort

SJW was not superior to placebo in one trial (n = 40, RCT, p/c, 12/52, Kobak et al, J Clin Psychopharmacol 2005;**25**:51–8).

Valproate

A small study showed complete ineffectiveness of valproate at up to 1500 mg/d (n = 16, mentioned by Jefferson, J Clin Psychiatry 2001; **62** [Suppl 1]:S50–S53).

1.26 TOURETTE'S SYNDROME (GILLES DE LA TOURETTE) *
see also OCD (1.18) and SIB (1.23)

The main diagnostic symptoms of this hereditary disorder include multiple tics, vocal tics (grunts, snarls, throat clearing and obscenities), stereotyped movements (jumping and dancing), overactivity, learning difficulties and emotional problems. The incidence is 1–5 per 10000 and is more common in males. It has an onset at 5–6 years, beginning with respiratory or vocal tics with grunting or barking noises. Psychiatric comorbidity is common, e.g. OCD, anxiety, depression and ADHD.

Role of drugs

If the condition is affecting the person's abilities to function, drug therapy may be useful. Low starting doses, gradual increases and adequate therapeutic trials are necessary.

Reviews: * general (Kurlan, New Engl J Med 2010;**363**:2332–8), in adults (Jankovic et al, Mov Disord 2010;**25**:2171–5), management (Bestha et al, Expert Opin Pharmacother 2010;**11**:1813–22), pharmacotherapies (Rajapakse and Pringsheim, Semin Pediatr Neurol 2010;**17**:254–60).

BNF listed

Haloperidol

Haloperidol 0.5–40 mg/d was the licensed drug of choice and remains a treatment option. Side-effects may be limiting and its efficacy has been questioned (n = 22, p/c, d/b, Sallee et al, Am J Psychiatry 1997;**154**:1057–62). See also pimozide and nicotine chewing gum.

Pimozide

Cochrane concludes that pimozide is effective, although the data is limited (s = 6, n = 162, RCT, Pringsheim and Marras, Cochrane Database Syst Rev 2009;**2**:CD006996). An ECG is essential monitoring (see 3.2.1).

● Unlicensed/some efficacy

Antipsychotics (see also BNF Listed) *

There are a number of studies showing a significant effect from risperidone, eg. a mean dose of 2.5 mg/d was clearly superior to placebo on global assessment of Tourette symptoms (n = 48, RCT, d/b, p/c, Dion et al, J Clin Psychopharmacol 2002;**22**:31–9), and a mean dose of 3.8 mg/d was at least as effective as pimozide (mean 2.9 mg/d), but much better tolerated (n = 50, d/b, 12/52, Bruggeman et al, J Clin Psychiatry 2001;**62**:50–6). Risperidone (mean 2.5 mg/d) may also be useful for the short-term management of tics in Tourette's (n = 34, RCT, d/b, p/c, 8/52, Scahill et al, Neurology 2003;**60**:1130–5). Sulpiride 200–400 mg/d has been used, as has amisulpride (n = 1, Fountoulakis et al, Ann Pharmacother 2004;**38**:901). Aripiprazole (mean 12 mg/d) reduced tics and explosive outbursts in 100% and 96% completers respectively (n = 37 [c = 29], open, retrospective, Budman et al, J Child Adolesc Psychopharmacol 2008;**18**:509–15), with low-doses seeming effective for Tourette's and tics (e.g. n = 15, open, 12/52, Seo et al, J Child Adolesc Psychopharmacol

2008;**18**:197–205). A pilot study suggested efficacy without weight gain or other major ADRs (n = 72, open, 8/52, Cui et al, *J Child Adolesc Psychopharmacol* 2010;**20**:291–8). 10–20 mg/d has been dramatically and rapidly effective in some patients (n = 11, Davies et al, *Hum Psychopharmacol* 2006;**21**:447–53; Bubl et al, *World J Biol Psychiatry* 2006;**7**:123–5), including late-onset Tourette's (n = 1, Ikenouchi-Sugita et al, *World J Biol Psychiatry* 2009;**10**:977–80; for review of aripiprazole in Tourette's see Kawohl et al, *World J Biol Psychiatry* 2008; **10**:827–31). In a small study, **olanzapine** (mean 14.5 mg/d) improved aggression and tics, albeit with significant weight gain (n = 10, RCT, s/b, 10/52, Stephens et al, *J Child Adolesc Psychopharmacol* 2004;**14**:255–66; n = 12, open, 6/12, McCracken et al, *J Child Adolesc Psychopharmacol* 2008;**18**:501–8) and it may be superior to pimozide (n = 4, d/b, c/o, 12/12, Onofrj et al, *J Neurol* 2000;**247**:443–6). **Quetiapine** (mean 175 mg/d) may have some efficacy in Tourette's (n = 12, retrospective, 8/52, Copur et al, *Clin Drug Invest* 2007;**27**:123–30), but may not be well tolerated (n = 12 [c = 9], open, 8–12/52, de Jonge et al, *J Clin Psychiatry* 2007; **68**:1148–50). **Review:** * antipsychotics in Tourette disorder (Cath et al, *Tijdschr Psychiatr* 2008;**50**:593–602).

Clonidine

Clonidine 0.1–0.6 mg/d may be as effective as haloperidol. Clonidine or methylphenidate alone or in combination are effective for ADHD with comorbid tics (n = 16, RCT, p/c, 16/52, TSSG, *Neurology* 2002;**58**:527–36; review by Goldberg, *EBMH* 2002;**5**:122), and clonidine 0.1 mg/d was effective in a trial vs levetiracetam (n = 12 [c = 10], RCT, d/b, c/o, 15/52, Hedderick et al, *Pediatr Neurol* 2009; **40**:420–5).

Lorazepam

Lorazepam 1.5–10 mg/d has been useful as adjuvant therapy.

Topiramate *

Topiramate has been used with some success (n = 29 [c = 20], RCT, d/b, p/c, 10/52, Jankovic et al, *J Neurol Neurosurg Psychiatry* 2010;**81**:70–3; see also n = 2, Abuzzhab and Brown, *Am J Psychiatry* 2001;**158**:968) and seems to have at least moderate efficacy for tics in TS (n = 41,

retrospective, Kuo et al, *Clin Neuropharmacol* 2010;**33**:32–4).

■ **Unlicensed/possible efficacy**

Cannabinoids

An RCT showed that THC doses of up to 10 mg/d showed significant trends in favour of THC on a variety of measures, with no reported adverse effects (n = 24, RCT, d/b, 6/52, Muller-Vahl et al, *J Clin Psychiatry* 2003;**64**:459–65), supporting an earlier survey of people with Tourette's who had tried marijuana, 82% reported a reduction or complete remission in motor and vocal tics, urges and OCD symptoms (n = 17, Muller-Vahl et al, *Acta Psychiatr Scand* 1998;**98**:502–6).

Fluoxetine

81% patients with OCD in Tourette's syndrome had improved symptoms on fluoxetine (n = 32, open, Como and Kurlan, *Neurology* 1991;**41**:872–4). A potential effect has been suggested in children with OCD symptoms in Tourette's (n = 11, Kyrlan et al, *Clin Neuropharmacol* 1993; **16**:167–72).

Methylphenidate

Methylphenidate can aggravate tics or be associated with their appearance (Klein, *Arch Gen Psychiatry* 1995;**52**:429–33), but some tics may be significantly worse, although generally these are not to the extent of contraindicating a trial, e.g. in ADHD with Tourette's (Gadow et al, *Arch Gen Psychiatry* 1995;**52**:444–55).

Nicotine

Transdermal nicotine (7 mg/d) has been shown to be superior to placebo as an adjunct to haloperidol (eg. n = 70 [c = 56], d/b, p/c, Silver et al, *J Clin Psychiatry* 2001;**62**:707–14). Nicotine chewing gum is an alternative and PRN usage may have a low risk and help to minimise this.

Ondansetron

In haloperidol-resistant Tourette's, ondansetron 24 mg/d significantly improved tic severity on one rating scale but not on others (n = 30, RCT, d/b, p/c, 3/52, Toren et al, *J Clin Psychiatry* 2005;**66**:499–503).

Pergolide

Pergolide (up to 300mcg/d) may be safe and effective in children with Tourette's disorder, chronic motor or vocal tic disorder (n=245, RCT, 6/52, Gilbert *et al, Neurology* 2000;**54**:1310–6).

Tetrabenazine

For a review of use see Porta *et al, Clin Drug Investig* 2008;**28**:443–59.

✷ Case reports

- **Buspirone** 30mg/d (n=1, Dursun *et al, Lancet* 1995;**345**:1366–7).
- **Duloxetine** 40mg/d (n=1, Niederhofer, *Prim Care Companion J Clin Psychiatry* 2010;**12**: PCC.09l00889).
- **Finasteride** 5mg/d (n=1, Bortolato *et al, Am J Psychiatry* 2007;**164**:1914–5).
- **Methadone** 110mg/d (n=1, Meuldijk and Colon, *Am J Psychiatry* 1992;**149**:139–40).
- **Naltrexone + codeine** sequentially (n=2, McConville *et al, Lancet* 1994;**343**:601).

◆ Others

Other drugs used include **paroxetine** (n=45, open, 8/52, Bruun and Budman, *J Clin Psychiatry* 1998;**59**:581–4), and **selegiline** (n=24, d/b, p/c, c/o, Feigin *et al, Neurology* 1996;**46**:965–8).

□ No efficacy

Levetiracetam

In a small but perfectly formed trial, levetiracetam (10mg/kg/d) was completely ineffective (n=12 [c=10],RCT,d/b,c/o,15/52,Hedderick *et al, Pediatr Neurol* 2009;**40**:420–5).

1.27 TRICHOTILLOMANIA

see also OCD (*1.18*)

Symptoms

Trichotillomania presents as impulsive pulling out of a person's own hair (scalp, eyebrows, and eyelashes, pubic, chest, etc), resulting in hair loss. It is associated with OCD, and can occur in the presence of learning disability, anxiety, depression, schizophrenia and borderline personality disorder. It may result in relief of tension, can be episodic or chronic, and is more common in females.

Role of drugs

A range of psychological and behaviour therapies are used and may be most effective when combined with pharmacotherapy. A significant review has concluded that clomipramine is effective, but that SSRIs are not (s=7, Bloch *et al, Biol Psychiatry* 2007;**62**:839–46), and trials need to be at least 8–10 weeks' duration to prove or disprove an effect in an individual case. HRT (habit reversal training) combined with sertraline is more effective than either approach alone (n=24, RCT, d/b, Dougherty *et al, J Clin Psychiatry* 2006;**67**:1086–92). Dermatological help is beneficial.

Reviews: * general (Duke *et al, Clin Psychol Rev* 2010;**30**:181–93; Chamberlain *et al, Neurosci Biobehav Rev* 2009;**33**:831–42; Sah *et al, Dermatol Ther* 2008;**21**:13–21), treatment (Bloch *et al, Biol Psychiatry* 2007;**62**:839–46).

+ Combinations

Antipsychotics + SSRI

There have been reports of symptom improvement when **olanzapine** 10mg/d was added to **fluoxetine** 40mg/d (n=1, Potenza *et al, Am J Psychiatry* 1998;**155**:1329–30) or citalopram (n=4, Ashton, *Am J Psychiatry* 2001;**158**:1929–30). Resistant trichotillomania has responded to **risperidone** augmentation of **fluvoxamine** (n=1, Gabriel, *Can J Psychiatry* 2001;**46**:285–6). **Haloperidol** has been used successfully as SSRI augmentation (n=9, open, Van Ameringen *et al, J Affect Disord* 1999; **56**:219–26).

● Unlicensed/some efficacy

Clomipramine

Several studies (s=7, Bloch *et al, Biol Psychiatry* 2007;**62**:839–46) have shown clomipramine in doses of around 180mg/d to be effective in some patients with trichotillomania.

Olanzapine * (see also combinations)

Olanzapine has shown robust efficacy (85% vs 17%) over placebo for a wide range of symptoms (n=25[c=25], RCT, d/b, p/c,

12/52, Van Ameringen et al, J Clin Psychiatry 2010;**71**:1336–43). Up to 10mg/d has produced a significant reduction in hair pulling and anxiety, with 22% achieving full remission (n=18, open, 3/12, Stewart and Nejtek, J Clin Psychiatry 2003;**64**:49–52), and it has been successfully used to augment fluoxetine (n=2, Srivastava et al, Aust NZ J Psychiatry 2005; **39**:112–3).

■ **Unlicensed/possible efficacy**

SSRIs

A major review concluded that SSRIs lack significant clinical effect (s=7, Bloch et al, Biol Psychiatry 2007;**62**:839–46), although there have been some positive reports, e.g. **citalopram** has a modest but significant effect (n=14, open, 12/52, Stein et al, Eur Arch Psychiatry Clin Neurosci 1997;**247**:234–6), as may **escitalopram** (n=1, Bhatia and Sapra, Eur Psychiatry 2004;**19**:239–40). **Fluoxetine** appears minimally effective (e.g. Winchel et al, J Clin Psychiatry 1992;**53**:304–8), the doses required are high (up to 80mg/d) and if response occurs, relapse is not uncommon and was no better than placebo in two studies (n=43, RCT, 12/52, van Minnen et al, Arch Gen Psychiatry 2003;**60**:517–22).

Lithium

80% patients tried on lithium showed reduced hair pulling and some hair regrowth, possibly via an effect on aggressive behaviour (n=10, open, 14/12, Christenson et al, J Clin Psychiatry 1991;**52**:116–20; see also Sharma and Corpse, Arch Women's Ment Health 2008;**11**:305–6).

✱ **Case reports**

- **Aripiprazole + clonazepam** (n=1,Virit et al, J Clin Pharm Ther 2009;**34**:723–5).
- **Bupropion** 300mg/d (n=1,Bhanji and Margolese, J Clin Psychiatry 2004;**65**:1283).
- **Inositol** (n=3, Seedat et al, J Clin Psychiatry 2001;**62**:60–1).
- **Oxcarbazepine** * 1200mg/d (n=1, Leombruni and Gastaldi, Clin Neuropharmacol 2010;**33**:107–8).
- **Quetiapine** (n=1, Khouzam et al, Psychiatry 2002;**65**:261–70).

- **Valproate** (n=1,Adewuya et al, J Child Adolesc Psychopharmacol 2008;**18**:533–6).

■ **Others**

Other drugs include **paroxetine** (n=1, Reid, Am J Psychiatry 1994;**151**:290), **pimozide** (e.g. J Clin Psychiatry 1992;**53**:123–6) and **trazodone** (e.g. Sunkureddi and Markovitz, Am J Psychiatry 1993;**150**:523–4).

1.28 CAFFEINISM

Caffeine is an antagonist at adenosine receptors, which increase dopamine activity, leading to increased activity. Tolerance develops very quickly to the stimulant effect, e.g. complete tolerance to sleep disruption from 400mg/d occurs in seven days. Caffeine consumption at 250–500mg/d is regarded as moderate use. Caffeinism is estimated to start at a consumption of between 600mg and 750mg/d, with above 1000mg/d well into the toxic range. Caffeine dependence displays features of a typical psychoactive substance dependence, i.e. withdrawal, continued use despite caffeine-induced problems, tolerance and persistent desire or unsuccessful attempts to cut down or control use.

Caffeine withdrawal

Caffeine withdrawal is a DSM-IV diagnosis and thus should be taken seriously. The 14 main withdrawal symptoms fall into three groups (Ozsungur et al, Psychopharmacology [Berl] 2009; **201**:541–8):

1. Fatigue and headache (52%) – more likely with high habitual use
2. Dysphoric mood, rebound drowsiness – more likely with high habitual use
3. Flu-like, somatic – no more likely with high habitual use than low use

(review by Dews et al, Food Chem Toxicol 2002; **40**:1257–61).

Symptoms of caffeinism (acute or chronic)

Adverse effects of low-to-moderate doses: Diuresis, increased gastric secretion, fine tremor, increased skeletal muscle stamina, mild anxiety, negative mood, palpitations and nervousness.

Adverse effects of high doses: Chronic insomnia, persistent anxiety, restlessness, tension, irritability, tremulousness, panic, poor concentration, confusion, disorientation, paranoia, delirium, tremor, muscle twitching, convulsions, vertigo, dizziness, tinnitus, auditory and visual hallucinations, facial flushing, hyperthermia, nausea, vomiting, abdominal discomfort and tachypnoea. High caffeine use is also associated with high daily cigarette use, and aggression, conduct disorder, ADHD and social problems in adolescents (n = 132, Martin et al, Scientific World Journal 2008;**8**:512–6).

Adverse consequences: There is some contradictory evidence about the effect of caffeine on people with mental health problems. Clearly, high doses can cause significant effects. Acute high doses (10 mg/kg) significantly increase arousal and have a psychotogenic effect in schizophrenics (n = 13, d/b, Lucas et al, Biol Psychiatry 1990;**28**:35–40). Caffeinism can precipitate or exacerbate psychoses and make these more resistant (n = 2, Zaslove et al, Br J Psychiatry 1991;**159**:565–7) to drug treatment, especially antipsychotics. The clinical signs of affective diseases can be modified. Caffeine 150 mg at bedtime has a marked effect on sleep latency, total sleep time and reduced sleep efficacy and REM periods. Consumption may be influenced by some genetic factors (n = 1934 twin study, Kendler and Prescott, Am J Psychiatry 1999;**156**:223–8). Conversely, there are reports of lack of correlation between caffeine consumption and anxiety and depression.

Methods of caffeine reduction

1. Recognition of the problems of excess caffeine consumption (>750 mg/d) and the likely benefits of reduction.
2. Identification of all current caffeine sources and the pattern of consumption.
3. Implement a planned gradual reduction, e.g. making weaker drinks, taken less often, increasing use of caffeine-free equivalent drinks (particularly at 'usual' drinking times of the day), using half-caffeine coffee, or mixing caffeine and decaffeinated coffee to give a lower strength.
4. Use of analgesia (caffeine-free, of course) for withdrawal headaches.
5. Setting a target for consumption, which will not need to be complete abstinence, e.g. caffeine drinks only at set times in the day, e.g. on rising, etc.

Calculating caffeine intake: *

Source	Caffeine content	
	per 100 ml	per container
Brewed coffee	55–85 mg	140–210 mg/cup
Instant coffee	35–45 mg	85–110 mg/cup
Decaf. coffee	2 mg	5 mg/cup
Cocoa	3 mg	7 mg/cup
Brewed tea	25–55 mg	55–140 mg/cup
Coca-cola	11 mg	36 mg/can
Pepsi cola	7 mg	22 mg/can
Milk chocolate		22 mg/100 g
Alka-Seltzer XS		40 mg/tablet
Red Bull (varies by country)		80 mg/250 ml
Relentless		160 mg/500 ml
Lucozade alert		120 mg/60 ml
Lucozade Energy		80 mg/500 ml

A cup is taken as being 250 ml

From 20 assorted commercial US tea samples (Chin et al, J Anal Toxicol 2008;**32**:702–4; although my experience of US tea is not impressive):

• Ordinary teas (white, green or black) ranged between 14–61 mg/serving (defined as 6–8 oz), but with no observable trend due to the variety
• Herbal teas: caffeine not detectable
• Decaffeinated teas all contained less than 12 mg/serving
• All contained more caffeine the longer they were brewed.

Additional information — specialty coffees

In American specialty coffees, the mean caffeine content of caffeinated coffees ranged from 5.2–12.2 mg/g for powder and 0.23–0.49 mg/g for decaffeinated coffee (Hackett et al, J Anal Toxicol 2008;**32**:695–701). One scoop of ground coffee is 7 g or 0.25 oz (content of a cup is thus 36–85 mg).

Reviews: * dependence (Ogawa and Ueki, Psychiatry Clin Neurosci 2007;**61**:263–8), caffeine and mental health (Lara, J Alzheimer's Dis 2010;**20**(Suppl 1):S239–48; Broderick and Benjamin, J Okla State Med Assoc 2004;**97**:538–42), caffeine craving questionnaire (West and Roderique-Davies, J Psychopharmacol 2008; **22**:80–91), withdrawal (Juliano and Griffiths, Psychopharmacology [Berl] 2004;**176**:1–29).

1.29 ELECTROCONVULSIVE THERAPY (ECT) *

ECT was first used in its current form

in 1938 (Linington and Harris, *Br Med J* 1988;**297**:1354–5). It is effective for rapid and short-term improvement in severe unipolar and bipolar depression (n = 220, Bailine *et al, Acta Psychiatr Scand* 2010;**121**:431–6) where other treatments have proven ineffective or life is threatened. The risks are higher in pregnancy, older people and in children. It is also used in mania (especially manic delirium), in TRS where it can help about one in two (54%) people, particularly for positive symptoms (n = 253, open, Chanpattana and Sackeim, *J ECT* 2010;**26**:289–98), more rarely catatonia and drug-resistant Parkinsonism. ECT is probably superior to, or at least as effective as, antidepressants and tends to be quicker-acting in severely depressed patients, although there remains some dispute about this. ECT may be better than antidepressants for the short-term treatment of acute depression (n = 256, s = 6, UK ECT Group, *Lancet* 2003; **361**:799–808; comment by Bauer, *EBMH* 2003; **6**:83). Combining maintenance ECT with antidepressants may improve outcomes (n = 58, retrospective chart review, Gagné *et al, Am J Psychiatry* 2000;**157**:1960–5).

Induction agents: **Propofol** is now widely used as it is well tolerated and short-acting with a quick recovery. It shortens seizure length by up to 30%, but seemingly without significant effect on the clinical outcome (n = 62, RCT, Bauer *et al, J ECT* 2009;**25**:85–90), although ECT courses may be prolonged. It may be associated with bradycardia and hypotension. **Etomidate** is short-acting, has a rapid recovery, less hypotension than propofol and may lengthen seizure duration compared to methohexital and propofol (Ilivicky *et al, Am J Psychiatry* 1995;**152**:957–8), but is painful at the injection site, has a high incidence of extraneous muscle movements, and rarely causes adrenocortical dysfunction with repeated doses, although it can be successful (n = 3, Benbow *et al, Psychiatric Bull* 2002;**26**:351–3). Inhaled **sevoflurane** has been used successfully as an induction agent for ECT and is equivalent to thiopental for induction, and significantly better for postictal orientation 20 minutes after treatment (n = 31, RCT, d/b, Rasmussen *et al, J ECT* 2007;**23**:236–8).

Post-ECT memory loss and agitation: High anticholinergic drug levels have been associated with a greater risk of post-ECT confusion (n = 20, Mondimore *et al, Am J Psychiatry* 1983; **140**:930–1). Oral thiamine 50–200 mg/d may lead to rapid resolution (3–5 days) of post-ECT confusion and memory loss, and so thiamine deficiency is implicated in post-ECT confusional state (n = 3, Linton *et al, Int J Geriatr Psychiatry* 2002;**7**:189–92). **Promethazine** 25–50 mg orally 1–2 hours before ECT has been used successfully for severe post-ECT agitation (n = 8, Vishne *et al, J ECT* 2005;**21**:118–21). **Piracetam** appears to have no effect in reducing post-ECT cognitive impairment either in short (n = 18, d/b, c/o, 3/7, Mindus *et al, Acta Psychiatr Scand* 1975; **51**:319–26) or longer courses (given during and after an ECT course), although it might slightly enhance ECT's clinical effect (n = 38, RCT, d/b, p/c, >2/52, Tang *et al, J ECT* 2002;**18**:130–7). Propofol has been used to help manage post-ictal agitation after ECT (n = 10, O'Reardon *et al, J ECT* 2006;**22**:247–52). **Donepezil** has been used successfully for cognitive deficits associated with maintenance ECT (see donepezil).

Reviews: comprehensive reviews (Lisanby, *N Engl J Med* 2007;**357**:1939–45; Scott, *Adv Psychiatr Treat* 2005;**11**:150–6), in the elderly (Flint and Gagnon, *Can J Psychiatry* 2002;**47**:734–41).

Drug considerations

There are no RCTs of ECT given with concurrent anticonvulsants and one thorough review suggests that there is no evidence that ECT and anticonvulsants cannot be used together (Sienaert and Peuskens, *J ECT* 2007;**23**:120–3).

Agomelatine

There is no experience on the use of agomelatine with ECT, but no pro- or anticonvulsant effects have been shown (MI).

Antipsychotics (see also clozapine)

Antipsychotics lower the seizure threshold and would be expected to lead to seizures at lower ECT doses. A review of ECT with antipsychotics in schizophrenia concluded that the combination appeared to be safe and effective (review by Braga and Petrides, *J ECT* 2005;**21**:75–83). ECT and **risperidone** Consta have been used successfully together (n = 1, Sengul *et al, J ECT* 2009;**25**:282–3).

Weekly ECT followed by maintenance as an adjunct to **sulpiride** (n = 17), **risperidone** (n = 26) and **olanzapine** (n = 27) showed long-term safety and some efficacy (especially with olanzapine), albeit with a high drop-out rate (n = 70 [c = 32], two years, Ravani et al, Psychiatr Danub 2009;**21**:179–86). There were also no apparent problems with ECT in a patient taking **olanzapine** and duloxetine (n = 1, Hanretta and Malek-Ahmadi, J ECT 2006;**22**:139–41). There were no significant adverse effects when ECT was used with **aripiprazole** (n = 4, Masdrakis et al, J ECT 2008;**24**:236–8).

Benzodiazepines

Benzodiazepines may lessen the improvement with unilateral ECT (n = 124, Jha and Stein, Acta Psychiatr Scand 1996;**94**:101–4), even several months after treatment is stopped, probably by raising the seizure threshold, having an effect on seizure duration, the number of sub-maximal seizures or by increasing the number of treatments needed.

Bupropion

Use with ECT has been reported (n = 2, Kellner et al, J Clin Psychopharmacol 1994;**14**:215–6), as has prolonged seizures when used with lithium and venlafaxine (n = 1, Conway and Nelson, J ECT 2001;**17**:216–8).

Caffeine

Caffeine 240mg IV has been used to augment seizure duration (reported by the ideally named Coffey et al, Am J Psychiatry 1990;**147**:579–85) or 300–1000mg orally (n = 30, Ancill and Carlyle, Am J Psychiatry 1992;**149**:137), as has 125mg IV during treatment (Jaffe and Dubin, Am J Psychiatry 1992;**149**:1610). Cases of cardiac dysrhythmia have been reported.

Carbamazepine

Logic would dictate that since carbamazepine is an anticonvulsant it would have an effect on reducing seizures. A small retrospective study showed that in seven patients taking either valproate or carbamazepine, seizure durations were slightly shorter but that this appeared to have no dramatic effect on either the efficacy or side-effects of ECT (n = 7, Zarate et al, Ann Clin Psychiatry 1997;**9**:19–25).

Ciprofloxacin

There is a case of prolonged seizures related to concurrent ciprofloxacin 1g/d (n = 1, Kisa et al, J ECT 2005;**21**:43–4).

Clozapine

The UK SmPCs recommend suspending clozapine for 24 hours pre-ECT to reduce the risk of unwanted or prolonged seizures (n = 1, Bloch et al, Br J Psychiatry 1996;**169**:253–4). However, some case series have been published. One showed that 2–20 sessions of ECT with clozapine (mean 518mg/d, range 200–900mg/d) to probably be safe and with short-term efficacy (72% showing marked initial improvement but only in 23% beyond 4/12) in resistant cases (n = 22, Havaki-Kontaxaki et al, Clin Neuropharmacol 2006;**29**:52–6). Comparison, combined ECT and clozapine improved TRS more than either alone (PANSS scores reductions 71% combination, 46% clozapine and 40% placebo) and there were no significant adverse effects with the combination (n = 18, p/c, Masoudzadeh and Khalilian, Pak J Biol Sci 2007;**10**:4287–90). Finally, the combination appeared particularly effective in schizoaffective patients (n = 43, Gazdag et al, Ideggyogy Sz 2006;**59**:261–7). Apart from mild cognitive disturbances, there were no negative consequences from 24 ECTs in someone taking high-dose clozapine (1600mg/d), although there were no positive consequences either (n = 1, Keller et al, J ECT 2009;**25**:280–1). However, not omitting doses is a risky strategy, especially with higher doses of clozapine where the seizure threshold may be significantly lower.

Donepezil

Donepezil has been used successfully for treating cognitive deficits from maintenance ECT (n = 1, Rao et al, J ECT 2009;**25**:216–8). Donepezil 5mg given from before ECT until three days after ECT finishes improves post-ECT cognitive function recovery time compared to placebo (n = 45, RCT, t/b, p/c, Prakash et al, J ECT 2006;**22**:163–8; n = 1, Logan and Stewart, J ECT 2007;**23**:28–9).

Duloxetine

There were no apparent problems with ECT

in a patient taking olanzapine and duloxetine (n = 1, Hanretta and Malek-Ahmadi, J ECT 2006; **22**:139–41).

Escitalopram

There is a report of ECT being well-tolerated with escitalopram 20 mg/d (n = 3, Masdrakis et al, J ECT 2008;**24**:289–91).

Flumazenil

Effective ECT was only possible in a benzo-diazepine-dependent depressed woman when the anticonvulsant effect of clonazepam was reversed by flumazenil 0.1 mg (n = 1, Berigan et al, Am J Psychiatry 1995;**152**:957).

Ibuprofen

Ibuprofen 600 mg/d 90 minutes before ECT may reduce the frequency and severity of post-ECT headache (n = 34, RCT, p/c, d/b, Leung et al, J Clin Psychiatry 2003;**64**:551–3), although Kessler thinks their data shows that it might actually increase seizure duration (Kessler, J Clin Psychiatry 2004;**65**:442).

Ketamine *

Use of ketamine as an anaesthetic may actually enhance the improvement in depression (n = 31, Okamoto et al, J ECT 2010;**26**:223–7).

Lamotrigine *

A retrospective case review suggested ECT is generally well tolerated and effective with lamotrigine, albeit with the occasional missed seizure (n = 19, Sienaert et al, J ECT 2011; **27**:148–52). Lamotrigine (mean 100 mg/d) also had no adverse effect on concurrent ECT in bipolar depression, with no rashes, no worsening cognitive function and clinically adequate ECT seizures (n = 9, Penland and Ostroff, J ECT 2006;**22**:142–7).

Lithium *

A recent prospective study has concluded that there are no differences in seizure variables, apnea time and recovery, but that the mean maximum heart rate and maximum systolic bp are lower with lithium and that post-ECT recovery time is directly correlated with serum lithium levels (n = 55, Thirthalli et al, World J Biol Psychiatry 2011;**12**:149–55). Although severe

memory loss, neurological abnormalities and a reduced antidepressant effect have been claimed, a retrospective study showed no increase in side-effects or other problems (e.g. n = 12 and review, Dolenc and Rasmussen, J ECT 2005;**21**:165–70), although there are case series, e.g. prolonged seizure, serotonin syndrome and focal seizures (n = 3, Sartorius et al, World J Biol Psychiatry 2005;**6**:121–4). It has been suggested that ECT facilitates lithium toxicity, possibly by releasing lithium from cells, producing a pure toxicity. Elderly patients may be more susceptible to this combination. Some sources recommend discontinuing lithium 48 hours before ECT to prevent this neurotoxicity and not re-starting for several days after the last treatment (Ferrier et al, Adv Psychiatr Treat 1995;**1**:102–10), although discontinuing lithium would risk discontinuation effects and be potentially dangerous (see lithium in 1.10).

MAOIs

A review has concluded that there is no dangerous interaction between MAOIs and ECT (n = 4, Dolenc et al, J ECT 2004;**20**:258–61).

Moxifloxacin

Moxifloxacin has been associated with prolonged seizures (n = 1, Reti and Davydow, J ECT 2007;**23**:289–90).

Mirtazapine *

An open study indicated that there were no problems with mirtazapine, either started before or during a course of ECT (n = 19, Söderström, poster, WCP, 1999, Germany). There are cases of successful and uneventful use (n = 2, Farah, Convul Ther 1997;**13**:116–7). Mirtazapine may even relieve post-ECT headaches and nausea, possibly by 5HT2 and 5HT3 antagonism (case series, Li et al, J ECT 2011;**27**:165–7).

Moclobemide

The SmPC recommends suspending moclo-bemide for 24 hours pre-ECT, although there is no data on its use with ECT.

Naloxone

Naloxone has no detectable effect (Rasmussen et al, Convuls Ther 1997;**13**: 44–6).

Paliperidone *

No problems have been detected in cardiac adverse events (n = 9, 83 ECTs, Masdrakis *et al*, *Gen Hosp Psychiatry* 2011;**33**:9–10).

Rivastigmine

There is a case of eight ECTs being successful with the person taking rivastigmine throughout (n = 1, Zink *et al*, *J ECT* 2002;**18**:162–4).

Selegiline *

Two cases suggested no problems with transdermal selegiline and ECT (n = 2, Horn *et al*, *Psychosomatics* 2010;**51**:176–8).

SSRIs

A small study showed a significantly longer seizure duration in patients taking SSRIs compared to other antidepressants (n = 13, Potokar *et al*, *Int J Psychiatr Clin Pract* 1997;**1**:277–80), although an earlier review did not support the theory that **fluoxetine** causes prolonged seizures (n = 12, Gutierrez-Esteinou and Pope, *Convul Ther* 1989;**5**:344–8). There are reports of prolonged seizures with ECT and **paroxetine** and in a rater-blinded comparison seizure length was twice as long in those taking paroxetine (n = 14, Curran, *Acta Psychiatr Scand* 1995;**92**:239–40). Prolonged seizures may occur with **fluvoxamine** and ECT and the SmPC recommends a four-day interval between stopping fluvoxamine and giving ECT. There is only limited experience with ECT and **sertraline** or **citalopram**.

Steroids

In chronic steroid users, additional 'stress doses' are sometimes given before general anaesthesia, but this appears unnecessary for prednisolone and ECT (n = 27, Rasmussen *et al*, *J ECT* 2008;**24**:128–30).

Sumatriptan

Sumatriptan may prevent post-ECT headaches (White *et al*, *Headache* 2006;**46**:692).

Theophylline

Theophylline (related to caffeine) at 100–400 mg IV has been reported to facilitate ECT seizures in previously resistant patients (n = 7, Leentjens *et al*, *Convuls Ther* 1996;**12**:232–7).

There are, however, reports of status epilepticus and increase in seizure duration with concomitant ECT.

Trazodone

A prolonged seizure duration has been reported (n = 1, Lanes and Ravaris, *Am J Psychiatry* 1993;**150**:525), although low-dose use did not produce any problems in one retrospective study (n = 100, Krahn *et al*, *J Clin Psychiatry* 2001;**62**:108–10).

Tricyclics

Combined tricyclic and ECT therapy is often used and seems to present no routine problems. Indeed, nortriptyline enhances the effect of ECT and reduces cognitive adverse effects (n < 319, RCT, Sackeim *et al*, *Arch Gen Psychiatry* 2009;**66**:729–37). The use of anaesthetics could enhance the risk of cardiac arrhythmias and hypotension.

Valproate

A small retrospective study showed that in patients taking either valproate seizure durations were slightly shorter but that this appeared to have no dramatic effect on the efficacy, or side-effects of ECT (n = 7, Zarate *et al*, *Ann Clin Psychiatry* 1997;**9**:19–25).

Venlafaxine

Venlafaxine seems to reduce the effect of ECT and tends to worsen cognitive adverse effects (n < 319, RCT, Sackeim *et al*, *Arch Gen Psychiatry* 2009;**66**:729–37). Venlafaxine at doses of up to 300 mg/d seems safe if propofol is the anaesthetic but the possibility of asystole cannot be excluded (n = 13, Gonzalez-Pinto *et al*, *J Neuropsychiatry Clin Neurosci* 2002; **14**:206–9).

Zopiclone

Reduced seizure length has been reported with 7.5–15 mg of zopiclone the previous night (n = 2, Tobiansky, *J Psychopharmacol* 1991; **5**:268–9) and so is best avoided.

Ziprasidone *

There are cases of safe and well tolerated use (n = 8, Masdrakis *et al*, *J ECT* 2010;**26**: 139–42).

2 SELECTING DRUGS, DOSES AND PREPARATIONS

Contents

TABLE 2.1.1: HYPNOTICS — RELATIVE SIDE-EFFECTS *

Class	Drug	Usual night dose mg/d	Adult max dose mg/d	Elderly max dose mg/d	Elimination half-life (hours) adult	Elimination half-life (hours) elderly	G/I upset	Hang-over	Depen-dence po-tential
Shorter-acting benzodiazepines									
1a	Loprazolam	1	2	7	10	24	○	●	●
1a	Lormetazepam	1	1.5+	<Ad	10	14	○	●	●
1a	Temazepam	10–20	40	20	5–11	14+	○	●	●●
Longer-acting benzodiazepines									
1b	Flunitrazepam (U)	1	2	1	35	35	○	●●	●
1b	Flurazepam	15	30	15+	47–95	?	○	●●●	●●
1b	Nitrazepam	5	10	5	18–36	40+	○	●●●	●
Chloral and derivatives									
2	Chloral betane	707	5 tabs	<Ad?	7–10	Same	●●●	●	●
2	Triclofos	1 g	2 g	1 g	?	?	●	?	?
Other hypnotics									
3	Clomethiazole#	N/A#	2 caps#	Same	4–5	Same	○	●	●●
4	Promethazine	25	50	–	10–19	10–19	○	●●	○
5	Zaleplon	10	10	5	2	3	○	○	○
6	Zopiclone	7.5	7.5	<Ad	3.5–6	8	●	●	●
7	Zolpidem	5	(10)	10	2(2–3)	Longer	○	○	○
8	Melatonin	2	2	2	3.5–4	3.5–4	○	○	○
9	Ramelteon (U)	8	8	8	1–2	1–2	○	○	○

Classes
1a = Shorter-acting or minimally-accumulating benzodiazepines
1b = Longer-acting or accumulating benzodiazepines
2 = Chloral and derivative
3 = Clomethiazole (chormethiazole)
4 = Antihistamine
5 = Pyrazolopyrimidine
6 = Imidazopyridine
7 = Cyclopyrrone
8 = Melatonin
9 = Melatonin receptor agonist

Side-effects frequency
●●● = Marked effect (severity will be dose-related)
●● = Moderate effect
● = Mild effect
○ = Little or nothing reported
? = No information available

Other abbreviations
Usual night dose = suggested usual dose for an adult in the UK SmPC
Adult max dose = suggested maximum adult hypnotic dose in the UK SmPC
Elderly max dose = suggested maximum elderly hypnotic dose in the UK SmPC
# = 1 capsule is therapeutically equivalent to 5 ml syrup. Indicated for severe insomnia in the elderly only
U = unlicensed in UK at time of writing

TABLE 2.1.2: ANTIDEPRESSANTS — RELATIVE SIDE-EFFECTS *

Drug	Adult max dose mg/d	Elderly max dose mg/d	Anti-cholinergic	Cardiac	Nausea ‡	Sedation	Overdose §	Pro-convulsant	Sexual dysfunction
Tricyclics									
Amitriptyline	200	75	●●●	●●●	●●	●●●	●●●	●●●	●●
Clomipramine	250	75	●●●	●●●	●●	●●	●	●●●	●●●
Dosulepin (dothiepin)	150	75	●●	●●●	○	●●●	●●●	●●●	●●
Doxepin	300	<Ad	●	●●	●	●	●●●	●●●	●●
Imipramine	300	50	●●	●●	●●	●	●●●	●●●	●●
Lofepramine	210	<Ad	●●	●	●	●	○	○	●●
Nortriptyline	150	50	●●	●	●	●	●●	●	●●
Trimipramine	300	<Ad	●●●	●●	●	●●	●●	●	●●●
SSRIs									
Citalopram	60	40	○	○	●●●	○	●	○	●●
Escitalopram	20	<20	○	○	●●●	○	○	○	●●
Fluoxetine	(20)	(60)	○	○	●●●	○	○	○	●●
Fluvoxamine	300	300	●	○	●●●	●	○	○	●
Paroxetine	50	40	○	○	●●	○	○	○	●●●
Sertraline	200	200	○	○	●●	○	○	○	●●
MAOIs									
Isocarboxazid	60	<Ad	●●	●●	●●	○	●●	○	●
Phenelzine	90	(90)	●	●	●●	●	●●●	○	●
Tranylcypromine	CA30	(30)	●	●	●●	●	●●●	○	●

2

TABLE 2.1.2: ANTIDEPRESSANTS — RELATIVE SIDE-EFFECTS (CONT) *

Drug	Adult max dose mg/d	Elderly max dose mg/d	Relative side-effects (most will be dose-related)						
			Anti-cholinergic	Cardiac	Nausea ‡	Sedation	Overdose §	Pro-convulsant	Sexual dysfunction
Others									
Agomelatine	50	50?	○	○	○	○	○	○	○
Bupropion/amfebutamone (U)	–	–	●	○	●	○	●●	●●●	○
Duloxetine	120	Caution	○	○	●●	●	?	?	●●
Flupentixol	3	2	●●	○	○	●	●	?	●
Mianserin	90+	<Ad	●	○	○	●●●	○	○	●
Mirtazapine	45	45	○	○	○	●●	○	●●	●●
Moclobemide	600	600	●	○	●	○	○	?	●
Reboxetine	12	NR	●	●	●	○	○	○	○
Trazodone	600	+300	●	●	●●●	●●	●	○	●●
Tryptophan	6g	6g	○	○	●	●●	●	○	○
Venlafaxine	375	Same	○	●●	●●	●	●●	●	●

Side-effects frequency (severity will be dose-related)

●●●	=	Marked effect
●●	=	Moderate effect
●	=	Mild effect
○	=	Little or minimal effect
?	=	No information or little reported
U	=	Unlicensed in UK for depression

Other abbreviations

‡	=	Typical serotonergic side-effect
Adult max dose	=	Maximum adult oral antidepressant dose in UK SmPC
Elderly max dose	=	Maximum elderly oral antidepressant dose as stated in UK SmPC. Most state that half the adult dose may be sufficient
Overdose §	=	Based on UK Fatal Toxicity Index (Henry et al, Br J Med 1995;**310**:221–48). For review of epidemiology and relative toxicity of antidepressant drugs in overdose see Henry (Drug Safety 1997;**16**:374–90, 92 refs)

TABLE 2.1.3: ANTIDEPRESSANTS — PHARMACOKINETICS AND RECEPTOR EFFECTS *

Drug	Major active metabolites	Half-life (hours)	Peak plasma conc (hours)	5-HT	Transmitter reuptake inhibition NA/NE	DA
Tricyclics						
Amitriptyline		8–24	6	+++	++++	+
	Nortriptyline	18–96	(4–5)	+	++++	+
Clomipramine		17–28	2.5	+++	+	–
	Desmethylclomipramine	>36	4–24	+	+++	–
Dosulepin (dothiepin)		14–40	3	+	+	+
	Desmethyldothiepin	22–60	2			–
Doxepin		8–24	4	+	+	–
	Desmethyldoxepin	30–72	–			–
Imipramine		4–18	2	+++	+	–
	Desipramine	12–24	(4–5)	+	++++	–
Lofepramine		1.6	1–2	+	++++	–
	Desipramine	12–24	(4–5)	+	++++	–
Nortriptyline		18–96	(4–5)	+	+++	–
Trimipramine	(Desmethyltrimipramine)	7–23	3	+	+	+
Selective serotonin reuptake inhibitors (SSRIs)						
Citalopram		33	2–4	++++	–	–
Escitalopram		30	2–4	++++	–	–
Fluoxetine		24–140	6–8	++++	–	+
	Norfluoxetine	168–216	–	+	–	–
Fluvoxamine	None	13–22	2–8	+++	–	–
Paroxetine	None	24	6	++++	+	–
Sertraline		25–36	4–10	+++	–	–
	Desmethylsertraline	66–109	8–12	+	–	–

TABLE 2.1.3: ANTIDEPRESSANTS — PHARMACOKINETICS AND RECEPTOR EFFECTS (CONT) *

Drug	Major active metabolites	Half-life (hours)	Peak plasma conc (hours)	Transmitter reuptake inhibition 5-HT	NA/NE	DA
Monoamine oxidase inhibitors						
Isocarboxazid	NK	N/K	2-3	←	←	←
Phenelzine	NK	1.5	2-3	←	←	←
Tranylcypromine	NK	2.5	2-3	←	←	←
Others						
Agomelatine	None	1-2	1-2	5HT2C antagonist	O	O
Bupropion (U)	Hydroxybupropion	3-16 (highly variable) 12-38	4	-	+	++
Duloxetine	NK	8-17	6	+++	+++	-
Flupentixol	NK	35	3-8	-	-	-
Mianserin	Desmethyl-8-hydroxy	12-29	1-3	O	O	+
Mirtazapine	None	20-40	1-3	+++	←	←
Moclobemide	None	1-2	1	O	+++	O
Reboxetine	NK	13	2	++# PPSA	+++	O
Trazodone	mCPP	3-7	½-2	+++§	O	O
Venlafaxine §	Desmethylvenlafaxine	1-2	5(2-7) 10(8-13)	+++§	+++§	+§

Abbreviations

++++ = Marked potency   ++ = Minor potency
+++ = Moderate potency   + = Minimal
                O = Nil

Other abbreviations

§ = Dose-dependent reuptake inhibiton (see C1)   ↑ = Cytoplasm levels increase
PPSA = Potent postsynaptic 5-HT agonist   5-HT = 5-hydroxytryptamine or serotonin
NA/NE = Noradrenaline or norepinephrine   # = Also potent central 5HT antagonist

TABLE 2.1.4: ANTIPSYCHOTICS — RELATIVE SIDE-EFFECTS *

Drug	Adult max dose mg/d	Elderly max dose mg/d	Relative side-effects (most will be dose related)								
			Anti-cholinergic	Cardiac	EPSE	Hypo-tension	Sedation	Minor O/D	Weight gain	Prolactin	Procon-vulsant
Phenothiazines											
Chlorpromazine	1000	<Ad	●●	●●	●●	●●●	●●●	●●	●●●	●●●?	●●●
Levomepromazine (methotrimeprazine)	1000	NR	●●	●●	●●?	●●●	●●●	●●	?	●●●?	●●●?
Promazine	800	<Ad	●	●●	●	●●●	●●●	●	?	●●?	●●?
Pericyazine	(300)	<Ad	●●	●●	●	●●	●●●	●	?	●●●?	●●?
Thioridazine	600	<Ad	●●	●●●	●	●●	●●●	●●	●●	●●●?	●●?
Perphenazine	24	<Ad	○	●●	●●	●	●●	●●	●●●	●●●?	●●?
Trifluoperazine	–	<Ad	●●●	●●	●●	●	●	●	?	●●●?	●
Others											
Benperidol	1.5	<Ad	?	?	?	●	●	?	?	●●●	●?
Haloperidol	30	30	●●	●●	●●●	●	●	●	●	●●●	●●?
Flupentixol	18	<Ad	●●	○	●●●	○	●	●●	●	●●?	●●?
Zuclopenthixol	150	<Ad	●●●	●	●●●	●	●●●	●●	?	●●●?	○?
Pimozide	20	<Ad	●●●	●●●	●	○○	○	●●	○	●●	●
Amisulpride	1200	1200	●●	○	●●	○○	●	●?	●●	●●	●?
Sulpride	2400	2400	●	○○	●●	○○	●	●●	●●	●●	○?
Depot and long-acting injections ◆											
Fluphenazine decanoate	100–2/52	<Ad	●●	●●	●●●	●	●●	●	●	●●●?	●
Pipotiazine palmitate	200–4/52	<Ad	○	●●	●●	●	●	?	?	●●●?	●●?
Haloperidol decanoate	300–4/52	<Ad	●	●	●●●	●	●	●	●	●●	●
Flupentixol decanoate	400–/52	<Ad	●●	○	●●	○	●	?	?	●●?	●?
Zuclopentixol decanoate	600–/52	<Ad	●●●	●	●●●	●	●●	●●	?	●●●?	○?

2

TABLE 2.1.4: ANTIPSYCHOTICS — RELATIVE SIDE-EFFECTS (CONT) *

Drug	Adult max dose mg/d	Elderly max dose mg/d ?	Relative side-effects (most will be dose related)								
			Anti-cholinergic	Cardiac	EPSE	Hypo-tension	Sedation	Minor O/D	Weight gain	Prolactin	Procon-vulsant
Depot and long-acting injections ◆											
Fluspirilene	20–1/52	<Ad	●●	●	●●●	●●	●●	?	?	●●?	●
Rispiridone Consta	50–2/52	25–2/52	○	○	●●	●●●	●?	?	●	●●	○
Olanzapine pamoate	300–2/52	See SmPC	●	○	○	○	●●	○	●●●	●●	●●
Paliperidone palmitate	150mg/month	Same (but see SmPC)	○	○	●	●	●●	○	●●	●●	○
Second generation/atypicals											
Aripiprazole	30	30	○	●	○	○	○	?	●	○	○
Asenapine (U)	(10)	(20)	○?	?	●?	●?	●●?	?	●?	?	?
Clozapine	900	(900)	●●	●●●	○	●●●	●●●	?	●●●	○	●●●
Olanzapine	20	20	●	○	○	●	●●	○	●●●	●	●●
Paliperidone	12	12	○	●	○	●●	●	○	●●	●●	●●
Quetiapine	800	<Ad	●●	●	●	●●	●●	●	●●	●	○
Rispiridone	(16)	4	●	○	●	●●●	●?	○	●●	●●	●
Sertindole	(20)	(20)	●●	●●●	●	●●	○	○	●●?	○	○
Zotepine (U)	300	150	●●	●●	●	●●	●	?	●●?	●●?	●●●
Ziprasidone (U)	–	–	○	●●	○	○	○	?	○	○	○

Side-effects frequency (severity will be dose-related)

●●● = Marked effect
●● = Moderate effect
● = Mild/transient effect

○ = Little or minimal effect
? = No information or little reported
U = Unlicensed in UK at time of writing

Other abbreviations

Adult max dose = Maximum adult oral antipsychotic dose as stated in UK SmPC or BNF. May be different for other indications

Elderly max dose = Maximum oral antipsychotic dose in the elderly as stated in UK SmPC or BNF
Most state that a starting dose of half to a quarter of the adult dose should be adequate, with smaller dose increments

◆ = 100–1/52 means 100mg every two weeks; 400–1/52 means 400mg every week, etc

TABLE 2.1.5: ANTIPSYCHOTICS — PHARMACOKINETICS AND RECEPTOR EFFECTS

Drug/group	Receptor blockade (5)										$5HT_{2a}:D_2$ affinity ratio	Half-life (hours)	Time to peak (oral) (2) hours	Main metabolite(s)
	D_1	D_2	D_3	D_4	$5HT_{1A}$	$5HT_{2A}$	M_1	α-1	α-2	H_1				
Phenothiazines														
Chlorpromazine	++	+	++	+		+++	++	+++	+	++	10:1	6(2–119)	3(IM 1–4, IV 2–4)	Many
Fluphenazine HCl Fluphenazine decanoate	++	+++	+++	++		++	+	++	O	+	1:2	FHCl 33 FD 14–27/7	FHCl 3	Some, unclear if active
Levomepromazine	++	++	+++	?		+++	+++	+++	O	+++	5:1	15–30	1–3	Some, unclear if active
Pericyazine (3)	++?	+?	++?	+?		+++?	+++?			++?		NK	NK	NK
Perphenazine	++	++	NK	?		+++	+	++	++	+++	2:1	10(8–12)	4–8	Some, unclear if active
Thioridazine	++	+	++	+		+++	+++	+++	+	+	5:1	21–24	NK	Mesoridazine
Trifluoperazine	++	++	NK	+		+++	+	+++	+	+	2:1	24	2–4	Several
Others														
Benperidol	+?	+++	+?	+?		+?	O?	+?	+?	++?	NK	8	2	1% unchanged in urine
Haloperidol HCl Haloperidol decanoate	++	+++	+++	+++	+	++	+	++	+	+	1:25	HHCl 21 (9–38) HD 21/7	2–6	Hydroxy-haloperidol
Flupentixol HCl Flupentixol decanoate												FHCl 22–36 FD 3–7/7(1)	FHCl 3–6 FD 3–10/7	Inactive
Zuclopenthixol HCl Zuclopenthixol decanoate Zuclopenthixol acetate	++	+++	+	NK		+++	++	++	NK	++	1:3	20	ZHCl 3–4 ZD 5–7 days ZA 24–48	Inactive
Sulpiride	O	+++	+	O		O	O	O	O	O	1:50	6–8	2–6	Nil
Amisulpride	O	+++	+++	O		O	O	O	O	O		12–17	1–4	Nil
Pimozide	+	+++	+++	+		+++	+	+++	+	O	1:5	53–55	6–8	Some, unclear if active
Fluspirilene	NK	NK	NK	NK	NK	NK	NK	NK	NK	NK	NK	32–>300	1–48	Inactive

2

TABLE 2.1.5: ANTIPSYCHOTICS — PHARMACOKINETICS AND RECEPTOR EFFECTS (CONT) *

Drug/group	Receptor blockade (5)										$5HT_{2A}:D_2$ affinity ratio	Half-life (hours)	Time to peak (oral) (2) hours	Main metabolite(s)
	D_1	D_2	D_3	D_4	$5HT_{1A}$	$5HT_{2A}$	M_1	α–1	α–2	H_1				
Second generation/Atypicals														
Aripiprazole	O	++++	O	O	PAg	AAnt	O	O	O	O	N/A	75(31–146)	3–7	None known
Asenapine (TBC)	++	+++	++	++	+++	+++	O	++	++	++	20:1?	6 [8]	0.5–1.5	Minor
Clozapine	++	+++	++	++	++	+++	+++	+++	++	+++	20–30:1	4–12	2–3	Norclozapine
Olanzapine	++	+++	++	++	+	+++	++	++	+	+++	50:1	30(21–54)	3–6	Inactive
Paliperidone	+	+++	+++	++	+	+++	O	+++	++	++		23	23–29	None known
Paliperidone palmitate *	+	+++	+++	+	+	+++	O	+++	++	++		29–45 days	13 days	None known
Quetiapine	O	++	+	+	++	++	O	++	O	+	1:1	7	1.5, XL 5–6hrs	N-desalkylquetiapine (t1/2 12hrs)
Risperidone	+	+++	++	++	++	+++	O	+++	+++	++	8–11:1	20–30	1–2 (7)	Hydroxyrisperidone
Sertindole	+	++++	++	++	+	+++	O	+++	O	+	100:1	55–90	10	Dehydrosertindole
Ziprasidone	+	+++	++	+	+++	+++	O	++	+	O	3:1	7	4–5	Many
Zotepine	++	+++	++	++	++	+++	+	+++	+	+++	4:1	14–24	1 and 10–12	Norzotepine (inactive)

Receptor binding: +++ = High affinity; ++ = Moderate; + = Low; O = Very low; NK = Not known; ? = Possible; PAg = Partial agonist with very high affinity; AAnt = Antagonist

Additional ref: Shiloh, Nutt and Weizman (2006) *Atlas of Psychiatric Pharmacotherapy*, Informa Healthcare (very colourful and useful)

1. Flupentixol decanoate's half-life is longer (up to 17 days) on continuous administration
2. Time to oral peak may vary with food
3. Receptor-binding studies for pericyazine have not been published, but it has been reported to have some differences to chlorpromazine
4. Sertindole, olanzapine and clozapine appear to have some D2 limbic selectivity
5. Inclusion of a receptor may give some guide to therapeutic action and adverse effects
6. There is a considerable degree of variation between published sources, depending upon how the results are presented, whether they are single studies or averages, the receptor sources, assay type, etc. These figures should be taken only as a guide, eg. there is little, or nothing published about fluspirilene or pericyazine
7. All oral preparations, including tablets, orodispersable and liquid
8. Biphasic half-life: 6hrs for the first 18hrs, then terminal half-life is 23hrs.

TABLE 2.1.6: ANXIOLYTICS — RELATIVE SIDE-EFFECTS *

Class	Drug	Usual dose mg/d	Adult max dose mg/d	Elderly max dose mg/d	Half-life (hours) adult (+ range)	Half-life (hours) elderly	Hang-over	Depen-dence po-tential
Shorter-acting benzodiazepines								
1a	Lorazepam	4	4	<Ad	12 (8–25)	Same	●●●	●●●
1a	Oxazepam	30	120	80	8 (5–15)	Same	●●●	●●
Longer-acting benzodiazepines								
1b	Chlordiazepoxide	30	100	<50	12 (6–30)	L	●●●	●●
1b	Clobazam	30	60	20	18 (9–77)	L	●	●●
1b	Diazepam	6	30	15	32 (21–50)	L	●●●	●●
Beta-blockers								
2	Oxprenolol	80	80	80	4# (3–6)	Same	○	○
2	Propranolol	80	120	–	2# (1–2)	Same	○	○
Other anxiolytics								
3	Buspirone	30	45	45	7 (2–11)	Same	○	○
4	Pregabalin	300	600	<600	6	L	○	○
5	Duloxetine	30	120	120	8-17	Same?	○	○
5	Venlafaxine	75	75	75	1-2	Same	○	○
6	Escitalopram	10	20	<Ad	30	L	○	○
6	Paroxetine	20	50	40	c24	c24	○	●

Classes:
1a = Shorter-acting or minimally-accumulating benzodiazepines
1b = Longer-acting or accumulating benzodiazepines. These also have metabolites which enhance their length of action
2 = Beta-blockers
3 = Azapirone (Azaspirodecanedione)
4 = Anticonvulsant
5 = SNRI
6 = SSRI

Side-effects frequency (severity will be dose-related)
●●● = Marked effect   ○ = Little or nothing reported
●● = Moderate effect   ? = No information available
● = Mild effect

Other abbreviations
Adult max dose = Suggested maximum oral dose in the UK SmPC. Most recommend treatment for up to four weeks
Elderly max dose = Suggested maximum oral dose in the elderly in the UK SmPC. Most state that half the adult dose should be adequate
\# = Pharmacological action longer than half-life suggests
L = Longer in elderly than younger adults
The data on this and the previous pages is based on a large number of papers. Note was taken of presentation of data, equivalence of dose used, etc. When non-comparable papers are excluded, there is a surprisingly high level of consistency on reported relative side-effects. Individuals response may, of course, vary widely. Many effects may be dose-related.

2.2 SWITCHING OR DISCONTINUING PSYCHOTROPICS

Switching psychotropics can be achieved using a variety of methods, varying in rate, overlap, gap and complexity. The main types are summarised in the graphs and comments. The remarks below specifically relating to antipsychotics are marked with #.

Switch 1: Drug-free interval
(Discontinue first drug, leave drug-free interval, introduce second drug.)
Advantages:
1. Minimises combined ADRs.
2. Relapse risk not too high, if the patient is relatively stable and the gap is not prolonged.
3. Minimal interaction potential.
4. Side-effects from the second drug are less likely to be confused with discontinuation effects from the first drug.
5. Anticholinergic drug doses can be titrated as needed. #
6. Ideal (but often impractical) for switches to clozapine to reduce additive myelosuppressive potential. #
7. Lowest medication error potential.
Disadvantages:
1. Takes time, which delays the desired relief of symptoms or side-effects. #
2. Potential for relapse or deterioration during the gap and changeover.
3. Early relapse before reaching a therapeutic dose might be interpreted as lack of efficacy of the second drug.

Switch 2: No interval
(Stop first drug, start second immediately.)
Advantages:
1. Straightforward.
2. Low medication error potential.
3. Appropriate for inpatient settings with better supervision.
4. Appropriate where an acute severe reaction to a drug has occurred, e.g. statutory abrupt withdrawal of clozapine due to a blood dyscrasia. #
5. Sometimes acceptable for high-risk switches to clozapine to reduce additive myelosuppressive potential, but retaining antipsychotic cover. #

TABLE 2.2.1: SWITCHING PSYCHOTROPICS

Switch 1: Drug-free interval (safest)

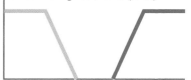

Switch 2: No interval (generally preferred)

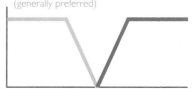

Switch 3: Partial overlap (usually acceptable)

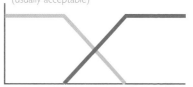

Switch 4a: Full overlap (risks NMS, serotonin syndrome and combined ADRs)

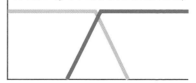

Switch 4b: Abrupt switch (risks discontinuation symptoms)

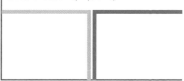

Switch 5: Incomplete (switch never finished, default polypharmacy, avoid)

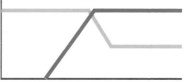

Disadvantages:

1. May raise unrealistic expectations from the patient and family of a rapid improvement on the second drug.
2. Combined ADRs, albeit short-lived.
4. Potential for drug interactions if the first drug has a long half-life, e.g. fluoxetine.
5. Rapid discontinuation of the first drug may produce higher relapse rates, e.g. antipsychotics.
6. Discontinuation effects from the first drug might be interpreted as side-effects of the second, e.g. some antipsychotics.

Switch 3: Partial overlap

(Add new drug, either at standard dose or quickly titrated upwards, while slowly tapering the first drug.)

Advantages:

1. Appropriate when symptom or side-effect relief is needed but there is a high risk or relapse or deterioration.
2. No sudden changes occur (which might destabilise the patient).
3. This switch may be unavoidable for depot to oral switches, where plasma levels of depot will decline slowly. #
4. Useful for switches from a high potency antipsychotic to a newer or lower potency antipsychotic where cholinergic rebound may occur. Either way, anticholinergic cover can be retained for several weeks. #

Disadvantages:

1. If the taper is too quick, two drugs may be given at sub-therapeutic doses.
2. Combined ADRs may occur.
3. Potential for drug interactions, especially with antidepressants.
4. Potential for medication errors if not planned fully in advance — involve carers and patient if patient is at home.
5. High potential for polypharmacy if the switch is never completed (see Switch 5). #

Switch 4: Full overlap *

(Add new drug to therapeutic dose and then slowly taper previous drug.)

Advantages:

1. Safest if relapse prevention is of greatest concern.
2. Most appropriate if the patient has recently

(e.g. < 3 months) recovered from acute relapse with the first drug.
3. Low risk of discontinuation effects of the first drug.
4. If depot to oral antipsychotic switch, this may be the lowest risk opportunity to assess compliance with oral drugs. #
5. Slow taper is possible and is better for drugs with a high anticholinergic activity.
6. Probably the safest switch for aripiprazole.

Disadvantages:

1. Combined ADRs may occur (but not necessarily with antipsychotics, Gardner *et al*, *Can J Psychiatry* 1997;**42**:430–1).
2. Potential severe reactions, e.g. NMS or serotonin syndrome.
3. Potential for drug interactions.
4. Potential for medication errors if not planned and completed fully.
5. High potential for polypharmacy if switch never completed (see switch 5 below).

Switch 5: Incomplete

(Add new drug to therapeutic dose and then never stop previous drug).

This can happen if the switch is started but the treatment plan is not passed on or the patient improves and there is a reluctance to discontinue the first drug and possibly destabilise the patient. Default polypharmacy' should be avoided. Long-term monotherapy is beneficial, as it is easier to judge accurately the effectiveness of any given drug, and medication regimens are simple and not confused by polypharmacy (extensive review, Weiden *et al*, *J Clin Psychiatry* 1998;**59**[Suppl 19]:36–49). Monotherapy should thus always be tried first and, if, at some time later, a rational, planned and assessed polypharmacy is tried, that is reasonable. See *1.21* for a discussion on combined antipsychotics.

2.2.1 SWITCHING OR DISCONTINUING ANTIPSYCHOTICS

Reviews:* switching for side-effects (Mukundan *et al*, *Cochrane Database Syst Rev* 2010;**12**; CD006629), strategies (Lambert, *J Clin Psychiatry* 2007;**68(Suppl 6)**:10–3), general (Buckley and Correll, *J Clin Psychiatry* 2008;**69**(Suppl 1):4–17, Correll, *CNS Spectr* 2010;**15**(4 Suppl 6):8–11).

2.2.1.1 GENERAL ADVICE ON SWITCHING ANTIPSYCHOTICS

Reasons for switching antipsychotics include (Weiden *et al, J Clin Psychiatry* 1997;**58**[Suppl 10]: S63–S72):

1. Persistent positive (distressing and disruptive) symptoms.
2. Persistent negative (restrictive and burdening) symptoms.
3. Relapse despite compliance.
4. Persistent distressing adverse effects such as EPS, akathisia, hyperprolactinaemia, poor self-image and sexual dysfunction.
5. Oral to depot or other formulation change.

Risks of discontinuing (or switching) antipsychotics (review and guidance, Keks *et al, CNS Drugs* 1995;**4**:351–6):

1. Cholinergic rebound (e.g. nausea, vomiting, restlessness, anxiety, insomnia, fatigue, malaise, myalgia, diaphoresis, rhinitis, paraesthesia, GI distress, headaches, nightmares) may occur on discontinuation, particularly if a second drug has less anticholinergic effect or if anticholinergics are withdrawn too soon. It can be severe but brief and predictable.
2. Withdrawal dyskinesias, e.g. extrapyramidal symptoms, rebound akathisia (may be confused with anxiety or psychosis), rebound dystonia and worsening tardive dyskinesia. These may partly be related to cholinergic rebound, and have been reported in mentally 'healthy' people taking metoclopramide as an antiemetic (Tranter and Healy, *J Psychopharmacol* 1998;**12**:401–6), and can be minimised by slow tapering.
3. Other discontinuation symptoms, e.g. NMS (Spivak *et al, Acta Psychiatr Scand* 1990; **81**:168–9).
4. Relapse or destabilisation — this may present an unacceptable risk to the patient. Relapse rates of up to 50% at six months after abrupt discontinuation have been reported (n = 1210, Viguera *et al, Arch Gen Psychiatry* 1997;**54**:49–55), and people with schizophrenia who switch antipsychotics have poorer outcomes, e.g. are more likely to use in-patient and crisis services (n = 651, open, 12/12, Faries *et al, BMC Psychiatry* 2009;**9**:54). Gradual

discontinuation reduces this risk (reviewed by Tranter and Healy, *J Psychopharmacol* 1998;**12**:401–6). True relapses tend to occur from 1–6 months after abrupt withdrawal of oral drugs and 3–6 months with depots, probably due to persistence of the drug at receptor level. There may be a particular problem with clozapine, where relapse or rebound psychosis can be more severe (e.g. Baldessarini *et al, Arch Gen Psychiatry* 1995; **52**:1071–2, see also *2.2.1.4*).

5. Anxiety or stress from the switch causing symptom flare-up.
6. Medication errors.
7. The replacement drug being less effective than the former, or having different but still unacceptable side-effects, resulting in premature abandonment and an inadequate trial of the new drug.

General principles for switching antipsychotics:

1. Ensure the optimum effect is obtained from the first drug (see CATIE study in *C1.21*)
2. Ensure a treatment target is set and measured (take care that the key aims of a switch are not easier and less risky to achieve by, e.g. dose or timing adjustment of the first drug).
3. Avoid switches:
   - coinciding with major life stress events
   - after a change in treatment team — allow full assimilation into the new team first
   - from a drug that was successfully used to treat a major relapse within the last 3–6/12
   - in patients previously non-compliant with oral drugs now stable for under a year on a depot (Weiden *et al, J Clin Psychiatry* 1997;**58**[Suppl 10]:63–72).
4. If possible, slowly taper the first antipsychotic, probably over at least eight weeks, as this reduces the risk of relapse and emergent extrapyramidal and psychotic symptoms.
5. Slowly taper any anticholinergic, which may also be allowed to continue for a time after the drug has been discontinued. Reintroduce if necessary for any emergent symptoms.
6. Monitor mental and physical state regularly (particularly during the first month).

Before switching to a newer antipsychotic:

1. Warn about possible ADRs (e.g. weight gain, short-term sedation, diabetes, implications of reduced prolactin inhibition).
2. Discuss the need for an adequate trial and the need to complete the switch.
3. Agree how to define success or failure, and the chances thereof.
4. Warn that the new drug is not perfect — that one also is swapping one set of side-effects for another.

2.2.1.2 SPECIFIC DRUG SWITCHES

NMS has been reported during many anti-psychotic switches.

1. Phenothiazine to phenothiazine

Get the predicted optimum dose equivalent right, then switches 2 or 3 are probably reasonable.

2. Phenothiazine to D2-blocker

Get the optimum dose equivalent, then switches 2 or 3 are reasonable, but beware of cholinergic rebound (nausea, vomiting, restlessness, anxiety, insomnia, fatigue, GI distress) and stronger D2-blockade leading to additional EPSE.

TABLE 2.2.2: SWITCHING ANTIPSYCHOTICS **

From \ To	Pheno-thiazines	D2 blockers	Typical depots	Aripip-razole[15]	Asena-pine[15]	Cloza-pine[15]	Olanza-pine[15]	Olanza-pine[15] pamoate	Paliperi-done palm	Risperi-done	Risperi-done consta	Quetia-pine[15]
Pheno-thiazines	RT (1)	RT (2)	RT (3)	RT (4)	RT (12)	Care (5,)	NOP (6)	NOP (13)	RT (15)	RT (7)	RT (8a)	RT (9a)
D2 blockers	RT (10)	RT (11)	RT (3)	RT (4)	RT (12)	Care (5)	NOP (6)	NOP (13)	RT (15)	RT (7)	RT (8a)	RT (9b)
Typical depots	RT (3)	RT (3)	RT (3)	RT (3,4)	RT (3,12)	Care (3,5)	RT (3,6)	NOP (3,13)	RT (15)	RT (3,7)	RT (3,8c)	RT (3,9c)
Aripiprazole[15]	RT (4)	RT (4)	RT (3,4)	-	RT (12)	Care (4,5)	RT (4,6)	NOP (13)	RT (15)	RT (4,7)	RT (4,8a)	NOP (4,9d)
Asenapine[15]	RT (12)	RT (12)	RT (3,12)	RT (4,12)	-	NOP (5,12)	RT (6,12)	NOP (12,13)	RT (15)	RT (7,12)	RT (8a,12)	RT (9,12)
Clozapine[15]	Care (5)	Care (5)	Care (3,5)	RT (4,5)	NOP (5,12)	-	Care (5,6c)	NOP (5,13)	RT (15)	RT (5,7)	RT (5,8a)	RT (5,9e)
Olanzapine[15]	NOP (6)	NOP (6)	NOP (3,13)	RT (4,6)	RT (6,12)	Care (5,6)	-	NOP (6,13)	RT (15)	RT (6,7)	RT (6,8a)	NOP (6,9f)
Olanzapine pamoate[15]	RT (13)	RT (13)	RT (3,13e)	RT (4,13)	RT (13,12)	RT (5,13)	RT (6,13)	-	RT (15)	RT (7,13)	RT (8,13)	RT (9,13)
Paliperidone palmitate	RT (15)	RT (15)	RT (15)	RT (15)	RT (15)	RT (15)	RT (15)	RT (15)		RT (15)	RT (15)	RT (15)
Risperidone	RT (14)	RT (14)	RT (3,14)	RT (4, 14)	RT (14,12)	Care (5, 14)	NOP (6a, 14)	NOP (13,14)	RT (15)	-	RT (8d, 14)	NOP (9g, 14)
Risperidone Consta	RT (8e)	RT (8e)	RT (3,8)	RT (4,8e,16)	RT (8e,12)	Care (5,8e)	RT (6,8, 15)	NOP (8a,13)	RT (15)	RT (7,8e)	-	RT (8e,9)
Quetiapine[15]	NOP (9,14)	NOP (9,14)	NOP (3,14)	RT (4,9,14)	RT (9,12,14)	Care (5,9,14)	NOP (6,9,14)	NOP (9,13,14)	RT (15)	RT (7, 9,14)	RT (8a,9,14)	-
Stopping	RT (17)	RT (17)	RT (17)	RT (17)	RT (17)	RT (17)	RT (17)	RT (17)	RT (17)	RT (17)	RT (17)	RT (17)

NOP = No obvious problems, although there is the definite risk of NMS with **all** switches
RT = Read text
Care = Great care needed, also read text

3. Switching to a typical depot

Studies have shown that this is usually relatively straightforward if done carefully, remembering that typical depots peak plasma levels may vary (see *Table 2.2.2*) and so reduce doses accordingly. Beware of additive EPSEs.

3a. Oral antipsychotic to typical depot:
Anecdotal evidence shows that the change can usually be made uneventfully (e.g. review in *Clin Pharmacokinet* 1985;**10**:315–33), although there are no formal studies. Converting to the same drug as a depot should present no great problems if doses are chosen carefully (e.g. switch 3, see also *2.2.1.4*).

3b. Changing from one typical depot to another typical depot:
No significant problems are usually experienced (Soni *et al*, *Acta Psychiatr Scand* 1992;**85**:354–9) and a direct exchange from one depot to another can often be made uneventfully (e.g. switch 3).

3c. Combined oral antipsychotic plus depot to depot alone:
This can be an unusually difficult procedure and relapses may occur more frequently with this change when compared to other changes. Relapses can occur, particularly in the first 3–4 months, when antipsychotic levels can be inadvertently sub-therapeutic (Soni *et al*, *Acta Psychiatr Scand* 1992;**85**:354–9). If the risk of relapse is high, any change should probably be done verging on the side of caution, e.g. increasing the depot dose, then reducing oral doses later.

3d. Oral fluphenazine to depot fluphenazine:
If transferring from oral fluphenazine, multiply the total daily oral dose by 1.2 and administer as fluphenazine decanoate IM every one to two weeks. Accumulation occurs and so the dosing interval may be increased to every three weeks or so after four to six weeks of therapy (review, Ereshefsky *et al*, *J Clin Psychiatry* 1984;**45**:50–9). Concomitant oral therapy should be limited to the initial period or during times of decompensation.

3e. Oral haloperidol to depot haloperidol:
If transferring from stabilised oral haloperidol to haloperidol depot, multiply the total daily oral dose by 15–20, to a maximum of 300mg monthly, preferably much lower. Accumulation occurs and so the decanoate dose should be decreased by 25% a month until the minimum effective dose is achieved. The average maintenance dose appears to be about 100mg every four weeks. Elderly patients or those stabilised on less than 10mg/d oral haloperidol should receive haloperidol decanoate in an IM dose that is 10–15 times the oral dose every four weeks. Concomitant oral therapy should be limited to the initial period or during times of decompensation.

3f. Altering the frequency of a typical depot:
Such a change should present no great problems, provided antipsychotic levels do not drop too low or rise too high. Computer modelling suggests that:

- If switching from weekly to fortnightly, add 25–40% to the last weekly dose, then go to fortnightly with double the weekly dose, e.g. 100mg/wk to 200mg/fortnight:

Week	1	2	3	4	5	6	7
Dose	100	100	125	-	200	-	200

- If switching from fortnightly to 4-weekly, add 50% to the last fortnightly dose then go to 4-weekly with double the weekly dose, e.g. 100mg/fortnight to 200mg/monthly:

Week	1	3	5	7	9	11	13
Dose	100	100	150	-	200		200

3g. Depot typicals to others:
Stop the depot and introduce the next anti-psychotic when the next depot dose would have been due, remembering that a slow decay in depot plasma levels may occur so beware of adding the new drug too quickly, e.g. 33% of people stopping fluphenazine decanoate had notable plasma levels 12/52 after last dose (Gitlin *et al*, *J Clin Psychopharmacol* 1988;**8**:53–6). Depots are occasionally given more often than strictly necessary.

3h. Typical depot to typical depot:
This is not usually a problem, with a direct switch often possible.

4. Switching to aripiprazole **

For most antipsychotics, it would seem that abrupt switching to aripiprazole can often be poorly tolerated, especially in people with milder rather than more severe symptoms (n=77, RCT, open, 12/52, Pae *et al*, *Clin Drug Invest* 2010;**30**:187–93). Aripiprazole strongly binds to dopamine receptors, with a long half-life, displacing almost every other antipsychotic, and stimulating receptors to about 30% activity. This abrupt change from minimal dopamine activity to 30% within hours can be acutely distressing and adversive. A cross-taper is most likely to be successful, starting aripiprazole at 5 mg/d (SmPC mentions 10mg/d) then increasing stepwise to 15 mg/d, and reducing the previous antipsychotic by 25% twice a week (n = 53 [c = 48], RCT, open, 14/52, Takeuchi et al, J Clin Psychopharmacol 2008; **28**:540–3; n = 77, RCT, open, 12/52, Pae et al, Eur Neuropsychopharmacol 2009;**19**:562–70). In a switching study, although all 3 switches from risperidone (n = 105) or olanzapine (n = 164) to aripiprazole (abrupt; immediate aripiprazole start with tapered reduction of first drug; or a 14-day cross-taper) were reportedly well tolerated (n = 269, 8/52, Byerly et al, Schizophr Res 2009;**107**:218–22), the data is inconsistent (e.g. 12/52, Ryckmans et al, Pharmacopsychiatry 2009; **42**:114–21):

- Switching from FGAs/D2 specific antipsychotics may have a lower success rate than SGAs and may be more difficult than thought, possibly because of higher receptor affinity with FGAs.
- Olanzapine and quetiapine may need a smoother switching process with a longer cross-taper (n = 45 [c = 31], 12/52, Lin et al, Chang Gung Med J 2009;**32**:409–16).

5. Switching to/from clozapine

5a. Switching to clozapine: Care would be needed with the increased risk of dyscrasias with phenothiazines and delayed clearance of depots (especially Risperdal Consta®, Janssen-Cilag and olanzapine pamoate). Ideally, a previous drug should be completely withdrawn before clozapine is started, including depots (e.g. switch 1), but this is rarely practical. Clozapine is markedly sedative and hypotensive, and care is needed with additive effects so start with the usual gradual dose titration but monitor carefully. Warn women about the possible normalisation of prolactin and the need for adequate oral contraception if necessary. Pharmacokinetic interactions are unlikely (see 4.2.2).

5b. Switching from clozapine (see also 17, discontinuing antipsychotics)
Converting clozapine to other antipsychotics seems particularly problematic (n = 30, RCT, Shiovitz et al, Schizophr Bull 1996;**22**:591–5). Relapse after clozapine discontinuation seems to be of a higher incidence, may be more rapid and withdrawal symptoms may be more severe than with other drugs (see 16, prolactin warning). For gradual discontinuation of clozapine, it is best simultaneously to introduce and escalate the doses of another antipsychotic.

6. Switching to/from oral olanzapine

There are no apparent problems with stopping olanzapine suddenly, so any switch from olanzapine should be possible. When switching to olanzapine, additive EPSE, hypotension and drug interactions are unlikely to occur and so switch 3 is usually suitable with care. Due to a lesser effect on prolactin, unexpected pregnancies have been reported a couple of months after a switch from typicals to olanzapine, despite no contraceptive

TABLE 2.2.3: SUMMARY OF ANTIPSYCHOTIC INJECTIONS *

Drug	Peak (days)	Usual frequency	Main duration	Depot half-life	Time to steady state from first dose
Flupentixol	7–10	2/52	2–4/52	7/7	10–12/52
Fluphenazine	1–2	2–4/52	3–4/52	14/7	6–12/52
Fluspirilene	1–2	1/52	1/52	?	5–6/52
Haloperidol	3–9	4/52	4/52	21–28/7	10–12/52
Pipothiazine	9–10	4/52	4/52	21–28/7	8–12/52
Zuclopenthixol	4–9	2/52	2–4/52	7/7	10–12/52
Risperidone	35	2/52	2–3/52	?	12/52
Olanzapine	2–4	2/52 or 4/52	4–6/52?	30 (13–42)/7	12/52
Paliperidone *	13	Monthly	3 months or longer	29-45/7	2–4 weeks

use for 4–5 years (n = 2, Neumann and Frasch, *Nervenarzt* 2001;**72**:876–8).

6a. Risperidone to oral olanzapine: In a comparison of four different typical/risperidone to olanzapine switches in partially remitted, stable schizophrenic out-patients, the most successful method was starting 10mg **olanzapine** then gradually discontinuing the original drug. The next most successful was gradual introduction/gradual discontinuation, and probably best for elderly/frail patients. Most drop-outs (usually sleep-related) were with abrupt discontinuation (switch 2) and gradual olanzapine introduction (n = 209, 82% completed, open, Kinon et al, J Clin Psychiatry 2000;**61**:833–40). In first-episode schizophrenics with residual symptoms from risperidone, a switch to olanzapine was effective in 30%, although 47% gained significant weight from baseline (n = 58 [c = 51], open, 12/52, Takahashi et al, J Clin Psychiatry 2006;**67**:1577–82; IS).

6b. Depots to oral olanzapine: There has been a three-month trial (which may have been of inadequate duration) of switching of clinically stable schizophrenics on depots, either continuing the depot or transferred to olanzapine over 4/52. After 3/12 those transferring to olanzapine were clinically improved and all preferred olanzapine, so a four-week switch is clinically viable (n = 26, RCT, open, 3/12, Godleski et al, J Clin Psychiatry 2003;**64**:119–22).

6c. Clozapine to oral olanzapine: In an open study of a clozapine to olanzapine switch by patients wishing to avoid blood monitoring, eight of 19 successfully completed the switch (using switch 4) and the others required restabilising on clozapine (n = 19, Henderson et al, J Clin Psychiatry 1998;**59**:585–8). In patients responsive to clozapine but suffering adverse effects, a slow cross-titration over at least two weeks to olanzapine may be successful in about 90% of patients (n = 20, open, 24/52, Littrell et al, J Clin Psychiatry 2000;**61**:912–5; Lilly part-funded).

6d.* Oral olanzapine to olanzapine LAI: The dose may be important:

- 10mg/d to 300mg 2/52 had 1.5% relapse rate (cf. 12% at 150mg 2/52; and 6% at 405 mg 4/52)
- 15mg/d to 150mg 2/52 had 9% relapse rate (cf. 3% at 300mg 2/52)

- 20mg/d to 150mg 2/52 had 19% relapse rate (cf. 9% at 300mg 2/52).

The conclusion is that switching needs an adequate LAI dose to minimise the potential for relapse (n = 1065, 24/52, Detke et al, Int Clin Psychopharmacol 2011;**26**:35–42).

6e. Others to olanzapine: One study showed that in resistant schizophrenia, switching to olanzapine may be successful (n = 25, open, five years, Karagianis et al, Curr Med Res Opin 2003;**6**:47–80). Both a direct switch (2) and tapered switch (3), over 2/52, had equivalent outcomes, both therapeutic (67–74% successful) and for adverse effects (n = 108, RCT, open, 6/52, Lee et al, J Clin Psychiatry 2002;**63**:569–76).

7. Switching to/from oral risperidone

Hypotension may occur, so gradual dose titration over at least 3/7 (or longer if possible) to 4mg/d is recommended. Additive hypotension with low potency drugs may occur during a switch. A sudden switch (along with gradual withdrawal of anticholinergics) may be successful in about 60% patients, but a more gradual switch and dose escallation is preferable (n = 36, Kirov et al, Acta Psychiatr Scand 1997;**95**:439–43). A review of switching to risperidone recommended reducing the existing antipsychotic dose, then overlapping risperidone with the existing therapy, rather than making an abrupt switch (Borison et al, Clin Ther 1996;**18**:592–607). Risperidone may be a suitable replacement if introduced before slow clozapine withdrawal, i.e. switch 4 (Zimbroff, Am J Psychiatry 1995;**152**:1102). There are few obvious other problems with stopping or switching risperidone (e.g. interactions), except the standard potential for NMS, prolactin altered and additive EPS if switching to a phenothiazine or D2-blocker. Switches 2 or 3 should be possible.

8. Switching to/from Risperdal Consta®(LAI)

8a. Switching to risperidone LAI: It is important to understand the release kinetics of Consta before deciding a switch strategy, i.e. therapeutic levels are not reached until week 4 (i.e. just before the third injection), but only reach optimum in weeks 5–6 (i.e. after the third injection). Assessment of the response to oral risperidone is strongly recommended before giving the first injection, then giving oral for 3–4 weeks, or more. Consta may have the best chance of success if the person has been shown to respond to oral risperidone first.

8b. Oral antipsychotics to risperidone LAI Continue for three weeks after starting Consta, then discontinue step-wise during week 4 (preferably through time-limited prescriptions to avoid polypharmacy). There has been a study of three **olanzapine** to risperidone switches:

1. Olanzapine stopped abruptly, risperidone started immediately and increased as usual.
2. Gradual 1; week 1 olanzapine reduced by 50% for a week and risperidone started; week 2 olanzapine stopped.
3. Gradual 2; week 1 olanzapine full dose, risperidone started; week 2 olanzapine 50%; week 3 olanzapine stopped.

Gradual 2 had the least drop-outs and the best outcomes (n = 123 [c = 97], RCT, open, 6/52, Ganguli et al, BMC Med 2008;**6**:17).

8c. Typical depot to risperidone LAI: Janssen Cilag recommend starting Risperdal Consta® one week before the last fortnightly injection, with an oral drug available if the risk of relapse is high. Or, switch on the depot due date, supplementing with oral risperidone for 3–4 weeks.

8d. Oral risperidone to risperidone LAI: Continue risperidone for three weeks, then gradually discontinue in week 4.

8e. Risperidone LAI to others: The last dose of Consta will finally stop releasing risperidone about six weeks later, so wait until then and introduce the new antipsychotic gradually from about day 42.

9. Switching to/from quetiapine

Quetiapine has a short receptor half-life so warn women about a possible normalisation of prolactin and the need for adequate oral contraception if necessary. A switching study to quetiapine XL from other antipsychotics (mostly conventionals and risperidone) used:

- Day 1: 300 mg plus 75% previous antipsychotic
- Day 2: 600 mg plus 50% previous;
- Day 3: 400–800 mg/d plus 25% of previous, then stop
- Day 4: 400–800 mg over four days.

63% of the completers achieved clinical benefit and tolerated the switch (n = 477 [c = 370], open, 12/52, Ganesan et al, Curr Med Res Opin 2008;**24**:21–32; MS).

9a. Phenothiazine to quetiapine: Switch 3 may be reasonable. Be aware of additional initial postural hypotension, so a slightly slower dose titration or additional monitoring might be prudent.

9b. D2-blocker to quetiapine: Switch 2 or 3 should be tolerable, as receptor blockade with quetiapine is quite different to that of standard D2-blockers.

9c. Typical depot to quetiapine: Switch 2 should be tolerable, starting quetiapine when the next depot dose is due.

9d. Aripiprazole to quetiapine: Quetiapine will not displace aripiprazole from receptors, so the onset of quetiapine's action will be dependent upon the rate at which aripiprazole dissociates from dopamine and serotonin receptors.

9e. Clozapine to quetiapine: Switches 2, 3 or 4 should be tolerable, depending on the reason for the switch.

9f. Olanzapine to quetiapine: Any switch should be acceptable.

9g. Risperidone to quetiapine: Switches 2 or 3 should be tolerable. An abrupt switch from risperidone (mean 1.4 mg/d) to quetiapine (mean 87 mg/d) in elderly people (mean age 82) with BPSD was well tolerated, with only three discontinuing (n = 67, open, Madhusoodanan and Bogunovic, Am J Alzheimer's Dis Other Demen 2006;**21**:169–74).

9h. Switching from quetiapine: There are few obvious problems with stopping or switching from quetiapine (except perhaps NMS), so switches 2 or 3 should be OK (for review see Weiden, J Psychopharmacol 2006;**20**:104–18).

10. Switching D2-blockers to phenothiazines

Switches 2 or 3 should be considered first.

11. Switching D2-blocker to D2 blocker

Consider switches 1–3 first, bearing in mind the potential for NMS and additional EPSE. For a general, waffly review on switching to or from amisulpride, see Peuskens (Curr Med Res Opin 2002;**18**[Suppl 3]:S23–S28).

12. Switching to/from asenapine

The US PI for asenapine recommends gradual discontinuation and minimising overlap with other antipsychotics.

13. Switching to/from olanzapine pamoate*

There is no systematic data on switching to or from olanzapine pamoate. Switching to it should present few problems as olanzapine pamoate takes 12 weeks to reach steady state, so some crossover, e.g. switches 2–4 would be viable. Switching from olanzapine pamoate requires a gradual switch, as olanzapine levels can persist for up to 6–8 months after discontinuation and close supervision is required for at least 2 months post-switch.

14. Switching to/from ziprasidone *

14a. Haloperidol to ziprasidone: This has a good completion rate with, surprisingly, some weight increase (n = 99 [c = 67, 68%], open, 12/52, Alptekin et al, Int Clin Psychopharmacol 2009;**24**:229–38).

14b. Olanzapine to ziprasidone: Again, this has a good completion rate, with some weight reduction (n = 82 [c = 71, 86%], open, 12/52, Alptekin et al, Int Clin Psychopharmacol 2009; **24**: 229–38).

14c. Risperidone to ziprasidone: This has an average completion rate, with some weight reduction (n = 104 [c = 62, 60%], open, 12/52, Alptekin et al, Int Clin Psychopharmacol 2009;**24**:229–38).

14d. Aripiprazole to ziprasidone:* Cross-tapering with aripiprazole reduced stepwise over 4/52, while ziprasidone is increased to up to 160mg/d maximum over same time has been used. Switching in non-responsive or intolerant patients improved depression, negative symptoms and metabolic symptoms, but this was balanced by sedation and raised prolactin (n = 19, open, 12/52, Kim et al, Clin Neuropharmacol 2010; **33**:121–5).

14e. First generation antipsychotics (FGA) to ziprasidone:* Three FGAs have been tried (the ziprasidone dose in all 3 was 40mg BD for 2/7, then titrated up to 80mg BD):

- Switch 1: Abrupt discontinuation of FGA on day 1 (n=18)
- Switch 2: FGA 50% from days 1–7, then stopped (n=18)
- Switch 3: FGA 100% days 1 and 2, 50% from days 3–7, then stopped (n=18).

The slowest switch (3) may have improved BPRS quicker, but all were statistically the same at the end-point (n = 54, open, RCT, 6/52, Stip et al, Prog Neuropsychopharmacol Biol Psychiatry 2010;**34**:997–1000).

15. Switching to/from paliperidone palmitate (Xeplion®) *

15a. Oral risperidone or paliperidone to paliperidone palmitate LAI: Discontinue oral same day or day before Xeplion® (Janssen Cilag) LAI starts using standard commencement (SmPC).

15b. Oral (other) antipsychotic to paliperidone palmitate: LAI:

- No previous exposure to paliperidone or risperidone: give a short course of oral risperidone or paliperidone to assure no idiosyncratic response to the molecule, then commence as per standard (SmPC).
- Previous tolerated exposure to paliperidone or risperidone: no short oral course is needed, commence as standard.
- Previous exposure to paliperidone or risperidone but no reponse or not tolerated: assuming compliance then Xeplion® is not suitable.

15c. Risperidone LAI to paliperidone palmitate: LAI: Start Xeplion® when the next Consta® dose is due and go straight to monthly (see Table 2.2.4 for dose equivalent).

15d. Another depot to paliperidone palmitate: LAI: Start Xeplion® when the next depot dose is due and go straight to monthly.

15e. Paliperidone palmitate LAI to oral antipsychotic: Start oral antipsychotic when the next depot dose is due, but titrate slowly as paliperidone levels can persist for up to 6 months.

15f. Paliperidone palmitate LAI to Consta®: Start Consta® when the next depot dose is due.

15g. Paliperidone palmitate LAI to another depot injection: There are no official recommendations, but start the new depot slowly to avoid additive ADRs and NMS as paliperidone levels can persist for up to 6 months.

16. Prolactin warning

Warn women about the possibility of currently raised prolactin (particularly with D2-blockers) causing amenorrhoea, and normalisation of prolactin with the new drug and, if necessary, the need for adequate oral contraception.

17. Discontinuing antipsychotics

Stopping an antipsychotic has three main risks; discontinuation symptoms, withdrawal/rebound psychosis, and relapse. Discontinuing gradually is the ideal and has the lowest incidence of these adverse outcomes. See individual drugs for their specific reports:

17a. Withdrawal symptoms

Cholinergic rebound (Lieberman, *Psychosomatics* 1981;**22**:253–4) from abrupt withdrawal of phenothiazine and other low-potency antipsychotics can include headache, restlessness, nausea, emesis, anorexia, diarrhoea, rhinorrhea, diaphoresis, myalgia, paraesthesia, anxiety (Dilsaver and Alessi, *Acta Psychiatr Scand* 1988; **77**:241–6) and rebound insomnia (n = 3, van Sweden, *Pharmacopsychiatry* 1987;**20**:116–9). When switching to high-potency antipsychotics, 85% suffer insomnia, anxiety and tensional restlessness (akathisia), again probably from cholinergic rebound (n = 26, Chouinard *et al*, *J Clin Psychiatry* 1984;**45**:500–2). Dramatic withdrawal-emergent cachexia (loss of weight, appetite, muscle atrophy, wasting) has also been reported in learning disabilities (n = 10, Mikkelsen *et al*, *N Engl J Med* 1988;**318**:929).

17b. Withdrawal psychosis

Rapid-onset psychosis (so-called 'supersensitivity psychosis') has been reported with antipsychotic withdrawal (incidence possibly 12–20%, peak 24–48 hours), but is less common with gradual compared to abrupt withdrawal (n = 2, Ekblom *et al*, *Psychopharmacology* [Berl] 1984;**83**:293–4), can occur even in bipolar patients (n = 1, Witschy *et al*, *Am J Psychiatry* 1984;**141**:105–6) and usually disappears rapidly on reinstitution. It may occur more with clozapine, possibly because of its short half-life (Baldessarini *et al*, *Arch Gen Psychiatry* 1995;**52**:1071–2).

17c. Relapse

Obviously, if an antipsychotic has been effective, discontinuation risks relapse. Relapse after gradual withdrawal may be heralded by anxiety, agitation, restlessness and insomnia (Dilsaver and Alessi, *Acta Psychiatr Scand* 1988;**77**:241–6). A number of studies and analyses (e.g. Moncrieff, *Acta Psychiatr Scand* 2006;**114**:3–13) have concluded that:

- About 25–50% relapse within 10–12 weeks (s = 66, n = 4365), 50% after 6/12 (s = 13, n = 1210)
- The relapse rate with slow discontinuation (32%) is half that of rapid discontinuation (65%)
- People who remain stable after 6/12 tend to remain relapse-free without medication (n = 1210, retrospective, Viguera *et al*, *Arch Gen Psychiatry* 1997;**54**:49–55).

17d. Discontinuing aripiprazole

Supersensitivity psychosis has been reported after tapering aripiprazole (n = 1, Chang *et al*, *Prog Neuropsychopharmacol Biol Psychiatry* 2009; **33**:388–9).

17e. Discontinuing clozapine

Sudden discontinuation of clozapine due to a blood dyscrasia is sometimes necessary and can lead to more difficult to treat psychosis in TRS, e.g. in a retrospective comparison, doses needed to be 43% higher on re-treatment (n = 43), compared to 12.5% lower if the person (n = 12) had stayed on clozapine (n = 55, Miodowniok et

Median and near maximal daily dose		
Drug	**ED 50**	**ED 85–95**
Oral:		
Chlorpromazine	150 mg	400–450 mg
Fluphenazine	–	< 6.9 mg
Haloperidol	0.5–2 mg	3.5–10 mg
Trifluoperazine	–	10–15 mg/d
Amisulpride	50 mg	200 mg
Aripiprazole	< 1.5	10 mg/d
Clozapine		> 400 mg
Olanzapine	9 mg	> 16 mg
Quetiapine	80–215 mg	150–600 mg
Risperidone	2 mg	4 mg
Sertindole	10 mg	12–20 mg
Depots		
Fluphenazine dec	–	25 mg/fortnight
Risperidone		
Consta	15 mg/mon	50 mg/mon

TABLE 2.2.4: ANTIPSYCHOTIC DOSE EQUIVALENTS *

Oral	mg/d (+ range)
Chlorpromazine	100mg (25–50mg IM or 250mg rectally)
Fluphenazine	2mg (1.25–5mg)
Levomepromazine	NK
Pericyazine	24mg
Perphenazine	8mg (7–15mg)
Promazine	100mg (50–200mg)
Trifluoperazine	5mg (2–8mg)
Benperidol	2mg
Haloperidol §	3mg (1–5mg), or 1.5mg IM/IV for doses up to 20mg
Flupentixol	2mg
Zuclopenthixol	25mg (25–60mg), up to a maximum of 150mg/d
Pimozide	2mg (25–60mg) up to 1a maximum of 50mg/d
Amisulpride	100mg (40–150mg)
Sulpiride	200mg (200–333mg)
Clozapine	100mg (30–150mg)
Olanzapine	NE
Quetiapine	NE
Paliperidone	NE
Risperidone	0.5-1mg (0.5–3mg)
Depots and LAIs *	**mg/week**
Flupentixol decanoate	10mg (8–20mg)
Fluphenazine decanoate	5–10mg (1–12.5mg)
Fluspirilene	2mg (NE)
Haloperidol decanoate	15mg (5–25mg)
Olanzapine pamoate *	Should only be used for people responding to oral olanzapine. See *Chapter 1* for oral to depot dose equivalent
Pipothiazine palmitate	10mg (5–12.5mg)
Risperidone Consta LAI	12.5mg (25mg/fortnight)
Zuclopenthixol decanoate	100mg (40–100mg)
Paliperidone palmitate *	6.25mg (around 25mg a month)

§ The bioavailability of oral haloperidol is about 50-60% of IM, with IV approximately equivalent to IM.

Key:

NE = Not fully established

90mg (75–100) = Recommended average dose + ranges quoted in the literature. The wider the range, the greater the uncertainty about the exact equivalent

> **The actual dose of a new drug required =**
>
> $$\frac{\text{Current total daily (oral) or weekly (depot) dose of the existing drug}}{\text{Equivalent dose stated for the existing drug in that form}} \times \text{equivalent dose of the new drug as stated in that table}$$

al, J Clin Psychiatry 2006;**67**:1204–8). After sudden withdrawal of 200 mg/d clozapine taken for 4/52 (in schizophrenia in remission),

- 39% (11/28) had no withdrawal symptoms
- 43% (12/28) had mild symptoms (agitation, headache, nausea)
- 14% (4/28) had moderate symptoms (nausea, vomiting, diarrhoea)
- 4% (1/28) had rebound psychosis requiring hospitalisation for manic episodes.

Most symptoms occurred within 24–36 hours and resolved over 3–7 days (n = 30 [c = 28], 7/7, open, Shiovitz *et al, Schizophr Bull* 1996;**22**:591–5).

A major mechanism of clozapine withdrawal symptoms is cholinergic rebound, within 24–48 hours of stopping, with reports of limb and neck dystonias, choreoform movements, dyskinesias lasting 5–14 days (n = 4, Ahmed *et al, J Clin Psychiatry* 1998;**59**:472–7), delirium (n = 3, Stanillla *et al, J Clin Psychiatry* 1997;**58**:252–5), and oculogyric crisis (n = 1, Mendhekar and Duggal, *J Neuropsychiatry Clin Neurosci* 2006;**18**:424–3). Other withdrawal symptoms reported include *de novo* OCD (n = 2, Poyurovsky *et al, Clin Neuropharmacol* 1998;**21**:97–100), Tourette-like tics (n = 1, Poyurovsky *et al, Clin Neuropharmacol* 1998;**21**:97–100), catatonia (after abrupt withdrawal, n = 1, Yeh *et al, Clin Neuropharmacol* 2004;**27**:216–8), rebound insomnia (n = 1, Staedt *et al, Eur Arch Psychiatry Clin Neurosci* 1996;**246**:79–82), severe akathisia with suicidal and autoaggressive behaviour (n = 1, Poyurovsky *et al, Int Clin Psychopharmacol* 1996;**11**:283-6) and NMS (n = 1, Margetic and Aukst-Margetic, *Prog Neuropsychopharmacol Biol Psychiatry* 2005;**29**:14507). Most dramatically resolve on recommencement, or use of anticholinergics (De Leon *et al, J Clin Psychiatry* 1994; **55**:119–20). They may occur in 25% clozapine patients (< 300 mg/d), but this is reduced significantly if switching to olanzapine (n = 106, RCT, d/b, p/c, Tollefson *et al, J Clin Psychopharmacol* 1999;**19**:435–43).

16f. Discontinuing haloperidol

Rebound psychosis (n = 1, Kahne, *Can J Psychiatry* 1989;**34**:227–9) and dyskinesia (n = 1, Sexson and Barak, *J Perinatol* 1989;**9**:170–2; n = 5, Riker *et al, Chest* 1997;**111**:1778–81) have been reported with haloperidol.

17g. Discontinuing olanzapine

Supersensitivity psychosis 48 hours after sudden olanzapine discontinuation has been reported (n = 3, Llorca *et al, Can J Psychiatry* 2001;**46**:87–8), as has myoclonus (as part of a possible serotonin syndrome caused by serotonin rebound) after a six-month course (n = 1, Nayudu and Scheftner, *J Clin Psychopharmacol* 2000;**20**:489–90).

17h. Discontinuing quetiapine

Acute withdrawal symptoms such as nausea, vomiting, insomnia, headache, diarrhoea, dizziness, chorea (Jiménez-Caballero *et al, Rev Neurol* 2004;**38**:1094) and irritability have been reported with acute cessation of high doses. In one case, these occurred within 24 hours of a dose reduction, where a very slow taper or ondansetron did not help, but prochlorperazine did (n = 1, Kim and Staab, *Am J Psychiatry* 2005; **162**:1020). The SmPC recommends withdraw over at least 1–2 weeks.

17i. Discontinuing risperidone

Risperidone discontinuation symptoms have included tics (Rowan and Malone, *J Am Acad Child Adolesc Psychiatry* 1997;**36**:162–3), dyskinesia during dose reduction (n = 1, Anand and Dewan, *Ann Clin Psychiatry* 1996;**8**:179–82), or abrupt discontinuation, (n = 1, Miller, *Ann Pharmacother* 2000;**34**:269), respiratory dyskinesia, e.g. involuntary movements of respiratory muscles, and grunting (n = 1, Ehrt *et al, J Clin Psychopharmacol* 2005;**25**:609) and akathisia (n = 2, Bertolín Guillén *et al, Actas Esp Psiquiatr* 2002;**30**:195–7).

Reviews: neuroleptic discontinuation syndromes (Tranter and Healy, *J Psychopharmacol* 1998;**12**: 401–6; Baldessarini and Viguera, *Arch Gen Psychiatry* 1995;**52**:189–92; Moncrieff, *Acta Psychiatr Scand* 2006;**114**:3–13).

2.2.1.3 ANTIPSYCHOTIC DOSE EQUIVALENTS

The antipsychotic dose(s) of each drug within each heading of this section are approximately equivalent to others under the same heading (e.g. perphenazine 24 mg/d is equivalent to chlorpromazine 300 mg/d and to flupentixol 60 mg 2/52), based on the references indicated. There is, however, a genuine lack of agreement about antipsychotic equivalents. This is mainly because the four methods of assessing antipsychotic equivalence (clinical studies, non-clinical/receptor binding studies, median effective doses and manufacturers' information) can produce up to a five-fold difference in the equivalents calculated. This is particularly true in the case of high-potency antipsychotics. Ranges quoted here are thus unweighted for individual variation and are valid, but imprecise. The five methods are:

1. Clinical studies — there aren't any.

2. Receptor binding — antipsychotics displace ligands from dopamine receptors (particularly D2) at a rate that to some extent correlates with their antipsychotic potency and so roughly equivalent antipsychotic doses can be calculated. However, some dose relationships, e.g. haloperidol, are unlikely to be linear and sedation and anxiety may not be directly related to dopamine blockade. High-potency drugs, e.g. haloperidol and fluphenazine, have the highest quoted variance, over 1000% in some cases, which may lead to prescribing in higher doses than necessary (Dewan and Koss, *Acta Psychiatr Scand* 1995;**91**:229–32). Additionally, higher doses of antipsychotics tend to be used to control disruptive behaviour rather than just to control psychotic symptoms (Peralta *et al*, *Acta Psychiatr Scand* 1994;**90**:354–7).

3. Median effective doses — median effective doses (ED50) and near maximal effective doses (ED85 to ED95) can be used (systematic review and meta-analysis, Davis and Chen, *J Clin Psychopharmacol* 2004;**24**:192–208; review by Woods, *EBMH* 2004;**7**:106).

4. Percentage of maximum dose — this has been proposed as an alternative, but is also imprecise, as maximum doses may not be equivalent, e.g. is flupentixol decanoate 400 mg a week really equivalent to 50 mg a week of fluphenazine decanoate? Defined daily doses (DDDs) are an alternative to CPZ equivalents, but do not really match up as they assume optimum doses are being used, which is not always the case (Rikcken *et al*, *J Clin Psychopharmacol* 2003;**23**:657–9).

Antipsychotic equivalence is specifically quoted here and the doses are as accurate as data allows, but to avoid any confusion you must consider the following:

1. Antipsychotic equivalence must not be confused with sedation, e.g. there may be no extra antipsychotic effect from haloperidol above 8–12 mg/d (see *1.10.4*). If using a sedating 'broad-spectrum' drug (e.g. a phenothiazine) and converting to a D2 receptor selective drug (e.g. flupentixol, sulpiride, etc), the use of conversion tables

may not thus be appropriate and may result in enhanced side-effects or over-dosage.

2. With some drugs there may not be a linear relationship between the dose and the antipsychotic effect.

3. Dose frequency with depots may be important as the first pass effect may reduce the effective doses of oral preparations.

4. Differing half-lives may complicate the calculations and final dose recommendation.

5. These equivalent doses are not necessarily equivalent in terms of maximum doses.

6. For the newer antipsychotics, therapeutic doses are better defined and so no equivalent doses are appropriate.

You should always check your answer against the SmPC to ensure an inappropriately high dose is not inadvertently considered (review, Atkins *et al*, *Psychiatr Bull* 1997;**21**:224–6).

Review: general (Remington *et al*, *Am J Psychiatry* 1998;**155**:1301–2).

2.2.1.4 POST-SWITCHING ANTIPSYCHOTIC ISSUES

(Based on an extensive review by Weiden *et al*, *J Clin Psychiatry* 1998;**59**[Suppl 19]:36–49.)

Assessing response:

1. For all drugs, aim for a minimum of three months at full therapeutic dosage.

2. Be cautious of any significant gains (e.g. reduced side-effects) within 6/52 of the last drug stopping, as drug concentrations at receptor level may outlast plasma levels (see haloperidol, *1.25*).

3. Even if gains occur, make sure a full therapeutic trial is achieved, as discontinuation of the previous drug will lead to a gradual loss of its side-effects (including cognitive impairment), which may be interpreted as improvement.

4. If therapeutic gains occur, it has been suggested to delay discontinuing any anticholinergic and/or antiakathisia drugs until during the second month.

5. Raised prolactin levels may take over 3/12 to resolve, so women need to be warned about this, and to ensure that they have adequate contraceptive cover.

6. If positive changes occur, caution the patient not to risk relapse by 'over-doing it'.

Managing a sub-optimum response to a switch:

1. No improvement by 6/52 — exclude non-compliance with the switch, substance misuse and inadequate dosage. Try to work towards 12/52 at full dose.
2. Some response by 6/52 — do not get too excited, continue to 12/52.
3. Partial response between 6/52 and 12/52 — consider an increase in dose, and try to go for a 6/12 trial.
4. Initial response followed by worsening of positive symptoms — check worsening is not actually improvement (e.g. previous positive symptoms hidden by the patient now surfacing), try to restabilise and aim for 12/52 at full dose.

Long-term issues:

1. With improvements in insight, increased psychosocial support and monitoring will be needed to reduce the risk of post-psychotic depression and self-harm.

2.2.2 SWITCHING BENZODIAZEPINES

Switching benzodiazepines may be advantageous for a variety of reasons, e.g. to a drug with a longer half-life before discontinuation. While there is broad agreement in the literature about equivalent doses, clonazepam has a wide variety of reported equivalences and particular care is needed with this drug. Inter-patient variability and differing half-lives means that the figures can never be exact and should be interpreted using your own pharmaceutical knowledge.

2.2.3 SWITCHING ANTICHOLINERGICS

See 6.7 about the overall indications for the use of anticholinergics. Equivalent doses are:

Orphenadrine	50mg
Procyclidine	2mg
Trihexyphenidyl (benzhexol)	2mg

2.2.4 SWITCHING DRUGS OF ABUSE OR DEPENDENCE

Switching drugs of abuse/dependence, usually to methadone, is a common strategy. *Table*

TABLE 2.2.5: BENZODIAZEPINE EQUIVALENT DOSES

See note in introduction regarding half lives

Diazepam	5mg (oral, im, or iv)
Alprazolam	0.5mg (0.25–0.5mg)
Chlordiazepoxide	15mg (10–25mg)
Clobazam	10mg
Clonazepam	0.5mg (0.25–4)
Flunitrazepam	0.5mg
Flurazepam	7.5–15mg
Loprazolam	0.5–1mg
Lorazepam	0.5–1mg at 4mg/d
	2mg at 5mg/d
Lormetazepam	0.5–1mg
Nitrazepam	5mg (2.5–20mg)
Oxazepam	15mg (10–40mg)
Temazepam	10mg

2.2.6 may be of some use, although caution is obviously necessary regarding, e.g. the potency of individual samples of street drugs.

Advice:

1. Most of these equivalent doses are based on **analgesic** equivalents, which may differ by a factor of 10 to the dose needed to suppress opiate withdrawal symptoms.
2. The dose relationship may be non-linear, especially at higher doses and above BNF limits.
3. Analgesic equivalents are mostly derived from single-dose studies, not long-term studies where a steady state has been achieved.
4. Total daily doses should be calculated.
5. These are definitely **not** starter doses, but may give an idea of a possible maximum. The person should be dose titrated and assessed, based on withdrawal symptoms and clinical response.
6. Analgesic equivalents for tramadol produce a much higher methadone equivalent. The tramadol dose here is based on a study showing tramadol 450mg/d is equivalent to 15mg/d methadone for suppressing opiate withdrawal symptoms (n = 70, RCT, d/b, Salehi *et al, J Res Med Sci* 2006;**11**:185–9). NB. SR, dispersable and liquid and tramadol may have different bioavailabilities.
7. Codeine is metabolised by 2D6 to active

TABLE 2.2.6: METHADONE EQUIVALENT DOSES

Narcotics

Drug	Total daily dose	Equivalent daily dose of methadone in mg	Range quoted	
			Lower	Upper
Buprenorhine injection	0.3mg	8	8	8
Buprenorphine S/L	0.2mg	5	5	8
Codeine linctus 15mg/5ml	1ml	0.2	0.2	0.2
Codeine phosphate	15mg	1	1	1
Dextropropoxyphene	32.5mg	2.145	2.145	2.145
Diamorphine BP injection	5mg	10	10	10
Diamorphine BP oral	10mg	10	10	20
Diconal tablets	1 tab	5	4	5
Dihydrocodeine	30mg	2.5	2	3
Fentanyl patches (**mcg/hr**)	25mcg/hr	2	1.65	2.5
Gee's Linctus	100ml	10	10	10
Hydromorphone oral	1mg	2.5	2.5	6.5
J Collis Brown's (**mls**)	100mls	10	10	10
Morphine BP injection	10mg	10	10	10
Morphine BP oral	15mg	10	10	10
MST tablets	10mg	3.25	3.25	3.25
Oxycodone	1mg	0.8	0.4	1.32
Palfium	5mg	5	5	10
Papaveretum	10mg	4.4		
Pentazocine	25mg	2	2	2
Pethidone injection/tablets	50mg	4.25	4	5
Tramadol	50mg	1.6	1.6	8.25

morphine, so any 2D6 slow or ultra-rapid metabolisers will affect the equivalent dose.

8. Some texts recommend that when changing from weaker to stronger opioids, reduce the dose by up to 30–50%, as there is often incomplete cross tolerance due to different binding profiles and also increased sedation.

9. Dihydrocodeine SR (DHC) is 95–100% absorbed so the total daily dose is the same for plain tablets (information from Napp).

2.2.5 SWITCHING ADHD TREATMENTS

Methylphenidate to atomoxetine:

Although this switch can be done quickly, a slower switch is generally recommended to minimise adverse effects, as they can be given together. About 50% of methylphenidate non-responders will respond to atomoxetine and 75% methylphenidate responders will also respond to

Switching methylphenidate preparations: *

IR-MPH, Equasym XL, Medikinet XL	Concerta XL equivalent dose
10mg/d	
15mg	18mg
20mg	
30mg	36mg
40mg	
45mg	54mg
50mg	72mg (unlicensed)

atomoxetine (Prasad and Steer, *Paediatr Drugs* 2008;**10**:39–47).

Week 1 = full-dose methylphenidate, plus atomoxetine 0.5mg/kg/d

Week 2 = half-dose methylphenidate, plus atomoxetine 1.2mg/kg/d

Week 3 = stop methylphenidate, atomoxetine 1.2 mg/kg/d

Ref: (n = 69 [c = 58], open, Quintana et al, Clin Ther 2007;**29**:1168–77).

2.2.6 SWITCHING ANTI-CHOLINESTERASES

Switching anticholinesterases:
Switching anticholinesterases may be necessary for tolerability, lack of efficacy, or long-term loss of efficacy. There is no data on the last point. There are subtle differences in receptor modulation between the anticholinesterases and so lack of response to one does not necessarily exclude response to another. There is no published data on the outcome of switching to donepezil.

Donepezil to galantamine:
One review suggested that the response rate to galantamine may be the same regardless of non-response to donepezil (Emre, Int J Clin Pract Suppl 2002;**127**:64–72) and is well tolerated (n = 4, Bartorelli et al, Curr Med Res Opin 2005;**21**:1809–18).

Donepezil to rivastigmine oral/patches:*
It has been reported that in donepezil non-response, around 50% will then respond to rivastigmine (n = 382, Auriacombe et al, Curr Med Res Opin 2002;**18**:129–38; n = 188, Bartorelli et al, Curr Med Res Opin 2005;**21**:1809–18). An immediate switch from donepezil 5–10 mg/d to rivastigmine patches 4.6 mg/24 hours may be well-tolerated and safe, but a slower switch might be appropriate with any pre-existing bradycardia or if concurrent beta-blockers are being taken, the incidence of nausea and vomiting being 4% and 1% respectively (open, Sadowsky et al, Am J Alzheimer's Dis Other Demen 2009;**24**:267–75). Abrupt switch from donepezil to oral rivastigmine (without washout) may be effective and well-tolerated (n = 146, open, 12/12, Figiel et al, Prim Care Companion J Clin Psychiatry 2008;**10**:363–7 and 291–8, MS; review of three switching studies; Sadowsky et al, Int J Clin Pract 2010;**64**:188–93).

Galantamine plain to galantamine XL:
A manufacturer's computer simulation suggests that an abrupt switch should be acceptable (Hing et al, Curr Med Res Opin 2005;**21**:482–8).

Galantamine to rivastigmine patches:
A review has concluded that galantamine can be switched abruptly to the patch, with nausea or vomiting in only 2–3% (Sadowsky et al, CNS Neurosci Ther 2010; **16**:51–60), and that response to rivastigmine can occur despite non-response to galantamine (n = 33, Bartorelli et al, Curr Med Res Opin 2005;**21**:1809–18).

Rivastigmine to galantamine:
One review has suggested that the response rate to galantamine may be the same regardless of non-response to other anticholinesterases (Emre, Int J Clin Pract Suppl 2002;**127**:64–72).

Rivastigmine oral to rivastigmine patches:*
A review has concluded that rivastigmine oral high dose can be switched abruptly to the 9.5 mg/24-hour patch, but low dose should be switched to 4.6 mg/24-hour for four weeks before increasing. The incidence of nausea and vomiting is 3% and 2% respectively (Sadowsky et al, CNS Neurosci Ther 2010;**16**:51–60). The first patch should be applied the day after the last oral dose:

Rivastigmine oral dose per day	Patch strength
3–6 mg	4.6 mg/24 hours
9 mg (not stable/poorly tolerated)	4.6 mg/24 hours
9 mg (stable and well-tolerated)	9.5 mg/24 hours
12 mg	9.5 mg/24 hours

Review: expert consensus (Gauthier et al, Curr Med Res Opin 2003;**19**:707–14).

2.2.7 SWITCHING OR DIS-CONTINUING ANTIDEPRESSANTS *

Switching from one antidepressant to another, either for reasons of side-effects, safety or lack of efficacy, can be problematical and present unexpected problems. Clinicians must be aware of these to eliminate avoidable adverse events. However, a meta-analysis of the three double blind switching studies failed to show that switching was superior to sticking (s = 3, d/b, Bschor and Baethge, Acta Psychiatr Scand 2010; **121**:174–9).

1. Agomelatine to/from others *

Agomelatine has no apparent significant problem with other antidepressants so should be able to be switched to and from with negligible risk (except fluvoxamine, which inhibits 1A2 and

2

raises levels significantly). It is recommended to be careful until more data is available (thorough review by McAllister-Williams *et al, Hum Psychopharmacol* 2010;**25**:95–102).

2. SSRI to/from TCA

Fluoxetine, paroxetine and fluvoxamine (but probably not citalopram, escitalopram and sertraline at standard doses) can double or triple tricyclic levels (particularly of amitriptyline,

---

Factors to consider before choosing an antidepressant switching regimen

- Speed at which the switch is needed, e.g. with less urgency a more cautious regimen can be used, e.g. drugs that can be used in combination. Faster switches can obviously be made, but additional monitoring is recommended.
- Current dose of the first drug.
- Individual drugs and their effects, neurotransmitter effects, kinetics, etc.
- Individuals' susceptibility to (additive) ADRs.

Potential problems

- Cholinergic rebound, e.g. headache, restlessness, diarrhoea, nausea and vomiting (Lieberman, *Psychosomatics* 1981;**22**:253–4) from withdrawal of drugs blocking cholinergic receptors, e.g. tricyclics.
- Antidepressant withdrawal or discontinuation symptoms (see *13*).
- Serotonin syndrome, for drugs affecting serotonin (see *6.9*).
- Drug-drug interactions e.g. changed drug levels from altered metabolism (see *4.3*).
- Discontinuation effects from the first drug being interpreted as side-effects of the second.

Switching drugs 'with care' means

- Drop and stop first drug.
- Leave a gap of a few days if possible.
- Warn the patient about potential complications and what to do about them, e.g. serotonin syndrome, cholinergic rebound, toxicity and discontinuation.

---

imipramine, nortriptyline and clomipramine), by CYP2D6 inhibition and so great care is needed. Prescribing both drugs together over a change-over period is not advised unless the drugs and doses are chosen carefully and specific care is taken. Ideally, 'drop-and-stop' before starting the next drug is recommended (switch 1 or 2).

Factors to be considered with an SSRI-tricyclic switch:

- Speed at which the switch is needed, e.g. faster switches can obviously be made, but additional monitoring, e.g. tricyclic levels and cardiac status is recommended.
- SSRI dose — CYP2D6 inhibition is dose-related for most drugs, e.g. paroxetine, fluoxetine.
- Tricyclic — stronger serotonin reuptake inhibitors are more likely to produce serotonin syndrome (e.g. clomipramine),
- Tertiary tricyclics (e.g. imipramine, amitriptyline, clomipramine) are also metabolised by CYP3A3/4 and CYP1A2, which are inhibited by fluvoxamine.
- P450 status of the patient ie slow or rapid metaboliser (see *4.2*).
- Individual susceptibility to tricyclic and SSRI side-effects.

Main potential problems (see introduction for more details):

- Cholinergic rebound from tricyclics.
- Tricyclic/SSRI discontinuation symptoms (see reference *13*).
- Serotonin syndrome (see *6.9*).
- Increased tricyclic levels via CYP2D6 inhibition by SSRIs (see *4.3.1*).

Suggested switch regimens:

Tricyclic to fluoxetine, paroxetine or fluvoxamine: Taper tricyclic dose to around 25–50 mg/d, start SSRI at usual starting dose and discontinue tricyclic over next 5–7 days. Be wary of serotonin syndrome, raised tricyclic levels by P450 inhibition, cholinergic rebound and tricyclic withdrawal.

Tricyclic to citalopram, escitalopram or sertraline: Taper tricyclic as above, but there is a much lower potential for interactions so problems are less likely and serotonin syndromes have been reported.

Fluoxetine to tricyclic: Drop fluoxetine to 20 mg/d, stop, wait several days for peak levels to fall, then add the tricyclic **cautiously at low**

dose and build up slowly. Care is needed for up to four weeks as the interaction potential via 2D6 inhibition may be prolonged (see *4.3.2*), e.g. an abrupt switch from fluoxetine 20mg/d to amitriptyline 50–100mg/d resulted in 14% dropping out due to adverse reactions, the rest tolerating the switch (Rutten *et al*, MI). Be wary of serotonin syndrome (especially with drugs such as clomipramine) and higher tricyclic levels via CYP2D6 inhibition.

Paroxetine to tricyclic: Leave a gap if possible or taper paroxetine to about 10mg/d, and introduce the tricyclic at low dose. After several days, discontinue paroxetine and increase tricyclic dose to therapeutic levels. Be wary of paroxetine withdrawal (see *17*), serotonin syndrome (especially with drugs such as clomipramine) and higher tricyclic levels via CYP2D6 inhibition.

Fluvoxamine to tricyclic: As paroxetine. Be wary of fluvoxamine withdrawal (rare, see *17*), serotonin syndrome (especially with drugs such as clomipramine) and higher tricyclic levels via CYP1A2 and 3A3/4 inhibition (especially with tertiary tricyclics).

Citalopram, escitalopram or sertraline to tricyclic: If necessary, reduce to minimum doses of citalopram (20mg/d), escitalopram (10mg) or sertraline (50mg/d). Stop the SSRI and introduce the tricyclic, titrating dose upwards as tolerated. With standard doses of these SSRIs, few problems should be seen. Be wary of SSRI withdrawal (rare, see reference *17*), serotonin syndrome (especially with, e.g. clomipramine) and higher tricyclic levels via CYP2D6 inhibition (low risk).

3. Trazodone to/from others

Trazodone to SSRIs: Trazodone and fluoxetine have been used together but the risks include enhanced sedation (e.g. n=8, Nirenberg *et al*, *J Clin Psychiatry* 1992;**53**:83), serotonin syndrome (n=1, George and Godleski, *Biol Psychiatry* 1996;**39**:384–5) and slightly raised trazodone levels (see *4.3.2.2*). A serotonin syndrome with low dose trazodone added to paroxetine (n=1, Reeves and Bullen, *Psychosomatics* 1995;**36**:159–60) would indicate the need for similar care. For citalopram, there is a report of lack of a pharmacokinetic interaction, with no changes in plasma levels (n=40+41 controls; Prapotnik *et al*, *Int J Clin Pharmacol Ther* 2004;**42**:120–4). There

---

How to use *Table 2.2.7*:

i. Look down the vertical column headed 'from' and find the drug, or drug group, the patient is currently taking.

ii. Follow that line along until you come to the column of the drug, or drug group to which you wish to change.

iii. The details there give the current known information. For further details look up the reference number quoted.

Example: Changing from tranylcypromine to a tricyclic requires a 14-day drug-free gap (reference 9), but changing from a tricyclic to tranylcypromine only requires a seven-day drug-free gap (reference 9).

is no information on changing from trazodone to sertraline but a gradual switch, with close observation would seem sensible (see *5*).

Trazodone to tricyclics: hypomania has been reported after an abrupt change to imipramine (n=2, Haggerty and Jackson, *J Clin Psychiatry* 1985;**5**:342–3), so care is needed.

4. Tricyclic to/from tricyclic

No significant problems have been reported but a gradual switch is recommended as per normal practice (switches 1, 2 or 3).

5. SSRI to/from another SSRI

Any combination of SSRIs could precipitate a serotonin syndrome (see *6.9*). Thus, careful observation initially and a gentle changeover is recommended. A washout period would further minimise the possibility of problems.

Fluoxetine to sertraline: be mindful of fluoxetine's long half-life, e.g. in outpatients abruptly switched from fluoxetine to sertraline (20mg:50mg respectively dose substitution), 63% were successful but 37% failed, including 18% with intolerable adverse effects (nervousness, jitters, diarrhoea, nausea and headache), suggestive of a serotonin-like syndrome (n=54, Stock and Kofoed, *Am J Hosp Pharm* 1994;**51**:2279–81).

TABLE 2.2.7: SWITCHING ANTIDEPRESSANTS *

NSPR = no significant problems reported, careful cross-taper; OP = occasional problems; SSP = serotonin syndrome possible

From \ To	MAOIs Hydrazines	MAOIs Tranylcypromine	Tricyclics	SSRIs Citalopram/escitalopram	SSRIs Fluvoxamine	SSRIs Fluoxetine	SSRIs Sertraline	SSRIs Paroxetine	Trazodone	Bupropion[10]	Moclobemide	Venlafaxine	Duloxetine[6]	Mirtazapine[6]	Agomelatine[13]	Reboxetine
Hydrazines	▓	14/7[7]	7–14/7[7]	14/7[7]	14/7[7]	14/7[7]	14/7[7]	14/7[7]	14/7[7] or care	7/7[9]	Read text[7]	14/7[11]	14/7[6]	2/52[7]	NSPR[1]	2/52[7]
Tranylcypromine	14/7[7]	▓	14/7[7]	14/7[7]	14/7[7]	14/7[7]	14/7[7]	14/7[7]	14/7[7]	7/7[9]	Read text[7]	14/7[11]	14/7[6]	2/52[7]	NSPR[1]	2/52[7]
Tricyclics	7/7[7]	7/7[7]	▓	Care[2]	Great care[2]	Great care[2]	Care[2]	Great care[2]	NSPR[10]	NSPR[9]	Read text[7,8]	Care[3]	SSP[5]	NSPR[11]	NSPR[1]	NSPR[12]
Citalopram/escitalopram	7/7[7]	7/7[7]	Care[2]	▓ SSP	SSP[5]	SSP[5]	SSP[5]	SSP[5]	Care	NSPR[9]	7/7[8]	Care[3]	SSP[5]	NSPR[11]	NSPR[1]	NSPR[12]
Fluvoxamine	4–5/7[7]	7–14/7[7]	Great care[2]	SSP[5]	▓	SSP[5]	SSP[5]	SSP[5]	Care	NSPR[9]	3/7[8]	Care[3]	Care SSP[5]	NSPR[11]	Care[1]	NSPR[12]
Fluoxetine	5/52[7]	5/52[7]	Great care for 28/7[2]	SSP[5]	SSP[5]	▓	SSP[5]	SSP[5]	Care	NSPR[10]	3/52[8]	Care[3]	SSP[5]	NSPR[11]	NSPR[1]	NSPR[12]
Sertraline	7–14/7[7]	7–14/7[7]	Great care[2]	SSP[5]	SSP[5]	SSP[5]	▓	SSP[5]	Care	NSPR[9]	7–13/7[8]	Care[3]	SSP[5]	NSPR[11]	NSPR[1]	NSPR[12]
Paroxetine	14/7[7]	14/7[7]	Great care[2]	SSP[5]	SSP[5]	SSP[5]	SSP[5]	▓	Care[6]	NSPR[9]	5/7[8]	Care[3]	SSP[5]	NSPR[11]	NSPR[1]	NSPR[12]
Trazodone	14/7[7]	14/7[7]	OP[3]	Care[3]	Care[3]	Care[3]	Care[3]	Care[3]	▓	NSPR[9]	NSPR	Care[3]	SSP[5]	NSPR[11]	NSPR[1]	NSPR[9]
Bupropion[10]	7/7[7]	7/7[7]	Care	NSPR[8]	NSPR[9]	NSPR[9]	NSPR[9]	NSPR[9]	NSPR[9]	▓	NSPR[9]	NSPR[9]	SSP[8]	NSPR[9,11]	NSPR[1]	NSPR[12]
Moclobemide	NSPR[7]	NSPR[7]	OP[8]	NSPR[8]	NSPR[8]	2/52[8]	NSPR[8]	NSPR[8]	NSPR[13]	NSPR	▓	NSPR[13]	SSP[8]	NSPR[9,11]	NSPR[1]	NSPR[12]
Venlafaxine	7/7[13]	7/7[13]	NSPR[3]	Care[13]	Care[13]	Care[13]	Care[13]	Care[13]	Care[13]	NSPR[13]	NSPR[13]	▓	SSP[6]	NSPR[11]	NSPR[1]	NSPR[12]
Duloxetine	5/7[6]	5/7[6]	SSP[6]	SSP[6] care	SSP[6]	SSP[6]	SSP[6]	SSP[6]	SSP[6]	SSP[6]	SSP[6]	SSP[6,13]	▓	NSPR[11]	NSPR[1]	NSPR[12]
Mirtazapine	7/7[7]	7/7[7]	NSPR[11]	NSPR[11]	NSPR[11]	NSPR[11]	NSPR[11]	NSPR[11]	NSPR[11]	NSPR[11]	NSPR[11]	NSPR[11]	NSPR	▓	NSPR[1]	NSPR[11]
Agomelatine[1]	NSPR[1]	NSPR[1]	NSPR[1]	NSPR[1]	Care[1]	NSPR[1]	NSPR[1]	NSPR[1]	NSPR[1]	NSPR[1]	NSPR[1]	NSPR[1]	NSPR[1]	NSPR[1]	▓	NSPR[1]
Reboxetine	1/52[12]	1/52[12]	NSPR[2]	NSPR[2]	NSPR[12]	NSPR[12]	NSPR[12]	NSPR[12]	NSPR[12]	NSPR[12]	NSPR[12]	NSPR[12]	NSPR[12]	NSPR[1]	NSPR[1]	▓
Just plain stopping[17]	Over 4/52[14]	Over 4/52[14]	Over 4/52[14]	Over 4/52[14]	Over 4/52[14]	Drop to 20mg/d then stop[14]	Over 4/52[14]	Over 4/52[14] or longer	Over 4/52[14]	Over 4/52[14]	Over 4/52[14]	Over 4/52[14] or longer	Over 4/52[14] or longer	Over 4/52[14]	NSPR[14]	Over 4/52[14]

Fluoxetine to paroxetine: abrupt switching has produced an increased level of side-effects such as insomnia, nausea, dry mouth, nervousness and tremor in the immediate switch group, when compared to a two-week washout, which was well tolerated (n = 240, d/b, Kreider et al, J Clin Psychiatry 1995;**56**:142–5; see also n = 9, Dominguez et al, J Clin Psychopharmacol 1996;**16**:320–3).

Fluvoxamine to paroxetine: there is a case of rapidly increased fluvoxamine levels when paroxetine was started during a switch, probably via 2D6 inhibition (n = 1, Hori et al, World J Biol Psychiatry 2009;**10**:620–2).

6. Duloxetine *

SSRIs/venlafaxine to duloxetine: Abruptly stopping an SSRI and starting **duloxetine** was as well-tolerated and safe as tapered SSRI discontinuation and immediate duloxetine starting (n = 368, RCT, 10/52, Perahia et al, J Clin Psychiatry 2008;**69**:95–105). See also 8. Patients switching from SSRIs or venlafaxine to duloxetine have been reported to have less nausea when starting than those starting de novo; immediate switching may be well-tolerated, although fluoxetine was surprisingly excluded from this Lilly study (n = 155, Wohlreich et al, Ann Clin Psychiatry 2005;**17**:259–68, MS) as it could pose particular problems, e.g. serotonin syndrome (n = 1, Liu et al, J Am Geriatr Soc 2009;**57**:2384).

7. MAOIs

MAOI to MAOI: A two-week gap is recommended, especially if switching to tranylcypromine (UK SmPC). Then starting tranyl-cypromine at half the usual dosage for one week. Careful observation is essential. An open study of switching MAOIs with less than a 14-day gap showed that only one patient suffered adverse events, probably tranylcypromine withdrawal or a mild serotonin syndrome and so a shorter gap may be feasible with full dietary control, good compliance and close monitoring (n = 8, Szuba et al, J Clin Psychiatry 1997;**58**:307–10), although deaths have been reported (e.g. n = 1, Bazire, Drug Intell Clin Pharm 1986;**20**:954–56).

SSRIs to MAOIs: The gap between stopping an SSRI and starting an MAOI depends upon the SSRI. The SmPC for tranylcypromine recommends leaving at least a 14-day gap after stopping other antidepressants, then starting tranylcypromine at half the usual dosage for one week.

Fluvoxamine to MAOI: Fluvoxamine has a short half-life and so isocarboxazid/phenelzine may be started 4–5 days after stopping fluvoxamine (4–5 x half-life), or seven days for tranylcypromine.

Paroxetine to MAOI: A two-week gap is recommended (SmPC).

Fluoxetine to MAOI: A serotonin syndrome has been reported when tranylcypromine was started six weeks after fluoxetine was stopped, due to the persistence of norfluoxetine (but not fluoxetine) in the blood (n = 1, Coplan and Gorman, Am J Psychiatry 1993;**150**:837). Since several reported interactions exist, it might be better to allow six weeks after stopping fluoxetine before starting an MAOI (Drug Ther Bull 1990;**28**:334). The isocarboxazid SmPC recommends a gap longer than two weeks.

Sertraline to MAOI: A one-week gap should elapse before starting an MAOI. A serotonergic syndrome has been reported with sertraline and tranylcypromine (see SSRI interactions 4.3.2). The SmPC states that at least a two-week gap between sertraline and MAOIs is needed.

Trazodone to MAOI: The literature recommends a one-week gap. A study of combined treatment did not show hypertensive reactions but an increase in side-effects, e.g. sedation and postural hypotension occurred (n = 13, Nierenberg and Keck, J Clin Psychopharmacol 1989;**9**:42).

Moclobemide to MAOI: Moclobemide has a half-life of 14 hours and so stopping it one day and starting an MAOI the next day is adequate.

Mirtazapine to MAOI: A one-week wash-out period is recommended by the manufacturers, although there are no reports of problems.

Trazodone to MAOI: The SmPC recommends a two-week gap after stopping trazodone before MAOIs.

Tricyclic to MAOI: A one-week gap is re-commended and is advisable particularly if imipramine, clomipramine or tranylcypromine are involved. Low doses of the MAOI are essential.

MAOI to SSRIs: A two-week gap has been recommended (e.g. fluoxetine SmPC), but longer may be safer as a severe serotonin syndrome has been reported with a two-week gap between stopping tranylcypromine and starting fluoxetine (n = 1, Ruiz, *Ann Emerg Med* 1994;**24**:983–5), although tranylcypromine has a relatively short action (i.e. reversible MAO inhibition).

MAOI to moclobemide: A gap is not needed between stopping an MAOI and starting moclobemide, provided MAOI dietary restrictions are maintained for 10–14 days.

MAOI to mirtazapine: A two-week wash-out period is recommended.

MAOI to trazodone: The SmPC recommends a two-week gap after stopping an MAOI before trazodone is started.

MAOIs to tricyclic: A 10–14-day gap is often recommended (isocarboxazid '1–2 weeks'), particularly if imipramine, clomipramine or tranylcypromine are involved. Using initial low doses of the tricyclic is essential.

8. Moclobemide to/from others

Moclobemide to duloxetine: Immediate switching from moclobemide 400 mg/d to duloxetine 60 mg/d has induced serotonin syndrome within an hour (n = 1, Jimenez-Genchi, *J Clin Psychiatry* 2006;**67**:1821–2).

Moclobemide to fluoxetine: The fluoxetine SmPC states that it can be started the day after moclobemide is stopped.

Moclobemide to tricyclic: Abrupt switching from moclobemide to tricyclics appears well-tolerated, but switching to clomipramine has caused problems.

SSRIs to moclobemide: The SmPC recommends a gap of 4–5 half-lives after stopping an SSRI before starting moclobemide, as serotonin syndromes have been reported (see *4.3.3.5*).

Citalopram/escitalopram to moclobemide: A seven-day gap is recommended.

Fluoxetine to moclobemide: With fluoxetine's long half-life, the gap should be as much as six weeks if five times the half-life of norfluoxetine is calculated. A three-week gap together with careful monitoring would seem a reasonably practical figure. However, in a study where up to 600 mg/d moclobemide was added to established fluoxetine therapy, there was no change in the number, intensity, or type of adverse events. Fluoxetine inhibited the metabolism of moclobemide but did not lead to excessive accumulation, with no evidence of a 'serotonin syndrome' (n = 18, RCT, p/c, Dingemanse *et al*,

Clin Pharmacol Ther 1998;**63**:403–13).

Fluvoxamine to moclobemide: A three-day gap is recommended (but see above).

Paroxetine to moclobemide: A five-day gap is recommended (but see above), although paroxetine's half-life can be longer in the elderly. A severe serotonin syndrome has been reported when moclobemide replaced paroxetine with no washout (n = 1, Wu and Deng, *J Chin Med Assoc* 2009;**72**:446–9).

Sertraline to moclobemide: With the long half-life of desmethylsertraline, the gap should be up to 13 days, but only seven days is recommended by the sertraline SmPC (but see above).

Tricyclic to moclobemide: A gap of 4–5 half-lives is recommended if the tricyclic concerned is a 5-HT reuptake inhibitor. However, healthy volunteers taking either clomipramine 100 mg/d or amitriptyline 75 mg/d for at least a week were swapped abruptly to moclobemide (150 mg first day, 300 mg/d thereafter) or placebo. There was no increase in the incidence or severity of side-effects or any significant pharmacokinetic interaction (n = 24, d/b, p/c, Dingemanse *et al*, *J Clin Psychopharmacol* 1995;**15**:41–8).

9. Bupropion

Bupropion is contraindicated with **MAOIs**, as animal studies show that acute bupropion toxicity is enhanced by phenelzine. Co-administration of bupropion with drugs that are metabolised by CYP2D6 (e.g. **tricyclics, paroxetine** and **fluoxetine**) should be approached with caution and initiated at the lower end of the dose range of the concomitant medication. If bupropion is added to the treatment regimen of a patient already receiving a drug metabolised by CYP2D6, the need to decrease the dose of the original medication should be considered, particularly for those with a narrow therapeutic index.

Fluoxetine to bupropion: In fluoxetine non-responders, a switch to bupropion yielded 35% responders and 25% partial responders (n = 29, 12 + 8/52, open, Fava *et al*, *Ann Clin Psychiatry* 2003;**15**:17–22).

10. Tryptophan to/from others

Adding tryptophan to existing therapy is far

more common than switching to tryptophan. Behavioural and neurological toxicity has been reported with concomitant high dose tryptophan and MAOIs, and so initial observation and care would seem advisable. With SSRIs, cases of central toxicity, agitation and nausea have occurred with the combination and are suggested as likely to occur with all SSRIs, and the possibility of a serotonergic syndrome should be considered.

11. Mirtazapine to/from others

Mirtazapine has multiple routes of metabolism (CYP2D6, 3A4 and 1A2), so switching problems will be unlikely in terms of P450 inhibition. The only recommendation is for MAOIs (see 7). Fluoxetine 20–40 mg/d has been switched abruptly to mirtazapine 15 mg/d, without problems (n = 40, Preskorn et al, Biol Psychiatry 1997;**41**:96S), although serotonin syndrome has been reported during a cross-over switch to venlafaxine (n = 1, Dimellis, World J Biol Psychiatry 2002;**3**:167).

12. SSRIs to/from reboxetine

Fluoxetine to reboxetine: In fluoxetine non-responders, abrupt switch to reboxetine was well-tolerated (n = 128, open, Fava et al, J Clin Psychopharmacol 2003;**23**:365–9).

13. Venlafaxine to/from others

MAOI to venlafaxine: A 14-day gap has been recommended between stopping MAOI and starting venlafaxine. This is appropriate as there are a number of reports of interactions, e.g. extreme agitation, diaphoresis, rapid respiration and raised CPK, e.g. after a 37.5 mg dose of venlafaxine seven days after phenelzine 45 mg/d was stopped, but did not occur a further 7/7 later (n = 1, Phillips and Ringo, Am J Psychiatry 1995;**15**:1400–1), and serotonin syndrome (e.g. n = 4, Diamond et al, Neurology 1998;**51**:274–6).

Venlafaxine to MAOI: The SmPC recommends at least a seven-day gap (see above).

Venlafaxine to other drugs: No information, although agomelatine and mirtazapine have no reported or theoretical problems.

Tricyclic to venlafaxine: The venlafaxine SmPC states that there is little problem between venlafaxine and tricyclics. There are no reports of any problems.

Other drugs to venlafaxine: No information, as above.

14. Withdrawal or discontinuation *

Adverse discontinuation events have been reported for many antidepressants. Such symptoms are not, however, indicative of dependence, which usually requires three of the following:

- tolerance
- withdrawal symptoms
- use greater than needed
- inability to reduce doses
- excessive time taken procuring drug
- primacy of drug-taking over other activities
- continued use despite understanding of adverse consequences.

Discontinuation symptoms usually start within 1–2 days of stopping, resolve within 2–24 hours of restarting the drug, and are more common with longer courses or higher doses. They can occur with missed doses and about 30% of patients on SSRIs have dosing lapses of two or more days, long enough to produce discontinuation symptoms in patients on some short-acting SSRIs (n = 82, 3/12, Meijer et al, Br J Psychiatry 2001;**179**:519–22), but not fluoxetine (Curr Prob 2000;**26**:11–2). Stopping antidepressants suddenly (over 1–7 days) means you are more likely to relapse and it will happen quicker (half the time it would take otherwise) than stopping more slowly (14 days or longer) (n = 398, mean 3-year follow-up, Baldessarini et al, Am J Psychiatry 2010;**167**:934–41) The UK Drug and Therapeutics Bulletin (1999;**37**:49–52) recommends:

- after less than eight weeks of treatment, withdraw over 1–2 weeks
- after 6–8 months of treatment, taper over a 6–8-week period
- after long-term maintenance treatment, reduce the dose by 25% every 4–6 weeks.

Options for the management of antidepressant withdrawal symptoms include:

1. Reduce the dose stepwise every week or so, stabilising between reductions, e.g. paroxetine 20 mg/d, 10 mg/d, then 10 mg

alternate days (but not less frequently). Use of the syrup, gradually diluted, may also be effective.

2. Transfer to a long half-life antidepressant, e.g. fluoxetine (care with switching), then reduce (clomipramine case, Benazzi, *Am J Psychiatry* 1999 **156**:661–2; venlafaxine case, Giakas and David, *Psychiatr Ann* 1997;**27**:85–92).

3. Treat the emerging syndrome symptomatically, e.g. nausea, headache and diarrhoea have been managed with ondansetron (n = 1, Raby, *J Clin Psychiatry* 1998;**59**:621–2) and ginger root (Schechter, *J Clin Psychiatry* 1998;**59**:431–2).

Reviews: recognition, prevention and management of antidepressant withdrawal syndromes (Haddad, *Drug Safety* 2001;**24**:183–97), general (Healy, *Prescriber* 2002;**13**:91–9).

Main withdrawal symptoms *

Tricyclics:* Cholinergic rebound, e.g. headache, restlessness, diarrhoea, nausea and vomiting (Lieberman, *Psychosomatics* 1981;**22**:253–4), flu-like symptoms, lethargy, abdominal cramps, sleep disturbance, delirium (n = 1, Alexander and Berce, *Aust N Z J Psychiatry* 2010;**44**:863) and movement disorders.

MAOIs: Psychosis, hallucinations, disorientation, catatonia, irritability, hypomania, nausea, sweating, palpitations, nightmares and delirium.

SSRIs:* Dizziness, vertigo/lightheadedness, nausea, fatigue, headache, sensory disturbance, 'electric shocks' in the head, insomnia, abdominal cramps, chills, flu-like symptoms, increased or more vivid dreaming, anxiety/agitation and volatility, but not caused by anything else, e.g. physical illness or other drugs. Dizziness without vertigo may be caused by a sudden decrease in serotonin in the VNC (vestibular nuclear complex, also damaged in BSE/CJD) which disrupts the neurones bilaterally (Smith and Darlington, *Acta Otolaryngol* 2010;**130**:981–3).

Review: SSRI withdrawal (Healy, *Prescriber* 2002; **13**:91–9).

Specific drugs

SSRIs: There have been a number of comparative studies between SSRIs. Interruption for 5–8 days of maintenance therapy produced few discontinuation symptoms with fluoxetine

(long half-life), some with sertraline and most with paroxetine (n = 242, RCT, d/b, 4/52, Rosenbaum *et al*, *Biol Psychiatry* 1998;**44**:77–87; MS). In another study, suddenly discontinuing fluoxetine showed slightly more dizziness and somnolence at weeks 2–4, but no difference at week 6, compared to continuous treatment (n = 395, RCT, 12/52, Zajecka *et al*, *J Clin Psychopharmacol* 1998;**18**:193–7; review, Kendrick, *EBMH* 1999;**2**:31). A third study of a five-day interruption showed increased symptoms after a second missed dose with paroxetine, with impaired functional performance at five days, sertraline with less pronounced changes, and fluoxetine with no significant symptoms (n = 107, RCT, Michelson *et al*, *Br J Psychiatry* 2000;**174**: 363–8).

Citalopram: Even rapid discontinuation appears only to produce mild and transient effects (n = 225, RCT, d/b, 10/52, Markowitz *et al*, *Int Clin Psychopharmacol* 2000;**15**:329–33).

Escitalopram: See citalopram. Electric shock-like sensations have been reported with escitalopram discontinuation (n = 1, Prakash and Dhar, *J Clin Psychopharmacol* 2008;**28**:359–60).

Fluoxetine: Fluoxetine has a long half-life and discontinuation problems are rare. There are reports of extreme dizziness 3–14 days after fluoxetine stopped (n = 1, Einbinder, *Am J Psychiatry* 1995;**152**:1235), of severe, dull, aching pain in the left arm after abrupt withdrawal, which remitted after reintroduction (n = 1, Lauterbach, *Neurology* 1994;**44**:983–4), and reversible delirium (Kasantikul, *J Med Assoc Thai-land* 1995;**78**:53–4).

Fluvoxamine: A slow withdrawal may be preferred (Szabadi, *Br J Psychiatry* 1992;**160**:283–4).

Paroxetine: Paroxetine has been associated with more discontinuation reports than other SSRIs. A retrospective chart analysis showed that about 10% of people may get a significant discontinuation syndrome. This is more common with rapid withdrawal in people who got adverse reactions early in treatment (n = 385, Himei and Okamura, *CNS Drugs* 2006;**20**:665–72). Case reports include fever, severe fatigue, headache, nausea, vomiting, agitation, electrical, shock-like sensations (Frost and Lal, *Am J Psychiatry* 1995;**152**:180) and nocturnal enuresis (n = 1, Polimeni *et al*, *J Clin Psychopharmacol* 2008;

28:589–91). It has presented as stroke (n = 2, Haddad et al, J Psychopharmacol 2001;**15**:139–41) and confused with dosulepin side-effects during a switch (n = 1, Haddad and Qureshi, Acta Psychiatr Scand 2000;**102**:466–8). This phenomenon may be more frequent because paroxetine has a short half-life and inhibits its own CYP2D6 metabolism. This dissipates much quicker than fluoxetine and sertraline (n = 45, RCT, open, Liston et al, J Clin Psychopharmacol 2002;**22**:169–73) and, as concentrations fall, metabolism is less inhibited and levels fall quicker, leading to a more rapid drop. Discontinuation symptoms tend to resolve in a few days or rapidly on reintroduction of paroxetine. The CSM recommends tapering if withdrawal symptoms occur, i.e. stop and then restart and taper over 12 weeks, with either half-tablet doses or alternate day (but not less frequently) therapy. However, even a four-week gradual dose reduction may not prevent significant symptoms of vertigo, light-headedness and gait instability, so care is needed (n = 5, Pacheco et al, Br J Psychiatry 1996;**169**:384).

Sertraline: Discontinuation reactions are relatively uncommon, e.g. fatigue, cramps, insomnia (which resolved on restarting and where tapering over 14 weeks was successful (Louie et al, Am J Psychiatry 1994;**151**:450–1), electrical shock-like sensations and postural hypotension (n = 1, Amsden and Georgian, Pharmacotherapy 1996; **16**:684–6). Abrupt sertraline 100 mg/d dis-continuation has been enhanced by buspirone 15 mg/d (n = 1, Carrazana et al, Am J Psychiatry 2001;**158**:966–7).

Other antidepressants

Agomelatine: No discontinuation symptoms have been seen and so no tapering is required on discontinuation (MI).

Duloxetine: The MHRA recommends that duloxetine should not be discontinued abruptly (MHRA Drug Safety Update 2007;1–9), and the UK SmPC states that duloxetine should be tapered over one to two weeks, reduced by a half on alternate days. Symptoms of abrupt withdrawal have been reported to occur in 44% people stopping duloxetine (cf. 23% for placebo), with dizziness (12%), nausea, headache, paraesthesia, vomiting, irritability, shock-like sensations (n = 1, Pitchot and Ansseau, Ann Clin Psychiatry 2008;**20**:175) and nightmares being the most common. Resolution occurs in a week in 65% (s = 6, Perahia et al, J Affect Disord 2005;**89**:207–12).

Mirtazapine: A withdrawal hypomania has been reported (n = 1, MacCall and Callender, Br J Psychiatry 1999;**175**:390; n = 1, Berigan, Prim Care Companion J Clin Psychiatry 2001; **3**:143).

Moclobemide: A discontinuation syndrome may present with influenza-like symptoms. Sertraline may not modify the symptoms, suggesting a different mechanism (n = 1, Curtin et al, J Psycho-pharmacol 2002;**16**:271–2).

Reboxetine: No withdrawal or discontinuation syndrome has been observed in studies with reboxetine, with few additional effects on abrupt withdrawal.

St John's wort: A withdrawal syndrome has been reported (Dean et al, Ann Pharmacother 2003; **37**:150).

Tryptophan: Many patients had their tryptophan stopped abruptly after it was withdrawn from the market in the UK without serious withdrawal problems, other than recurrence of depression.

Venlafaxine: If used for more than six weeks, withdrawal over at least a week is recommended by the SmPC, which describes withdrawal reactions from abrupt cessation, dose reduction or tapering of venlafaxine. These can include fatigue, nausea, vomiting, dizziness, dry mouth, diarrhoea, insomnia, nervousness, confusion, paraesthesia, sweating, vertigo, headache (e.g. n = 1, Mayr and Bonelli, Ann Pharmacother 2003;**37**:1145–6), electric shock-like symptoms (e.g. n = 2, Reeves et al, Pharmacother 2003;**23**:678–81), suicidal ideation (n = 2, Stone et al, J Clin Psychopharmacol 2007; **27**:94–5), delusions and psychosis (n = 1, Koga et al, Acta Psychiatr Scand 2009;**120**:329–31), and mania (n = 1, Fava and Mangelli, Int J Neuropsychopharmacol 2003;**6**:89–90). Other symptoms include abdominal distension and congested sinuses (n = 1, resolving within 12 hours of restarting, Farah and Lauer, Am J Psychiatry 1996;**153**:576), gastrointestinal upset (which responded to reintroduction and then slow reduction over 1–4 weeks, n = 3, Louie et al, Am J Psychiatry 1996;**153**:1652) and classic SSRI-type discontinuation symptoms (e.g. confusion, headache, agitation, abdominal distension and sweating) occurring 16 and 20

2

hours after stopping (n = 2, Agelink et al, Am J Psychiatry 1997;**154**:1473–4; review of similarity to SSRI symptoms, n = 13, Boyd, Med J Aus 1998;**169**:91–2). Discontinuation effects may also adversely effect driving abilities (Campagne, Med Gen Med 2005;**7**:22). An outpatient study showed that seven of the nine patients discontinuing sustained-release venlafaxine reported the emergence of adverse reactions, compared to two of the nine stopping placebo (n = 9, d/b, p/c, Fava et al, Am J Psychiatry 1997;**154**:1760–2). It may be resolved by sertraline (n = 1, Luckhaus and Jacob, Int J Neuropsychopharmacol 2001;**4**:43–4).

3 PSYCHOTROPICS IN PROBLEM AREAS

Contents

3.1 BREAST-FEEDING

	LOWER RISK	MODERATE RISK	HIGHER RISK
Antipsychotics	Quetiapine[2] Sulpiride[5] Zuclopenthixol[4]	Amisulpride[5] Flupentixol[4] Haloperidol[6] Phenothiazines LD[7]	Aripiprazole[2] Asenapine[2] Clozapine[3] Olanzapine[2] Paliperidone[1] Pimozide[8] Phenothiazines HD[7] Risperidone[1] Ziprasidone[2]
Antidepressants	Flupentixol LD[4] Moclobemide[16] Tricyclics[12] (most) Tryptophan[16]	Agomelatine[11] Mianserin[16] Mirtazapine[11] SSRIs[9] St John's wort[16] Trazodone[13]	Doxepin?[12] Duloxetine[10] MAOIs[15] Reboxetine[14] Venlafaxine[10]
Anxiolytics and hypnotics	Benzodiazepines LD[17] Beta-blockers LD[20] Chloral[21] Temazepam LD[17] Zolpidem[19]	Benzodiazepines HD[17] Clomethiazole[21]	Buspirone[18] Hydroxyzine[18] Melatonin[21] Ramelteon[21] Zaleplon[19] Zopiclone[19]
Anticonvulsants	Carbamazepine[22] Phenytoin[24] Valproate[23]	Acetazolamide[28] Benzodiazepines[17] Gabapentin[26] Vigabatrin[27]	Ethosuximide[28] Lacosamide[27] Lamotrigine[26] Levetiracetam[27] Oxcarbazepine[22] Phenobarbital[25] Pregabalin[27] Rufinamide[27] Tiagabine[27] Topiramate[27] Zonisamide[27]
Others	Methadone[35]	Anticholinergics[30] Atomoxetine[34] Buprenorphine[35] Disulfiram[31] Methylphenidate[34] Sodium oxybate[33]	Acamprosate[31] Anticholinesterases[29] Bupropion[36] Lithium?[32] Memantine[29] Modafinil[33]

GENERAL PRINCIPLES FOR MEDICATION IN BREAST FEEDING

1. All psychotropics pass into milk, so no decision is risk-free. Milk levels are usually around 1% of maternal plasma levels, but there have been few formal studies.

2. Breast milk is more acidic than plasma, so basic compounds may be retained in milk and concentrations accumulate. Protein binding may also be a factor (in general, drug binding to milk proteins is less than to plasma proteins). The higher lipid content of the hind milk (second half of feed)

makes it likely to have a higher drug concentration than the first half (fore milk).

3. Drugs should be avoided if the infant is premature, or has renal, hepatic, cardiac or neurological impairment. Neonates (and particularly premature infants) are at greater risk from exposure to drugs via breast milk, because of an immature excretory function and the consequent risk of drug accumulation.

4. Avoid sedating drugs and those with long half-lives. Avoid drugs known to cause serious toxicity in adults or children. Drugs licensed for use in infants do not generally pose a hazard. Avoid new drugs if a therapeutically equivalent alternative is available that has been more widely used.

5. It is best to avoid long-acting preparations, especially those of drugs likely to cause serious side-effects (e.g. antipsychotic agents), as it is difficult to time feeds to avoid significant amounts of drug in breast milk.

6. Choose a regimen and route of administration which presents the minimum amount of drug to the infant. Since nearly all psychotropics can be given as a once-daily dose, this should be implemented as a single daily dose just before the infant's longest sleep period feed (e.g. for peak milk concentrations after oral administration: see *Tables 2.3.1* and *2.5.1*).

7. If a mother was taking a drug during pregnancy, it will not usually be necessary to switch drugs during breast-feeding, as the amount to which the infant is exposed will be less than that *in utero*.

8. Adverse effects will often be dose-related, so use the minimum effective maternal dose.

9. Polypharmacy may lead to enhanced adverse effects in the infant. Avoiding interacting drugs that raise plasma levels (even if asymptomatically) is essential. Multiple drug regimens may pose an increased risk, especially when adverse effects such as drowsiness are additive.

10. Drug effects on the development of the infant's brain are not clear and so monitor biochemical and behavioural parameters, especially if the infant shows signs of possible psychotropic side-effects (eg. sedation, tremulousness, colic) and take appropriate action, e.g. dose reduction, drug change, etc.

11. Avoid unnecessary drug use and limit the use of over-the-counter (OTC) products.

A robust assessment of the balance of benefit to risk for a mother–child pair requires data both on the drug's passage into breast milk and its effects in infants: there is rarely enough information available about new drugs to allow such an assessment to be made.

Reviews: * general and extensive (tripathi and Majumder, *Mens Sana Monogr* 2010;**8**:83–95), mood stabilisers in breast-feeding (Gentile, *Bipolar Disord* 2006;**8**:207–20), bipolar disorder treatments in puerperium (Dodd and Berk, *Curr Drug Saf* 2006;**1**:25–33), practical recommendations for treating mood disorders during lactation (Eberhard-Gran *et al*, *CNS Drugs* 2006;**20**:187–98).

3.1.1 ANTIPSYCHOTICS

Review: general (which concludes there is little difference between the available antipsychotics, and safety is not proven so chose the best one, except for avoiding clozapine and olanzapine; Gentile, *J Clin Psychiatry* 2008;**69**:666–73).

1. The UK SmPCs for **risperidone** and **paliperidone** state that women should not breast-feed. In two cases the milk:plasma ratio for risperidone was <0.5 with a relative infant dose lower than the 10% level of concern (n = 2, Ilett *et al*, *Ann Pharmacother* 2004;**38**:273–6), and in another milk levels were 10 times higher than in the maternal serum but no adverse effects were seen in the infant and development was normal (n = 1, Aichhorn *et al*, *J Psychopharmacol* 2005;**19**:211–3; see also Hill *et al*, *J Clin Psychopharmacol* 2000;**20**:285–6).

2. * There is one reported human case, where **aripiprazole** milk levels were about 20% of maternal levels (15 mg/d producing 14 ng/ml in milk) giving a relatively low potential level to the infant (n = 1, Schlotterbeck *et al*, *Int J Neuropsychopharmacol* 2007;**10**:433). It is excreted into rat milk. **Asenapine** is excreted in milk in animal studies but until human data is available it should be used only with great caution in breastfeeding (US PI). **Olanzapine** is excreted in breast milk, with infants exposed to about 1% of a maternal dose of olanzapine (below the 10% nominal level of concern), with few adverse effects (eg. n = 7, Gardiner *et al*, *Am J Psychiatry* 2003;**160**:1428–31) and a comparative study failed to show any long-term consequences from breast-feeding with olanzapine (n = 88 [c = 37], Gilad *et al*, *Breastfeed Med* 2011;**6**:55–8). However,

in a breast-fed infant whose mum was taking olanzapine, plasma levels at four months were relatively high but declined to undetectable over the next four months, probably due to maturing of the hepatic systems (n = 1, Whitworth *et al*, *J Psychopharmacol* 2008;**22**:923–4), but even at 15 mg/d levels can be undetectable in the infant aged 5/12 (n = 1, Lutz *et al*, *Ther Drug Monit* 2008; **30**:399–401). The UK SmPC recommends not breast-feeding while taking olanzapine. For **quetiapine**, there are several reports suggesting a low risk. A case series showed undetectable levels in milk, with low or undetectable levels in the infant's serum, the authors concluding that quetiapine posed only a low-level risk (n = 6, Misri *et al*, *J Clin Psychopharmacol* 2006;**26**:508–11). In another, milk levels at an oral dose of 200 mg/d were at a maximum of 0.43% of the weight-adjusted maternal dose and fell to pre-dose levels within two hours, appearing to be too small for significant pharmacological effects (n = 1, Lee *et al*, *Am J Psychiatry* 2004;**161**:1715–6) and an infant's plasma concentration was 6% of the mother's serum level and was exposed to less than 0.1% of the maternal dose, supporting the use of quetiapine following an appropriate risk:benefit analysis (n = 1, Rampono *et al*, *Ann Pharmacother* 2007;**41**:711–4). **Sertindole** is excreted in rat's milk but no human data exists so should not be used, as it would be expected to be excreted in milk. There is little data on **ziprasidone** apart from a case report (n = 1, Schlotterbeck *et al*, *Int J Neuropharmacol* 2009;**12**:437–8).

3.   **Clozapine** is contraindicated as animal studies suggest it is excreted into milk and so it risks agranulocytosis in the infant. In the close study of one mother, there was some accumulation of clozapine in breast milk (possibly due to higher lipid concentrations), and so doses must be kept low (Barnas, *Am J Psychiatry* 1994;**151**:945) and the infant's plasma monitored if breast-feeding is essential. There are reports indicating that infants experience sedation if mothers take clozapine and breast-feed.

4.   A study showed that 0.6 mcg/kg or 1–2% of the maternal **flupentixol** dose might reach the infant and thus is probably safe at low dose, e.g. <2 mg/d (n = 6, Matheson and Skjaeraasen, *Eur J Clin Pharmacol* 1988;**35**:217–20). The **zuclopenthixol** UK SmPC states that breast-feeding can be continued during treatment as less

than 1% of the weight-related maternal dose (in mg/kg) reaches the infant, but observe (especially during the first four weeks) for adverse effects.

5.* A mother taking **sulpiride** 100 mg/d is likely to give the child less than 1 mg/d. No adverse effects have been reported at higher doses (n = 28, p/c, d/b, 4/52, Ylikorkala *et al*, *Br Med J* 1982;**285**:249–51) but it is not recommended (UK SmPC). There is a single case of **amisulpride** 200 mg/d producing a dose to the infant of 6% of maternal dose and plasma levels 4% of the mother's level (n = 1, Ilett *et al*, *Ther Drug Monit* 2010;**32**:704–7).

6.   **Haloperidol** is excreted into breast milk but levels are probably low, although infant levels may be the same as adults. Some element of delayed development has been detected (n = 5, Yoshida *et al*, *Psychol Med* 1998;**28**:81–91) and so the infant must be monitored carefully.

7.   High doses of **phenothiazines** can produce drowsiness in the infant. **Chlorpromazine** has an inconsistent milk/plasma ratio, and drowsiness and lethargy are possible but not inevitable. With careful monitoring it should be safe, although some element of delayed development has been suggested (n = 3, Yoshida *et al*, *Psychol Med* 1998;**28**:81–91). In one case report the amount of **perphenazine** passed to an infant was about 0.1% of the adult dose in terms of mcg/kg body weight (Olesen *et al*, *Am J Psychiatry* 1990;**10**:1378–9), and this drug may become 'trapped' in milk due to its physiochemical properties.

8.   **Pimozide** may be excreted into breast milk and use is not recommended (SmPC).

3.1.2 ANTIDEPRESSANTS

Breast-feeding has many benefits, and the amount of antidepressant in milk varies according to the drug and what part of the milk is assayed, but maternal use at normal doses does not usually lead to substantial levels in the neonate, although they should be monitored for feeding difficulties, weight gain, and sleep or state changes (review by Yonkers, *Am J Psychiatry* 2007;**164**:1457–9). Infants have significantly lower weight if the mother has a depression lasting longer than two months (n = 78, naturalistic, 18/12, Hendrick *et al*, *J Clin Psychiatry* 2003;**64**:410–2), so there is a risk of **not** treating depression. In a review wryly entitled a 'pooled analysis of antidepressant levels in… breast milk' the conclusion was that fluoxetine produces the highest proportion (22%) of infant levels above 10% of the average maternal level, citalopram next at 17%, and that nortriptyline, paroxetine and sertraline may be the preferred choices, with citalopram relatively safe if doses are minimised (s = 67, Weissman *et al*, *Am J Psychiatry* 2004;**161**:1066–78).

Reviews: extensive (s = 31, Lanza di Scalea and Wisner, *Clin Obstet Gynaecol* 2009;**52**:483–97).

9.* Treatment with the **SSRIs** seems to be compatible with breast-feeding, although fluoxetine should probably best be avoided during lactation, unless also used during pregnancy. SSRIs can delay secretory activation by around 15 hours postpartum so might delay onset of breast-feeding (n = 431, Marshall *et al*, *J Clin Endocrin Metabol* 2010;**95**:837–46).

Citalopram, escitalopram and **demethylcitalopram** are excreted into milk. In one study, the mean combined dose (4.4–5.1% as citalopram equivalents) transmitted to infants was below the 10% notional level of concern, and infant levels appear low or undetectable (n = 11, Heikkinen *et al*, *Clin Pharmacol Ther* 2002;**72**:184–91). Another showed infant plasma concentrations to be very low or absent, with no adverse effects (n = 7, Rampono *et al*, *Br J Clin Pharmacol* 2000;**50**:263–8), and a prospective, observational, cohort study was unable to show any significant clinical events in mothers who took citalopram and breast-fed (n = 43, Lee *et al*, *Clin Pharmacol Ther* 2002;**71**:43). In eight women taking **escitalopram** 10 mg/d, the total dose reaching the infants was about 5% with no apparent adverse effects and, in the infants tested (n = 5), plasma levels were mostly below that detectable (Rampono *et al*, *Br J Clin Pharmacol* 2006;**62**:316–22). These data support the safety of the use of **citalopram** in breast-feeding women, provided doses are optimised.

Fluoxetine (s = 11, n = 190, Burt *et al*, *Am J Psychiatry* 2001;**158**:1001–9) plasma levels in the infant may range from undetectable to 340 ng/ml, but with no clear associations between maternal dose, age and plasma levels, so there is clearly some significant interpatient variability and adverse effects have been observed in breast-fed infants, e.g. colic. Plasma levels peak in breast milk at about eight hours post-dose and are dose-related, with 20 mg/d or less producing low infant serum levels (n = 19, Hendrick *et al*, *Biol Psychiatry* 2001;**15**:775–82), and probably less than 10% of the adult therapeutic dose of fluoxetine reaches the infant, below the notional level of concern (e.g. n = 10 pairs, Suri *et al*, *Biol Psychiatry* 2002;**52**:446–51), with no developmental effects likely (n = 4, Yoshida *et al*, *Br J Psychiatry* 1998;**172**:175–9). Mean estimated infant exposures are 2.4–3.8% of the maternal plasma level (n = 11 + 10 controls, Heikkinen *et al*, *Clin Pharmacol Ther* 2003;**73**:330–7). Considering the potential for accumulation, careful monitoring of the infants is mandatory, especially in neonates exposed to these drugs *in utero* (n = 14, Kristensen *et al*, *Br J Clin Pharmacol* 1999;**48**:521–7).

Fluvoxamine levels in milk and infant plasma appear low in the few reported cases. The estimated daily intake by an infant is probably about 0.5% of the maternal dose (e.g. 100 or 200 mg/d), so it is thought to be of little risk, with no concerns about development up to 21 months (e.g. n = 2, Kristensen *et al*, *J Hum Lact* 2002;**18**:139–43; n = 1, Hägg *et al*, *Br J Clin Pharmacol* 2000;**49**:286–8).

Paroxetine has been well studied and maternal doses of 10–50 mg/d are found in milk, but at highly variable levels (sample n = 108, range 2–101 ng/ml). In 25 mother–infant sample sets, paroxetine was detected in all but one milk sample, but undetectable (i.e. < 0.1 ng/ml) in the infant's serum, with no adverse events reported (n = 24, Misri *et al*, *J Clin Psychiatry* 2000;**61**:828–32; n = 6, open, Ohman *et al*, *J Clin Psychiatry* 1999;**60**:519–23). Hindmilk concentrations may be 78% higher than foremilk (n = 16, Stowe *et al*, *Am J Psychiatry* 2000;**257**:185–9).

Sertraline and metabolite generally appear only at low levels in the infant (probably less than 2% of the maternal dose per day; n = 10, Dodd *et al*, *Hum Psychopharmacol* 2000;**15**:161–4), unlikely to cause any significant adverse effects (n = 8, Kristensen *et al*, *Br J Clin Pharmacol* 1998;**45**:453–7). Peak sertraline levels occur in milk at around 8–9 hours after the last dose, and discarding this peak reduces the infant's intake by 18% (n = 26, 186 samples, Stowe *et al*, *J Clin Psychiatry* 2003;**64**:73–80). Higher levels have been reported rarely (Wisner *et al*, *Am J Psychiatry* 1998;**155**:690–2), as have rare withdrawal reactions in breast-fed children after

3

the mother has abruptly stopped sertraline (Kent and Laidlaw, *Br J Psychiatry* 1995;**167**:412–3), implying that sertraline may appear in breast milk at levels sufficient to suppress withdrawal after birth, especially at higher doses, e.g. 200 mg/d (e.g. n = 12, Stowe *et al*, *Am J Psychiatry* 1997;**154**:1255–60).

10. * **Venlafaxine** milk levels peak at eight hours, with infant venlafaxine/desvenlafaxine plasma levels 37% of the maternal plasma levels, and highly variable but in excess of the notional 10% safety level (n = 13, Newport *et al*, *J Clin Psychiatry* 2009;**70**:1304–10). The UK SmPC notes that breast-fed infants who cry, are irritable and have abnormal sleep patterns may have discontinuation effects. The risk:benefit of continuing or discontinuing must be considered carefully, but there may be enough in milk to attenuate withdrawal symptoms (Koren *et al*, *J Obstet Gynaecol Can* 2006;**28**:299–302). Venlafaxine may be metabolised by infants, with no detectable adverse effects or apparent developmental issues (n = 2, Hendrick *et al*, *Am J Psychiatry* 2001;**158**:2089–90). **Duloxetine** is excreted weakly into human breast milk The estimated daily infant dose on a mg/kg basis is approximately 0.14% of the maternal dose but it is not recommended in the SmPC.

11. In a careful study of breast-feeding mothers, a maximum of 1.5% of the adult **mirtazapine** dose (median 38 mg/d) reached the infants and of the four infants tested, only one had detectable plasma levels, well below the notional level of concern (n = 8, Kristensen *et al*, *Br J Clin Pharmacol* 2006;**6 3**:322–7). However, much higher levels have been reported, with one case where the infant had plasma levels approaching the adult range, with the authors suggesting close monitoring (n = 1, Toon *et al*, *J Clin Psychopharmacol* 2009;**29**:191–2). Hindmilk levels are slightly higher than foremilk (n = 1, Klier *et al*, *Am J Psychiatry* 2007;**164**:348–9). There is no data on **agomelatine** in breast milk, although it is excreted into rat milk, so should not be used in lactating mothers until more information is available (MI).

12. **Tricyclic antidepressants** should be used with care, but it does not seem warranted that breast-feeding should be discontinued completely (except for doxepin), as only about 1% of the maternal dose of tricyclics reaches the infant, with only minute amounts in the infant serum

with no acute toxic effects and no evidence of developmental delay (n = 10, Yoshida *et al*, *J Affect Disord* 1997;**43**:225–37). For **imipramine**, a milk/plasma ratio of 0.05–0.08, based on high dose samples, would lead to 0.1% of the maternal daily dose appearing in milk. **Amitriptyline**/nortriptyline levels in the infant are probably very low (Breyer-Pfaff, *Am J Psychiatry* 1995;**152**:812–3). Two studies showed no detectable **nortriptyline** in the infant serum, despite some unusually high maternal plasma levels, although two infants had detectable levels of 10–hydroxy metabolites. None of the infants showed any adverse effects and so the risk could be considered very low (n = 12, Wisner and Perel, *Am J Psychiatry* 1996; **153**:295). Sertraline and nortriptyline were of equivalent efficacy in postpartum depression, with very low or undetectable levels in infant serum (n = 109 [c = 95], RCT, d/b, 8/52, Wisner *et al*, *J Clin Psychopharmacol* 2006;**26**:453–60). In two studies of a five-year follow-up of children who had received **dosulepin** via breast milk, no detectable adverse effects on cognitive development were detectable (compared to a variety of controls, n = 66 controls, Buist and Janson, *Br J Psychiatry* 1995;**167**:370–3), and the drug is unlikely to be a significant hazard for the infant (n = 5, Ilett *et al*, *Br J Clin Pharmacol* 1992;**33**:635–9). Case reports suggest that the infant may only receive up to 3.7% of the mother's **clomipramine** dose (n = 1, Pons *et al*, *Clin Pharmacokinetics* 1994;**27**:270–89), with no adverse effects (n = 4, Wisner *et al*, *J Clin Psychiatry* 1995;**56**:17–20). **Doxepin** has a longer-acting metabolite N-desmethyldoxepin, which may accumulate in breast-fed infants, causing severe drowsiness and near fatal respiratory depression (n = 1, Matheson *et al*, *Lancet* 1985;ii:1124; n = 1, Frey *et al*, *Ann Pharmacother* 1999;**33**:690–3). However, other reports failed to detect any effects in the infant with maternal doxepin doses of 150 mg/d (e.g. Kemp *et al*, *Br J Clin Pharmacol* 1995;**20**:497–9; Wisner *et al*, *Am J Psychiatry* 1996;**153**:1132) and so metabolic differences could explain these.

The general recommendation is to observe the child carefully for sedation and respiratory depression. A tricyclic with a short half-life for itself (and any active metabolites) would appear to be the best option. It has been recommended that amitriptyline and imipramine are the preferred tricyclics.

13. With **trazodone**, a 50mg single-dose study showed that 1% passed into the milk (n = 6, Verbeck et al, Br J Clin Pharmacol 1986;**22**:367–70). More information on, e.g. metabolites is needed, but it would appear to be of low risk. Drowsiness and poor feeding have been reported (n = 1, Yapp et al, Ann Pharmacother 2000;**34**:1269–72; n = 2, Dodd et al, Clin Psychopharmacol 2000;**20**:717–8). Caution is thus advised.

14. Although **reboxetine** is excreted in breast milk, the amount excreted is low and so it is no longer contraindicated (SmPC).

15. Minimal data is available for the **MAOIs**. **Tranylcypromine** is excreted in breast milk but levels are not thought to be significant. Some sources state that MAOI levels in milk are too small to affect the child, but this has not been supported by any studies other than with tranylcypromine.

16. In six lactating women, 0.06% of a single dose of **moclobemide** was excreted unchanged in the milk. It would seem unlikely this amount would produce adverse effects in the baby (Pons et al, Br J Clin Pharmacol 1990;**29**:27–31). **Mianserin** 40–60mg/d may produce only low milk and infant plasma levels with no untoward effects (Buist et al, Br J Clin Pharmacol 1993;**36**:133–4). In a prospective study, there were no significant problems in infants whose mothers took **St John's wort** while breast-feeding; there was no decrease in milk production or infant weight over the first year (n = 33 + 134 controls, Lee et al, J Clin Psychiatry 2003;**64**:966–8), and in a thorough study, hyperforin was only detected at low levels in milk, with infant exposure 0.9–2.5% of the maternal dose, thus it is comparable with other psychotropics and appears relatively safe (n = 5, Klier et al, J Clin Psychiatry 2006;**67**:305–9). However, if possible, it should probably be avoided in breast-feeding (review by Dugoua et al, Can J Clin Pharmacol 2006;**13**:268–76). There are no known problems with **tryptophan**.

3.1.3 ANXIOLYTICS AND HYPNOTICS

17. Since **benzodiazepines** are excreted in breast milk, they should probably not be given to lactating mothers. Repeated doses of long-acting benzodiazepines can produce lethargy and weight loss but low and single doses are probably of low risk, provided the infant is monitored for drowsiness. Oxazepam seems to be preferable to diazepam in lactating women but, as with all anxiolytic benzodiazepines, infants should be observed for signs of sedation and poor suckling. **Diazepam, oxazepam, lorazepam, lormetazepam, nitrazepam** and **flunitrazepam** have all been shown in breast milk. Infant **temazepam** levels have been reported to be below detection levels at maternal doses of 10–20mg/d and no adverse effects have been seen (Lebedevs et al, Br J Clin Pharmacol 1992;**33**:204–6). Very little **midazolam** appears to reach breast milk (n = 5, Nitsun et al, Clin Pharmacol Ther 2006;**79**:549–57).

18. **Buspirone** should be avoided, based on excretion studies in rats, although there is no specific human data to show adverse effects. It is not known if **hydroxyzine** is excreted in human milk (UK SmPC), so its use is not recommended.

19. **Zaleplon** is excreted in breast milk and should not be administered to breast-feeding mothers, although the actual amount likely to be transferred may be very low, e.g. 0.017% of the maternal dose (n = 5, Darwish et al, J Clin Pharmacol 1999;**39**:670–4). **Zopiclone** is contra-indicated in breast-feeding, as it is excreted in appreciable amounts (up to 50% of maternal levels: n = 12, Matheson et al, Br J Clin Pharmacol 1990;**30**:267–71). Single occasional doses of 7.5mg are probably of low risk as accumulation is unlikely. The AAPCD considers **zolpidem** compatible with breast-feeding, as it is found only in minute amounts in milk due to its low lipophilic properties and rapid onset and excretion. In one study of women taking a (high) stat dose of 20mg, 3.8–19% of zolpidem was excreted into breast milk, nearly all within three hours of the dose, so 5–10mg should be relatively low risk (n = 5, Pons et al, Eur J Clin Pharmacol 1989;**37**:245–8). A low dose at bedtime and avoiding breast-feeding for the next 2–3 hours would minimise the potential effect on an infant.

20. For **beta-blockers**, the amounts excreted into breast milk are probably too small to affect the baby (<0.1% of maternal doses), but could produce bradycardia and hypoglycaemia in high doses.

21. **Clomethiazole** is excreted in insignificant amounts, based on IV and oral studies in pre-eclampsia (Acta Psychiatr Scand 1986;**73**[Suppl 329]:185–8). An infant might ingest active amounts and, although the sedative effects of this could be relevant, they are unlikely to be harmful. **Chloral hydrate** is excreted in breast milk and

3

the sedation caused in the infant makes this a precaution, although only minimal sedation after large feeds has been reported (*Adv Drug React Bull* 1976;Dec:212). The American Academy of Pediatrics recommends that chloral can safely be used in lactating mothers, as do the authorities in many European countries. **Melatonin** is probably secreted into human breast milk and so use in lactating mothers is not recommended (SmPC). **Ramelteon** is excreted into milk in animal studies but human data is not available yet.

3.1.4 ANTICONVULSANTS *

Breast-feeding should be encouraged as bonding is especially important in epileptic mothers. Extensive reviews conclude that:

* carbamazepine, valproate and phenytoin are compatible with breast-feeding
* ethosuximide, phenobarbital and primidone are potentially unsafe and close clinical monitoring of the infant is recommended
* data on the newer drugs is too sparse for reliable recommendations
* occasional or short-term treatment with benzodiazepines could be considered compatible with breast-feeding, although maternal diazepam treatment has caused sedation in suckling infants after short-term use. During long-term use of benzo-diazepines, infants should be observed for signs of sedation and poor suckling
* there are no differences in IQs and no negative effect on cognitive outcomes in children also exposed *in utero* for carbamazepine, lamotrigine, phenytoin or valproate (n = 199, 3 years, Meador *et al*, *Neurology* 2010;**75**:1954–60).

Reviews: general (Sabers and Tomson, *Curr Opin Neurol* 2009;**22**:157–61; Hägg and Spigset, *Drug Safety* 2000; **22**:425–40, 88 refs).

22. **Carbamazepine** has been classed by the AAPCD as compatible with breast-feeding, as levels have been found to be relatively low. This is, however, based only on case reports in epilepsy, with few reports when used as a mood stabiliser. The half-life is longer in infants, with levels in milk ranging from 7–95% of the mother's serum, but probably usually around 10%, on the cusp of the notional level of concern. There are cases of adverse effects in the infant (n = 1, Merlob *et al*,

Ann Pharmacother 1992;**26**:1563–5; n = 1, Frey *et al*, *Eur J Pediatr* 1990;**150**:136–8) and several of poor feeding. The mother should be informed of the potential signs of hepatic dysfunction and CNS effects (review, Chaudron and Jefferson, *J Clin Psychiatry* 2000;**161**:79–90). **Oxcarbazepine** is excreted into breast milk, the breast milk/plasma ratio for drug and metabolite being about 0.5, similar to carbamazepine (n = 1, Bulla *et al*, *Eur J Clin Pharmacol* 1988;**34**:311–3). It is currently contraindicated.

23. **Valproate** has been classified by the AAP as compatible with breast-feeding, based on case reports in epilepsy. Infant serum levels usually range from 5–12% but can range from undetectable to 40% of the mother's serum level (n = 16, van Unruh *et al*, *Ther Drug Monit* 1984;**6**:272–6). In six mother–infant pairs, where infant exposure was exclusively during breast-feeding, mothers had valproate levels in the usual range for bipolar (39–79 mcg/mL) but the infants had low levels (0.7–1.5 mcg/mL), thus presenting a relatively low risk compared to the risk of relapse in the mother (n = 6, Piontek *et al*, *J Clin Psychiatry* 2000;**61**:170–2). Valproate thus appears relatively safe, although with the small but finite risk of haematological effects (Stahl *et al*, *J Pediatr* 1997;**130**:1001–3). Care and careful counselling is needed for higher doses (review, Chaudron and Jefferson, *J Clin Psychiatry* 2000;**161**:79–90).

24. Small quantities of **phenytoin** are excreted in breast milk (SmPC), peaking at three hours, and have been considered clinically safe.

25. Larger doses of **phenobarbital** and **primidone** may accumulate in breast milk and cause unacceptable drowsiness.

26. Extensive passage of **lamotrigine** into breast milk occurs, and as lamotrigine is metabolised by glucuronidation (which is immature in neonates), and may lead to accumulation in the infant. Infant plasma levels have been reported to be 18% (peak four hours after the maternal dose; n = 30, Newport *et al*, *Pediatrics* 2008;**122**:223–31), 23–33% (milk to maternal serum ratio a consistent 0.6; review, Chaudron and Jefferson, *J Clin Psychiatry* 2000;**161**:79–90) and 30% (range 20–43%; n = 4, Liporace *et al*, *Epilepsy Behav* 2004;**5**:102–5), but with huge interindividual variations. **Gabapentin** crosses into breast milk but appears of lower risk. In six mother–baby pairs, gabapentin levels were estimated to be 12%

of the mother's plasma level, but with no adverse effects detected (n = 6, Ohman et al, Epilepsia 2005;**46**:1621–4) and in a single mother–infant pair, the infant plasma level was 0.4mg/L (6% of maternal plasma level) and absolute dose 3% of mother's dose (n = 1, Kristensen et al, J Hum Lact 2006;**22**:426–8).

27. It is not known if **lacosamide** is excreted in breast milk (SmPC). Animal studies indicate **levetiracetam** is excreted into breast milk and, since unusually high levels can occur (Pennell, Neurology 2003;**61**[6 Suppl 2]:S35–S42), breast-feeding is not recommended. **Pregabalin** is excreted into milk in animal studies but no human data exists, so is not recommended (SmPC). No information is available for **rufinamide** (UK SmPC). **Topiramate** and **tiagabine** are not recommended as no human information is currently available, although there is one healthy outcome with topiramate (n = 1, Gentile, Clin Drug Investig 2009;**29**:139–41). A small study suggested that the quantity of **vigabatrin** ingested through milk is small, at around 1–3% of the daily dose (n = 2, Tran et al, Br J Clin Pharmacol 1998;**45**:409–11). **Zonisamide** appears in breast milk, 41–57% being transferred, with a half-life in the two infants of 61–107 hours respectively (n = 2, Kawada et al, Brain Dev 2002;**24**:95–7), similar to the mother's plasma level. The UK SmPC recommends avoiding breast-feeding during therapy and for a month afterwards.

28. **Ethosuximide** is excreted in breast milk, with detectable infant levels and should not be used.

3.1.5 OTHERS

29. There is no information available on **donepezil**, **galantamine** and **rivastigmine**, so they should not be used in breast-feeding mothers. Human data is lacking but **memantine** is lipophilic and so is probably excreted into breast milk.

30. There is no data for **anticholinergics** but the UK SmPC for **orphenadrine** notes that as there is no information available, mothers should not breast-feed.

31. No information is available to date on **disulfiram** in breast milk and so use must be with great caution. There is the possibility of interactions with alcohol in paediatric medicines (see 4.7.1). **Acamprosate** is excreted in the milk of lactating animals and so the literature states that use in

breast-feeding is a contraindication. No human data is available.

32. **Lithium** has been classified by the AAP as contraindicated in breast-feeding since 1989 but this is based on limited information. A recent systematic study, however, has shown relatively low milk and lower infant plasma levels with no serious or persistent adverse events noted, the authors suggesting that there is a need to reassess this widespread contraindication, provided careful monitoring is carried out (n = 10 mother-infant pairs, Viguera et al, Am J Psychiatry 2007;**164**:342–5). Breast milk levels may be approximately 40% (range 24–72%), with infant serum having levels 5–200% of the mother's serum concentrations. There have been case reports of adverse events (e.g. hypotonia and lethargy, possibly due to reduced renal clearance), although many of these may have been multifactorial. There is wide interindividual variability of the dose reaching an infant, and so informed choice, with careful monitoring (e.g. TDM of milk or infant plasma), considering poorer renal excretion and fluid balance/electrolytes and use of low doses, may help if the risk of bipolar relapse is high if stopping lithium (Moretti et al, Ther Drug Monit 2003;**25**:364–6).

Review: Chaudron Jefferson, J Clin Psychiatry 2000; **161**:79–90.

33. **Modafinil** is contraindicated in breast-feeding. **Sodium oxybate** is not recommended but there is no human data available (SmPC).

34. In one report, no **methylphenidate** was detectable in breast milk 20–21 hours after the last dose of a plain tablet (probably because methylphenidate's short half-life of 2–3 hours), so breast-feeding before a morning dose should have a low risk (n = 1, Spigset et al, Am J Psychiatry 2007;**164**:348). The UK SmPC recommends caution for **atomoxetine**.

35. **Methadone** is now generally recommended, regardless of dose, as compatible with breast-feeding, based on three studies. Methadone concentrations in milk were unrelated to maternal dose, may peak about three hours post-dose but are small at 21–314ng/ml (n = 12, Jansson et al, J Hum Lact 2007;**23**:184–90). This is insufficient to prevent the development of a neonatal absence syndrome (n = 8 pairs, Begg et al, Br J Clin Pharmacol 2001;**52**:681–5) and even methadone doses as high as 50–105 mg/d

3

(plus eight matched formula-fed infants) give low infant levels. Levels increase gradually over 30 days, there are no significant effects from breast-feeding on neurobehavioural outcomes (n = 8 + 8, 30/7, Jansson et al, Pediatrics 2008; **121**: 106–14; see also n = 4, 6/52, Jansson et al, Breastfeed Med 2008; **3**: 34–7), and a retrospective chart analysis showed that breast-feeding by drug-dependent mothers reduced neonatal abstinence syndrome (NAS), delayed onset of NAS, and decreased the need for pharmacological interventions, regardless of gestation and type of drug. Methadone maintenance also reduces the risk of poor quality street drugs being used, and stopping opiates is also dangerous as withdrawal reactions can damage the fetus more than methadone (for effect on the child in the first year, Abdel-Latif et al, Pediatrics 2006; **117**: 1163–9). In breast-feeding mums, **buprenorphine** and norbuprenorphine levels are detectable in the infant's urine but the infant-exposed dose in mg/kg has been calculated at under 1%, supporting the use of buprenorphine during breast-feeding (n = 7, Lindemalm et al, J Hum Lact 2009; **25**: 199–205; see also n = 1, 10 samples, Grimm et al, Ther Drug Monit 2005; **27**: 526–30), although it is actually contraindicated in breast-feeding (UK SmPC).

36. **Bupropion** and metabolites accumulate in breast milk at higher levels than the mother's plasma (SmPC caution) and there is a report of an infant developing seizures from bupropion ingested via breast milk (n = 1, Prescrire Int 2005; **14**: 144), although other reports indicate that bupropion is not detectable in the infant's plasma (n = 1, Briggs et al, Ann Pharmacother 1993; **27**: 431–3; n = 2 pairs, Baab et al, J Clin Psychiatry 2002 **63**: 910–1).

3.2 CARDIOVASCULAR DISEASE

	LOWER RISK	MODERATE RISK	HIGHER RISK
Antipsychotics	Quetiapine[2] Sulpiride[5]	Amisulpride[5] Aripiprazole[2] Flupentixol[4] Olanzapine[2] Paliperidone[1] Phenothiazines[7] Risperidone[1] Zuclopenthixol[4]	Clozapine[3] Haloperidol[6] Pimozide[8] Ziprasidone[2]
Antidepressants	Agomelatine[14] Duloxetine[10] Mianserin[16] Mirtazapine[11] St John's wort[16] SSRIs[9] Trazodone[13] Tryptophan[16]	Moclobemide[16] Reboxetine[14] Venlafaxine[10]	MAOIs[15] Tricyclics (especially dosulepin)[12]
Anxiolytics and hypnotics	Benzodiazepines[17] Buspirone[18] Melatonin[21] Ramelteon[21] Zaleplon[19] Zolpidem[19] Zopiclone[19]	Beta-blockers[20] Chloral hydrate[21] Clomethiazole[21] Pregabalin[27]	
Anticonvulsants	Benzodiazepines[17] Gabapentin[26] Lamotrigine[26] Levetiracetam[27] Tiagabine[27] Topiramate[27] Vigabatrin[27] Valproate[23]	Barbiturates[25] Carbamazepine[22] Lacosamide[27] Oxcarbazepine[22] Paraldehyde[28] Phenytoin[24] Pregabalin[27]	Fosphenytoin[24]
Others	Acamprosate[31] Memantine[29]	Anticholinergics[30] Anticholinesterases[29] Atomoxetine[34] Buprenorphine[37] Bupropion[36] Dexamfetamine[35] Lithium[32] Methadone[37] Methylphenidate[34] Modafinil[33] Sodium oxybate[33]	Disulfiram[31]

3

GENERAL PRINCIPLES IN CARDIAC DISEASE

(adapted from *Maudsley Guidelines*)

1. Polypharmacy should be avoided where possible, particularly with drugs likely to effect cardiac rate and electrolyte balance.

2. Awareness of QT prolongation is increasing, and so care is essential with drugs likely to increase the QT interval.

3. Avoid drugs specifically contraindicated.

4. Start low and go slow is, as ever, good advice. Rapid dose escalation should be avoided.

Psychotropics in specific cardiac conditions

Angina

Avoid drugs causing orthostatic hypotension, which may exacerbate angina. Avoid drugs causing tachycardia, e.g. phenothiazines, clozapine and risperidone. Trazodone and tricyclics are best avoided, although most other antidepressants are thought to be of relatively low risk.

Arrhythmias

SSRIs are first choice antidepressants because of their lack of antiarrhythmic/proarrhythmic potential. Avoid phenothiazines, butyrophenones and pimozide. Sulpiride and olanzapine seem of low risk.

Congestive heart failure (CHF)

For chronic stable CHF, avoid beta-blockers and take care with drugs causing orthostatic hypotension, e.g. phenothiazines, clozapine, risperidone and tricyclics. For acute CHF, the cause will indicate which drugs are safer to use.

Hypertension

Drugs causing orthostatic hypotension should be monitored closely. Avoid MAOIs. Hypertension can occur with venlafaxine (high dose), clozapine and sometimes with tricyclics and antipsychotics.

Myocardial infarction (MI)

If essential, use SSRIs (except perhaps fluvoxamine) or agomelatine. Avoid high-dose antipsychotics and phenothiazines. Butyrophenones, thioxanthenes and benzamides are safer.

Reviews: cardiac effects of psychotropics (Kovacs and Arora, *Am J Ther* 2008;**15**:474–83; Mackin, *Hum Psychopharmacol* 2008;**23**(Suppl 1):3–14).

QTc prolongation

Many antipsychotics are known to affect cardiac conduction, with a class IA antiarrhythmic-like effect. One way this manifests itself is by lengthening of the QT interval. This may then lead onto torsade de pointes, which may be asymptomatic or, in rare cases, lead on to ventricular fibrillation and sudden death. The QT interval shortens with increased heart rate, and so a rate-correct value QTc is usually used. A QTc prolonged to about 450ms is considered of some concern, and above about 500ms to be of an unquantifiable risk of leading to torsade de pointes, which may be fatal, and should prompt review and possibly action. QTc varies markedly throughout the day, and so serial readings are necessary for accurate assessments.

Risk factors for antipsychotic-induced QTc prolongation:

- Recent introduction of an antipsychotic, dose increase or high doses (including overdose).
- Receiving other medicines associated with QT prolongation, including, e.g. some antiarrhythmic drugs, vasodilators, tricyclics, macrolide and fluoroquinolone antibiotics, antimalarials, ketoconazole, methadone and antihistamines.
- Underlying cardiac disease, e.g. heart-failure, angina and cardiac myopathy.
- Bradycardia, or second or third-degree heart block.
- Personal or family history of QTc prolongation, ventricular arrhythmias or torsade de pointes.
- Severe renal or hepatic impairment.
- Elderly or malnourished.
- History of heavy alcohol consumption or substance misuse.
- Electrolyte imbalance, especially hypokalaemia and hypomagnesaemia.
- Undergoing restraint and/or severe stress.
- Slow drug metabolisers.
- Female (QT prolongation may occur more frequently).

If a prolonged QT interval is predictable, monitoring of electrolytes and ECG may be indicated, but interpretation is dependent upon the timing (time since last dose, diurnal variation, postprandial state).

Reviews * QT alterations with psychotropics (Alvarez and Pahissa, *Curr Drug Saf* 2010;**5**:97–104).

3.2.1 ANTIPSYCHOTICS *

A massive retrospective cohort study showed the risk of sudden cardiac death was roughly double with antipsychotics (FGAs and SGAs were similar), although the effect wore off when they were stopped (n = 276907, Ray *et al, N Engl J Med* 2009;**360**:225–35; comment by Taylor, *EBMH* 2009;**12**:92). The ten-year incidence of CHD in CATIE showed:

- increased risk with olanzapine (0.5)
- increased risk with quetiapine (0.3)
- reduced risk with perphenazine (-0.5)
- reduced risk with risperidone (-0.6)
- reduced risk with ziprasidone (-0.6%)

(n = 1125, 18/12–10 years, part of CATIE, Daumit *et al, Schizophr Res* 2008;**105**:175–87).

Reviews: QTc, torsade de pointes and sudden death (Haddad and Anderson, *Drugs* 2002;**62**:1649–71), QTc prolongation (Taylor, *Acta Psychiatr Scand* 2003;**107**:85–95; 136 refs).

1. * **Risperidone** should be used with caution due to orthostatic hypotension; low doses slightly drop bp and increase heart rate. It is best to introduce it slowly over several weeks. In the Medicaid cohort study (n = 95,632 + 29,086 controls, Hennessy *et al, Br Med J* 2002;**325**:1070–2), risperidone was the only drug that had higher rates than haloperidol for cardiac arrest and ventricular arrhythmia, especially at lower dose. The authors concluded that this was due to the frailest patients being given lowest doses. Serious cardiac effects at standard doses seems to be uncommon (n = 107, Page *et al, J Clin Psychopharmacol* 2010;**30**:387–90). **Paliperidone** should be used with care in people with a familial history of CV disease or QT interval, or co-prescribed with drugs thought to prolong the QTc interval (SmPC), although it has the same effect on QTc as quetiapine (n=109, RCT, d/b, p/c, Hough *et al, Int Clin Psychopharmacol* 2011;**26**:25–34; MS).

2. * **Aripiprazole** may cause orthostatic hypotension and the UK SmPC now lists QT prolongation, ventricular arrhythmias, sudden unexplained death, cardiac arrest, torsades de pointes and bradycardia as unwanted effects. Orthostatic hypotension and syncope have been reported with **asenapine** (US PI), especially early in treatment and so should be used carefully with any other drugs with cardiac effects, those likely to prolong the QTc interval and in people with

cardiac risk factors (n = 148, p/c, Chapel *et al, J Clin Pharmacol* 2009;**49**:1297–308). QTc prolongation of 2–5 msec has been shown but with none going over 500 msec. Postural hypotension has been seen infrequently with **olanzapine**. Blood pressure monitoring is recommended periodically in patients over 65. One study showed that olanzapine (mean 14 mg/d) produced fasting triglyceride levels raised by a mean of 60 mg/dL (37%) (n = 25, 12/52, Osser *et al, J Clin Psychiatry* 1999;**60**:767–70), which, since triglycerides are a significant risk factor for exacerbation of CHD, needs care. An increase in the QTc interval has only been seen rarely, e.g. data from four RCTs showed the risk of QTc >450 msec was approximately the same as at baseline, suggesting a minimal effect on QTc prolongation and hence fatal arrhythmias (n = 2700, Czekalla *et al, J Clin Psychiatry* 2001;**62**:191–8). UK SmPC now cautions about the use of olanzapine with drugs known to increase the QTc interval. The SmPC for **quetiapine** recommends caution with drugs known to prolong the QTc interval and in patients with CV disease or conditions predisposing to hypotension. Trials have not shown sustained changes in the QTc interval but some sources list quetiapine as a moderate risk. Orthostatic hypotension is more common in the elderly, especially initially. **Sertindole** lengthens the QT interval and is contraindicated in people with a history of significant cardiovascular disease, congestive heart failure, cardiac hypertrophy, arrhythmia or bradycardia (< 50 bpm) and congenital prolonged QT (>450 msec in men, >470 msec in women), although a counter-balancing mechanism may reduce the risk (Lindstrom *et al, Int J Neuropsychopharmacol* 2005;**8**:615–29). **Ziprasidone** causes a well-publicised, dose-related prolongation of QTc interval (mean 10 msec), so should not be used in anyone with a known prolonged interval, recent MI or heart failure (review, Taylor, *CNS Drugs* 2003;**17**:423–30).

3. **Clozapine** has well-established CV side-effects, e.g. tachycardia and postural hypotension (particularly early in treatment). The literature (e.g. Layland *et al, Med J Aust* 2009;**190**:190–2) has warned that:

- patients who develop clozapine-induced cardiomyopathy should not be re-exposed to clozapine (data mining study, Coulter *et al, Br Med J* 2001;**322**:1207–9)

- it should only be started if severe heart disease has been excluded through a full history, examination and possibly an ECG
- myocarditis most commonly occurs in the first two months
- persistent tachycardia at rest, especially during first two months, should be followed up and the patient observed for other signs of cardiomyopathy/myocarditis
- it should be discontinued in anyone where cardiomyopathy or myocarditis is suspected
- ECG changes should be referred to a cardiologist for evaluation.

Studies of clozapine-associated myocarditis and cardiomyopathy (from Australian database of 8000, Kilian et al, Lancet 1999;**354**:1841–5; n = 41 [10 fatal], La Grenade et al, NEJM 2001;**345**:224–5) have shown that:

- the median onset is 17 days (mean 6/12)
- 90% occur within dose range of 100–450mg/d (50% recovered but 10% died)
- symptoms are diverse and non-specific and a high degree of suspicion must be maintained (n = 116, Haas et al, Drug Saf 2007;**30**:47–57)
- it can occur in young healthy adults.

A 10-year naturalistic study showed patients on clozapine were also at risk of death from cardiovascular disease secondary to obesity, diabetes, hypertension and hyperlipidaemia (n = 96, 10 years, Henderson et al, J Clin Psychiatry 2005;**66**:1116–21). Prolonged QTc is also known with clozapine. Risk factors included increased age (but less so if there was a normal ECG with other antipsychotics). It is dose-dependent, often corrects itself with time, occurs mostly during the initial stages of treatment, is mostly benign, and pathological prolongation of QTc is rare (n = 61, Kang et al, J Clin Psychiatry 2000;**61**:441–6).

4. There is a caution on the use of **flupentixol** in susceptible individuals (hypokalaemia, hypomagnesia, genetic disposition), or in people with a history of CV disorders (UK SmPC). Cardiac disease is a precaution for **zuclopenthixol**.

5. * **Amisulpride** overdose frequently results in QTc prolongation and torsades de pointes (n = 83, Isbister et al, J Clin Psychopharmacol 2010;**30**:391–5), and it is contraindicated with drugs that could cause torsade de pointes. There are no specific problems with **sulpiride** but prolonged QT and torsade de pointes have

been reported (n = 1, Huang et al, Int J Cardiol 2007;**118**:100–2; n = 1, Chang et al, Am J Emerg Med 2009;**27**:1016).

6. **Haloperidol** is now contraindicated in patients with clinically significant cardiac disorders or used with other QT-interval prolonging drugs (SmPC). Prolonged QT-interval has been reported (n = 596, Reilly et al, Lancet 2000;**35**:1048–52).

7. * Chlorpromazine and levomepromazine significantly lengthened QTc (n = 1017, Ozeki et al, Prog Neuropsychopharmacol Biol Psychiatry 2010;**34**:401–5) and some ECG abnormalities have been reported with other **phenothiazines**, e.g. tachycardia, T-wave abnormalities, ST depression, QT prolongation and right bundle branch block. **Levomepromazine** causes orthostatic hypotension that can, on occasion, be prolonged and profound.

8. **Pimozide** is contraindicated in QT prolongation, history of cardiac arrhythmias or torsades de pointes.

3.2.2 ANTIDEPRESSANTS *

Studies suggest that depressed patients:

- Are at 4–5-fold greater risk of cardiac mortality, but depression in the week preceding an MI is not (n = 588, mean 6.7 years, Dickens et al, Psychosom Med 2008;**70**:450–5; comment by Martens and de Jonge, EBMH 2009;**12**:8; n = 5936, mean 5.6yrs, Nabi et al, Heart 2010;**96**:1645–50).
- Are less likely to follow recommendations to reduce their cardiac risk during recovery from an MI (n = 204, Ziegelstein et al, Arch Intern Med 2000;**160**:1818–23).
- Are less likely to comply with antihypertensives (n = 496, one year, Wang et al, J Gen Intern Med 2002;**17**:504–11).
- Are at greater risk of new cardiac events within the first year after a heart attack (n = 528; 12/12, Kaptein et al, Psychosom Med 2006;**68**:662–8; comment by Huffman, EBMH 2007;**10**:42).
- May have a four times greater mortality over a seven-year follow-up if they have severe depression or fail to improve over 6/12 following ACS (acute coronary syndrome), so depression needs to be treated aggressively (n = 369, seven years, Glassman et al, Arch Gen Psychiatry 2009; **66**:1022–9;

n = 5936, mean 5.6 years, Nabi *et al, Heart* 2010;**96**:1645–50).

- With more severe depression may have this as an independent risk factor for increased CHD mortality in older adults free of CHD at baseline (n = 660, mean 12 years, Ahto *et al, Int J Ger Psychiatry* 2007;**22**:757–63; comment by Gump, *EBMH* 2008;**11**:56).

- Are 2.7 times more likely to die from ischaemic heart disease than those who do not, and although antidepressants do not seem to help cardiac outcomes (n = 19649, six years, Surtees *et al, Am J Psychiatry* 2008;**165**:515–23), they do help depressive outcomes (s=11, Thombs *et al, JAMA* 2008; **300**:2161–71), and may significantly benefit without increasing the risk of cardiac events (meta-analysis, s = 4, n = 798, RCT, d/b, p/c, Dowlati *et al, Can J Psychiatry* 2010;**55**:91–9), as untreated depression may be a greater risk than antidepressants (n = 1005, O'Connor *et al, Arch Intern Med* 2008;**168**:2232–7).

Treating depression is thus logical but not supported by the two largest studies (CBT +/- SSRIs, n = 2481, RCT, 6/12, ENRICHD, Berkman *et al, JAMA* 2003;**289**:3106–16; MIND-IT, n = 331, RCT, 18/12, van Melle *et al, Br J Psychiatry* 2007;**190**:460–6; for caveats see Carney and Freedland, *Br J Psychiatry* 2007;**190**:467–8), although treatment is associated with modest improvements (s=11, Thombs *et al, JAMA* 2008;**300**:2161–71).

However, only depression developing after a major cardiac event was associated with an increased risk of morbidity and mortality, but risk was substantial, i.e. seven times as high (n = 489, 12/12, Parker *et al, Biol Psychiatry* 2008;**64**:660–6).

Overall, sertraline, fluoxetine, citalopram, bupropion and mirtazapine appear safe after an MI; use of sertraline and response to citalopram and mirtazapine may improve mortality; paroxetine and citalopram appear safe in coronary artery disease, and tricyclics should be avoided (Taylor, *Acta Psychiatr Scand* 2008; **118**:434–42).

Reviews: depression after acute coronary syndrome (Carney and Freedland, *Am J Psychiatry* 2009;**166**:410–7), antidepressant cardiac side-effects (Sala *et al, Curr Opin Investig Drugs* 2006; **7**:256–63).

9.* Despite some reported cases of cardiac effects (e.g. a plasma-level related potential for conduction problems, e.g. AV block, QTc prolongation, etc; n = 114, Rodriguez de la Torre *et al, Ther Drug Monit* 2001;**23**:435–40), the **SSRIs** are generally considered safer to use in cardiac disease, with robust data accumulating to support this. Meta-analyses show that SSRIs are clearly more effective than placebo with no difference in drop-outs (s = 4, n = 798, p/c, 9–24/52, Dowlati *et al, Can J Psychiatry* 2010;**55**:91–9) and show lower relapse and readmission rates than without in acute coronary syndrome (s = 5, n = 801, Mazza *et al, J Psychopharmacol* 2010;**24**:1785–92).

The SADHART-CFH study showed **sertraline** was safe in patients with significant CHF, although may not be statistically significantly better than placebo (n=469, RCT, d/b, p/c, 12/52, O'Connor *et al, J Am Coll Cardiol* 2010;**56**:692-9). Other studies have shown it not to increase cardiac events in depressed patients with unstable angina or recent MI, and may even cut cardiac deaths post-MI by about 10% (n = 369, RCT, Glassman *et al, JAMA* 2002;**288**:701–9; review by Parissis *et al, Expert Opin Pharmacother* 2007;**8**:1529–37; see also n = 1080 + 4356, three years, Sauer *et al, Circulation* 2003;**108**:32–6).

Several open trials have indicated **fluoxetine** up to 60 mg/day to have no significant adverse cardiac effects in patients with pre-existing CHF, conduction disease and/ or ventricular arrhythmia (e.g. n = 27, average age 73, open, 7/52, Roose *et al, Am J Psychiatry* 1998;**155**:660–6). Fluoxetine 20 mg/d has produced a modest reduction in bp, and patients with pre-existing, stable cardiovascular disease (including hypertension) showed no significant bp change (n = 796, 12/52, Amsterdam *et al, J Clin Psychopharmacol* 1999;**19**:9–14). Rare cases of, e.g. atrial fibrillation, bradycardia and syncope have been reported. **Paroxetine** may increase cholesterol (LDL-C) concentrations by around 11%, which might increase the risk of CHD in vulnerable individuals (n = 18, Lara *et al, J Clin Psychiatry* 2003;**64**:1455, IS). **Citalopram,** and presumably **escitalopram**, have no significant reported effect on blood pressure, cardiac conduction or heart rate, but exacerbation of pre-existing bradycardia has been reported (e.g. Myth *et al, Acta Psychiatr Scand* 1992;**86**:138–45), as has occasional postural dizziness (review

3

by Rasmussen *et al*, *J Clin Psychopharmacol* 1999;**19**:407–15).

10.* **Venlafaxine** has a dose-dependent effect on supine diastolic blood pressure, clinically significant at high doses (200–300 mg/d), probably as a result of noradrenergic potentiation (3% incidence at less than 100 mg/d [n = 17, Emul *et al, J Psychopharmacol* 2009;**23**:163–7], 7% for 150–200 mg/d and 13% above 300 mg/d). However, high dose venlafaxine (mean 346 mg/d, range 225–525) did not produce any significant effects on ECG parameters, although 12.5% developed hypertension and a dose-related association with heart rate (n = 37, Mbaya *et al, Hum Psychopharmacol* 2007;**22**:129–33). Indeed, a nested case-control study showed that venlafaxine (n = 19268) is not associated with an excess risk of cardiac events compared to fluoxetine, dosulepin or citalopram in depression or anxiety (n = 207384, Martinez *et al, Br Med J* 2010;**340**:249). In the UK, venlafaxine is no longer subject to excessive MHRA and SmPC restrictions, as:

- It is only contraindicated in patients with an identified high risk of a serious cardiac ventricular arrhythmia or with uncontrolled hypertension (but is **not** contraindicated in controlled hypertension).
- There is a caution for use in established cardiac disease that may increase the risk of ventricular arrhythmias. No baseline ECG is needed but regular bp is recommended.

Duloxetine causes no QTc prolongation or major cardiac effects (n = 128, Wohlreich *et al, Depress Anxiety* 2007;**24**:41–52, MS), but is contraindicated in uncontrolled hypertension (SmPC; *MHRA Drug Safety Update* 2007;1–9). In rare studies of supra-therapeutic doses, duloxetine up to 400 mg/d produced rises in bp and pulse (which might precipitate prehypertensive people to become hypertensive), but did not have severe clinically important ADRs (related studies: n = 117, RCT, d/b, p/c, c/o, 16/7, Derby *et al, J Cardiovasc Pharmacol* 2007;**49**:384–93; n = 117, RCT, d/b, p/c, Zhang *et al, J Cardiovasc Pharmacol* 2007;**49**:146–53, MS). Exacerbation of stable heart failure has been reported with duloxetine and/or venlafaxine (n = 2, Colucci and Berry, *Ann Pharmacother* 2008; **42**:882–7).

11.* A meta-analysis showed that **mirtazapine** was clearly more effective for depression in cardiac disease than placebo, with no difference in drop-outs (s = 4, n = 798, p/c, 9–24/52, Dowlati *et al, Can J Psychiatry* 2010;**55**:91–9). No ECG changes have been observed in reported trials, or bp and heart rate changes in a depressed in-patient trial (n = 251, RCT, 6/12, Zivkov and Jongh, *Hum Psychopharmacol* 1995;**10**:173–80). **Agomelatine** appears to have no cardiac effects, e.g. no QTc changes, ECG abnormalities, or other parameters (SmPC), although there is a single case of fully reversible QTc prolongation with agomelatine (n = 1, Kozian and Syrbe, *Psychiatr Prax* 2010;**37**:405–7).

12.* **Tricyclics** produce orthostatic hypotension (and hence occasional myocardial infarction), have antiarrhythmic actions (quinidine-like) in high dose and antimuscarinic actions (raising heart rate) and a large cross-sectional survey showed a modest risk of CVD with tricyclics, although an HR of 1.35 is non-significant in a non-RCT (n = 14784 [4.9% on antidepressants], Hamer *et al, Eur Heart J* 2011;**32**:437–42). On average, starting tricyclics increases the QTc interval by 6.9 msec (including amitriptyline 8.5 ms and nortriptyline 35 msec) (n = 8222, van Noord *et al, J Clin Psychopharmacol* 2009;**29**:9–15). Thus, tricyclics should only be used with extreme caution in patients with ischaemic heart disease, ventricular arrhythmia, angina, recent MI and hypertension. Indeed, a study indicated that the odds ratio for developing IHD was significantly raised for patients who had *ever* received a TCA (even adjusting for other factors), with a further specific, significant and dose-related association with **dosulepin** (n = 922 with IHD, 5516 controls, Hippisley-Cox *et al, Br Med J* 2001;**323**:666–9). In patients with recurrent chest pain but normal coronary angiograms, **imipramine** therapy over 9–33 months produced no symptoms of a pro-arrhythmic effect, a slightly prolonged corrected QT interval and reduced chest pain (n = 58, Cannon *et al, NEJM* 1994;**330**:1411–7). Conversely, 150 mg/d of **amitriptyline** increased heart rate from 78 bpm to 93 bpm, and all other heart rate analysis parameters significantly worsened (n = 48, Rechlin *et al, Psychopharmacology* 1994;**116**:110–4). **Nortriptyline** has significant effects on cardiac vagal function and should only be used with care in IHD (n = 44, Yeragani *et al, Neuropsychobiology* 2002;**46**:125–35), especially in men who may be more susceptible to its cardiac side-effects (n = 78, 6/52, Pomara *et al, Prog Neuropsychopharmacol Biol Psychiatry* 2001;**25**:1035–48). **Doxepin-**

induced torsade de pointes tachycardia has been reported (n = 1, Alter et al, Ann Intern Med 2001;**135**:384–5).

13. Reversible ventricular tachycardia (n = 1, Vitullo et al, Chest 1990;**98**:247–8) and QT prolongation has been reported with **trazodone** overdose (n = 1, Service and Waring, Clin Toxicol [Phila] 2008;**46**:71–3; n = 1, Dattilo and Nordin, J Clin Psychiatry 2007;**68**:1309–10), but is generally considered of low risk.

14. **Reboxetine** increased baseline heart rate in 20% of patients in short-term trials. Orthostatic hypotension occurs with increasing frequency at higher doses.

15. **Isocarboxazid, phenelzine** and **tranylcypromine** are contraindicated in severe cardiac disease.

16. Many cases of hypertension have been reported with **moclobemide**, so monitoring bp may be useful. Occasional hypertension with tyramine in patients with pre-existing labile hypertension has also occurred, and so caution in cardiac disease would be sensible. **St John's wort** does not seem to affect heart rate variability 75 mg/d (n = 12, RCT, d/b, c/o, 14/7 per arm, Siepmann et al, Br J Clin Pharmacol 2002;**54**:277–82). There are no apparent problems with **mianserin** and **tryptophan**.

3.2.3 ANXIOLYTICS AND HYPNOTICS

Anxiety and depression are inter-related predictors of ventricular arrhythmias in people with coronary artery disease and so treatment of these may be important (n = 940, Watkins et al, Psychosom Med 2006;**68**:651–6; comment by Rutledge and Linke, EBMH 2007;**10**:43).

17. **Benzodiazepines** are relatively safe but contraindicated in acute pulmonary insufficiency. One study in elderly patients showed that temazepam (up to 30 mg/d) caused a fall in systolic blood pressure and an increase in heart rate (n = 12, Ford, Br J Clin Pharmacol 1990;**29**:61–7).

18. **Buspirone** may have some cardiac effects, e.g. rare cases of hypertension and tachycardia.

19. There are no apparent problems with **zaleplon, zolpidem** and **zopiclone**.

20. The use of **beta-blockers** would depend upon the nature of the cardiac disease. In a prospective study of people with end-stage severe HF (61% with MDD), beta-blockers had a significant effect on reducing mortality but only if used with SSRIs, and had a negative effect if used with SNRIs or TCAs (n = 250 [c = 83], 18/12, Tousoulis et al, J Card Fail 2008;**14**:456–64).

21. **Clomethiazole** is contraindicated in acute pulmonary insufficiency and should be used with care in chronic pulmonary insufficiency. **Chloral** is contraindicated in severe cardiac disease. No problems are anticipated for **melatonin** (SmPC; s = 2, n = 43, RCT, Zaslavskaia et al, Klin Med (Mosk) 2008;**86**:64–7).

3.2.4 ANTICONVULSANTS

22. * CV effects from **carbamazepine** are uncommon but reports exist of cardiac conduction changes, hypertension and AV block (n = 1, Labrecque et al, Am J Psychiatry 1992;**149**:572–3), enough to make a pacemaker ineffective (n = 1, Ambrosi et al, Lancet 1993;**342**:365). Carbamazepine causes a rise in cholesterol, HDL and LDL levels (n = 52 + 80 controls, Svalheim et al, Acta Neurol Scand Suppl 2010;**190**:30–3). Patients on **oxcarbazepine** with cardiac insufficiency and secondary heart failure should have regular weight measurements to help detect any fluid retention and care is needed in patients with pre-existing conduction disturbances (UK SmPC).

23. * **Valproate** appears to have no adverse effects on ECG, it might even have some preventive or stabilising effects on ventricular conduction (n = 55, Kurt et al, J Psychopharmacol 2009;**23**:328–33) and may decrease the risk of MI in people with epilepsy (n = 155089, 10 years, Olesen et al, Pharmacoepidemiol Drug Saf 2011;**20**:146–53).

24. **Phenytoin** has many cardiac effects and is a third-line treatment in cardiac arrhythmias. It is, however, contraindicated in sinus bradycardia, sino-atrial block, second and third-degree A-V block and patients with Adams-Stokes syndrome. Severe cardiovascular ADRs have been reported with **fosphenytoin** IV, including asystole, VF and cardiac arrest, mostly within 30 minutes of an injection (see SmPC for full details).

25. IV **barbiturates** can cause hypotension. As there is no evidence that **primidone** causes QT-prolongation (and may actually shorten it), it may be a drug of choice in QT-prolongation (Christidis et al, Seizure 2006;**15**:64–6).

26. * There is no evidence of any problems with **gabapentin** in cardiac disease. A study showed

that **lamotrigine** 100–400 mg/d had no QTc prolonging effect (n = 152, d/b, p/c, c/o, 11/52, Dixon et al, Br J Clin Pharmacol 2008;**66**:396–404), or raise its lipid levels over six months (n = 73 + 80 controls, Svalheim et al, Acta Neurol Scand Suppl 2010;**190**:30–3) but ECG monitoring is recommended in cases of overdose (Buckley et al, Lancet 1993;**342**:1552–3). **Levetiracetam** does not affect lipid levels over six months (n = 52 + 80 controls, Svalheim et al, Acta Neurol Scand Suppl 2010;**190**:30–3).

27. No significant changes in ECG, blood pressure or heart rate have been noted in clinical trials with **topiramate, vigabatrin** and **tiagabine**. There is now a caution for the use of **pregabalin** in severe CHF (SmPC) and there are cases of exacerbation of heart failure in people with clinically stable CHF taking pregabalin for neuropathic pain (n = 3 and review, Page et al, J Cardiovasc Med (Hagerstown) 2008;**9**:922–5). The UK SmPC for **rufinamide** states it may shorten the QTc interval. Prolongations in PR interval have been observed with **lacosamide** and so caution is necessary in severe cardiac disease (SmPC).

28. There have been reports of hypotension and tachycardia in young children given IV **paraldehyde** (Sinal and Crowe, Pediatrics 1976;**57**:158).

3.2.5 OTHERS

29. The use of **anticholinesterases** has been associated with increased rates and risk of hospitalisation for bradycardia (n = 627, Park-Wyllie et al, PloS Med 2009;**6**:e1000157), syncope, bradycardia, pacemaker insertion, and hip fractures in older adults with dementia (n = 81,302, Gill et al, Arch Intern Med 2009;**169**:867–73). Heart block has been reported with **donepezil**, and so the UK SmPC has recommended considering this before prescribing (Curr Prob Pharmacovig 1999;**25**:7). **Rivastigmine** appears to have a favourable cardiac safety profile (s = 4, n = 2149, d/b, p/c, 26/52, Morganroth et al, J Clin Pharmacol 2002;**42**:558–68) and a modest reduction in mean heart rate of 1.5–2 bpm, but no bradycardia or ECG abnormalities (n = 661, Ballard et al, Int J Clin Pract 2006;**60**:639–45). **Galantamine** would appear relatively safe but caution is advised in people with cardiovascular conditions, e.g. sick sinus syndrome or other supraventricular cardiac conduction disturbances.

There is little data on **memantine** in cardiac disease and use should be only with caution as it has been reported to cause bradycardia (n = 36, Gallini et al, Pharmacoepidemiol Drug Saf 2008;**17**:877–81).

30. **Anticholinergics** should be used with caution, particularly in those with a tendency to tachycardia. Sinus bradycardia has been reported with **benzatropine** (Voinov et al, Am J Psychiatry 1992;**149**:711) and **benzhexol/trihexyphenidyl** (n = 1, Blumensohn et al, Drug Intell Clin Pharm 1986;**20**:786–7).

31. **Disulfiram** is C/I in cardiac failure, coronary artery disease, previous history of CVA and hypertension, and can be cardiotoxic in overdose (n = 1, Jerónimo et al, Arq Bras Cardiol 2009;**92**:16–18). The Antabuse-alcohol reaction can cause cardiac arrest even in healthy adults. There are no known problems with **acamprosate**.

32. **Lithium** rarely causes clinical problems, although cardiac failure and sick sinus syndrome are contraindications. Usually benign cardiovascular side-effects may occur in 20–30% patients. The main problems with lithium can be T-wave flattening (or possibly inversion), ventricular ectopics, congestive myopathy, bradycardia (Farag et al, Lancet 1994;**343**:1371), ECG changes and conduction disturbances, e.g. sinus node dysfunction (Terao et al, Acta Psychiatr Scand 1996;**93**:407–8). On average, starting lithium increases the QTc interval by 18.6 msec (n = 8222, van Noord et al, J Clin Psychopharmacol 2009;**29**:9–15). An analysis, however, (n = 827, Ahrens et al, J Affect Disord 1995;**33**:67–75) showed that deaths from cardiac-related causes were no different in people taking lithium than in the general population, and so, despite the above reported problems, lithium can be considered to have no significant risk in this situation (reviewed by Ananth, Lithium 1993; **4**:167–79). A pre-treatment ECG is very useful, especially in the elderly.

33. **Modafinil** is contraindicated in severe hypertension and arrhythmia and used with caution in patients with concurrent heart disease. Monitor heart rate and bp if used in moderate hypertension (MI; discussion by Heitmann et al, Clin Pharmacol Therapy 1999;**65**:328–35). **Sodium oxybate** contains a significant dose of sodium (0.75 g in 4.5 g dose) and so dietary restriction of sodium might be considered in hypertension and heart failure (SmPC).

34. The EMEA (2009) recommends screening for c/v problems before prescribing and periodically, as stimulant and non-stimulant medication are associated with minor but statistically significant changes in heart rate and bp (n = 125, Wilens et al, J Clin Psychiatry 2005;**66**:253–9). The SmPCs for **methylphenidate** recommend caution in people with severe hypertension, and bp monitoring should be carried out in all patients. Ongoing therapy at relatively high dose methylphenidate (1.5 mg/kg/d) can produce a small but significant increase in bp, especially during the first six weeks (n = 114[c = 57], open, 6/12, Hammerness et al, J Pediatr 2009;**155**:84–9). **Atomoxetine** is associated with modest increases in bp (mean < 5 mmHg) and pulse (mean < 10 bpm), which stabilise over two years (UK SmPC). Recent UK MHRA guidance is that atomoxetine should be used with caution in those with prolonged QT or a family history of QT prolongation, and care when used with other drugs that produce QT prolongation, drugs that can cause electrolyte disturbances and CYP2D6 inhibitors. Atomoxetine may produce a dramatic rise in blood pressure in people with central autonomic failure, even at very low doses (n = 3, RCT, p/c, c/o, Shibao et al, Hypertension 2007;**50**:47–53).

35. There is little evidence of developing hypertension with **dexamfetamine**, although regular bp testing has been recommended (ASDA, Sleep 1994;**17**:348–51). In adult ADHD, cardiovascular effects from amphetamine XR preps at < 60 mg/d were minimal (n = 223, < 24/12, Weisler et al, CNS Spectr 2005;**10**(suppl 20):35–43).

36. **Bupropion** may cause small rises in supine blood pressure (n = 58, RCT, Kiev et al, Ann Clin Psychiatry 1994;**6**:107–15), but tends not to cause significant conduction complications, or to exacerbate ventricular arrhythmias and has a low rate of orthostatic hypotension (n = 36, open, Roose et al, Am J Psychiatry 1991;**148**:512–6). However, infrequent occurrences of orthostatic hypotension, tachycardia, stroke and vasodilation have been reported. In mild untreated hyper-

tension, bupropion up to 400 mg/d has no effect on blood pressure (n = 300, RCT, d/b, p/c, 4/52, Thase et al, J Clin Psychopharmacol 2008; **28**:302–7).

37. **Methadone** can lengthen the QT interval and the CSAT (Center for Substance Abuse Treatment Cardiac Expert Panel) Consensus Guidelines has made five recommendations:
1. Inform patients of the risk of arrhythmia.
2. Enquire about any history of heart disease, arrhythmia or syncope.
3. Carry out pre-treatment ECG to measure QTc, repeated at 30 days and annually, with additional ECGs if the dose exceeds 100 mg/d or if unexplained syncope or seizures occur.
4. If QTc is 451–499 ms, discuss with client and monitor more frequently. If QTc > 500 ms discontinue or reduce dose (although there appears to be no recommendation if the QTc is exactly 500 ms).
5. Clinicians must be aware of interactions with other QT-prolonging or interacting drugs, e.g. 3A4 inhibitors.

(Krantz et al, Ann Intern Med 2009;**150**:387–95, 417–8; George et al, Curr Drug Abuse Rev 2008;**1**:297–302; Stringer et al, Am J Health Syst Pharm 2009;**66**:825–33; n = 109, Fonseca et al, Drug Alcohol Depend 2009;**99**:327–32).

However, to put it in perspective, a Finnish study showed that 4.6% of methadone-treated patients had a QTc > 500 msec, but that the maximum mortality attributable to QTc prolongation was low at 0.06 per 100 patient-years (n = 200, Anchersen et al, Addiction 2009;**104**:993–9). **Buprenorphine** is associated with less QTc prolongation than methadone (n = 165, RCT, d/b, 17/52, Wedam et al, Arch Intern Med 2007;**167**:2469–75), with some reports of no QTc prolongation with Suboxone (n = 50, 2–4/52, Baker et al, Ann Pharmacotherapy 2006;**40**:392–6). It has been used safely in a patient with methadone-induced torsades de pointes (n = 1, Krantz et al, Pharmacotherapy 2005;**25**:611–4).

3

3.3 DIABETES

	LOWER RISK	MODERATE RISK	HIGHER RISK
Antipsychotics	Amisulpride[5] Aripiprazole[2] Asenapine[2] Butyrophenones[6] Paliperidone[1] Pimozide[8] Risperidone[1] Sulpiride[5] Ziprasidone[2]	Phenothiazines[7] Quetiapine[2] Thioxanthenes[4]	Clozapine[3] Olanzapine?[2]
Antidepressants	Agomelatine[14] Duloxetine[10] Moclobemide[16] Reboxetine[14] SSRIs[9] Trazodone[13] Tryptophan[16] Venlafaxine[10]	Fluoxetine[9] Mianserin[16] Mirtazapine[11] Tricyclics[12]	MAOIs[15]
Anxiolytics and hypnotics	Benzodiazepines[17] Buspirone[18] Chloral[21] Clomethiazole[21] Melatonin[21] Zaleplon[19] Zolpidem[19] Zopiclone[19]	Beta-blockers[20]	
Anticonvulsants	Barbiturates[25] Benzodiazepines[17] Carbamazepine[22] Ethosuximide[28] Gabapentin[26] Lamotrigine[26] Oxcarbazepine[22] Pregabalin[26] Rufinamide[27] Vigabatrin[27]	Acetazolamide[28] Phenytoin[24] Topiramate[27] Tiagabine[27] Zonisamide[27] Valproate[23]	Lacosamide[26]
Others	Acamprosate[31] Anticholinergics[30] Anticholinesterases[29] Atomoxetine[33] Buprenorphine[35] Lithium[32] Memantine[29] Methadone[35] Methylphenidate[33] Modafinil[33]	Bupropion[34] Disulfiram[31] Sodium oxybate[33]	

GENERAL PRINCIPLES IN DIABETES

1. Use drugs least likely to promote loss of diabetic control or alter glucose levels.
2. Warn that some side-effects may be interpreted as hypoglycaemia.
3. Check the family history.
4. Monitor weight and glucose parameters.

3.3.1 ANTIPSYCHOTICS *

People with schizophrenia are more liable to develop diabetes, with antipsychotics adding to that risk (n = 99, RCT, d/b, Saddichha et al, Acta Psychiatr Scand 2008;**117**:342–7). In a study of 30% of the Danish population, 3.5% developed diabetes, and this was 1.17-1.57 times more likely with olanzapine, clozapine and risperidone, but not with amisulpride, quetiapine, aripiprazole (n=345242,937, Kessing et al, Br J Psychiatry 2010;**197**:266-71). In non-diabetic schizophrenics, glucose tolerance tests show elevated plasma glucose (compared to placebo or FGAs) at all time points for olanzapine, partly raised for clozapine and only raised with risperidone compared to untreated non-schizophrenics, indicating an adverse effect by some atypicals on glucose regulation (n = 79, Newcomer et al, Arch Gen Psychiatry 2002;**59**:337–45). In diabetics, antipsychotics can worsen metabolic control and double the need for insulin, especially in the first two years (n = 2585, Spoelstra et al, J Clin Psychiatry 2004;**65**:674–8). In people aged over 65 with pre-existing diabetes, initiating any antipsychotic is associated with increased risk for hospitalisation for hyperglycaemia (n = 13817, Lipscombe et al, Arch Int Med 2009;**169**:1282–9).

1. There appears to be only a modest effect from **risperidone** on blood biochemistry (n = 38 632, Veterans, Sernyak et al, Am J Psychiatry 2002;**159**:561–6). **Paliperidone** has only a few rare reports of glucose-related adverse events (SmPC).

2. **Aripiprazole** is not thought to have any problems in diabetes (see n=345,937, Kessing et al, Br J Psychiatry 2010;**197**:266-71) although hyperglycaemia as an ADR has been added to the UK SmPC. The incidence of hyperglycaemia in trials with **asenapine** (US PI) is less than 1% and so some care would be prudent, although it is only a precaution. **Olanzapine** seems to be the most likely of the SGAs to cause or exacerbate diabetes (see introduction), e.g. a cohort study indicated that the incidence of new-onset diabetes was about 1%, but 20% higher with olanzapine than risperidone, and 90% higher in the first three months of treatment (n = 33 946, three years, Caro et al, J Clin Psychiatry 2002;**63**:1135–9). In 5000 patients with baseline non-fasting glucose levels of ≤ 7.8/L, the incidence of raised glucose (≥ 11 mmol/L, suggestive of diabetes) was 1% (cf 0.9% placebo). Raised levels (8.9–11 mmol/L; suggestive of hyperglycaemia) were 2% with olanzapine (cf 1.6% placebo) and so hyperglycaemia or exacerbation of pre-existing diabetes is in the 'very rare' spontaneous event (< 0.01%) category in the UK SmPC. Olanzapine is also associated with the metabolic syndrome via e.g. weight gain, elevated levels of insulin, leptin and lipids (triglycerides and cholesterol), e.g. olanzapine (mean 14 mg/d) can produce fasting triglyceride levels raised by a mean of 60 mg/dL (37%) (n = 25, 12/52, Osser et al, J Clin Psychiatry 1999;**60**:767–70), which needs care since triglycerides are a risk factor for precipitation or exacerbation of diabetes. Insulin resistance is possibly the predominant mechanism, as the insulin secretory response to hyperglycaemic challenge is significantly decreased by olanzapine (e.g. n = 26, RCT, 14/7, Chiu et al, J Clin Psychopharmacol 2006;**26**:504–7). Routine quarterly glucose monitoring is recommended with olanzapine, regardless of pre-existing diabetes (n = 590, Wirshing et al, J Clin Psychiatry 2002;**63**:856–65; reviews by Eder-Ischia et al, Essent Psychopharmacol 2005;**6**:112–7; Koller and Doraiswamy, Pharmacotherapy 2002;**22**:841–52). There is evidence for a slightly increased risk of diabetes with **quetiapine** (n = 38 632, Veterans, Sernyak et al, Am J Psychiatry 2002;**159**:561–6). **Sertindole** may modify insulin and glucose responses and may require adjustments to hypoglycaemic drug doses. Short-term treatment with **ziprasidone** appears to have little effect on glucose levels, and it may actually lower serum cholesterol and triglyceride levels (n = 37, 6/52, open, Kingsbury et al, J Clin Psychiatry 2001; **62**:347–9).

3. Elevated glucose levels (in up to 23% in people with no PMH, n = 121, Sernyak et al, J Clin Psychiatry 2003;**64**:605–8) and diabetes have been shown with **clozapine**, and a dose-related effect noted, indicating a probable influence on insulin secretion and a causal relationship

3

(n = 384, FDA MedWatch, Koller et al, Am J Med 2001;**111**:716–23). Clozapine may impair glucose control, independent of changes in insulin sensitivity and BMI (n = 20, open, 4/12, Howes et al, Am J Psychiatry 2004;**161**:361–3).Clozapine is also well-known to cause metabolic syndrome, e.g. weight gain and lipid abnormalities (e.g. raised serum triglycerides) which are significant risk factors for developing diabetes (n = 82, naturalistic, five years, Henderson et al, Am J Psychiatry 2000; **157**:975–81). Augmentation with quetiapine has been suggested as a possible management option (n = 65, open, 10/12, Reinstein et al, Clin Drug Invest 1999;**18**:99–104). Routine glucose monitoring is recommended with clozapine, regardless of pre-existing diabetes (n = 590, Wirshing et al, J Clin Psychiatry 2002;**63**:856–65; review by Mir and Taylor, Int Clin Psychopharmacol 2001;**16**:63–74).

4. Lack of relationship between serum levels of **zuclopenthixol** (n = 9) and plasma insulin has been shown (Melkersson et al, J Clin Psychiatry 1999;**60**:783–91). The UK SmPC for **flupentixol** notes that control of diabetes may be impaired and that an adjustment in antidiabetic therapy may be necessary.

5. There are no apparent problems with **sulpiride** and **amisulpride**.

6. There are no apparent problems with **haloperidol**.

7. A case-control study of cases of newly-treated diabetes indicated a modest and significant increased risk with **chlorpromazine** and **perphenazine** (n = 7227 + 6780, Wang et al, J Clin Psychopharmacol 2002;**22**:236–43), but lack of relationship between serum levels of perphenazine (n = 12) and plasma insulin has been shown (Melkersson et al, J Clin Psychiatry 1999;**60**:783–91). Many phenothiazines cause weight gain and appetite stimulation which wouldn't help diabetic control.

8. There are no known problems with **pimozide**.

3.3.2 ANTIDEPRESSANTS *

Although diabetes is a major risk factor for depression and vice versa, depression needs to be resolved as well for diabetes to improve (s = 14, n = 1724, RCT, van der Feltz-Cornelius et al, Gen Hosp Psychiatry 2010;**32**:380–95). The presence of pain in type 2 diabetes inhibits antidepressant response so needs auxiliary treatment (n = 387,

open, 16/52, Anderson et al, Diabetes Care 2010;**33**:485–9), the presence of depression reduces glycaemic control and adherence (n = 866, 12/12, Dirmaier et al, Psychother Psychosom 2010;**79**:172–8), but the presence of DM has no effect on the response of MDD to antidepressants (n = 2876, Bryan et al, Gen Hosp Psychiatry 2010;**32**:33–41). In the short-term, SSRIs may even decrease serum glucose levels by up to 30% and cause anorexia (reducing body weight), and in the short-term may enable people with diabetes to control hunger and eat better, via their serotonergic effects, but tricyclics have the opposite effects (n = 60[c = 43], RCT, d/b, 8/52, Ghaeli et al, J Clin Psychopharmacol 2004;**24**:386–8). Indeed, in insulin-dependent diabetics, insulin use increases by 16%, but remains unchanged if treated with tricyclics and reduced by 13% if treated with an SSRI (n = 133, two years, Knol et al, Pharmacoepidemiol Drug Saf 2008;**17**:577–86).

There is, however, an increased incidence of diabetes with long-term (two years) anti-depressant use (same for tricyclics and SSRIs) at moderate to high dose, but not with lower doses or shorter-use (n = 2243 + 8963 controls, Andersohn et al, Am J Psychiatry 2009;**166**:591–8). The five-year absolute risk for developing diabetes is:

- 1.1% for non-users/general population
- 1.7% for standard use of antidepressants
- 2.3% for higher doses of antidepressants
- but no effect in people taking metformin

(n = 151,347, Kivimäki et al Diabetes Care 2010; **33**:2611–6).

Reviews: * treatment of depression in diabetes mellitus (s = 14, n = 1724, RCT, van der Feltz-Cornelis et al, Gen Hosp Psychiatry 2010;**32**:380–95), general (Lustman, Curr Psychiatry Rep 2008;**10**:495–502).

9. No dose changes are recommended with **citalopram/escitalopram**. Citalopram has no significant effect on insulin sensitivity in women of reproductive age (n = 32, RCT, open, 8/52, Kauffman et al, Gynecol Endocrinol 2005;**21**:129–37), and no changes in glycaemic control were seen in another trial (Sindrup et al, Clin Pharmacol Ther 1992;**52**:547–52). People with diabetes may become hypoglycaemic during **fluoxetine** treatment (Drug Ther Bull 1990;**28**:33) and its side-effects, e.g. tremor, nausea, sweating and

anxiety may be mistaken for hypoglycaemia. Fluoxetine has been shown to effectively reduce the severity of depression in people with diabetes with a trend towards better glycaemic control (n = 60, RCT, p/c, 8/52, Lustman *et al*, *Diabetes Care* 2000;**23**:618–23). Most problems have been reported with the more common type 2 diabetes rather than the insulin dependent type 1 disease. If fluoxetine is used, warn about this effect, noting a possible loss of hypoglycaemic awareness (n = 1, Sawka *et al*, *J Pediatr* 2000;**136**:394–6) and regularly check serum glucose levels. There is a case of **fluvoxamine**-induced acute hyperglycaemia in a patient with diabetes (n = 1, Oswald *et al*, *Int J Neuropsychopharmacol* 2003;**6**:85–7). Little is reported with **paroxetine**. There have been no major reports of problems with **sertraline**, and maintenance dosing seems safe and effective in diabetes with a positive effect on the diabetes itself (n = 152, RCT, d/b, p/c, Lustman *et al*, *Arch Gen Psychiatry* 2006;**63**:521–9), especially in younger people (n = 152, d/b, p/c, Williams *et al*, *Diabetes Care* 2007;**30**:801–6). There are, however, cases of hypoglycaemia associated with sertraline (e.g. n = 1, Takhar and Williamson, *Can J Clin Pharmacol* 1999;**6**:12–4; n = 1, Pollak *et al*, *Ann Pharmacother* 2001;**35**:1371–4) and raised glucose levels in a person with diabetes (n = 1, Sansome and Sansome, *Int J Psychiatr Med* 2003;**33**:103–5).

10. There is no published evidence of problems with **venlafaxine** or **duloxetine**.

11. **Mirtazapine** does not seem to influence glucose homeostasis (n = 14, Laimer *et al*, *J Clin Psychiatry* 2006;**67**:421–4) and glucose tolerance may improve but insulin sensitivity remains unchanged (n = 10, Hennings *et al*, *Exp Clin Endocrinol Diabetes* 2010;**118**:98–100). Mirtazapine causes increased appetite which might be counter-productive. The mirtazapine UK SmPC recommends care, a class labelling precaution.

12. **Tricyclics** may adversely affect diabetic control as they increase serum glucose levels by up to 150%, increase carbohydrate craving and reduce the metabolic rate, but are generally considered safe unless the diabetes is very brittle. Nortriptyline tends to worsen glycaemic control (n = 68, RCT, d/b, p/c, 8/52, Lustman *et al*, *Psychosom Med* 1997;**59**:241–50).

13. There are no apparent problems with **trazodone**.

14. There are no apparent problems with **reboxetine** or **agomelatine**.

15. **MAOIs** may decrease serum glucose levels by up to 35% due to a direct influence on gluconeogenesis (Goodnick *et al*, *J Clin Psychiatry* 1995; **56**:128–36). Diabetes is a UK SmPC precaution for **isocarboxazid**.

16. There is a case of **mianserin** dose-related hyperglycaemia in a non-diabetic woman (Marley and Rohan, *Lancet* 1993;**342**:1430–1). **Moclobemide** 600 mg/d did not modify the effect of glibenclamide on plasma glucose and insulin levels in healthy individuals (Amrein *et al*, *Psychopharmacology* 1992;**106**:S24–S31).

3.3.3 ANXIOLYTICS AND HYPNOTICS

17. There is a case of a person with diabetes presenting with a reduction in insulin requirements after discontinuing **clonazepam** (n = 1, Wagner *et al*, *Diabetes Care* 1999;**22**:2099).

18. There are no apparent problems with **buspirone**.

19. There are no apparent problems with **zaleplon**, **zolpidem** and **zopiclone**.

20. **Propranolol** may prolong the hypoglycaemic response to insulin and may effect hypoglycaemic episodes.

21. There are no apparent problems with **ramelteon**, **melatonin**, **clomethiazole** or **chloral hydrate**.

3.3.4 ANTICONVULSANTS

22. There is an isolated report of **carbamazepine**-induced urinary retention in two patients with diabetes, where withdrawal improved the condition (Steiner and Birman, *Neurology* 1993; **43**:1855–6). There are no apparent problems with **oxcarbazepine**.

23. **Valproate** may give false positives in urine tests for diabetes. Protein binding of valproate may be lower in diabetes (Doucet *et al*, *Eur J Clin Pharmacol* 1993;**45**:577–9).

24. Hypoglycaemia has been reported with **phenytoin** and glucose metabolism can be affected. Protein binding of phenytoin may be lower in diabetes (Doucet *et al*, *Eur J Clin Pharmacol* 1993;**45**:577–9).

25. There are no apparent problems with **phenobarbital** or **primidone**.

3

26. There are no apparent problems with **lamotrigine** or **pregabalin**. Blood glucose fluctuations have been reported with **gabapentin** (e.g. n = 1, Penumalee *et al, Am J Kid Dis* 2003; **42**:E3–5).

27. No information is available on **topiramate, zonisamide** and **tiagabine** and no problems noted for **rufinamide**. There is no information on **lacosamide** (UK SmPC)

28. There are no apparent problems with **ethosuximide**. Hyperglycaemia has been reported with **acetazolamide** in diabetics and prediabetics, but probably not in non-diabetic patients, so some care may be necessary.

3.3.5 OTHERS

29. There are no apparent problems with **donepezil** or **galantamine**, but diabetes mellitus is a precaution for **rivastigmine**. No effect with **memantine** has been reported.

30. There are no known problems with the **anticholinergic agents**.

31. The literature for **disulfiram** recommends caution in diabetes mellitus. There are no apparent problems with **acamprosate**.

32. There is no problem with **lithium** in diabetes, but many patients on lithium develop polyuria and polydipsia, a diabetes insipidus-like syndrome via an effect on cAMP and vasopressin. This can be controlled by ensuring an adequate fluid and salt intake. There is a case of increased clearance of lithium in a patient with persistent hyperglycaemia, probably due to the subsequent osmotic diuresis increasing renal clearance (n = 1, Cyr *et al, Ann Pharmacother* 2002; **36**:427–9). Lithium may also increase insulin secretion.

33. There are no apparent problems with **methylphenidate** or **atomoxetine** but a transient loss of appetite may occur. There is no information on **sodium oxybate** and no apparent problems with **modafinil**.

34. Animal studies suggest some risks with **bupropion** and so caution is needed with use in people with type 2 diabetes (El-Dakhakhny *et al, Arzneimittel-forschung* 1996; **46**:667–9).

35. There are no precautions for the use of **buprenorphine** in diabetes (UK SmPC), or **methadone**, although the sugar-free liquid would be the presentation of choice for the latter.

3.4 EPILEPSY

	LOWER RISK	MODERATE RISK	HIGHER RISK
Antipsychotics	Amisulpride[5] Aripiprazole[2] Asenapine[2] Haloperidol[6] Pimozide[8] Risperidone?[1]	Olanzapine[2] Phenothiazines (most)[7] Quetiapine[2] Sertindole 2 Sulpiride[5] Ziprasidone[2] Zuclopenthixol[4]	Chlorpromazine[7] Clozapine[3]
Antidepressants	Agomelatine[14] MAOIs[15] Moclobemide?[16] Reboxetine[14] SSRIs[9] Tryptophan[16]	Duloxetine[10] Mianserin[16] Mirtazapine[11] Trazodone[13] Tricyclics (most)[12] Venlafaxine[10]	
Anxiolytics and hypnotics	Benzodiazepines[17] Beta-blockers[20] Chloral[21] Clomethiazole[21] Melatonin[21] Ramelteon[21] Zaleplon[19] Zolpidem[19] Zopiclone[19]	Buspirone[18]	
Others	Acamprosate[24] Anticholinergics[23] Methylphenidate[26] Modafinil[26]	Anticholinesterases[22] Atomoxetine[26] Disulfiram[24] Lithium[25] Memantine[22]	Bupropion[27] Sodium oxybate [26]

3

GENERAL PRINCIPLES FOR PRESCRIBING IN EPILEPSY (Pisani *et al*, *Drug Safety* 2002;**25**: 91–110, 166 refs)

Risk factors for psychotropic-induced seizures:

- History of epilepsy (including febrile seizures) in the patient or their family.
- Neurological abnormalities (including brain injury, angioma cavernous, blood-brain barrier abnormality).
- Cerebral arteriosclerosis.
- Elderly.
- Reduced drug clearance.
- Pre-existing EEG alterations.
- Physical illness (eg malignant hypertension).
- Polypharmacy.

Practical recommendations in pre-existing epilepsy:

- Use psychotropics with anticonvulsant properties where possible (e.g. carbamazepine, lamotrigine, benzodiazepines or valproate).
- Avoid high-risk drugs.
- Start low and go slow, monitoring plasma levels and EEG where possible.
- Keep dosing simple and avoid polypharmacy.

3.4.1 ANTIPSYCHOTICS

General principles

1. Keep the daily dose as low as possible; the proconvulsive effect may be dose-related.

2. Take extra care where risk factors exist, including head trauma, previous seizure history and concomitant drugs (especially other antipsychotics). The most susceptible patients are those with a history of epilepsy, any condition that predisposes to epilepsy and those withdrawing from central depressants, e.g. benzodiazepines and alcohol.

3. Use lowest risk drugs unless essential.

4. Use a slow rate of introduction and withdrawal. Anticonvulsant cover may be appropriate.

5. Dose changes should be small and gentle.

6. Avoid antipsychotics having more antihistaminic, antiserotonergic, sedative and antiadrenergic effects, which may have a greater seizure threshold lowering effect.

Reviews: interventions for psychosis in epilepsy (Farooq and Sherin, *Cochrane Database Syst Rev* 2008;**4**:CD006118), general (Kanner, *Semin Neurol* 2008;**28**:279–88).

1. There is little adverse information about **risperidone**. Pre-marketing trials showed a seizure incidence of 0.3% (n = 2607) and it has been used successfully for psychosis in epilepsy (n = 1, Mahgoub, *J Neuropsychiatry Clin Neurosci* 2007;**19**:347–8). The SmPC for **paliperidone** urges caution in people with risk factors or a history of seizures.

2. In pre-marketing trials, seizures occurred in only 0.1% patients taking **aripiprazole**, but should probably still be used with caution in epilepsy. Seizures have been reported in one patient on **asenapine** in trials (n = 851; 0.3%), compared with none with placebo (n = 706), and in long-term trials in five (n = 1953; 0.3%), so some care would be prudent but it is not an obvious problem (US PI). The literature for **olanzapine** states that it should be used cautiously in patients with a history of seizures. Unexplained seizures (i.e. patients without reported risk factors) occurred in 0.9% patients during pre-marketing trials (n = 2500). There may be a slightly higher risk of seizures in people over 65. The incidence of seizures during **quetiapine** trials has been equivalent to placebo but a short review suggested that it is associated with new-onset seizures in patients with seizurogenic conditions (Yalug *et al, J Neuropsychiatry Clin Neurosci* 2007;**19**:341–2). **Sertindole** should be used with caution in patients with a history of seizures. Seizures occurred in 0.4% patients during

pre-marketing trials with **ziprasidone** (many with confounding factors), but it would be wise to use with caution in epilepsy.

3. **Clozapine** can cause dose-related seizures, the risk rising from 1% (< 300 mg/d), through 2.7% (300–600 mg/d) to 4.4% (> 600 mg/d). EEG changes occur in 75% people on clozapine, with up to 40% having paroxysmal discharges (reviewed by Pacia and Devinsky, *Neurology* 1994;**44**:2247–9). A more rapid dose-titration increases the risk. Valproate is the routine anticonvulsant cover of choice, at clozapine doses of 600 mg/d or more. See also *4.2.4* and *6.3*.

4. **Zuclopenthixol** may have only mild-to-moderate effects, with few adverse reports, and may be one of the drugs of choice, although the UK SmPC now notes that it should only be used with caution in epilepsy. There is no mention in the **flupentixol** SmPC.

5. There are no known problems with **amisulpride**, except in overdose (n = 1, Tracqui *et al, Hum Exp Toxicol* 1995;**14**:294–8). **Sulpiride** may be a reasonable choice, with a few cases of convulsions reported and only minimal EEG effects but the UK SmPC warns about reducing the seizure threshold so care is recommended in unstable epilepsy.

6. **Haloperidol** may have only mild-to-moderate effects, and may be a lower risk drug.

7. **Fluphenazine** may have a low proconvulsive effect, although status epilepticus has been reported (n = 1, Leksowski, *Psychiatr Pol* 1983; **17**:445–7). The incidence of seizures with **chlorpromazine** may be 9% at doses above 1 g/d and 0.5% at less than 1 g/d and is best avoided.

8. **Pimozide** may have a low effect as, although it may enhance spike activity at low dose, it may not do so at higher dose (Oliver *et al, Arch Gen Psychiatry* 1982;**39**:206–9). Epilepsy is not mentioned in the UK SmPC.

3.4.2 ANTIDEPRESSANTS

Unless a large scale trial is carried out (unlikely), the safest antidepressant in epilepsy will remain unknown. All patients require an individual assessment of their risk factors and recognition that there is a dose-dependent relationship between antidepressants and seizures. A **slow rate of introduction** reduces the risk. **Lamotrigine** has proved useful for interictal depression (n = 13, open, Kalogjera-Sackellares and Sackellares, *Epilepsy Behav* 2002;**3**:510–6), as well as in bipolar depression. In a post-hoc analysis of patients with MDD and TLE, antidepressants were effective, with no serious ADRs and no increase in seizures with citalopram, reboxetine and mirtazapine (n = 75, RCT, Kuhn *et al*, *Epilepsy Behav* 2003;**4**:674–9). The risk of depression is doubled in seizure sufferers (13% vs 7%) (n = 130,880, Fuller-Thomson and Brennenstuhl, *Epilepsia* 2009;**50**:1051–8).

Reviews: depression in epilepsy (Seethalakshmi and Krishnamoorthy, *Epileptic Disord* 2007;**9**:1–10; Mula *et al*, *Expert Opin Pharmacother* 2008;**9**: 3159–68).

9. Serotonin function is unlikely to be of major importance in the genesis of seizures and so **SSRIs** are likely to have a low proconvulsive effect (review by Kondziella and Asztely, *Acta Neurol Scand* 2009;**119**:75–80). **Citalopram** and escitalopram have not been reported to interact with anticonvulsants or to have a proconvulsive effect, and citalopram has been used for interictal depression without an increase in seizure frequency or severity (n = 43, 8/52, Hovorka *et al*, *Epilepsy Behav* 2000;**1**:444–7; n = 75, RCT, Kuhn *et al*, *Epilepsy Behav* 2003;**4**:674–9). **Fluoxetine** has a probable seizure incidence of 0.2%, similar to other antidepressants, and may even have a positive effect (n = 17, open, add-on, Favale *et al*, *Neurology* 1995;**45**:1926–7). **Fluvoxamine** probably has a low proconvulsive effect, although this has been disputed (Vincenti, *Lancet* 1990;**336**:947) and there have been some literature reports of fits. **Paroxetine** appears to have a minimal potential for producing seizures at clinically useful doses (Sedgwick *et al*, *J Psychopharmacol* 1987;**1**:31–4; Milne and Goa, *Drugs* 1991;**41**:450–77). With **sertraline**, seizures occurred in early clinical trials at a similar frequency to placebo and only in people with a history of seizures, and it has been effective for depression in children and adolescents with epilepsy, with increased fits in only 6% (n = 36, Thomé-Souza *et al*, *Epilepsy Behav* 2007;**10**:417–25).

10. Seizures have been reported in 0.26% of patients treated with **venlafaxine** during clinical trials and so a slow introduction and withdrawal is recommended. For **duloxetine**, there is a UK SmPC caution for epilepsy but no reported problems as such.

11. One grand mal seizure has been reported

in a patient with a history of seizures receiving **mirtazapine** at a high dose of 80 mg/d during a trial. More definite information would be needed before a cause-effect link could be made. Care and monitoring would thus be standard.

12. All **tricyclics** seem to lower the seizure threshold, with **amitriptyline** reputed to be the most proconvulsive and **doxepin** possibly of lowest risk. TDM of tricyclics minimises the risk of toxicity (review by Preskorn and Fast, *J Clin Psychiatry* 1992;**53**:160–2).

13. The literature for **trazodone** now includes a caution in epilepsy, and a warning to avoid abrupt changes in dose.

14. **Reboxetine** may be particularly useful in epilepsy with a low interaction potential and a spontaneous incidence of seizures of < 0.2% (n = 1500), with no seizures in overdose. There are no apparent problems with **agomelatine**.

15. **MAOIs** are generally not considered epileptogenic at therapeutic doses and the UK SmPC for **isocarboxazid** notes a varying effect, with some people having decreased seizures and others increased seizures. MAOI-induced myoclonic jerks and serotonin syndrome can occasionally be interpreted as seizures.

16. There have been no reports of problems with **moclobemide** or **tryptophan** in epilepsy to date. **Mianserin** is often quoted as being relatively safe in epilepsy (n = 40, Edwards and Glen-Bott, *Br J Clin Pharmacol* 1983;**15**:299S–311S). One study of 84 overdoses of 1 g or more showed no convulsions (*Curr Med Res Opin* 1980;**6**:44).

3.4.3 ANXIOLYTICS AND HYPNOTICS

17. Animal studies show **buspirone** to have no anticonvulsant activity. The literature states buspirone to be contraindicated in epilepsy but there is no evidence that it is actually epileptogenic.

18. A weak anticonvulsant activity for **zopiclone** has been shown (Julou *et al*, *Pharmacol Biochem Behav* 1985;**23**:653–9). **Zolpidem** is not reported to have any anticonvulsant activity. There is no data on **zaleplon**.

19. There are no apparent problems with the **beta-blockers**.

20. There are no apparent problems with **melatonin** or **ramelteon**. **Chloral hydrate** and **clomethiazole** have anticonvulsant properties.

3.4.4 OTHERS

21. **Cholinomimetics** may have some potential for causing seizures so care is needed with **donepezil** in pre-existing seizure activity, although 10mg/d had no adverse effects on seizures in one trial (n = 23, RCT, s/b, p/c, c/o, 3+3/12, Hamberger *et al, Epilepsia* 2007;**48**:1283–91). Care should be exercised with the use of **rivastigmine** in patients predisposed to seizures. There has been no increase in the incidence of seizures with **galantamine** in clinical trials. A single case report with **memantine** suggests it should only be used with caution.

22. There are no problems reported with the **anticholinergic** agents.

23. The literature for **disulfiram** recommends caution in epilepsy. The manufacturers report no known problems with **acamprosate** in epilepsy.

24. **Lithium** has a marked epileptogenic activity in overdose, but probably has no effect at standard dose. **Carbamazepine** and **valproate** may be suitable alternatives.

25. * **Methylphenidate** is not associated with a significant risk of seizures at therapeutic doses, e.g. there was no association between methylphenidate and seizure risk in children aged 6–17 years with ADHD and no prior seizures (n < 34727, McAfee *et al, Curr Drug Saf* 2008;**3**:123–31), and it is generally considered safe for seizure-free children with epilepsy although there are a few reports of exacerbation (Kaufmann *et al, J Child Neurol* 2009;**24**:727–33). The incidence of seizures during clinical trials is 0.1–0.2%, not significantly different to placebo and similar to population-based data (review by Wernicke *et al, Dev Med Child Neurol*

2007;**49**:498–502) and so it may have a good risk:benefit ratio (Hamoda *et al, Expert Rev Neurother* 2009;**9**:1747–54; review by Koneski and Casella, *Arq Neuropsiquiatr* 2010;**68**:107–14). The MHRA guidance is that **atomoxetine** should be introduced with caution in patients with a history of seizures and discontinuing considered if seizures start or increase in frequency. However, the incidence during clinical trials was 0.1–0.2%, not significantly different to placebo and similar to population-based data (Wernicke *et al, Dev Med Child Neurol* 2007;**49**:498–502) and there was no association between atomoxetine and the seizure risk in children aged 6–17 years with ADHD and no prior seizures (n < 34727, McAfee *et al, Curr Drug Saf* 2008;**3**:123–31). **Sodium oxybate** has been reported to cause seizures and use is not recommended in epilepsy (SmPC). There are no apparent problems with **modafinil**.

26. **Bupropion** has some epileptogenic activity (literature warning: *Curr Prob Pharmacovig* 2001; **27**:5). The risk of seizures is about 0.4%, and it appears plasma level-related. Doses should not exceed 450mg/d (although new-onset seizures can occur at therapeutic doses up to 450mg/d, e.g. Pesola and Avasarala, *J Emerg Med* 2002;**22**:235–9), no single dose should be above 200mg and doses should not be increased at more than 150mg/d. It should be contraindicated in people with a history of seizures and concurrent eating disorder, known CNS tumor, and if abruptly withdrawing from benzodiazepines or alcohol. Other risk factors include concomitant use with any drug known to lower the seizure threshold, alcohol abuse, history of head trauma, diabetes treated with hypoglycaemics or insulin, and the use of stimulants or anorectics.

3.5 GLAUCOMA (narrow-angle)

	LOWER RISK	MODERATE RISK	HIGHER RISK
Antipsychotics	Asenapine[3] Butyrophenones[3] Paliperidone[3] Risperidone[3] Sulpiride[3] Thioxanthenes[2]	Aripiprazole[3] Clozapine[2] Phenothiazines[1] Sertindole 2 Ziprasidone[3] Zotepine[3]	Olanzapine[2]
Antidepressants	Agomelatine[5] Bupropion[5] Flupentixol[5] MAOIs[5] Moclobemide[5] Trazodone[5] Tryptophan[5]	Duloxetine[5] Mirtazapine[5] SSRIs[5] Venlafaxine[5]	Tricyclics[4]
Others	Acamprosate[8] Benzodiazepines[6] Clomethiazole[6] Disulfiram[8] Gabapentin[7] Lithium[8] Lofexidine[8] Memantine[8] Melatonin[8] Naltrexone[8] Phenobarbital[7] Phenytoin[7] Rufinamide[7] Tiagabine[7] Valproate[7] Z hypnotics[6]	Caffeine[8] Carbamazepine[7] Dexamfetamine[8] Lacosamide[7] Methylphenidate[8]	Atomoxetine[8] Anticholinergics[8] Topiramate[7]

3

Narrow-angle glaucoma (also called angle closure glaucoma) occurs in eyes with a narrow anterior chamber angle, where drainage of the aqueous fluid through the anterior chamber angle is reduced or blocked. Drugs with anticholinergic properties have the potential to either induce narrow-angle glaucoma or to worsen it, although the degree of anticholinergic effects is of greater importance (review by Lam *et al, Curr Opin Ophthalmol* 2007;**18**:146–51).

GENERAL RECOMMENDATIONS
Patients with shallow anterior chamber and/ or narrow angles, or with previously diagnosed glaucoma may be treated with drugs with anticholinergic properties, provided intraocular pressure is monitored, an ophthalmologist is involved and information is given on the symptoms of acute narrow-angle closure, with a recommendation to stop the drug and seek medical attention immediately should those symptoms occur. In a patient with a shallow anterior chamber and narrow angles, an ophthalmologist would normally perform an iridotomy or some type of drainage surgery to allow drug use. Treatment with miotic therapy, e.g. pilocarpine may not necessarily protect the patient with narrow angles against drug-induced angle closure, so monitoring is essential.

The main symptoms of acute narrow-angle

glaucoma are blurred vision, 'coloured halos' around bright lights, intense pain, lacrimation, lid oedema, red eye, nausea and vomiting (review by Quigley, *Lancet* 2011;**377**:1367–77). The incidence rises with age due to the ageing process, e.g. thickening of the lens, and most acute attacks occur in people who are unaware they have narrow iridocorneal angles. The peak effect from a drug on intraocular pressure can occur within 5–24 hours (or sooner).

Reviews: * ocular ADRs of psychotropics, including glaucoma (Richa and Yazbek, *CNS Drugs* 2010;**24**:501–26), drug-induced acute angle-closure glaucoma (Lachkar and Bouassida, *Curr Opin Ophthalmol* 2007;**18**:129–33), risk factors (Coleman and Kodjebacheva, *Open Ophthalmol J* 2009;**3**:38–42).

3.5.1 ANTIPSYCHOTICS

1. **Phenothiazines** have some anticholinergic effects so the potential for problems exists. Screening for glaucoma has been recommended before initiating therapy, although several studies have shown no detectable narrow-angle glaucoma in, e.g. 100 patients taking **thioridazine**, 98 on **fluphenazine** and 99 on **chlorpromazine** (Applebaum, *Arch Ophthalmol* 1963;**69**:578–80). Thus, there is a need for routine care (see introduction). There are a few case reports of single high-dose injection of IV or IM chlorpromazine producing a transient decrease in intraocular pressure (mentioned in review by Bristow and Hirsch, *Drug Saf* 1993;**8**:136–48).

2. Other antipsychotics with similar anticholinergic effects would include **clozapine**, **flupentixol**, **zotepine** and **zuclopenthixol**. Olanzapine is contraindicated in narrow-angle glaucoma.

3. Antipsychotics with little or no anticholinergic effect must still be considered to have a potential for problems, albeit probably at a low level, e.g. **sulpiride**, **haloperidol**, **risperidone** and **paliperidone**. Asenapine has no appreciable effect on muscarinic cholinergic receptors and so exacerbation of glaucoma is unlikely (US PI). No information is available on **ziprasidone** or **aripiprazole** but nothing would be expected.

3.5.2 ANTIDEPRESSANTS

4. **Tricyclics** generally have a greater anti-cholinergic effect than phenothiazines, although most of the data is so old it should be pensioned off soon. If patients are at risk of narrow-angle glaucoma, pre-treatment examination by an ophthalmologist is recommended. Patients with a narrow anterior chamber angle who are receiving glaucoma treatment or who have had laser treatment should have few problems provided care (see introduction) is taken (Oshika, *Drug Saf* 1995;**12**:256–63). There is a report of patients with narrow angles developing acute-angle closure glaucoma with **imipramine** (n = 4, Ritch et al, *Arch Ophthalmol* 1994;**112**:67–8), and with **clomipramine** (Schlingemann et al, *Lancet* 1996;**347**:465). A survey by Reid and Blouin (*Psychosomatics* 1976;**17**:83–5) showed no abnormal intraocular pressures in patients taking tricyclics, even in combination with **phenothiazines**. A postal survey of ophthalmologists and psychiatrists indicated that occasional, probably drug-induced cases had been seen, most frequently associated with **amitriptyline** (review by Lieberman and Stoudemire, *Psychosomatics* 1987;**28**:145–8). See general recommendations.

5. * Antidepressants that can cause dilation of the pupil include the **SSRIs**, **mirtazapine**, **moclobemide**, **trazodone** (case of aggravated angle-closure glaucoma with low-dose trazodone: Pae et al, *Psych Clin Neurosci* 2003;**57**:127–8) and **MAOIs**. An extensive and arcane review has summarised six cases of angle-closure glaucoma with **paroxetine** (three in older people [aged 70–91] outside the normal life-period presentation; and three in younger people), one case with **fluvoxamine** (n = 1, Jimenez-Jimenez et al, *Ann Pharmacother* 2001;**35**:1565–6), and two with **citalopram** (in younger women, n = 1, Croos et al, *BMC Ophthalmol* 2005;**5**:23; n = 1, Massaoutis et al, *Br J Ophthalmol* 2007;**91**:1086–7). There is a new UK SmPC warning, uveal effusions and bilateral angle-closure glaucoma with **escitalopram** (n = 1, Zelefsky et al, *Am J Ophthalmol* 2006;**141**:1144–7). There are cases with **fluoxetine** (Ahmad, *DICP Ann Pharmacother* 1991;**25**:436; n = 1, Aveyard et al, *Prog Neurol Psychiatry* 2010;**14**:8–10), and none with **sertraline** (review by Costagliola et al, *Curr Neuropharmacol* 2008;**6**:293–310). There is limited experience with **reboxetine** but the literature recommends close supervision. Raised intraocular pressure or narrow-angle glaucoma is a warning in the UK SmPC for **venlafaxine**, and

bilateral acute narrow-angle glaucoma has been reported as developing rapidly with venlafaxine (n = 1, Ng et al, Med J Aust 2002;**176**:241). Mydriasis has been reported with **duloxetine**, so caution is necessary in patients with raised intraocular pressure or at risk of acute narrow-angle glaucoma. No problems are expected with **agomelatine**. **Bupropion** has no effect on intraocular pressure or other parameters (Ghibellini et al, J Clin Pharmacol 2009;**49**:489–95).

3.5.3 HYPNOTICS

6. No problems are expected with the **benzodiazepines**, **zaleplon**, **zopiclone**, **zolpidem**, **melatonin** or **ramelteon**.

3.5.4 ANTICONVULSANTS

7. * There are no reported problems with any of the mood stabilisers, anxiolytics, hypnotics or anticonvulsants (no information on **lacosamide** yet), except **topiramate**, which has a particular problem. Although one study showed no evidence of topiramate-induced angle narrowing (n = 20, 4/52, Leung et al, Eye [Lond] 2009;**23**:2079–81), there are numerous reports of reversible acute secondary narrow-angle glaucoma (n = 86, Fraunfelder et al, Ophthalmology 2004;**111**:109–11; n = 1, Sachi and Vijaya, J Postgrad Med 2006;**52**:72–3) occurring within a month of starting treatment, bilateral angle-closure glaucoma (e.g. n = 1, Cruciani et al, Clin Ter 2009;**160**:215–6; n = 1, Singh et al, Kathmandu Univ Med J (KUMJ) 2007;**5**:234–6; n = 1, Levy et al, Can J Ophthalmol 2006;**1**:221–5; n = 1, Mansoor and Jain, Acta Ophthalmol Scand 2005;**83**:27–8; n = 1, Coats, J AAPOS 2003;**7**:303; discussion of possible mechanisms: Craig et al, Am J Ophthalmology 2004;**137**:193–5), possibly enhanced by combination with citalopram

(n = 1, Spaccapelo et al, Cases J 2009;**2**:87). The UK SmPC notes that symptoms usually start within the first month and include decreased visual acuity and/or ocular pain. If this occurs, topiramate should be discontinued as soon as clinically feasible and appropriate measures to reduce intraocular pressure introduced (see also Curr Probs 2002;**28**:4; review by van Issum et al, Eur J Ophthalmol 2010; in press).

3.5.5 OTHERS

8. **Amfetamine** causes a transient rise in intraocular pressure, which is not associated with closure of the angle. **Caffeine** has been reported to cause a transient rise in intraocular pressure, which is not associated with closure of the angle. Average daily intakes of more than 180 mg/d caffeine (not a lot by the author's standards) may cause a clinically significant elevation of intraocular pressure (n = 28, Avisar et al, Ann Pharmacother 2002;**36**:992–5). **Methylphenidate** causes a transient rise in intraocular pressure but this is not associated with closure of the angle. There is a case of uneventful use of methylphenidate in a man with ADHD and primary open-angle glaucoma well-controlled by pilocarpine and betaxolol (Bartlik et al, Arch Gen Psychiatry 1997;**54**:188–9), but methylphenidate 60 mg/d has precipitated severe glaucoma requiring surgery (n = 1, Lu et al, J Chin Med Assoc 2006;**69**:589–90). The UK SmPC lists glaucoma as a contraindication for **atomoxetine**. **Anticholinergics** are contraindicated in narrow-angle glaucoma. There is a case of angle-closure glaucoma after discontinuing **donepezil** (n = 1, Enzenauer and Bowers, J Geront A Biol Sci Med Sci 2005;**60**:1083). Glaucoma is not mentioned in the literature for **memantine**. There is no association with use of **ginkgo biloba** over last 12/12 and having glaucoma (Khoury et al, J Glaucoma 2009; **18**:543–5).

3.6 HEPATIC IMPAIRMENT

	LOWER RISK	MODERATE RISK	HIGHER RISK
Antipsychotics	Amisulpride[5] Aripiprazole[2] Flupentixol[4] Haloperidol[6] Paliperidone[1] Pimozide[8] Sulpiride[5] Ziprasidone[2] Zuclopenthixol[4]	Asenapine[2] Clozapine[3] Olanzapine[2] Risperidone[1] Phenothiazines[7] Quetiapine[2] Risperidone[1] Sertindole[2]	
Antidepressants	Mianserin[16] Paroxetine[9] Tryptophan[16]	Duloxetine[10] Mirtazapine[11] Moclobemide[16] Reboxetine[14] SSRIs[9] St John's wort[16] Trazodone[13] Tricyclics[12] Venlafaxine[10]	Agomelatine[14] Lofepramine[12] MAOIs[15]
Anxiolytics and hynpotics	Lorazepam LD[17] Melatonin[21] Oxazepam LD[17] Ramelteon[21] Temazepam LD[17]	Buspirone[18] Clomethiazole[21] Zaleplon[19] Zolpidem[19] Zopiclone[19]	Benzodiazepines (esp LA)[17] Chloral[21] Propranolol[20]
Anticonvulsants	Carbamazepine[22] Gabapentin[26] Pregabalin[27] Topiramate?[27] Vigabatrin[27]	Acetazolamide[28] Benzodiazepines[17] Lamotrigine[26] Levetiracetam[27] Oxcarbazepine[22] Paraldehyde[28] Rufinamide[27] Tiagabine[27]	Barbiturates[25] Ethosuximide[28] Fosphenytoin[24] Phenytoin[24] Valproate[23]
Others	Buprenorphine[36] Donepezil[29] Lithium[32] Memantine[29]	Acamprosate[31] Anticholinergics[30] Atomoxetine[34] Bupropion[35] Disulfiram[31] Galantamine[29] Methadone[36] Methylphenidate[34] Modafinil[33] Rivastigmine[29]	

LD = low dose   HD = high dose
SA = short-acting   LA = long-acting

GENERAL PRINCIPLES FOR PRESCRIBING IN HEPATIC IMPAIRMENT (adapted from *Maudsley Guidelines*)

1. The greater the degree of hepatic impairment, the greater the degree of impaired drug metabolism, and the greater the risk of drug toxicity, as people may be more sensitive to common or predictable side-effects.
2. Start low, go slow, and monitor LFTs regularly (e.g. weekly).
3. LFTs do not necessarily correlate well with metabolic impairment, although they can give a reasonable indication.
4. Care is needed with drugs with a high first-pass clearance effect.
5. In severe liver disease, avoid drugs with the marked sedation and/or constipation.

Child-Pugh is a measure of the severity and prognosis of cirrhosis, and is calculated from the severity of ascites and encephalopathy, bilirubin, albumin and clotting times:
Review: * general (Verbeeck, *Eur J Clin Pharmacol* 2008;**64**:1147–61).

Child-Pugh grade	A	B	C
Child-Pugh score	5–6	7–9	10–15
Description	Cirrhosis but functioning liver	Significant functional compromise	Decompensation of liver

3.6.1 ANTIPSYCHOTICS

1. Unbound **risperidone** levels increase in hepatic impairment and so initial doses and dose increments should be halved, and 4 mg/d not exceeded. Risperidone-induced jaundice (n = 1, Oyewole et al, *Int J Geriatr Psychiatry* 1996;**11**:179) and rapid onset hepatotoxicity (n = 1, Phillips et al, *Ann Pharmacother* 1998;**32**:843) have been reported. **Paliperidone** is not extensively metabolised by the liver so no dose adjustments are needed in moderate hepatic impairment (n = 20, Boom et al, *Int J Clin Pharmacol Ther* 2009;**47**:606–16), but no data is available in

severe impairment so caution is recommended (SmPC).
2. No changes in dose with **aripiprazole** seem necessary with mild, moderate or severe hepatic impairment. A single dose study showed that although the Cmax was lower in hepatic impairment there were no significant adverse effects (n = 25, Mallikaarjun et al, *Clin Pharmacokinet* 2008;**47**:533–42). **Asenapine** is not recommended in severe hepatic impairment (Child-Pugh C) as seven-fold increases in plasma levels have been shown. No asenapine dose changes are necessary in Child-Pugh A or B (US PI) as plasma levels are only increased by about 12%. **Olanzapine** should be started at a lower dose, e.g. 5 mg/d. Transient, asymptomatic elevations in ALT and AST have been noted and monitoring of these in patients with risk factors (e.g. hepatic impairment, concomitant hepatotoxic drugs) may be appropriate. A lower starting dose of 150 mg/4 weeks should be considered for **olanzapine pamoate** in people with moderate (Child-Pugh A or B) hepatic impairment (SmPC) and only increased with caution. The **quetiapine** SmPC now says oral clearance is reduced by 25% in hepatic impairment, so start at 50 mg/d and increase at 50 mg/d according to response and tolerability. Discontinue if jaundice develops (Thyrum et al, *Prog Neuropsychopharmacol Biol Psychiatry* 2000; **24**:521–33). **Sertindole** is contraindicated in severe hepatic failure. **Ziprasidone** is extensively metabolised and an extended half-life has been shown in Child-Pugh A or B, but dose adjustment is not necessary in mild-to-moderate impairment (n = 30, open, Everson et al, *Br J Clin Pharmacol* 2000;**49**(S3):21–6).
3. **Clozapine** is contraindicated in severe hepatic disease and so lower doses, regular plasma level monitoring and LFT monitoring would be necessary if used. There are reported cases of toxic hepatitis, with AST levels dramatically raised, eosinophilia developing early and full LFT normalisation within 4–5 weeks of stopping (e.g. Thatcher et al, *Am J Psychiatry* 1995;**152**:296–7).
4. * No dosage adjustments are necessary for **flupentixol** or **zuclopenthixol**, although both undergo hepatic metabolism. The UK SmPC for flupentixol now states that it has not been studied but that increased cerebral sensitivity has been reported with other antipsychotics.
5. **Sulpiride** and **amisulpride** are virtually un-

metabolised with little or no biliary excretion. There is a low incidence of liver toxicity reported, with a transient rise in serum transaminase the only reported effect. Dosage adjustments are thus unnecessary (SmPC).

6. There are no apparent problems with **haloperidol**, although the UK SmPC states liver disease to be a caution.

7. **Phenothiazines** (particularly chlorpromazine) may cause hepatocanalicular cholestasis and there have been suggestions of immunological liver damage. They should be avoided where possible in hepatic dysfunction. Onset is usually during the first month of therapy. Coma may be precipitated due to increased cerebral neuronal sensitivity.

8. **Pimozide** should be used with caution in hepatic impairment (UK SmPC).

3.6.2 ANTIDEPRESSANTS

9. **Citalopram** and **escitalopram** are metabolised extensively by the liver, with three major metabolites. Doses at the lower end of the therapeutic range should be used (n = 1000, Milne and Goa, *Drugs* 1991;**41**:450–77), although no liver enzyme abnormalities were noted in this study. In hepatic impairment, alternate day dosing of **fluoxetine** is recommended. Patients with cirrhosis show higher plasma levels of fluoxetine and **norfluoxetine** and longer half-lives occur, and a 50% reduction in dose is recommended, especially if a low albumin is present. **Fluvoxamine** should be started at 50 mg/d and monitored carefully, as raised hepatic enzymes have been reported. **Paroxetine** appears to be the safest option, using doses at the lower end of the therapeutic range, although cases of hepatitis (Benbow and Gill, *Br Med J* 1997;**314**:1387) and hepatotoxicity have been reported (n = 3, Azaz-Livshits *et al*, *Pharmacopsychiatry* 2002;**35**:112–5). **Sertraline** is extensively metabolised by the liver and is contraindicated in significant hepatic dysfunction. One study showed a 2.5–fold increase in half-life and a 1.6–fold increase in sertraline/desmethylsertraline peak levels in stable chronic cirrhosis (n = 20, Demolis *et al*, *Br J Clin Pharmacol* 1996;**42**:394–7; n = 1, Persky and Reinus, *Dig Dis Sci* 2003;**48**:939–44).

10. **Venlafaxine** clearance is reduced by about 35% in mild-to-moderate hepatic impairment, and so doses should be reduced by about 50% (UK SmPC), although there is much interpatient variability (Anon, *J Clin Psychiatry* 1993;**54**:119–26) and it is not recommended in severe hepatic impairment. **Duloxetine** is contraindicated in hepatic impairment (UK SmPC). Moderate liver disease (Child-Pugh B) increases the half-life 2.3-fold and AUC 3.7-fold. The FDA in 2006 noted that duloxetine can cause hepatitis and jaundice, and people with pre-existing liver disease may be at risk of additional problems. There is no data in mild or severe hepatic insufficiency.

11. **Mirtazapine** clearance is reduced by 33% in moderate hepatic impairment (n = 16, single-dose study, Murdoch *et al*, *Br J Clin Pharmacol* 1993;**35**:76P), and so dosage reduction may be necessary. Transient asymptomatic raised liver enzymes (e.g. SGTP) have been noted in a few patients in early clinical trials.

12. Most **tricyclics** have a high first-pass clearance by the liver, and so lower starting doses are necessary. Increased sedation with tricyclics is likely to be due to decreased metabolism, e.g. **amitriptyline** plasma levels may be doubled or tripled in patients with cirrhosis and should be avoided. Increased blood levels may also occur with reduced plasma protein-binding if albumin levels are lower, as protein-binding is high with many tricyclics. Particular care is obviously needed if albumin levels are low. SSRIs, such as paroxetine, would appear to be easier to use than tricyclics in liver disease. Cholestatic jaundice has occasionally been noted with tricyclics. **Lofepramine** is contraindicated in severe liver disease.

13. **Trazodone** should be used with care in severe hepatic impairment, as hepatoxicity has been reported (n = 1, Rettman and McClintock, *Ann Pharmacother* 2001;**35**:1559–61).

14. **Reboxetine's** half-life and plasma levels appear to rise in severe hepatic insufficiency and dose adjustment may be necessary. A starting dose of 2 mg BD is recommended (n = 12, Tran *et al*, *Clin Drug Invest* 2000;**19**:473–7). **Agomelatine** is contraindicated in hepatic impairment (i.e. cirrhosis or active liver disease).

15. **MAOIs** are hepatotoxic and may precipitate coma. Patients may also be more sensitive to side-effects. If essential, start with a low dose, increase gradually and observe carefully. **Isocarboxazid** is contraindicated in any degree of impaired hepatic function.

16. **Moclobemide's** clearance can be reduced and half-life increased in cirrhosis and so

doses should be reduced by 25–33% to avoid accumulation (Stoeckel et al, Acta Psychiatr Scand 1990;**360**[Suppl]:94–7). There are no apparent problems with **mianserin** and **tryptophan**. **St John's wort** levels may rise in moderate cirrhosis, but absorption is decreased in mild cirrhosis (n = 16, Johne et al, Clin Pharmacol Ther 2002;**71**:P95). Hepatotoxicity has been reported (n = 1, Domínguez Jiménez et al, Gastroenterol Hepatol 2007;**30**:54–5).

3.6.3 ANXIOLYTICS AND HYPNOTICS

17. The metabolism of **diazepam** and **chlordiazepoxide** is impaired in liver disease. The half-lives of the metabolites desmethylchlordiazepoxide and demoxepam are also reported to be prolonged to up to 346 hours and 150 hours respectively (n = 1, Barton et al, Med Tox Adv Drug Exp 1989;**4**:73–6) which may induce coma, and may be detectable two months after stopping treatment in patients with hepatic encephalopathy (Meier et al, Gastroenterology, 1991;**101**:274–5). Impaired metabolism has also been reported with **alprazolam**, **clobazam** and **midazolam** (significantly impaired in cirrhosis, as it is metabolised by at least three different P450 enzymes, Wandel et al, Br J Anaesthesia 1994;**73**:658–61). The metabolism of **lorazepam**, **temazepam** and **oxazepam** is unchanged and in low dose these are probably the benzodiazepines of choice.

18. **Buspirone** plasma levels are higher in patients with hepatic failure, with a good correlation between steady-state buspirone levels and serum albumin (open, Barbhaiya et al, Eur J Clin Pharmacol 1994;**46**:41–7). Caution is recommended with a history of hepatic impairment and it should not be used in severe hepatic disease.

19. Elimination of **zopiclone** can be reduced with hepatic dysfunction, producing enhanced adverse effects (n = 17, open, Parker and Roberts, Br J Clin Pharmacol 1983;**16**:259). A lower dose of 3.75 mg to 7.5 mg (but no higher) can be used with caution in hepatic disease. Plasma protein binding of **zolpidem** is reduced in hepatic impairment (n = 42, open, Pacifici, Int J Clin Pharmacol Toxicol 1988;**26**:439–43) and it is contraindicated in severe hepatic insufficiency. Reduced doses are recommended in cirrhosis and other hepatic impairment (where half-life may rise to 10 hours). Hepatoxicity has been reported (n = 1, Karsenti

et al, Br Med J 1999;**318**:1179). **Zaleplon** is contraindicated in severe hepatic insufficiency and the dose reduced to 5 mg in mild-to-moderate hepatic impairment.

20. * **Propranolol's** metabolism is impaired in decompensated liver disease and by portal systemic shunting. Propranolol use significantly shortens survival vs. placebo (5/12 vs. 20/12) in cirrhosis and ascites and so it should not be used (n = 151, 8/12, Sersté et al, Hepatology 2010;**52**:1017–22).

21. **Clomethiazole** clearance is reduced by 50% in moderate-to-severe heptic impairment, but with sedation not significantly enhanced in the majority (n = 24, Centerholt et al, Eur J Clin Pharmacol 2003;**59**:1117–22). In severe liver disease a tenfold increase can occur, so reduce oral doses, e.g. a third of normal, and note that sedation can mask the onset of hepatic coma. **Chloral hydrate** is contraindicated in marked hepatic impairment. No problems are expected with **melatonin** or **ramelteon**.

3.6.4 ANTICONVULSANTS

Review: optimising anticonvulsants in hepatic dysfunction (Lalerda et al, Neurology 2006;**67**[12 Suppl 4]:S28–33).

22. Serious problems with **carbamazepine** are rare, but jaundice, hepatitis and liver function disorders have been reported, and so use should be with caution. Although **oxcarbazepine** is rapidly and extensively metabolised, no dose adjustments are generally needed in mild-to-moderate hepatic impairment. It has not been studied in severe hepatic impairment.

23. **Valproate** is contraindicated in active liver disease, as it can be hepatotoxic and liver failure can occur in about one in 10 000 cases. The risk is higher early on in therapy and lessens after a couple of months (review by Eadie et al, Med Tox 1988;**3**:85–106). Electron-microscopy shows lipid droplets and a scarcity of cytoplasmic cells and normal mitochondria have been reported (n = 1, Caparros-Lefebvre et al, Lancet 1993;**341**:1604). Hepatotoxicity occurs mostly in children and presents as worsening epilepsy, drowsiness and with biochemical and/or clinical evidence of liver failure. Some fatal cases have been reported. Care needs to be taken if valproate is used in children, especially if used with other anticonvulsants. Valproate use

3

may be possible in patients with hepatitis C, provided ALT is closely monitored (n = 564, Felker et al, Am J Psychiatry 2003;**160**:174–8).

24. **Phenytoin** is highly protein bound and extensively metabolised and so accumulation and toxicity may occur in severe liver disease. Use reduced doses and monitor for toxicity. In uraemia, protein-binding may be reduced but active/free levels remain unchanged so therapeutic control may be possible at plasma levels below the usual range. Severe cardiovascular ADRs have been reported with **fosphenytoin** IV (see 3.2.4), and a reduction in loading dose and/or infusion rate by 10–25% is recommended in hepatic impairment.

25. Increased cerebral sensitivity and impaired **barbiturate** metabolism may precipitate coma.

26. **Gabapentin** is virtually unmetabolised and so dose adjustments are unnecessary. No adjustment to initial and maintenance doses of **lamotrigine** is necessary for Child-Pugh grade A but should be reduced by 50% in moderate (Child-Pugh grade B) hepatic impairment, and by 75% in severe (Child-Pugh grade C) impairment (n = 36, Marcellin et al, Br J Clin Pharmacol 2001; **51**:410–4).

27. No dose adjustment is needed with **lacosamide** in mild-to-moderate hepatic impairment, but there is no information on use in severe hepatic impairment (SmPC). No dose adjustment of **levetiracetam** is necessary in Child-Pugh grade A and B, but in grade C start with half the normal dose as total clearance is reduced by about 57% (n = 16, Brockmoller et al, Clin Pharmacol Ther 2005;**77**:29–41). However, levetiracetam (dose 250 mg/d titrated to tolerance and response) was effective and produced no worsening of LFTs in epileptics with liver disease (n = 14 [c = 10], open, 3/12, Bilo et al, Clin Neuropharmacol 2008;**31**:221–5). No dose adjustments are necessary for **pregabalin** in hepatic impairment. No information is available for **rufinamide** but the UK SmPC recommends slower dose titration in mild-to-moderate hepatic impairment and to avoid in severe hepatic impairment. **Tiagabine** is metabolised by the liver. Initial doses in mild-to-moderate hepatic impairment should be lower, and so use in severe hepatic impairment is not recommended (n = 13, open, 8/7, Lau et al, Epilepsia 1997;**38**:445–51). **Topiramate** is not extensively metabolised and about 60% is

excreted unchanged via the kidneys. In moderate-to-severe liver disease, clearance is reduced by about 26%, although the resultant changes in plasma levels have been considered clinically insignificant by the manufacturers. **Vigabatrin** can cause decreased LFT levels but there is no evidence of hepatic toxicity. **Zonisamide** has not been studied in hepatic impairment so caution is needed.

28. The UK SmPC for **ethosuximide** now requires extreme caution in impaired hepatic function. **Acetazolamide** should be used with caution. **Paraldehyde** elimination is slower in hepatic failure and so lower doses may be needed.

3.6.5 OTHERS

29. **Donepezil** 5 mg/d can be safely given in mild-to-moderate (Child-Pugh grade A or B) hepatic impairment (n = 35 [c = 32], Reyes et al, Br J Clin Pharmacol 2004;**58**[Suppl 1]:9–17, MS), and a 5 mg single-dose study indicated that compromised hepatic function did not significantly alter its kinetics (n = 20, Tiseo et al, Br J Clin Pharmacol 1998;**46**[Suppl 1]:51–5). **Rivastigmine** is contraindicated in severe liver impairment. **Galantamine** is not affected by mild hepatic impairment but clearance is reduced by 23% in moderate impairment and so care is necessary in moderate-to-severe impairment (n = 25, open, Zhao et al, J Clin Pharmacol 2002;**42**:428–36). Start with 4 mg/d, increasing slowly to a maximum of 8 mg BD. In severe impairment (Child-Pugh grade C), galantamine is contraindicated (due to current lack of safety data). There is no data on **memantine** in hepatic impairment but since it is metabolised only to a minor extent to inactive metabolites, mild-to-moderate hepatic impairment is unlikely to have a significant effect.

30. All the literature for the **anticholinergics** urges some caution in hepatic disease.

31. The literature for **disulfiram** recommends caution in liver disease. Although some evidence of further raised LFTs was noted, an open trial showed disulfiram was safe in patients with elevated LFTs and/or evidence of hepatitis C virus, provided LFTs were monitored regularly (n = 57, Saxon et al, J Clin Psych 1998;**59**:313–6). The literature for **acamprosate** states that use in severe hepatic failure (Child-Pugh grade C)

is a contraindication, but the pharmacokinetics are not altered in mild-to-moderate hepatic dysfunction and this is only an SmPC caution.

32. There are no problems with **lithium** in liver disease.

33. **Modafinil's** maximum dose of 400 mg/d should only be used in the absence of hepatic impairment. The starting dose of **sodium oxybate** should be halved in hepatic impairment as the elimination half-life is increased (UK SmPC).

34. There is no data on **methylphenidate** (UK SmPC). The UK SmPC recommends possible **atomoxetine** dose modification in hepatic impairment and rare (one in 50 000) cases have been reported of severe acute hepatitis with markedly elevated hepatic enzymes and bilirubin (MHRA warning).

35. **Bupropion** is extensively metabolised and there are rare reports of abnormal LFTs, liver damage and hepatotoxicity, with some metabolite half-lives prolonged in cirrhosis. Reduced initial doses and close monitoring are required, as a prolonged half-life has been reported in hepatic failure (n = 16, open, DeVane et al, J Clin Psychopharmacol 1990; **10**:328–32).

36. Cases of QT interval prolongation and torsades de pointes have been reported during treatment with **methadone** (particularly at doses > 100 mg/d) and liver disease (a risk factor for prolonged QTc) is a UK SmPC caution. **Buprenorphine** is primarily metabolised by glucuronidation (Tegeder et al, Clin Pharmacokinet 1999;**37**:17–40) and so should have a low risk in mild-to-moderate hepatic impairment, although it is contraindicated in severe hepatic insufficiency as this may, in itself, possibly be associated with hepatic events (UK SmPC).

3

3.7 OLD AGE

	Lower risk	Moderate risk	Higher risk
Antipsychotics	Amisulpride[5] Aripiprazole[2] Paliperidone[1] Risperidone[1] Sulpiride[5] Ziprasidone[2]	Asenapine[2] Butyrophenones[6] Olanzapine[2] Quetiapine[2] Sertindole[2] Thioxanthenes[4]	Clozapine[3] Phenothiazines[7] Pimozide[8]
Antidepressants	Agomelatine[14] Duloxetine[10] Lofepramine[12] Mirtazapine[11] Moclobemide[16] SSRIs[9] Tryptophan[16] Venlafaxine[10]	Flupentixol[4] MAOIs[15] Mianserin[16] Nortriptyline[12] Reboxetine[14] Trazodone[13]	Tricyclics[12]
Anxiolytics and hynpotics	Alprazolam[17] Buspirone[18] Clobazam[17] Lorazepam[17] Melatonin[21] Oxazepam[17] Oxprenolol[20] Ramelteon[21] Zaleplon[19] Zopiclone[19]	Clomethiazole[21] Benzodiazepines, short-acting[17] Flunitrazepam[17] Flurazepam[17] Propranolol[20] Temazepam[17] Zolpidem[19]	Benzodiazepines, long-acting[17]
Anticonvulsants	Clobazam[17] Rufinamide[27] Tiagabine[27]	Barbiturates[25] Carbamazepine[22] Clonazepam[17] Gabapentin[26] Lamotrigine[26] Levetiracetam[27] Oxcarbazepine[22] Piracetam?[27] Pregabalin[27] Topiramate[27] Valproate[23]	Acetazolamide[28] Benzodiazepines (most)[17] Fosphenytoin[24] Paraldehyde[28] Phenytoin[24] Vigabatrin[27]
Others	Anticholinesterases[29] Bupropion[35] Memantine[29] Modafinil[33] Sodium oxybate [33]	Buprenorphine[36] Lithium[32] Methadone[36]	Acamprosate?[31] Anticholinergics[30] Methlyphenidate[34]

GENERAL PRINCIPLES FOR PRESCRIBING IN OLD AGE (adapted from *Maudsley Guidelines*)

1. Increased sensitivity to drugs occurs due to age-related changes in pharmacokinetics (ADME and protein binding) and pharmacodynamics (e.g. neuronal changes, and receptor binding). The over 70s have about twice as many ADRs as under 50s, e.g. postural hypotension, enhanced sedation with, and increased sensitivity to, anticholinergic side-effects (see 8).

2. Hepatic changes (e.g. reduced metabolism) and reduced renal clearance will affect many drugs.

3. The lowest effective dose should be used (so 'start low and go slow'), avoid polypharmacy and monitor effects (both positive and negative) regularly and frequently.

4. Avoid drugs with sedative and hypotensive effects, which can increase the under-rated risks of falls. A meta-analysis concluded that psychotropics are associated with a small increase in falls (s = 40, Leipzig *et al*, *J Am Geriatr Soc* 1999;**47**:30–9; reviewed by Shorr, *EBMH* 1999; **2**:95).

5. Use drugs only when necessary, decide a treat-ment aim, keep therapy simple, use the smallest effective doses and discontinue gradually if no apparent benefit can be seen, as accumulation of a drug can lead to the subtle and insidious development of side-effects.

6. Most drugs are highly lipophilic and an increased fat to lean body mass ratio, in addition to decreased metabolism and excretion, means that half-lives usually increase.

7. Consider other factors, e.g. potential poor compliance due to social or physical reasons, or use of OTC medicines.

8. Avoid drugs with anticholinergic effects. These can increase the risk of cognitive decline and dementia (HR=1.65), although discontinuing decreases the risk (n = 6912, four years, Carrière *et al*, *Arch Intern Med* 2009;**169**:1317–24).

9. Monitor more carefully with pre-existing diabetes, as in people aged >66 initiating *any* antipsychotic has been associated with an increased risk of hospitalisation for hyperglycaemia (n = 13817, Lipscombe *et al*, *Arch Int Med* 2009; **169**:1282–9).

Review: geriatric psychopharmacology (Turnheim, *Exp Gerontol* 2003;**38**:843–53).

3.7.1 ANTIPSYCHOTICS

The EMEA 2008 review of antipsychotics in elderly people with dementia concludes that:

- conventional antipsychotics are associated with excess mortality
- conventional antipsychotics are associated with excess mortality compared to atypicals
- no conclusion can be drawn on individual antipsychotics

The case against antipsychotics in the elderly:

- there is an increased risk of femur fracture in elderly institutionalised patients (n = 7393, Liperoti *et al*, *J Clin Psychiatry* 2007;**68**:929–34) and a 60% increased risk of pneumonia (n = 22944, Knol *et al*, *J Am Geriatr Soc* 2008; **56**:661–6) with antipsychotic use
- a one-year study showed that in patients with AD in residential care treated with antipsychotics, those that carried on had a survival probability of 70% compared to 77% in the switch-to-placebo group, clinically significant. In the follow-on study, the two-year survival was 46% vs 71%, and three-year was 30% vs 59%, even more marked (n = 128, RCT, p/c, 12/12, Ballard *et al*, *Lancet Neurol* 2009;**8**:151–7)
- the **haloperidol** SmPC now states that in elderly people with dementia-related psychosis, the risk of death with SGAs is 1.6–1.7 times higher than with placebo (4.5% vs 2.6%) vs placebo, mostly cardiovascular or infections (s = 17, mean, 10/52, UK SmPC).

The evidence for the safety of antipsychotics in old age includes:

- a Medicaid analysis was unable to show that 'atypicals' (including risperidone) were more likely to cause CVEs than haloperidol or benzodiazepines (n = 8 million, Finkel *et al*, *Int Psychogeriatr* 2005;**17**:617–29)
- a prospective nursing home study failed to show that antipsychotics increased mortality in dementia (n = 273, 12/12, Suh *et al*, *Int Psychogeriatr* 2005;**17**:429–41)
- a large study showed the risk of death (all causes) in elderly people taking FGAs comparable to and possibly higher than that associated with SGAs (n = 37241, 180/7, Schneeweiss *et al*, *CMAJ* 2007;**176**:627–32).

The useful case in the middle: *

- Three new large cohort studies suggest that

3

the risk of CVAEs is higher in the first four weeks (OR 9.9) but falls to baseline after three months, and so chronic use is not associated with CVAEs (n = 26157, Kleijer *et al, J Psychopharmacol* 2009;**23**:909–14; n = 134,448, Sacchetti *et al, J Psychopharmacol* 2010;**24**:1131–32). The increased mortality occurs with higher doses e.g. haloperidol, n = 2217, > 1 mg/d; olanzapine, n = 3384, > 2.5 mg and risperidone, n = 8249, > 1 mg/d, but not with quetiapine, n = 4277 (5 years, Rossom *et al, J Am Geriatr Soc* 2010;**58**:1027–34). This may be due to dehydration and poor mobilisation (Ballard and Corbett, *CNS Drugs* 2010;**24**:729–39), so ensuring adequate hydration and movement in the first month is essential.

Antipsychotics can relieve psychotic symptoms in older adults but pre-treatment assessment, repeated every 3–6 months, is recommended to detect common side-effects such as postural hypotension, anticholinergic effects and Parkinsonism. Single daily doses are usually appropriate once stable (as, indeed, they are in younger adults). Doses should be reviewed regularly, and a periodic reduction in dose (e.g. by 10–25% every four weeks) for some patients may be indicated.

Reviews: * general (Trifiro and Spina, *Curr Drug Metab* 2011; in press), FGAs in elderly (Bouman and Pinner, *Adv Psychiatr Treat* 2002;**8**:49–58), SGAs in the elderly (Burke and Tariot, *Expert Opin Pharmacother* 2009;**10**:2407–14), psychosis in the elderly with Parkinsonism (Hasnain *et al, Am J Med* 2009;**122**:614–22).

1. * **Risperidone** is partially metabolised to an active metabolite and so lower doses may be needed only if hepatic impairment is present (see *3.6.1*). Significant age-related differences have been noted, with higher plasma levels in patients over 40 years, and with a 30% increase per decade of life (n = 129, Aichhorn *et al, J Psychopharmacol* 2005;**19**:395–401). The same would apply to **paliperidone** (review by Madhusoodanan and Zaveri; *Curr Drug Saf* 2010;**5**:149–52), but any renal impairment might require lower doses (see *3.9.1.1*).

2. * In older adults with bipolar disorder, **aripiprazole** appears to be fairly well tolerated and have some efficacy (n = 20, open, 12/52, Sajatovic *et al, J Clin Psychiatry* 2008;**69**:41–6) and no dose

adjustments are necessary in the elderly (review of use in late-life schizophrenia; Rado and Janicak, *Clin Interv Aging* 2010;**5**:253–8). There is a class warning for **asenapine** in dementia-related psychosis (US PI), and it is likely to cause postural hypotension in the elderly as plasma levels may be 30–40% higher than younger adults. The UK CSM recommends not using **olanzapine** in elderly demented people with behavioural problems, due to an increased risk of stroke (2% vs 1% on placebo), although the absolute risk is low, and the alternatives are not risk-free. The restriction does not apply to elderly demented people *without* behavioural problems, where a lower starting dose of 5 mg/d may be appropriate, as the mean elimination half-life is 50% longer and clearance slightly reduced in otherwise healthy elderly patients. Periodic blood pressure monitoring is recommended and there may be a slightly higher risk of seizures in people over 65. Transient sedation and somnolence were more marked in the elderly in pre-marketing trials. **Olanzapine pamoate** is not recommended for use in the elderly unless oral olanzapine has been used uneventfully before (SmPC), and should not be used for people over 75. The UK SmPC for **quetiapine** has been updated with a warning that quetiapine is not approved for the treatment of patients with dementia-related psychosis due to an approximately three-fold increased risk of cerebrovascular adverse events seen in RCTs with some antipsychotics in the dementia population. The mean clearance in elderly patients is 30–50% lower than healthy adults, so the starting dose should be 25 mg/d, with dose increments of 25–50 mg/d. Somnolence (32%), dizziness (13%) and postural hypotension (13%) are the most common side-effects in old age. Quetiapine (mean 200 mg/d, range 50–800 mg/d) can be effective and safe in elderly in-patients, but there is a wide and diagnosis-dependent (e.g. higher in functional psychosis) dosing range (n = 100 [c = 91], Yang *et al, J Psychopharmacol* 2005;**19**:661–6). **Sertindole** requires a slower dose titration and perhaps lower final doses. There are no dose changes needed for **ziprasidone**.

3. **Clozapine** may be safe, reasonably well-tolerated (with slower dose titration) and effective in the elderly (n = 133, Barak *et al, Compr Psychiatry* 1999;**40**:320–5) at doses as low as 50–100 mg, with 6.25–50 mg/d suggested as the optimal dosage (review by Hoeh *et al, J Geriatr*

Psychiatry Neurol 2003;**16**:213–8). There may be an increased incidence of agranulocytosis, so great care should be taken (review by Gareri *et al*, *Expert Opin Drug Saf* 2008;**7**:525–38).

4. * **Zuclopenthixol** and **flupentixol** should be used with caution in renal disease. The UK SmPC for zuclopenthixol now has a generic warning about use in BPSD. The UK SmPC for flupentixol recommends caution in people with risk factors for stroke, and lower dose increases and maximum (1.5 mg) may be needed due to altered kinetics.

5. Plasma levels for **amisulpride** in the elderly are similar to adults but the elderly may respond to lower plasma levels (n = 395, Müller *et al*, *J Psychopharmacol* 2009;**23**:278–86). Single doses of **sulpiride** are well tolerated and show a similar pharmacokinetic profile in healthy elderly and young subjects (n = 20, open, Hamon-Vilcot *et al*, *Eur J Clin Pharmacol* 1998;**54**:405–9). However, the UK SmPCs now include a mention of increased mortality with sulpiride in elderly people with dementia.

6. The **haloperidol** SmPC now states that in elderly people with dementia-related psychosis, the risk of death with SGAs is 1.6–1.7 times higher than with placebo (4.5% vs 2.6%), mostly cardiovascular or infections (s = 17, mean, 10/52, UK SmPC). Although the causes of death were varied, most of the deaths appeared to be either cardiovascular (e.g. heart failure, sudden death) or infections (e.g. pneumonia). An increased severity of side-effects including EPSE, sedation, hypotension and respiratory depression may occur and so lower starting doses are indicated.

7. It is generally recommended that 33–50% of the adult dose of **phenothiazines** should be used for elderly patients, who are more susceptible to Parkinsonian side-effects (n = 120, open, Caligiuri *et al*, *J Clin Psychopharmacol* 1999; **19**:322–8), and which are often then harder to manage. **Chlorpromazine** should be avoided. **Levomepromazine** is not recommended for use in people over 50 unless the risk of hypotension has been assessed.

8. Half the usual starting dose of **pimozide** should be used.

3.7.2 ANTIDEPRESSANTS

Depression increases mortality in the elderly with cardiac disease, so it should not be ignored, especially if long-standing and severe (n = 652, Geerlings *et al*, *Psychol Med* 2002;**32**:609–18). Drugs with anticholinergic side-effects may further harm an already compromised cholinergic system. SSRIs and tricyclics (but not other antidepressants) may increase the risk of non-vertebral fractures in the elderly, although the number of cases was very small (n = 7983, >55 years of age [mean 77 years of age], Ziere *et al*, *J Clin Psychopharmacol* 2008;**28**:411–7; comment by Diem, *EBMH* 2009;**12**:26). To put it into perspective, one review states that the magnitude of the risk of falling with an antidepressant is about the same as the excess risk found in people with untreated depression (Darowski *et al*, *Drugs Aging* 2009;**26**:381–94).

9. * **SSRIs** have obvious advantages over other antidepressants in the elderly but have some risks, including hyponatraemia, weight loss (review: Herrmann, *Can J Clin Pharmacol* 2000;**7**:91–5) and increased risk of falls and osteoporotic fractures in the over 50s (n = 5008, 137 on SSRIs, Richards *et al*, *Arch Int Med* 2007;**167**:188–94). A prolonged **citalopram** half-life (up to 3.8 days) and raised steady-state plasma levels may be due to reduced metabolism, with side-effects more prevalent in the elderly, particularly bradycardia, nausea, sweating and headache (n = 1344, >6/52, Barak *et al*, *Prog Neuropsychopharmacol Biol Psychiatry* 2003;**27**:545–8). Dose reduction (by up to 50%) has been suggested, but normal adult doses have been used in many studies with no apparent problem and a meta-analysis concluded citalopram in late-life depression is equivalent to other antidepressants with similar tolerability (s = 7, n = 1288, Seitz *et al*, *Int J Geriatr Psychiatry* 2010;**25**:1296–1305). For **escitalopram**, an initial dose of 5 mg daily for the first two weeks of treatment is recommended, increasing to 10 mg/d (UK SmPC). It is well-tolerated in older adults (mean 68 years), albeit not superior to placebo (n = 268 [c = 205], RCT, d/b, p/c, 12/52, Bose and Gandhi, *Am J Geriatr Psychiatry* 2008; **16**:14–20), although in responders it reduces relapse (n = 225 [c = 171], open extension, one year, Kasper *et al*, *Neuropsychobiology* 2006; **54**:152–9). Escitalopram was also modestly effective for GAD in older people, but not significantly (n = 177 [c = 170], RCT, p/c, d/b, 12/52, Lenze *et al*, *JAMA* 2009;**301**:295–303).

3

The half-life of **fluoxetine** appears not to be significantly different in the elderly. In an open study of depressed and physically ill hospitalised elderly patients with multiple pathology and polypharmacy, fluoxetine was claimed to be a safe and effective antidepressant in this difficult to treat cohort (n = 20, open, Evans and Lye, *J Clin Exp Gerontol* 1992;**14**:297–307). No pharmacokinetic differences have been seen with **fluvoxamine** in the elderly and so no dose alterations are necessary and 200 mg/d seems as equally well-tolerated and effective in old age depression as sertraline 150 mg/d (n = 93, RCT, d/b, 7/52, Rossini *et al*, *J Clin Psychopharmacol* 2005;**25**:471–5). Initially, lower doses of 10 mg/d are recommended for **paroxetine**, as blood levels with 20 mg/d in the elderly can be similar to those of 30 mg/d in younger people (review in old age Holliday and Plosker, *Drugs Aging* 1993;**3**:278–99). **Sertraline's** clearance may be slightly reduced and half-life increased in elderly volunteers, but this does not seem to warrant dosage adjustment (n = 44, open, 30/7, Ronfeld *et al*, *Clin Pharmacokin* 1997;**32**[Suppl 1]:S22–S30), and it seems safe and effective in the elderly even with significant comorbid medical status (n = 752, RCT, d/b, p/c, 8/52, Sheikh *et al*, *J Am Geriatr Soc* 2004;**52**:86–92; review by Kurzthaler and Fleischhacker, *EBMH* 2004;**7**:82).

10. **Venlafaxine** clearance is reduced by about 15% in the elderly, probably due to reduced renal function, but dosage adjustment is not generally considered necessary (Anon, *J Clin Psychiatry* 1993;**54**:119–26). However, venlafaxine (up to 150 mg/d) may be less well tolerated and possibly less safe than sertraline (up to 100 mg/d) in elderly frail populations (n = 32, RCT, d/b, Oslin *et al*, *J Clin Psychiatry* 2003;**64**:875–82; comment by Schneider, *EBMH* 2004;**7**:47). Postural hypotension may be more common. **Duloxetine's** half-life is about 25% longer in the elderly, but no dose adjustment is necessary and 60 mg/d was shown to have no adverse effects on cognition and depression in elderly (65–89) patients (n = 311, RCT, d/b, p/c, Wise *et al*, *Int J Clin Pract* 2007;**61**:1283–93). A pooled analysis of the sub-set of people over 65 taking part in larger trials for GAD showed duloxetine 60–120 mg/d to be effective, but with a high discontinuation rate due to ADRs (s = 4, n = 73, RCT, d/b, p/c, < 10/52, Davidson *et al, Hum Psychopharmacol* 2008;**23**:519–26).

11. **Mirtazapine** dosage is the same in the elderly as younger adults, although the manufacturers recommend care with dosage increments, e.g. 15–45 mg/d has equivalent efficacy to sub-therapeutic amitriptyline 30–90 mg/d, but with relatively fewer cardiac effects (n = 115, d/b, Hoyberg *et al, Acta Psychiatr Scand* 1996;**93**:184–90). It appears to be slightly quicker acting and better tolerated than paroxetine in elderly depressed patients (n = 255, RCT, d/b, 8 + 16/52, Schatzberg *et al, Am J Geriatr Psychiatry* 2002;**10**:541–50).

12. Reduced initial doses of **tricyclics** are recommended, with perhaps slightly lower final doses, depending upon tolerance, as cognitive, anticholinergic and central effects are enhanced in the elderly. **Clomipramine** is as well-tolerated in patients 56–70 years old as in younger adults, although postural hypotension and anticholinergic side-effects are more common (n = 150, Stage *et al, Acta Psychiatr Scand* 2002;**105**:55–9). Single night-time doses of **dosulepin** have been used in the elderly with no increase in side-effects. Higher serum levels occur with standard doses of **imipramine** (reviewed by Hicks *et al, J Clin Psychiatry* 1981;**42**:374–85), with reduced clearance and doubled half-life (open, Benetello *et al, Int J Clin Pharmacol Res* 1990;**10**:191–5). Elderly patients may respond to lower doses of **lofepramine** but in depressed elderly in-patients, low dose lofepramine (70 mg/d) appears no better than placebo, indicating that full, or at least higher, doses are necessary (n = 63. 4/52, Tan *et al, Br J Clin Pharmacol* 1994;**37**:321–4). **Nortriptyline** kinetics appear the same in the elderly as the young, although individual variation is high and the elderly may respond to lower doses (Kanba *et al, Prog Neuropsychopharmacol Biol Psychiatry* 1992;**16**:301–9). ECG changes may occur so care is needed in cardiovascular disease.

13. Single daily dosing of **trazodone** (except when used as a hypnotic) may not be appropriate in the elderly. 150 mg/d may be the optimum dose in the elderly, as higher plasma levels (n = 97, Prapotnik *et al, Int J Clin Pharmacol Ther* 2004;**42**:120–4) and a longer half-life occur in the elderly.

14. The incidence of side-effects with **reboxetine** is no greater in the elderly than in younger people, although the half-life may be doubled (Holm and Spencer, *CNS Drugs* 1999;**12**:65–83), and peak plasma levels are also over twice that in younger people (n = 12, Bergmann *et al, Eur*

J Drug Metab Pharmacokinet 2000;**25**:195–8). The starting dose should probably be 2 mg BD. A delayed lowering of potassium levels and some treatment-emergent tachycardia has been reported. Frail elderly may need dose reductions. The UK SmPC does not recommend use in the elderly, due to lack of safety data rather than the presence of negative data. No problems are expected with **agomelatine**.

15. **MAOIs** are often considered to be more toxic in the elderly, mainly due to postural hypotension and dizziness, but they can be highly effective in resistant depression in the elderly (review by Volz and Gleiter, *Drugs Aging* 1998:**13**:341–55).

16. **Moclobemide** is considered to be safe, effective and having a seemingly beneficial effect on a range of cognitive functions (n = 694, d/b, p/c, Roth et al, *Br J Psychiatry* 1996;**168**:149–57). **Mianserin** elimination is highly variable and often prolonged in the elderly (n = 27, open, Begg et al, *Br J Clin Pharmacol* 1989;**27**:445–51).There are no apparent problems with **tryptophan**.

3.7.3 ANXIOLYTICS AND HYPNOTICS *

A meta-analysis showed that improvements in sleep with the use of sedatives are significant in the elderly, albeit of small magnitude, but that ADRs and the risk of falls are clinically relevant (s = 24, n = 2417, RCT, Glass et al, *Br Med J* 2005; **331**:1169). Benzodiazepines and Z-hypnotics significantly impair body balance and standing steadiness after a single dose, aggravated by alcohol, but that tolerance partially develops with time (s = 57, Mets et al, *Sleep Med Rev* 2010;**14**:259–67).

Review: management of insomnia in elderly (Bain, *Am J Geriatr Pharmacother* 2006;**4**:168–92).

17. * All **benzodiazepines** should be used with care in the elderly, as side-effects are likely to be enhanced, e.g. sedation, disturbances in gait, daytime drowsiness, cognitive impairment, hypotension, memory impairment and reduced psychomotor performance. For example, the risk of falls and hip fracture with BDZs is higher on initiation with higher doses, and when other BDZs or hypnotics are also used (n = 103,188, Zint et al, *Pharmacoepidemiol Drug Saf* 2010;**19**:1248–55). Half-lives are generally lengthened, sometimes only in men, although there is considerable interpatient variability. Prolonged half-lives in the elderly have been reported with **clonazepam, clobazam, flunitrazepam, nitrazepam, flurazepam, chlordiazepoxide, clorazepate, bromazepam, diazepam** and **midazolam**. **Temazepam** is relatively safe over 8/52 and CBT may slightly improve the response (n = 60, RCT, 8/52, Morin et al, *Hum Psychopharmacol* 2003;**18**:75–82). Normal adult doses of **oxazepam** can be used as there are apparently no clinically significant pharmacokinetic changes in the elderly (n = 17, RCT, c/o, Dreyfuss et al, *J Clin Psychiatry* 1986;**47**:511–4). If used as a hypnotic, **lorazepam** doses should probably be slightly reduced. **Loprazolam** appears well-tolerated in the elderly, with a half-life similar to young adults, although peak levels are prolonged (n = 12, Dorling and Hindmarsh, *Drugs Exp Clin Res* 2001;**27**:151–9).

18. There do not appear to be any significant changes in the pharmacokinetics of **buspirone** in the elderly and so dose adjustments are not considered necessary (n = 48, open, Gammans et al, *J Clin Pharmacol* 1989;**29**:72–8).

19. Normal adult doses of **zopiclone** can be used (Goa and Heel, *Drugs* 1986;**32**:48–65). **Zolpidem** 5 mg is an effective hypnotic in the elderly, with no consistent memory or performance effects, or daytime drowsiness (n = 221, Roger and Attali, *Clin Therap* 1993;**15**:127–36), but doses of 10 mg or above slightly reduce REM sleep (n = 30, Scharf et al, *J Clin Psychiatry* 1991;**52**:77–83). Zolpidem causes less cognitive, memory and equilibrium adverse effects then zopiclone and lormetazepam and should be the preferred hypnotic in the elderly (n = 48, RCT, d/b, p/c, c/o, Allain et al, *Eur J Clin Pharmacol* 2003;**59**:179–88). There appear to be no problems with **zaleplon** in the elderly.

20. Increased **propranolol** side-effects have been reported in the elderly and so reduced initial doses are generally recommended. No dose reduction is necessary for **oxprenolol**.

21. **Clomethiazole** doses should be reduced, as the half-life can be at least doubled and plasma levels up to five times normal can occur (Dehlin, *Acta Psychiatr Scand* 1986;**73**[Suppl 329]:112–5). No problems are expected with **melatonin** or **ramelteon**.

3.7.4 ANTICONVULSANTS

For anticonvulsants, it is best to avoid renally

excreted drugs (e.g. **gabapentin**), as the renal excretion of some drugs may be significantly reduced in the elderly compared with younger people. Hepatically metabolised drugs, e.g. **carbamazepine** and **lamotrigine** are not influenced by age and are to be preferred.

Reviews: management of epilepsy in old age (Brodie et al, *Lancet Neurol* 2009;**8**:1019–30; Marasco and Ramsay, *Consult Pharm* 2009;**24** (Suppl A):17–22).

22. No significant changes have been shown with **carbamazepine** in the elderly, including ECG (n = 108 [c = 75], RCT, d/b, 40/52, Saetre *et al, Epilepsia* 2009;**50**:1841–9), and so dose requirements are likely to be the same as adults or perhaps slightly lower (n = 171, Bondareva *et al, J Clin Pharm Ther* 2006;**31**:211–21). Although the AUC with **oxcarbazepine** may be 30–60% higher in the elderly, tolerability is comparable to that in adults (n = 52 cf. 1574 adults, Kutluay *et al, Epilepsy Behav* 2003;**4**:175–80). No dose recommendations exist, other than gradual dose titration (n = 48, van Heiningen *et al, Clin Pharmacol Ther* 1991;**50**:410–9), a lower dose if the patient has compromised renal function, and monitoring as it may cause hyponatraemia (review by Sommer *et al, Expert Opin Drug Saf* 2007;**6**:133–45).

23. **Valproate's** half-life may be doubled in the elderly and an extensive study of elderly nursing home residents on stable regimens, concluded that valproate doses may need to be lower (by around 25%) in women, but higher in either gender with concurrent carbamazepine or phenytoin and if the syrup is used (n = 146, Birnbaum *et al, Ther Drug Monit* 2007;**29**:571–5). CNS side-effects and nausea are correlated with total and unbound levels, and thus are likely to be increased in older people (n = 6, s/b, Felix *et al, J Clin Psychopharmacol* 2003;**23**:471–8).

24. Reduced doses of **phenytoin** may be needed with the elderly, e.g. by about 20% (n = 92, open, Bauer and Blouin, *Clin Pharmacol* 1982;**31**:301–4). Careful monitoring is necessary, especially in those with hypoalbuminaemia or renal disease, as these individuals may have an increased level of side-effects and risk of toxicity, including cardiac arrhythmias. It may be that reduced doses are only needed with monotherapy, as opposed to anticonvulsant polypharmacy (review by Bachmann and Belloto, *Drugs Aging* 1999;**15**:235–50). Severe

cardiovascular ADRs have been reported with **fosphenytoin** IV (see *3.2*), and a reduction in the loading dose and/or infusion rate by 10–25% in the elderly is recommended.

25. The half-lives of **phenobarbital** and **primidone** are longer in the elderly due to reduced metabolism and so reduced doses should be used.

26. **Lamotrigine** is hepatically metabolised and this is influenced by genetic factors rather than age. An increased volume of distribution in the elderly has been shown to increase the half-life of lamotrigine, thus increasing the chance of side-effects, and so reduced doses may be needed. When used in elderly patients with newly diagnosed epilepsy and no pre-existing AV conduction defects, lamotrigine had no significant effects on the ECG (n = 108 [c = 75], RCT, d/b, 40/52, Saetre *et al, Epilepsia* 2009;**50**:1841–9). In older epileptics suffering ADRs from existing AEDs, either adding lamotrigine or switching to lamotrigine has been associated with improved tolerability and effectiveness, especially as monotherapy (n = 62, open, Evans *et al, Am J Geriatr Pharmacother* 2007;**5**:112–9). **Gabapentin** clearance is reduced in old age, probably via reduced renal clearance, although it seems to cause less cognitive impairment than carbamazepine in healthy adults (n = 34, RCT, c/o, Martin *et al, Epilepsia* 2001;**42**:764–71) but may cause ataxia (review by Sommer *et al, Expert Opin Drug Saf* 2007;**6**:133–45). It has been successful and well-tolerated as add-on therapy for neuroleptics or valproate in geriatric mania (n = 7, open, Sethi *et al, J Geriatr Psychiatry Neurol* 2003;**16**:117–20).

27. * No dose reduction is needed with **lacosamide** in old age, although the AUC may be increased by 30–50%, especially if renally impaired, but experience is limited (SmPC). **Levetiracetam** seems well-tolerated in the elderly, e.g. it has been successful in 72% patients with new-onset seizures in advanced Alzheimer's (n = 25 [c = 24], open, Belcastro *et al, Eur J Neurol* 2007;**14**:1176–8), with only headache and tremor occurring more frequently (n = 3352, Cramer *et al, Epilepsy Res* 2003;**56**:135–45). Older adults (55–88 years) may, however, require 40% lower doses than younger adults to achieve the same serum levels (n = 308, retrospective, one year, Hirsch *et al, Epilepsia* 2007;**48**:1351–9), especially in renal impairment (see *3.9.4*). **Topiramate** seems effective in epilepsy in elderly

people, but up to 50% discontinue because of cognitive ADRs (Sommer and Fenn, *Clin Interv Aging* 2010;**5**:89–99). The half-life of **piracetam** is extended in the elderly (n = 10, open, Platt *et al*, *Arzneimittel Forschung* 1985;**35**:533–5). Reduced **pregabalin** doses may be necessary due to decreased renal function (see *3.9.4*), but it seems safe and effective for anxiety in older people (mean 72 years) within two weeks (n = 273, RCT, d/b, p/c, 8/52, Montgomery *et al*, *Br J Psychiatry* 2008;**193**:389–94). Although evidence is limited for **rufinamide**, dose adjustments are not required in people over 65 (UK SmPC). There is no need to adjust the dose of **tiagabine** on the basis of age, although slightly higher plasma levels may occur in the elderly (n = 24, Snel *et al*, *J Clin Pharmacol* 1997;**37**:1015–20). **Vigabatrin** is renally excreted and reduced doses are recommended for Ccr < 60 ml/min and avoided in the elderly.

28. Lower **acetazolamide** doses are indicated (n = 12, open, Chapron *et al*, *J Clin Pharmacol* 1989;**29**:348–53).

3.7.5 OTHERS

29. There are no specific problems with **donepezil** and **rivastigmine**, provided the dose titration guidelines are followed. **Galantamine** levels are about 30–40% higher in elderly patients than healthy young individuals. **Memantine** has a usual maximum dose of 20 mg/d.

30. Confusion can be induced in the elderly by further compromising brain cholinergic activity. An initial low dose is recommended for **trihexyphenidyl** (SmPC now says use with extreme caution in elderly) and **orphenadrine**. Clearance of **procyclidine** should be reduced in the elderly (UK SmPC) and so BD dosing may be more appropriate than TDS dosing (n = 6, RCT, p/c, Whiteman *et al*, *Eur J Clin Pharmacol* 1985; **28**:73–8).

31. **Acamprosate** should not be used in the elderly (UK SmPC), due more to a lack of data rather than specific reported problems.

32. * Reduced **lithium** clearance occurs in the elderly through reduced renal function and increased volume of distribution (review by Sproule *et al*, *Drugs Aging* 2000;**16**:165–77), so doses should be reduced by as much as 50%. The elderly may also develop symptoms of lithium toxicity at standard therapeutic blood levels (Nakra and Grossberg, *J Geriatr Drug Ther* 1987;**2**:47–63), but lithium can be safely used in the elderly if monitored closely and frequently. Just to prove it, a study in octogenarians showed lithium can be well tolerated provided serum levels and renal and thyroid function are monitored regularly (n = 12, Fahy and Lawlor, *Int J Geriatr Psychiatry* 2001;**16**:1000–3). Hypothyroidism can also occur. A review of the use of lithium in old age concluded that although not easy to use, lithium remains a safe, practical and effective option if properly used and monitored (Shulman, *Drugs Aging* 2010;**27**:607–15).

33. In the elderly, a **modafinil** starting dose of 100 mg/d is recommended. **Sodium oxybate** may cause cognitive impairment so care might be needed (SmPC).

34. There is no data for **methylphenidate**, but it has been used for depression in the elderly. There is no information on **atomoxetine** (UK SmPC).

35. * **Bupropion** can be effective and well-tolerated in the elderly (n = 100, RCT, Weihs *et al*, *J Clin Psychiatry* 2000;**61**:196–202) and bupropion ER 150–300 mg/d appeared effective and well-tolerated treatment for MDD in adults 65 years or older (n = 418 [c = 414], d/b, p/c, 10/52, Hewett *et al*, *J Psychopharmacol* 2010; **24**:521–9).

36. Caution is recommended with repeated doses of **methadone,** but there are no recommendations for **buprenorphine**.

3

3.8 PREGNANCY

	LOWER RISK (FDA=A)	MODERATE RISK (FDA=B OR C)	HIGHER RISK (FDA=D OR X)
Antipsychotics		Aripiprazole[2] Butyrophenones[6] Clozapine[3] Olanzapine[2] Paliperidone[1] Phenothiazines[7] Quetiapine[2] Risperidone[1] Sulpiride[5] Thioxanthenes[4] Ziprasidone[2]	Sertindole[2]
Antidepressants	Flupentixol?[4] Tryptophan?[16]	Agomelatine[14] Duloxetine[10] MAOIs[15] Mianserin[16] Mirtazapine[11] Moclobemide[16] SSRIs (except paroxetine)[9] St John's wort[16] Trazodone[13] Tricyclics[12] Venlafaxine[10]	Paroxetine[9] Reboxetine[14]
Anxiolytics and hynpotics	Chloral[21] Clomethiazole[21] Melatonin[21] Zolpidem[19]	Beta-blockers[20] Buspirone[18] Chlordiazepoxide[17] Clonazepam[17] Oxazepam[17] Promethazine[21] Zaleplon[19] Zopiclone[19]	Alprazolam[17] Hydroxyzine[17] Lorazepam[17] Ramelteon[21] Temazepam[17]
Anticonvulsants		Acetazolamide[28] Clonazepam?[17] Gabapentin[26] Lamotrigine[26] Levetiracetam[27] Oxcarbazepine[22] Paraldehyde[28] Pregabalin[27] Tiagabine[27]	Benzodiazepines[17] Carbamazepine[22] Ethosuximide[28] Fosphenytoin[24] Lacosamide[27] Phenobarbital[25] Phenytoin[24] Rufinamide[27] Topiramate[27] Valproate[23] Vigabatrin[27] Zonisamide[27]

Others		Acamprosate[31]	Lithium[32]
		Anticholinergics[30]	Methadone HD[34]
		Anticholinesterases[29]	
		Atomoxetine[35]	
		Buprenorphine[34]	
		Bupropion[36]	
		Dexamfetamine[35]	
		Disulfiram[31]	
		Memantine[29]	
		Methylphenidate[35]	
		Modafinil[33]	
		Methadone LD[34]	
		Sodium oxybate[33]	

The **FDA** has established five categories to indicate a drug's potential for teratogenicity, and, where known, these are noted in the text:

A Controlled studies in women fail to show a risk in the first trimester and the risk of fetal harm seems remote.

B Either animal tests do not show a risk but there are no human studies, **or** animal studies show a risk but human studies have failed to show a risk to the fetus.

C Either animal studies show teratogenic or embryocidal effects but there are no controlled studies in humans, **or** there are no studies in either animals or humans.

D Definite evidence of a risk to the fetus exists, but the benefits in certain circumstances (e.g. life-threatening situations) may make use acceptable.

X Fetal abnormalities have been shown in animals or humans or both and the risk outweighs any possible benefits.

The **Australian (ADEC) pregnancy category definitions** (in brief) are:

A Drug has been taken by a large number of pregnant women with no proven increase in malformations or other direct or indirect harmful effects on the fetus.

B1 Drug has been taken by a limited number of pregnant women with no proven increase in malformations or other direct or indirect harmful effects on the fetus. Animal studies have not shown evidence of fetal damage.

B2 As B1, but animal studies are inadequate or lacking, but other evidence shows no evidence of fetal damage.

B3 As B1, but animal studies have shown evidence of an increased occurrence of fetal damage of uncertain significance.

C Drugs that have caused or are suspected of causing an increase in fetal malformations or irreversible damage.

D As 'C', but also may be expected to cause an increase in fetal malformations or irreversible damage, and have adverse pharmacological effects.

X High risk of causing permanent damage so should not be used in pregnancy or where there is a possibility of pregnancy.

Where known, both the FDA and ADEC categories are quoted.

Further information should be sought on individual drugs to balance the risk-benefit ratio in a particular individual patient. The FDA and ADEC risk classification systems may not always be a reliable source of information (Addis *et al*, *Drug Saf* 2000;**23**:245–53).

Reproductive toxicity falls into five domains (Wisner *et al*, *Am J Psychiatry* 2000;**157**:1933–40):

1. Intrauterine fetal death/miscarriage.
2. Physical malformations.
3. Growth impairment.
4. Behavioural toxicity (post-birth).
5. Neonatal toxicity, e.g. withdrawal or direct adverse effects.

For the record, spontaneous major or gross malformations (usually defined as incompatible with life or requiring surgical correction) occur in 2–3% of pregnancies and spontaneous abortions in about 10–20% of clinically recognised pregnancies. In the first trimester, teratogenicity is

3

the main drug risk, and growth retardation and neurological damage may occur in the second and third trimesters. After birth, drug withdrawal effects may occur. Although there are a few reports that pregnancy may protect against the risk of, e.g. bipolar disorder, other papers show an increased risk (reviewed by Viguera and Cohen, *Psychopharmacol Bull* 1998;**34**:339–46).

Assessing risk: Recent retrospective studies are more useful pointers to risk than the length of time a drug has been on the market or anecdotal case reports.

GENERAL PRINCIPLES FOR PRESCRIBING IN PREGNANCY (adapted from *Maudsley Guidelines*)

Planning for possible pregnancy provides time for informed decisions. In bipolar disorder, pregnancy and the postpartum periods can be considered as separate risk periods, and treatment plans may need to be different for each. See also an additional section under anticonvulsants (*3.8.4*).

Pre-conception

1. For planned conception, discuss the risks and benefits of discontinuing or continuing medication, e.g. relapse, teratogenicity, etc, the unpredictability of the pre-conceptual duration, and that no decision is risk-free. Avoiding all drugs during the first trimester is the ideal but may risk relapse. Other options include continuing at the lowest possible dose (or switching to a drug with the shortest possible half-life) until a positive pregnancy test, or continuing throughout pregnancy at the lowest viable dose.
2. Consider the risk of pregnancy even if not currently planned, e.g. carry out a pregnancy test before starting teratogenic drugs in a woman of child-bearing potential. As up to 50% of pregnancies are unplanned:
   - document the woman's birth control method
   - document the potential risks for exposure to drug(s) during pregnancy
   - encourage proper nutrition, exercise and vitamin supplementation
   - note any other substances taken (e.g. excess caffeine, alcohol and natural products)

- educate the patient about the risks
- inquire about any pregnancy plans and emphasise the need for a pre-pregnancy consultation.

3. For drugs of known significant risk or where there is little data, consider switching to a lower-risk drug before conception.
4. Avoid polypharmacy, as synergistic teratogenicity can occur (up to 16% with multiple AEDs, n = 172, Kaneko *et al*, *Epilepsia* 1988;**29**:459–67).

Pregnancy

1. Avoid all drugs during the first trimester if possible. The maximum teratogenic potential is from days 17–60 (2–9 weeks) after conception, and decisions must balance the relative versus absolute risk.
2. Behavioural teratogenesis and subtle functional disturbances (e.g. learning difficulties, neurological deficits and developmental delay), and an effect on labour and delivery may occur in the second and third trimesters.
3. Use the lowest possible (maintenance) dose and monitor effects (adverse and desired) carefully. Maintain a low threshold for reintroduction or dose increase.
4. In many cases, the risk of relapse (and subsequent higher dose drug use) will be higher than the risk of fetal damage.
5. The pharmacokinetics of drugs may change during pregnancy and so doses may need to be adjusted (see e.g. lithium, tricyclics).
6. Discontinuation effects have been reported in the newborn (e.g. benzodiazepines, antidepressants and opiates) and these psychotropics should, if possible, be gradually reduced or withdrawn over the weeks before delivery is due.

Unexpected pregnancy

If a woman discovers or reports that she is pregnant while taking a drug:
1. Don't panic.
2. If before day 17, consider immediate stopping or temporary discontinuation.
3. If after day 60, the major risk has passed and so decisions are less urgent.

4. Institute immediate nutritional supplements (e.g. folic acid).

5. Reduce the dose if possible, at least during the high risk period.

6. Discontinue any non-essential treatments, particularly any that might be at sub-therapeutic doses.

7. Do not stop lithium abruptly (see point 32), and beware of stopping some SSRIs and anticonvulsants.

8. Seek specific specialist advice, and discuss the risk of the possible consequences of relapse versus the published risk to the fetus.

Reviews: * neurodevelopmental effects of pre-natal exposure to psychotropics (Gentile, *Depress Anxiety* 2010;**27**:675–86), general (Kohen, *Adv Psychiatr Treat* 2004;**10**:59–66, 55 refs), psychotropics in pregnancy in bipolar disorder (Nguyen et al, *Adv Ther* 2009;**26**:281–94; Dodd and Berk, *Curr Drug Saf* 2006;**1**:25–33; Yonkers et al, *Am J Psychiatry* 2004;**161**:608–20).

3.8.1 ANTIPSYCHOTICS

An extensive Swedish study (1995–2005) showed no difference in the MCM rate between women taking antipsychotics or not, a consistent finding with other large studies, although the rate was higher in women also taking anticonvulsants (infants n = 973,767, Reis and Kallen, *J Clin Psychopharmacol* 2008;**28**:279–88; comment by Einarson and Einarson, *EMBH* 2009;**12**:29), although there may be an may increase in infant birth weight and risk of larger gestational age (n = 108, Newham et al, *Br J Psychiatry* 2008;**192**:333–7). Low folate intake and low serum folate levels have been shown in women taking SGAs, increasing the risk of neural tube defects (Koren et al, *Am J Psychiatry* 2002;**159**:136–7) and so dietary advice and folate supplements pre-conception are **essential**. The placental passage ratio for transfer (based on umbilical cord cf. maternal plasma) for the major antipsychotics is:

- olanzapine 72% (highest)
- haloperidol 66%
- risperidone 49%
- quetiapine 24% (lowest).

Reviews: * general (Einarson and Boskovic, *J Psychiatr Pract* 2009;**15**:183–92; McCauley-Elsom et al, *J Psychiatr Ment Health Nurs* 2010;**17**:97–

104), systematic review (Gentile, *Schizophr Bull* 2010;**36**:518–44).

1. **Risperidone** (FDA = C; ADEC = B3) has no reported teratogenicity in animal tests. A prospective cohort study showed no increase in malformations in women who took risperidone (n = 49, McKenna et al, *J Clin Psychiatry* 2005;**66**:444–9; comment by Howard, *EBMH* 2005;**8**:115). There are several published reports of normal pregnancies and postnatal development with oral or Risperidone Consta throughout pregnancy (e.g. n = 1, Kim et al, *Prog Neuropsychopharmacol Biol Psychiatry* 2007;**30**:543–5; two successive pregnancies; n = 1, Mendhekar and Lohia, *J Neuropsychiatry Clin Neurosci* 2008;**20**:485–6; n = 1, Rodríguez-Salgado, *Actas Esp Psiquiatr* 2008;**36**:366–8). **Paliperidone** (FDA=C) is not teratogenic in animal studies but some reversible developmental effects have been seen, so is not recommended, but should not be stopped abruptly during pregnancy (SmPC).

2. There is limited adequate data on **aripiprazole** (FDA = C), although data is currently unremarkable. Healthy children have been born with aripiprazole throughout pregnancy (e.g. n = 1, Doulgeraki et al, *Eur Psychiatry* 2007;**22**(suppl 1):S206); n = 1, Mervak et al, *Arch Women's Ment Health* 2008;**11**:249–50), and with aripiprazole 10–15mg/d from 0–8 weeks and then 20 weeks to term (n = 1, Mendhekar et al, *Bipolar Disord* 2006;**8**:299–300), although there was a lactation failure in this last case, possibly due to aripiprazole-induced regulation of prolactin. **Asenapine** (FDA = C) is not teratogenic in animal studies but human data is not yet available (US PI).

Olanzapine (FDA = C; ADEC=B3): from 516 documented pregnancies to May 2008 (MI) 65.1% were normal, 10.3% premature, 8.7% spontaneous abortions, 8.3% had perinatal complications, 4.7% MCMs and 2.9% others, all within normal ranges (n = 23, Goldstein et al, *J Clin Psychopharmacol* 2000;**20**:399–403). A prospective cohort study also showed no increase in malformations in women who took olanzapine (n = 60, McKenna et al, *J Clin Psychiatry* 2005;**66**:444–9; comment by Howard, *EBMH* 2005;**8**:115). Use should only be when the potential benefit outweighs the potential risk. In a woman who took olanzapine throughout pregnancy, the newborn's plasma levels were about a third of the mother's (11ng/ml vs 25–34ng/ml), with normal development over the first six months (n = 1, Aichhorn et

3

al, J Psychopharmacol 2008;**22**:923–4). There is a tendency for lower birth rates and SCBU admissions with olanzapine (n = 54, New-port *et al, Am J Psychiatry* 2007;**164**:1214–20).

Quetiapine (FDA = C): the literature recommends using only if the benefits justify the risk but the available data shows no major cause for concern. A prospective cohort study showed no increase in malformations in women who took quetiapine (n = 36, McKenna *et al, J Clin Psychiatry* 2005;**66**:444–9; comment by Howard, *EBMH* 2005;**8**:115). There are cases of up to 400 mg/d (n = 1, Tényi *et al, Am J Psychiatry* 2002;**159**:674; n = 1, Taylor *et al, Am J Psychiatry* 2003;**160**:587–8) and 1200 mg/d (starting from week 21, n = 1, Cabuk *et al, Arch Women's Ment Health* 2007;**10**:235–6) taken throughout pregnancy without complications and with normal development at six months. Other reports note a low placental transfer (n = 21, Newport *et al, Am J Psychiatry* 2007;**164**:1214–20) and uneventful use with risperidone (n = 4, Gentile *et al, Ann Pharmacother* 2004;**38**:1265–71). There are no adequate human studies during pregnancy with **ziprasidone** (FDA = C). **Sertindole** is contraindicated in pregnancy, but no teratogenic activity has been shown.

3.* Women are more likely to conceive on **clozapine** (FDA = B; ADEC = C) than most other antipsychotics due to an absence of raised prolactin. In a review of nearly 200 cases, the authors cite a 6% malformations incidence (Nguyen and Lalonde, *Encephale* 2003;**29**:119–24) and clear accumulation of clozapine has been shown in the infant, possibly due to higher albumin concentrations (n = 1, Barnas, *Am J Psychiatry* 1994;**151**:945). No clear conclusion can be drawn, although combined with animal studies it would appear clozapine is not a major teratogen, but not recommended in pregnancy as such.

4. **Thioxanthenes**: **Flupentixol** (ADEC = C) passes across the placenta and fetal levels are about a quarter of the mother's levels (n = 5, open, Kirk and Jorgensen, *Psychopharmacology* 1980;**72**:107–8). There is no positive evidence of teratogenicity, although the UK SmPC does not recommend its use. Studies in three species have not shown malformations. The UK SmPC now states that **zuclopenthixol** should not be used during pregnancy unless the benefit outweighs the theoretical risk to the fetus. Animal studies

have not shown any increase in fetal effects but lethargy, tremor, hyperexcitability and low Apgar scores have been reported (SmPC).

5. **Sulpiride** has been used as an antinauseant in pregnancy. Limited human data has shown some possible adverse effects but these are probably not drug-related and animal studies have not shown direct or indirect adverse effects (the UK SmPC now recommends appropriate monitoring of the neonate). **Amisulpride** shows no animal reproductive toxicity, but is contraindicated in pregnancy in humans.

6. **Butyrophenones**: The safety of **haloperidol** (FDA = C; ADEC = C) in pregnancy has not been fully established, but a prospective study showed there was no significant increase in MCMs (cf. control group) even if taken in the first trimester (although there were two limb defects), but there was a higher incidence of therapeutic termination, preterm birth and low birth weight (n = 188, Diav-Citrin *et al, J Clin Psychiatry* 2005;**66**:317–22). There is a case of dyskinesia in a newborn after haloperidol monotherapy (n = 1, Collins and Comer, *Am J Health Syst Pharm* 2003;**60**:2253–5).

7. **Phenothiazines**: (ADEC: chlorpromazine = C, promazine = C, trifluoperazine = C, fluphenazine = C)

Most of the teratogenicity data on phenothiazines is based on low doses and thus not necessarily applicable to higher dose use. The phenothiazines are considered by some to be of low risk, although the potential for hypotension, sedation and anticholinergic effects means that any use must be with extreme care. Severe MCMs were not significantly different in the studies of 543 women taking low-dose phenothiazines, other than **prochlorperazine** (FDA = C) for nausea (Miklovich and van den Berg, *Am J Obstet Gynecol* 1976;**125**:244–8), and in 1309 mothers mostly taking prochlorperazine (prospective, Slone *et al, Am J Obstet Gynecol* 1977;**128**:486–8). The largest study of 315 pregnancies where phenothiazines were taken in the first trimester, showed a statistically significant difference in the malformation rate of 3.5% in the aliphatic (**chlorpromazine** and **promazine**) phenothiazine-treated group (11 malformed infants), compared with 1.6% in the control group. There was no apparent trend in the type of abnormality and the risk is still considered low. There was no difference with the other phenothiazines, which appear to have an incidence of malformations similar to the background incidence (*Teratology* 1977;**15**:57–64). Although **levomepromazine** (methotrimeprazine) is an aliphatic phenothiazine, it has generally been considered safe for both mother and fetus if used occasionally in low dose later in pregnancy. A follow-up of **trifluoperazine** pregnancies showed no teratogenic effects (Moriarity, *Can Med Assoc J* 1963;**88**:97). In the neonate, lethargy and extra-pyramidal symptoms have been reported, as has respiratory depression when given in high dose (above 500mg chlorpromazine equivalents) close to term.

Postnatal development: A lack of impaired mental or physical development has been shown at two and seven years in a follow-up study (n = 16, Ayd, *Int Drug Ther Newsletter* 1976;**11**:5). 8. Animal studies of **pimozide** have shown no teratogenicity but use is not advisable (SmPC).

3.8.2 ANTIDEPRESSANTS *

It is still unclear which is worse; untreated ante-natal depression (e.g. higher incidence of SIDS, poor engagement and self-care) or antidepressant exposure during pregnancy (e.g. neonatal syndrome from antidepressant exposure), so no decision is risk-free (summary by Freeman, *J Clin Psychiatry* 2007;**68**:1277–8).

Overall, the adverse effects of all classes of anti-depressants in general in pregnancy have been reported as:

- In women aged 15–45 who had used an antidepressant for at least a month in the year before pregnancy, there was no association with an increased risk of MCMs compared to no antidepressants (n = 2329, 21/12, Ramos *et al, Br J Psychiatry* 2008;**199**:344–50; comment by Howard, *EBMH* 2009;**12**:28).
- In first trimester exposure to antidepressants, MCMs were 3.2% in antidepressant group and 3.3% in matched controls, so there was no association with increased MCM (n = 2486, Einarson *et al, Can J Psychiatry* 2009;**54**:242–6).
- No consistent link with MCMs if used in the first trimester, but with third trimester use there is an increased risk of perinatal complications (n = 2201, Davis *et al, Pharma-*

coepidemiol Drug Saf 2007;**16**:1086–94).

- In mothers who took a tricyclic [n = 80], fluoxetine [n = 55] or nothing [n = 84] (Nulman *et al, NEJM* 1997;**336**:258–62) there seems to be no effect on the neurological development or intelligence of their children (see 20 below).
- Third trimester exposure to antidepressants was not associated with a significant increase in postpartum haemorrhage (n = 28863 [PPH n = 2460 vs 26403 controls], Salkeld *et al, J Clin Psychopharmacol* 2008;**28**:230–4; comment by Heerdink, *EBMH* 2008;**11**:125).
- A systematic review showed no difference in child outcome (cognition, motor and behaviour) with prenatal exposure to antidepressants, although two studies showed a difference in motor function (s = 12, Gentile and Galbally, *J Affect Disord* 2011;**128**:1–9).

A 2009 US report on the management of depression during pregnancy recommends:

Women thinking of getting pregnant:

- If mild or no symptoms for 6/12 or longer consider tapering and discontinuation before becoming pregnant.
- This may not be appropriate if the depression is severe or recurrent (including psychosis, bipolar, history of suicide).
- Women with suicidal or acute psychosis should be referred to secondary care for 'aggressive' treatment.

Pregnant women currently taking antidepressants:

- Psychiatrically stable women who want to stay on medication may be able to after discussion with a psychiatrist/obstetrician.
- Women who want to discontinue may attempt tapering, and stopping if no symptoms recur.
- Women with recurrent depression, or who have symptoms despite antidepressants, may be helped by psychological therapies as a replacement or augmentation.
- Women with severe depression (with e.g. suicidal attempts, weight loss) should remain on antidepressants.

Pregnant women who are depressed and not currently on antidepressants:

- Psychotherapy may be helpful if the woman prefers to avoid antidepressants.

3

- If preferring antidepressants, choose carefully based on, e.g. trimester, history of depression, comorbidity.

All pregnant women:

- Seek psychiatric help urgently if suicidal or psychotic symptoms develop.

(Yonkers et al, Gen Hosp Psychiatry 2009;**31**:403–13; Yonkers et al, Obstet Gynecol 2009;**114**:703–13).

Reviews: * general (Osborne and O'Keane, Prog Neurol Psychiatry 2009;**13**:6–12; Bérard et al, CMAJ 2010;**182**:1079), risks of untreated depression (Bonari et al, Can J Psychiatry 2004;**49**:726–35), depression during pregnancy and postpartum (Cohen et al, CNS Spectr 2004;**9**:209–16).

9. * **SSRIs:** (FDA: citalopram = C, escitalopram = C, fluoxetine = C, fluvoxamine = C, paroxetine = D, sertraline = C, ADEC: citalopram = C, fluoxetine = C, paroxetine = B3, sertraline = B3) There is a significant body of data on SSRIs in pregnancy:

First trimester use:

- A prospective, multicentre cohort study of 267 women exposed to an SSRI (**fluvoxamine**, **sertraline** or **paroxetine**) during pregnancy and 267 controls, exposure to SSRIs at recommended doses did not appear to be associated with increased teratogenicity (relative risk 1.06, 95% CI, 0.43–2.62) or higher rates of miscarriage, stillbirth or prematurity (prospective, Kulin et al, JAMA 1998;**279**:609–10).

- A prospective controlled study of SSRIs in the first trimester showed a higher rate of abnormalities with **paroxetine** (5.2%, n = 410) and **fluoxetine** (4.7%, n = 314) compared to placebo (2.5%, n = 1467), particularly cardiovascular abnormalities; 2%, 2.8%, 0.6% respectively (n = 2191, Diav-Citrin et al, Br J Clin Pharmacol 2008;**66**:695–705).

- A case-control study of first-trimester exposure to paroxetine showed no increase in heart defects overall but a possible association with atrial septum defects (n = 1293, Bakker et al, Birth Defects Res A Clin Mol Teratol 2010;**88**:94–100). However, another review suggested that while cardiovascular malformations with SSRIs might be possible, there are many methodological weaknesses in the data and

is not proven (Tuccori et al, Postgrad Med 2010;**122**:49–65).

- First trimester use of SSRIs has been associated with two-fold higher risk of mild nonsyndromic heart defects (n = 235 + 67636, Merlob et al, Birth Defects Res A Clin Mol Teratology 2009;**85**:837–41).

- In a population-based cohort study, the incidence of septal heart defects was 0.5% (n = 2315) in unexposed children, 0.9% (n = 12) with SSRIs, and 2.1% (n = 4) in children exposed to more than one SSRI, with the risk being greater with **sertraline** and **citalopram** in the first trimester (n = 493113, Pedersen et al, Br Med J 2009; **339**:b3569).

- Two reviews concluded little or no increase in the rates of MCMs, low birth weight and preterm births, although high-dose **fluoxetine** (40–80 mg/d) may be associated with a risk of lower birth weight (n = 138, Hendrick et al, Am J Obstet Gynaecol 2003;**188**:812–15), and there was a slight increased risk of septal defects with **sertraline** (n = 2062 + 213712 controls, Kornum et al, Clin Epidemiol 2010;**2**:29–36).

- The overall rate of MCMs is 1.4%, similar to that seen in the general population, e.g. there were no general increases in heart defects and other birth defects with first-trimester exposure to SSRIs. There was a slight association of **sertraline** with omphalocele and septal defects, and between paroxetine and right ventricular obstruction defects, but these specific defects are rare and the absolute risk is small (n = 15,709, Louik et al, N Engl J Med 2007;**356**:2675–83).

Second and third trimesters: *

- One study showed an increased incidence of gestational hypertension in pregnant women taking SSRIs (19% vs 9%), especially if used in the third trimester, although a causal link was not established (n = 5731, Toh et al, Am J Psychiatry 2009;**166**:320–8).

- In a prospective study, exposure to SSRIs was associated with an increased risk of pre-term delivery, a lower 5-minute Apgar score and SCBU admission (n = 329, + 4902 controls, Lund et al, Arch Pediatr Adolesc Med 2009;**163**:949–54).

- There is an association between SSRI

use after 20 weeks' gestation and PPHN (persistent pulmonary hypertension in the newborn), with the absolute risk being around 1%, but not with other antidepressants or use up to 20 weeks (n = 1213, Chambers et al, N Engl J Med 2006;**354**:579–87).

- SSRI use in later pregnancy may also be associated with persistent pulmonary hypertension in the newborn (PPHN), with an extra 3–4 cases per 1000 pregnancies (Kallen and Olausson, Pharmacoepidemiol Drug Saf 2008;**17**:801–6; Anon, Drug Safety Update 2010;**3**:2).

- In a retrospective study, apparent prenatal SSRI exposure, slightly earlier delivery (0.9 week) and decreased birth weight (175 g) were noted and third trimester exposure to SSRIs was associated with a 0.29 decrease in mean Apgar scores at five minutes (n = 185, controls n = 185, Simon et al, Am J Psychiatry 2002;**159**:2055–61). Caution is advised and use should only be if clearly needed.

- Having untreated depression in pregnancy increases the risk of pre-term birth and low birth-weight (meta-analysis, s = 27, Grote et al, Arch Gen Psychiatry 2010;**67**:1012–24).

Birth:

- A Canadian study has concluded that the risk of adverse neonatal outcomes (e.g. gestation duration and low birth rate, but not length of hospital stay, convulsions or feeding difficulties) is more related to the duration of SSRI exposure during pregnancy, rather than the timing of the exposure, a confusing finding (n = 3500, one year, Oberlander et al, Br J Psychiatry 2008; **192**:338–43; comment by Gentile, EBMH 2009;**12**:27).

- Serotonergic drugs may increase the risk of CNS serotonergic adverse effects (tremor, restlessness, rigidity), but these subside quickly without treatment and may be due to serotonergic hyperstimulation rather than withdrawal (prospective, n = 40, p/c, Laine et al, Arch Gen Psychiatry 2003;**60**:720–6).

- Neonatal withdrawal symptoms (irritability, constant crying, shivering, increased tonus, eating and sleeping difficulties and con-vulsions) have been reported after in utero exposure to **paroxetine** (n = 3), **citalopram** (n = 1) and **fluoxetine** (n = 1), four requiring

calming with chlorpromazine (Nordeng et al, Acta Paediatrica 2001;**90**:288–91).

Postnatal development:

- In a retrospective study, apparent prenatal SSRI exposure was not associated with malformation or any developmental delay (n = 185, controls n = 185, Simon et al, Am J Psychiatry 2002;**159**:2055–61).

Citalopram and **escitalopram** (review by Gentile, Clin Drug Investig 2008;**28**:735–9): of 125 women who took citalopram in the first trimester (including 71 who also took it throughout pregnancy), there were 86% normal live births, 11% spontaneous abortions, 1.5% elective terminations and 1.5% stillbirths, plus one male infant born with MCMs and there was an overall increased risk of admission to a SCBU (n = 125, Sivojelezova et al, Am J Obstet Gynecol 2005;**193**:2004–9). Occasionally, slightly increased doses of citalopram may be needed in pregnancy (n = 11, Heikkinen et al, Clin Pharmacol Ther 2002;**72**:184–91).

Fluoxetine: There is a mass of safety data on fluoxetine-exposed pregnancies reported in prospective cohort-controlled studies and surveys. Based on published studies, use in the first trimester is not associated with a significantly increased risk of major malformations (see introduction to 3.8.9). Studies have shown first-trimester exposure produces no statistical differences in pregnancy outcome, age or weight, but a slight tendency to miscarriage with both drug groups (SSRI 14.8%, TCA 12.2%, no drug 7.8%; n = 312, Pastuszak et al, JAMA 1993;**269**:2246–8; Goldstein and Marvel, JAMA, 1993;**270**:2177–8), but miscarriage rates double that in the control group (n = 228, Chambers et al, NEJM 1996;**335**:1010–5). A prospective study showed a possible association between cardiovascular abnormalities and first-trimester exposure to fluoxetine (n = 314, risk 2.8%), but not quite with paroxetine (n = 410, risk 2%), compared to controls (n = 1467, risk 0.6%) (Diav-Citrin et al, Br J Clin Pharmacol 2008;**66**:695–705). The UK MHRA has issued warning of an increase in cardiac defects with fluoxetine taken early in pregnancy. The background rate of cardiac defects is 1%, fluoxetine is associated with increase to about 1.5% pregnancies, roughly same as paroxetine. However, the MHRA noted that there was no increase in non-cardiac defects

3

and no consistent defects, and to consider that untreated depression in pregnancy can cause low birth weight, pre-term delivery and low Apgar scores (Reefhuis et al, NEJM 2006;**354**:2188–90; s = 7, MHRA, Drug Safety Update 2010;**3**:8). Relatively low plasma fluoxetine levels have been reported in pregnancy, which might lead to therapeutic failure at standard doses, with infant fluoxetine and norfluoxetine plasma levels 65% and 72% respectively at birth (n = 11 + 10 controls, Heikkinen et al, Clin Pharmacol Ther 2003;**73**:330–7).

Postnatal development: A careful prospective study of children (assessed between 18 and 86 months) whose mothers had taken either fluoxetine (n = 55) or no drug (n = 84) showed fluoxetine to have had no effect on global IQ, language development or behavioural development (n = 139, Nulman et al, NEJM 1997;**336**:258–62). Further data on exposure to fluoxetine throughout pregnancy shows no detectable adverse affect on cognition, language development or temperament, whereas untreated depression was associated with poorer cognitive and language achievement in their children (TCA n = 46, fluoxetine n = 40, control n = 36; open, Nulman et al, Am J Psychiatry 2002; **159**:1889–95).

Paroxetine: A review from respected authors of the use of paroxetine in early pregnancy concludes that the data is inconsistent and inconclusive (s = 25, Gentile and Bellantuono, J Clin Psychiatry 2009;**70**:414–22; see also meta-analysis showing no increased risk of cardiac malformations from first trimester exposure; s = 9, n = 97,656, O'Brien et al, J Obstet Gynaecol Can 2008;**30**:696–70). although a mild-to-moderate association could not be excluded (n = 182 exposed infants, Davis et al, Pharmacoepidemiol Drug Saf 2007;**16**:1086–94). Another study suggested that first trimester exposure to paroxetine does not appear to be associated with increased cardiac effects (paroxetine 0.7%, unexposed group 0.7%) unlike antidepressants in general (n = 2061, 1.5%), when the usual population incidence is around 1% (n = 1174, Einarson et al, Am J Psychiatry 2008; **165**:749–52). However, the UK SmPC now states that paroxetine use in the first trimester is associated with increased risk of cardiovascular defects (increase from about 1% to less than 2%), but the MHRA does not recommend stopping paroxetine abruptly if a woman is pregnant as this could precipitate discontinuation symptoms, but to discuss the risks and benefits at the next appointment. When used in the third trimester, paroxetine may cause a high rate of neonatal complications, probably due to a withdrawal syndrome, e.g. a careful prospective study showed 22% neonates had complications (9 = respiratory distress, 2 = hypoglycaemia) requiring intensive treatment and hospitalisation, although all symptoms had disappeared within 1–2 weeks (n = 55 + controls; Costei et al, Arch Pediatr Adolesc Med 2002;**156**:1129–32; more severe case, Morag et al, J Toxicol Clin Toxicol 2004; **42**:97–100). Finally, in women who are extensive or ultra-rapid 2D6 metabolisers, paroxetine levels steadily decrease throughout pregnancy at 0.3 mcg/L per week, whereas in intermediate and poor metabolisers plasma paroxetine levels increase by 0.82 mcg/L per week. Accumulation can thus occur in some women, which might have adverse consequences (n = 74, Ververs et al, Clin Pharmacokinet 2009;**48**:677–83).

Review: (n = 22, Wurst et al, Birth Defects Res A Clin Mol Teratol 2010;**88**:159–70).

Sertraline: (see also introduction) has been included in a number of studies, e.g. in a prospective, multicentre cohort study of 267 women exposed to an SSRI (fluvoxamine, sertraline or paroxetine) during pregnancy and 267 controls, exposure to SSRIs at recommended doses did not appear to be associated with increased teratogenicity (relative risk 1.06, 95% CI, 0.43–2.62) or higher rates of miscarriage, stillbirth or prematurity. Gestational ages and birth weights were similar among offspring of both groups of women (n = 534, Kulin et al, JAMA 1998;**279**: 609–10). Sertraline levels and AUC remain fairly constant throughout pregnancy and postpartum, although they fall slightly in the third trimester (n = 11, Freeman et al, J Clin Psychopharmacol 2008;**28**:646–53).

10. Prospective data on 150 **venlafaxine** (FDA = C; ADEC = B2) pregnancies showed 125 live births, 18 spontaneous abortions, seven therapeutic abortions and two major malformations, suggesting that the base-rate of malformations does not rise above the spontaneous rate but, as with the SSRIs, the spontaneous abortion rate is slightly higher (venlafaxine n = 150; SSRIs n = 150; controls n = 150; Einarson et al, Am J Psychiatry 2001;**158**:1728–30).

It is no longer contraindicated in pregnancy in the UK SmPC, although there is a warning of the potential for withdrawal symptoms in the neonate (e.g. n = 1, de Moor et al, Ned Tijdschr Geneeskd 2003;**147**:1370–2). The UK SmPC now notes PPHN has been reported for SSRIs and, although there are no reports for venlafaxine, it cannot be ruled out as it is also an SSRI. Neonatal discontinuation signs start as soon as infant plasma levels decline; respiratory symptoms tend to start early and may contribute to PPHN (n = 5, Boucher et al, Ther Drug Monit 2009;**31**:404–9). Animal studies with **duloxetine** (FDA = C) suggest some adverse behavioural effects in one animal species. There is no adequate human data, but one uneventful use from the middle of the second trimester (n = 1, Briggs et al, Ann Pharmacother 2009;**43**:1898–902). However, a case has been reported of neonatal withdrawal syndrome similar to SSRIs (e.g. jitteriness, poor muscle tone, weak cry, respiratory distress, hypoglycaemia, low Apgar score and seizure) lasting several weeks but with normal development at two years (n = 1, Eyal and Yaeger, Am J Psychiatry 2008;**165**:651).

11. For **mirtazapine** (FDA = C; ADEC = B3) a recent comprehensive and prospective study has shown no increase in the baseline rate of major malformations but a slight increase in spontaneous abortions (19% vs 17% vs 11%) and preterm births (10% vs 7% vs 2%) (n = 104 mirtazapine, vs n = 104 other antidepressants vs. control group, Djulus et al, J Clin Psychiatry 2006;**67**:1280–4). Animal tests do not show any teratogenicity or fetal harm. There are two cases of recurrent hypothermia lasting for 10 days in identical twins born to mother who took mirtazapine throughout pregnancy (n = 2, Sokolover et al, Can J Clin Pharmacol 2008;**15**:188–90). When used for depression, anxiety and hyperemesis gravidarum in seven pregnancies, all women improved and all babies were born healthy at term (n = 7, Saks, Arch Women's Ment Health 2001;**3**:165–170; see also n = 2, Kesim et al, Teratology 2002;**66**:204).

12. **Tricyclic antidepressants:** (FDA: clomipramine = C, desipramine = C, doxepin = B, maprotiline = B, trimipramine = C; ADEC: amitriptyline = C, clomipramine = C, dosulepin = C, doxepin = C, imipramine = C, nortriptyline = C, trimipramine = C)

In the most recent retrospective study, prenatal tricyclic exposure was not associated with MCMs, developmental delay or any adverse perinatal outcomes (n = 209, controls n = 209, Simon et al, Am J Psychiatry 2002;**159**:2055–61), confirming an earlier meta-analysis (n = 414 from 414 000 live births), although withdrawal symptoms were noted.

In pregnancy, mild toxicity in the infant has been seen with **imipramine**, e.g. respiratory distress, hypotonia, irritability, tremors, convulsions and jerky movements (e.g. n = 2, Ware and DeVane, J Clin Psychiatry 1990;**51**:482–4). Phenobarbital can improve these symptoms, which can persist for a total duration of up to two weeks. **Amitriptyline** and **imipramine** are considered the tricyclics of choice, based on cumulative data on their relative safety.

Discontinuation effects have been noted in the neonate, sometimes requiring active treatment, e.g. clomipramine discontinuation causing a jittery/twitchy infant (n = 1, Schimmel et al, Clin Toxicol 1991;**29**:479–84) and a lethargic and cyanotic baby, who had abnormal movements, feeding difficulties and fetal seizures (Bromiker and Kaplan, JAMA 1994;**272**:1722–3), both of whom settled when clomipramine was started.

Postnatal development: A careful study of children (assessed between 18 and 86 months) whose mothers had taken either a tricyclic (n = 84) or no drug (n = 80) showed tricyclics to have no adverse effect on global IQ, language development or behavioural development compared to no drug (n = 164, Nulman et al, NEJM 1997;**336**:258–62). Further data shows no adverse affect on cognition, language development or temperament, whereas untreated depression is associated with poorer cognitive and language achievement in their children (tricyclic n = 46, fluoxetine n = 40, control n = 36, open, Nulman et al, Am J Psychiatry 2002; **159**:1889–95).

13. For **trazodone** (FDA = C) at very high doses (15+ times the maximum human dose), there appears to be some fetal resorption and MCMs in animals but little human data exists.

14. No teratogenic effects have been noted with **reboxetine** (and so it is no longer contraindicated). For **agomelatine**, little human data exists so it should be avoided in pregnancy.

15. **MAOIs:** (FDA: all = C, ADEC: isocarboxazid = B3, phenelzine = B3, tranyl-cypromine = B2)

3

There are no reports of human teratogenicity with **phenelzine** or **tranylcypromine**, although it has been suggested that the risk may be roughly doubled if tranylcypromine is taken in the first trimester (AAPCD, *Pediatrics* 1982;**69**:241–3). Growth retardation and fetal toxicity have been reported. If at all possible, MAOIs should be avoided due to maternal toxicity and lack of published safety data. MAOIs may also interact with drugs used in labour (see also *4.3.4*).

16. There is no evidence of teratogenicity with **mianserin** (ADEC = B2) in animals except at toxic doses, but little human data is available. No firm data is available on the use of **moclobemide** in pregnancy, but there is a case of 300 mg/d taken throughout pregnancy with no problems and normal development within the first 14 months (n = 1, Rybakowski, *Pharmacopsychiatry* 2001;**34**:82–3). No human data is available for **tryptophan**, but it is a naturally occurring substance in food. In **St John's wort**-exposed pregnancies (n = 54), the MCM rate was 5%, comparable to other antidepressants (4%, n = 54) and controls (0%, n = 54), not considered statistically different from each other (n = 162, Moretti *et al, Reprod Toxicol* 2009;**28**:96–9).

3.8.3 ANXIOLYTICS AND HYPNOTICS

Review: general (Vythilingum, *Curr Psychiatry Rep* 2008;**10**:331–5)

17. **Benzodiazepines**: (FDA: alprazolam = D, chlordiazepoxide = C, clonazepam = D, diazepam=D, lorazepam = D, oxazepam=D, temazepam = X; ADEC: clonazepam = C, diazepam=C, flunitrazepam=C, lorazepam=C, oxazepam=C, temazepam=C)
Assessment of 104 000 births in the USA has shown a higher incidence of teratogenicity in women taking a variety of benzodiazepines, but multiple alcohol and illicit substance exposure could account for this (Bergman *et al, Lancet* 1992;**340**:694–6). For individual BDZs, a population-based case-control study indicated that **nitrazepam, medazepam, alprazolam** and **clonazepam** taken during pregnancy did not present a detectable teratogenic risk (n = 38,151, Eros *et al, Eur J Obstet Gynecol Reprod Biol* 2002; **101**:147–54). With **chlordiazepoxide**, there was slight increase in MCMs with use in the second to third months, but no specific type or pattern was

seen, and so the risk is unlikely to be substantial (n = 469, Czeizel *et al, Neurotoxicol Teratol* 2004;**26**:593–8). **Clobazam** is known to cross the placenta and benzodiazepine withdrawal symptoms in the neonate have been suggested but no teratogenicity has been reported. For **diazepam**, studies show a varying risk of oral clefts, with the worst case scenario bringing the risk to seven in 1000. Doses of 30 mg or more of diazepam IM or IV during the last 15 hours of labour can induce neonatal respiratory depression and feeding problems, although 10 mg given IV within 10 minutes of birth has been shown not to affect Apgar scores (n = 23, open, McAllister, *Br J Anaesth* 1980;**52**:423–7). As with other benzodiazepines, withdrawal symptoms in the neonate have been seen (n = 3, Rementeria and Bhatt, *J Pediatr* 1977;**90**:123–6). As **lorazepam** crosses the placenta, the floppy baby syndrome and respiratory depression can occur, especially if IV doses are used close to birth. Oral use during later pregnancy may show delayed feeding in full-term infants, but premature infants may have lower Apgar scores and respiratory depression (n = 53, open, Whitelaw *et al, Br Med J* 1981;**282**:1106–8).

The UK CSM has noted the danger of benzodiazepine use during pregnancy or labour due to the effects on the neonate, such as hypothermia, hypotonia, respiratory depression and withdrawal symptoms (*Curr Prob* 1997; **23**:10). Shorter-acting benzodiazepines on a 'when required' basis may be acceptable later in pregnancy, but the first trimester should be avoided if possible. After birth, benzodiazepine withdrawal symptoms have been noticed in the neonate with many benzodiazepines. The 'floppy baby' syndrome, as it is often termed, includes facial features and CNS dysfunction and can occur particularly with higher doses (eg. > 30 mg diazepam equivalent per day) of longer-acting benzodiazepines (n = 8, Laegreid *et al, J Pediatrics* 1989;**114**:126–31).

Overdoses:

- **Alprazolam**: In cases of attempted suicide by overdose (7.5–100 mg, mean 30 mg) there was no significantly higher rate of MCMs, although only 10 live births were assessed and an association cannot be excluded for one multiple abnormality (n = 10, Gidai *et al, Toxicol Ind Health* 2008; **24**:53–60).

- **Chlordiazepoxide**: In women who took large overdoses of CDZ during pregnancy, there was no evidence of a higher rate of MCMs but a dose-dependent intrauterine growth retardation was seen, with lower birth weight newborns (n = 88, live births = 35, Gidal *et al, Toxicol Ind Health* 2008;**24**:41–51).

- **Diazepam**: In women who attempted suicide by diazepam in overdose, doses of 25–800mg produced 13.4% MCMs (cf. 7.1% matched controls), but the overdoses taken during the first trimester critical periods did not show excess abnormalities, suggesting the MCMs were unrelated to diazepam (n = 229; 112 live births, Gidai *et al, Toxicol Ind Health* 2008;**24**:29–39).

- **Nitrazepam**: * in pregnant women attempting suicide with very high doses of nitrazepam (mean 204 mg), 30% children had congenital abnormalities (cf. 10% controls), although most were reported to be mild malformations (n = 43, Gidai *et al, Pharmacoepidemiol Drug Saf* 2010;**19**: 175–82).

18. There is no evidence of teratogenicity from **buspirone** (FDA = B; ADEC = B1) but effects on survival and weights have been noted in some, but not all, animal tests. **Hydroxyzine** is contraindicated in early pregnancy as very high-dose animal tests induced fetal abnormalities (UK SmPC).

19. **Zopiclone** has not been contraindicated in pregnancy. Animal tests have shown no abnormalities and the limited human data is unremarkable. Little information is currently available on **zaleplon** (FDA = C). **Zolpidem** (FDA = C; ADEC = B3) crosses the placenta but clears rapidly from the fetal circulation, and there is a (statistically) non-significant increase in pre-term delivery (27% vs 13%) and low birth weight (16% vs 5%) from regular zolpidem compared to matched controls (n = 45, Juric *et al, Arch Women's Ment Health* 2009;**12**:441–6). In an unusual case, maternal use of high-dose zolpidem (at least 1000 mg over at least one month) was studied; cord levels were less than the mean maternal plasma levels likely from a single 5 mg dose, and the neonate was alert and with no apparent withdrawal symptoms over the first 48 hours (n = 1, Askew, *Pharmacotherapy* 2007;**27**:306–8). None of these three hypnotics are contraindicated in pregnancy and short-term

'when required' use of zolpidem would appear to present only minimal risk.

20. **Beta-blockers**: (FDA: propranolol = C; ADEC = C)

Beta-blockers are not generally considered teratogens but a connection between **propranolol** use in pregnancy and tracheosophageal fistulas and intrauterine growth retardation has been proposed but not substantiated. Direct effects of beta-blockade on the fetus would also occur, e.g. bradycardia. Use in the second and third trimesters may aggravate or produce neonatal hypoglycaemia. Fetal and neonatal bradycardia may occur, especially in pregnancies already complicated by placental insufficiency (e.g. severe maternal hypertension). Due to direct cardiac effects, hypoglycaemia and apnoea from beta-blockers, it may be prudent to discontinue treatment 1–2 weeks before delivery.

21. Maternally administered **chloral** (ADEC = A) appears relatively safe as no increase in MCMs was seen in a study of 71 women who took chloral in the first four months of pregnancy, or to 358 women who took chloral at some time in pregnancy (Heinonen *et al, Birth Defects and Drugs in Pregnancy*, Publishing Sciences Group 1977:336–7). The UK SmPC states that **clomethiazole** (ADEC = A) should not be used, particularly in the first and third trimesters, although it has been used widely for pre-eclampsia. Platelet aggregation in the neonate has been reported with **promethazine** (FDA = C; ADEC = C). In pregnant women attempting suicide by taking up to 1780 mg promethazine, there was no evidence of teratogenicity, lower IQ or development, although the total MCM rate was very high in the cohort (n = 32 from 1044 overdoses, Petik *et al, Toxicol Ind Health* 2008;**24**:87–96). **Melatonin** has no apparent teratogenic effects but use is not recommended at the moment (SmPC).

3.8.4 ANTICONVULSANTS

Pregnant women with epilepsy are at increased risk of complications and 25–33% have an increased risk of seizures. One of the main reasons for this increase is the marked alterations in plasma protein-binding of drugs as pregnancy progresses, resulting in declining plasma levels. A number of prospective and retrospective studies have shown that there are a wide range of risks associated with anticonvulsants (some used as mood stabilisers) used throughout pregnancy. Polytherapy carries additional risks, e.g. it is associated with a (partly reversible) decline in body dimension (n = 963, Swedish survey, Wide *et al, Epilepsia* 2000;**41**:854–61), including the risk of pre-term delivery, lower birthweight, length and head circumference (n = 193, controls n = 24094, Hvas *et al, Br J Obstet Gynaecol* 2000; **107**:896–902).

Postnatal development: Some specific effects on postnatal development of children exposed to anticonvulsants during pregnancy, e.g. a higher frequency of educational needs statements (10.3% drug exposed cf. 5.7% non-drug-exposed), especially for **valproate** (30%), and polypharmacy, (n = 400 school-age children: 150 exposed to monotherapy, 74 to polytherapy and 176 to none; Adab *et al, J Neurol Neurosurg Psychiatry* 2001; **70**:15–21) and phenytoin (n = 76 exposed, c/w 71 unexposed, Wide *et al, Acta Paediatrica* 2002;**91**:409–14). One review concluded developmental delay was seen in 24% of AED exposed children (cf. 11% non-exposed siblings), childhood medical problems in 31% (cf. 13% of non-exposed siblings) and behaviour disorders in 20% (cf. 5% of non-exposed), concluding that prenatal antiepileptic drug exposure is associated with developmental delay and later childhood morbidity, in addition to MCMs (n = 129 mothers, 293 children, Dean *et al, J Med Genet* 2002;**39**:251–9). Facial dysmorphism has been described in patients with uncontrolled seizures, as well as with phenytoin, phenobarbital, primidone, valproate, benzodiazepines and carbamazepine.

Summary of the risks of pregnancy in women with epilepsy:

- 25–33% increase in maternal seizure frequency
- 10% risk of vaginal bleeding
- 7% risk of neonatal haemorrhage if no vitamin K is given
- 10% risk of infant facial dysmorphism
- 4–6% risk of major malformations (30% of which are oral facial defects)
- 1–2% risk of spina bifida with valproate
- 0.5–1% risk of spina bifida with carbamazepine.

(Yerby, *Epilepsia* 1992;**33**[Suppl 1]:S23–S27.)

UK epilepsy and pregnancy register

A prospective study (n = 3607, Morrow *et al, J Neurol Neurosurg Psychiatry* 2006;**77**:193–8) has shown that only 4.2% of children born to mothers with epilepsy and taking AEDs had MCMs, subdivided as follows:

- 6% polytherapy exposures had MCMs
- 3.7% monotherapy exposures had MCMs
- more polytherapies with MCM had valproate than those that did not include valproate.

Relative risks of MCMs with monotherapy:

- 2.2% carbamazepine (least risk)
- 3.2% lamotrigine (> 200 mg/d had higher risk)
- 6% valproate (higher with > 1000 mg/d at 9%).

Summary of risk minimisation strategies:

1. Pre-conception:

- Education of the patient as to the risks and benefits of continued treatment. This should be documented and supported with written information (n = 300, survey, Fairgrieve *et al, Br Med J* 2000;**321**:674–5).
- Adequate oral contraceptive dosage (see individual drugs' interactions, 4.5) until conception is planned, e.g. 50 mcg of ethinylestradiol.
- Start regular multivitamins with folate (4–5 mg/d from before oral contraceptives are stopped, until at least 12 weeks of gestation) to reduce the chance of spina bifida, cardiovascular birth defects and oral clefts, especially with folic acid antagonists e.g. carbamazepine, phenytoin, phenobarbital (n = 6932, Hernandez-Diaz *et al, NEJM* 2000;**343**:1608–14).
- Minimise the exposure to drugs with known associated risks, e.g. phenobarbital, valproate, carbamazepine and benzodiazepines.
- Seizure control with the lowest dose monotherapy (Vajda *et al, Epilepsia* 2010;**51**:805–10) should be targeted.
- Diagnosis should be verified and the need for anticonvulsants confirmed.

2. After conception:

- Education of the patient about risk minimisation, e.g. vitamin supplementation.

3. Seizure control without toxicity during pregnancy:

- Do not change drugs if the patient is stabilised.

- Continue multivitamins with folate.
- Frequent monitoring of free anticonvulsant concentrations and dose adjustment if necessary.
- Monotherapy should be continued if possible.
- Vitamin K should be given during last week of pregnancy if possible.
- Ultrasound and AFPs should be carried out.

Reviews: * extensive (Hill et al, Expert Rev Neurother 2010;**10**:943–59), teratogenicity (Tomson and Battino, Neurol Clin 2009;**27**:993–1002), general (Iniesta and Winterbottom, Prescriber 2010;**21**:61–6; Crawford, Drug Saf 2009; **32**:293–307; Pennell, Epilepsia 2008; **49**(Suppl 9):43–55; Hovinga and Pennell, Int Rev Neurobiol 2008;**83**:241–58; Sabers and Tomson, Curr Opin Neurol 2009;**22**:157–61), mood stabilisers (Galbally et al, Aust N Z J Psychiatry 2010;**44**:967–77), postnatal development (Meador et al, N Engl J Med 2009;**360**:1597–605).

22. **Carbamazepine** * (FDA = D; ADEC = D) is now considered to have a higher risk. However, a recent literature review and analysis concludes that the incidence of MCMs with carbamazepine monotherapy in the first trimester is 3.3% (specifically spina bifida) but still rare, and smaller than with valproate (s = 8, n = 2680, Jentink et al, Br Med J 2010;**341**:6581). The UK epilepsy and pregnancy register showed that carbamazepine monotherapy may also have a low risk of major malformations (n = 3607, Morrow et al, J Neurol Neurosurg Psychiatry 2006; **7**:193–8). The literature recommends the need for counselling and screening for neural tube defects, which can detect 90–95% of neural tube defects if carried out with AFP levels at 16–18 weeks. In late pregnancy, routine vitamin K to mothers and the neonates is usually recommended.

Postnatal development: A meta-analysis has shown no difference in verbal IQ but performance IQ slightly lower (s = 7, n = 67 + n = 494 controls, Banach et al, Drug Saf 2010;**33**:73–9).

Oxcarbazepine (FDA = D) is closely related to carbamazepine and data indicate that oxcarbazepine may cause serious birth defects, and there is significant transfer through the placenta in humans (n = 12, Myllynen et al, Epilepsia 2001;**42**:1482–5). However, a large study from Argentina suggested that oxcarbazepine had a lower risk of teratogenicity than older AEDs (n = 114, Meischenguiser et al, Epilepsy Behav 2004;**5**:163–7). There is a significant decrease in ratio of plasma levels of oxcarbazepine MHD and dose in the first (26%), second (37%) and third (38%) trimesters, leading to seizures in eight patients (n = 10 [13 pregnancies], Petrenaite et al, Epilepsy Res 2009;**84**:245–9; n = 1956, EURAP Study Group, Neurology 2006;**66**:354–60), and so higher doses may be needed as levels drop to 72% in the first trimester, 74% in the second trimester and down to 64% in the third trimester, rising to 108% after pregnancy (n = 7, Christensen et al, Neurology 2006;**67**:1497–9). Careful monitoring throughout pregnancy and immediately afterwards is essential (n = 5, Mazzucchelli et al, Epilepsia 2006;**47**:504–9).

23. * **Valproate** (FDA = D; ADEC = D) crosses the placenta easily and is now well-established as both teratogenic and causing developmental problems and should not be used in women of child-bearing potential. There is undoubtedly a pharmacogenetic component to teratogenic and neurodevelopmental effects (Duncan, Curr Opin Neurol 2007;**20**:175–80):

- First trimester: *

Exposure to valproate during pregnancy associated with:

- spina bifida (OR 12–16)
- atrial septal defect (OR 2.5)
- cleft palate (OR 5.2)
- hypospadias (OR 4.8)
- polydactyly (OR 2.2)
- craniosynostenosis (OR 6.8).

However, the absolute risk remains low at 0.1–0.7% (n = 1565 from n = 98075, Jentink et al, N Engl J Med 2010;**362**:2185–93).

In the first trimester there is an increased relative risk of 7.3 of major malformations after first trimester exposure to valproate (10.7% had major malformations cf. 2.9% controls; n = 149, n = 1048 controls, Wyszynski et al, Neurology 2005;**64**:961–5). These include facial dysmorphia, hypospadias, limb malformations and spina bifida. However, dysmorphic features, developmental delay and structural anomalies may only be found in children exposed to maternal valproate doses above 1000 mg/d (n = 69, Mawer et al, Seizure 2002;**11**:512–8), an important observation. The FDA issued a warning (December 2009) that neural tube defects occur one in 20 babies if the mother

3

took valproate during first 12/52 of pregnancy (cf. one in 1500 in general population) and that folic acid before and during first trimester reduces the risk (although not everyone thinks this is proven, Jentink et al, Pharmacoepidemiol Drug Saf 2010;**19**:803–7), as, indeed, might co-prescribing with lamotrigine (s = 14, Vajda et al, Epilepsia 2010;**51**:805–10).

- Second/third trimester: reduced mean birth-weight-adjusted mean head circumference has been shown, although the significance of this is unknown, but has not been shown for phenytoin, clonazepam, lamotrigine and gabapentin (n = 900000, Almgren et al, Seizure 2009;**18**:672–5).

- Birth: The literature now states that there have been rare reports of haemorrhagic syndrome in neonates whose mothers took valproate in pregnancy.

- Postnatal development: * A meta-analysis has shown IQ significantly lower with valproate taken throughout pregnancy (s = 7, n = 67 + n = 494 controls, Banach et al, Drug Saf 2010;**33**:73–9), e.g. exposure to valproate in utero is more likely to lead to an IQ below 69 and a poorer memory compared to exposure to other AEDs or none (n = 249, Vinten et al, Neurology 2005;**64**:949–54; n = 309, Meador et al, N Engl J Med 2009;**360**:1597–605), a seven times higher incidence cf. the control group of autism (6.3% vs 0.9%) if valproate is used as monotherapy (n = 620 mothers, n = 632 live births, Bromley et al, Neurology 2008;**71**:1923–24), a higher than expected incidence of education needs statements (n = 400 school-age children: 150 exposed to monotherapy, 74 to polytherapy and 176 to none, Adab et al, J Neurol Neurosurg Psychiatry 2001;**70**:15–21), and some evidence of reduced verbal intelligence in children exposed to valproate and AED polytherapy during pregnancy compared to matched controls (n = 323; valproate n = 13, polytherapy n = 30, Gaily et al, Neurology 2004;**13**:28–32; see also n = 400, Adab et al, J Neurol Neurosurg Psychiatry 2001;**70**:15–21).

- Polycystic ovary syndrome (PCOS): There is an association between valproate and PCOS which may have some effect on reproductive capacity (n = 32, O'Donovan et al, J Clin Psychiatry 2002;**63**:322–30; review by Genton et al, Epilepsia 2001;**42**:295–304), but this may just be because valproate causes weight gain, a risk factor for PCOS.

The UK MHRA noted in September 2003 (Curr Prob Pharmacovig 2003;**29** [Sept]:6) that:

- specialist consultation should be sought for women likely to become pregnant on valproate
- if used in pregnancy, use the lowest effective dose (below 1000 mg/d)
- monotherapy
- use divided daily doses (2–3 times a day)
- give as an MR prep to reduce peak levels
- 5 mg folic acid should be started as soon as contraception is discontinued.

(Ornoy, Reprod Toxicol 2009;**28**:1–10).

NICE has recommended (Bipolar Guidelines, 2006) that valproate should not be used in women of child-bearing potential.

Review: general (Duncan, Curr Opin Neurol 2007;**20**:175–80).

24. **Phenytoin** (FDA = D; fosphenytoin = D; ADEC: phenytoin = D) crosses the placenta freely and teratogenicity is well-established, particularly the 'fetal hydantoin syndrome', e.g. growth retardation, microcephaly, mental retardation, facial defects, and others (review: Ozkinay et al, Turk J Pediatr 1998;**40**:273–8). The full syndrome occurs in about 8–10% of children born to mothers who took phenytoin in the first trimester (n = 88, Rodriguez-Palomares et al, Arch Med Res 1995; **26**:371–7), and a part syndrome in a further 30% of children (controlled prospective study, n = 34, Nulman et al, Am J Med Genet 1997; **68**:18–24). It appears not to be dose-related (n = 88, Rodriguez-Palomares et al, Arch Med Res 1995;**26**:371–7). It has also been noted that epileptic fathers taking phenytoin have increased rates of malformed children (Friis, Acta Neurol Scand 1983;**94**[Suppl]:39–43).

The kinetics of phenytoin change in pregnancy: elimination increases and plasma levels fall steadily as the pregnancy progresses, but free (i.e. active) levels may be unchanged in pregnancy and so care with plasma level interpretation is needed (review of phenytoin, Eadie et al, Eur J Clin Pharmacol 1992;**43**:389–92).

Risk reduction with phenytoin: where documented, seizures are proven to be controlled by phenytoin, the risks of withdrawal may be greater than with the continued use of phenytoin, with the following precautions:

1. **Use of minimal effective doses.** At least monthly blood level monitoring (including free levels) during pregnancy (and for up to six months after) is essential.

2. **Use of folic acid 5 mg/d** from before conception, which has a **significant** and highly important protective effect (n = 66 retrospective, n = 22 prospective, Biale and Lewenthal, *Eur J Obstet Gynecol Reprod Biol* 1984;**18**:211). The neural tube closes around the time of the first missed period and so folic acid supplements need to be started **before** pregnancy is detected. However, not everyone agrees that folic acid supplementation reduces the risk, as other mechanisms may be responsible other than folic acid metabolism (n = 1935, Morrow *et al, J Neurol Neurosurg Psychiatry* 2009;**80**:506–11), but it is a low risk strategy either way.

3. **Vitamin K supplementation.** Phenytoin inhibits the synthesis of vitamin K-dependent clotting factors and neonatal haemorrhage may occur., and so early vitamin K supplementation in at-risk pregnancies is recommended and to the neonate after birth.

Postnatal development: One study has indicated a negative neurodevelopmental effect from phenytoin. In a controlled study of *in utero* exposure, 34 children born to mothers taking phenytoin and 36 children born to mothers taking carbamazepine were compared to matched controls. Allowing for other variables, the phenytoin children had a significantly lower mean IQ and language ability, the carbamazepine children being similar to controls (Scolnik *et al, JAMA* 1994;**271**:767).

25. **Phenobarbital** (FDA = D) has been implicated as a teratogen (see introduction to *3.8.4*), although in many reported cases it has been as part of a combination therapy. Minor digital deformities as well as hip and facial abnormalities have been reported. In a study of pregnant women who attempted suicide by a barbiturate overdose, single very large doses did not appear to have any teratogenic, growth retardation or development adverse effects (n = 367, Timmermann *et al, Toxicol Ind Health* 2008;**24**:109–19; n = 88,

Timmermann *et al, Pharmacoepidemiol Drug Saf* 2009;**18**:815–25). Withdrawal symptoms, such as seizures and irritability have occurred in the neonate, some delayed by up to two weeks after birth. Neonatal bleeding in the first 24 hours has been reported, as has respiratory depression. However, antenatal phenobarbital exposure does not appear to affect the neurodevelopmental outcome of premature infants at 18–22 months of age (n = 578, Shankaran *et al, Am J Obstet Gynecol* 2002;**187**:171–7).

Postnatal development: There is some evidence of a direct neurotoxic effect by phenobarbital on developing fetal neurons, which may be responsible for some cognitive or CNS abnormalities. Prenatal exposure to combined phenobarbital and phenytoin (n = 172), compared to controls (n = 168), produced smaller head size at birth and persistent learning problems (12%) compared to controls (1%) in one study (Dessens *et al, Acta Paediatrica* 2000;**89**:533–41). In the longer-term, a smaller head circumference and an impaired cognitive development has been suggested in two studies (n = 122, van der Pol *et al, Am J Obstet Gynecol* 1991;**164**:121–8).

26. For **lamotrigine** (FDA = C; ADEC = B3), teratogenicity data in 2006 suggested an increase in the risk of oral clefts, but more recent data showed that the MCM level for lamotrigine was 2.3%, with an increased risk of isolated cleft palate or cleft lip deformity (n = 684, Holmes *et al, Neurology* 2008;**70**:2152–8), but there was no evidence of a specific increased risk of isolated orofacial clefts compared to other lamotrigine-associated malformation (n = 72 live births, Dolk *et al, Neurology* 2008;**71**:714–22). Previously, the incidence of major malformations with first-trimester exposure had been reported to be 1.8% (eg. n = 51, Sabers *et al, Acta Neurol Scand* 2004;**109**:9–13). When used as an anticonvulsant, extreme care is needed as plasma levels change throughout pregnancy:

- First trimester: LTG clearance increases by 197%, reducing levels by about 20% (n = 11, Franco *et al, Ther Drug Monit* 2008;**30**:544–7)
- Second trimester: clearance is increased by 236%
- Third trimester: clearance is increased by 248%
- Delivery: clearance is increased by 264%.

The average lamotrigine dose increase necessary

3

to maintain therapeutic plasma levels was 250%. (n = 9, Fotopoulou *et al*, *Epilepsy Res* 2009; **85**:60–4; see also n = 6, Tomson *et al*, *Neurology* 2006;**67**:1297–9; n = 11, Petrenaite *et al*, *Epilepsy Res* 2005;**65**:185–8; n = 1956, EURAP Study Group, *Neurology* 2006;**66**:354–60). Levels revert rapidly to normal after delivery so reduce doses again immediately (e.g. n = 1, Nordmo *et al*, *Ann Pharmacother* 2009; **43**:1893–7). In six mother–baby pairs, fetal **gabapentin** (FDA = C, ADEC = B1) levels were estimated to be 0.2–1.3 mg/kg/d (1.3–3.8% of mother's dose), with no adverse effects detected (n = 6, Ohman *et al*, *Epilepsia* 2005;**46**:1621–4), and there were no MCMs in the 11 babies born to mothers taking gabapentin in the first trimester in the Southampton PMSS (n = 3100, Wilton and Shakir, *Epilepsia* 2002;**43**:983–92).

27. **Lacosamide** should not be used in pregnancy unless clearly indicated (SmPC). Although some animal studies show reproductive toxicity, early results from the UK Epilepsy and Pregnancy Register show that in 117 infants exposed to **levetiracetam** (FDA = C), three (2.7%) had MCMs. Although all three had also been exposed to other AEDs (n = 117, Hunt *et al*, *Neurology* 2006;**67**:1876–9), it should not be used unless clearly necessary. In another study, the infant dose was equivalent to 2.4 mg/kg/d, equivalent to 7.9% of weight-normalised maternal dose, with plasma concentrations in the infant around 13% of mother's plasma levels (n = 15, Abou-Khalil, *Epilepsy Curr* 2008;**8**:62–3). Limited data suggests that a significant fall in levetiracetam levels may occur during pregnancy (Tomson and Battino, *Clin Pharmacokinet* 2007;**46**:209–19). Animal studies have shown some animal reproductive toxicity with **pregabalin** (FDA = C) at high dose, but the human risk is not known (SmPC). The UK SmPC recommends avoiding **rufinamide** in pregnancy and ensuring adequate contraception measures during treatment as the incidence of malformations is 2–3 times greater than the general spontaneous rate (UK SmPC). No human data is available on **tiagabine** (FDA = C; ADEC = B3) in pregnancy and so use should only be where clearly indicated. **Topiramate** (FDA = C; ADEC = B3) crosses the placenta and levels may rise in the first trimester by around 32%, by 81% in the second and by 75% in the third trimester, with significant interindividual variation (n = 10,

Ohman *et al*, *Epilepsy Res* 2009;**87**:124–9), so TDM and assessing doses is advised to avoid the risk of increased seizures (n = 12, Westin *et al*, *Epilepsia* 2009;**50**:480–5). Preliminary experience from the UK Epilepsy and Pregnancy Register showed 31 (17%) abnormalities from 178 live births, including 16 with MCMs (n = 203, Hunt *et al*, *Neurology* 2008;**71**:272–6). The incidence of oral clefts was 2.2%, about 11 times the background rate. Another study of 52 pregnancies had 41 live births with reduced birth weight, but no increase in structural defects (n = 52, Ornoy *et al*, *Reprod Toxicol* 2008;**25**:388–9). **Vigabatrin** is contraindicated in pregnancy. **Zonisamide** is transferred to the infant via the placenta, the transfer rate being 92% (n = 2, Kawada *et al*, *Brain Dev* 2002;**24**:95–7), and adequate contraception in women is necessary during treatment and for one month afterwards. A significant increase in clearance at the end of the second trimester may occur and increased doses may be appropriate (n = 1, Oles and Bell, *Ann Pharmacother* 2008; **42**:1139–41).

28. For **acetazolamide** (FDA = C; ADEC = B3), animal tests indicate that it is teratogenic and can increase miscarriages when taken at toxic doses. If use is essential, maternal electrolyte balance should be monitored. There are reported cases of malformations with **ethosuximide** (ADEC = D) alone, and some when combined with other drugs, but no cause-effect relationship has been proven. Little data is available for **paraldehyde** (FDA = C).

3.8.5 OTHERS

29. Very high doses of **donepezil** (FDA = C; ADEC = B3) may have some minor effects in pregnancy but no teratogenicity has been detected. The safety of **rivastigmine** (FDA = B) in pregnancy has not been established. There is no data on **galantamine** (FDA = B) in pregnancy, although animal studies show a slight delay in fetal and neonatal development. Human data is lacking with **memantine** (FDA = B), but animal data suggests potentially reduced interuterine growth.

30. **Anticholinergics**: (FDA: procyclidine = C, orphenadrine = C, ADEC: benzatropine = B2, procyclidine = A)
There is little data available on these drugs. A 'small left colon syndrome' has been reported in children whose mothers who took benzatropine

and other psychotropic drugs late in pregnancy (n = 2, Falterman and Richardson, *J Paediatr* 1980;**92**:308–10), although a cause-effect relationship was not established. The UK SmPC notes that there no studies with **orphenadrine** and so it should only be used if there is no safer alternative.

31. For **disulfiram** (FDA=C, ADEC = B2) there have been isolated reports of MCMs (e.g. Gardner and Clarkson, *N Z Med J* 1981;**93**:184–6), although other drugs were often taken and the symptoms were similar to the fetal alcohol syndrome. In animals, disulfiram has been shown to be embryotoxic. The risk-benefit ratio for the risks of alcoholism against disulfiram for the fetus must be assessed carefully. The UK SmPC for **acamprosate** (FDA = C) states that use in pregnancy is a contraindication, but animal studies have not shown any evidence of teratogenicity.

32. **Lithium** (FDA = D; ADEC = D) completely equilibrates across the placenta. Some studies show that the overall MCM rates with lithium (2.8%) are similar to control rates (2.4%), and suggest that lithium is not an important human teratogen if used with adequate screening (including level II ultrasound and fetal echocardiography) to detect Ebstein's anomaly (n = 148, prospective Jacobson *et al*, *Lancet* 1992;**339**:530–3; see also n=225, Yacobi and Ornoy, *Isr J Psychiatry Relat Sci* 2008;**45**:95–106). The risk of Ebstein's anomaly (a rare congenital downward displacement of the tricuspid valve into the right ventricle) exists if lithium is taken during weeks two to six post-conception. Ebstein's anomaly is often quoted as 20 times more common with lithium, but remains rare as the risk allegedly rises from one in 20 000 to one in 1000, although it is unclear from where these oft-quoted figures come. However, this risk must be weighed against the 50% chance of relapsing if lithium is stopped abruptly. An important study (n = 101, retrospective, Viguera *et al*, *Am J Psychiatry* 2000;**157**:179–84) noted that:

- the heart is formed very early, so stopping lithium when pregnancy is confirmed is too late anyway
- the relapse rates in the 40 weeks after lithium discontinuation are similar for pregnant (52%) and non-pregnant (58%) women, but much higher than the year before discontinuation (21%), so stopping lithium raises the risk of release 2–3-fold but

pregnancy itself is relatively 'risk neutral'
- women who remained stable over the first 40 weeks after lithium discontinuation were 2.9 times more likely to relapse than non-pregnant women during weeks 41–62 (70% vs 24%)
- the relapse rates are much higher in rapid rather than gradual lithium discontinuation
- the > 50% relapse rate in the first 40 weeks is high, and the risk from consequentially needed drugs is high
- there were no major malformations in the children born to the women (n = 9) who continued lithium throughout pregnancy
- an unstudied option might be to stop lithium gradually as soon as pregnancy is known, then reintroduce it in the third trimester.

NICE (Antenatal and Postnatal Mental Health Guideline, 2007) recommends:

- advising a woman to stop lithium if she is planning a pregnancy, is well and not at high risk of relapse
- if a woman taking lithium becomes pregnant, is well and not at high risk of relapse, lithium should be stopped gradually over four weeks, and then informed that this may not remove the risk of cardiac defects in the fetus (although the author of this book fails to fully comprehend the logic of this bearing in mind the Viguera study mentioned above)
- if the woman is not well or at high risk of relapse, NICE recommends switching to an antipsychotic, stopping lithium and restarting in the second trimester, or continuing lithium if at high risk of relapse (for which rapid withdrawal would be a risk factor).

During pregnancy: Renal clearance is increased and so higher doses are needed, but then lithium clearance reduces markedly near the end of term, doses may need to be reduced by up to 30–50% in the last few weeks (or a few doses omitted close to delivery) and plasma levels monitored carefully and frequently (n = 10 + 32, Newport *et al*, *Am J Psychiatry* 2005;**162**:2162–70). NICE recommends monitoring levels every four weeks until the 36th week, then weekly, then within the first 24 hours after childbirth, with doses adjusted according to those serum levels, and adequate fluid intake maintained.

Postnatal development: A study of healthy children born to mothers who took lithium

3

during the first trimester did not reveal any increased frequency of physical or mental anomalies among the lithium children compared to their non-lithium exposed siblings over 5–10 years (n = 60, Schou, *Acta Psychiatr Scand* 1976;**54**:193–7; see also Pinelli et al, *Am J Obstet Gynecol* 2002;**187**:245–9).

Reviews: Llewellyn et al, *J Clin Psychiatry* 1998; **59**[Suppl 6]:S57–S64; Yonkers et al, *CNS Drugs* 1998;**9**:261–9.

33. **Modafinil** (FDA = C) is contraindicated in pregnancy. Pre-clinical studies have shown no teratogenicity but more information is required. There is limited data on **sodium oxybate** (FDA = B), with no evidence of malformations or toxicity after second and third trimester exposure, but there is no data in the first trimester and so it is not recommended (SmPC).

34. **Methadone** (ADEC = C) maintenance throughout pregnancy is associated with reduced risk of poor quality street drug use, earlier and better antenatal care and improved treatment retention (n = 2993, Burns et al, *Addiction* 2007; **102**:264–70) than tapered withdrawal (n = 175, Jones et al, *Am J Addict* 2008;**17**:372–86).

- First trimester: with potential illicit drug-using mothers, teratogenicity with methadone will obviously be very difficult to ascertain, but there does not appear to be a clear association with malformations (e.g. study by Newman et al, *Am J Obstet Gynecol* 1975;**121**:233–7). Stopping opiates abruptly is dangerous, as withdrawal reactions can damage the fetus more than methadone.

- Second/third trimester: methadone clearance can be increased, with trough plasma levels dropping to 58%, which may require higher doses (n = 9, Wolff et al, *Eur J Clin Pharmacol* 2005;**61**:763–8). In a study of methadone maintenance in pregnancy, head circumference and birth weight were slightly lower compared to controls (n = 32, Brown et al, *Am J Obstet Gynecol* 1998;**179**:459–63).

- NAS (neonatal abstinence syndrome): symptoms include tremor, irritability, hyperactivity, jitteriness, shrill cry, vomiting, diarrhoea and convulsions. About 45% of infants develop NAS with maternal methadone requiring treatment (median stay 10/7), and the incidence can be reduced by breast-feeding (n = 450, Dryden et al, *BJOG*

2009;**116**:665–71). Although logically dose-related, high-dose methadone appears not to be associated with an increased risk of NAS compared to lower doses (e.g. n = 159, Simmat-Durand et al, *Eur J Obstet Gynecol Reprod Biol* 2009;142:119–23), but rather to overall maternal drug use (n = 81, McCarthy et al, *Am J Obstet Gynecol* 2005;**193**:606–10; see also breast-feeding, *3.1*). Each 1 mg increase in methadone dose taken before delivery adds an extra 0.18 days to neonatal abstinence syndrome duration or, to put it another way, each 5.5 mg adds a day to the NAS (n = 68, retrospective, Lim et al, *Am J Obstet Gynecol* 2009;**200**:e1–5). With average methadone doses of 117 mg/d, 68% developed NAS but with no correlation between maternal dose and rate of NAS. However, higher doses associated with reduced illicit opiate abuse at delivery (n = 330, offspring n = 388, Seligman et al, *J Pediatr* 2010;**157**:428–33). At lower doses, there was a linear relationship between dose and infant ADRs (n = 32 + 42 controls, Wouldes and Woodward *Neurotoxicol Teratol* 2010;**32**:406–13). There has been a suggestion that NAS is higher with 40 mg/d methadone than 20 mg/d, and > 40 mg/d than 40 mg/d, but there was no significant association so methadone dose is only one factor in development of NAS (meta-analysis, s = 29, Cleary et al, *Addiction* 2010;**105**:2071–84).

- NAS: buprenorphine vs methadone. The incidence of NAS may be higher with buprenorphine than methadone (67% vs 58%, n = 41 [c = 38], Bakstad et al, *Eur Addict Res* 2009;**15**:128–34) or vice versa (methadone 78% vs 40%, n = 47, Kakko et al, *Drug Alcohol Depend* 2008;**96**:69–78), although may be lower if buprenorphine is started pre-conception. Cochrane concluded that there was no proven significant difference between the available opiate agonists with regard to NAS and birth weight, but the data sample was small (s = 3, n = 96, Minozzi et al, *Cochrane Database Syst Rev* 2008;**2**:CD006318).

- Although use of methadone and buprenorphine has problems, compared to controls the incidence of low birth weight pre-term births (31% vs 8%) and growth restriction show the risk of not doing anything, although pre-eclampsia appears rare in SMs (n = 247 vs 741, 4 years, Pinto *et al, Eur J Obstet Gynecol Reprod Biol* 2010; **150**:137–41).

- Immediate postnatal: * maternal drug-exposed infants usually show excessive early weight loss. This peaks at day 5 and is more marked in formula-fed infants (n = 354, Dryden *et al, Arch Dis Child Fetal Neonatal Ed* 2011; in press). There might also be a six times higher mortality in infants (especially of SIDS) of mothers on methadone maintenance than all other mothers (Burns *et al, Drug Alcohol Rev* 2010; **29**:551–6).

- Postnatal development: * long-term developmental outcome seems unaffected by methadone (Kaltenbach and Finnegan, *Neurotoxicol Teratol* 1987;**9**:311–3; effect in the first year see van Baar *et al, Arch Dis Child* 1989;**64**:235–40). There may be an eyesight risk for children of mothers taking methadone in pregnancy, e.g. acuity (95%), nystagmus (70%), delayed visual maturation (50%), strabismus (30%), refractive errors (30%), and cerebral visual impairment (25%), although the underlying causes are unclear (n = 20, Hamilton *et al, Br J Ophthamol* 2010; **94**:696–700).

Buprenorphine (FDA = C; ADEC = C) may have some advantages over methadone in pregnancy

- Second/third trimester: buprenorphine may cause less suppression of spontaneous motor activity in fetuses compared to methadone (n = 13, Jansson *et al, Neurotoxicol Teratol* 2011;**33**:204–3). In weeks 24–29, buprenorpine has a higher retention rate than methadone, but higher additional opioid use with an earlier onset of NAS occurring with methadone (mean 60 hours) than buprenorphine (72 hours) (n = 18 [c = 14], RCT, d/b, Fischer *et al, Addiction* 2006;**101**:275–81). There is evidence for increased buprenorphine renal elimination in the third trimester, but with significant intrasubject differences (n = 9, Kacinko *et al, Clin Chem* 2009;**55**:1177–87).

- NAS (neonatal abstinence syndrome): buprenorphine is associated with a shorter NAS hospital stay than with oral morphine (n = 24, open, Kraft *et al, Addiction* 2011;**106**:574–80). Infants exposed to buprenorphine require significantly less morphine (mean 1.1 mg vs 10.4 mg), hospital stays are shorter by 43%, and NAS duration is shorter by 41% than those exposed to methadone, although the incidence of NAS was the same (n = 175 [c = 131], RCT, d/b, Jones *et al, N Engl J Med* 2010;**363**:2320–31). High-dose buprenorphine (n = 159) throughout pregnancy (cf. to methadone), surprisingly showed that there was no relationship between dose and duration or severity of NAS (n = 251, Simmat-Durand *et al, Eur J Obstet Gynecol Reprod Biol* 2008;**142**:119–23).

Review: * extensive review of methadone, naltrexone and buprenorphine (Farid *et al, Curr Neuropharmacol* 2008;**6**:125–50), opioids (Winklbaur *et al, Curr Opin Psychiatry* 2008; **21**:255–9).

35. No teratogenic effects have been reported in women who took **dexamfetamine** (FDA = C) before knowing they were pregnant (Guilleminault, *Sleep* 1993;**16**:199–201). There is little information available for **methylphenidate** (FDA = C; ADEC = B2) and the few reported cases are unremarkable, but the literature advises caution. The UK SmPC recommends use of **atomoxetine** (FDA = C) only where the benefit justifies the potential risk (short review of evidence for all ADHD treatments: Humphreys *et al, Can Fam Physician* 2007;**53**:1153–5).

36. * There have been reports of a higher than expected incidence of neonatal malformations with **bupropion** (FDA = C), e.g. there is a very slight increased risk (OR 2.6) of left outflow tract heart defects with first trimester use (n = 6853 + 5869, Alwan *et al, Am J Obstet Gynecol* 2010;**203**:52.e1–6), but a large US study (1995–2004) showed that exposure to bupropion in the first trimester (n = 1213) and second and third trimesters (n = 1049) was not associated with an increased risk of cardiovascular or other malformations, compared to other antidepressant (n = 4743) first trimester exposures (Cole *et al, Pharmacepidemiol Drug Saf* 2007;**16**:474–84).

3

3.9 RENAL IMPAIRMENT (SEE ALSO BNF)

	LOWER RISK (FDA=A)	MODERATE RISK (FDA=B OR C)	HIGHER RISK (FDA=D OR X)
Antipsychotics	Asenapine[2]	Aripiprazole[2] Butyrophenones[6] Clozapine[3] Olanzapine[2] Phenothiazines[7] Pimozide[8] Quetiapine[2] Thioxanthenes[4] Ziprasidone[2]	Amisulpride[5] Paliperidone[1] Risperidone[1] Sertindole 2 Sulpiride[5] Zotepine[2]
Antidepressants	Agomelatine[14] Mianserin[16] Moclobemide[16] Tricyclics[12] Trazodone[13] Tryptophan[16]	Duloxetine[10] MAOIs[15] Mirtazapine[11] Reboxetine[14] SSRIs[9]	Fluoxetine[9] Venlafaxine[10]
Anxiolytics and hynpotics	Benzodiazepines (some)[17] Zaleplon[19] Zopiclone[19]	Benzodiazepines[17] Beta-blockers[20] Clomethiazole[21] Hydroxyzine[18] Melatonin[21] Zolpidem[19]	Buspirone[18] Chloral[21]
Anticonvulsants	Phenytoin[24] Rufinamide[27] Tiagabine[27]	Barbiturates[25] Benzodiazepines[17] Carbamazepine[22] Fosphenytoin[24] Lacosamide[27] Lamotrigine[26] Piracetam[27] Topiramate[27] Zonisamide[27]	Acetazolamide[28] Ethosuximide[28] Gabapentin[26] Levetiracetam[27] Midazolam[17] Oxcarbazepine[22] Pregabalin[27] Valproate[23]
Others	Anticholinesterases[29] Sodium oxybate [33]	Anticholinergics[30] Atomoxetine[35] Bupropion[34] Disulfiram[31] Memantine[29] Modafinil[33]	Acamprosate[31] Lithium[32] Methylphenidate [35]

Grade	GFR ml/min	Serum creatinine micromo/L
Mild	20–50	150–300
Moderate	10–20	300–700
Severe	<10	>700

GENERAL PRINCIPLES FOR PRESCRIBING IN RENAL IMPAIRMENT (adapted from *Maudsley Guidelines*)

1. The greater the renal impairment, the greater the potential for accumulation of drugs. Adverse effects such as postural hypotension, sedation and confusion may be more common.
2. Serum creatinine may not be raised in the elderly, although renal impairment may be present.
3. Care is needed with drugs or active metabolites predominantly cleared by the kidney, e.g. antidepressants and antipsychotics (except substituted benzamides).
4. Start low and go slow, adjusting doses to tolerance.
5. Care is needed with drugs with marked anticholinergic activity, which may cause urinary retention and interfere with U&E measurements.

3.9.1 ANTIPSYCHOTICS

Lower doses of all antipsychotics should be used, due to increased cerebral sensitivity and EPS.

1. * **Risperidone** elimination is reduced in renal disease and so initial doses and dose increments should be halved, up to a maximum of about 4 mg/d. Haemodialysis has resulted in reduced risperidone levels, leading to relapse (n = 1, Railton et al, *Ther Drug Monit* 2005;**27**:558–61). In mild renal impairment (Ccr 50–79 ml/min), start with **paliperidone** 3 mg/d and increase carefully. If 30–49 ml/min stay at 3 mg/d, if 10–29 ml/min, use 3 mg on alternate days and it is not recommended for < 10 ml/min. No dose adjustment is needed for **paliperidone palmitate** in mild-to-moderate renal impairment, but there is no data on severe impairment (Gopal et al, *Curr Med Res Opin* 2010; **26**:377–87).

2. Dose adjustment with **aripiprazole** is not necessary even in severe renal impairment, e.g. although the Cmax for a single dose of aripiprazole 15 mg was 40% higher in severe renal impairment, there were no significant adverse effects (n = 13, Mallikaarjun et al, *Clin Pharmacokinet* 2008;**47**:533–42). For **asenapine**, 50% is renally excreted but no dose alterations are necessary in renal impairment (US PI).

Olanzapine is excreted primarily (57%) via the renal pathway and 30% in faeces. A lower olanzapine starting dose of 5 mg/d may be appropriate in renal impairment. If creatinine clearance is < 10 ml/min, there is only a slight (11%) increase in half-life and 17% reduction in clearance. For **olanzapine pamoate,** a lower starting dose of 150 mg/4 weeks should be considered in people with renal impairment (SmPC). The UK SmPC for **quetiapine** now states that oral clearance is reduced by 25% in renal impairment, so start at 50 mg/d (25 mg/d in severe) and increase at 50 mg/d according to response and tolerability (e.g. n = 8, Thyrum et al, *Prog Neuropsychopharmacol Biol Psychiatry* 2000;**24**:521–33). Only 4% of an oral dose of **sertindole** is excreted via the kidneys. Clearance is unchanged by deteriorating renal function and in dialysis and usual doses can be used even in patients with severe renal impairment. Only 1% of a **ziprasidone** dose is excreted unchanged via urine (20% excreted as metabolites), so dosage adjustment is not required in renal impairment.

3. **Clozapine** is contraindicated in severe renal disease. Start at 12.5 mg/d and increase slowly in mild-to-moderate renal failure.

4. * The BNF now recommends **zuclopenthixol** is used at half-dose in renal impairment. The UK SmPC notes that **flupentixol** has not been studied in renal impairment but increased cerebral sensitivity reported with other antipsychotics.

5. **Sulpiride** is mainly cleared by the kidneys and its half-life can range from 6–25 hours, depending upon renal function. Reduce the dose by 35–70% or extend the dosage interval by a factor of 1.5 to 3 if necessary (n = 24, open, Bressolle et al, *Clin Pharmacokinet* 1989;**17**:367–73). **Amisulpride** is principally cleared unchanged through the kidneys, so care is needed in moderate-to-severe renal insufficiency (GFR 10–30 ml/min). It is not appreciably removed during haemodialysis.

6. There are no apparent problems with **haloperidol**, although the literature recommends caution as some accumulation might occur.

7. There is little information on **phenothiazines**, but excretion may be slower and accumulation may occur, causing sedation or postural hypotension. **Levomepromazine** should be used with care in renal disease, and chlorpromazine avoided.

8. The UK SmPC for **pimozide** recommends caution in renal impairment.

3

3.9.2 ANTIDEPRESSANTS *

Depression in renal impairment needs treating as there is a 3x greater risk of death in depressed people with stage 5 diabetic chronic kidney disease cf. non-depressed people (n = 110, 5 years, Young et al, Gen Hosp Psychiatry 2010;**32**: 119–24).

Review: antidepressants in chronic kidney disease (Raymond et al, Nephrol Nurs J 2008;**35**: 257–63).

9. * Renal clearance accounts for about 20% of total **citalopram** elimination, and although half-life increases slightly, no reduction of citalopram dosage is warranted in patients with moderately impaired renal function, but a slight reduction in severe renal failure may be prudent (open, Joffe et al, Eur J Clin Pharmacol 1998;**54**:237–42). Haemodialysis has an insignificant effect on plasma levels (n = 12, open, Spigset et al, Eur J Clin Pharmacol 2000;**56**:699–703). Dosage adjustment with **escitalopram** is not necessary in patients with mild or moderate renal impairment. Caution is advised in patients with severely reduced renal function (Ccr < 30 ml/min). The UK SmPC for **fluoxetine** notes that when taken 20 mg/day for two months by patients with severe renal failure (GFR < 10 ml/min) requiring dialysis, there was no difference in plasma levels of fluoxetine or norfluoxetine compared to controls with normal renal function. **Fluvoxamine** should be used with care, starting at 50 mg/d and increasing only slowly. Plasma levels of fluvoxamine are reduced by about 22% by haemodialysis, so higher doses might be needed (n = 7, Kamo et al, Psychiatr Clin Neurosci 2004;**58**:133–7). In moderate renal impairment, reduce the initial dose of **paroxetine** to 10 mg/d and increase only if necessary. **Sertraline** seems to be safe, effective and improves QoL in chronic peritoneal dialysis (n = 25, 12/52, Atalay et al, Int Urol Nephrol 2010;**42**:527–36), although not recommended by the SmPC.

10. About 1–10% of a **venlafaxine** dose is cleared unchanged by the kidney and 30% renally excreted as the major metabolite. Total clearance is reduced by about 35% in mild-to-moderate renal impairment (GFR 10–30 ml/min) and so doses should be reduced by about 25–50%, although there is much inter-patient variability in renal impairment (Anon, J Clin Psychiatry 1993;**54**:119–26). A study (12 with renal impairment, eight on dialysis and 18 matched controls) showed that clearance was reduced by about 55% in moderate-to-severe renal disease, and the authors suggested a 50% reduction in venlafaxine dose, given once a day, where GFR was less than 30 ml/min (n = 38, open, Troy et al, Clin Pharmacol Therapeut 1994;**56**:14–21). Daily doses should also be reduced by 50% in dialysis and doses withheld until after dialysis is complete. Venlafaxine is not recommended in severe renal failure. No dose adjustment is needed for **duloxetine** in mild-to-moderate renal disease (Ccr 30–80 ml/min), but is contraindicated in severe (Ccr < 30 ml/min) renal disease where plasma levels are doubled.

11. **Mirtazapine** clearance was reduced by 33% in moderate and by 50% in severe renal failure, but not in mild renal impairment in a single dose study (n = 40, Bengtsson et al, Hum Psychopharmacol 1998;**13**:357–65). Care with higher doses is recommended. Mirtazapine is largely unaffected by haemodialysis as, since 85% is protein-bound, only 15% is likely to be dialysed (n = 1, Schlotterbeck et al, Pharmacopsychiatry 2008;**41**:259–60).

12. **Tricyclics** should be started at low dose and increased slowly, with divided doses. Avoid **lofepramine** in severe renal impairment, as 50% is renally excreted.

13. No dosage adjustment is necessary for **trazodone**.

14. **Reboxetine's** half-life and plasma levels appear to rise (up to two-fold) in severe renal impairment, where dose adjustment may be necessary. In a single-dose study, a reduction in starting dose to 2 mg BD in patients with moderate-to-severe renal dysfunction has been suggested (n = 18, open, Coulomb et al, J Clin Pharmacol 2000; **40**: 482–7). No dose adjustments are needed with **agomelatine**.

15. No dosage adjustments are usually necessary for the **MAOIs**, although **isocarboxazid** should be used with caution with impaired renal function to prevent accumulation.

16. Dosage adjustments in renal disease are not necessary for **moclobemide** (n = 12, open, Stoeckel et al, Acta Psychiatr Scand 1990;**360**[Suppl]:S94–S97), **mianserin** or **tryptophan**.

3.9.3 ANXIOLYTICS AND HYPNOTICS

17. Low dose anticonvulsant use of **benzo-diazepines** may be acceptable, as higher doses

produce an increase in CNS sedative side-effects. **Chlordiazepoxide** can be given in normal doses and is not affected by haemodialysis (review, Bennett et al, Am J Kidney Dis 1983;**3**:155). In severe renal failure, doses of **oxazepam** should be reduced to 75%. In end-stage renal failure and haemodialysis, **clobazam** and metabolite concentrations appear no different to those with normal renal function, so there may be no need to change doses in any degree of renal failure or in haemodialysis (n = 1, Roberts and Zoanetti, Ann Pharmacother 1994;**28**:966–7). Accumulation of metabolites of **midazolam** may be responsible for prolonged sedation, not reversible by flumazenil (n = 5, Bauer et al, Lancet 1995;**346**:145–7).

18. * **Buspirone** plasma levels have been shown to be higher in patients with renal failure, with a good correlation between steady-state levels and serum albumin (n = 54, open, Barbhaiya et al, Eur J Clin Pharmacol 1994;**46**:41–7). It is contraindicated in moderate or severe renal impairment. Reduce the dose of **hydroxyzine** by a half in renal impairment (UK SmPC).

19. Plasma protein-binding of **zolpidem** is reduced in renal failure (n = 54, open, Pacifici, Int J Clin Pharmacol Ther Toxicol 1988;**26**:439–43). The half-life may be doubled but no dosage adjustments are recommended in mild renal dysfunction. The pharmacokinetics of **zaleplon** and **zopiclone** are not significantly different in renal impairment, and dose alteration is not required.

20. In severe renal disease, plasma levels of **beta-blockers** may be higher and so starting doses should be lower. Beta-blockers may also reduce renal blood flow and adversely affect renal function.

21. Caution is needed with **clomethiazole** in chronic renal disease. **Chloral** is contraindicated in moderate to marked renal impairment. **Melatonin** has not been studied in renal impairment (SmPC), but 3 mg/d improves sleep-wake rhythm in people undergoing haemodialysis (c = 20, RCT, d/b, p/c, c/o, 3×6/52, Koch et al, Br J Clin Pharmacol 2009; **67**:68–75).

3.9.4 ANTICONVULSANTS

Review: optimising AEDs in renal dysfunction (Lalerda et al, Neurology 2006;**67**(12 Suppl 4): S28–33).

22. **Carbamazepine** rarely causes renal disturbances, although it has been suggested that doses should be reduced by 25% in severe renal failure. The UK SmPC has renal impairment as a precaution. For **oxcarbazepine** in renal impairment (Ccr < 30 ml/min), start at half the usual dose (300 mg/day), increasing no more frequently than at weekly intervals. In patients with pre-existing renal conditions associated with low sodium or in patients treated concomitantly with sodium-lowering drugs (e.g. diuretics, desmopressin) as well as NSAIDs, serum sodium levels should be monitored carefully.

23. **Valproate** is eliminated mainly through the kidneys and the literature states that it may be necessary to decrease dosage in renal insufficiency. There are two cases of valproate used successfully in renal failure of haemodialysis (n = 2, Gupta and Annadatha, Clin Pract Epidemol Ment Health 2008;**4**:21).

24. No specific dose adjustments are required for **phenytoin**, but protein-binding is altered in uraemia, which can be problematic in accurately assessing serum levels. Severe cardiovascular ADRs have been reported with **fosphenytoin** IV in renal impairment (see 3.2), and so a reducing loading dose and/or infusion rate by 10–25% is recommended.

25. **Phenobarbital** causes increased sedation and the dosage interval should be no more frequently than 12–16 hours in severe renal failure. Large doses of **primidone** should be avoided. Active metabolites of **amylobarbital** accumulate in severe renal disease.

26. * **Gabapentin** is mainly excreted unchanged in the urine and the UK SmPC now recommends dose reductions as follows:

Creatine clearance	Gabapentin dosage and frequency
≥80 ml/min	300–1200 mg TDS
50-79 ml/min	200–600 mg TDS
30–49 ml/min	100–300 mg BD
15–29 ml/min	300 mg on alternative days, up to 200 mg/d TDS
<15 ml/min	300 mg on alternative days, up to 100 mg/d TDS

Patients undergoing haemodialysis should

receive a gabapentin loading dose of 300–400 mg, plus 200–300 mg for every four hours of dialysis with no treatment on dialysis-free days (see SmPC for full details). Gabapentin toxicity in renal impairment is often unrecognised, leading to unnecessary morbidity (n = 729, Zand et al, Am J Med 2010;**123**:367–73). A reduced maintenance dose of **lamotrigine** is usually recommended in severe renal impairment, but the dose probably needs little adjustment in mild-to-moderate impairment (n = 21, Wootton et al, Br J Clin Pharmacol 1997;**43**:23–7), and even in end-stage renal failure, although the major glucuronide metabolite levels may increase eight-fold due to reduced renal clearance.

27. No dose adjustment is needed with **laco-samide** in mild-to-moderate renal impairment, but 250 mg/d is the maximum in severe renal impairment (SmPC) as the AUC is increased by about 30%. Supplements are needed in haemodialysis. Since 66% of a dose of **levetiracetam** is excreted unchanged in the urine, dose reductions are necessary in impaired renal function as follows (UK SmPC):

Renal function	Creatinine clearance	Levetiracetam maximum dose
Normal	80 ml/min	500–1500 mg BD
Mild	50–79 ml/min	500–1000 mg BD
Moderate	30–49 ml/min	250–750 mg BD
Severe	< 30 ml/min	250–500 mg BD
End-stage renal disease, undergoing dialysis	–	500–1000 mg OD

Following dialysis, a 250–500 mg supplemental dose is recommended.

Piracetam is excreted unchanged via the kidneys and dose adjustments may be needed in renal impairment (review: Tacconi and Wurtman, Adv Neurol 1986;**43**:675–85). **Pregabalin** is mainly excreted unchanged by the kidney, clearance being directly proportional to creatinine clearance (n = 50, Randinitis et al, J Clin Pharmacol 2003;**43**:277–83), so doses in renal impairment

must be individually calculated (see SmPC), as a few cases of reversible renal failure have been reported. Supplementary doses are necessary after every four-hour haemodialysis (SmPC). No dose adjustment is needed for **rufinamide** in people with severe renal impairment (UK SmPC) as it is almost entirely metabolised, but levels are reduced by about 30% by haemodialysis. There are no apparent problems with **tiagabine** (n = 25, Cato et al, Epilepsia 1998;**39**:43–7). About 60–70% of a **topiramate** dose is excreted unchanged via the kidneys. Time to steady state may be 10–15 days in severe renal impairment instead of 4–8 days with normal renal function. Dose titration may thus need to be more careful. Supplemental doses of 50% of the daily dose should be given on haemodialysis days. There is an increased risk of renal stone formation, via its carbonic anhydrase inhibition; carbonic anhydrase being a known inhibitor of renal crystallisation. Care is needed to ensure adequate fluid throughput, especially in patients with known disposition to this problem (Wasserstein et al, Epilepsia 1995;**36**[Suppl 3]: S153). **Vigabatrin** is renally excreted and so reduced doses are recommended with a Ccr < 60 mL/min. **Zonisamide** and metabolite are excreted renally and should not be used in acute renal failure or where serum creatinine is significantly raised. Zonisamide AUC is increased by 35% in people where Ccr < 20 ml/min. It may cause symptomatic renal calculus.

28. The UK SmPC for **ethosuximide** now requires use only with extreme caution in impaired renal function, and doses should be reduced by at least 25% in severe renal failure.

3.9.5 OTHERS

29. No change in dose is necessary with **donepezil** in mild-to-moderate renal impairment and a 5 mg single-dose study indicated that even moderate-to-severe renal impairment did not significantly alter donepezil kinetics (open, n = 22, Tiseo et al, Br J Clin Pharmacol 1998;**46**[Suppl 1]:S56–S60). There are no reported problems with **rivastigmine**. No dosage reduction of **galantamine** is necessary for creatinine clearance greater than 9 ml/min. In severe impairment (< 9 ml/min) galantamine is contraindicated (due to a lack of safety data). **Memantine** can be used in renal failure with no dosage adjustments, although

5 mg BD is recommended in severe renal failure (n = 32 [c = 31], Periclou *et al*, *Clin Pharmacol Ther* 2006;**79**:134–43).

30. The literature recommends some caution in renal disease with the **anticholinergics**. **Orphenadrine** is mainly excreted in the urine.

31. The SmPC for **disulfiram** recommends caution in renal disease. The UK SmPC contraindicates **acamprosate** in renal insufficiency (serum creatinine >120 micromol/L).

32. * **Lithium** is contraindicated in severe renal impairment. Progressive renal failure is much less common with the lower doses now used. The prevalence of chronic renal disease (plasma creatinine > 150 micromol/l) is about 1.2% with lithium, the main risk factor being duration of therapy (n = 3369, mean 10 years, Bendz *et al*, *Kidney Int* 2010;**77**:219–24). The main symptoms are polyuria and polydipsia (Le Roy *et al*, *Encephale* 2009;**35**:605–10), thus:

- avoid acute episodes of toxicity
- ensure regular plasma monitoring to get the optimum dose
- use a single daily dose at night.

A review of lithium and chronic kidney disease (Kripalani *et al*, *Br Med J* 2009;**339**:b2452) notes that the renal markers that should prompt nephrology advice and stopping lithium include:

- fall in GFR to below 45 ml/min/1.732 body surface, a rapidly falling rate or heavy proteinuria
- a steady or persistent fall in GFR (rather than a single measurement)

- stages 4 and 5 of chronic kidney disease.

ESDR (end stage renal disease) occurs in < 1% people taking lithium for more than 15 years, and classifies as being extremely rare (n = 114, mean 16 years, Tredget *et al*, *J Affect Disord* 2010; **126**:436–40). If use is unavoidable, use alternate-day dosing, very low doses (25–75% normal), and frequently estimate levels (e.g. 125 mg on alternate days, n = 1, Gash *et al*, *J Affect Disord* 1995;**34**:51–3; use in chronic renal failure n = 1, Belgamwar *et al*, *Gen Hosp Psychiatry* 2010;**32**:341.e3–5) and with haemodialysis in end-stage renal disease (n = 1, Knebel *et al*, *Am J Psychiatry* 2010;**167**:1409–10).

Review: lithium nephrotoxicity (Grünfeld and Rossier, *Nat Rev Nephrology* 2009;**5**:270–6).

33. The maximum **modafinil** dose of 400 mg/d should only be used in the absence of renal impairment. **Sodium oxybate** contains a significant dose of sodium (0.75 g in 4.5 g dose) and so dietary restriction of sodium might be considered, but since the kidney is not involved in excretion no dose reduction is thought to be necessary (SmPC).

34. **Bupropion** and metabolites are almost exclusively (85%) excreted through the kidneys and so, in renal failure, the initial dose should be reduced and close monitoring for toxicity carried out.

35. For **atomoxetine**, 80% of a dose is excreted in urine and the UK SmPC recommends possible dose reduction in renal impairment. The SmPCs for **methylphenidate** note that there is no experience of use in renal failure.

3

3.10 SLEEP APNEA (APNOEA)

	LOWER RISK (BUT SEE TEXT)	MODERATE RISK (BUT SEE TEXT)	HIGH RISK
Antipsychotics	All others[1]	Aripiprazole[2] Clozapine[2] Olanzapine[2] Quetiapine[2]	
Antidepressants		Most antidepressants[3] Mirtazapine[4]	
Anxiolytics and hynpotics	All[6], including benzo-diazepines[5]	Midazolam[5]	
Anticonvulsants	All others[7]	Vigabatrin[8]	
Others	All others[11]	Anticholinesterases[9] Lithium[10]	

Sleep apnea (SA) can have several forms, of which obstructive sleep apnea (OSA) is predominant (75% cases). It is defined as periods of stopping breathing while asleep, clinically significant if lasting for more than 10 seconds and more than 10 times an hour. Symptoms include loud snoring, daytime sleepiness, irritability, changes in mood or behaviour (n = 79, Peng et al, Chin Med Sci J 2004;**19**:262–5), unexplained fatigue and tiredness (n = 64, Jackson et al, Sleep Breath 2010; in press), anxiety and depression (n = 1408, Peppard et al, Arch Intern Med 2006;**166**:1709–15; 0.8% population have both, with a 20% comorbidity, Schröder and O'Hara, Ann Gen Psychiatry 2005;**4**:13). It naturally occurs in about 4% men and 2% women, and is associated with being overweight, smoking, age and having type 2 diabetes (n = 90, Lecube et al, PLoS One 2009;**4**:e4692). OSA is more common (10%) in psychiatric outpatients than the general population (3%) (n = 330, Nasr et al, Ann Clin Psychiatry 2010;**22**:29–32), especially in people with depression (22%), anxiety (17%), PTSD (12%) psychosis (5%) and bipolar (3.3%) (n = 4,060,504, Sharafkhaneh et al, Sleep 2005;**28**:1405–11).

First-line treatment of OSA is continuous positive airway pressure (CPAP). Severity is measured using the Respiratory Disturbance Index (RDI) or the apnea-hypopnea index (AHI; higher score is worse).

Treating OSA with CPAP has resulted in remission of psychosis (n = 1, Karanti and Landén, Psychopharmacol Bull 2007;**40**:113–7), TRS (n = 1, Boufidis et al, Int J Psychiatry Med 2003;**33**:305–10), depression (n = 50, Schwartz et al, Chest 2005;**128**:1304–9), suicidal ideation (n = 1, Krahn et al, J Clin Sleep Med 2008;**4**:64–5), and tonsillectomy has resolved recurrent psychosis (n = 1, Lee et al, Aust N Z J Psychiatry 1989;**23**:571–3). However, CPAP is not risk-free, as psychotic mania (n = 1, Lahera Forteza and González Aguado, Actas Esp Psiquiatr 2007;**35**:406–7; n = 1, Bergé et al, Psychosomatics 2008;**49**:447–9; n = 1, Trakada et al, Psychopharmacol Bull 2008;**41**:89–92), and psychosis (n = 1, Chiner et al, Eur Respir J 2001;**17**:313–5) have been reported.

If OSA is being properly managed with CPAP (or BiPAP as an alternative), then prescribing any drug should have no more problems than in a person without OSA. However, as not everyone can tolerate CPAP, the potential effects on respiration or sleep architecture need to be considered.

Reviews: sleep disturbances in depression (Neylan, J Clin Psychiatry 1995;**56**(Suppl 2):56–61), general (Madani and Madani, Oral Maxillofac Surg Clin North Am 2009;**21**:369–75).

3.10.1 ANTIPSYCHOTICS *

Obesity, male gender and chronic antipsychotics appear to be risk factors for OSA and so overweight patients should be evaluated for OSA (n = 364, Winkelman, J Clin Psychiatry

2001;**62**:8–11). Logically, antipsychotics causing sedation and weight gain can exacerbate or precipitate OSA (Wirshing et al, J Clin Psychiatry 2002;**63**:369–70). SGAs have been associated with a greater risk of severe OSA (n = 68, Rishi et al, Clin Neuropharmacol 2010;**33**:109–13). ECT is a viable alternative for mania (n = 1, Bastiampillai et al, J ECT 2011;**27**:15–6).

1. There is no information on **risperidone, paliperidone, zuclopenthixol, flupentixol, sulpiride, amisulpride, phenothiazines** or **pimozide**. There is a case of 10 mg/d **haloperidol** having no adverse effect on OSA (n = 1, Sobel et al, Am J Psychiatry 1985;**142**:775–6).

2. There is a case of OSA caused by **aripiprazole** in a man with psychotic depression (n = 1, Kohen and Sarcevic, Am J Ther 2009;**16**:197–8). There are cases of severe exacerbation of OSA in obese patients treated with **quetiapine**, one in combination with previously tolerated lorazepam, and so use should only be with full monitoring (n = 2, Freudenmann et al, Pharmacopsychiatry 2008;**41**:119–21). There is no information on **olanzapine** nor **clozapine**, although weight gain would be detrimental.

3.10.2 ANTIDEPRESSANTS *

Depression can be a symptom of OSA and standard antidepressants can exacerbate the symptoms. The diagnosis of OSA is more common when antidepressants and antihypertensives are co-prescribed (n = 212,972, Farney et al, Chest 2004;**125**:1279–85). Many people with residual depressive symptoms may have OSA and treatment with CPAP may improve these residual symptoms, probably due to improvement in daytime sleepiness (n = 17, Habukawa et al, Sleep Med 2010;**11**:552–7). People with OSA and daytime sleepiness are more likely to have depression (n = 53, Ishman et al, Laryngoscope 2010;**120**:2331–5).

3. **SSRIs** disrupt sleep architecture so are best avoided if possible or short-acting SSRIs used as morning doses. Intuitively avoiding **fluoxetine** with its long half-life would be appropriate. There are, however, some suggestions that boosting serotonin with SSRIs can have modest benefits on OSA during non-REM sleep, and a trial showed fluoxetine plus ondansetron to be well-tolerated and improved AHI compared

to placebo (n = 35, RCT, p/c, 4/52, Prasad et al, Sleep 2010;**33**:982–9). **Paroxetine** 20 mg/d seems to reduce apnea or improve breathing in non-REM sleep but not during REM sleep (n = 20[c = 17], RCT, d/b, p/c, 16/52, Kraiczi et al, Sleep 1999;**22**:61–7). For **tricyclics**, abrupt **amitriptyline** withdrawal has precipitated OSA, probably due to cholinergic rebound, which may be detrimental to OSA (n = 1, Musa, J Clin Pharmacol 1988;**28**:1038–9). A case series suggested that **imipramine** 25–50 mg/d may improve OSA, especially COSA (n = 31, Rubin et al, Eur Neurol 1986;**25**:81–5). **Trazodone** has increased arousal threshold in OSA, allowing higher CO2 levels to be tolerated (n = 9, RCT, p/c, d/b, c/o, 2/7, Heinzer et al, Eur Respir J 2008;**31**:1308–12). There is no information on **reboxetine, venlafaxine, duloxetine, MAOIs, moclobemide, mianserin** or **tryptophan**. There is no information on **agomelatine** but it does not cause drowsiness and improves sleep architecture so would seem a potentially good option.

4. A small but careful study showed that 4.5–15 mg/d **mirtazapine** reduces AHI scores by a half in adults with OSA, but did not recommend it as a treatment for OSA as such (n = 12, RCT, d/b, p/c, c/o, 3/52, Carley et al, Sleep 2007;**30**:35–41). In non-depressed stroke patients who refused CPAP, mirtazapine has had a mixed effect, improving RDI in six but deteriorating it in four, so monitor carefully (n = 10, 9/52, Brunner, Sleep Breath 2008; **12**:281–5). However, two studies with different designs failed to show an improvement in OSA with mirtazapine 7.5–45 mg/d, but caused excessive sedation and weight gain which may worsen OSA (s = 2, n = 64[c = 46], RCT, d/b, p/c, Marshall et al, Sleep 2008;**31**:824–31).

3.10.3 ANXIOLYTICS AND HYPNOTICS *

Insomnia and OSA frequently co-occur. 39–58% of people with OSA also have insomnia and 29–67% people with insomnia also have OSA (s = 12, Luyster et al, J Clin Sleep Med 2010;**6**:196–204) and so it is essential to ensure when treating insomnia that OSA has been excluded as a cause (e.g. n = 90, Sivertsen et al, J Clin Sleep Med 2009;**5**:349–54).

Review: comorbid insomnia and OSA inc

3

differential diagnosis (Luyster et al, J Clin Sleep Med 2010;**6**:196–204).

5. **Benzodiazepines**: these are associated with sleep breathing disorders and so intuitively probably will not help. **Flumazenil** has no effect, either positive or negative (n = 10, RCT, s/b, p/c, c/o, Schönhofer and Köhler, Eur Respir J 1996;**9**:1816–20). **Temazepam** 15–30 mg/d may cause no change in RDI in mild apnoea (n = 15, RCT, p/c, Camacho and Morin, Sleep 1995;**18**:644–5). **Nitrazepam** 5–10 mg/d had no significant effect in mild-to-moderate OSA (n = 14 [c = 11], RCT, d/b, p/c, 3/52, Höijer et al, Eur Respir J 1994;**7**:2011–5). **Midazolam** 15 mg orally has caused rapid and life-threatening sedation and apnea in someone with OSA (n = 1, Bezel et al, Schweiz Med Wochenschr 1987;**117**:579–83) and there is a case of OSA induced by **clonazepam** (n = 1, Schuld et al, J Sleep Res 1999;**8**:321–2). In patients with treated arterial hypertension and obesity (BMI > 25), BDZ use was not associated with an increase in apnea indices (n = 30, Nunes et al, Int J Cardiol 2007;**114**:416–8).

6. OSA is a whole night problem and so very short-acting hypnotics such as **zolpidem** would probably be preferred, e.g. zolpidem 10 mg at night had no effect on API, nor did it impair the efficacy of CPAP in severe OSA (n = 16, RCT, d/b, p/c, c/o, 3/52, Berry and Patel, Sleep 2006;**29**:1052–6) but improved sleep continuity (n = 20, open, 9/52, Quadri et al, J Clin Sleep Med 2009;**5**:122–9) possibly because of its short duration of effect. **Zaleplon** may be an alternative (Coyle et al, J Clin Sleep Med 2005;**1**:97). In one study, 41% of chronic **zopiclone** users had OSA as the probable underlying cause (n = 90, Sivertsen et al, J Clin Sleep Med 2009;**5**:349–54). There is no information on **buspirone**, but no problem would be expected. **Beta-blockers** have no consistent associations with changes in sleep architecture in untreated OSA (n = 1779, Smith et al, J Clin Sleep Med 2006;**2**:156–62). There is no information on **clomethiazole**. **Melatonin** has no relevant adverse effects, nor acts by causing sedation and so might be a good choice.

3.10.4 ANTICONVULSANTS *

There is little published on AEDs and OSA, but comorbidity may occur in 10% adult epileptics, 20% children with epilepsy and in 30% with drug-resistant epilepsy (Manni and Terzaghi, Epilepsy Res 2010;**90**:171–7). There is a case of carbamazepine and tiapride being successfully used for AWS in someone with OSA (n = 1, Gartenmaier et al, Pharmacopsychiatry 2005;**38**:96–8).

7. There is no information on **carbamazepine, valproate, phenytoin, gabapentin, lamotrigine, ethosuximide, lacosamide, levetiracetam, piracetam, pregabalin, tiagabine** or **zonisamide**. **Topiramate** initiation in bipolar disorder has led to marked improvement in OSA (n = 1, Weber, Am J Psychiatry 2002;**159**:872–3). In hypersomnia, **phenobarbital** withdrawal has improved alertness but unmasked OSA (n = 1, Takhar and Bishop, J Psychiatry Neurosci 2000; **25**:321–4).

8. Rapid weight gain from **vigabatrin** has precipitated OSA (n = 1, Lambert and Bird, Seizure 1997;**6**:233–5).

3.10.5 OTHERS *

9. **Anticholinesterases**: there is a strong association between severe OSA and severe dementia (n = 235, Ancoli-Israel et al, J Am Geriatr Soc 1991;**39**:258–63), which may be as high as 43% (n = 61, Reynolds et al, J Clin Psychiatry 1985;**46**:257–61). It is not known if anticholinesterases have an effect but increased acetylcholine (see 11) might be detrimental.

10. There are possible cases with an association between OSA and **lithium** in treatment-resistant mania (n = 4, Strakowski et al, J Clin Psychiatry 1991;**52**:156–8).

11. Excess acetylcholine increases REM sleep, which may be detrimental to OSA (n = 1, Musa, J Clin Pharmacol 1988;**28**:1038–9), so **anticholinergics** might in theory not be detrimental. **Modafinil** seems safe in OSA as it can maintain the effects of CPAP if interrupted (n = 21, RCT, d/b, c/o, Williams et al, Am J Respir Crit Care Med 2010;**181**:825–31). When used for excessive sleepiness, it can lead to improvements in daytime functioning in OSA (s = 2, n = 480, RCT, p/c, Weaver et al, J Clin Sleep Med 2009;**5**:499–505). **Sodium oxybate** 4.5 g at night has significantly reduced AHI (n = 48, p/c, 3/52, George et al, Sleep Breath 2010; in press) and 9 g at night had no detrimental effect in mild-to-moderate OSA, but should still be used with caution (n = 60 [c = 42], RCT, d/b, c/o, p/c, George et al, Sleep Med 2010;**11**:38–42). There is no information on **disulfiram, acamprosate, bupropion, atomoxetine** or **methylphenidate**.

4 DRUG INTERACTIONS

Absolute classification of interactions is impossible. Many factors, e.g. age, concurrent illness, P450 status, etc are important. Single case reports merely suggest a possible interaction. To give some guidance, interactions with the drugs in **CAPITAL LETTERS** are those that could be:

- potentially hazardous
- where dosage adjustment may be needed
- well-established and documented
- rare but important.

How to use this section:

1. Look up the psychiatric drug or group.
2. Look up the group of the interacting drug.
3. If no entry there, look up the actual drug.
4. If still no entry, little has been reported

4.1 ANXIOLYTICS AND HYPNOTICS

Reviews: clinically important drug interactions with zopiclone, zaleplon and zolpidem (Hesse et al, CNS Drugs 2003;**17**:513–32), pharmacokinetics and pharmacodynamics (Drover, Clin Pharmaco-kinet 2004;**43**:227–38).

4.1.1 BENZODIAZEPINES

Benzodiazepines are mainly metabolised by CYP2C19 and CYP3A3/4.
Review: Herbal medication interactions with midazolam (Tweddell and Boyle, Dent Update 2009;**36**:175–8)
Acamprosate + benzodiazepines
See acamprosate (4.6.1).
Agomelatine + benzodiazepines
See agomelatine (4.3.3.1).
ALCOHOL + BENZODIAZEPINES
See alcohol (4.7.1).
Alosetron + alprazolam
Alosetron, a 5–HT3 receptor antagonist, has no effect on the kinetics of alprazolam (n = 12, RCT, open, D'Souza et al, J Clin Pharmacol 2001; **41**:452–4).
Amfetamines + benzodiazepines
Amfetamine significantly reverses the sedative and memory-impairing effects of triazolam (n = 20, p/c, d/b, c/o, Mintzer and Griffiths, J Psychopharmacol 2003;**17**:17–29, 146).
Amiodarone + clonazepam
Amidarone has been reported to cause clonazepam toxicity at low dose (n = 1, Witt et al, Ann Pharmacother 1993;**27**:1463–4).

Antacids + benzodiazepines
Benzodiazepine absorption is slightly delayed by antacids, but total absorption remains the same.
Anticholinergics + benzodiazepines
Benzodiazepine absorption may be delayed by anticholinergics, but the AUC remains unchanged.
Anticoagulants + benzodiazepines
Lack of an interaction has been demonstrated and benzodiazepines. Isolated cases of adverse reactions have been reported, e.g. no interaction has been reported with warfarin but is theoretically possible (mentioned in Sayal et al, Acta Psychiatr Scand 2000;**102**:250–5).
Antihistamines + benzodiazepines
Enhanced sedation is possible.
Antihypertensives + benzodiazepines
Enhanced hypotension is possible.
Antipsychotics + benzodiazepines
See individual drugs and antipsychotics (4.2.1).
Antiretrovirals + benzodiazepines
Maraviroc levels have not been measured, but although midazolam levels change slightly no significant interaction is expected.
Atomoxetine + benzodiazepines
See atomoxetine (4.6.4).
Atropine + benzodiazepines
No interaction is thought to occur.
Baclofen + benzodiazepines
Enhanced sedation can occur.
Barbiturates + benzodiazepines
Enhanced sedation and increased benzodiazepine clearance may occur via CYP3A4 induction. Dose adjustment may be necessary.
Beta-blockers + benzodiazepines
Propranolol and metoprolol produce a small but significant reduction in diazepam clearance. Propranolol and labetolol have no effect on oxazepam (n = 6, Sonne et al, Br J Clin Pharmacol 1990;**29**:33–7) and metoprolol has no effect on lorazepam (n = 12, open, Scott et al, Eur J Clin Pharmacol 1991;**40**:405–9).
Buprenorphine + benzodiazepines
Buprenorphine does not inhibit the metabolism of flunitrazepam and so any interaction is likely to be pharmacodynamic rather than metabolic, although deaths have been reported with con-comitant buprenorphine and benzodiazepines (n = 6, Reynaud et al, Addiction 1998;**93**:1385–92).
Buspirone + benzodiazepines
See buspirone (4.1.2).

CALCIUM-CHANNEL BLOCKERS + BENZODIAZEPINES *

Diltiazem significantly increases diazepam levels, probably via CYP3A4 inhibition (n = 13, RCT, d/b, c/o, Kosuge et al, Drug Metab Dispos 2001;**29**:1284–9, UK SmPC 2010). Both diltiazem and verapamil significantly raise midazolam levels and half-life, via 3A4 inhibition, increasing sedative side-effects, and a 50% midazolam dose reduction has been recommended (n = 9, RCT, d/b, c/o, 2/7, Backman et al, Br J Clin Pharmacol 1994;**37**:221–5).

Cannabis + benzodiazepines

See cannabis (4.7.2).

Carbamazepine + benzodiazepines

See carbamazepine (4.5.1).

Charcoal, activated + benzodiazepines

25 g of activated charcoal given 30 minutes after diazepam 5 mg reduces diazepam AUC by 27%, but not the peak levels. Concurrent gastric lavage does not provide any additional reductions (n = 9, RCT, Lapatto-Reiniluoto et al, Br J Clin Pharmacol 1999;**48**:148–53).

Citalopram + benzodiazepines

See citalopram/escitalopram (4.3.2.1).

Clarithromycin + benzodiazepines

Higher dose clarithromycin (2.5 g/d) may increase the availability of midazolam, probably via CYP3A4 inhibition (n = 16, open, 8/7, Gorski et al, Clin Pharmacol Ther 1998;**64**:133–43).

CLOZAPINE + BENZODIAZEPINES

See clozapine (4.2.4).

Cyclophosphamide + benzodiazepines

Cyclophosphamide toxicity has been suggested in animals but not reported in humans.

Dehydroepiandrosterone + benzodiazepines

Alprazolam rapidly and significantly increases dehydroepiandrosterone levels (n = 38, Kroboth et al, J Clin Psychopharmacol 1999;**19**:114–24).

Dextropropoxyphene + alprazolam

Increased sedation can occur with alprazolam.

Digoxin + benzodiazepines

Lack of interaction has been shown.

Disulfiram + benzodiazepines

See disulfiram (4.6.8).

Escitalopram + benzodiazepines

See citalopram/escitalopram (4.3.2.1).

Ethambutol + diazepam

Lack of interaction has been shown.

Fluoxetine + benzodiazepines

See fluoxetine (4.3.2.2).

Fluvoxamine + benzodiazepines

See fluvoxamine (4.3.2.3).

Food + benzodiazepines

Food delays the absorption of benzodiazepines; only significant if rapid onset of action is needed.

Gabapentin + benzodiazepines

See gabapentin (4.5.3).

Gingko biloba + benzodiazepines *

GB may inhibit CYP3A4 and increase midazolam's AUC by 25–30%, possibly significantly (n = 14, 2/52, Robertson et al, Curr Med Res Opin 2008;**24**:591–9), but there appears to be no interaction with diazepam in healthy Chinese subjects (n = 12, Zuo et al, Eur J Clin Pharmacol 2010;**66**:503–9).

Grapefruit juice + benzodiazepines

200ml normal-strength grapefruit juice increases plasma triazolam levels, and repeated consumption produces a greater increase (n = 12, RCT, Lilja et al, Eur J Clin Pharmacol 2000;**56**:411–5).

H2-blockers + benzodiazepines

Cimetidine inhibits the CYP3A4 metabolism of long-acting benzodiazepines, but not lorazepam, oxazepam and temazepam. The effect is probably negligible. Ranitidine may slightly reduce the absorption of diazepam, probably clinically insignificantly (n = 30, RCT, open, 3/7, O'Connor-Semmes et al, Clin Pharmacol Ther 2001;**70**:126–31).

Heparin + benzodiazepines

A transient rise in benzodiazepine levels could occur (n = 14, open, Desmond et al, Br J Clin Pharmacol 1980;**9**:171–5).

Indometacin + diazepam

Increased dizziness may occur (d/b, Nuotto and Saariolho, Pharmacol Toxicol 1988;**62**:293–7).

Isoniazid + benzodiazepines

Isoniazid reduces the clearance of diazepam but not of oxazepam (n = 9, Ochs et al, Clin Pharmacol Ther 1981;**29**:671–8).

Itraconazole/ketoconazole/posaconazole + benzodiazepines

Increased chlordiazepoxide oral bioavailability and midazolam AUC can occur, up to eight-fold higher (e.g. n = 10, RCT, 12/7, Lam et al, J Clin Pharmacol 2003;**43**:1274–82). Midazolam levels were significantly higher with itraconazole 200mg/d for four days, the effect being detectable up to four days after cessation of treatment (n = 9, open, Backman et al, Eur J Clin Pharmacol 1998;**54**:53–8). Posaconazole is a

4

less potent inhibitor of 3A4 than ketoconazole but can cause an up to 2.4-fold increase in midazolam levels (n = 12, open, Krishna *et al*, *Clin Ther* 2009;**31**:286–98).

Lamotrigine + benzodiazepines
See lamotrigine (*4.5.5*).

LEVODOPA + BENZODIAZEPINES
Levodopa can be antagonised by diazepam, nitrazepam and chlordiazepoxide (Yousselson *et al*, *Ann Intern Med* 1982;**96**:259–60): observe for worsening of symptoms.

Lithium + benzodiazepines
See lithium (*4.4*).

MAOIs + benzodiazepines
See MAOIs (*4.3.4*).

Melatonin + benzodiazepines
See melatonin (*4.1.4*).

Methadone + benzodiazepines
See methadone (*4.6.10*).

Metronidazole + benzodiazepines
Lack of interaction has been reported.

Mianserin + benzodiazepines
See mianserin (*4.3.3.3*).

Mirtazapine + benzodiazepines
See mirtazapine (*4.3.3.4*).

Moclobemide + benzodiazepines
See moclobemide (*4.3.3.5*).

Modafinil + benzodiazepines
See modafinil (*4.6.12*).

Muscle relaxants + benzodiazepines
Variable relatively minor effects have been reported (n = 113, Driessen *et al*, *Acta Anaesthesiol Scand* 1986;**30**:642–6). Diazepam may hasten the onset and prolong the duration of action of vecuronium (n = 20, RCT, Yuan *et al*, *Chung Hua I Hsueh Tsa Chih (Taipei)* 1994;**54**:259–64), but midazolam appears not to do this (n = 10, Husby *et al*, *Acta Anaesthesiol Scand* 1989;**33**:280–2).

Nimodipine + benzodiazepines
Lack of a clinically significant interaction during chronic oral administration has been reported (n = 24, RCT, c/o, 3×5/7, Heine *et al*, *Br J Clin Pharmacol* 1994;**38**:39–43).

Olanzapine + benzodiazepines
See olanzapine (*4.2.4*).

Ondansetron + benzodiazepines
Lack of interaction has been shown with temazepam (n = 24, RCT, d/b, c/o, 2/7, Preston *et al*, *Anesthesia* 1996;**51**:827–30).

Opioids + benzodiazepines

Synergism (e.g. n = 95, RCT, d/b, Kissin *et al*, *Anesth Analg* 1990;**71**:65–9) and changes in haemodynamic status have been reported, as has a fatal interaction with clonazepam and oxycodone, although the mechanism is unclear (n = 1, Burrows *et al*, *J Forensic Sci* 2003; **48**:683–6).

Oral contraceptives + benzodiazepines
OCs may increase the effects of longer-acting benzodiazepines, probably of minimal significance.

Paraldehyde + benzodiazepines
Enhanced sedation would be expected.

Paroxetine + benzodiazepines
See paroxetine (*4.3.2.4*).

Passiflora incarnata + benzodiazepines
See valerian + benzodiazepines.

Phenytoin + benzodiazepines
See phenytoin (*4.5.9*).

Physostigmine + benzodiazepines
Physostigmine may reverse diazepam-induced sleep (Speeg *et al*, *J Neurochem* 1980;**34**:856–5) and midazolam-induced somnolence (Ho *et al*, *Ma Tsui Hsueh Tsa Chi* 1991;**29**:643–7).

Pregabalin + benzodiazepines
See pregabalin (*4.5.11*).

Probenecid + lorazepam
Administration of probenecid with lorazepam can lead to a more rapid onset and prolonged effect and so lorazepam doses should be reduced by 50% (SmPC 2009).

Progabide + clonazepam
Lack of interaction has been reported.

Propofol + benzodiazepines
Propofol increases the half-life of midazolam by 61%, probably by inhibiting CYP3A4 (n = 24, RCT, Hamaoka *et al*, *Clin Pharmacol Ther* 1999;**66**:110–7).

Proton–pump inhibitors + benzodiazepines
Omeprazole and esomeprazole (review: Steinijans *et al*, *Int J Clin Pharmacol Ther* 1996; **34**:S31–S50), can reduce diazepam clearance by up to 50% (n = 12, 1/52, Andersson *et al*, *Eur J Clin Pharmacol* 1990;**39**:51–4), AUC (28%), Cmax (31%) and half-life (41%) probably by 3A4 inhibition, whereas pantoprazole does not and is a safer alternative (n = 24, RCT, d/b, c/o, Drewelow *et al*, *Arzneimittelforschung* 2010;**60**:483–91).

Quetiapine + benzodiazepines
See quetiapine (*4.2.6*).

Reboxetine + benzodiazepines
See reboxetine (*4.3.3.6*).

Rifampicin + benzodiazepines

CYP3A4 induction by rifampicin can lead to reduced diazepam (n=21, 7/7, Ohnhaus, *Clin Pharmacol Ther* 1987;**42**:148) and midazolam levels (n=9, 9/7, Backman *et al, Eur J Clin Pharmacol* 1998;**54**:53–8).

Ritonavir + benzodiazepines

The UK SmPC now contraindicates ritonavir with clorazepate, diazepam, estazolam, flurazepam, oral (parenteral is just a warning) midazolam and triazolam due to the risk of extreme sedation and respiratory depression.

Rivastigmine + benzodiazepines

See rivastigmine (*4.6.3.3*).

Rufinamide + benzodiazepines

See rufinamide (*4.5.12*).

Selegiline + benzodiazepines

Selegiline transdermal system (STS) had no effects on the pharmacokinetics of alprazolam (open, RCT, c/o, Azzaro *et al, J Clin Pharmacol* 2007;**47**:146–58).

Sertindole + benzodiazepines *

See sertindole (*4.2.8*).

Sertraline + benzodiazepines

See sertraline (*4.3.2.5*).

Smoking + benzodiazepines

See smoking (*4.7.4*).

Sodium oxybate + benzodiazepines

See sodium oxybate (*4.6.13*).

St John's wort + benzodiazepines

See St John's wort (*4.3.3.10*).

Tiagabine + benzodiazepines

See tiagabine (*4.5.13*).

Tricyclics + benzodiazepines

Enhanced sedation has been reported and would be expected. Reduced hydroxylation of clomipramine has been reported and dose reduction may be necessary (*Pharmaceutisch Weekblad* 1992;**14**[4] Suppl D:D3).

Valerian + benzodiazepines

Tremor, dizziness and fatigue have been reported in someone on lorazepam after taking valerian officinalis and Passiflora incarnate (n=1, Carrasco *et al, Phytother Res* 2009;**23**:1795–6).

Valproate + benzodiazepines *

Valproate displaces diazepam from plasma protein-binding sites and so doses may need to be reduced. Valproate increases lorazepam levels by up to 20–40% (SmPC change 2009) via reduced lorazepam clearance (n=1, Lee *et al, Seizure* 2002;**11**:124–5) and coma has been reported. Valproate increases clonazepam clearance by 14% and reduces valproate clearance by 18% (n=317, Yukawa *et al, J Clin Pharm Ther* 2003;**28**:497–504), probably of minimal significance (n=4, Wang and Wang, *Ther Drug Monit* 2002;**24**:532–6).

Venlafaxine + benzodiazepines

See venlafaxine (*4.3.3.9*).

Xanthines + benzodiazepines

Xanthines, e.g. theophylline, aminophylline and caffeine antagonise the sedative (and possibly anxiolytic) effects of benzodiazepines (e.g. midazolam 12mg is moderately antagonised by 250mg caffeine, n=114, Mattila *et al, Int J Clin Pharmacol Ther* 2000;**38**:581–7). This can be useful in the treatment of benzodiazepine overdose, but care must be taken if a patient on a benzodiazepine has theophylline stopped, as respiratory depression could then occur.

Ziprasidone + benzodiazepines

See ziprasidone (*4.2.9*).

4.1.2 BUSPIRONE

Buspirone is metabolised by CYP3A4 and has an active metabolite 6-hydroxybuspirone (n=13, Dockens *et al, J Clin Pharmacol* 2006;**46**:1308–12).

Alcohol + buspirone

See alcohol (*4.7.1*).

Benzodiazepines + buspirone

Two studies with diazepam have shown only a minimal enhanced sedation. Alprazolam appears not to interact with buspirone (n=24, 7/7, Buch *et al, J Clin Pharmacol* 1993;**33**:1104–9).

Beta-blockers + buspirone

Buspirone appears not to displace propranolol from plasma-binding sites (review: Gammans *et al, Am J Med* 1986;**80**[Suppl 3B]:41–51).

Calcium–channel blockers + buspirone

Verapamil and diltiazem increase buspirone plasma concentrations three-fold and five-fold respectively, probably by CYP3A4 inhibition, potentially enhancing the side-effects of buspirone (n=9, RCT, p/c, c/o, Lamberg *et al, Clin Pharmacol Ther* 1998;**63**:640–5).

Cimetidine + buspirone

Lack of interaction has been reported (n=10, open, Gammans *et al, Pharmacotherapy* 1987; **7**:72–9).

Citalopram + buspirone

See citalopram/escitalopram (*4.3.2.1*).

4

Clozapine + buspirone

Near fatal gastrointestinal bleeding and hyperglycaemia occurring one month after buspirone was added to a stable clozapine regimen has been reported, but no firm explanation found (n = 1, Good, *Am J Psychiatry* 1997;**154**:1473).

Erythromycin + buspirone

Erythromycin and itraconazole may increase plasma buspirone levels dramatically, probably via CYP3A4 inhibition, with increased side-effects noted (n = 8, Kivisto *et al*, *Clin Pharmacol Ther* 1997;**62**:348–54).

Escitalopram + buspirone

See citalopram/escitalopram (*4.3.2.1*).

Fluoxetine + buspirone

Reduced anxiolytic effect, dystonia, akathisia (e.g. n = 1, Metz, *Can J Psychiatry* 1990;**35**:722–3) have been reported.

Fluvoxamine + buspirone

Fluvoxamine 100 mg/d raises buspirone levels, probably via CYP3A4 inhibition, but this is of limited significance (n = 10, RCT, Lamberg *et al*, *Eur J Clin Pharmacol* 1998;**54**:761–6).

Grapefruit juice + buspirone

200 ml double-strength grapefruit juice raised peak buspirone plasma levels four-fold, probably via CYP3A4 inhibition or delayed gastric emptying, so avoid buspirone and, at least, large amounts of grapefruit juice, or adjust doses (n = 10, RCT, Lilja *et al*, *Clin Pharmacol Ther* 1998;**64**:655–60).

Itraconazole + buspirone

See erythromycin + buspirone (above).

MAOIs + BUSPIRONE

See MAOIs (*4.3.4*).

NSAIDs + buspirone

GI side-effects and headache may be slightly more common with the combination (n = 150, Kiev and Domantay, *Curr Ther Res* 1989;**46**:1086–90).

Phenytoin + buspirone

Buspirone does not appear to displace phenytoin from plasma-binding sites (review: Gammans *et al*, *Am J Med* 1986;**80**[Suppl 3B]:41–51).

Rifampicin + buspirone

The buspirone UK SmPC now states that rifampicin decreases buspirone plasma levels, probably via CYP3A4 induction. Significant changes in psychomotor tests have been noted and so dose adjustment may be necessary (n = 10, Lamberg *et al*, *Br J Clin Pharmacol* 1998; **45**:381–5).

Ritonavir + buspirone

Severe EPSE have appeared after ritonavir was added to buspirone (n = 1, Clay and Adams, *Ann Pharmacother* 2003;**37**:202–5).

St John's wort + buspirone

There is a possible case of serotonin syndrome (n = 1, Dannawi, *J Psychopharmacol* 2002; 16:401).

Terfenadine + buspirone

No interaction occurs (n = 10, RCT, p/c, c/o, 3/7, Lamberg *et al*, *Pharmacol Toxicol* 1999;**84**:165–9).

Trazodone + buspirone

There are some isolated reports of raised SGPT/ALT levels and a case of serotonin syndrome (n = 1, Goldberg and Huk, *Psychosomatics* 1992;**3**:235).

Warfarin + buspirone

Buspirone does not appear to displace warfarin from plasma-binding sites (review: Gammans *et al*, *Am J Med* 1986;**80**[Suppl 3B]:41–51).

Zidovidine + buspirone

The combination has been used safely (n = 2, Batki, *J Clin Psychopharmacol* 1990;**10**[Suppl 3]: 111S–5S).

4.1.3 CHLORAL HYDRATE

Chloral is probably metabolised by CYP2E1.

ALCOHOL + CHLORAL HYDRATE

See alcohol (*4.7.1*)

Fluvoxamine + chloral hydrate

See fluvoxamine (*4.3.2.3*).

Furosemide + chloral hydrate

Diaphoresis, facial flushing and agitation occurred with chloral hydrate and IV furosemide, which stopped when the chloral was discontinued (n = 1, Dean *et al*, *Clin Pharm* 1991;**10**:385–7).

MAOIs + chloral hydrate

See MAOIs (*4.3.4*).

Methadone + chloral hydrate

See methadone (*4.6.10*).

Phenytoin + chloral hydrate

See phenytoin (*4.5.9*).

Nicoumalone + chloral hydrate

An enhanced anticoagulant effect can occur. See also warfarin + chloral hydrate.

Warfarin + chloral hydrate

The anticoagulant effects of warfarin are increased slightly by chloral hydrate, probably by plasma protein displacement (BCDSP, *N Engl J Med* 1972;**286**:53–5). This can be important if chloral hydrate is given as a PRN hypnotic.

4.1.4 MELATONIN

Melatonin is metabolised by 1A2 and possibly 2C9/19 to a minor extent (Facciola et al, Eur J Clin Pharmacol 2001;**56**:881–8) and induces 3A4, possibly 2C19, but has no effect on 1A2.

Alcohol + melatonin
Alcohol reduces the effect of melatonin (SmPC).

Antipsychotics + melatonin
Muzzy-headedness has been reported with thioridazine and melatonin (SmPC).

Benzodiazepines + melatonin
Melatonin can enhance the sedative effects (SmPC).

Carbamazepine + melatonin
Carbamazepine may decrease melatonin levels (SmPC) via 1A2 induction.

Cimetidine + melatonin
Cimetidine may raise melatonin levels (SmPC).

Citalopram/escitalopram + melatonin
See citalopram/escitalopram (4.3.2.1).

Estrogens + melatonin
Estrogens (e.g. oral contraceptives or HRT) may increase melatonin levels (SmPC).

FLUVOXAMINE + MELATONIN
The UK SmPC states that fluvoxamine may raise melatonin levels, with AUC 17–fold higher and Cmax 12-fold higher (SmPC) (e.g. n = 5, open, Hartter et al, Clin Pharmacol Ther 2000;**67**:1–6), and so combining the treatments improved sleep (n = 1, Grozinger et al, Arch Gen Psychiatry 2000; **57**:812–3).

Methoxypsoralen + melatonin
Melatonin levels can be raised (SmPC).

Quinolones + melatonin
Quinolones may increase melatonin levels via 1A2 inhibition (SmPC).

Rifampicin + melatonin
Rifampicin may decrease melatonin levels (SmPC) via 1A2 induction.

Smoking + melatonin
Smoking may decrease melatonin levels (SmPC) via 1A2 induction.

Tricyclics + melatonin
Increased feelings of tranquillity have been reported with imipramine and melatonin (SmPC).

Zaleplon + melatonin
Melatonin can enhance the sedative effects of zaleplon (SmPC).

Zolpidem + melatonin
Melatonin can enhance the sedative effects of zolpidem (SmPC).

Zopiclone + melatonin
Melatonin can enhance the sedative effects of zopiclone (SmPC).

4.1.5 ZALEPLON

Zaleplon is primarily metabolised by aldehyde oxidase, and a small amount by CYP3A4 to inactive metabolites. As with other such drugs, use with other CNS-depressants needs care.

Alcohol + zaleplon
See alcohol (4.7.1).

Antipsychotics + zaleplon
Additive psychomotor effects may occur with thioridazine (n = 12, RCT, Hetta et al, Eur J Clin Pharmacol 2000;**56**:211–7).

Carbamazepine + zaleplon
Co-administration may reduce zaleplon's efficacy through CYP3A4 induction.

Cimetidine + zaleplon
Raised zaleplon levels can occur with cimetidine, via aldehyde oxidase and CYP3A4 inhibition.

Digoxin + zaleplon
Lack of interaction has been shown (n = 20, Sanchez-Garcia et al, Am J Health Syst Pharm 2000;**57**:2267–70).

Erythromycin + zaleplon
Raised zaleplon levels can occur, via 3A4 inhibition.

Ibuprofen + zaleplon
Lack of significant interaction has been shown (n = 17, open, Sanchez–Garcia et al, Am J Health Syst Pharm 2000;**57**:1137–41).

Ketoconazole + zaleplon
Raised zaleplon levels can occur, via 3A4 inhibition.

Melatonin + zaleplon
See melatonin (4.1.4).

Opioids + zaleplon
Enhanced euphoria is possible.

Phenobarbital + zaleplon
Reduced zaleplon levels can occur, via CYP3A4 induction.

Rifampicin + zaleplon
A four-fold reduction in zaleplon levels can occur, via CYP3A4 induction.

Warfarin + zaleplon
No interaction occurs.

4

4.1.6 ZOLPIDEM

Zolpidem is mainly metabolised by CYP3A4 and has no effect on 1A2, 2B6, 2C9, 2D6 and 3A4. Enhanced sedation would be expected with concurrent use with any CNS depressant.

Alcohol + zolpidem
See alcohol (4.7.1).

Antipsychotics + zolpidem
Excessive sedation has been reported with chlorpromazine (n = 6, d/b, single-dose, Desager et al, Psychopharmacol 1988;**96**:63–6).

Bupropion + zolpidem
See bupropion (4.6.6).

Caffeine + zolpidem *
While antagonism would be expected, 300 mg caffeine did not antagonise the sedative effects of zolpidem given during the day (n = 45+, d/b, p/c, Mattila et al, Eur J Clin Pharmacol 1998;**54**:421–5), and there are even cases of paradoxically enhanced sedation (discussion of possible mechanisms; Myslobodsky, Curr Drug Targets 2009;**10**:1009–20).

Clarithromycin + zolpidem
Clarithromycin has no effect on the kinetics or dynamics of zolpidem (n = 10, c/o, Farkas et al, Clin Pharmacol Ther 2009;**85**:644–50).

Food + zolpidem
The rate of absorption of zolpidem is slowed significantly by food.

H2-blockers + zolpidem
Lack of a significant interaction has been shown with cimetidine and ranitidine (n = 6, c/o, 18/7, Hulhoven et al, Int J Clin Pharmacol Res 1988;**8**:471–6).

Itraconazole/fluconazole/ketoconazole + zolpidem
Single doses of itraconazole or fluconazole slightly lengthen the half–life of zolpidem (n = 12, RCT, Greenblatt et al, Clin Pharmacol Ther 1998;**64**:661–71). However, itraconazole 200 mg/d for four days had no marked effect on the pharmacokinetics of zolpidem, although central effects were slightly increased (n = 10, Luurila et al, Eur J Clin Pharmacol 1998;**54**:163–6).

Melatonin + zolpidem
See melatonin (4.1.4).

Oral Contraceptives + zolpidem
Zolpidem clearance is slightly higher and half-life slightly shorter in women using OCs (n = 16, Olubodun et al, J Clin Pharmacol 2002;**42**:1142–6).

Rifampicin + zolpidem
Rifampicin significantly reduces zolpidem's plasma levels and therapeutic effect, via CYP3A4 induction (n = 8, RCT, Villikka et al, Br J Clin Pharmacol 1997;**43**:629–34).

Smoking + zolpidem
Zolpidem's half–life may be 30% shorter in smokers than non–smokers, of low clinical significance (due to CYP1A2 induction; n = 16, Olubodun et al, J Clin Pharmacol 2002; **42**:1142–6).

Sodium oxybate + zolpidem
See sodium oxybate (4.6.13).

SSRIs + zolpidem
SSRIs may enhance zolpidem-associated hallucinations (n = 5, Elko et al, J Toxicol Clin Toxicol 1998;**36**:195–203; n = 1 Coleman and Ota, J Forensic Sci 2004;**49**:392–3). One study showed a minimal pharmacokinetic interaction between **fluoxetine** and regular zolpidem in healthy women, with no significant psychomotor function changes, although zolpidem's half-life increased slightly (n = 29, 5/52, Allard et al, Drug Metab Dispos 1998;**26**:617–22). Visual hallucinations and amnesia triggered by **fluvoxamine** have been reported (n = 1, Kito and Koga, Int Psychogeriatr 2006;**18**:749–51). The combination with **sertraline** may lead to a shorter onset of action and an increased effect from zolpidem (n = 28, RCT, Allard et al, J Clin Pharmacol 1999;**39**;184–91).

St John's wort + zolpidem *
In most people SJW reduces zolpidem AUC and Cmax by 30% but can slightly increase it in a few (n = 3) people (n = 14, 14/7, Hojo et al, J Clin Pharm Ther 2011; in press).

Valproate + zolpidem
Somnambulism has been reported with the combination in a 47-year-old male (n = 1, Sattar et al, Ann Pharmacother 2003;**37**:1429–33).

4.1.7 ZOPICLONE

Zopiclone is mainly metabolised by CYP3A4 to active metabolites, with 2C8 a minor metaboliser. It is excreted via the urine (80%) and faeces (16%).

Alcohol + zopiclone
See alcohol (4.7.1).

Aspirin + zopiclone
Lack of interaction has been shown.

Caffeine + zopiclone

Caffeine moderately antagonises the psycho-motor impairment caused by zopiclone (d/b, Mattila et al, Pharmacol Toxicol 1992; **70**:286–9).

Erythromycin + zopiclone

Erythromycin accelerates zopiclone absorption, leading to a more rapid onset, which could be clinically significant in the elderly (n = 10, Aranko et al, Br J Clin Pharmacol 1994;**38**:363–7).

Itraconazole + zopiclone

Itraconazole significantly increased zopiclone plasma levels by 28% and half-life by 40%, but had no clinically significant effect (n = 10, d/b, p/c, c/o, Jalava et al, Eur J Clin Pharmacol 1996;**51**:331–4).

Melatonin + zopiclone

See melatonin (4.1.4).

Ranitidine + zopiclone

Lack of interaction has been shown.

Rifampicin + zopiclone

Rifampicin significantly reduces zopiclone plasma levels and therapeutic effect, via CYP3A4 induction (n = 8, RCT, Villikka et al, Br J Clin Pharmacol 1997;**43**:471–4).

Tricyclics + zopiclone

One study showed decreased levels of trimipramine and zopiclone, of minimal significance (n = 10, RCT, Caille et al, Biopharm Drug Dispos 1984;**5**:117–25).

4.2 ANTIPSYCHOTICS

Aripiprazole (4.2.2), asenapine (4.2.3) clozapine (4.2.4), olanzapine (4.2.5), quetiapine (4.2.6), risperidone/paliperidone (4.2.7), sertindole (4.2.8) and ziprasidone (4.2.9) also have their own sections

4.2.1 ANTIPSYCHOTICS — GENERAL *

There are few specific interactions reported for some antipsychotics, other than additive sedation. Phenothiazines have multiple metabolites and multiple metabolism, 1A2 seems the prominent enzyme (Wójcikowski et al, Biochem Pharmacol 2010;**80**:1252–9). Sulpiride has no significant effect on 1A2, 2C9, 2C19, 2D6 2E1 or 3A4 enzymes (Niwa et al, Biol Pharm Bull 2005;**28**:188–91). **Haloperidol** is metabolised by 3A4, 2D6 and by glucuronidation, and is susceptible to interaction with drugs affecting these enzymes. Use of haloperidol with other drugs known to prolong the QTc interval is not

recommended (UK SmPC, 2009), e.g:

- Class 1A (quinidine, disopyramide, procainamide)
- Class III (e.g. amiodarone, sotalol, dofetilide)
- Some antimicrobials (moxifloxacin, IV erythromycin)
- Tricyclics, other neuroleptics (e.g. pimozide, phenothiazines), bretylium, quinine, mefloquine.

ACE inhibitors + antipsychotics

An enhanced hypotensive effect with severe postural hypotension has been reported, e.g. captopril plus chlorpromazine (White, Arch Int Med 1986;**146**:1833–4).

Activated charcoal + phenothiazines

Decreased antipsychotic absorption is likely.

ALCOHOL + ANTIPSYCHOTICS

See alcohol (4.7.1).

Amfetamines + antipsychotics

The antipsychotic effects of phenothiazines can be antagonised by amfetamines, although haloperidol and other antipsychotics can be used to treat amfetamine-induced psychosis.

Amiodarone + phenothiazines

The literature notes an increased risk of ventricular arrhythmias with phenothiazines. A small but potentially significant QTc prolongation (but not ventricular arrhythmia) has been seen with amiodarone and haloperidol (n = 49, Bush et al, Am J Health Syst Pharm 2008;**65**:2232–6).

Antacids + antipsychotics

Antacids may reduce chlorpromazine and possibly haloperidol serum levels. Sulpiride absorption may be reduced by sucralfate or aluminium-containing antacids. Separate doses by a couple of hours minimises the effect.

Anticholinergics + antipsychotics

Anticholinergics may reduce the efficacy of antipsychotics, probably by lowering the serum levels of oral and depot antipsychotics (n = 25, Bamrah et al, Br J Psychiatry 1986;**149**:726–33). Additive anticholinergic effects, e.g. acute intestinal pseudo-obstruction have been reported with benzatropine and haloperidol (n = 1, Sheikh et al, Am J Gastroenterol 2001;**96**:934–5). The UK SmPC now recommends anticholinergics are not used with **olanzapine.**

ANTICONVULSANTS + ANTIPSYCHOTICS

Antipsychotics lower the seizure threshold and may thus antagonise anticonvulsant actions. See also individual anticonvulsants (4.5).

4

ANTIHISTAMINES + ANTIPSYCHOTICS

Loratadine and fexofenadine are currently considered suitable, although there are three unproven reports of arrhythmia with loratadine.

Antihypertensives + phenothiazines

Combined hypotensive effect may occur.

Antimalarials + chlorpromazine

One study showed markedly increased chlorpromazine levels with anti-malarials, e.g. chloroquine and 'Fansidar' (open, Makanjuola *et al*, *Trop Geogr Med* 1988;**40**:31–3).

Aripiprazole + antipsychotics (other)

See aripiprazole (*4.2.2*).

Ascorbic acid + fluphenazine

An isolated case exists of reduced fluphenazine levels (Dysken *et al*, *JAMA* 1979;**241**:2008) with 1 g/d of ascorbic acid.

BARBITURATES + ANTIPSYCHOTICS

Additive sedative effects can occur acutely with this combination, and death has been reported (n = 1, Hino *et al*, *Leg Med* (Tokyo) 1999;**1**:48–51). Barbiturates may induce the metabolism of many antipsychotics, e.g. haloperidol levels are reduced by 40–75%. Antagonism of the anticonvulsant effects may also occur.

Benzodiazepines + antipsychotics

Enhanced sedation and impaired psychomotor function can occur (see *1.1*) and death has been reported after an overdose of triazolam and promazine in an older woman (n = 1, Rossi *et al*, *Med Sci Law* 2009;**49**:65–8).

Beta-blockers + antipsychotics

Generally, raised antipsychotic plasma levels occur, of possible clinical significance, e.g. chlorpromazine levels may rise by up to 100–500% with propranolol (Peet *et al*, *Lancet* 1980;**ii**:978), although pindolol has no significant effect on haloperidol levels (n = 26, open, Greendyke and Gulya, *J Clin Psychiatry* 1988;**49**:105–7).

Betel nut + antipsychotics

Betel nut (*Areca catechu*), which contains the cholinergic alkaloid arecoline, has been reported to cause EPSE, bradykinesia, stiffness and akathisia with flupentixol and fluphenazine (n = 1, Deahl, *Mov Disord* 1998;**4**:330–3).

Bromocriptine + antipsychotics

A predictable reversal of the antipsychotic effect may occur. Antipsychotics may also antagonise the hypoprolactinaemic and antiparkinsonian effects of bromocriptine.

Calcium-channel blockers + antipsychotics

Increased antipsychotic plasma levels or enhanced hypotension might occur (review by Markowitz *et al*, *Ann Pharmacother* 1995;**29**:603–9).

Cannabis + antipsychotics

See cannabis (*4.7.2*).

CARBAMAZEPINE + ANTIPSYCHOTICS

See carbamazepine (*4.5.1*).

Citalopram + antipsychotics

See antipsychotics + citalopram/escitalopram (*4.3.2.1*).

CLARITHROMYCIN + ANTIPSYCHOTICS

There are reports of an increased risk of arrhythmias with phenothiazines and the combination should be avoided. Death has been reported when clarithromycin was added to pimozide in a man with a documented prolonged QT interval (n = 1, Flockhart *et al*, *J Clin Psychopharmacol* 2000;**20**:317–24).

Clonidine + antipsychotics

Animal studies have shown phenothiazines and haloperidol (but not pimozide) to antagonise the hypotensive effect of clonidine. Severe hypotension and delirium have been reported (review by Markowitz *et al*, *Ann Pharmacother* 1995;**29**:603–9).

CLOZAPINE + ANTIPSYCHOTICS

See clozapine (*4.2.4*).

Cocaine + antipsychotics

See cocaine (*4.7.3*).

Desferrioxamine + prochlorperazine

Prolonged unconsciousness may occur.

Diazoxide + chlorpromazine

Enhanced hypoglycaemia has been reported (n = 1, Aynsley-Green and Illig, *Lancet* 1975;**2**:658).

Disopyramide + antipsychotics

Increased anticholinergic effects may occur.

Disulfiram + antipsychotics

See disulfiram (*4.6.8*).

Domperidone + antipsychotics

There is an enhanced risk of EPSE.

Donepezil + antipsychotics

See donepezil (*4.6.3.1*).

Erythromycin + antipsychotics

See clarithromycin + antipsychotics.

Escitalopram + antipsychotics

See citalopram/escitalopram (*4.3.2.1*).

FLUOXETINE + ANTIPSYCHOTICS *

Severe EPSE have been reported with fluoxetine and **haloperidol** (n = 1, Tate, *Am J Psychiatry* 1989;**146**:399–400), dystonia with **fluphenazine**, and stupor; confusion (n = 1, Hansen–Grant et al, Am J Psychiatry 1993;**150**:1750–1), and severe bradycardia and drowsiness (n = 1, Friedman, Can J Psychiatry 1994;**39**:634) with pimozide. Zuclopenthixol levels are increased by around 93% by fluoxetine, in a dose-dependent manner (n = 923 samples, Davies et al, Acta Psychiatr Scand 2010;**122**:44–53), and has caused laryngeal dystonia (n = 1, Hood et al, Australas Psychiatry 2010;**18**:174–6). The probable mechanism is CYP2D6 inhibition so the combination should be avoided if possible (Ahmed et al, Can J Psychiatry 1993;**38**:62–3). Citalopram, escitalopram and sertraline would be suitable alternatives.

Fluvoxamine + antipsychotics
See fluvoxamine (4.3.2.3).

Ginseng + haloperidol
Ginseng may potentiate the effects of haloperidol (Mitra et al, Indian J Exp Biol 1996; **34**:41–7).

H2-blockers + antipsychotics
Chlorpromazine levels may be reduced by 30% by cimetidine (Howes et al, Eur J Clin Pharmacol 1983;**24**:99–102), but not ranitidine.

Haloperidol + chlorpromazine
Chlorpromazine may significantly increase haloperidol levels, probably via CYP2D6 inhibition (n = 43, Suzuki et al, Ther Drug Monit 2001;**23**:363–8).

Hydroxyzine + phenothiazines
The effect of phenothiazines may be decreased (Ross and Priest, Dis Nerv Syst 1970;**31**:412).

Hypoglycaemics + chlorpromazine
Chlorpromazine can induce hyperglycaemia and disrupt the control of diabetes (Schwarz and Munoz, Am J Psychiatry 1968;**125**:253).

Indometacin + haloperidol
Profound drowsiness and confusion can occur with the combination (Bird et al, Lancet 1983;i:830–1).

Itraconazole + haloperidol
Itraconazole 200mg/d for seven days significantly increases haloperidol and metabolite levels, leading to increased side-effects, presumably due to CYP3A4 inhibition (n = 13, Yasui et al, J Clin Psychopharmacol 1999;**19**:149–54).

LEVODOPA + ANTIPSYCHOTICS
The therapeutic effect of levodopa is antagonised by antipsychotics and vice versa. Levodopa may worsen antipsychotic-induced EPSE.

Levomepromazine + zuclopenthixol *
Zuclopenthixol levels are increased by around 46% by levomepromazine, in a dose-dependent manner (n = 923 samples, Davies et al, Acta Psychiatr Scand 2010;**122**:44–53).

Lithium + antipsychotics
See antipsychotics + lithium (4.4).

MAOIs + antipsychotics
See antipsychotics + MAOIs (4.3.4).

Melatonin + antipsychotics
See melatonin (4.1.4).

Memantine + antipsychotics
See memantine (4.6.9).

Methadone + sulpiride
The sulpiride SmPC now states that it should be used with caution with drugs that can prolong QTc, e.g. methadone and halofantrine.

Metirosine + antipsychotics
An enhanced risk of EPSE exists.

Metoclopramide + antipsychotics
An enhanced risk of EPSE exists.

Minocycline + phenothiazines
Pigmented galactorrhoea has been reported with the combination (n = 1, Basler and Lynch, Arch Dermatol 1985;**121**:417).

Naltrexone + phenothiazines
Severe drowsiness may occur with chlorpromazine.

Olanzapine + antipsychotics (other)
See olanzapine (4.2.5).

Oral contraceptives + chlorpromazine
There is a report of a combined OC raising chlorpromazine levels six-fold (n = 1, Chetty and Miller, Ther Drug Monit 2001; **23**:556–8).

Orlistat + haloperidol
A small trial suggested a lack of interaction (n = 8, open, 8/52, Hilger et al, J Clin Psychopharmacol 2002;**22**:68–70).

Oxcarbazepine + antipsychotics
See oxcarbazepine (4.5.7).

Paroxetine + antipsychotics *
See antipsychotics + paroxetine (4.3.2.4).

Pethidine + phenothiazines
Increased CNS toxicity and hypotension can occur (n = 10, open, c/o, Stambaugh and Wainer, J Clin Pharmacol 1981;**21**:140–6).

PHENYTOIN + ANTIPSYCHOTICS
Phenytoin may reduce haloperidol levels by 40–75%, probably via enzyme induction (n = 30, open, Linnoila et al, Am J Psychiatry 1980;**137**:819). Chlorpromazine may increase phenytoin levels by up to 50% (n = 27, open, Sands et al, Drug Intell Clin Pharm 1987;**21**:267–72), although other studies

4

show a nil or opposite effect. Antipsychotics lower the seizure threshold and may antagonise the anticonvulsant effect of phenytoin.

Piperazine + chlorpromazine
The validity of a single case of convulsions with the combination has been queried by a small study (Sturman, *Br J Pharmacol* 1974;**50**:153–5).

Polymyxin + phenothiazines
The neuromuscular blocking effects of polymyxin antibiotics may be increased by phenothiazines with prolonged respiratory depression possible (Pohlmann, *JAMA* 1966;**196**:181).

Procarbazine + antipsychotics
Enhanced sedation is possible.

Quetiapine + antipsychotics (other)
See quetiapine (*4.2.6*).

Reboxetine + antipsychotics
See reboxetine (*4.3.3.6*).

RIFAMPICIN + HALOPERIDOL
Rifampicin may reduce haloperidol serum levels by a third (n = 17, Kim et al, *J Clin Psychopharmacol* 1996;**16**:247–52), a clinically significant effect. Care would be needed if rifampicin were stopped.

SERTINDOLE + ANTIPSYCHOTICS *
See sertindole (*4.2.8*).

Sertraline + antipsychotics
See sertraline (*4.3.2.5*).

Smoking + antipsychotics
See smoking (*4.7.4*).

Suxamethonium + promazine
Prolonged apnoea has been reported (n = 1, Regan and Aldrete, *Anesth Analg* 1967;**46**:315–8).

Sucralfate + antipsychotics
See antacids + antipsychotics (*4.2.1*).

Tea or coffee + antipsychotics
Typical antipsychotics precipitate out of solution to form a tannin complex with tea and coffee, almost certainly of minimal clinical significance (Bowen et al, *Lancet* 1981;**i**:1217–8).

Tetrabenazine + antipsychotics
A single predictable case exists of enhanced EPSE in a Huntington's patient (Moss and Stewart, *Can J Psychiatry* 1986;**31**:865–6).

Trazodone + antipsychotics
See trazodone (*4.3.3.7*).

Tricyclics + antipsychotics
See tricyclics (*4.3.1*).

Valproate + antipsychotics
No interaction occurs with **aripiprazole** (Citrome et al, *Int J Neuropsychopharmacol* 2002;**5**[Suppl 1]:S187). **Chlorpromazine** may inhibit valproate's

metabolism and so monitoring of valproate levels may be useful (open, Ishizaki et al, *J Clin Psychopharmacol* 1984;**4**:254–61). Valproate has no significant effect on the plasma levels of **haloperidol** (n = 27, 4/52, Hesslinger et al, *J Clin Psychopharmacol* 1999;**19**:310–5) or **risperidone** and 9–hydroxyrisperidone (e.g. n = 12, Yoshimura et al, *Pharmacopsychiatry* 2007;**40**:9–13), but there are cases of dose-related generalised oedema with risperidone and valproate (n = 2, Sanders and Lehrer, *J Clin Psychiatry* 1998;**59**:689–90). Although valproate is often used as anticonvulsant cover for higher doses of clozapine, a careful study showed valproate to produce a 15% drop in clozapine levels and a 65% drop in norclozapine levels (n = 7, Longo and Salzman, *Am J Psychiatry* 1995;**152**:650), although raised clozapine levels have been reported (n = 1, Costello and Suppes, *J Clin Psychopharmacol* 1995;**15**:139–41). Since norclozapine is more toxic than clozapine, this may be a useful effect with careful manipulation of the dose. Clozapine may, of course, also lower the seizure threshold and antagonise the anticonvulsant effect of valproate.

Venlafaxine + antipsychotics
See venlafaxine (*4.3.3.9*).

Warfarin + antipsychotics
An interaction is theoretically possible (see Sayal et al, *Acta Psychiatr Scand* 2000;**102**:250–5).

Zaleplon + antipsychotics
See zaleplon (*4.1.5*).

Zolpidem + antipsychotics
See zolpidem (*4.1.6*).

4.2.2 ANTIPSYCHOTICS — ARIPIPRAZOLE *

Aripiprazole is metabolised mainly by CYP2D6 (n = 80, Kim et al, *Br J Clin Pharmacol* 2008;**66**:802–10) and 3A4, but not CYP1A1, 1A2 or 2C9/19. It has no effect on CYP2C9, 2C19, 2D6 and 3A4. 3A4 inducing drugs lower aripiprazole levels by about 60%, while 3A4 inhibitors increase levels by about 45% (samples = 361, Waade et al, *Ther Drug Monit* 2009;**31**:233–8). The UK SmPC now says caution is necessary with drugs known to cause QTc prolongation or electrolyte imbalance.

Alcohol + aripiprazole
See alcohol (*4.7.1*).

Antipsychotics (other) + aripiprazole
There is a theoretical interaction with potent

D2 antagonists such as older neuroleptics and risperidone with aripiprazole. Aripiprazole has a very high affinity for D2 receptors and would displace almost any other antipsychotic from these receptors. There is a case of asymptomatic QTc prolongation with aripiprazole and haloperidol (n = 1, Leo et al, J Clin Psychiatry 2008;**69**:327–8). See also combinations in Chapter 1.23.

CARBAMAZEPINE + ARIPIPRAZOLE
See antipsychotics + carbamazepine (4.5.1).

Citalopram + aripiprazole
See antipsychotics + citalopram (4.3.2.1).

Dextromethorphan + aripiprazole
Lack of interaction has been shown.

Duloxetine + aripiprazole *
See aripiprazole + duloxetine (4.3.3.2).

Escitalopram + aripiprazole
See antipsychotics + escitalopram (4.3.2.1).

Fluoxetine + aripiprazole *
Pooled data from 2 trials shows no substantial effect from adjunctive aripiprazole on fluoxetine and norfluoxetine kinetics (n=55, d/b, p/c, Boulton et al, J Psychopharmacol 2010;**24**:537-46; MS).

H2-blockers + aripiprazole
Lack of significant interaction has been shown with famotidine.

Itraconazole + aripiprazole
Although itraconazole is a potent CYP3A4 inhibitor, it made no clinically significant difference to aripiprazole levels in one study (n = 24, Kubo et al, Drug Metab Pharmacokinet 2005;**20**:55–64).

Ketoconazole + aripiprazole
Ketoconazole decreases aripiprazole metabolism and so aripiprazole doses should be decreased by a half during co-administration.

Lamotrigine + aripiprazole
See aripiprazole + lamotrigine (see 4.5.5).

Lithium + aripiprazole
See antipsychotics + lithium (4.4).

Omeprazole + aripiprazole
Lack of interaction has been shown.

Paroxetine + aripiprazole
See antipsychotics + paroxetine (4.3.2.4).

Quinidine + aripiprazole
Quinidine decreases aripiprazole metabolism and so aripiprazole doses should be halved.

Smoking + aripiprazole
See smoking (4.7.4)

Sertraline + aripiprazole
See antipsychotics + sertraline (4.3.3.9).

Tamoxifen + aripiprazole
There is a case of tardive dyskinesia occurring with the combination (n = 1, Evcimen et al, Am J Psychiatry 2007;**164**:1436–7).

Valproate + aripiprazole
See valproate + antipsychotics (4.2.1).

Venlafaxine + aripiprazole
See antipsychotics + venlafaxine (4.3.3.9).

Warfarin + aripiprazole
Lack of interaction has been shown.

4.2.3 ANTIPSYCHOTICS — ASENAPINE
Asenapine is primarily metabolised by UGT1A4 and 1A2.

Cimetidine + asenapine
Lack of interaction has been shown (US PI).

Carbamazepine + asenapine
See antipsychotics + carbamazepine (4.5.1).

Fluvoxamine + asenapine
See antipsychotics + fluvoxamine (4.3.2.3).

Imipramine + asenapine
Lack of interaction has been shown (US PI).

Paroxetine + asenapine
Lack of interaction has been shown (US PI).

Valproate + asenapine
Lack of interaction has been shown (US PI).

Smoking + asenapine
Lack of interaction has been shown (US PI).

4.2.4 ANTIPSYCHOTICS — CLOZAPINE
See 4.2.1 for other, more general interactions

The major metabolic route of clozapine is to norclozapine, which is more stable but more toxic to stem cells (Gerson et al, Br J Haematology 1994;**86**:555–61). CYP1A2 is the major metabolising enzyme, with 2D6, 3A4, 2C9/19 and FMO enzymes also involved (Urichuk et al, Curr Drug Metab 2008;**9**:410–8).
Review: general (Chetty and Murray, Curr Drug Metab 2007;**8**:307–13).

ACE inhibitors + clozapine
Clozapine plus diltiazem or enalapril (Aronowitz et al, J Clin Psychopharmacol 1994;**14**:429–30) have been reported to produce additional hypotension. There is also a well-documented case of a clinically important rise in clozapine and norclozapine levels with lisinopril (n = 1, Abraham et al, Am J Psychiatry 2001;**158**:969).

Alcohol + clozapine
See antipsychotics + alcohol (4.7.1).

Amiodarone + clozapine

Raised clozapine levels have been reported with concurrent amiodarone (n = 1, Stevens *et al*, *Psychosomatics* 2008;**49**:255–7).

ANTIBIOTICS/FUNGALS/VIRALS + CLOZAPINE*

Antibiotics reported to cause leucopenia/neutropenia may enhance the likelihood of clozapine-induced neutropenia and should, if possible, be avoided. It should be noted however, that respiratory infections can themselves inhibit CYP1A2, raising clozapine levels, and so antibiotics may not always be the cause of apparent interactions (Leon, *J Clin Psychiatry* 2004;**65**:1144–5).

Where possible, choose antibiotics from the first list and be aware of the potential for problems if drugs from the second list must be used.

1. Antibiotics LESS likely to cause neutropenia (safer to use): penicillins (all except benzylpenicillin G), all tetracyclines, aminoglycosides, macrolides, clarithromycin, some anti-TBs (ethambutol, pyrazinamide, streptomycin), clofazimide, hexamine, sodium fusidate, spectinomycin, colistin, polymixin B and cycloserine.

2. Antibiotics MORE likely/CAN cause leucopenia and/or neutropenia (less safe to use): cephalosporins and cephamycins, clindamycin, lincomycin, sulphonamides (mandatory precaution in SmPC) and trimethoprim, some anti-TBs (capreomycin, isoniazid [n = 1, Angelini *et al*, *J Clin Psychopharmacol* 2009;**29**:190–1], rifampicin), co-trimoxazole, dapsone, metronidazole, tinidazole, nitrofurantoin, **chloramphenicol**, erythromycin, vancomycin, teicoplanin and the 4-quinolones (ciprofloxacin, nalidixic acid, etc). For example, clozapine levels have fallen by nearly 50% when **ciprofloxacin** was stopped, probably due to CYP1A2 inhibition (n=1, Markowitz *et al*, *Am J Psychiatry* 1997;**153**:881) and doubled a few days after ciprofloxacin added, presumably by 1A2 and 3A4 inhibition (n = 2, Brouwers *et al*, *Clin Drug Invest* 2009;**29**:59–63). Raised clozapine levels and seizures have been reported seven days after **erythromycin** 250 mg/d was added to clozapine 800 mg/d, with levels falling by 50% when erythromycin was stopped (Funderburg *et al*, *Am J Psychiatry* 1994;**151**:1840) and increased toxicity, e.g. somnolence and leukocytosis (n = 1, Cohen *et al*, *Arch Intern Med* 1996;**156**:675–7). There is a case of a 600% reduction in clozapine levels 2–3 weeks after rifampicin was started, probably via 1A2 and 3A4 induction (n = 1, Joos *et al*, *J Clin Psychopharmacol* 1998;**18**:83–5).

3. Antifungals: **itraconazole** 200 mg/d had no effect on plasma clozapine and norclozapine levels (RCT, n = 7, 7/7, Raaska and Neuvonen, *Eur J Clin Pharmacol* 1998; **54**:167–70), and **ketoconazole** also has no effect on clozapine (Lane *et al*, *Drug Metabol Drug Interact* 2001;**18**:263–78).

3. Antivirals: Although absolute neutrophil counts can be significantly different when oseltamivir is used in people taking clozapine, this is not considered significant and stopping clozapine is not warranted (n=32, Demler and Trigoboff, *Psychiatry (Edgmont)* 2009;**11**:29-33).

Anticholinergics + clozapine

See antipsychotics (*4.2.1*).

Antihypertensives + clozapine

Potentiation of the antihypertensive effects may occur. This can be particularly important during the upward dose titration period.

ANTIPSYCHOTICS (other) + CLOZAPINE

A 15% reduction in clozapine levels has been reported with **aripiprazole** (n = 94, Englisch and Zink, *Prog Neuropsychopharmacol Biol Psychiatry* 2008;**32**:1386–92). **Amisulpride** has no apparent effect on plasma clozapine concentrations (Bergemann *et al*, *J Clin Psychopharmacol* 2005;**25**:494–7). There is an enhanced risk of agranulocytosis with some antipsychotics, e.g. **phenothiazines**, which would additionally be complicated by the long-term nature of any given as a depot. Examples include thrombocytopenia with **fluphenazine** and clozapine (n = 1, Mihaljevic-Peles *et al*, *Nord J Psychiatry* 2001;**55**:449–50) and significantly lower clozapine plasma levels with **levomepromazine** (n = 2, Bugamelli *et al*, *Prog Neuropsychopharmacol Biol Psychiatry* 2007;**31**:567–70). Elevated **haloperidol** levels have been reported in combination with clozapine (n = 1, Allen, *J Clin Pharmacol* 2000;**40**:1296–7), as have myoclonic and GTC seizures (n = 1, Haberfellner, *Eur Psychiatry* 2002;**17**:55–6). Although there have been case reports, e.g. (n = 18, Raaska *et al*, *Eur J Clin Pharmacol* 2002;**58**:587–91; n = 1, Kontaxakis *et al*, *Prog Neuropsychopharmacol Biol Psychiatry* 2002;**26**:407–9), a study was unable to show any kinetic interactions between **risperidone** and clozapine (n = 20, Chetty *et al*, *Br J Clin Pharmacol* 2009;**68**:574–9). The mechanism cannot be explained by inhibition of CYP1A2, 2D6 or 2C19 (n = 8, Eap *et al*, *Ther Drug Monit* 2001;**23**:228–

31). See also antipsychotics + quetiapine (4.2.6) and combinations (1.23).

BENZODIAZEPINES + CLOZAPINE

There are rare cases of severe hypotension and respiratory depression (e.g. n = 3, Friedman et al, N Engl J Med 1991;**325**:518–9), sudden death after IV lorazepam (n = 1, Klimke and Klieser, Am J Psychiatry 1994;**151**:780), sedation (n = 2, Cobb et al, Am J Psychiatry 1991;**148**:1606–7) and delirium with lorazepam (n = 3, Jackson et al, Ann Clin Psychiatry1995;**7**:139–41). Monitor for enhanced sedation and take particular care when a clozapine dose is being increased.

Buspirone + clozapine

See buspirone (4.1.2).

Caffeine + clozapine

Caffeine and clozapine are both metabolised by CYP1A2 and so some competitive inhibition of metabolism may occur. Caffeine, in doses of 400–1000 mg, inhibits the metabolism of clozapine to an extent that might be significant in some people (n = 12, RCT, open, Hagg et al, Br J Clin Pharmacol 2000;**49**:59–63), e.g. mean serum trough levels of clozapine increased by about 26% have been reported, probably of minor clinical significance in most patients (n = 12[c = 6], RCT, d/b, Raaska et al, Basic Clin Pharmacol Toxicol 2004;**94**:13–8), causing drowsiness and siallorrhoea, with clozapine levels halving when caffeine was stopped (n = 1, Odom–White and de Leon, J Clin Psychiatry 1996;**57**:175–6).

Cannabis + clozapine

See antipsychotics + cannabis (4.7.2).

CARBAMAZEPINE + CLOZAPINE

See antipsychotics + carbamazepine (4.5.1).

Citalopram + clozapine

See antipsychotics + citalopram/escitalopram (4.3.2.1).

Clonidine + clozapine

See clonidine + antipsychotics (4.2.1).

Cocaine + clozapine

See antipsychotics + cocaine (4.7.3).

Cytotoxic agents + clozapine

Although there is an increased risk of neutropenia, there may be no need to discontinue clozapine. Patients receiving chemotherapy should be assessed on an individual basis and special monitoring should be carried out, e.g. monitor for symptoms of infection, increase frequency of testing schedule and establish thresholds for stopping those treatments, in collaboration with medical and haematological specialists.

Digoxin + clozapine

The SmPC for clozapine advises caution with highly bound drugs, which would include digoxin. Monitor and adjust doses as necessary.

Escitalopram + clozapine

See antipsychotics + citalopram/escitalopram (4.3.2.1).

FLUOXETINE + CLOZAPINE

Fluoxetine produces significant increases in plasma clozapine and norclozapine levels, with some inter-individual variation (n = 80, open, Centorrino et al, Am J Psychiatry 1996; **153**:820–2). There are many case reports (e.g. n = 6, Centorrino et al, Am J Psychiatry 1994;**151**: 123–5), including death (n = 1, Ferslew et al, J Forensic Sci 1998;**43**:1082–5) and uncontrollable myoclonic jerks (n = 1, Kingsbury and Puckett, Am J Psychiatry 1995;**152**:473–2). The mechanism is possibly CYP2D6 inhibition. The risk of clozapine toxicity must be considered and measuring clozapine levels may be useful.

FLUVOXAMINE + CLOZAPINE

This is an important and significant interaction. Fluvoxamine inhibition of CYP1A2 leads to clozapine levels increased by up to 900% and AUC by 40% (e.g. n = 1, Armstrong and Stephans, J Clin Psychiatry 1997;**58**:499) although peak levels may remain unchanged (n = 9, Wang et al, J Clin Pharmacol 2004;**44**:785–92). So predictable is the effect that fluvoxamine has been used to counteract 1A2 induction by smoking, which can lead to clozapine non-response (n = 3, Bender and Eap, Arch Gen Psychiatry 1998;**55**:1048–50) in 1A2 ultra-rapid metabolisers. Close pharmacokinetic monitoring is thus necessary, as the effect can be dramatic over a few days in some patients even with very low doses, e.g. 10–20 mg/d fluvoxamine.

Grapefruit juice + clozapine

Grapefruit juice has no effect on clozapine levels (n = 15, open, 12/52, Lane et al, Drug Metabol Drug Interact 2001;**18**:263–78).

H2-blockers + clozapine

Clozapine levels may rise by over 50% with cimetidine (n = 1, Czymanski et al, J Clin Psychiatry 1991;**52**:21). Ranitidine is a safer alternative.

Influenza vaccine + clozapine

Influenza vaccine has no effect on clozapine levels (n = 14, Raaska et al, Eur J Clin Pharmacol 2001;**57**:705–8).

4

Lamotrigine + clozapine

Lamotrigine 200 mg/d has no effect on stable clozapine levels (n = 11, 8/52, Spina *et al*, *Ther Drug Monit* 2006;**28**:599–602), but an unexplained three-fold increase in clozapine levels was seen two weeks after lamotrigine 100 mg/d was added to a stable clozapine 400 mg/d regimen (n = 1, Kossen *et al*, *Am J Psychiatry* 2001;**158**:1930).

Lithium + clozapine

See antipsychotics + lithium (4.4).

MAOIs + clozapine

See antipsychotics + MAOIs (4.3.4).

Mirtazapine + clozapine

See mirtazapine (4.3.3.4).

Oral contraceptives + clozapine

Elevated plasma clozapine levels have been reported with norethindrone, resolving on OC discontinuation (n = 1, Gabbay *et al*, *J Clin Psychopharmacol* 2002;**22**:621–2).

Orlistat + clozapine

A small trial suggested lack of interaction (8/52, Hilger *et al*, *J Clin Psychopharmacol* 2002;**22**:68–70).

Oxcarbazepine + clozapine

See antipsychotics + oxcarbazepine (4.5.7).

PAROXETINE + CLOZAPINE

Paroxetine produces significant increases in plasma clozapine and norclozapine levels (n = 60, open, Centorrino *et al*, *Am J Psychiatry* 1996;**153**:820–2), and so the risk of clozapine toxicity must be considered carefully. NMS with no leukocytosis and normal CPK has also been reported with the combination (n = 1, Gambassi *et al*, *Aging Clin Exp Res* 2006;**18**:266–70).

Penicillamine + clozapine

There is an enhanced risk of agranulocytosis (mandatory precaution in SmPC).

Phenobarbital + clozapine

Elevated plasma clozapine levels (requiring dose reduction) have been reported after discontinuation of phenobarbital, presumably from removal of CYP1A2 induction (n = 1, Lane *et al*, *J Clin Psychiatry* 1998;**59**:131–3).

Phenylbutazone + clozapine

There is an enhanced risk of agranulocytosis (mandatory precaution in SmPC).

PHENYTOIN + CLOZAPINE

Serum concentrations of clozapine may be markedly reduced by phenytoin (n = 2, Miller *et al*, *J Clin Psychiatry* 1991;**52**:23) via CYP1A2 induction, so monitor for reduced effect.

Proton pump inhibitors + clozapine

A switch from omeprazole to pantoprazole does not alter average clozapine plasma levels, although some individual increases may be seen (n = 13, Mookhoek and Loonen, *Br J Clin Pharmacol* 2002;**53**:545P).

Pyrazolone analgesics + clozapine

There is an enhanced risk of agranulocytosis (mandatory precaution in SmPC).

Quetiapine + clozapine

See quetiapine (4.2.6).

Reboxetine + clozapine

See reboxetine (4.3.3.6).

SERTRALINE + CLOZAPINE

Sertraline may produce significant increases in plasma clozapine and norclozapine levels, with some inter-individual variation (n = 80, Centorrino *et al*, *Am J Psychiatry* 1996;**153**:820–2) and sudden death has been reported, probably as a result of cardiac arrhythmia (n = 1, Hoehns *et al*, *Ann Pharmacother* 2001;**35**:826–6). The risk of clozapine toxicity must be considered.

SERTINDOLE + CLOZAPINE *

See sertindole (4.2.8).

Smoking + clozapine

See antipsychotics + smoking (4.7.4).

Topiramate + clozapine

See antipsychotics + topiramate (4.5.13).

Tricyclics + clozapine

See antipsychotics + tricyclics (4.3.1).

Valproate + clozapine

See valproate + antipsychotics (4.2.1).

Venlafaxine + clozapine

See venlafaxine (4.3.3.9).

Warfarin + clozapine

The SmPC for clozapine advises caution with highly bound drugs, including warfarin (mentioned in Sayal *et al*, *Acta Psychiatr Scand* 2000;**102**:250–5), so monitor and adjust doses.

4.2.5 ANTIPSYCHOTICS — OLANZAPINE

See *4.2.1* for other, more general, interactions

Olanzapine is metabolised by CYP1A2 and 2D6, 2D6 and 3A4 (Urichuk *et al*, *Curr Drug Metab* 2008;**9**:410–8), with little or no effect on 1A2, 2D6, 2C19, 2C9 and 3A4 at normal doses. It is highly bound to albumin (90%) and alpha 1-acid glycoprotein (77%), and interactions may be possible through this mechanism. Olanzapine also undergoes N-glucuronidation by UGT1A4.

Olanzapine is approximately 60% excreted in urine and 30% in faeces. Fixed doses appear to give higher levels in women. The UK SmPC now cautions about the use of olanzapine with drugs known to increase the QTc interval.

Review: extensive, of pharmacokinetics and pharmacodynamics (Callaghan *et al*, *Clin Pharmacokinetics* 1999;**37**:177–93, 56 refs).

Alcohol + olanzapine
See antipsychotics + alcohol (*4.7.1*).

Antacids + olanzapine
Antacids have no effect on olanzapine bio–availability.

Anticholinergics + olanzapine
The UK SmPC now recommends that anti-cholinergics are not used with olanzapine.

Antipsychotics (other) + olanzapine
An interaction has been suggested with **halo–peridol** (Gomberg, *J Clin Psychopharmacol* 1999;**19**:272–3) and NMS has been reported (n = 1, Mujica and Weiden, *Am J Psychiatry* 2001;**158**:650–1). Seizures have been reported with **quetiapine** and olanzapine (n = 1, Hedges and Jeppson, *Ann Pharmacother* 2002;**36**:437–9). Unchanged olanzapine levels with **flupentixol** were mentioned in one study (Bergemann *et al*, *Pharmacopsychiatry* 2004; **37**:63–8).

Benzodiazepines + olanzapine
Single dose studies show no effect of olanzapine on the metabolism of **diazepam**. Mild increases in heart rate, sedation and dry mouth were noted, but no dose adjustment is considered necessary. Unchanged olanzapine levels with **lorazepam** were mentioned in one study (Bergemann *et al*, *Pharmacopsychiatry* 2004; **37**:63–8). Concomitant IM olanzapine and IM BDZs are contraindicated (UK SmPC) and must be separated by at least one hour. There is one case report of significant hypotension (down to 66/30 within four hours) lasting 12 hours in a patient given olanzapine IM with lorazepam 2 mg IM 30 minutes later (n = 1, Zacher and Roche–Desilets, *J Clin Psychiatry* 2005;**66**:1614–5).

Carbamazepine + olanzapine
See antipsychotics + carbamazepine (*4.5.1*).

Charcoal (activated) + olanzapine
Activated charcoal reduces olanzapine bio–availability by 50–60%.

Cimetidine + olanzapine
There is no effect on olanzapine bioavailability.

Ciprofloxacin + olanzapine
Raised olanzapine levels have been reported, possibly caused by ciprofloxacin (n = 1, Marko-witz and DeVane, *J Clin Psychophamacol* 1999; **19**:289–91).

Duloxetine + olanzapine
There is a case of urinary retention with the combination, resolving when duloxetine was switched to venlafaxine (n = 1, Englisch *et al*, *Clin Neuropharmacol* 2008;**31**:308–9).

Lamotrigine + olanzapine
Lamotrigine 200 mg/d for 8/52 produced a statistically significant but probably clinically insignificant rise in stable olanzapine levels (n = 11, Spina *et al*, *Ther Drug Monit* 2006;**28**:599–602).

Lisinopril + olanzapine *
There is a case of women taking olanzapine for bipolar who developed acute pancreatitis 3/12 after starting lisinopril (n = 1, Bracamonte *et al*, *Am J Health-Syst Pharm* 2010;**67**:214-6).

Lithium + olanzapine
See antipsychotics + lithium (*4.4*).

MAOIs + olanzapine
See antipsychotics + MAOIs (*4.3.4*).

Mirtazapine + olanzapine
See olanzapine + mirtazapine (*4.3.3.4*).

Opioids + olanzapine
Opioid-induced delirium has been reported with the combination (n = 2, Estfan *et al*, *J Pain Symptom Manage* 2005;**29**:330–2).

Oxcarbazepine + olanzapine
See antipsychotics + oxcarbazepine (*4.5.7*).

Probenecid + olanzapine
Probenecid appears to decrease olanzapine glucuronidation (n = 12, RCT, d/b, c/o, Markowitz *et al*, *Clin Pharmacol Ther* 2002;**71**:30–8).

Reboxetine + olanzapine
See antipsychotics + reboxetine (*4.3.3.6*).

Rufinamide + olanzapine
See olanzapine + rufinamide (*4.5.12*).

Selegiline + olanzapine
Selegiline transdermal system (STS) had no effects on the pharmacokinetics of olanzapine (open, RCT, c/o, Azzaro *et al*, *J Clin Pharmacol* 2007;**47**:146–58).

Smoking + olanzapine
See antipsychotics + smoking (*4.7.4*).

SSRIs + olanzapine
Fluvoxamine (but not **sertraline**) inhibits the metabolism of olanzapine, probably via CYP1A2 (n = 165, Weigmann *et al*, *Ther Drug Monit*

4

2001;**23**:410–13; Bergemann *et al, Pharmaco-psychiatry* 2004;**37**:63–8), with 100 mg/d raising peak levels by 49%, AUC by 70%, half–life by 40% and steady-state olanzapine levels by 12–112% and so care is needed (e.g. n = 12, Wang *et al, J Clin Pharmacol* 2004;**44**:785–92). Use of fluvoxamine 25 mg/d has allowed a 26% reduction in olanzapine dose for the same plasma level, or could have increased OLZ levels by 25% without increasing the dose (n = 10, 6/52, open, Albers *et al, J Clin Psychopharmacol* 2005;**25**:170–4). This could be a useful trick for keeping olanzapine doses within BNF limits with the MHA commissioners around. Higher doses of **fluoxetine** may slightly increase olanzapine levels, probably via CYP2D6 inhibition (n = 15, Gossen *et al, AAPS PharmSci* 2002;**4**:E11). Melancholic depression has been reported with fluoxetine and olanzapine (n = 1, Nelson and Swartz, *Ann Clin Psychiatry* 2000;**12**:167–70), although the combination has been licensed in the USA for bipolar and acute treatment-resistant depression but not relapse prevention.

Topiramate + olanzapine
See antipsychotics + topiramate (*4.5.14*).

Tricyclics + olanzapine
See antipsychotics + tricyclics (*4.3.1*).

Valproate + olanzapine *
Valproate lowers the plasma levels of olanzapine (Bergemann *et al, J Clin Psychopharmacol* 2006; **26**:432–4) by about 18% at doses of up to 2g/d, not apparently of clinical significance (n=18, Spina *et al, Ther Drug Monit* 2009;**31**:758-63).

Warfarin + olanzapine
Single dose studies show no effect of olanzapine on the metabolism of warfarin, although it could be possible (mentioned in Sayal *et al, Acta Psychiatr Scand* 2000;**102**:250–5).

Xanthines + olanzapine
Lack of interaction has been shown with aminophylline and theophylline (n = 19, RCT, Macias *et al, Pharmacotherapy* 1998;**18**:1237–48).

4.2.6 ANTIPSYCHOTICS — QUETIAPINE *
See *4.2.1* for other, more general, interactions

Quetiapine is metabolised primarily by CYP3A4. The quetiapine UK SmPC now contraindicates it with 3A4 inhibitors and advises caution when used with drugs known to increase the QTc interval or cause electrolyte imbalances.

Alcohol + quetiapine
See alcohol (*4.7.1*).

Antipsychotics (other) + quetiapine
Haloperidol 15 mg/d and **risperidone** 6 mg/d have no effect on quetiapine levels (n = 36, RCT, 9/7, Potkin *et al, J Clin Psychopharmacol* 2002;**22**:121–30). Lower quetiapine doses when used with **clozapine** have been recommended in a TDM service analysis (n = 1179, Castberg *et al, J Clin Psychiatry* 2007;**68**:1540–5). See also *4.2.4*.

Antiretrovirals + quetiapine *
The UK SmPC states that caution is necessary with antiretrovirals, as quetiapine levels can rise via CYP3A4 induction by, e.g. **fosamprenavir**, **indinavir**, **nelfinavir** and **ritonavir**. There are many case reports e.g. rapid but reversible weight gain and sedation with **atazanavir/ritonavir** (n = 2, Pollack *et al, Pharmacother* 2009; **29**:1386–91), and deep coma and sustained hypotension with lamuvidine, ritonavir, atazanavir, and tenofovir (n=1, Hantson *et al, Drug Metab Lett* 2010;**4**:7-8).

Baclofen + quetiapine
There is a case of cranial diabetes insipidus after an overdose of baclofen and quetiapine (n = 1, Silverstone and Scott, *Anaesth Intensive Care* 2009;**37**:319–20).

Barbiturates + quetiapine
Lower levels of quetiapine would be expected, due to CYP3A4 induction by barbiturates.

Benzodiazepines + quetiapine
Single doses of lorazepam and diazepam are unaffected by quetiapine.

Carbamazepine + quetiapine
See antipsychotics + carbamazepine (*4.5.1*).

Cimetidine + quetiapine
No interaction occurs (n = 13, open, Strakowski *et al, J Clin Psychopharmacol* 2002;**22**:201–5).

Clarithromycin + quetiapine
There is a case of major increase in quetiapine plasma levels when clarithromycin was started (n = 1, Schulz–Du Bois *et al, Pharmacopsychiatry* 2008;**41**:258–9).

Erythromycin + quetiapine
Raised quetiapine levels are likely via CYP3A4 inhibition.

KETOCONAZOLE + QUETIAPINE
Ketoconazole 200 mg/d increases quetiapine plasma levels 3.5-fold, by CYP3A4 inhibition, potentially clinically significant (n = 12, Grimm *et al, Br J Clin Pharmacol* 2006;**61**:58–69).

Lithium + quetiapine
See antipsychotics + lithium (4.4).

Lovastatin + quetiapine
A prolonged QTc interval has been reported with the combination (n=1, Furst et al, Biol Psychiatry 2002;51:264–5).

MAOIs + quetiapine
See antipsychotics + MAOIs (4.3.4).

Methadone + quetiapine
See quetiapine + methadone (4.6.10).

Phenytoin + quetiapine
Lower levels of quetiapine would be expected, due to CYP3A4 induction by phenytoin.

Reboxetine + quetiapine
See antipsychotics + reboxetine (4.3.3.6).

Rifampicin + quetiapine
Lower levels of quetiapine would be expected, due to CYP3A4 induction by rifampicin.

Smoking + quetiapine
See quetiapine + smoking (4.7.4).

SSRIs + quetiapine *
Fluoxetine 60mg/d has no significant effect on quetiapine kinetics (n=26, RCT, Potkin et al, J Clin Psychopharmacol 2002;22:174–82) although rhabdomyolysis has been reported (n=1, Himmerrich et al, J Clin Psychopharmacol 2006;26:676–7) and restless legs with paroxetine (n=1, Chou et al, Prog Neuropsychopharmacol Biol Psychiatry 2010;34:1139-40). Lower quetiapine doses when used with fluvoxamine have been recommended in a TDM service analysis (n=1179, Castberg et al, J Clin Psychiatry 2007;68:1540–5).

Topiramate + quetiapine
See antipsychotics + topiramate (4.5.13).

Tricyclics + quetiapine
Imipramine 150mg/d has no significant effect on quetiapine (n=26, RCT, Potkin et al, J Clin Psychopharmacol 2002;22:174–82) but quetiapine has caused a falsely elevated estimation of nortriptyline levels (n=1, Schussler et al, Am J Psychiatry 2003;160:589).

Valproate + quetiapine *
There are cases of cervical dystonia (n=1, Habermeyer et al, J Clin Psychopharmacol 2007;27:396–7) and delirium (n=2, Huang and Wei, Gen Hosp Psychiatry 2010;32:46).

Warfarin + quetiapine
No interaction is likely to occur routinely (mentioned in Sayal et al, Acta Psychiatr Scand 2000;102:250–5), but an isolated case has been reported (n=1, Rogers et al, J Clin Psychopharmacol 1999;19:382–3).

4.2.7 ANTIPSYCHOTICS — RISPERIDONE AND PALIPERIDONE *
See 4.2.1 for other, more general, interactions

Risperidone is metabolised by 3A4 (n=130, Du et al, J Psychopharmacol 2010;24:1115–20) and by 2D6 to 9-hydroxy-risperidone n=218, Mannheimer et al, Ther Drug Monit 2008;30:565–9) where CYP2D6 genotype affects response (Novalbos et al, J Clin Psychopharmacol 2010;30:504–11).

Reviews: P450 metabolism (Berecz et al, Curr Drug Targets 2004; 5:573–9).

Aripiprazole + risperidone/paliperidone
See antipsychotics (other) + aripiprazole (4.2.2).

Caffeine + risperidone/paliperidone
Caffeine appears to have no effect on plasma risperidone levels (n=136, Kakihara et al, Int Clin Psychopharmacol 2005;20:71–8).

CARBAMAZEPINE + RISPERIDONE/ PALIPERIDONE
See antipsychotics + carbamazepine (4.5.1).

Citalopram/escitalopram + risperidone/ paliperidone
See citalopram/escitalopram (4.3.2.1).

Clindamycin + risperidone/paliperidone
Abnormal movements have been seen when clindamycin was added to risperidone in a girl with autism (n=1, Malone and Harvery, J Child Adolesc Psychopharmacol 2008;18:221–2).

CLOZAPINE + RISPERIDONE/PALIPERIDONE
See antipsychotics + clozapine (4.2.4).

Dexamfetamine + risperidone
There is a report of an acute dystonic reaction when dexamfetamine was stopped from the combination (e.g. n=1, Keshen and Carandang, J Child Adolesc Psychopharmacol 2007;17:867–70).

Donepezil + risperidone/paliperidone
See antipsychotics + donepezil (4.6.3.1).

Duloxetine + risperidone *
See risperidone + duloxetine (4.3.3.2).

FLUOXETINE + RISPERIDONE/PALIPERIDONE
Fluoxetine 20mg/d has caused a 75% increase in risperidone levels over four weeks, resulting in side-effects in 30% (n=10, Spina et al, J Clin Psychopharmacol 2002;22:419–23) and there have been reports of severe EPSE, urinary retention (n=1, Bozikas et al, J Psychopharmacol 2001;15:142–3)

4

and nasal bleeding (n=1, Mowla *et al*, *Pharmacopsychiatry* 2009;**42**:204–5).

Fluvoxamine + risperidone/paliperidone

See antipsychotics + fluvoxamine (*4.3.2.3*).

Galantamine + risperidone/paliperidone

See antipsychotics + galantamine (*4.6.3.2*).

Gingko biloba + risperidone/paliperidone

Priapism has been reported (n=1, Lin *et al*, *Mayo Clin Proc* 2007; **82**: 1289–90).

Itraconazole + risperidone/paliperidone

One week of itraconazole 200mg/d raised risperidone and metabolite levels by around 70–75%, presumably via 3A4 inhibition, returning to normal over the next week (n=19, 2/52, Jung *et al*, *Clin Pharmacol Ther* 2005;**78**:520–8).

Lamotrigine + risperidone/paliperidone

Increasing lamotrigine from 175mg/d to 225mg/d produced a rise in risperidone levels from 70ng/ml to 412ng/ml in one patient also on clozapine, although the mechanism was unknown (n=1, Bienentreu and Kronmüller, *Am J Psychiatry* 2005;**162**:811–2). Others have disputed this (n=15+211 controls, Castberg and Spigset, *J Clin Psychiatry* 2006;**67**:1159) as lamotrigine 200mg/d for 8/52 had no effect on stable risperidone levels in another study (n=10, Spina *et al*, *Ther Drug Monit* 2006;**28**:599–602).

Lithium + risperidone/paliperidone

See antipsychotics + lithium (*4.4*).

Methadone + risperidone/paliperidone

See methadone (*4.6.10*).

MAOIs + risperidone/paliperidone

See antipsychotics + MAOIs (*4.3.4*).

Mirtazapine + risperidone/paliperidone

See mirtazapine (*4.3.3.4*).

Oxcarbazepine + risperidone/paliperidone

See antipsychotics + oxcarbazepine (*4.5.7*).

Paroxetine + risperidone/paliperidone

Paroxetine causes a dose-dependent rise in risperidone and metabolite levels (up to double with paroxetine 40mg/d), and so risperidone dose reduction might be needed should side–effects occur (e.g. n=12, open, 12/52, Saito *et al*, *J Clin Psychopharmacol* 2005;**25**:527–32; n=1, Barnhill *et al*, *Pharmacopsychiatry* 2005;**38**: 223–5). There seems to be no clinically relevant interaction with single doses of paliperidone (RCT, c/o, Berwaerts *et al*, *Pharmacopsychiatry* 2009;**42**:158–63).

Phenothiazines + risperidone/paliperidone

Levomepromazine has no effect on risperidone

plasma levels (n=20, 2/52, Yoshimura *et al*, *Pharmacopsychiatry* 2005;**38**:98–100).

Phenytoin + risperidone/paliperidone

Severe EPSE have been reported (n=1, Sanderson, *J Clin Psychiatry* 1996;**57**:177).

Probenecid + risperidone/paliperidone

Probenecid has no effect on risperidone kinetics (n=12, RCT, d/b, c/o, Markowitz *et al*, *Clin Pharmacol Ther* 2002;**71**:30–8).

Quetiapine + risperidone/paliperidone

See antipsychotics + quetiapine (*4.2.6*).

Reboxetine + risperidone/paliperidone

See antipsychotics + reboxetine (*4.3.3.6*).

RIFAMPICIN + RISPERIDONE/PALIPERIDONE

Rifamipin reduces risperidone AUC by 72% and reduces Cmax by 50%, probably by 3A4 and 2D6 induction (n=10, RCT, open, c/o, 2x5/7, Mahatthanatrakul *et al*, *J Clin Pharm Ther* 2007; **32**:161–7).

Ritonavir/indinavir + risperidone/ paliperidone

Addition of ritonavir/indinavir to risperidone has led to severe EPSE, dystonia (n=1, Kelly *et al*, *Ann Pharmacother* 2002;**36**:827–30) and reversible coma (n=1, Jover *et al*, *Clin Neuropharmacol* 2002; **25**:251–3), probably via risperidone toxicity.

Selegiline + risperidone/paliperidone

Selegiline transdermal system (STS) had no effects on the pharmacokinetics of risperidone (open, RCT, c/o, Azzaro *et al*, *J Clin Pharmacol* 2007;**47**:146–58).

Sertraline + risperidone/paliperidone *

High doses of sertraline (150mg/d) can elevate risperidone levels by about 40%, presumably via 2D6 inhibition (n=11, open, Spina *et al*, *Ther Drug Monit* 2004;**26**:386–90), and priapism has been reported (n=1, Salawu *et al*, *Ann African Med* 2010;**9**:195). Risperidone has no effect on sertraline kinetics (n=10, 4/52, Yoshimura *et al*, *Hum Psychopharmacol* 2008;**23**:707–13).

Smoking + risperidone/paliperidone

See antipsychotics + risperidone (*4.7.4*).

Topiramate + risperidone/paliperidone

See antipsychotics + topiramate (*4.5.14*).

Tricyclics + risperidone/paliperidone

See antipsychotics + tricyclics (*4.3.1*).

Valproate + risperidone/paliperidone

See antipsychotics (*4.2.1*).

Venlafaxine + risperidone/paliperidone

See antipsychotics + venlafaxine (*4.3.3.9*).

4.2.8 ANTIPSYCHOTICS — SERTINDOLE
See *4.2.1* for other, more general, interactions

Sertindole is extensively metabolised by CYP2D6 and 3A4 and is a weak 2D6 and 3A4 inhibitor. It is contraindicated in patients also receiving drugs known to prolong the QT interval (see C3).

Aluminium-magnesium antacids + sertindole
There is no effect on sertindole absorption.

ANTIARRHYTHMICS + SERTINDOLE
Sertindole is contraindicated with drugs known to prolong the QT interval, eg. class Ia and III antiarrhythmics, eg. quinidine, amiodarone, sotalol, dofetilide, etc.

ANTIPSYCHOTICS (other) + SERTINDOLE
Sertindole is contraindicated with antipsychotics known to prolong the QT interval.

Benzodiazepines + sertindole
Sertindole has no significant effect on alprazolam (n = 14, open, Wong *et al*, *Psychopharmacol* [Berl] 1998;**135**:236–41).

Calcium-channel blockers + sertindole
Minor, non-significant increases in sertindole levels have been detected with calcium-channel antagonists via CYP3A4 inhibition.

CARBAMAZEPINE + SERTINDOLE
Carbamazepine can reduce sertindole levels 2–3-fold by CYP3A4 induction, so higher maintenance doses might be needed.

CIMETIDINE + SERTINDOLE
Sertindole is contraindicated with cimetidine due to CYP3A4 inhibition. Ranitidine would be a suitable alternative.

Citalopram + sertindole
No interaction via CYP2D6 appears to occur.

Escitalopram + sertindole
See citalopram above.

FLUOXETINE + SERTINDOLE
Plasma levels of sertindole are increased 2–3-fold via CYP2D6 inhibition, so lower maintenance doses might be needed or use of a non-2D6 inhibiting antidepressant.

HIV PROTEASE INIBITORS + SERTINDOLE
Sertindole is contraindicated with drugs such as indinavir due to 3A4 inhibition.

ITRACONAZOLE/KETOCONAZOLE + SERTINDOLE
Sertindole is contraindicated with systemic itraconazole and ketoconazole due to CYP3A4 inhibition.

LITHIUM + SERTINDOLE
See antipsychotics + lithium (*4.4*).

MACROLIDES + SERTINDOLE
QT prolongation potential makes this combination a contraindication. Minor, non-significant increases in sertindole levels have also been detected with **erythromycin** and other macrolides, via CYP3A4 inhibition.

MAOIs + sertindole
See antipsychotics + sertindole (*4.3.4*).

PAROXETINE + SERTINDOLE
Plasma levels of sertindole are increased 2–3-fold via CYP2D6 inhibition, so lower maintenance doses might be needed or use of a non-2D6 inhibiting antidepressant. There is a case of sertindole enhancing paroxetine withdrawal symptoms (Walker-Kinnear and McNaughton, *Br J Psychiatry* 1997;**170**:389).

PHENYTOIN + SERTINDOLE
Phenytoin can reduce sertindole levels 2–3-fold by 3A4 induction, so higher maintenance doses might be needed.

Propranolol + sertindole
No interaction via 2D6 seems to occur.

QUINIDINE + SERTINDOLE
Plasma levels of sertindole are thought to be increased 2–3-fold via 2D6 inhibition, so use is contraindicated. Sertindole is contraindicated with eg. quinidine.

QUINOLONE ANTIBIOTICS + SERTINDOLE
The QT prolongation potential makes the combination with, eg. gatifloxacin a contraindication.

Sertraline + sertindole
No interaction via CYP2D6 appears to occur.

TRICYCLICS + SERTINDOLE
Sertindole is contraindicated with drugs known to prolong the QT interval, eg. some tricyclics. No interaction via CYP2D6 appears to occur with the tricyclics.

4.2.9 ANTIPSYCHOTICS — ZIPRASIDONE

Ziprasidone is partly metabolised by CYP3A4 (with a minor amount from 1A2), plus around 65% via aldehyde reductase. It has no effect on CYP1A2, 2C9/19, 2D6 or 3A4. It is 99% plasma bound. Due to the QTc-prolonging effect, ziprasidone should not be used with drugs also likely to prolong the QTc interval, e.g. sotalol, quinidine, other class Ia and III anti-arrhythmics, phenothiazines, tricyclics, pimozide, mefloquine and dolasetron (see SmPC).

Antacids + ziprasidone
Lack of interaction has been shown with 30ml

4

Maalox (n = 11, RCT, Wilner *et al*, *Br J Clin Pharmacol* 2000;**49**[S3]:57–60).

Anticholinergics + ziprasidone
Lack of interaction has been shown with benzatropine.

Benzodiazepines + ziprasidone
Lack of interaction with lorazepam has been shown.

Beta-blockers + ziprasidone
Lack of interaction has been shown with propranolol.

Carbamazepine + ziprasidone
See antipsychotics + carbamazepine (*4.5.1*).

Cimetidine + ziprasidone
Lack of interaction has been shown (n = 11, RCT, Wilner *et al*, *Br J Clin Pharmacol* 2000;**49**[S3]: 57–60).

Dextromethorphan + ziprasidone
Lack of interaction has been shown (Wilner *et al*, *Br J Clin Pharmacol* 2000;**49**(S3):43–8).

Ketoconazole + ziprasidone
Ketoconazole decreases ziprasidone AUC by about 35%, requiring slightly raised doses.

Levodopa + ziprasidone
Ziprasidone may antagonise the effects of levodopa and other dopaminergic agents.

Lithium + ziprasidone
See antipsychotics + lithium (4.4).

Oral contraceptive + ziprasidone
Lack of interaction has been shown with combined OCs (n = 19, d/b, p/c, c/o, Muirhead *et al*, *Br J Clin Pharmacol* 2000;**49**[S3]:49–56).

Smoking + ziprasidone
See antipsychotics + smoking (*4.7.4*).

Warfarin + ziprasidone
Lack of interaction has been shown.

4.3 ANTIDEPRESSANTS

Review: significant drug interactions with antidepressants in the elderly (Spina and Scordo, *Drugs Aging* 2002;**19**:299–320, 95 refs).

4.3.1 TRICYCLIC ANTIDEPRESSANTS

Tricyclics are metabolised by a range of P450 enzymes, e.g. CYP1A2, 2D6 and 3A3/4. Some tricyclics have several metabolic routes, which may vary with concentration and where another might take over should one be inhibited.

Acamprosate + tricyclics
See acamprosate (*4.6.1*).

Acetazolamide + tricyclics
An interaction is unlikely to occur.

Adrenaline + tricyclics
Tricyclics may potentiate the effects of adrenaline injection increasing the risk of hypertension and cardiac arrhythmias (SmPC).

ALCOHOL + TRICYCLICS
See alcohol (*4.7.1*).

Amiodarone + tricyclics
The literature notes an increased risk of ventricular arrhythmias with tricyclics.

Anaesthetics + tricyclics
Halothane and pancuronium should be used with care with tricyclics with strong anticholinergic actions. Enflurane may be a safer alternative.

Anticholinergics + tricyclics
Enhanced anticholinergic effects may occur, especially in the elderly.

Antihistamines + tricyclics
Enhanced sedation and anticholinergic effects are possible.

Antipsychotics + tricyclics
Tricyclic levels may be up to twice as high if **haloperidol** is also taken, e.g. with desipramine, nortriptyline and imipramine. Tricyclic levels may also rise with phenothiazines, e.g. **perphenazine** increased nortriptyline levels by about 25%, probably by CYP2D6 inhibition (n = 25, Mulsant *et al*, *J Clin Psychopharmacol* 1997;**17**:318–21). No significant interaction has been reported with the **thioxanthenes**, although raised imipramine levels with **flupentixol** have occurred (n = 1, Cook *et al*, *Can J Psychiatry* 1986;**31**:235–7). Single dose studies show no effect of **olanzapine** on the metabolism of imipramine (n = 9, open, Callaghan *et al*, *J Clin Pharmacol* 1997;**37**:971–8) although seizures have been reported with olanzapine and clomipramine (Deshauer *et al*, *J Clin Psychopharmacol* 2000;**20**:283–4). Lower olanzapine levels with trimipramine, but unchanged levels with amitriptyline were mentioned in one study (Bergemann *et al*, *Pharmacopsychiatry* 2004;**37**:63–8). Up to 100 mg/d amitriptyline may have no effect on **risperidone** (n = 12, open, Sommers *et al*, *Int Clin Psychopharmacol* 1997;**12**:141–5) but risperidone may raise **maprotiline** levels, not a thing you would want to do accidentally (Normann *et al*, *J Clin Psychopharmacol* 2002;**22**:92–4).

Asenapine + imipramine
See imipramine + asenapine (*4.2.3*).

Aspirin + imipramine
Imipramine plasma levels may rise and ADRs increase when aspirin is added to imipramine (n = 20, Juarez–Olguin et al, Clin Neuropharmacol 2002;**25**:32–6).

Atomoxetine + tricyclics
See atomoxetine (4.6.4).

Baclofen + tricyclics
A patient with MS lost muscle tone when nortriptyline and imipramine were added to baclofen (n = 1, Silverglat, JAMA 1981;**246**:1659).

BARBITURATES + TRICYCLICS
Barbiturates can reduce the serum levels of amitriptyline, protriptyline and nortriptyline by 14–60%, via CYP3A4 induction. Pentobarbital may affect nortriptyline metabolism within two days, both when starting (induction) and on discontinuation (n = 6, von Bahr et al, Clin Pharmacol Ther 1998;**64**:18–26). Use an alternative to barbiturates or monitor tricyclic levels.

Benzodiazepines + tricyclics
See benzodiazepines (4.1.1).

Beta-blockers + tricyclics
Enhanced maprotiline toxicity has been reported, labetolol increases imipramine plasma levels by 28% (n = 12, RCT, p/c, c/o, Hermann et al, J Clin Pharmacol 1992;**32**:176–83) and there are cases of propranolol possibly raising imipramine levels in children (n = 2, Gillette and Tannery, J Am Acad Child Adolesc Psychiatry 1994;**33**:223–4), possibly via 2D6 inhibition. This would appear to be a rare but possible interaction.

Buprenorphine + amitriptyline
No enhanced CNS or respiratory depression have been seen (n = 12, d/b, p/c, c/o, Saarialho–Kere et al, Eur J Clin Pharmacol 1987; **33**:139–46).

Bupropion + tricyclics
See bupropion (4.6.6).

Calcium-channel blockers + tricyclics
Amitriptyline clearance was reduced by diltiazem and verapamil in one study, with adverse effects increased (n = 32, Hermann et al, J Clin Pharmacol 1992;**32**:176–83). Diltiazem may increase nor–triptyline concentrations (n = 1, Krahenbuhl et al, Eur J Clin Pharmacol 1996;**49**:417–9). Enhanced cardiac side-effects are also possible.

Cannabis + tricyclics
See antidepressants + cannabis (4.7.2).

CARBAMAZEPINE + TRICYCLICS
See carbamazepine (4.5.1).

Charcoal, activated + tricyclics
5–10g may reduce the absorption of tricyclics by up to 75% if given within 30 minutes and may be an effective treatment for overdose, even up to two hours after the overdose is taken (open, Dawling et al, Eur J Clin Pharmacol 1978;**14**:445–7).

Cholestyramine + doxepin
Plasma levels of doxepin may be reduced to a third by cholestyramine (n = 1, Geeze et al, Psychosomatics 1988; **29**:233–5).

CLONIDINE + TRICYCLICS
Tricyclics can be expected to antagonise the hypotensive effects of clonidine (e.g. Hui, J Am Geriatr Soc 1983;**31**:164–5).

Cocaine + tricyclics
See antidepressants + cocaine (4.7.3).

Codfish + clomipramine
In the never-ending quest for completeness, it is (probably) worth reporting that a generalised urticaria (Naranjo 'probable') has occurred after someone ate codfish while taking clomipramine 75–100mg/d (n = 1, Gallelli et al, Pharmacopsychiatry 2006;**39**:154–6).

Co-trimoxazole + tricyclics
Relapse has been reported when co-trimoxazole was added to a tricyclic (n=5, L'Encephale 1987;**8**:123–6).

Dextropropoxyphene + doxepin
There are reports of doxepin plasma levels raised by up to 150% with dextropropoxyphene, via 2D6 inhibition.

Disopyramide + tricyclics
Increased anticholinergic effects may be seen (Hartel et al, Clin Pharmacol Ther 1974;**15**:551–5) and the BNF notes an increased risk of ventricular arrhythmias.

Disulfiram + tricyclics
Amitriptyline may enhance the effects of disulfiram (MacCallum, Lancet 1969;**i**:313) and tricyclic levels may be increased by about 30% by CYP1A2 inhibition (n = 2, Ciraulo et al, Am J Psychiatry 1985;**142**:1373–4).

Duloxetine + tricyclics
See duloxetine (4.3.3.2).

Fibre + tricyclics
There are several cases of a high fibre diet reducing tricyclic levels by up to a third (and hence to inactive levels), e.g. with doxepin. This might explain non-response in some patients.

Fluconazole + tricyclics
Inhibition of CYP3A4 by fluconazole has

resulted in cases of elevated, toxic nortriptyline levels (n = 1, Gannon, *Ann Pharmacother* 1992; **26**:1456–7) and syncope (Robinson *et al*, *Ann Pharmacother* 2000;**34**:1406–9). Delirium (Duggal, *Gen Hosp Psychiatry* 2003;**25**:297–8) has occurred with amitriptyline and fluconazole.

Glyceryl trinitrate + tricyclics
See nitrates + tricyclics (below).

H2-blockers + tricyclics
CYP1A2 inhibition by **cimetidine** may decrease the metabolism and increase the half-life and plasma levels of tricyclics, e.g. amitriptyline (by 37–80%, Curry *et al*, *Eur J Clin Pharmacol* 1985;**29**:429–33), doxepin (by 30%, n = 10, RCT, Abernethy and Todd, *J Clin Psychopharmacol* 1986;**6**:8–12), imipramine (by over 100%, n = 12, RCT, d/b, p/c, c/o, Wells *et al*, *Eur J Clin Pharmacol* 1986;**31**:285–90) and nortriptyline (by 20%, Henauer and Hollister, *Clin Pharmacol Ther* 1984;**35**:183–7). Other H2-blockers, e.g. **ranitidine**, do not appear to interact this way (n = 6, open, Sutherland *et al*, *Eur J Clin Pharmacol* 1987;**32**:159–64).

Hypoglycaemics + tricyclics
Enhanced hypoglycaemia has been reported with doxepin and nortriptyline (n = 2, True *et al*, *Am J Psychiatry* 1987;**144**:1220–1), so monitor blood glucose regularly.

Levodopa + tricyclics
A small reduction in the effect of levodopa may be seen (open, Morgan *et al*, *Neurology* 1975; **25**:1029), of minimal clinical significance.

Levothyroxine + tricyclics
This is usually a synergistic interaction (see *1.14*) but a few isolated cases of tachycardia and hypothyroidism have been reported.

Lithium + tricyclics
Although formerly well used some adverse reactions have been reported, e.g. myoclonus (Devanand *et al*, *J Clin Psychopharmacol* 1988;**8**:446), neurotoxicity with motor symptoms and seizures (e.g. Austin *et al*, *J Clin Psychiatry* 1990;**51**:344) and NMS with amoxapine (n = 1, Gupta and Racaniello, *Ann Clin Psychiatry* 2000;**12**:107–9).

MAOIs + TRICYCLICS
See MAOIs (*4.3.4*).

Melatonin + tricyclics
See melatonin (*4.1.4*).

Methadone + tricyclics
See methadone (*4.6.10*).

Methyldopa + desipramine
The hypotensive effect of methyldopa may be decreased, with possible tachycardia and CNS stimulation (Van Spanning *et al*, *Int J Clin Pharmacol Biopharm* 1975;**11**:65–7).

Methylene blue + clomipramine *
See methylene blue + paroxetine (*4.3.2.4*).

Methylphenidate + tricyclics
See methylphenidate (*4.6.11*).

Mirtazapine + tricyclics
See mirtazapine (*4.3.3.4*).

Moclobemide + tricyclics
See moclobemide (*4.3.3.5*).

Modafinil + tricyclics
See modafinil (*4.6.12*).

Morphine + tricyclics
Tricyclics may increase the bioavailability of morphine and potentiate the analgesic effect, usually beneficial (Ventafridda *et al*, *Lancet* 1987;**i**:1204).

Nitrates (sublingual) + tricyclics
Tricyclic-induced dry mouth may reduce the dissolution of sublingual nitrates.

Olanzapine + tricyclics
See olanzapine (*4.2.5*).

Oral contraceptives/estrogens + tricyclics
Akathisia (n = 3, Krishnan *et al*, *Am J Psychiatry* 1984;**141**:696–7), reduced tricyclic effectiveness and enhanced tricyclic toxicity have been reported. Best to monitor the tricyclic closely.

Orlistat + tricyclics
A small trial suggested lack of interaction with clomipramine (n = 8, 8/52, Hilger *et al*, *J Clin Psychopharmacol* 2002;**22**:68–70).

Phenindione + tricyclics
An enhanced risk of bleeding may occur.

Phenylbutazone + tricyclics
Tricyclic absorption may be delayed or reduced by phenylbutazone (Consolo *et al*, *Eur J Pharmacol* 1970;**10**:239–42).

PHENYTOIN + TRICYCLICS
See phenytoin (*4.5.9*).

Quetiapine + tricyclics
See quetiapine (*4.2.6*).

Quinine/quinidine + tricyclics
Raised nortriptyline levels may occur quinidine and quinine (n = 10, Steiner *et al*, *Clin Pharmacol Ther* 1988; **43**:577–81), via 2D6 inhibition. Best to monitor tricyclic levels.

Reboxetine + tricyclics
See reboxetine (*4.3.3.6*).

SERTINDOLE + TRICYCLICS *
See sertindole (*4.2.8*).

Smoking + tricyclics

See smoking (4.7.4).

Sodium oxybate + tricyclics

See sodium oxybate (4.6.13).

SSRIs + TRICYCLICS

Tricyclics are predominantly metabolised by CYP2D6, and SSRIs produce a dose-related inhibition of this enzyme. Fluoxetine, paroxetine and fluvoxamine all cause significant inhibition at therapeutic doses, whereas citalopram/escitalopram and sertraline cause little clinically significant 2D6 inhibition at standard doses. Citalopram (and presumably escitalopram) has no effect on some tricyclic levels (n=5, Baettig et al, Eur J Clin Pharmacol 1993;**44**:403–5), although desipramine (but not imipramine) levels may rise slightly (e.g. n=1, Ashton, J Clin Psychiatry 2000;**61**:144). Fluoxetine may double or triple tricyclic levels, e.g. with amitriptyline (e.g. fatal, n=1, Preskorn and Baker, JAMA 1997; **277**:1682; n=29, open, Vandel et al, Pharmacol Res 1995; **31**:347–53), clomipramine (n=4, Vandel et al, Neuropsychobiology 1992;**25**:202–7), imipramine (Leroj and Walentynowicz, Can J Psychiatry 1996;**41**:318–9), even if the tricyclic is used after an extended interval (Extein, Am J Psychiatry 1991;**148**:1601–2). Tricyclic doses should be reduced by up to 75% if used with fluoxetine (n=3, Wester-Meyer, J Clin Pharmacol 1991;**31**:388–92). Fluvoxamine increases amitriptyline (n=22, Vezmar et al, J Pharmacol Sci 2009;**110**:98–104), clomipramine (n=1, Bertschy et al, Eur J Clin Pharmacol 1991;**40**:119–20) and imipramine levels (Maskall and Lam, Am J Psychiatry 1993; **50**:1566), also by inhibiting both hydroxylation and N-demethylation (Hartter et al, Psychopharmacology 1993;**110**:302–8). Paroxetine significantly reduces the metabolism of amitriptyline and imipramine (e.g. Skjelbo and Brosen, Br J Clin Pharmacol 1992;**34**:256–61), resulting in enhanced tricyclic toxicity. Sertraline 50 mg/d may produce a 31–60% increase in desipramine levels (n=18, RCT, 7/52, Preskorn et al, J Clin Psychopharmacol 1994;**14**:90–8) but a 200–300% increase has been seen (e.g. n=12, RCT, open, Kurtz et al, Clin Pharmacol Ther 1997;**62**:145–56). Serotonin syndrome has been reported with many SSRI-tricyclic combinations (see 5.14).

St John's wort + tricyclics

See St John's wort (4.3.3.10).

Sucralfate + amitriptyline

One small study showed a marked reduction in amitriptyline absorption (Fed Proc 1986;**45**:205).

Tea or coffee + tricyclics

Studies have shown that some tricyclics (e.g. amitriptyline and imipramine) precipitate out of solution to form a tannin complex with tea and coffee (J Pharm Sci 1984;**73**:1056–8). The clinical significance is thought to be minimal (Bowen et al, Lancet 1981;**i**:1217–8).

TERBINAFINE + TRICYCLICS

Terbinafine, a potent 2D6 inhibitor, may triple desipramine plasma levels (n=1, O'Reardon et al, Am J Psychiatry 2002;**159**:492) and induce imipramine (e.g. n=1, Teitelbaum and Pearson, Am J Psychiatry 2001;**158**:2086) and nortriptyline toxicity (n=1, van der Kuy et al, Ann Pharmacother 2002;**36**:1712–4). A significant rise may occur in amitriptyline levels, an effect that may, extraordinarily, last for up to three to six months after stopping terbinafine (n=1, Castberg et al, Ther Drug Monit 2005;**27**:680–2).

Valproate + tricyclics

See antidepressants + valproate (4.5.15).

VASOCONSTRICTOR SYMPATHOMIMETICS + TRICYCLICS

A greatly enhanced response, e.g. hypertension and arrhythmias, to norepinephrine and phenylephrine in patients taking tricyclics has been shown in many reports. Doxepin may have a lesser effect. Local anaesthetics with epinephrine appear safe. Moderate doses of cold cures containing sympathomimetics should present little risk in healthy patients.

Venlafaxine + tricyclics

Venlafaxine increases imipramine levels, showing a consistent but probably clinically modest effect (n=8, Albers et al, Psychiatr Res 2000;**6**:35–43). Serotonin syndrome has been reported with venlafaxine and amitriptyline (n=1, Postgrad Med J 2000;**76**:254–6) and a GTC fit with venlafaxine and trimipramine (n=1, Schlienger et al, Ann Pharmacother 2000;**34**:1402–5).

Warfarin + tricyclics

Normally there is no problem, but occasional control problems have been reported with lofepramine (see Sayal et al, Acta Psychiatr Scand 2000;**102**:250–55).

Yohimbine + tricyclics

Tricyclics can potentiate the blood pressure changes caused by yohimbine, especially if blood

4

pressure is already raised (mentioned in Fugh-Berman, *Lancet* 2000;**355**:134–8).

Zopiclone + tricyclics

See zopiclone (*4.1.8*).

4.3.2 SSRIs (SELECTIVE SEROTONIN REUPTAKE INHIBITORS)

Drug interactions involving the P450 system have been described for all SSRIs, but there are significant differences in the isoenzymes inhibited and the degree of inhibition.

The *in vitro* inhibition of 2D6 on a molar basis is: paroxetine (most potent), norfluoxetine, fluoxetine, sertraline, fluvoxamine and escitalopram/citalopram (least potent). *In vivo* is probably broadly similar. Fluoxetine and paroxetine are probably similar in 2D6 inhibition, but with some variation (n = 31, RCT, using multiple-dose fluoxetine 60 mg/d, fluvoxamine 100 mg/d, paroxetine 20 mg/d, or sertraline 100 mg/d; Alfaro *et al*, *J Clin Psychopharmacol* 1999;**19**:155–63).

Review: overview and review of SSRI interactions and P450 effects (Hemeryck and Belpaire, *Curr Drug Metab* 2002;**3**:13–37).

4.3.2.1 CITALOPRAM AND ESCITALOPRAM

Citalopram is a weak inhibitor of CYP2D6 and is metabolised mainly by 3A4 (also 2D6 and 2C19). A review (Brosen and Naranjo, *Eur Neuropsychopharmacol* 2001;**11**:275–83) concludes that citalopram is neither a source nor a cause of clinically important drug–drug interactions. Escitalopram would be expected to have similar characteristics.

Acenocoumarol + citalopram/escitalopram

There is a reported case of interaction (n = 1, Borras-Blasco *et al*, *Ann Pharmacother* 2002; **36**:345).

Alcohol + citalopram/escitalopram

See alcohol (*4.7.1*).

Alimemazine (trimeprazine) + citalopram/escitalopram

See antipsychotics + citalopram/escitalopram.

Antipsychotics + citalopram/escitalopram *

Pooled data from two trials shows no substantial effect from adjunctive **aripiprazole** on escitalopram kinetics (n = 163, d/b, p/c, Boulton *et al*, *J Psychopharmacol* 2010;**24**:537–46; MS) although urinary obstruction has

been reported in an elderly patient taking citalopram and aripiprazole (n = 1, Padala *et al*, *J Clin Psychopharmacol* 2006; **26**:667–8).

Levomepromazine may increase plasma levels of citalopram by about a third (Milne and Goa, *Drugs* 1991;**41**:450–77), possibly via enzyme inhibition and of minimal clinical significance. There has been no detectable effect from citalopram on the plasma levels of other antipsychotics (n = 90, d/b, Syvalahti *et al*, *J Intern Med Res* 1997;**25**:24–32), e.g. citalopram 40 mg/d had no effect on the plasma levels of **clozapine** (n = 8, 200–400 mg/d), **risperidone** (n = 7, 4–6 mg/d) in patients with chronic schizophrenia (8/52, Avenoso *et al*, *Clin Drug Investigation* 1998;**16**:393–8), although torsades de pointes with risperidone and citalopram has been reported (n = 1, Blaschke *et al*, *Pharmacopsychiatry* 2007;**40**:294–5). Despite this, the FDA has issued a warning about citalopram raising **clozapine** levels by clinically significant levels.

Atomoxetine + citalopram/escitalopram

See SSRIs + atomoxetine (*4.6.4*).

Benzodiazepines + citalopram/escitalopram

Lack of interaction has been shown between citalopram and the CYP3A4 substrate triazolam (n = 18, open, Nolting and Abramowitz, *Pharmacother* 2000; **20**:750–5) and citalopram does not prolong the half-life of alprazolam (Hall *et al*, *J Clin Psycho-pharmacol* 2003;**23**:349–57).

Beta-blockers + citalopram/escitalopram

Escitalopram is a weak 2D6 inhibitor, but can increase metoprolol's AUC by 89% (Preskorn *et al*, *J Clin Psychopharmacol* 2007;**27**:28–34).

Buspirone + citalopram/escitalopram

Hyponatraemia and serotonin syndrome has been reported (Spigset and Adielsson, *Int Clin Psychopharmacol* 1997; **12**:61–3).

Carbamazepine + citalopram/escitalopram

Carbamazepine may reduce the proportion and concentration of the escitalopram isomer (n = 6, Steinacher *et al*, *Eur Neuropsychopharmacol* 2002;**12**:255–60). Citalopram has no effect on carbamazepine kinetics (n = 12, open, Moller *et al*, *J Clin Psychophamacol* 2001;**21**:493–9).

Charcoal + citalopram/escitalopram

25 g activated charcoal given 30 minutes after citalopram reduced citalopram AUC by 51%, and peak levels by over 50%. Concurrent gastric lavage did not provide any additional reductions (n = 9, RCT, Lapatto-Reiniluoto *et al*, *Br J Clin Pharmacol* 1999;**48**:148–53).

Ciclosporin + citalopram/escitalopram
Citalopram has no effect on ciclosporin kinetics (Liston et al, Psychosomatics 2001;**42**:370–2).

Cimetidine + citalopram/escitalopram
Cimetidine increases escitalopram levels but this is unlikely to be clinically significant (n = 16, RCT, p/c, Malling et al, Br J Clin Pharmacol 2005;**60**:287–90).

Cyproheptadine + citalopram *
A death has been reported after intoxication of these two serotonergic agents (n=1, Hargrove and Molina, J Anal Toxicol 2009;**33**:564-7).

Digoxin + citalopram/escitalopram
Steady state citalopram 40mg/d had no effect on the kinetics of single doses of digoxin 1mg (n = 11, open, c/o, 50/7, Larsen et al, J Clin Pharmacol 2001;**41**:340).

Donepezil + citalopram/escitalopram
See SSRIs + donepezil (4.6.3.1).

Duloxetine + citalopram/escitalopram
See SSRIs + duloxetine (4.3.3.2).

Fluconazole + citalopram/escitalopram
Serotonin syndrome has been reported with this combination, probably via 2C19 inhibition (n = 2, Levin et al, Gen Hosp Psychiatry 2008;**30**:372–7).

Fluvoxamine + citalopram/escitalopram
Fluvoxamine may increase the ratio of escitalopram to R-citalopram, enhancing its action (n = 7, open, Bondolfi et al, Psychopharmacol [Berl] 1996;**128**:421–5).

Itopride + escitalopram
Tardive dyskinesia has been reported after long–term co-administration of escitalopram and the D2 antagonist antinauseant itopride (n = 1, Park et al, Prog Neuropsychopharmacol Biol Psychiatry 2009;**33**: 380–1).

Ketoconazole + citalopram/escitalopram
Single doses of ketoconazole have no effect on citalopram (n = 18, RCT, d/b, c/o, Gutierrez and Abramowitz, Pharmacotherapy 2001;**21**:163–8).

Lamotrigine + citalopram/escitalopram
Myoclonus has been reported with the combination (n = 1, Rosenhagen et al, J Clin Psychopharmacol 2006;**26**:346–7).

Linezolid + citalopram/escitalopram *
In people taking SSRIs, serotonin syndrome may occur around nine days after the introduction of linezolid (longer the older you are); symptoms may resolve in three days or longer (eg. n = 12, Morales–Molina et al, J Antimicrob Chemother 2005;**56**:1176–8; n = 1, McClean et al, Ir J Med Sci 2011;**180**:285–6).

Lithium + citalopram/escitalopram
No pharmacokinetic interaction was noted in one study (n = 24, open, Gram et al, Ther Drug Monit 1993;**15**:18–24).

MAOIs + citalopram/escitalopram
See MAOIs (4.3.4).

Melatonin + citalopram/escitalopram
Citalopram may slow the metabolism of exogenous melatonin (n = 15, RCT, d/b, p/c, 21/7, Huuhka et al, Methods Find Exp Clin Pharmacol 2006;**28**:447–50).

Methylene blue + citalopram/escitalopram *
See methylene blue + paroxetine (4.3.2.4).

Metoclopramide + citalopram/escitalopram
See metoclopramide + fluvoxamine (4.3.2.3).

Moclobemide + citalopram/escitalopram
See SSRIs + moclobemide (4.3.3.5).

NSAIDs + citalopram/escitalopram
See NSAIDs + fluoxetine (4.3.2.2).

Omeprazole + citalopram/escitalopram
Omeprazole increases escitalopram levels but this is unlikely to be clinically significant (n = 16, RCT, p/c, Malling et al, Br J Clin Pharmacol 2005;**60**:287–90).

Oxcarbazepine + citalopram/escitalopram
See oxcarbazepine (4.5.7).

Perhexiline + citalopram/escitalopram
Perhexiline toxicity with citalopram has been reported (n = 1, Nyfort–Hansen, Med J Aust 2002;**176**:560–1).

Propafenone + citalopram/escitalopram
There is a case of citalopram enhancing propafenone's side-effects such as dizziness, and mimicking coronary artery disease (n = 1, Garcia, Am J Geriatr Pharmacother 2008;**6**:96–9).

Rasagiline + escitalopram
Lack of significant interaction has been shown, although the AUC for rasagiline was increased by 42% (n = 12, 17/7, Hilli et al, Prog Neuropsychopharmacol Biol Psychiatry 2009; **33**:1526–32). Confusion and hallucinations have also been reported (n = 1, Bandrés et al, Farm Hosp 2009;**33**:173–5).

Ritonavir + citalopram/escitalopram
No pharmacokinetic interaction occurs (n = 21 [c = 18], RCT, open, c/o, Gutierrez et al, Clin Ther 2003;**25**:1200–10).

Selegiline + citalopram/escitalopram
One study showed the lack of a clinically significant interaction (n = 18, RCT, Laine et al, Clin Neuropharmacol 1997;**20**:419–33).

4

Sertindole + citalopram/escitalopram*
See sertindole (4.2.8).

Sibutramine + citalopram/escitalopram *
Hypomania has been reported with this combination (n = 1, Benazzi, *J Clin Psychiatry* 2002;**63**:165). A serotonin syndrome is also possible.

St John's wort + citalopram/escitalopram
See SSRIs + St John's wort (4.3.3.10).

Sympathomimetics + citalopram/escitalopram
Augmentation of amfetamines is theoretically possible (see sympathomimetics + fluoxetine).

Tamoxifen + citalopram/escitalopram *
A nested case-control study showed that long-term citalopram does not reduce tamoxifen's breast cancer protective effect (n=732, Lash *et al, Acta Oncol* 2010;**49**:305-12).

Topiramate + citalopram/escitalopram
See citalopram + topiramate (4.5.14).

Tramadol + citalopram/escitalopram
Serotonin syndrome has been reported with tramadol 50mg/d and citalopram 10mg/d in a patient with a slow 2D6 and 2C19 metaboliser (n = 1, Mahlberg *et al, Am J Psychiatry* 2004;**161**:1129).

Trazodone + citalopram/escitalopram
No pharmacokinetic interaction occurs (n=41, Prapotnik *et al, Int J Clin Pharmacol Ther* 2004; **42**:120–4).

Tricyclics + citalopram/escitalopram
See SSRIs + tricyclics (4.3.1).

Triptans + citalopram/escitalopram
The literature notes an increased risk of CNS toxicity with sumatriptan and recommends avoiding the combination. See also triptans + fluoxetine (4.3.2.2).

Warfarin + citalopram/escitalopram
Citalopram 40mg/d may produce a small increase in prothrombin time (n=12, Preskorn *et al, Br J Clin Pharmacol* 1997;**44**:199–202), but this is probably clinically insignificant (Sayal *et al, Acta Psychiatr Scand* 2000;**102**:250–5).

Zolpidem + citalopram/escitalopram
See SSRIs + zolpidem (4.1.7).

4.3.2.2 FLUOXETINE
Fluoxetine is 95% protein bound and substantially inhibits CYP2D6 and probably 2C9/10, moderately inhibits 2C19 and weakly inhibits 3A3/4 and has a higher incidence of interactions with drugs metabolised by these enzymes. Norfluoxetine is a potent CYP3A4 inhibitor and a moderate inhibitor of 2D6.

Alcohol + fluoxetine
See alcohol (4.7.1).

Alosetron + fluoxetine
There is no significant effect from the 5-HT3 antagonist alosetron on fluoxetine kinetics (n = 12, D'Souza *et al, J Clin Pharmacol* 2001;**41**:455–8).

Amfetamines + fluoxetine
See sympathomimetics + fluoxetine.

ANTIPSYCHOTICS + FLUOXETINE *
See antipsychotics (4.2.1), aripiprazole (4.2.2), asenapine (4.2.3), clozapine (4.2.4), olanzapine (4.2.5), quetiapine (4.2.6), risperidone and paliperidone (4.2.7) and sertindole (4.2.8).

Atomoxetine + fluoxetine
See SSRIs + atomoxetine (4.6.4).

Beta-blockers + fluoxetine *
Bradycardia may occur in people taking fluoxetine and metoprolol, possibly due to CYP2D6 inhibition. Atenolol, sotalol (n = 2, Proudlove, *Lancet* 1993;**341**: 967) and nebivolol (Lindamood *et al, J Clin Pharmacol* 2011;**51**:575–85) may be suitable alternatives. Fluoxetine may inhibit the metabolism of R-carvedilol (rather than S-carvedilol), but this appears to have little clinical significance (n = 10, RCT, d/b, c/o, 28/7, Graff *et al, J Clin Pharmacol* 2001;**41**:97–106).

Benzodiazepines + fluoxetine
Fluoxetine may slightly increase the plasma levels of some benzodiazepines (e.g. **diazepam**: n = 10, Lemberger *et al, Clin Pharmacol Ther* 1988;**43**:412–9), although probably not **midazolam** (n = 10, RCT, 12/7, Lam *et al, J Clin Pharmacol* 2003;**43**:1274–82). Desmethyldiaze-pam levels may be lower, which may explain the lack of additive psychomotor impairment (Ciraulo and Shader, *J Clin Psychopharmacol* 1990;**10**:213–7). Fluoxetine increases **alprazolam's** half-life by 16% (Hall *et al, J Clin Psychopharmacol* 2003;**23**:349–57) due to decreased clearance. The clinical significance is minor.

Bupropion + fluoxetine
See bupropion (4.6.6).

Buspirone + fluoxetine
See buspirone (4.1.2).

Calcium-channel blockers + fluoxetine
Oedema, weight gain and headache have occurred with verapamil and fluoxetine (n = 2, Sternbach, *J Clin Psychopharmacol* 1991;**11**:390).

Lowering doses is recommended if an interaction is suspected.

Cannabis + fluoxetine
See antidepressants + cannabis (4.7.2).

Carbamazepine + fluoxetine
Two studies have shown that fluoxetine and norfluoxetine inhibit carbamazepine metabolism, increasing levels by up to 25% (n = 14, Gidal *et al*, *Ther Drug Monit* 1993;**15**:405–9), but a small study showed fluoxetine 20mg/d to have no effect on carbamazepine levels (n = 8, open, Spina *et al*, *Ther Drug Monit* 1993;**15**:247–50). A toxic serotonin syndrome has been reported (n = 1, Dursun *et al*, *Lancet* 1993;**342**:442–3).

Ciclosporin + fluoxetine
Ciclosporin plasma concentrations were nearly doubled by fluoxetine 20mg/d in one report, probably by CYP3A4 inhibition (n = 1, Holton and Bonser, *Br Med J* 1995;**311**:422).

Clarithromycin + fluoxetine
Acute delirium has been reported when clarithromycin was added to fluoxetine (e.g. n = 1, Tracy and Johns Cupp, *Ann Pharmacother* 1996;**30**:1199–200), probably via CYP3A4 inhibition.

Cocaine + fluoxetine
See antidepressants + cocaine (4.7.3).

Cyproheptadine + fluoxetine
Patients treated with cyproheptadine for fluoxetine-induced anorgasmia may relapse (n = 3, Feder, *J Clin Psychiatry* 1991;**52**:163–4), and interaction has been reported in a bulimic patient (n = 2, Goldbloom and Kennedy, *J Clin Psychiatry* 1991;**52**:261–2).

Dextromethorphan + fluoxetine
Visual hallucinations lasting 6–8 hours occurred in a patient taking fluoxetine 20mg/d who also took a cough mixture containing dextromethorphan (n=1, Achamallah, *Am J Psychiatry* 1992;**149**:1406), as has a serotonin syndrome (n = 1, Navarro *et al*, *Gen Hosp Psychiatry* 2006; **28**:78–80).

Digoxin + fluoxetine
There is no apparent increased risk of digoxin toxicity after initiation of paroxetine, fluoxetine, sertraline and fluvoxamine compared to tricyclics and benzodiazepines (n = 3144, Juurlink *et al*, *Br J Clin Pharmacol* 2005;**59**:102–7).

Donepezil + fluoxetine
See SSRIs + donepezil (4.6.3.1).

Duloxetine + fluoxetine
See SSRIs + duloxetine (4.3.3.2).

Lamotrigine + fluoxetine
Delirium has occurred within two weeks of a lamotrigine dose being increased from 200mg/d to 400mg/d in a lady taking fluoxetine 40mg/d (n = 1, Chistyyakova and Amos, *Am J Psychiatry* 2008;**165**:918–9).

Lithium + fluoxetine
See lithium (4.4).

LSD + fluoxetine
GTC convulsions occurred in one patient who took a double dose of LSD while on fluoxetine 20mg/d, having previously taken single doses of LSD uneventfully (n = 1, Achamallah, *Am J Psychiatry* 1992;**149**:843–4).

MAOIs + FLUOXETINE
See MAOIs (4.3.4)

Methadone + fluoxetine
See methadone (4.6.10).

Methylene blue + fluoxetine *
See methylene blue + paroxetine (4.3.2.4).

Methylphenidate + fluoxetine
See fluoxetine + methylphenidate (4.6.11).

Metoclopramide + fluoxetine
Fluoxetine increases metoclopramide plasma levels, increasing Cmax by 42% and half-life by 53% (n = 24, c/o,Viase *et al*, *Biopharm Drug Dispos* 2006;**27**:285–9). See also fluvoxamine.

Mirtazapine + fluoxetine
See mirtazapine (4.3.3.4).

Moclobemide + fluoxetine
See SSRIs + moclobemide (4.3.3.5).

Morphine + fluoxetine
Fluoxetine may mildly enhance the analgesic effects of morphine and reduce its side-effects (n = 15, d/b, Erjavec *et al*, *J Clin Pharmacol* 2000; **40**:1286–95).

NSAIDs + SSRIs
There is a three-fold increase in upper GI bleeding, although the absolute risk remains low, e.g. NNH = 411 for SSRIs alone, NNH = 106 for an SSRI plus NSAID (s = 4, n = 153,000, Loke *et al*, *Aliment Pharmacol Ther* 2008;**27**:31–40). So, use NSAIDs and SSRIs together with caution in the over 80s, in those with a history of GI bleeding and in those taking aspirin or other NSAIDs (*Drug Ther Bull* 2004;**42**:17–8).

Olanzapine + fluoxetine
See SSRIs + olanzapine (4.2.5).

Oral contraceptives + fluoxetine
Lack of interaction has been shown (n = 1698, Koke *et al*, *Am J Obstet Gynecol* 2002;**187**:551–5).

4

Pentazocine + fluoxetine

Rapid toxicity has been reported, although an interaction was not proven (n = 1, Hansen et al, Am J Psychiatry 1990;**147**:949–50).

PHENYTOIN + FLUOXETINE

See phenytoin (4.5.9).

Quetiapine + fluoxetine

See SSRIs + quetiapine (4.2.6).

Reboxetine + fluoxetine

See reboxetine (4.3.3.6).

RISPERIDONE + FLUOXETINE

See risperidone (4.2.7).

Rivastigmine + fluoxetine

See rivastigmine (4.6.3.3).

Selegiline + fluoxetine

There are isolated cases of toxic reactions, e.g. hypomania, hypertension and shivering (n = 1, Suchowersky and de Vries, Can J Psychiatry 1991;**35**:571–2), ataxia (n = 1, Jermain et al, Ann Pharmacother 1992;**26**:1300) and hypertension (Montastruc et al, Lancet 1993;**341**:555).

SERTINDOLE + FLUOXETINE *

See sertindole (4.2.8).

Sertraline + fluoxetine

See sertraline (4.3.2.5).

Sibutramine + fluoxetine *

Serotonin syndrome is possible.

St John's wort + fluoxetine

See SSRIs + St John's wort (4.3.3.10).

Sympathomimetics + fluoxetine

An interaction has been suggested by reports of extreme restlessness, agitation and psychotic symptoms apparently caused by fluoxetine augmentation of amfetamines (n = 2, Barrett et al, Br J Psychiatry 1996;**168**:253).

Tamoxifen + fluoxetine *

See tamoxifen + paroxetine (4.3.2.4).

Tolterodine + fluoxetine

Fluoxetine inhibits the 2D6 metabolism of tolterodine (n = 13, open, Brynne et al, Br J Clin Pharmacology 1999;**48**:553–63).

Tramadol + fluoxetine

Serotonin syndrome and mania have been reported (n = 1, Kesavan and Sobala, J Roy Soc Med 1999;**92**:474–5; n = 1, Gonzalez–Pinto et al, Am J Psychiatry 2001; **158**:964–5).

Trazodone + fluoxetine

No pharmacokinetic interaction occurs (n = 16, Prapotnik et al, Int J Clin Pharmacol Ther 2004; **42**:120–4), although trazodone toxicity (e.g. Neirenberg et al, J Clin Psychiatry 1992;**53**:83) and

myoclonus have been reported (n = 1, Darko et al, Vet Hum Toxicol 2001;**43**:214–5).

TRICYCLICS + FLUOXETINE

See SSRIs + tricyclics (4.3.1).

Triptans + fluoxetine *

The literature notes an increased risk of CNS toxicity with all SSRIs and recommends avoiding the combination. However, the American Headache Society position statement reviews 25 published cases and concludes that none satisfied the Hunter Serotonin Toxicity Criteria, so the evidence for limiting SSRIs with triptans is lacking, although some caution is still prudent (Evans et al, Headache 2010;**50**:1089–99). The evidence is that activation of 5HT2A is the predominant cause, so there is neither clinical nor theoretical reason to suggest serious SS from triptans and SSRIs (Gillman, Headache 2010;**50**:264–72) and denies a highly effective drug for a disabling (for a day or so) and painful condition (and the author is speaking here from personal experience). Triptans with low lipid solubility and a short half-life (e.g. sumatriptan, rizatriptan or zolmitriptan) may in theory be a safer choice than others (e.g. frovatriptan, which has a long half-life).

Tryptophan + fluoxetine

Central toxicity has been reported (n = 5, Steiner and Fontaine, Biol Psychiatry 1986;**21**:1067–71).

Valproate + fluoxetine

Valproate levels may rise by up to 50% if fluoxetine is added, although the mechanism is not established (e.g. Lucena et al, Am J Psychiatry 1998;**155**:575), and reduced valproate levels have also been reported (Droulers et al, J Clin Psychopharmacol 1997;**17**:139–40).

Venlafaxine + fluoxetine

Serotonin syndrome has been reported when venlafaxine was started immediately after fluoxetine was discontinued (n = 1, Bhatara et al, Ann Pharmacother 1998;**32**:432–6), as have severe anticholinergic side–effects (n = 4, Benazzi, J Clin Psychopharmacol 1999;**19**:96–8).

WARFARIN + FLUOXETINE

An in vitro study indicated fluoxetine has a potentially significant effect on warfarin (Schmider et al, Br J Clin Pharmacol 1997;**44**:495–8). Raised INR has been reported within ten days of starting fluoxetine (n = 2, Woolfrey et al, Br Med J 1993; **307**:241) and two patients on warfarin with stable INRs experienced dramatic increases in

INR when fluoxetine 20 mg/d was added (n = 2, Hanger and Thomas, *N Z Med J* 1995;**108**:157). There is also a case report of an elderly man prescribed warfarin, diazepam and fluoxetine who developed an elevated INR and died from a cerebral haemorrhage (n = 1, Dent and Orrock, *Pharmacotherapy* 1997;**17**:170–2).

Zolpidem + fluoxetine
See SSRIs + zolpidem (*4.1.6*).

4.3.2.3 FLUVOXAMINE
Fluvoxamine is 80% protein bound and strongly inhibits CYP1A2, 2D6, 3A4 and 2C19 (and possibly 2C8 weakly) and may have a high incidence of interactions with drugs metabolised by these enzymes (n = 20, *Clin Pharmacol Ther* 1998;**64**:257–68). It is probably only metabolised by CYP2D6 to fluvoxamino alcohol, then by alcohol dehydrogenase (Miura and Ohkubo, *Xenobiotica* 2007;**37**:169–79).

AGOMELATINE + FLUVOXAMINE
See agomelatine (*4.3.3.1*).

Alcohol + fluvoxamine
See alcohol (*4.7.1*).

AMINOPHYLLINE + FLUVOXAMINE
See theophylline + fluvoxamine.

Antipsychotics + fluvoxamine
Fluvoxamine is a 1A2 inhibitor and asenapine plasma levels may rise by up to 29% (US PI). Seizures have been reported with levomepromazine and fluvoxamine (n = 1, Grinshpoon et al, *Int Clin Psychopharmacol* 1993;**8**:61–2), although levomepromazine does not appear to increase fluvoxamine levels (n = 15, Yoshimura et al, *Int Clin Psychopharmacol* 2000;**15**:233–5). Fluvoxamine 100 mg/d had no effect on plasma levels of risperidone 3–6 mg/d but 200 mg/d increased concentrations by 26% (n = 11, open, 8/52, D'Arrigo et al, *Pharmacol Res* 2005;**52**:497–501). Neurotoxicity (e.g. confusion, diaphoresis and myoclonus) has been reported within two days of fluvoxamine being added to risperidone (n = 1, Reeves et al, *Ann Pharmacother* 2002; **36**:440–3). Fluvoxamine produces a dose-dependent increase in haloperidol levels, 150 mg/d raising levels by 60%, although this was without additional side-effects at 6 mg/d (n = 12, Yasui-Furukori et al, *Psychopharmacol [Berl]* 2003; **171**:223–7). See also clozapine (*4.2.4*).

Benzodiazepines + fluvoxamine
Plasma concentrations of bromazepam are doubled by fluvoxamine, but lorazepam is unaffected (van Harten et al, mentioned in *Clin Pharmacokinet* 1993;**24**:203–20). A study showed that fluvoxamine 100 mg/d increased alprazolam plasma levels by 100%, and so reduced doses of alprazolam should be used (n = 60, Fleishaker and Hulst, *Eur J Clin Pharmacol* 1994;**46**:35–9), and the effect may be 30% greater in non-smokers compared to smokers (n = 49, Sugahara et al, *Eur J Clin Pharmacol* 2009:**65**:699–704). A slight increase (66%) in midazolam (n = 10, RCT, 12/7, Lam et al, *J Clin Pharmacol* 2003;**43**:1274–82) and quazepam levels (n = 12, RCT, d/b, c/o, p/c, 14/7, Kanda et al, *J Clin Pharmacol* 2003;**43**:1392–7) has been reported.

Beta-blockers + fluvoxamine
Lack of significant interaction has been shown with atenolol. Propranolol plasma levels can be raised by fluvoxamine by up to 500%, but apparently without major clinical effect (reviewed by Benfield and Ward, *Drugs* 1988;**32**:313–34).

Buspirone + fluvoxamine
See buspirone (*4.1.2*).

Caffeine + fluvoxamine
Even low-dose fluvoxamine (10–20 mg/d) inhibits the metabolism of caffeine, presumably via 1A2 inhibition (n = 10, Christensen et al, *Clin Pharmacol Ther* 2002;**71**:141–52), and half-life may rise from five hours to 22 hours (Slaughter and Edwards, *Ann Pharmacother* 1995;**29**:619–24), unlikely to be significant (n = 10, Spigset, *Eur J Clin Pharmacol* 1998;**54**:665–6). Caffeine decreases plasma levels of fluvoxamine but not its effects (n = 12, RCT, 11/7, d/b, p/c, c/o, Fukasawa et al, *Ther Drug Monit* 2006; **28**:308–11).

Carbamazepine + fluvoxamine
One small study showed fluvoxamine 100 mg/d to have no effect on carbamazepine levels (n = 15, RCT, Spina et al, *Ther Drug Monit* 1993;**15**:247–50), although increased carbamazepine levels and toxicity have been reported (e.g. Martinelli et al, *Br J Clin Pharmacol* 1993;**36**:615–6).

Chloral + fluvoxamine
Lack of interaction has been reported (Wagner et al, *Adv Pharmacother* 1986;**2**:34–56).

Ciclosporin + fluvoxamine
There is a report of ciclosporin levels elevated by the introduction of fluvoxamine to a ciclosporin-treated allograft recipient, probably via CYP3A4 inhibition. Intensive monitoring of the serum creatinine and ciclosporin level was

4

recommended, along with appropriate dose reductions (n = 2, Vella and Sayegh, *Am J Kidney Dis* 1998;**31**:320–3).

Citalopram/escitalopram + fluvoxamine
See citalopram/escitalopram (*4.3.2.1*).

CLOZAPINE + FLUVOXAMINE
See clozapine (*4.2.4*).

Digoxin + fluvoxamine
See digoxin + fluoxetine (*4.3.2.2*).

Donepezil + fluvoxamine
See SSRIs + donepezil (*4.6.3.1*).

DULOXETINE + FLUVOXAMINE
See SSRIs + duloxetine (*4.3.3.2*).

Enoxacin + fluvoxamine
Enoxacin appears to increase the sleepiness caused by fluvoxamine (n = 10, RCT, d/b, c/o, 11/7, Kunii *et al*, *Ther Drug Monit* 2005;**27**:349–53).

Glimepiride + fluvoxamine
Fluvoxamine may produce a modest increase in glimepiride plasma concentrations (n = 12, RCT, d/b, c/o, 4/7, Niemi *et al*, *Clin Pharmacol Ther* 2001;**69**:194–200).

Lansoprazole + fluvoxamine
Fluvoxamine increases lansoprazole levels 2–3-fold in extensive (but not poor) metabolisers, probably by 2C19 inhibition (n = 18, RCT, p/c, Yasui-Furukori *et al*, *J Clin Pharmacol* 2004; **44**:1223–9; n = 18, Muira *et al*, *Br J Clin Pharmacol* 2005;**60**:61–8).

Lidocaine + fluvoxamine
Lidocaine metabolism is reduced by fluvoxamine, leading to potential toxicity (n = 8, RCT, d/b, p/c, c/o, Isohanni *et al*, *Basic Clin Pharmacol Toxicol* 2006;**99**:168–72), although the effect of the interaction lessens as liver function worsens (n = 30, RCT, d/b, c/o, Orlando *et al*, *Clin Pharmacol Ther* 2004;**75**:80–8).

Lithium + fluvoxamine
Although lack of interaction has been reported (Hendrickx and Floris, *Curr Ther Res* 1991;**49**:106–10), case reports exist of serotonin syndrome (n = 1, Ohman and Spigset, *Pharmacopsychiatry* 1993;**26**:263–4), irresistible somnolence (n = 1, Evans and Marwick, *Br J Psychiatry* 1990;**156**:286) and diurnal somnolence (n = 1, Marchesi *et al*, *Pharmacopsychiatry* 2005;**38**:145–6).

MAOIs + FLUVOXAMINE
See MAOIs (*4.3.4*).

MELATONIN + FLUVOXAMINE
See melatonin (*4.1.4*).

Methadone + fluvoxamine
See methadone (*4.6.10*).

Metoclopramide + fluvoxamine
The combination metoclopramide with **fluoxetine**, **sertraline** (n = 1, Fisher and Davies, *Ann Pharmacother* 2002;**36**:67–71) or **fluvoxamine** may increase the incidence of serotonin syndrome (SmPC). Acute dystonia has been associated with the combination (n = 1, Palop *et al*, *Ann Pharmacother* 1999;**33**:382).

MIRTAZAPINE + FLUVOXAMINE
See mirtazapine (*4.3.3.4*).

Moclobemide + fluvoxamine
See SSRIs + moclobemide (*4.3.3.5*).

NICOUMALONE + FLUVOXAMINE
The anticoagulant effects may be enhanced by fluvoxamine.

NSAIDs + FLUVOXAMINE
See NSAIDs + fluoxetine (*4.3.2.2*).

Olanzapine + fluvoxamine
See olanzapine (*4.2.5*).

Oxycodone + fluvoxamine
Serotonin syndrome has been reported with the combination (n = 1, Karunatilake and Buckley, *Ann Pharmacother* 2006;**40**:155–7).

PHENYTOIN + FLUVOXAMINE
See phenytoin (*4.5.9*).

Pipamperone + fluvoxamine
ECG changes have occurred as a result of acute overdose with this combination (Gallerani *et al*, *Clin Drug Invest* 1998;**15**:64–8).

Quetiapine + fluvoxamine
See quetiapine (*4.2.6*).

Quinidine + fluvoxamine
Fluvoxamine significantly inhibits the 3A4 clearance of quinidine (n = 6, open, Damkier *et al*, *Eur J Clin Pharmacol* 1999; **55**:451–6).

Ramosetron + fluvoxamine
Fluvoxamine increases ramosetron Cmax and AUC 1.42-fold and 2.78-fold respectively (open, 11/7, Kadokura *et al*, *Eur J Clin Pharmacol* 2008; **64**:691–5).

Reboxetine + fluvoxamine
See reboxetine (*4.3.3.6*).

Risperidone + fluvoxamine
See antipsychotics + risperidone (*4.2.7*).

Rosiglitazone + fluvoxamine
There appears no significant interaction, although rosiglitazone levels may rise in some people (n = 23, open, c/o, Pedersen *et al*, *Br J Clin Pharmacol* 2006;**62**:682–9).

Sibutramine + fluvoxamine *
Serotonin syndrome is possible.

Sildenafil + fluvoxamine
Fluvoxamine increases sildenafil AUC by 40% and half–life by 19%, probably via CYP3A4 inhibition (n = 12, Hesse et al, J Clin Psychopharmacol 2005; **25**:589–92).

Smoking + fluvoxamine
See smoking (4.7.4).

St John's wort + fluvoxamine
See SSRIs + St John's wort (4.3.3.10).

Sympathomimetics + fluvoxamine
Augmentation of amfetamines is theoretically possible (see also fluoxetine, 4.3.2.2).

THEOPHYLLINE + FLUVOXAMINE
Several cases of theophylline toxicity have been reported (eg. Devane et al, Am J Psychiatry 1997;**154**:1317–18), probably via CYP1A2 inhibition. The literature recommends avoiding the combination (Curr Prob 1994;**20**:12).

TIZANIDINE + FLUVOXAMINE
Fluvoxamine increases tizanidine's AUC 33-fold and peak levels 12-fold, a dramatic and important interaction (n = 10, RCT, d/b, c/o, 4/7, Granfors et al, Clin Pharmacol Ther 2004;**75**:331–41).

Tolbutamide + fluvoxamine
Fluvoxamine 150 mg/d may increase tolbutamide levels by about 20% (n = 14, RCT, Madsen et al, Clin Pharmacol Ther 2001;**69**:41–7).

Topiramate + fluvoxamine
There is a case of rapidly reversible tremor and myoclonus with the combination (n = 1, Oulis et al, Clin Neuropharmacol 2008;**31**:366–7).

TRICYCLICS + FLUVOXAMINE
See SSRIs + tricyclics (4.3.1).

Triptans + fluvoxamine
See triptans + fluoxetine (4.3.2.2).

Tryptophan + fluvoxamine
Central toxicity has been suggested with fluvoxamine (n = 5, Steiner and Fontaine, Biol Psychiatry 1986;**21**:1067–71).

Valproate + fluvoxamine
Augmentation of fluvoxamine has been claimed with valproate (Corrigan, Biol Psychiatry 1992; **31**:1178–9).

WARFARIN + FLUVOXAMINE
An in vitro study indicated fluvoxamine has the most potent effect on warfarin of the SSRIs (Schmider et al, Br J Clin Pharmacol 1997;**44**:495–8), e.g. it can increase warfarin levels by up to 65%, increasing prothrombin time (Benfield and Ward, Drugs 1986;**32**:313–34; n = 1, Limke et al, Ann Pharmacother 2002;**36**:1890–2). Elevated INR

has occurred up to two weeks after fluvoxamine was stopped, a prolonged effect (n = 1, Yap and Low, Singapore Med J 1999; **40**:480–2).

Zolpidem + fluvoxamine
See SSRIs + zolpidem (4.1.7).

4.3.2.4 PAROXETINE
Paroxetine is 95% protein bound and probably the most potent SSRI inhibitor of CYP2D6, although this is rapidly reversible. It does not appear to inhibit any other P450 enzyme. The main metabolite has approximately one third the CYP2D6 inhibition potency of paroxetine.

Agomelatine + paroxetine
See agomelatine (4.3.3.1).

Alcohol + paroxetine
See alcohol (4.7.1).

Anticholinergics + paroxetine
See SSRIs + anticholinergics (4.6.2).

Antipsychotics + paroxetine *
Lack of interaction has been shown between paroxetine and **haloperidol** (Cooper et al, Acta Psychiatr Scand 1989;**80**[Suppl 350]:53–5), thiothixene (a thioxanthene; n = 10, Guthrie et al, J Clin Pharm Ther 1997;**22**:221–6) and with **asenapine** (US PI). Pooled data from two trials shows no substantial effect from adjunctive **aripiprazole** on paroxetine kinetics (n = 38, d/b, p/c, Boulton et al, J Psychopharmacol 2010;**24**:537–46; MS). **Zuclopenthixol** levels are increased by around 78% by paroxetine, in a dose-dependent manner (n = 923 samples, Davies et al, Acta Psychiatr Scand 2010;**122**:44–53). See also clozapine (4.2.4) and quetiapine (4.2.6).

Atomoxetine + paroxetine
See SSRIs + atomoxetine (4.6.4).

Benzodiazepines + paroxetine
Lack of interaction has been shown, e.g. with **oxazepam** (Cooper et al, Acta Psychiatr Scand 1989;**80**[Suppl 350]: 53–5) and **alprazolam** (n = 25, d/b, p/c, c/o, 4×15/7, Calvo et al, J Clin Psychopharmacol 2004;**24**:268–76), but NMS has been reported with paroxetine 20 mg/d and alprazolam 1.2 mg/d (n = 1, Naranjo = 6, Tanii et al, Prog Neuropsychopharmacol Biol Psychiatry 2006;**30**:1176–8). Serotonin syndrome has been reported in a person taking maintenance paroxetine after a single dose **clonazepam** (Rella and Hoffman, J Toxicol Clin Toxicol 1998;**36**:257–8).

Beta-blockers + paroxetine *
CYP2D6 inhibition by paroxetine leads to

4

metoprolol levels raised 3–5-fold, which might lead to greater beta-blockade and lost cardioselectivity (n = 10, Stout et al, J Clin Pharmacol 2011;**51**:389–96) and complete AV block has been reported with the combination (n = 1, Onalan et al, Mayo Clin Proc 2008;**83**:595–9). Raised paroxetine levels after the addition of pindolol have been reported, probably via 2D6 inhibition (n = 1, Olver and Burrows, Int J Psych Clin Pract 1998;**2**:225–7). Paroxetine has no effect on **carvedilol** kinetics (n = 12, RCT, c/o, Stout et al, J Cardiovasc Pharmacol Ther 2010;**15**:373–9).

Bupropion + paroxetine
See bupropion (4.6.6).

Carbamazepine + paroxetine
Lack of significant interaction has been shown (n = 20, s/b, p/c, c/o, 23/7, Andersen et al, Epilepsy Res 1991;**10**:201–4), although hyponatraemia has been reported (n = 1, Sempere I Verdu et al, Aten Primaria 2004;**33**:473–4).

Cimetidine + paroxetine
Cimetidine may inhibit the first-pass metabolism of paroxetine, increasing bioavailability by up to 50% (Bannister et al, Acta Psychiatr Scand 1989; **80**[Suppl 350]:102–6), so use ranitidine instead.

CLOZAPINE + PAROXETINE
See clozapine (4.2.4).

Dextromethorphan + paroxetine
Paroxetine would be expected to increase dextromethorphan levels via CYP2D6 inhibition (see reported case with fluoxetine, 4.3.2.2).

Digitalis + paroxetine
Digitalis toxicity five days after starting paroxetine has been reported (n = 1, Yasui-Fukukori and Kaneko, Lancet 2006;**367**:788), although this may just have been hospital-induced compliance (Bateman et al, Lancet 2006;**368**:1962–3).

Digoxin + paroxetine
See digoxin + fluoxetine (4.3.2.2).

Donepezil + paroxetine
See SSRIs + donepezil (4.6.3.1).

Duloxetine + paroxetine
See SSRIs + duloxetine (4.3.3.2).

Ecstasy (MDMA) + paroxetine
In people treated with paroxetine 20 mg/d, the physiological and psychological effects of ecstasy were significantly attenuated, which could lead users to take higher (and hence toxic) doses to achieve the same effects (n = 12, RCT, d/b, p/c, c/o, 2 × 3/7, Farré et al, J Pharmacol Exp Ther 2007;**323**:954–62).

Flecainide + paroxetine *
Paroxetine inhibits flecainide's metabolism which may be related to 2D6 genotype (n = 21, open, Lim et al, Clin Ther 2010;**32**:659–66) and flecainide toxicity has led to delirium (n = 1, Tsao and Gugger, Ann Pharmacother 2009;**43**:1366–9).

Galantamine + paroxetine
See galantamine (4.6.3.2).

Interferon alfa + paroxetine
A previous good response to paroxetine and trazodone was reversed by interferon alfa, which has anti-serotonergic actions (n = 1, McAllister-Williams et al, Br J Psychiatry 2000;**176**:93).

Lithium + paroxetine
There are some cases of a possible serotonin syndrome (n = 17, Fagiolini et al, J Clin Psycho-pharmacol 2001;**21**:474–8).

Methadone + paroxetine
Steady-state plasma methadone levels may rise with paroxetine, but only in poor 2D6 metabolisers (n = 10, 12/7, Begre et al, J Clin Psychopharmacol 2002;**22**:211–5).

Methylene blue + paroxetine *
Postoperative serotonin syndrome has been reported after methylene blue was used in someone taking paroxetine (systematic review of SSRIs, n = 25, Ng and Cameron, Psychosomatics 2010;**51**:194–200).

Methylphenidate + paroxetine *
See paroxetine + methylphenidate (4.6.11).

Metoclopramine + paroxetine
See metoclopramide + fluvoxamine (4.3.2.3).

Mirtazapine + paroxetine
See mirtazapine (4.3.3.4).

Moclobemide + paroxetine
See SSRIs + moclobemide (4.3.3.5).

MAOIs + PAROXETINE
See MAOIs (4.3.4).

NSAIDs + SSRIs
See NSAIDs + fluoxetine (4.3.2.2).

Oral contraceptives + paroxetine
Lack of interaction has been shown (Boyer and Blumhardt, J Clin Psychiatry 1992;**53**[Suppl 2]: 132–4).

Oxycodone + paroxetine *
Paroxetine has no clinical effect on oxycodone (n = 12, p/c, Kummer et al, Eur J Clin Pharmacol 2011;**67**:63–71).

Phenytoin + paroxetine
Paroxetine bioavailability may be decreased

slightly (Andersen et al, Epilepsy Res 1991:**10**: 201–4).

Phenobarbital + paroxetine

Paroxetine bioavailability may be decreased slightly, resulting in a 25% decrease in plasma concentrations (Bannister et al, Acta Psychiatr Scand 1989;**80**[Suppl 350]:102–6). No inter-action occurs with amylobarbital (Cooper et al, Acta Psychiatr Scand 1989;**80**[Suppl 350]:53–5).

Risperidone + paroxetine

See risperidone (4.2.7).

SERTINDOLE + PAROXETINE *

See sertindole (4.2.8).

Sibutramine + paroxetine *

Serotonin syndrome is possible.

St John's wort + paroxetine

See SSRIs + St John's wort (4.3.3.10).

Sympathomimetics + paroxetine

Augmentation of amfetamines is theoretically possible (see sympathomimetics + fluoxetine 4.3.2.2).

Tamoxifen + paroxetine *

Tamoxifen and paroxetine may increase the risk of recurrence of breast cancer, but no increase with other other SSRIs (including fluoxetine), venlafaxine and mirtazapine (n = 2430, < 14 years, Kelly et al, Br Med J 2010;**340**:c693; s = 7, Desmarais and Looper, J Clin Psychiatry 2009; **70**:1688–97), although bupropion might (Drug Safety Update 2010;**4**:A1).

Terbinafine + paroxetine

Terbinafine 150mg/d increases the Cmax of paroxetine 2-fold and increases half-life 48% from 15–23 hours (n = 12, 2×6/7, Yasui-Furukori et al, Eur J Clin Pharmacol 2007;**63**:51–6).

TRICYCLICS + PAROXETINE

See SSRIs + tricyclics (4.3.1).

Triptans + paroxetine

The literature notes an increased risk of CNS toxicity and recommends avoiding sumatriptan and paroxetine, although almost complete lack of interaction has been shown with rizatriptan and paroxetine (n = 12, RCT, 14/7, Goldberg et al, J Clin Pharmacol 1999;**39**:192–9). See also fluoxetine (4.3.2.2).

Valproate + paroxetine

No significant interaction occurs (n = 20, s/b, p/c, c/o, 23/7, Andersen et al, Epilepsy Res 1991; **10**:201–4).

Warfarin + paroxetine

An in vitro study indicated that all SSRIs have an effect on warfarin (Schmider et al, Br J Clin Pharmacol 1997;**44**:495–8), e.g. up to a three-point rise in INR has been reported in several patients (mentioned by Askinazi, Am J Psychiatry 1996;**153**:135–6).

Zolpidem + paroxetine

See SSRIs + zolpidem (4.1.6).

4.3.2.5 SERTRALINE

Sertraline is 98% protein bound and has a minor but dose-related inhibition of CYP2D6 but has little, if any, effect on CYP1A2, 2C9/10, 2C19 or 3A3/4. At 50–100 mg/d, it is a low incidence of interactions with drugs metabolised by 2D6. It is metabolised mainly by 3A4 but also other P450 enzymes, plus monoamine oxidase and UGT2B7 (Obach et al, Drug Metab Disp 2005;**33**:262–70).

Alcohol + sertraline

See alcohol (4.7.1).

Anticholinergics + sertraline

See SSRIs + anticholinergics (4.6.2).

Antipsychotics + sertraline *

There were no changes in a range of anti-psychotic levels when sertraline 50–100 mg/d was added (n = 48, RCT, d/b, p/c, 6/52, Pierson et al, Can J Psychiatry 2006;**51**:715–8). Sertraline (up to 200 mg/d) may cause pimozide levels to rise by 35%, but with no prolonged QTc (n = 15, Alderman, Clin Ther 2005;**27**:1050–63). Pooled data from two trials shows no substantial effect from aripiprazole on sertraline (n = 90, d/b, p/c, Boulton et al, J Psychopharmacol 2010;**24**:537–46;MS),although life-threatening myxedema coma (responding to dexamethasone and IV levothyroxine) has been reported (n = 1, Church and Callen, Ann Pharmacother 2009;**43**:2113–6). See also individual antipsychotics + SSRIs.

Atomoxetine + sertraline

See SSRIs + atomoxetine (4.6.4).

Ayurvedic medicines + sertraline

There is a case of a patient twice suffering relapses after starting Ayurvedic herbal mixtures, probably due to either Terminalia chebula or Commiphora wighteii (n = 1, Prasad et al, J Psychopharmacol 2009;**23**:216–9).

Benzodiazepines + sertraline

Sertraline has no significant effect on diazepam and other benzodiazepines (n = 20, RCT, d/b, p/c, c/o, Gardner et al, Clin Pharmacokinetics 1997;

31[Suppl 1]:43–9; review: Warrington, *Int Clin Psychopharmacol* 1991;**6**[Suppl 2]:11–21).

Beta-blockers + sertraline

No pharmacodynamic interaction has been found with atenolol (e.g. n = 10, RCT, Ziegler and Wilner, *J Clin Psychiatry* 1996;**57**[Suppl 1]:12–15), but sertraline can increase metoprolol AUC by 48–67% (17/7, Preskorn et al, *J Clin Psychopharmacol* 2007;**27**:28–34).

Bupropion + sertraline

See bupropion (*4.6.6*).

Carbamazepine + sertraline

Lack of significant interaction has been reported, but there are cases where sertraline 100 mg/d increased carbamazepine (600 mg/d) plasma levels, probably via 3A4 inhibition (d/b, p/c, Joblin, *N Z Med J* 1994;**107**:43; Lane, *N Z Med J* 1994;**107**:209). Non-response to sertraline has been due to low plasma levels associated with carbamazepine use, possibly via CYP3A4 induction (n = 2, Khan et al, *J Clin Psychiatry* 2000; **61**:526–7).

Clozapine + sertraline

See clozapine (*4.2.4*).

Digoxin + sertraline

See digoxin + fluoxetine (*4.3.2.2*).

Dolasetron + sertraline

A serotonin syndrome has been reported with the combination (n = 1, Sorscher, *J Psycho-pharmacol* 2002;**16**:191).

Donepezil + sertraline

See SSRIs + donepezil (*4.6.3.1*).

Duloxetine + sertraline

See SSRIs + duloxetine (*4.3.3.2*).

Erythromycin + sertraline

Serotonin syndrome has been reported with the combination, possibly via CYP3A4 inhibition (n = 1, Lee and Lee, *Pharmacother* 1999;**19**:894–6).

Fluoxetine + sertraline

A possible serotonin syndrome has been reported (see switching antidepressants, *2.2.5*).

Indometacin + sertraline *

There is a case of serotonin syndrome with the combination (n = 1, Coster et al, *J Clin Psychopharmacol* 2010;**30**:468–70).

Lamotrigine + sertraline

See lamotrigine (*4.5.5*).

Linezolid + sertraline

A case of serotonin syndrome has been reported (n = 1, Clark et al, *Pharmacotherapy* 2006;**26**:269–76).

Lithium + sertraline

See SSRIs + lithium (*4.4*).

MAOIs + SERTRALINE

See MAOIs (*4.3.4*).

Methylene blue + sertraline *

See methylene blue + paroxetine (*4.3.2.4*).

Methylphenidate + sertraline

See sertraline + methylphenidate (*4.6.11*).

Metoclopramide + sertraline

See metoclopramide + fluvoxamine (*4.3.2.3*).

Mirtazapine + sertraline

See SSRIs + mirtazapine (*4.3.3.4*).

Moclobemide + sertraline

See SSRIs + moclobemide (*4.3.3.5*).

NSAIDs + sertraline

See NSAIDs + fluoxetine (*4.3.2.2*).

Olanzapine + sertraline

See SSRIs + olanzapine (*4.2.5*).

Oxycodone + sertraline

Visual hallucinations and tremor have been reported with the combination (n = 1, Rose-braugh et al, *J Clin Pharmacol* 2001;**41**:224).

Phenytoin + sertraline

Lack of significant interaction has been shown (n = 30, RCT, Rapeport et al, *J Clin Psychiatry* 1996;**57**[Suppl 1]:24–8), but dramatically raised phenytoin levels have been reported after the addition of sertraline (n = 2, Haselberger et al, *J Clin Psychopharmacol* 1997;**17**:107–9), as has a significant reduction in sertraline levels by phenytoin (Pihlsgard and Eliasson, *Eur J Clin Pharmacol* 2002;**57**:915–6). Monitoring levels would seem sensible.

Risperidone + sertraline

See risperidone (*4.2.7*).

Sertindole + sertraline *

See sertindole (*4.2.8*).

Sibutramine + sertraline *

Serotonin syndrome is possible.

St John's wort + sertraline

See SSRIs + St John's wort (*4.3.3.10*).

Sumatriptan + sertraline

The literature notes an increased risk of CNS toxicity and recommends avoiding the combination. See also fluoxetine (*4.3.2.2*).

Sympathomimetics + sertraline

Augmentation of amfetamines is theoretically possible (see sympathomimetics + fluoxetine, *4.3.2.2*).

Tamoxifen + sertraline *

See tamoxifen + paroxetine (*4.3.2.4*).

Tolbutamide + sertraline

In a parallel-group study, 200 mg/d sertraline produced a 16% decrease in tolbutamide clearance, possibly via inhibition of CYP2C9 (e.g. n = 25, RCT, Tremaine et al, Clin Pharmacokinet 1997; **31** [Suppl 1]:31–6).

Tramadol + sertraline

Serotonin syndrome has been reported when a tramadol dose was increased with concomitant sertraline (n = 1, Mason and Blackburn, Ann Pharmacother 1997;**31**:175–7).

Tricyclics + sertraline

See SSRIs + tricyclics (4.3.1).

Venlafaxine + sertraline

Acute liver damage possibly related to sertraline and venlafaxine ingestion has been reported (n = 1, Kim et al, Ann Pharmacother 1999;**3**:381–2).

Warfarin + sertraline

An in vitro study indicated that, of the SSRIs, sertraline had the least potent effect on warfarin (Schmider et al, Br J Clin Pharmacol 1997;**44**:495–8), with only a modest and clinically significant increase in prothrombin time (n = 12, RCT, 22/7, Apseloff et al, Clin Pharmacokinet 1997;**32**[Suppl 1]:37–42). However, prothrombin time can be increased by 9% (Wilner et al, Biol Psychiatry 1991;**29**:354S–355S) and up to a three-point rise in INR has been reported in several patients (mentioned by Askinazi, Am J Psychiatry 1996;**153**:135–6).

Zolpidem + sertraline

See SSRIs + zolpidem (4.1.6).

4.3.3 OTHER ANTIDEPRESSANTS

4.3.3.1 AGOMELATINE

Agomelatine is metabolised by CYP1A2 (90%) and CYP9/19 (10%). 2D6 and 3A4 are not involved.

Alcohol + agomelatine

The SmPC states that concurrent use is not advisable but there is no kinetic interaction, and only a very minor effect on one of 23 psychometric tests (MI).

Benzodiazepine + agomelatine

Lack of kinetic interaction has been shown (SmPC) and there is no interaction between concomitant agomelatine 50 mg/d and lorazepam 2.5 mg for seven days (MI).

CIPROFLOXACIN + AGOMELATINE

This combination is an SmPC contraindication.

Fluconazole + agomelatine

Fluconazole does not affect the pharmacokinetics of agomelatine (SmPC).

FLUVOXAMINE + AGOMELATINE

Fluvoxamine (a 1A2 and 2C9 inhibitor) may increase agomelatine Cmax and AUC 47-fold and 61-fold respectively, although agomelatine was still well tolerated (SmPC).

Lithium + agomelatine

Lack of significant interaction has been shown (SmPC), although agomelatine exposure was insignificantly increased.

Paroxetine + agomelatine

Paroxetine does not affect the pharmacokinetics of agomelatine (SmPC).

Smoking + agomelatine

Smoking induces 1A2 and reduces agomelatine bioavailability by 33%, seen as insignificant (MI).

Theophylline + agomelatine

Lack of interaction has been shown (SmPC).

4.3.3.2 DULOXETINE

Duloxetine is 95% protein bound and metabolised by 1A2 (but probably does not inhibit it), is a moderate inhibitor and substrate for 2D6 (s = 2, Skinner et al, Clin Pharmacol Ther 2003;**73**:170–7) but has no effect on 3A4. Caution is recommended with sedative drugs, e.g. alcohol, benzodiazepines, antipsychotics and sedative antihistamines. Elimination is primarily renal, after extensive metabolism by multiple oxidative pathways, methylation and conjugation (review of kinetics, Wernicke et al, Expert Opin Drug Saf 2005;**4**:987–93).

Antacids + duloxetine

Lack of interaction has been shown with a single 40 mg dose of duloxetine (UK SmPC).

Aripiprazole + duloxetine *

Duloxetine does not seem to affect the plasma levels of aripiprazole (n=7, Hendset et al, Ther Drug Monit 2010;**32**:787–90).

Beta-blockers + duloxetine

Duloxetine is a 2D6 inhibitor, and can increase metoprolol AUC by 180% (Preskorn et al, J Clin Psychopharmacol 2007;**27**:28–34).

CIPROFLOXACIN + DULOXETINE

This combination is a UK SmPC contraindication due to the potential for raised duloxetine levels from 1A2 inhibition by ciprofloxacin.

ENOXACINE + DULOXETINE

This combination is a UK SmPC contraindication due to the potential for raised duloxetine levels from 1A2 inhibition by enoxacine.

4

H2-blockers + duloxetine

Lack of interaction has been shown with a single 40 mg dose of duloxetine (UK SmPC).

MAOIs + DULOXETINE

This combination is a UK SmPC contraindication, due to the risk of serotonin syndrome. Do not use duloxetine within 14 days of stopping an MAOI, or use an MAOI until five days after stopping duloxetine.

Moclobemide + duloxetine

The UK SmPC recommends caution, due to the risk of serotonin syndrome, when duloxetine is used with moclobemide.

Olanzapine + duloxetine

See duloxetine + olanzapine (4.2.5).

Oral contraceptives + duloxetine

There is no reason to suspect an interaction would occur, but there are no formal studies.

Pethidine + duloxetine

Due to the risk of serotonin syndrome, duloxetine should only be used with care with pethidine.

Risperidone + duloxetine *

Duloxetine does not seem to affect the plasma levels of risperidone (n = 8, Hendset et al, Ther Drug Monit 2010;**32**:787–90).

SMOKING + DULOXETINE

Smokers may have duloxetine plasma levels 50% lower than non-smokers (UK SmPC).

SSRIs + DULOXETINE

Due to the risk of serotonin syndrome, duloxetine should only be used with care with SSRIs. **Fluvoxamine** may decrease duloxetine's clearance by 77% and increase AUC six-fold, and this combination is a UK SmPC contraindication because of the potential for duloxetine toxicity.

St John's wort + duloxetine

The UK SmPC recommends caution when duloxetine is used with St John's wort.

Theophylline + duloxetine

Duloxetine had no effect on theophylline in a study in male patients (UK SmPC).

Tolterodine + duloxetine

There is no significant interaction (n = 16, RCT, d/b, c/o, 2 × 5/7, Hua et al, Br J Clin Pharmacol 2004;**57**:652–6).

Tramadol + duloxetine

Due to the risk of serotonin syndrome, duloxetine should only be used with care with tramadol.

Tricyclics + duloxetine

Due to the risk of serotonin syndrome, duloxetine should only be used with care with tricyclics.

Triptans + duloxetine

Due to the risk of serotonin syndrome, duloxetine should only be used with care with triptans.

Tryptophan + duloxetine

Due to the risk of serotonin syndrome, duloxetine should only be used with care with tryptophan.

Venlafaxine + duloxetine

Due to the risk of serotonin syndrome, duloxetine should only be used with care with venlafaxine.

Warfarin + duloxetine

Duloxetine has been shown to have no significant effect on the kinetics of steady-state warfarin (n = 30, 14/7, Chappell et al, J Clin Pharmacol 2009;**49**:1456–66), although there are cases of duloxetine causing severe elevation of INR when combined with warfarin (n = 3, Glueck et al, JAMA 2006;**295**:1517–8).

4.3.3.3 MIANSERIN

ALCOHOL + MIANSERIN

See alcohol (4.7.1).

Benzodiazepines + mianserin

Enhanced sedation may occur.

Carbamazepine + mianserin

Plasma levels of mianserin may be halved by carbamazepine, probably via 3A4 induction (n = 12, Eap et al, Ther Drug Monit 1999;**21**:166–70).

Warfarin + mianserin

There is normally no problem but occasional control difficulties have been reported (Warwick and Mindham, Br J Psychiatry 1983;**143**:308).

4.3.3.4 MIRTAZAPINE

Mirtazapine does not inhibit CYP2D6, 1A2 nor 3A and so interactions via these enzymes are unlikely. Mirtazapine is mainly metabolised by CYP2D6 and 1A2 (Montgomery, Int Clin Psychopharmacol 1995;**10**[Suppl 4]:37–45) and if one enzyme is inhibited, the other takes over, so mirtazapine appears less susceptible to P450 interactions. It is 85% protein bound, has linear kinetics from 15–75 mg/d, and 100% is excreted via the urine and faeces.

Review: Clinical pharmacokinetics (Timmer et al, Clin Pharmacokinet 2000;**38**:461–74).

Alcohol + mirtazapine

See alcohol (4.7.1).

Atomoxetine + mirtazapine

See atomoxetine (4.6.4).

Benzodiazepines + mirtazapine

The combination of diazepam and mirtazapine,

not surprisingly, produces an additive sedative effect (n = 12, RCT, d/b, c/o, Mattila *et al*, *Pharmacol Toxicol* 1989;**65**:81–8).

Carbamazepine + mirtazapine

Mirtazapine has no significant effect on carbamazepine levels but carbamazepine decreases mirtazapine levels by 60%, probably by CYP3A4 induction, and mirtazapine doses may need to be increased (RCT, 4/52, Sitsen *et al*, *Eur J Drug Metab Pharmacokinet* 2001;**26**:109–21).

Cimetidine + mirtazapine

Mirtazapine has no effect on cimetidine but mirtazapine levels may be higher (probably by CYP3A4 inhibition), but not enough to require dose reduction (n = 12, d/b, p/c, c/o, Sitsen *et al*, *Eur J Clin Pharmacol* 2000;**56**:389–94).

Clozapine + mirtazapine

Lack of significant interaction has been shown (n = 9, 6/52, Zoccali *et al*, *Pharmacol Res* 2003; **48**:411–4).

Fluoxetine + mirtazapine

Fluoxetine 20–40 mg/d caused a clinically in-significant 32% increase in mirtazapine (15 mg/d) plasma levels after an abrupt switch (n = 40, Preskorn *et al*, *Biol Psychiatry* 1997;**41**:96S), although mania has been reported with mirtazapine augmentation of fluoxetine (n = 1, Ng, *Depress Anxiety* 2002;**15**:46–7) and immediately after a switch from fluoxetine, suggesting a combined effect (n = 1, Liu *et al*, *J Psychopharmacol* 2009;**23**:220–2).

FLUVOXAMINE + MIRTAZAPINE

Fluvoxamine 50–100 mg/d may increase mirtazapine serum levels 3–4-fold, a significant effect (n = 2, Anttila *et al*, *Ann Pharmacother* 2001;**35**:1221–3) and a serotonin syndrome has been reported (n = 1, Demers and Malone, *Ann Pharmacother* 2001;**35**:1217–20).

Levodopa + mirtazapine

Psychosis has been reported when mirtazapine was added to a stable levodopa regimen (n = 1, Normann *et al*, *Pharmacopsychiatry* 1997;**30**: 263–5).

Lithium + mirtazapine

No pharmacokinetic interaction has been detected between lithium 600 mg/d and mirtazapine 30 mg (n = 12, 10/7, Sitsen *et al*, *J Clin Psychopharmacol* 2000;**14**:172–6).

MAOIs + mirtazapine

The UK SmPC cautiously recommends a two-week gap between stopping an MAOI and

starting mirtazapine.

Olanzapine + mirtazapine

Lack of significant interaction has been shown (n = 7, 6/52, Zoccali *et al*, *Pharmacol Res* 2003; **48**:411–4), although status epilepticus has been reported when olanzapine was added to mirtazapine (n = 1, Spyridi *et al, Int J Clin Pharmacol Ther* 2009;**47**:120–3).

Paroxetine + mirtazapine

Mirtazapine had no effect on the kinetics of paroxetine and the combination was better tolerated than either alone, suggesting a lack of clinically relevant interaction (n = 24, RCT, c/o, 6/7 per arm, Ruwe *et al*, *Hum Psychopharmacol* 2001;**16**:449–59).

Phenytoin + mirtazapine

A multiple dose study showed that mirtazapine had no effect on the steady-state kinetics of phenytoin, but that phenytoin reduced mirtazapine levels by a mean of 46%, probably clinically significant (n = 17, RCT, open, Spaans *et al*, *Eur J Clin Pharmacol* 2002;**58**:423–9).

Risperidone + mirtazapine

Mirtazapine 30 mg/d has no effect on risperidone 2–6 mg/d (e.g. n = 8, 6/52, Zoccali *et al*, *Pharmacol Res* 2003;**48**: 411–4).

Sertraline + mirtazapine

Hypomania has been reported when mirtazapine 15 mg/d was used to augment sertraline 250 mg/d, which had been only partially effective (n = 1, Soutullo *et al*, *J Clin Psychiatry* 1998;**59**:320).

Smoking + mirtazapine

See mirtazapine + smoking (4.7.4).

Tacrolimus + mirtazapine

Rapid onset of hypotension with raised tacrolimus levels has been reported when mirtazapine was added (n = 1, Fraile *et al*, *Nephrol Dial Transplant* 2009;**24**:1999–2001).

Tamoxifen + mirtazapine *

See tamoxifen + paroxetine (4.3.2.4).

Tricyclics + mirtazapine

Amitriptyline causes clinically insignificant increases in mirtazapine plasma levels and vice versa (n = 24, Sennef *et al*, *Hum Psychopharmacol* 2003;**38**:91–101).

Venlafaxine + mirtazapine *

Serotonin syndrome has been reported during a cross-over (n = 1, Dimellis, *World J Biol Psychiatry* 2002;**3**:167), as has angiodema (n = 1, Lin and Chen, *Gen Hosp Psychiatry* 2010;**32**:341)

4

and when both were also combined with tramadol (n = 1, Houlihan, *Ann Pharmacother* 2004;**38**:411–3). See also *1.14* for rational use of this combination.

Warfarin + mirtazapine

No interaction is known or suspected, but there is insufficient information to confirm this at present (Sayal et al, *Acta Psychiatr Scand* 2000;**102**:250–5).

4.3.3.5 MOCLOBEMIDE

Moclobemide is metabolised by CYP2C19, and inhibits 2D6, 2C19 and 1A2. Due to serotonin syndrome, co-administered moclobemide with drugs that enhance serotonin, such as 5-HT re-uptake inhibitors and many other antidepressants is not recommended.

Alcohol + moclobemide

See alcohol (*4.7.1*).

Benzodiazepines + moclobemide

No significant interaction occurs (Zimmer et al, *Acta Psychiatr Scand* 1990;**360**:84–6).

Bupropion + moclobemide

See MAOIs + bupropion (*4.6.6*).

Carbamazepine + moclobemide

Carbamazepine 400mg/d can reduce moclo-bemide levels by about 35% (n = 21, open, 4/52, Rakic Ignjatovic et al, *Br J Clin Pharmacol* 2009; **67**:199–208).

CIMETIDINE + MOCLOBEMIDE

Cimetidine may reduce the clearance and prolong the half-life of moclobemide, so start with lower doses and monitor closely (n = 8, open, Schoerlin et al, *Clin Pharmacol Ther* 1991;**49**:32–8)

Digoxin + moclobemide

Lack of interaction has been reported (Berlin and Lecrubier, *CNS Drugs* 1996;**5**:403–13).

Duloxetine + moclobemide

See duloxetine (*4.3.3.2*).

Ecstasy/MDMA + moclobemide

Deaths have been reported, with the victims apparently taking moclobemide in an attempt to enhance the effects of MDMA (n = 4, Vuori et al, *Addiction* 2003;**98**:365–8).

Ibuprofen + moclobemide

Moclobemide is alleged to potentiate the effect of ibuprofen, but lack of interaction has been reported (Berlin and Lecrubier, *CNS Drugs* 1996; **5**:403–13).

Metoprolol + moclobemide

Concurrent metoprolol and moclobemide results

in further lowering of blood pressure, although postural hypotension was not reported (Zimmer et al, *Acta Psychiatr Scand* 1990;**360**:84–6).

Nifedipine + moclobemide

No significant interaction occurs, apart from some slight reduction in blood pressure (Zimmer et al, *Acta Psychiatr Scand* 1990;**360**:84–6).

Opiates + moclobemide

Moclobemide is alleged to potentiate the effect of opiates, and dose reductions of morphine and fentanyl may be considered necessary.

Oral contraceptives + moclobemide

No significant interaction has been detected (Zimmer et al, *Acta Psychiatr Scand* 1990;**360**: 84–6).

Pethidine + moclobemide

This is now an SmPC contraindication.

SELEGILINE + MOCLOBEMIDE

Selegiline is an MAO-B inhibitor and if combined with an MAO-A inhibitor, such as moclobemide, could produce full MAO inhibition (albeit reversible). The combination is not recommended but, if the two need to be used together, full MAOI dietary precautions might be required. The combination is now an SmPC contraindication.

SSRIs + moclobemide

A fatal serotonin syndrome has been reported with moclobemide and **citalopram** (n = 1, Dams et al, *J Anal Toxicol* 2001;**25**:147–51) but disputed (Isbister et al, *J Anal Toxicol* 2001;**25**:716–7). Headaches and fatigue (review, Dingemanse, *Int Clin Psychopharmacol* 1993;**7**:167–80), excitation, insomnia and dysphoria have been reported with **fluvoxamine** and moclobemide (n = 36, open, 6/52, Ebert, *Psychopharmacology* 1995;**119**:342–4). In a study where up to 600mg/d moclobemide was added to established **fluoxetine** therapy, there was no change in the number, intensity or type of adverse events. Fluoxetine markedly inhibited the metabolism of moclobemide, but did not lead to excessive accumulation or any indication of development of a serotonin syndrome (n = 18, RCT, open, Dingemanse et al, *Clin Pharmacol Ther* 1998;**63**:403–13). A serotonin syndrome would also be a possibility with the combination and the UK SmPC for moclobemide contraindicates the combination. A fatal case, following overdose of **paroxetine** and moclobemide and subsequent serotonin syndrome, has been reported (Singer and Jones, *J Anal Toxicol* 1997;**21**:518–20).

Sympathomimetics + moclobemide

The UK SmPC recommends avoiding this combination. Phenylephrine may slightly raise blood pressure in people taking high dose (600 mg/d) moclobemide (Amrein et al, Psychopharmacology 1992;**106**:S24–S31), but ephedrine produces a greater rise in bp (Dingemanse, Int Clin Psychopharmacol 1993;**7**:167–80). Another study noted no clinically significant interaction, although the pressor effect may be slightly enhanced (review: Zimmer et al, Acta Psychiatr Scand 1990; **360**:84–6).

Tricyclics + moclobemide

The UK SmPC contraindicates the combination if the tricyclic (or metabolite) is a serotonin reuptake inhibitor, e.g. clomipramine or imipramine. Serotonin syndrome has been reported with moclobemide and clomipramine, imipramine (Brodribb et al, Lancet 1994;**343**:475–6) and after moclobemide plus either citalopram or clomipramine overdoses (n = 5, fatal, Neuvonen et al, Lancet 1993;**342**:1419), where aggressive therapy may be needed. Lack of interaction has been noted with amitriptyline 150 mg/d (e.g. n = 21, Amrein et al, Psychopharmacology 1992; **106**:S24–S31).

Triptans + moclobemide

The literature notes an increased risk of CNS toxicity with **sumatriptan** or **zolmitriptan** and moclobemide (e.g. Morales Asin, Neurologia 1998;**13**[Suppl 2]:25–30), and that lower doses should be used, although a small study suggested combined use with **sumatriptan** was safe with care (n = 14, open, Blier and Bergeron, J Clin Psychopharmacol 1995;**15**:106–9). Moclobemide may significantly potentiate the effects of **rizatriptan** and the combination is not recommended (n = 12, RCT, Van Haarst et al, Br J Clin Pharmacol 1999;**48**:190–6). Moclobemide increases the plasma concentration of **almotriptan** but the combination appears well tolerated (n = 12, RCT, open, c/o, Fleishaker et al, Br J Clin Pharmacol 2001;**51**:437–41) and it may be the triptan of choice.

Tyramine + moclobemide

Moclobemide does not appear to significantly potentiate the pressor effects of tyramine. Dietary restrictions are generally not required, but patients should avoid eating excessive amounts of tyramine-containing foods, especially if they have pre-existing hypertension. Minor pressor effects are not seen until about 100 mg tyramine (Zimmer et al, Acta Psychiatr Scand 1990;**360**:84–6). Even 150 mg tyramine is suggested by some as being safe (Acta Psychiatr Scand 1990;**360**[Suppl]:78–80). The combination has been used to treat severe postural hypotension (e.g. n = 1, Karet et al, Lancet 1994;**344**:1263–5) and for clozapine-induced hypotension, allowing dose increases to an active therapeutic level (n = 1, Taylor et al, Br J Psychiatry 1995;**167**:409–10).

Venlafaxine + moclobemide

See venlafaxine (4.3.3.9).

Valproate + moclobemide

Valproate 1 g/d has no effect on moclobemide levels (n = 21, open, 4/52, Rakic Ignjatovic et al, Br J Clin Pharmacol 2009;**67**:199–208).

Warfarin + moclobemide

No interaction has been reported, but moclobemide inhibits CYP1A2 and 2C19 and so the potential for warfarin potentiation exists (Sayal et al, Acta Psychiatr Scand 2000;**102**:250–5).

4.3.3.6 REBOXETINE

Reboxetine is predominantly metabolised in vitro via CYP2D6 and 3A4 (n = 51, Kuhn et al, Int J Clin Pharmacol Ther 2007;**45**:36–46). Reboxetine inhibits both CYP2D6 and CYP3A4, but has shown no effect on the in vivo clearance of drugs metabolised by these enzymes. Reboxetine does not inhibit CYP1A2, CYP2C9, CYP2C19, and CYP2E1. Reboxetine should be co-prescribed with caution with potent inhibitors of CYP3A4. Reboxetine is extensively (97%) bound to plasma proteins (particularly the alpha-1 acid glycoprotein fraction) and may interact with drugs with a high affinity for this fraction, e.g. dipyridamole, propranolol, methadone, imipramine, chlorpromazine (see antipsychotics below) and local anaesthetics.

Alcohol + reboxetine

See alcohol (4.7.1).

Antipsychotics + reboxetine

An interaction is possible (see above). Reboxetine has no effect on **clozapine** or **risperidone** plasma levels (n = 7, Spina et al, Ther Drug Monit 2001;**23**;675–8).

Benzodiazepines + reboxetine

Lack of interaction has been reported, although some mild-to-moderate drowsiness and transient increases in heart rate have been noted.

4

Carbamazepine + reboxetine

Low serum concentrations of reboxetine have been reported with concurrent carbamazepine (n = 1, Helland and Spigset, *J Clin Psychopharmacol* 2007;**27**:308–10).

Dipyridamole + reboxetine

An interaction is possible (see introduction).

Disopyramide + reboxetine

The SmPC advises caution with the combination.

Diuretics + reboxetine

There may be an increased risk of hypokalaemia with loop diuretics or thiazides (BNF).

Erythromycin + reboxetine

The literature advises caution with the combination.

Flecainide + reboxetine

The literature advises caution with the combination.

Fluoxetine + reboxetine

There are no statistically significant effects of reboxetine on fluoxetine or norfluoxetine pharmacokinetics, and a minimal clinical impact is suggested (n = 30, RCT, d/b, p/c, 8/7, Fleishaker *et al*, *Clin Drug Investigat* 1999;**18**:141–50), although urinary retention has been reported (n = 1, Benazzi, *Can J Psychiatry* 2000;**45**:936).

Fluvoxamine + reboxetine

The literature advises caution with combination.

Ketoconazole + reboxetine

Ketoconazole decreases the clearance of reboxetine, with no adverse effects, but some caution may be advisable (n = 11, open, Herman *et al*, *Clin Pharmacol Therapeut* 1999;**66**:374–9)

Lidocaine + reboxetine

An interaction is possible (see introduction), and with other local anaesthetics. The literature advises caution with the combination.

MAOIs + reboxetine

This has not been evaluated so best to avoid and leave a two-week gap after an MAOI and one week after reboxetine before switching to the other.

Methadone + reboxetine

An interaction is possible (see introduction).

Phenobarbital + reboxetine

Low serum concentrations of reboxetine have been reported with concurrent phenobarbital (n = 1, Helland and Spigset, *J Clin Psychopharmacol* 2007;**27**:308–10).

Potassium-losing diuretics + reboxetine

See diuretics (introduction to *4.3.3.6*).

Propafenone + reboxetine

The literature advises caution with the combination.

Propranolol + reboxetine

An interaction is possible (see introduction).

Tricyclics + reboxetine

An interaction is possible (see introduction).

Triiodothyronine + reboxetine *

Noradrenergic adverse effects have been reported with the combination (n = 1, Cooper-Kazaz *et al*, *J Clin Psychopharmacol* 2010; **30**:211–2).

Warfarin + reboxetine

No interaction is known or suspected, but there is insufficient information to confirm this at present (Sayal *et al*, *Acta Psychiatr Scand* 2000; **102**:250–5).

4.3.3.7 TRAZODONE

Trazodone is metabolised by CYP2D6 and inhibits 3A4.

ALCOHOL + TRAZODONE

See alcohol (*4.7.1*).

Antipsychotics + trazodone

Enhanced hypotension may occur when trazodone was added to either **chlorpromazine** or **trifluoperazine** (n = 2, Asayesh, *Can J Psychiatry* 1986;**31**:857–8).

Buspirone + trazodone

See buspirone (*4.1.2*).

Carbamazepine + trazodone

See carbamazepine (*4.5.1*).

Citalopram/escitalopram + trazodone

See citalopram (*4.3.2.1*).

Clarithromycin + trazodone

Clarithromycin increases the AUC and half-life of trazodone, enhancing sedative effects (n = 10, c/o, Farkas *et al*, *Clin Pharmacol Ther* 2009;**85**:644–50).

Cocaine + trazodone

See antidepressants + cocaine (*4.7.3*).

Digoxin + trazodone

Cases of digoxin toxicity exist with trazodone (n = 2, Rauch and Jenike, *Psychosomatics* 1984;**25**: 334–5).

Fluoxetine + trazodone

See fluoxetine (*4.3.2.2*).

Gingko biloba + trazodone

Coma has been reported with concomitant use in an Alzheimer's patient (n = 1, Galluzzi *et al*, *J Neurol Neurosurg Psychiatry* 2000;**68**:679–80).

Interferon alfa + trazodone

See interferon alfa + paroxetine (*4.3.2.4*).

MAOIs + trazodone
See MAOIs (4.3.4).

Phenytoin + trazodone
See phenytoin (4.5.9).

Venlafaxine + trazodone
See venlafaxine (4.3.3.9).

Warfarin + trazodone
INR and PT can fall when trazodone is added to warfarin, and rise when trazodone is stopped, and so caution is necessary (adjust doses and/or monitor), especially if trazodone is used as a PRN hypnotic (e.g. n = 1, Jalili and Dehpour, *Arch Med Res* 2007;**38**:901–4).

4.3.3.8 TRYPTOPHAN

Duloxetine + tryptophan
See duloxetine (4.3.3.2).

Fluoxetine + tryptophan
See fluoxetine (4.3.2.2).

Fluvoxamine + tryptophan
See fluvoxamine (4.3.2.3).

MAOIs + tryptophan
See MAOIs (4.3.4).

4.3.3.9 VENLAFAXINE
Venlafaxine is metabolised by CYP2D6 to O-desmethylvenlafaxine, a major active metabolite and by CYP3A4 to N-desmethylvenlafaxine. Other, minor, metabolic pathways exist. Venlafaxine has a low potential for CYP2D6 and 3A4 inhibition (Ball et al, *Br J Clin Pharmacol* 1997;**43**:619–26) and does not appear to have a significant effect on other P450 enzymes. 2D6 polymorphism has no effect on desvenlafaxine metabolism, but has significant and predictable effects on venlafaxine (n = 14, open, c/o, Preskorn et al, *J Clin Psychopharmacol* 2009;**29**:39–43).

Alcohol + venlafaxine
See alcohol (4.7.1).

Anticholinergics + venlafaxine
See anticholinergics (4.6.2).

Antipsychotics + venlafaxine *
The UK SmPC notes that venlafaxine causes a 70% increase in haloperidol AUC and 88% increase in peak levels, so care is needed as urinary retention has been reported with **haloperidol** (Benazzi, *Pharmacopsychiatry* 1997;**30**:27). Pooled data from two trials shows no substantial effect from adjunctive **aripiprazole** on venlafaxine and metabolite kinetics (n = 152, d/b, p/c, Boulton et al, *J Psychopharmacol* 2010;**24**:537–46; MS). Increased

clozapine levels and adverse effects have also been reported, although one study showed that even moderate doses of venlafaxine had no significant effect on clozapine plasma levels (n = 11, Repo–Tiihonen et al, *Neuropsychobiol* 2005;**51**:173–6). Steady-state venlafaxine had no significant effect on the kinetics of a single 1 mg dose of **risperidone**, although some enzyme inhibition led to slightly raised risperidone plasma levels (n = 30, open, Amchin et al, *J Clin Pharmacol* 1999;**39**:297–309).

Atomoxetine + venlafaxine
See atomoxetine (4.6.4).

Benzodiazepines + venlafaxine
A study showed that diazepam 10 mg had no significant effect on venlafaxine or metabolite kinetics, but venlafaxine slightly increased diazepam clearance. No clinically significant interaction thus seems likely (n = 17, Troy et al, *J Clin Pharmacol* 1995;**35**:410–9).

Bupropion + venlafaxine
See bupropion (4.6.6).

Carbamazepine + venlafaxine
Carbamazepine 200–400 mg does not appear to effect venlafaxine plasma levels (mean 200 mg/d) and metabolite (n = 10, open, 8/52, Ciusani et al, *J Psychopharmacol* 2004;**18**:559–66).

Cimetidine + venlafaxine
A 45% reduction in venlafaxine clearance via reduced first-pass metabolism can result in increased venlafaxine levels and patients should be monitored for dose-related side-effects, e.g. nausea and bp changes. The major metabolite, O-desmethylvenlafaxine, is unaffected.

Co-amoxiclav + venlafaxine
Serotonin syndrome has been reported after single doses of co-amoxiclav during venlafaxine therapy (n = 1, Connor, *J R Soc Med* 2003;**96**:233–4).

Duloxetine + venlafaxine
See duloxetine (4.3.3.2).

ERYTHROMYCIN + VENLAFAXINE
Potent CYP3A4 inhibitors (e.g. ketoconazole, erythromycin) should only be prescribed with venlafaxine if strictly indicated (UK SmPC).

Fluoxetine + venlafaxine
See fluoxetine (4.3.2.2).

INDINAVIR + VENLAFAXINE
A study has shown that venlafaxine reduces indinavir's peak plasma levels by 36% and AUC by 28%, a potentially clinically significant

4

effect (n = 9, Levin *et al, Psychopharmacol Bull* 2001;**35**:62–71).

Ketoconazole + venlafaxine

Ketoconazole increases venlafaxine's AUC and Cmax by about 30% in CYP3A4 extensive metabolisers, but the effect appears erratic in poor metabolisers, variably increasing AUC (0–206%) and Cmax (0–119%), so it's a good job they're relatively rare (n = 21, open, Lindh *et al, Eur J Clin Pharmacol* 2003;**59**:401–6).

Linezolid + venlafaxine

Serotonin syndrome has been reported with the combination (n = 1, Jones *et al, J Antimicrob Chemother* 2004;**54**:289–90; n = 1, Bergeron *et al, Ann Pharmacother* 2005;**39**:956–61).

Lithium + venlafaxine

Venlafaxine has been shown to have no significant effect on lithium kinetics in a single dose study (open, Troy *et al, J Clin Pharmacol* 1996;**36**:175–81), but there are cases of raised lithium levels and of serotonin syndrome (e.g. Mekler and Woggon, *Pharmacopsychiatry* 1997; **30**:272–3; n = 1, Naranjo = probable, *J Clin Pharm Ther* 2006;**31**:397–400). Lithium reduces the renal clearance of venlafaxine but without apparent clinical significance.

MAOIs + VENLAFAXINE *

Wyeth state that venlafaxine and MAOIs should not be used together and recommend a 14-day gap after stopping an MAOI before starting venlafaxine, and a seven-day gap after stopping venlafaxine before starting an MAOI. This may not be enough in some people as hypotension has been reported four weeks after phenelzine was discontinued (Yates *et al, Ther Adv Psychopharmcol* 2011;[in press]). There are many reported cases of severe reactions, e.g. extreme agitation, diaphoresis, rapid respiration and raised CPK levels (n = 1, Phillips and Ringo, *Am J Psychiatry* 1995;**152**:1400–1), hypomania, heavy perspiration, shivering and dilated pupils (n = 1, Klysner *et al, Lancet* 1995;**346**:1298–9), and serotonin syndrome (e.g. n = 1, Weiner *et al, Pharmacother* 1998;**18**:399–403). Follow the manufacturer's recommendations carefully.

Mirtazapine + venlafaxine

See mirtazapine (*4.3.3.4*).

Moclobemide + venlafaxine

The UK SmPC for venlafaxine states very cautiously that venlafaxine and moclobemide should not be used together and that serious adverse reactions may occur. It recommends a 14-day gap after stopping moclobemide before starting venlafaxine, and a seven-day gap after venlafaxine before moclobemide is used. This seems overcautious, although a serotonin syndrome has been reported (n = 1, Fisher and Davies, *Ann Pharmacother* 2002;**36**:67–71).

Propafenone + venlafaxine

An organic psychosis has been reported, with raised venlafaxine levels (n = 1, Pfeffer and Grube, *Int J Psychiatr Med* 2001;**31**:427–32).

Selegiline + venlafaxine

The UK SmPC for venlafaxine states that the combination should not be used and that serious adverse reactions may occur. It recommends a 14-day gap after stopping selegiline before starting venlafaxine, and a seven-day gap after venlafaxine before selegiline is used.

Sertraline + venlafaxine

See sertraline (*4.3.2.5*).

Sour date nut + venlafaxine

A severe serotonin syndrome with anaphylactic features has been reported with combined sour date nut (jujube) and venlafaxine 37.5 mg/d (n = 1, Stewart, *Am J Psychiatry* 2004; **161**:1129–30).

Tamoxifen + venlafaxine *

See tamoxifen + paroxetine (*4.3.2.4*).

Trazodone + venlafaxine *

A serotonin syndrome has been reported (n = 1, McCue and Joseph, *Am J Psychiatry* 2001; **158**:2088–9), as has fulminant hepatic failure (n = 1, Detry *et al, Transplant Proc* 2009;**41**:3435–6).

Tricyclics + venlafaxine

See tricyclics (*4.3.1*).

Verapamil + venlafaxine

A fatality has been reported (n = 1, Kusman *et al, J Forensic Sci* 2000;**45**:926–8).

Warfarin + venlafaxine

Potentiation of the anticoagulant effects of warfarin has been reported, including increased PT or INR (UK SmPC).

4.3.3.10 ST JOHN'S WORT

Although not approved for depression in the UK, this section has been included because concerns about its interactions are frequently raised. Minor serotonin, norepinephrine and dopamine reuptake inhibition activity has been detected from St John's wort (SJW) and might thus potentiate any antidepressants, and so any combinations should in theory be avoided, particularly at high dose. SJW, when taken at recommended doses for depression, is unlikely to inhibit CYP2D6 or 3A4 activity (n=7, open, Markowitz et al, Life Sci 2000;**66**:133–9), but is probably a CYP3A4 and 2C9 inducer (n=2, Ruschitzka et al, Lancet 2000;**355**:548–9). SJW increases the expression of P-glycoprotein, which may have implications for drug interactions (n=22, Hennessy et al, Br J Clin Pharmacol 2002; **53**:75–82). There are reports of serotonin syndrome with SJW and antidepressants in elderly patients (n=5, Lantz et al, J Geriatr Psychiatry Neurol 1999;**12**:7–10). SJW is widely used as self-medication so remember to ask about it (up to 15% have used it recently, and 7% may be taking it at any one time; n=101, Redvers et al, Psychiatr Bull 2001;**25**:254–6).

Review: general interactions (Borrelli and Izzo, AAPS J 2009;**11**:710–27).

Alitretinoin + St John's wort
The SmPC for alitretinoin states that the combination should not be used with SJW.

Androgens + St John's wort
Short-term administration of SJW does not significantly alter circulating androgen levels in men and women, although 5-alpha-reduced-androgen levels may drop (n=12, 14/7, Donovan et al, Phytother Res 2005;**19**:901–6).

ANTIRETROVIRALS + ST JOHN'S WORT
SJW may induce the metabolism of antiretrovirals, reducing efficacy, and so should not be taken together (CSM warning, 2000). The UK SmPC now says **atazanavir** is contraindicated with any products containing SJW, with a similar warning for **maraviroc** (UK SmPC). SJW may reduce the levels of **indinavir** (AUC reduced by 57%), reducing efficacy, and so these should not be taken together (n=8, Piscitelli et al, Lancet 2000; **355**:547). The same would probably be true for other protease inhibitors, e.g. ritonavir and saquinavir. Suddenly stopping SJW may require dose adjustment of any anti-HIV drug.

Benzodiazepines + St John's wort
SJW halves **alprazolam's** half-life (n=12, open, Markowitz et al, JAMA 2003;**290**:1519–20) but there was no significant interaction between stat doses of alprazolam 1mg and the Esbericum brand of SJW (n=28, RCT, p/c, Arold et al, Planta Med 2005;**71**:31–7). SJW significantly reduces **quazepam** plasma levels (n=13, RCT, p/c, c/o, 14/7, Kawaguchi et al, Br J Clin Pharmacol 2004;**58**:403–10).

Bupropion + St John's wort *
St John's wort can decrease bupropion and hydrobupropion plasma levels, probably via 2B6 induction (n=18, Lei et al, Xenobiotica 2010;**40**:275-81).

Buspirone + St John's wort
See buspirone (4.1.2).

Caffeine + St John's wort
There was no significant interaction between stat doses of caffeine 100mg and the Esbericum brand of SJW (n=28, RCT, p/c, Arold et al, Planta Med 2005;**71**:331–7).

Carbamazepine + St John's wort
Carbamazepine reduces hypericum levels by 30%, probably clinically insignificant (n=33, RCT, p/c, 7/7, Johne et al, Eur J Clin Pharmacol 2004;**60**:617–22). SJW may have no effect on carbamazepine clearance (n=8, 5/52, Burstein et al, Clin Pharmacol Ther 2000;**68**:605–12), but the CSM (2000) has warned that SJW may induce the metabolism of carbamazepine, increasing the risk of seizures, and so should not be taken together. Suddenly stopping SJW may require dose adjustment of carbamazepine so check levels before and after stopping SJW.

Ciclosporin + St John's wort
SJW causes rapid (within three days) and significant (60%) reduction in ciclosporin plasma levels and may alter the metabolite ratio as well (n=11, open, 14/7, Bauer et al, Br J Clin Pharmacol 2003;**55**:203–11), so these should not be taken together (CSM warning, 2000; Moschella and Jaber, Am J Kidney Dis 2001;**38**:1105–7). Heart transplant rejection due to SJW has been reported (n=2, Ruschitzka et al, Lancet 2000;**355**:548).

Cimetidine + St John's wort
Cimetidine increases hypericum levels by 25%, probably clinically insignificant (n=33, RCT, p/c, 7/7, Johne et al, Eur J Clin Pharmacol 2004;**60**:617–22).

Digoxin + St John's wort
SJW reduces digoxin's AUC by up to 25%, and so avoid the combinations (n=25, 10/7, s/b, p/c, Johne et al, Clin Pharmacol Ther 1999;**66**:338–45; Cheng, Arch Intern Med 2000;**160**:2548), although stat doses are probably safe (n=28, RCT, p/c, Arold et al, Planta Med 2005;**71**:331–7). Suddenly stopping SJW may also require dose adjustment of digoxin.

4

Duloxetine + St John's wort
See duloxetine (4.3.3.2).

Fexofenadine + St John's wort
SJW may inhibit the metabolism of fexofenadine (open, c/o, Wang et al, Clin Pharmacol Therapeutics 2002;**71**:414–20).

Ibuprofen + St John's wort
SJW appears to have no significant effect on ibuprofen (n = 8, 21/7, Bell et al, Ann Pharmacother 2007;**41**:229–34).

MAOIs + St John's wort
Minor MAOI activity has been detected from SJW, which might potentiate existing MAOI therapy, and should be avoided, particularly at high dose.

Methadone + St John's wort
SJW induces methadone metabolism, decreasing levels by up to 47% and may precipitate withdrawal symptoms (n = 4, Eich-Hochli et al, Pharmacopsychiatry 2003;**36**:35–7).

Finasteride + St John's wort
SJW induces the metabolism of finasteride and reduces its AUC and half-life (n = 12, 2/52, Lundahl et al, Eur J Pharm Sci 2009; **36**:433–43).

Lacosamide + St John's wort
See St John's wort + lacosamide (4.5.4).

Methylphenidate + St John's wort
See St John's wort + methylphenidate (4.6.11).

Omeprazole + St John's wort
SJW may produce 'enormously' decreased omeprazole levels (n = 12, RCT, c/o, Wang et al, Clin Pharmacol Ther 2004;**75**:191–7).

Oral contraceptives + St John's wort
The UK CSM has recommended that since SJW reduces the effectiveness of oral contraceptives, the two should not be taken together (n = 2 pregnancies, Pharm J 2002;**268**:198) and reduced efficacy has been shown (n = 12, open, Hall et al, Clin Pharmacol Ther 2003;**74**:525–35). However, a small study showed no loss of efficacy of Loestrin 1/20® (Galen), with no significant change in serum androgen levels (n = 15, open, Fogle et al, Contraception 2006;**74**:245–8).

Oxycodone + St. John's wort *
SJW reduces oral oxycodone levels (AUC decreases 50%) and shortens the half-life (n=12, RCT, p/c, c/o, 15/7, Nieminen et al, Eur J Pain 2010;**14**:854-9).

Phenobarbital + St John's wort
SJW may induce the metabolism of phenobarbital, increasing the risk of seizures, and so should not be taken together (CSM warning, 2000). Suddenly stopping SJW may require dose adjustment of phenobarbital so check levels before and after stopping SJW.

Phenytoin + St John's wort
SJW may induce the metabolism of phenytoin, increasing the risk of seizures, and so should not be taken together (CSM warning, 2000). Suddenly stopping SJW may require dose adjustment of phenytoin so check levels before and after stopping SJW.

Prednisone + St John's wort
Lack of interaction has been shown (n = 8, 28/7, Bell et al, Ann Pharmacother 2007;**41**:1819–24).

Rasagiline + St John's wort *
Combined use (14 day gap required) is a contraindication (UK SmPC, 2010).

SSRIs + St John's wort
Minor serotonin reuptake inhibition activity has been detected from SJW which might potentiate existing SSRI therapy and so should, in theory, be avoided, particularly at high dose.

Statins + St John's wort
SJW may decrease simvastatin and atorvastatin (but not pravastatin) plasma levels (n = 16, d/b, c/o, 14/7, Fujimura et al, Clin Pharmacol Ther 2002;**71**:63). Reduced (rosuva)statin efficacy has been reported with SJW (n = 1, Gordon et al, Am J Med 2009;**122**:e1–2).

Tacrolimus + St John's wort
SJW induces tacrolimus metabolism via 3A4, which may lead to organ rejection (n = 10, Hebert et al, J Clin Pharmacol 2004;**44**:89–94).

Theophylline + St John's wort
SJW may induce the metabolism of theophylline, reducing efficacy, and so these should not be taken together (CSM warning, 2000), although suddenly stopping SJW may require dose adjustment of theophylline (n = 1, Nebel et al, Ann Pharmacother 1999;**33**:502). Check theophylline levels before and after stopping SJW. One study showed no significant changes from 14 days SJW and a single dose of theophylline (n = 12, open, RCT, c/o, 15/7, Morimoto et al, J Clin Pharmacol 2004;**44**:95–101), so there may be interindividual variation.

Tolbutamide + St. John's wort
There was no significant interaction between stat doses of tolbutamide 500 mg and the Esbericum brand of SJW (n = 28, RCT, p/c, Arold et al, Planta Med 2005;**71**:331–7).

Tricyclics + St John's wort
Minor serotonin and norepinephrine reuptake

inhibition activity has been detected from SJW, which might thus potentiate existing tricyclic therapy, and so should, in theory, be avoided, particularly at high dose. Amitriptyline and nortriptyline levels reduced by 22% have been reported (n = 12, Johne et al, *J Clin Psychopharmacol* 2002;**22**:46–54).

Triptans + St John's wort
The CSM has warned that SJW may increase the serotonergic effects of sumatriptan, naratriptan, rizatriptan and zolmitriptan, with increased adverse effects so avoid the combination.

Tyramine + St John's wort
There is not thought to be an interaction (mentioned by Cupp, *Am Fam Physician* 1999;**59**: 1239–45).

Verapamil + St John's wort
SJW significantly reduces verapamil bioavailability (AUC 50–60% decreased) via increased first-pass gut metabolism (n = 8, open, Tannergren et al, *Clin Pharmacol Ther* 2004;**75**:298–309).

Warfarin + St John's wort
SJW may induce the metabolism of warfarin, reducing efficacy, and so these should not be taken together (CSM warning, 2000). Suddenly stopping SJW may require dose adjustment of warfarin so check INR before and after stopping SJW and adjust doses as necessary.

Zolpidem + St John's wort *
See St John's wort + see zolpidem (*4.1.6*).

4.3.4 MONOAMINE OXIDASE INHIBITORS (MAOIs)

Review of MAOI interactions; Berlin and Lecrubier, *CNS Drugs* 1996;**5**:403–13.

Adrenaline + MAOIs
See norepinephrine + MAOIs.

ALCOHOL + MAOIs
See alcohol (*4.7.1*).

Amantadine + MAOIs
Hypertension occurred in one patient taking amantadine 48 hours after starting phenelzine (n = 1, Jack and Daniel, *Arch Gen Psychiatry* 1984;**41**:726), with reported safe use of both (n = 1, Greenberg and Meyers, *Am J Psychiatry* 1985;**142**:273).

AMFETAMINE + MAOIs
See dexamfetamine + MAOIs.

Anaesthetics + MAOIs
With proper monitoring, general and local anaesthesia can be given safely with MAOIs (n = 27, el-Ganzouri et al, *Anesth Analg* 1985;**64**:592–6), although occasional cases of reactions have been reported (e.g. Sides, *Anesthesia* 1987;**42**:633–5). This is generally considered safe, although care with analgesics and sympathomimetics is needed.

Anticholinergics + MAOIs
Enhanced anticholinergic effects have been postulated.

Anticoagulants + MAOIs
An enhanced anticoagulant effect has been shown in animals.

Antipsychotics + MAOIs
Unexplained deaths with levomepromazine exist, but are probably not related to a drug interaction. The combination is a risk factor for NMS and may enhance anticholinergic and EPSEs. Enhanced sedation could occur. There is a case of serotonin syndrome with **phenelzine** and **quetiapine** (n = 1, Kohen et al, *CNS Spectr* 2007;**12**:396–8).

Aspartane + MAOIs
Recurrent headaches following aspartane ingestion have been reported (n = 1, Ferguson, *Am J Psychiatry* 1985;**142**:271).

ATOMOXETINE + MAOIs
See atomoxetine (*4.6.4*).

Atracurium + MAOIs
A single case report exists of atracurium-induced hypertension (n = 1, Sides, *Anesthesia* 1987;**42**:633–5).

Barbiturates + MAOIs
Barbiturate sedation may be prolonged. Although little human data exists, be aware of the potential toxicity as one fatality has been reported.

Benzodiazepines + MAOIs
Although there are isolated cases of MAOI toxicity, oedema and hepatotoxicity (e.g. Young and Walpole, *Med J Aust* 1986;**144**:166–7), this is normally considered a safe combination.

Beta-blockers + MAOIs
Propranolol used with MAOIs has caused severe hypertension (Risch et al, *J Clin Psychiatry* 1982;**43**:16) and slight bradycardia (n = 1, Reggev and Vollhardt, *Psychosomatics* 1989;**30**:106–8), although not invariably so (review: Davidson et al, *J Clin Psychiatry* 1984;**45**:81–4). Best to monitor bp carefully, especially in the elderly.

Bretylium + MAOIs
Bretylium may increase the heart rate with

4

MAOIs, but it is only dangerous if other sympathomimetics are present. There are no case reports.

Bupropion + MAOIs

See bupropion (4.6.6).

BUSPIRONE + MAOIs

There are four unpublished reports of increased bp and possible CVA, although the combination has been used safely.

Caffeine + MAOIs

Case reports exist of increased jitteriness with caffeine taken while on MAOIs (Berkowitz et al, Eur J Pharmacol 1971;**16**:315).

Carbamazepine + MAOIs

Carbamazepine is structurally related to the tricyclics and so an interaction has been postulated. There have been case reports of raised carbamazepine levels but a lack of inter-action with **tranylcypromine** (Lydiard et al, J Clin Psychopharmacol 1987;**7**:360) and **phenelzine** (Yatham et al, Am J Psychiatry 1990;**147**:367).

Chloral hydrate + MAOIs

There are two poorly documented case reports of fatal hyperpyrexia and hypertension with chloral hydrate and **phenelzine**. This is not thought to be an important interaction.

Citalopram + MAOIs

There are many reported cases of serotonin syndrome (see 1.32) with other SSRIs and MAOIs and so care is needed (review: Graber et al, Ann Pharmacother 1994;**28**:732–5).

Clozapine + MAOIs

See clozapine (4.2.4).

Patient information: warning signs of a reaction

If a patient experiences any of the following symptoms, expecially after eating, taking drugs of any type or if unexpected or severe, a reaction should be suspected and appropriate medical attention sought immediately: headache (especially at the back of the head), lightheadedness or dizziness, flushing of the face, pounding of the heart, numbness or stiffness in the neck, photophobia, chest pain or nausea and vomiting. It usually occurs about two hours after the ingestion of the compound.

Cocaine + MAOIs

See cocaine (4.7.3).

Cyproheptadine + MAOIs

An isolated case exists of hallucinations with cyproheptadine and phenelzine (Hahn, Am J Psychiatry 1987;**144**:1242–3).

DEXAMFETAMINE + MAOIs

There is a case report of a death with phenelzine and dexamfetamine (Lloyd and Walker, Br Med J 1965;ii:168–9) and one with amfetamine.

Dextromethorphan + MAOIs

Case reports exist with cough mixtures containing dextromethorphan but, since all also contained sympathomimetics, these are questionable. Two were fatal so care is advised. Dizziness and muscle spasms have been reported (Harrison et al, J Clin Psychiatry 1989;**50**:64–5), as has a serotonin syndrome (Nierenberg et al, Clin Pharmacol Ther 1993;**53**:84–8).

Dextropropoxyphene + MAOIs

Dextropropoxyphene plus **phenelzine** has been reported to produce sedation (n=1, Garbutt, Am J Psychiatry 1987;**144**:251–2), severe hypotension, ataxia and impaired coordination (n=1, Zornberg and Hegarty, Am J Psychiatry 1993;**150**:1270).

Treatment for MAOI hypertensive crisis:

- Phenotamine 2–10mg by slow IV infusion (adults), repeated if necessary.
- Chlorpromazine 50–100mg IM can be used as an alternative, as can diazoxide (50–100mg by IV injection). Repeat after 10 minutes if necessary.
- Alternative advice might be to bite open a 10mg capsule of nifedipine, swallow the contents with water (Am J Psychiatry 1991;148:1616) then go immediately to a hospital casualty department. Due to serious adverse events (stroke, hypotension etc), s/l nifedipine should only be used with care (Grossman et al, JAMA 1996;276:1328–31). NB: nifedipine is light-sensitive and should not be left in bright light.
- Cool any fever with external cooling.

Blood pressure should be monitored frequently.

Disulfiram + MAOIs

See disulfiram (4.6.8).

DOPAMINE/DOXAPRAM + MAOIs

Animal studies show a clear interaction, with side-effects enhanced by MAOIs. The manufacturers recommend that dopamine or doxapram can be used if their initial dose is reduced to one tenth the normal dose and great care is taken.

DULOXETINE + MAOIs

See duloxetine (4.3.3.2).

Ecstasy/MDMA + MAOIs

Hypertensive crisis has been reported with MDMA/ecstasy and phenelzine (n = 1, Smilkstein et al, J Toxicol Clin Toxicol 1987;**25**:149–59) as has muscle tension, coma, hypertension and delirium (n = 2, Kaskey, Am J Psychiatry 1992;**192**:411–2).

Escitalopram + MAOIs

See citalopram + MAOIs.

FLUOXETINE + MAOIs

There are several reported interactions (e.g. Sternbach, Lancet 1988;ii:850–1), including four deaths. A gap must also be left when switching from one to the other (see 2.2.5).

FLUVOXAMINE + MAOIs

There is an SmPC recommendation to allow a two-week gap between therapies. There are many reports of serotonin syndrome with other SSRIs and MAOIs and so care is needed with this combination.

Ginseng + MAOIs

There are cases of headache, tremor (Shader and Greenblatt, J Clin Psychopharmacol 1985;**5**:65) and mania (Jones and Runikis, J Clin Psychopharmacol 1987;**7**:201–2) with ginseng and phenelzine.

Hypoglycaemics + MAOIs

An enhanced hypoglycaemic effect with insulin and sulphonylureas has been noted.

Indoramin + MAOIs

The SmPC for indoramin states this to be a contraindication, as indoramin antagonises alpha-receptors, thus competing with norepinephrine for post-synaptic alpha-receptors, which could cause vasoconstriction and raised blood pressure. No case reports are known.

Isoprenaline + MAOIs

This is a postulated interaction with some evidence that no interaction occurs. No case reports exist.

LEVODOPA + MAOIs

Low dose levodopa with carbidopa or ben-serazide seems safe but higher doses should be avoided, as should levodopa on its own (Clin Pharmacol Ther 1975;**18**:273).

Lithium + MAOIs

Lack of an interaction has been reported (n = 4, Fein et al, Am J Psychiatry 1988;**145**:249–50).

MAOIs + MAOIs

There is some evidence that different MAOIs may interact with each other, especially if abruptly changed, e.g. isocarboxazid to tranylcypromine (n = 1, Bazire, Drug Intell Clin Pharm 1986;**20**: 54–5) and phenelzine to isocarboxazid (Safferman and Masiar, Ann Pharmacother 1992;**26**:337–8). Tranyl-cypromine is metabolised to an amfetamine and an internal autoreaction (i.e. interacts with itself) has been postulated (n = 1, Gunn et al, Br Med J 1989;**298**:964).

Methadone + MAOIs

Lack of an interaction has been reported (Mendelson, Med J Aust 1979;**1**:400).

Methyldopa + MAOIs

There is a single case report of hallucinations with methyldopa and pargyline.

METHYLPHENIDATE + MAOIs

A less severe interaction than with amfetamines would be expected. A single case of headaches and hyperventilation has been reported.

Mirtazapine + MAOIs

See mirtazapine (4.3.3.4).

Modafinil + MAOIs

There is a report of safe use of tranylcypromine and modafinil for refractory narcolepsy (n = 1, Clemons et al, Sleep Med 2004; **5**:509–11).

Morphine + MAOIs

This is mainly extrapolation from pethidine. Two cases exist of hypotension and loss of consciousness with IV morphine (Barry, Anaesth Intens Care 1979;**7**:194), responsive to naloxone. Low dose morphine and other narcotics, e.g. codeine and fentanyl are probably safe. Methadone may be a suitable alternative. If opiates are used, it is best to start at a third or half the normal dose of opiate and titrate carefully, noting blood pressure and levels of consciousness. See also pethidine.

NEFOPAM + MAOIs

The manufacturers of nefopam recommend avoiding this combination.

Norepinephrine + MAOIs

Although unlikely to cause problems if care is used, norepinephrine is potentially dangerous by injection and/or if other sympathomimetics are present.

4

Oxcarbazepine + MAOIs

See oxcarbazepine (4.5.7).

Oxymetazoline/xylometazoline + MAOIs

There is thought to be little systemic effect when these drugs are used nasally, but this has not been formally studied.

Paraldehyde + MAOIs

Enhanced CNS sedation and respiratory depression have been suggested.

Paroxetine + MAOIs

Nothing has been reported but see other SSRIs in this MAOI section.

PETHIDINE + MAOIs

This is a well-documented, rapid, severe and potentially fatal interaction, although not inevitable (Evans-Prosser, *Br J Anaesth* 1968;**40**:279–82).

Rasagiline + MAOIs *

Combined use (14-day gap required) is a contra-indication (UK SmPC, 2010).

Reboxetine + MAOIs

See reboxetine (4.3.3.6).

Salbutamol + MAOIs

No interaction occurs.

Sertindole + MAOIs *

See sertindole (4.2.8).

SERTRALINE + MAOIs

The manufacturers suggest a one-week washout period after sertraline before an MAOI is used. Several cases of suspected serotonergic syndrome have been reported, so care is essential (e.g. cases and review, Graber *et al, Ann Pharmacother* 1994;**28**:732–5).

St John's wort + MAOIs

See St John's wort (4.3.3.10).

Sulphonamides + MAOIs

An isolated case exists of adverse effects with sulphafurazole and phenelzine (Boyer and Lake, *Am J Psychiatry* 1983;**140**:264–5).

Suxamethonium + MAOIs

There are three cases of enhancement of suxamethonium by phenelzine (Bodley *et al, Br Med J* 1969;**3**:510–2).

SYMPATHOMIMETICS + MAOIs

Hypertension has been reported with many indirectly acting sympathomimetic amines, e.g. ephedrine, metaraminol, pseudoephedrine and phenylpropanolamine. Phenylephrine is found in many OTC cough and cold remedies and can cause a massive rise in blood pressure with MAOIs. Use in nasal sprays and drops is not recommended, although there are no case reports.

Tetrabenazine + MAOIs

Reports exist of a central excitation and hypertension with tetrabenazine.

Trazodone + MAOIs

There are many reported cases of serotonin syndrome with SSRIs and MAOIs (see C5) and so care is needed with combination (n = 1, Graber *et al, Ann Pharmacother* 1994;**28**:732–5).

TRICYCLICS + MAOIs

The combination of tranylcypromine and **clomipramine** has caused four deaths and there has been a fatality between tranylcypromine and a single dose of **imipramine** (n = 1, Birkenhager and van den Broek, *Eur Psychiatry* 2003;**18**:264–5). There are cases of excitation, seizures, hyperpyrexia and a serotonin syndrome after a clomipramine overdose (325–750 mg) with phenelzine (Nierenberg *et al, Clin Pharmacol Ther* 1993;**53**:84–8). Other MAOI/tricyclic combinations have been used with extreme care (Graham *et al, Lancet* 1982;**ii**:440). The dangers could have been exaggerated and the combination may be relatively event-free if the following precautions are taken:

- avoid imipramine, desipramine, clomipramine and tranylcypromine
- prefer amitriptyline
- use oral doses only
- start both drugs simultaneously at low dose, increase slowly and monitor closely.

See also combinations in depression (1.14) for a review of the potentially beneficial effects.

TRIPTANS + MAOIs

The SmPCs recommend sumatriptan is not used with MAOIs, or for two weeks after an MAOI has stopped. The UK SmPC contraindicates MAOIs with rizatriptan.

Tryptophan + MAOIs

There are cases of hypomania (n = 2, Goff, *Am J Psychiatry* 1985;**142**:1487–8), behavioural and neurological toxicity with high doses of tryptophan, mostly with tranylcypromine (n = 8, Pope *et al, Am J Psychiatry* 1985;**142**:491–2), which may respond to propranolol (Guze and Baxter, *J Clin Psychopharmacol* 1986;**6**:119–20). Potentiation of the therapeutic effect is well known so monitor carefully.

TYRAMINE + MAOIs

Ingestion of dietary tyramine, levodopa or a sympathomimetic drug by a patient on an MAOI can produce a hypertensive crisis, e.g. headache, rapid and prolonged rise in blood pressure, intracranial haemorrhage, acute cardiac failure and death. The effect is probably only seen with slow acetylators, as fast acetylators seem able to handle tyramine and other monoamines better. The effect is hugely variable, but 8 mg tyramine can produce a 30 mmHg rise in bp in about 50% people, and 25 mg and above is potentially dangerous (Blackwell and Mabbitt, *Lancet* 1965;**1**:938–40; Berlin *et al*, *Clin Pharmacol Ther* 1989;**46**:344–51). In a normal person, bp rises within 10–20 minutes (range 0–60) of tyramine ingestion, peaking at 20–110 minutes, prolonged if an MAOI is taken. For advice on dietary tyramine, see the following section.

VENLAFAXINE + MAOIs

See venlafaxine (*4.3.3.9*).

Warfarin + MAOIs

No interaction is known, although tranylcypromine inhibits CYP2C19 and so some minor potential exists (Sayal *et al*, *Acta Psychiatr Scand* 2000;**102**:250–5).

Xylometazoline + MAOIs

See oxymetazoline + MAOIs.

FOOD

Reviews: Cheese and drink tyramine contents (Berlin and Lecrubier, *CNS Drugs* 1996;**5**:403–13), 'The making of a user–friendly MAOI diet' (Gardner *et al*, *J Clin Psychiatry* 1996;**57**:99–104), dietary restrictions (Rapaport, *J Clin Psychiatry* 2007;**68**[suppl 8]:42–6).

1. General principles

Freshness of food is vital. If there is any sign of spoilage then avoid. Avoid foods that are matured or might be 'spoiling'. Generally, the more 'convenience' the food, the safer it is, e.g. packet soups are generally safe. Although many foods have only small amounts of tyramine, it is possible to have local concentrations, which might give a reaction.

2. Tyramine-containing foods to avoid

The following may be useful guidelines:

- Dairy products

Hard cheeses and soft cheeses must be avoided. Special care is needed with salty, bitter tasting, refrigerated cheese. Foods containing cheese (e.g. pizzas and pies, see below) must also be avoided and are a known cause of inadvertent ingestion and death. However, cottage cheese, cream cheeses (e.g. Philadelphia), Ricotta and processed cheese contain only minute amounts of tyramine and large quantities would be needed to produce a reaction.

- Fruit and vegetables

Broad bean pods (but not the beans) and banana skins (occasionally cooked as part of whole unripe bananas in a stew) must be avoided. Avocado has been reported to produce a reaction and should be avoided if possible.

- Game, meat and fish

Pickled or salted dried herrings and any hung or badly stored game, poultry or other meat that might be 'spoiling' must be avoided. NB. the original reports with pickled herrings may have been due to spoilage in the brine surrounding the fish, and are probably safe.

- Meat products

Avoid chicken liver pâté, liver pâté and any other liver that is not fresh. Avoid aged and cured meats (e.g. salami, mortadella, pastrami). Fresh chicken liver, fresh beef liver and fresh pâté should be safe.

- Pizzas

Commercially available pizzas from large chain outlets seem safe (analysis by Shulman and Walker, *J Clin Psychiatry* 1999;**60**:191–3; comment by Feinberg and Holzer, reply by Shulman and Walker, *J Clin Psychiatry* 2000;**61**:145–6), and even those with double orders of cheese appear safe. Gourmet pizzas from smaller outlets may have higher tyramine contents, especially if mature cheeses are used.

- Soy and soybean

Some samples of soy sauce and soybean preparations may have very high tyramine levels. Either avoid entirely or a 10 ml maximum is recommended (Shulman and Walker, *J Clin Psychiatry* 1999;**60**:191–3):

> **Soy sauce** (Pearl River, etc) — some have high quantities, ie. up to 3.4 mg/15 ml, and so double or triple helpings could be well above the threshold for a reaction
> **Soybean curd** (e.g. Tofu) — some have high quantities, especiall y if kept

4

refrigerated for seven days or longer, i.e. up to 5 mg per 300 mg helping, and so double or triple helpings could well be above the threshold for a reaction.

- Yeast and meat extracts

'Oxo', 'Marmite', 'Bovril' and other meat or yeast extracts must be avoided. Gravy made with 'Bisto' is safe (all contain less than 0.0022 mg/g tyramine and a full, half-pint of gravy would contain less than 0.05 mg tyramine). Gravy made from juices of the roast or fresh meat should be safe. Brewers yeast (Shulman *et al, J Clin Psychopharmacol* 1989;**9**:397–402) and bread are safe.

3. Foods known to contain some tyramine where excessive consumption is not advisable, albeit unlikely

Plums, matured pork, sauerkraut, spinach.

4. Foods thought to contain only minute amounts of tyramine

Banana pulp (skins unsafe), chocolate (one anecdotal report of headache), cottage cheese, cream cheese, eggplant, fruit juices, octopus, peanuts, raspberries (minor reports of raised tyramine), sausages, soy milk, tomato, vinegar, yoghurt (commercial), Worcester sauce, eg. Lee and Perrins and others (very low, Shulman and Walker, *J Clin Psychiatry* 1999;**60**:191–3).

5. Other foods with isolated reports

Chicken nuggets, chapatti, protein dietary supplement, sea kale.

6. Alcoholic drinks

Patient instructions usually state that all alcoholic and some non-alcoholic drinks must be avoided. Real ales may contain up to 110 mg/L, with reports of hypertensive crisis after 0.6 pint (79 brand study, Tailor *et al, J Clin Psychopharmacol* 1994;**14**:5–14). There is some evidence that low or non-alcoholic beers can contain significant amounts of tyramine (Murray *et al, Lancet* 1988;**i**,167–8), shown by three reactions to less than two-thirds of a pint of alcohol-free and 'de-alcoholised' beer (n = 3, Thakore *et al, Int Clin Psychopharmacol* 1992;**7**:59–60). There is a large variation in other beers, so take in moderation (i.e. 1–2 bottles a day maximum), prefer canned beers from major brewers and take care with de-alcoholised beers. The maximum reported level in Chianti wine is 12 mg/L, likely to be dangerous only in overdose. The following may, however, be of use where a particular patient wishes to drink.

Avoid:
- Chianti
- Home-made beers and wines
- Real ales
- Red wines

True moderation (e.g. one unit):
- White wines
- Non-alcoholic beers and lagers

Safest:
- Gin, vodka, other clear spirits

Red wines contain phenolic flavanoids, which inhibit the enzymes which metabolise catecholamines, including tyramine (*Br Med J* 1990;**301**:544).

Over-the-counter medicines

Each patient should be warned about the possibility of interactions with over-the-counter medicines. The general advice for patients is:

1. Only buy medicines from a pharmacy

Do not use medicines from supermarket shelves, drug stores or newsagents. Do not take medicines given to you by friends or relatives. Do not take medicines taken before the MAOI was prescribed until advice has been sought.

2. Carry an MAOI card and show it to any doctor, dentist or pharmacist who may treat you.

3. Take special care over any medicines for coughs, colds, 'flu, hay fever, asthma and catarrh.

4.4 LITHIUM

Lithium may interact with other drugs, particularly via changes in renal excretion.

Reviews: interactions with serotonergic agents (may increase prevalence of lithium-induced polyuria; n = 75, 4/12, open, Movig *et al, Br J Psychiatry* 2003;**182**:319–23).

ACE INHIBITORS + LITHIUM

There are many cases of lithium toxicity with ACE inhibitors (n = 9, open, DasGupta *et al, J Clin Psychiatry* 1992;**53**:398–400), especially in the elderly (n = 20, Finley *et al, J Clin Psychopharmacol* 1996;**16**:68–71), so either monitor very carefully (review: Lehmann and Ritz, *Am J Kidney Dis* 1995;**25**:82–7) or use an alternative, e.g. beta-blockers. ACE inhibitors are most likely to increase lithium toxicity within a month of starting (Juurlink *et al, J Am Geriatr Soc* 2004;**52**:794–8;

review by Jacoby, *EBMH* 2004;**7**:120) and there is a case of a five-fold increase in lithium levels after switching from fosinopril to lisinopril, the authors recommending monitoring carefully for four to six weeks after any such change (n = 1, Meyer *et al*, *Int Clin Psychopharmacol* 2005;**20**:115–8).

Acetazolamide + lithium

Lithium excretion may be increased or, less likely, possibly decreased by acetazolamide (n = 2, Gay *et al*, *Encephale* 1985;**11**:261–2), probably of minimal importance.

Agomelatine + lithium

See agomelatine (*4.3.3.1*).

Alcohol + lithium

See alcohol (*4.7.1*).

Amfetamines + lithium

Lithium may suppress amfetamine 'highs' (n = 3, Flemenbaum, *Am J Psychiatry* 1974;**131**:820–1).

AMINOPHYLLINE + LITHIUM

See theophylline + lithium.

Amiodarone + lithium

The literature notes an increased risk of hypothyroidism with the combination.

Antacids + lithium

See sodium + lithium.

Antibiotics + lithium

Antibiotics may lead to raised lithium levels (cases within n = 102, Wilting *et al*, *Bipolar Disord* 2005;**7**:274–80).

Antipsychotics + lithium

Although generally considered a potentially useful combination, cases of mostly reversible neurotoxicity were reported in the 1980s, particularly with haloperidol (although these may have been undiagnosed NMS), encephalopathy, enhanced EPSE, neurotoxicity or irreversible brain damage. One review suggested that all these symptoms are consistent with lithium toxicity alone, the antipsychotic affecting fluid balance mechanisms and lithium intracellular concentrations (Knorring, *Hum Psychopharmacol* 1990;**5**:287–92). The main risk factors seem to be if high doses of both drugs are used and signs of impending toxicity are ignored.

There are, however, numerous reports for individual drugs. **Chlorpromazine** levels may be lowered by up to 40% by lithium, with enhanced EPSE and rarely neurotoxicity. Combined lithium and **clozapine** appears safe within moderate dose limits and without co-prescription of serotonergic or 1A2-inhibiting drugs (n = 44,

Bender *et al*, *Int J Neuropsychopharmacol* 2004;**7**:59–63), although there are reports of NMS and reversible neurotoxicity (n = 1, Blake *et al*, *J Clin Psychopharmacol* 1992;**12**:297–9), including one where lithium levels were below 0.5 mEq/L (n = 1, Lee and Yang, *Chung Hua I Hsueh Tsa Chih (Taipei)* 1999;**62**:184–7). Cases of diabetic ketoacidosis have also been reported (e. g. n = 1, Peterson and Byrd, *Am J Psychiatry* 1996;**153**:737–8), and so glucose monitoring might be indicated with this particular combination. While a short study showed a low risk of pharmacokinetic interaction between **risperidone** and lithium (n = 13, open, 9/7, Demling *et al*, *Pharmacopsychiatry* 2006;**39**:230–1) there are reports of delirium (n = 1, Chen and Cardasis, *Am J Psychiatry* 1996;**153**:1233–4), possible NMS (e.g. Bourgeois and Kahn, *J Clin Psychopharmacol* 2003; **23**:315–7), diabetic ketoacidosis, rabbit syndrome (n = 1, Mendhekar, *Can J Psychiatry* 2005;**50**:369), encephalopathy (e.g. n = 1, Boora *et al*, *Acta Psychiatr Scand* 2008;**117**:394–6) and myocardial infarction (n = 1, Ananth *et al*, *J Clin Psychiatry* 2004;**65**:724). Lower **olanzapine** levels were mentioned in one study (Bergemann *et al*, *Pharmacopsychiatry* 2004;**37**:63–8), NMS is possible (n = 1, Berry *et al*, *Pharmacother* 2003; **23**:55–9) and severe delirium and EPSE have occurred in an elderly patient (n = 1, Tuglu *et al*, *J Korean Med Sci* 2005; **20**:691–4).

Amisulpride 200 mg/d (n = 24, RCT, d/b, p/c, Canal *et al*, *Int J Neuropsychopharmacol* 2003; **6**:103–9), **aripiprazole** (n = 22, 2/52, Citrome *et al*, *J Clin Pharmacol* 2005;**45**:89–93) and **quetiapine** have no significant effect on lithium kinetics (n = 10, open, 4/52, Potkin *et al*, *Clin Ther* 2002;**24**:1809–23), although slightly increased lithium levels have been reported and increased risk of EPSEs with **sulpiride** (SmPC 2009) and rapidly developing delirium when **quetiapine** was added to lithium (n = 1, Miodownik *et al*, *Clin Neuropharmacol* 2008;**31**:176–9). Lack of interaction has been shown with **ziprasidone** (n = 25, RCT, Apseloff *et al*, *Br J Clin Pharmacol* 2000;**49**[S3]:61–4), although lithium toxicity (n = 2, Miodownik *et al*, *Clin Neuropharmacol* 2005;**28**:295–7) and NMS (n = 1, Borovicka *et al*, *Ann Pharmacother* 2006;**40**:139–42) have been reported.

Baclofen + lithium

Cases of aggravation of movement disorder in

4

Huntington's disease exist (n=2, Anden et al, Lancet 1973;ii:93).

Benzodiazepines + lithium

There have been several anecdotal reports of reactions, e.g. hypothermia (Naylor et al, Br Med J 1977;**2**:22) and, although a neurotoxic syndrome has been reported (n=5, Koczerginski et al, Int Clin Psychopharm 1989;**4**:195–9), routine use of this usually beneficial combination suggests it to be safe.

Beta-blockers + lithium

Bradycardia with propranolol and lithium has been reported (n=1, Becker, J Clin Psychiatry 1989;**50**:473), although propranolol and nadolol (n=1, Dave and Langbart, Ann Clin Psychiatry 1994;**6**:51–2) have been used uneventfully for lithium-induced tremor.

Bumetanide + lithium

Although studies have shown a minimal effect, bumetanide may cause lithium toxicity (Kerry et al, Br Med J 1980;**281**:371).

Calcium-channel blockers + lithium

Cases of enhanced effect and toxicity with unchanged plasma levels have been reported with verapamil (Price and Giannini, J Clin Pharmacol 1986;**26**:717–9), as have reduced lithium levels (Weinrauch et al, Am Heart J 1984;**108**:1378–80). Acute EPSE and bradycardia have been reported with diltiazem (n=1, Binder et al, Arch Intern Med 1991;**151**:373–4).

Angiotensin II antagonists + lithium

There are cases of lithium toxicity after eight weeks with **candesartan** (n=1, Zwanzger et al, J Clin Psychiatry 2001; **62**:208–9), after five weeks of **losartan** 50mg/d (n=1, Blanche et al, Eur J Clin Pharmacol 1999;**52**:501) and with **valsartan** (n=1, Su et al, Psychiatry Clin Neurosci 2007;**61**:204).

Cannabis + lithium

See cannabis (4.7.2).

Carbamazepine + lithium

See carbamazepine (4.5.1), plus 'combinations' in bipolar disorder (1.10) for a review of some beneficial effects.

Cisplatin + lithium

Reports exist of lithium levels decreased by up to 64% (e.g. Vincent et al, Cancer Chemother Pharmacol 1995;**35**:533–4).

Clonidine + lithium

Lithium may reduce the hypotensive effect of clonidine (Goodnick and Meltzer, Biol Psychiatry 1984;**19**:883–9), so monitor carefully.

Cocaine + lithium

See cocaine (4.7.3).

Corticosteroids + lithium

An isolated case exists of lithium reducing the effect of corticosteroids on the kidneys (Stewart et al, Clin Endocrinol 1987;**27**:63).

Co-trimoxazole + lithium

Two cases exist of enhanced toxicity with reduced levels (N Z Med J 1984;**97**:729–32).

COX-2 inhibitors + lithium

See NSAIDs + lithium.

Dextromethorphan + lithium

Serotonin syndrome has been reported with the combination in a patient also taking fluoxetine (n=1, Navarro et al, Gen Hosp Psychiatry 2006; **28**:78–80).

Digoxin + lithium

Lack of interaction has been shown (n=6, open, Cooper et al, Br J Clin Pharmacol 1984;**18**:21–5).

Dipyridamole + lithium

Lack of interaction has been shown (Wood et al, Br J Clin Pharmacol 1989;**27**:749–56).

Disulfiram + lithium

See disulfiram (4.6.8).

Domperidone + lithium

An enhanced risk of EPSE exists.

Fluoxetine + lithium

The incidence of problems may be low (n=110, open, Bauer et al, J Clin Psychopharmacol 1996; **16**:130–4) and lack of significant pharma-cokinetic interaction has been shown (n=10, open, Breuel et al, Int J Clin Pharmacol Ther 1995; **33**:415–9). The combination may, however, be poorly tolerated (n=14, open, Hawley et al, Int Clin Psychopharmacol 1994;**9**:31–3), with reports of serotonin syndrome (n=1, Muly et al, Am J Psychiatry 1993;**150**:1565), absence seizures (n=1, Sacristan et al, Am J Psychiatry 1991;**148**:146–7) and acute confusion or lithium toxicity (Int J Geriatr Psychiatry 1992;**7**:687–8; review by Levinson et al, DICP Ann Pharmacother 1991;**25**:657–61).

Furosemide + lithium

Studies have shown a minimal effect and furosemide to be the safest diuretic with lithium (e.g. n=13, RCT, Crabtree et al, Am J Psychiatry 1991;**148**:1060–3). Loop diuretics are most likely to increase lithium toxicity within a month of starting (Juurlink et al, J Am Geriatr Soc 2004;**52**:794–8; review by Jacoby, EBMH 2004; **7**:120).

Gabapentin + lithium
Although both are exclusively eliminated by renal excretion, a single-dose study showed that the pharmacokinetics of lithium are not altered by gabapentin (n = 13, Frye *et al*, *J Clin Psychopharmacol* 1998;**18**:461–4).

Herbal diuretics + lithium
A clear case of life-threatening lithium toxicity (4.5 mmol/L) induced by a herbal diuretic preparation has been reported (n = 1, Pyevich and Bogenschutz, *Am J Psychiatry* 2001;**158**:1329).

Hypoglycaemics + lithium
Lithium has been used to improve glucose metabolism and assist the effects of oral hypoglycaemics and insulin (n = 38, Hu *et al*, *Biol Trace Elem Res* 1997;**60**:131–7).

Iodides + lithium
Enhanced antithyroid and goiter effects of lithium have been reported.

Ispaghula husk + lithium
A single case exists of reduced lithium levels (Perlman, *Lancet* 1990;**335**:416).

Lamotrigine + lithium
Lamotrigine does not cause a significant change in the pharmacokinetics of lithium (n = 20, RCT, 6/7, Chen *et al*, *Br J Clin Pharmacol* 2000;**50**:193–6).

Levodopa + lithium
Lithium has been used to treat levodopa-induced psychiatric side-effects, e.g. psychosis and mania (n = 1, Braden, *Am J Psychiatry* 1977;**134**:808). Reversible Creutzfeldt-Jakob-like syndrome has also been reported (n = 1, Broussolle *et al*, *J Neurol Neurosurg Psychiatry* 1989;**52**:686–7).

Levofloxacin + lithium
A case has been reported of severe lithium toxicity (with plasma levels more than doubled) two days after starting levofloxacin in a stable bipolar patient (n = 1, Takahashi *et al*, *J Clin Psychiatry* 2000;**61**:949–50).

MAOIs + lithium
See MAOIs (*4.3.4*).

METHYLDOPA + LITHIUM
Many cases of rapidly appearing lithium toxicity with normal plasma levels have been reported (e.g. Yassa, *CSAJ* 1986;**134**:141–2).

Metoclopramide + lithium
Enhanced risk of EPSE and of neurotoxicity exists.

Metronidazole + lithium
Metronidazole-induced lithium toxicity has been reported (n=1, Teicher *et al*, *JAMA* 1987;**257**:3365–6).

Mirtazapine + lithium
See mirtazapine (*4.3.3.4*).

Neuromuscular blocking agents + lithium
A few cases of enhanced blockade have been reported with neostigmine (e.g. Martin and Kramer, *Am J Psychiatry* 1982;**139**:1326–8). Animal studies indicated the possibility of an interaction and so the last dose or two of lithium could be omitted before the use of an NMBA.

NON-STEROIDAL ANTI-INFLAMMATORY DRUGS/COX-2 INHIBITORS + LITHIUM
This is a well-known interaction, probably due to inhibition of renal prostaglandin PGE2 and reduced blood flow. Lithium levels should be monitored frequently if the combination is to be used.

Reviews: NSAIDs and COX-2 inhibitors (Phelan *et al*, *J Clin Psychiatry* 2003;**64**:1328–34).

Avoid:
- Indometacin: lithium levels increased by 61% have been reported (e.g. n = 10, open, Reimann *et al*, *Arch Gen Psychiatry* 1983;**40**:283–6).

Extra care:
- Ibuprofen: studies show a variable effect, with a 25% increase in lithium levels possible (e.g. n = 9, open, Ragheb, *J Clin Psychiatry* 1987;**48**:161–3; Bailey *et al*, *South Med J* 1989;**82**:1197). As ibuprofen is available over-the-counter, this interaction should be considered carefully.
- Diclofenac: lithium levels may rise by up to 23% (n = 5, Reimann and Frolich, *Clin Pharmacol Ther* 1981;**30**:348–52).
- Piroxicam: several cases exist of a slow-onset (e.g. several months) lithium toxicity (e.g. n = 1, Walbridge and Bazire, *Br J Psychiatry* 1985;**147**:206–7).

Care:
- Azapropazone: the literature notes the possibility of raised lithium levels.
- Celecoxib: several interactions have been reported (e.g. Gunja *et al*, *Intern Med J* 2002;**32**:494), one being life-threatening (Slordal *et al*, *Br J Clin Pharmacol* 2003;**55**:413–4).
- Etodolac: the UK SmPC says serum levels of lithium may be increased.
- Ketoprofen: raised lithium levels have been reported (n = 1, Singer *et al*, *Therapie* 1981;**36**:323–6).

4

- **Ketorolac:** lithium levels nearly doubled by ketorolac have been reported (n = 5, Cold *et al, J Clin Psychopharmacol* 1998;**18**:33–7).
- **Mefenamic acid:** acute lithium toxicity, possibly with renal damage, has been reported (n = 2, MacDonald and Neale, *Br Med J* 1988;**297**:1339).
- **Meloxicam:** 15 mg moderately increases plasma lithium, so monitor plasma levels closely (n = 16, Turck *et al, Br J Clin Pharmacol* 2000;**50**:197–204).
- **Naproxen:** short-term naproxen has little effect on lithium levels (n = 12, Levin *et al, J Clin Psychophamacol* 1998;**18**:237–40), although one study showed some increased lithium levels (n = 7, Ragheb and Powell, *J Clin Psychopharmacol* 1986;**6**:150–4).
- **Phenylbutazone:** doubled lithium levels have been reported (see Ragheb, *J Clin Psychopharmacol* 1990;**10**:49–50).
- **Rofecoxib:** 50 mg/d can increase lithium levels (n = 10, Sajbel *et al, Pharmacotherapy* 2001;**21**:380; n = 1, Lundmark *et al, Br J Clin Pharmacol* 2002;**53**:403–4; n = 1, Bravo *et al, Ann Pharmacother* 2004;**38**:1189–93).
- **Tiaprofenic acid:** increased serum lithium levels (requiring a dose reduction) occurred in a woman taking fosinopril and lithium to which tiaprofenic acid was added (n = 1, Alderman and Lindsay, *Ann Pharmacother* 1996;**30**:1411–3).

Least risk:

- **Aspirin:** 4 g/d for seven days had no effect on lithium levels in one study (n = 10, open, Reimann *et al, Arch Gen Psychiatry* 1983; **40**:283–6), and other studies have only shown a mildly variable effect (e.g. Ragheb, *J Clin Psychiatry* 1987;**48**:425).
- **Sulindac:** reports show either a slightly reduced level of lithium (n = 2, Furnell and Davies, *Drug Intell Clin Pharm* 1986;**19**:374–6), no effect (n = 4, Ragheb and Powell, *J Clin Psychiatry* 1986;**47**:33–4) or raised levels (n = 2, Jones and Stoner, *J Clin Psychiatry* 2000;**61**:527–8).

Oxcarbazepine + lithium

See oxcarbazepine (*4.5.6*).

Phenytoin + lithium

There are several reports of lithium neurotoxicity, without increased lithium levels (e.g. Raskin, *J Clin Psychopharmacol* 1984;**4**:120).

Potassium iodide + lithium

An additive effect may cause hypothyroidism.

Psyllium + lithium

See Ispaghula husk + lithium.

Quetiapine + lithium

See quetiapine (*4.2.6*).

SERTINDOLE + LITHIUM *

See sertindole (*4.2.8*).

Smoking + lithium

See smoking (*4.7.4*).

Sodium + lithium

Excess sodium (e.g. as bicarbonate in antacids) can reduce lithium levels (e.g. McSwiggan, *Med J Aust* 1978;**1**:38–9) and sodium restriction can lead to lithium intoxication (e.g. Baer *et al, J Psychiatr Res* 1971;**8**:91–105).

Spironolactone + lithium

A rise in lithium levels has been reported (Baer *et al, J Psychiatr Res* 1971;**8**:91–105), as has synergism (see combinations, *1.10*).

SSRIs + lithium

See citalopram/escitalopram (*4.3.2.1*), fluoxetine (*4.3.2.2*), fluvoxamine (*4.3.2.3*) and paroxetine (*4.3.2.4*). No interaction has been seen yet with sertraline.

Tetracyclines + lithium

Cases of lithium intoxication (e.g. McGennis, *Br Med J* 1978;**2**:1183) have been reported, so monitor lithium regularly.

THEOPHYLLINE + LITHIUM

Theophylline may reduce lithium levels by 20–30% (Cook *et al, J Clin Psychiatry* 1985;**46**:278–9) as may aminophylline, probably by increased excretion. An increased lithium dose can counteract this so monitoring of levels is essential, especially if theophylline is then stopped. The interaction has been made use of to treat lithium toxicity.

THIAZIDE DIURETICS + LITHIUM

Thiazides reduce the renal clearance of lithium and levels can rise within a few days. Thiazides should only be used where unavoidable and where strict monitoring is used, although it is possible that the effect on lithium is not always dramatic. The combination has occasionally been used in patients where large doses of lithium do not produce therapeutic levels.

- **Bendroflumethiazide:** a 24% reduction in lithium excretion has been shown, (Petersen *et al, Br Med J* 1974;**2**:143–5), as has lithium toxicity (n = 1, Vipond *et al, Anesthesia* 1996;**51**:1156–8).

- **Co-amilozide:** single case report (Dorevitch and Baruch, *Am J Psychiatry* 1986;**143**:257–8).
- **Hydrochlorthiazide:** the effect may only be minor (n = 13, RCT, Crabtree *et al*, *Am J Psychiatry* 1991;**148**:1060–3).
- **Hydroflumethiazide:** one study showed a 24% reduction in lithium excretion (Petersen *et al*, *Br Med J* 1974;**2**:143–5).
- **Triamterene:** increased lithium clearance may occur (n = 8, open, Wetzels *et al*, *Nephrol Dial Transplant* 1989;**4**:939–42).

Topiramate + lithium

Toxic lithium levels have been reported with higher (800mg/d) doses of topiramate, but not with 500mg/d (Pinninti and Zelinski, *J Clin Psychopharmacol* 2002;**22**:340; Abraham and Owen, *J Clin Psychopharmacol* 2004;**24**:565–7).

Tricyclics + lithium

See tricyclics (*4.3.1*).

Trimethoprim + lithium

Lithium toxicity has been reported following addition of trimethoprim (n = 1, de Vries, *Ned Tijdschr Geneeskd* 2001;**145**:539–40).

Triptans + lithium

The literature notes an increased risk of CNS toxicity with sumatriptan.

Venlafaxine + lithium

See venlafaxine (*4.3.3.9*).

Warfarin + lithium

No interaction is suspected or reported (Sayal *et al*, *Acta Psychiatr Scand* 2000;**102**:250–5).

Ziprasidone + lithium

See ziprasidone (*4.2.9*).

4.5 ANTICONVULSANTS

Combining anticonvulsants is a common and essential strategy and so knowledge of interactions is vital, both when adding drugs (or increasing doses) or stopping drugs (or decreasing doses).

Reviews: detailed review of pharmacokinetic interactions between AEDs (Hachad *et al*, *Ther Drug Monit* 2002;**24**:91–103), AED–OC interactions (Crawford, *CNS Drugs* 2002; **16**:263–72; concludes that a woman taking carbamazepine, oxcarbazepine, phenobarbital, phenytoin or topiramate would need an OC with at least 50mcg ethinylestradiol, or Depot Provera given every 10 weeks rather than 12), AEDs and antimicrobials (Desai, *Epilepsia* 2008;49(Suppl

6):47–9), AEDs and chemotherapeutics (Yap *et al*, *Clin Ther* 2008; **30**:1385–407), P450 interactions with AEDs (Mula, *Curr Drug Metab* 2008;**9**:730–7) and AEDs with other drugs (Díaz *et al*, *Neurologist* 2008;**14** [6 suppl 1]:S55–65).

4.5.1 CARBAMAZEPINE

Carbamazepine is principally metabolised by CYP3A4 (also CYP2C8), but is also a potent inducer of CYP3A4 and other oxidative mechanisms in the liver. This auto-induction takes up to four weeks to occur, although it is virtually complete after a week. Carbamazepine (CBZ) is metabolised to carbamazepine epoxide (CBZ-E), which may be more toxic than carbamazepine itself and so alteration of the CBZ:CBZ-E ratio by another drug would alter toxicity. Carbamazepine is extensively plasma protein-bound. Major diurnal variations in plasma levels occur, which can be as much as 90% during polytherapy compared to monotherapy (Hoppener *et al*, *Epilepsia* 1980;**21**:341–50).

Acetazolamide + carbamazepine

CYP3A4 inhibition may raise carbamazepine levels (mentioned in Spina *et al*, *Clin Pharmacokinet* 1996;**31**:198–214).

Alcohol + carbamazepine

See alcohol (*4.7.1*).

ANTIPSYCHOTICS + CARBAMAZEPINE

Antipsychotics lower the seizure threshold, antagonising carbamazepine's anticonvulsant effects and there are also a variety of other well-documented interactions. Carbamazepine reduces **aripiprazole** and metabolite levels by about 70%, probably by CYP3A4 induction, so aripiprazole doses may need to be doubled with carbamazepine, and halved if carbamazepine is discontinued (n = 9 [c = 6], 8/52, Citrome *et al*, *J Clin Psychopharmacol* 2007;**27**:279–83), although one study did not find a loss of efficacy despite the dramatic plasma level drop (n = 18, Nakamura *et al*, *Ther Drug Monit* 2009;**31**:575–8). Lack of interaction has been shown with **asenapine** (US PI). There are cases of **clozapine** levels increasing by up to 100% after carbamazepine was stopped (Raitasuo *et al*, *Am J Psychiatry* 1993;**150**:169. There is also the very real enhanced risk of agranulocytosis (mandatory precaution in SmPC), so carbamazepine and clozapine should not be used together (n = 1, Gerson, *Lancet* 1991;

4

338:262–3). Carbamazepine reduces **haloperidol** levels, with 240mg/d halving haloperidol levels (n = 11, Yasui–Furukori et al, *J Clin Psychopharmacol* 2003;**23**:435–40), in a dose-dependent manner, resulting in worsening symptoms and outcome (e.g. n = 27, 4/52, Hesslinger et al, *J Clin Psychopharmacol* 1999;**19**:310–5). More importantly, a significantly extended QT interval has been shown, probably by increased haloperidol metabolite concentrations. Care is thus needed (n = 2, Iwahashi et al, *Am J Psychiatry* 1996;**153**: 135). Carbamazepine increases **olanzapine** clearance by 44% and reduces half-life by 20% (n = 47, Linnet and Olesen, *Ther Drug Monit* 2002;**24**:512–7), probably by CYP1A2 induction, but dose adjustment is not needed as olanzapine has a wide therapeutic index (n = 11, Lucas et al, *Eur J Clin Pharmacol* 1998; **54**:639–43). Carbamazepine 600–800mg/d may decrease **quetiapine** plasma levels by 80%, presumably by CYP3A4 induction, potentially clinically significant (n = 18, Grimm et al, *Br J Clin Pharmacol* 2006;**61**:58–69; n = 2, Hasselstrom and Linnet, *Ther Drug Monit* 2004;**26**:486–91), and there is a case of undetectable quetiapine levels with carbamazepine (n=1, Nickl–Jockschat et al, *Clin Neuropharmacol* 2009;**32**:55). Toxic levels of CBZ-E (the toxic CBZ metabolite) raised 3–4-fold have been reported with concurrent quetiapine (n = 2, Fitzgerald and Okos, *Pharmacother* 2002; **22**:1500–3). The UK SmPC now notes that quetiapine can increase the levels of the metabolite CBZ-epoxide. Carbamazepine may halve plasma levels of **risperidone** and 9-hydroxyrisperidone, probably via 2D6 and 3A4 induction (n = 34, Spina et al, *Ther Drug Monit* 2000;**22**:481–5; n = 11, Ono et al, *Psychopharmacol (Berl)* 2002;**162**:50–4), and there are cases of EPSE after carbamazepine was discontinued (n = 2, Takahashi et al, *Clin Neuropharmacol* 2001;**24**:358–60). Alternatively, risperidone 1mg/d may increase steady-state carbamazepine levels by 10% over 24 hours and 20% over two weeks (n = 8, Mula and Monaco, *Clin Neuropharmacol* 2002;**25**:97–100). Carbamazepine causes a 37% reduction in **paliperidone** levels, mostly due to a dose-related increase in renal clearance due to induction of renal P-gp (UK SmPC). Carbamazepine decreases **ziprasidone** AUC by about 35%, which may require slightly raised doses (n = 25,

RCT, 4/52, Miceli et al, *Br J Clin Pharmacol* 2000;**49**[S3]:65–70).

Antiretrovirals + carbamazepine

The UK SmPC notes the possibility of reduced plasma **indinavir**, **rotinavir** and **saquinavir** levels, probably by 3A4 induction. Carbamazepine toxicity has been reported when **lopinavir/ ritonavir** and then **nelfinavir** were added separately to carbamazepine, both increasing CBZ plasma levels by 53%, where reducing CBZ dose by 33% solved the problem (n = 1, Bates and Herman, *Ann Pharmacother* 2006;**40**:1190–5). Indeed, even a single dose of carbamazepine reduced the half-life of nevirapine (n = 36, open, L'homme et al, *J Acquir Immune Defic Syndr* 2006;**43**:193–6). Raised carbamazepine levels and toxicity (including hepatic) have been reported with **ritonavir** (n = 1, Kato et al, *Pharmacother* 2000; **20**:851–4; Antonio et al, *Ann Pharmacother* 2001;**35**:125–6). **Darunavir** may increase carbamazepine AUC by 45% and a 25–50% dose reduction of carbamazepine is recommended (UK SmPC). Carbamazepine significantly reduces **efavirenz** levels and efavirenz significantly reduces carbamazepine (but not CBZ-E) levels (RCT, c/o, open, 6/52, Ji et al, *J Clin Pharmacol* 2008;**48**:948–56).

Benzodiazepines + carbamazepine

Concurrent clonazepam and carbamazepine results in a 22% increase in clonazepam clearance and a 20% decrease in carbamazepine clearance (n = 183, Yukawa et al, *J Clin Psychopharmacol* 2001;**21**:588–93), so slightly higher benzodiazepine doses may be needed (Baba et al, *Br J Clin Pharmacol* 1990;**29**:766–9). Carbamazepine toxicity has occurred after the addition of clobazam (Genton et al, *Epilepsia* 1998;**39**:1115–8), probably related to progressive increases in norclobazam.

Bupropion + carbamazepine

See bupropion (4.6.6).

Caffeine + carbamazepine

Carbamazepine induces the CYP1A2 metabolism of caffeine (n = 5, Parker et al, *Br J Clin Pharmacol* 1998;**45**:176–8).

CALCIUM-CHANNEL BLOCKERS + CARBAMAZEPINE

Verapamil increases carbamazepine plasma levels by 50%, via CYP3A4 inhibition (n = 43, open, Bahls et al, *Neurology* 1991;**41**:740–2) as does **diltiazem** (postoperative ophthalmoplegia and ataxia, n = 1, Wijdicks *et al, J Neuroophthalmol* 2004;**24**:95), suggesting a substantial risk of toxicity. The antihypertensive effect of **nilvadipine** (n = 1, Yasui-Furukori and Tateishi, *J Clin Pharmacol* 2002;**42**:100–3) and **isradipine** may be reduced. Since no interaction occurs with **nifedipine** (n = 43, open, Bahls *et al, Neurology* 1991;**41**:740–2), it is the calcium-channel blocker of choice, although the BNF notes the efficacy of **nifedipine** may be reduced, so care is needed.

Charcoal, activated + carbamazepine

Carbamazepine absorption may be almost completely stopped if activated charcoal is given five minutes after ingestion, with a lesser effect if given after an hour (Neuvonen and Elonen, *Eur J Clin Pharmacol* 1980;**17**:51–7).

Chinese medicines + carbamazepine

Paeoniae Radix, a traditional Chinese medicine, may increase carbamazepine absorption (in rats, Chen *et al, Biol Pharm Bull* 2002;**25**:532–5).

CICLOSPORIN + CARBAMAZEPINE

Ciclosporin metabolism is accelerated by carbamazepine, to give reduced plasma levels.

Cisplatin + carbamazepine

The UK SmPC notes that cisplatin might decrease carbamazepine plasma levels.

Citalopram + carbamazepine

See citalopram/escitalopram (*4.3.2.1*).

CLARITHROMYCIN + CARBAMAZEPINE

See erythromycin + carbamazepine.

Cocaine + carbamazepine

See cocaine (*4.7.3*).

CORTICOSTEROIDS + CARBAMAZEPINE

Corticosteroid CYP3A4 metabolism is accelerated by carbamazepine, giving a reduced effect (n = 15, open, Bartoszek *et al, Clin Pharmacol Ther* 1987;**42**:424–32).

DANAZOL + CARBAMAZEPINE

Danazol inhibits carbamazepine metabolism (n = 6, open, Zielinski *et al, Ther Drug Monit* 1987;**9**:24–7), so monitor levels and observe for side-effects.

Dantrolene + carbamazepine

Carbamazepine toxicity has been reported when dantrolene and oxybutinin were added to a stable carbamazepine dose (n = 1, Vander *et al, Spinal Cord* 2005;**43**:252–5).

DEXTROPROPOXYPHENE + CARBAMAZEPINE

Dextropropoxyphene enhances carbamazepine toxicity via CYP3A4 inhibition (e.g. *Neurology* 1987;**37**[Suppl 1]:87) and levels may rise by

44–77% or even more (4-fold over 24 hours; n = 1, Allen, *Postgrad Med J* 1994;**70**:764). Monitor closely if used together, especially in the elderly (n = 84, open, Bergendal *et al, Eur J Clin Pharmacol* 1997;**53**:103–6).

Digoxin + carbamazepine

An isolated case exists of bradycardia with digitalis and carbamazepine but not with digoxin.

Disulfiram + carbamazepine

See disulfiram (*4.6.8*).

Diuretics + carbamazepine

Hyponatraemia may uncommonly occur with furosemide or thiazides (n = 2, Yassa *et al, J Clin Psychiatry* 1987;**48**:81–3; n = 1, Ranta and Wooten, *Epilepsia* 2004;**45**:879).

Doxorubicin + carbamazepine

The UK SmPC notes that doxorubicin might decrease carbamazepine plasma levels, and vice versa.

DOXYCYCLINE + CARBAMAZEPINE

Doxycycline metabolism is accelerated by carbamazepine, reducing efficacy and halving half-life (Penttila *et al, Br Med J* 1974;**2**:470–2). Other tetracyclines appear not to interact.

Enteral feeds + carbamazepine

Carbamazepine suspension absorption has been shown to be slightly slowed and reduced during nasogastric feeding (n = 8, RCT, c/o, Bass *et al, Epilepsia* 1989;**30**:364–9), so take care with dosing after enteral feeding is stopped.

Escitalopram + carbamazepine

See citalopram/escitalopram (*4.3.2.1*).

Ethosuximide + carbamazepine

See ethosuximide (*4.5.2*).

Etretinate + carbamazepine

One girl treated with the combination only responded to etretinate when her carbamazepine was withdrawn (n = 1, Mohammed, *Dermatology* 1992;**185**:79).

ERYTHROMYCIN + CARBAMAZEPINE

A rapid 100–200% rise in carbamazepine levels has been reported with oral (n = 4, Wroblewski *et al, JAMA* 1986;**255**:165–7; n = 1, Tatum and Gonzalez, *Hosp Pharm* 1994;**29**:45) and with IV erythromycin (Mitsch, *Drug Intell Clin Pharm* 1989;**23**:878–9), probably via CYP3A4 inhibition. Monitor levels or use an alternative antibiotic. A review of the interaction concluded that the greatest risk is with high doses of both drugs, and least with clarithromycin (Pauwels, *Pharmacol Res* 2002;**45**:291–8), although clarithromycin

4

can raise CBZ levels significantly, leading to toxicity (n = 10, Gélisse *et al, Rev Neurol [Paris]* 2007;**163**:1096–9) and hyponatraemia (n = 1, Kanbay *et al, South Med J* 2007;**100**:222).

Fluconazole + carbamazepine

Fluconazole-induced carbamazepine toxicity has been reported (n = 1, Nair and Morris, *Ann Pharmacother* 1999;**33**:790–2), with elevated CBZ levels (n = 1, Finch *et al, South Med J* 2002; **95**:1099–2000; Ulivelli *et al, J Neurol* 2004;**251**: 622–3).

Fluoxetine + carbamazepine

See fluoxetine (*4.3.2.2*).

Fluvoxamine + carbamazepine

See fluvoxamine (*4.3.2.3*).

Gabapentin + carbamazepine

See gabapentin (*4.5.3*).

Gestrinone + carbamazepine

The UK SmPC states that carbamazepine may reduce the activity of gestrinone.

Grapefruit juice + carbamazepine

300 ml grapefruit juice increased carbamazepine levels by 40% and AUC by 41%, probably by CYP3A4 inhibition (n = 10, RCT, Garg *et al, Clin Pharmacol Ther* 1998; **64**:286–8).

Griseofulvin + carbamazepine

A reduced griseofulvin level by enzyme induction may occur (see Albengres *et al, Drug Saf* 1998; **18**:83–97).

H2-BLOCKERS + CARBAMAZEPINE

Studies have shown a transient 20% rise in carbamazepine levels with **cimetidine** (n = 8, open, 7/7, Dalton *et al, Epilepsia* 1986;**27**:553–8), reduced clearance, prolonged half-life (n = 12, open, 8/52, Webster *et al, Eur J Clin Pharmacol* 1984;**27**:341–3) and inhibition of non-renal elimination (n = 8, RCT, c/o, Dalton *et al, Epilepsia* 1985;**26**:127–30) via CYP3A4 inhibition. Studies show no interaction with **ranitidine** (e.g. n = 8, RCT, Dalton *et al, Drug Intell Clin Pharm* 1985;**19**:941–4), which would thus appear a safer option.

Herbal tea + carbamazepine

For completeness, I thought you'd like to know that rats drinking herbal tea may have raised carbamazepine levels (Thabrew *et al, Drug Metabol Drug Interact* 2003;**19**:177–87).

Honey + carbamazepine

Yes, I was surprised when I saw this too, but you'll be relieved to find there is no interaction (n = 10, RCT, c/o, 1/52, Malhotra *et al, Methods Find Exp Clin Pharmacol* 2003;**25**:537–40).

Imatinib + carbamazepine

Mean trough levels of imatinib are reduced up to 2.9-fold by carbamazepine (n < 224, p/c, Pursche *et al, Curr Clin Pharmacol* 2008;**3**:198–203).

Influenza vaccine + carbamazepine

A transient 10% increase in carbamazepine levels occurred in one study (n = 55, open, Jann and Fidone, *Clin Pharm* 1986;**5**:817–20), and there is a report of carbamazepine toxicity after influenza vaccination (n = 1, Robertson, *Pediatr Neurol* 2002;**26**:61–3).

ISONIAZID + CARBAMAZEPINE

Rapid carbamazepine toxicity may occur via 3A4 inhibition by isoniazid in this potentially serious interaction (Valsalan and Cooper, *Br Med J* 1982;**285**:261–2). It may be potentiated by cimetidine (n = 1, Garcia *et al, Ann Pharmacother* 1992;**26**:841–2). Monitor carefully for toxicity.

Isotretinoin + carbamazepine

Isotretinoin may slightly reduce carbamazepine plasma levels and alter the CBZ:CBZ-E ratio (n = 1, Marsden *et al, Br J Dermatol* 1988;**119**: 403).

Itraconazole + carbamazepine

Sub-therapeutic itraconazole levels may occur with carbamazepine, so monitor for lack of efficacy (n = 12, open, Tucker *et al, Clin Infect Dis* 1992;**14**:165–74).

Lacosamide + carbamazepine

See lacosamide (*4.5.4*).

Lamotrigine + carbamazepine

See lamotrigine (*4.5.5*).

Lapatinib + carbamazepine

Carbamazepine decreases lapatinib AUC, Cmax and absorption by 72%, 59% and 28% respectively, probably by CYP3A4 induction, but with no change in half-life (n = 24, 20/7, Smith *et al, Br J Clin Pharmacol* 2009;**67**:421–6).

Levetiracetam + carbamazepine

See levetiracetam (*4.5.6*).

Levothyroxine (thyroxine) + carbamazepine

Levothyroxine metabolism is accelerated by carbamazepine, increasing the thyroxine requirements in hypothyroidism.

Lithium + carbamazepine *

Although the combination is often used in rapid-cycling bipolar disorder, neurotoxicity may rarely occur without increased plasma levels (Marcoux, *Ann Pharmacother* 1996;**30**:547). While this is mostly in patients with pre-existing brain damage (n = 5, Shukla *et al, Am J Psychiatry*

1984;**141**:1604–6), there is a case of EPSE with therapeutic CBZ and lithium, which went when the CBZ was stopped (n = 1, Palma *et al, Clin Neuropharmacol* 2010;**33**:102–3). An additive anti-thyroid effect can occur, lowering T4 and free T4 levels (n = 23, open, Post *et al, Am J Psychiatry* 1990;**147**:615–20) and there is a case of lithium intoxication due to carbamazepine-induced renal failure (n = 1, Mayan *et al, Ann Pharmacother* 2001;**35**:560–2). Monitor carefully and regularly for signs of toxicity.

MAOIs + carbamazepine
See MAOIs (4.3.4).

Mefloquine + carbamazepine
The SmPC states that mefloquine may antagonise the anticonvulsant effect of carbamazepine.

Melatonin + carbamazepine
See melatonin (4.1.4).

Methadone + carbamazepine
See methadone (4.6.10).

Methylphenidate + carbamazepine
See methylphenidate (4.6.11).

Metoclopramide + carbamazepine
There is a report of apparent carbamazepine neurotoxicity occurring after metoclopramide 30 mg/d was added, which resolved when metoclopramide was stopped (n = 1, Sandyk, *Br Med J* 1984;**288**:830).

Metronidazole + carbamazepine
Plasma carbamazepine levels rose by 60% in one case when metronidazole was added, resulting in symptoms of toxicity (n = 1, Patterson, *Ann Pharmacother* 1994;**28**:1304).

Mianserin + carbamazepine
See mianserin (4.3.3.3).

Miconazole + carbamazepine
An isolated case report of an adverse response has appeared (n = 1, *Therapie* 1982;**37**:437–41).

Mirtazapine + carbamazepine
See mirtazapine (4.3.3.4).

Moclobemide + carbamazepine
See moclobemide (4.3.5).

Modafinil + carbamazepine
See modafinil (4.6.12).

Neuromuscular blocking agents + carbamazepine
Studies show reduced responses and recovery times to NMBAs (*Anaesthesiology* 1989;**71**:A784), e.g. vecuronium doses need to be significantly higher in patients on maintenance carbamazepine (n = 8, open, Whalley and Ebrahim, *Br J Anaesth*

1994;**72**:125–6) and recovery times can be 40–60% faster with atracurium and pancuronium (n = 53, open, Tempelhoff *et al, Anesth Analg* 1990;**71**:665–9).

Nicotinamide + carbamazepine
The UK SmPC notes that high-dose nicotinamide can raise CBZ/CBZ-epoxide in adults.

NICOUMALONE + CARBAMAZEPINE
The metabolism of nicoumalone is accelerated by carbamazepine to give a reduced effect.

ORAL CONTRACEPTIVES + CARBAMAZEPINE *
The CYP3A4 metabolism of OCs is accelerated by carbamazepine to give a **reduced contraceptive effect.** In women taking enzyme-inducing AEDs (eg. carbamazepine, phenobarbital or phenytoin), the choice of a Combined Oral Contraceptive requires 50–60 mcg/d estrogen (ethinylestradiol, EE). In UK there is no suitable product at the time of writing, but this dose can be achieved by a daily combination of:

- Leostrin 20® and Loestrin 30® daily (norethisterone)
- Mercilon® and Marvelon® (desogesterol)
- Femodette® and Femodene® (gestodene)
- Sunya 20/75® and Katya 30/75® (gestodene).

Alternatively, two tablets daily of, e.g. Microgynon 30®, Ovranette®, Loestrin 30®, Marvelon®, Femodene® or Katya 30/75® can be used, but provide 60 mcg ethinyloestradiol. The NELM (National Electronic Library for Medicines, UKMI Q&A 43.4, Sept 2010) recommend three success packets without a pill-free interval (PFI), followed by a shorter four-day PFI, as well as additional non-hormonal contraception. This is unlicensed and there is no evidence to support this. Depot Provera given every 10 rather than 12 weeks has been suggested (Crawford, *CNS Drugs* 2002;**16**:263–72).

Orlistat + carbamazepine
A small trial suggested lack of interaction (n = 8, open, 8/52, Hilger *et al, J Clin Psychopharmacol* 2002;**22**:68–70).

Oxcarbazepine + carbamazepine
See oxcarbazepine (4.5.7).

Oxybutynin + carbamazepine
See dantrolene + carbamazepine.

Paracetamol + carbamazepine *
Co-administration with carbamazepine may reduce the bioavailability of paracetamol (UK SmPC), and hepatotoxicity (n = 1, Parikh *et al, Intern Med J* 2004;**34**:441–2) and acute liver

and renal failure have been reported (n=1, Jickling et al, *Epilept Disord* 2009;**11**:329-32).

Paroxetine + carbamazepine
See paroxetine (*4.3.2.4*).

Phenobarbital + carbamazepine
Phenobarbital induces carbamazepine CYP3A4 metabolism, slightly reducing plasma levels (Christianssen and Dam, *Acta Neurol Scand* 1973;**49**:543–6). Carbamazepine may raise phenobarbital levels but not by a clinically significant amount (d/b, c/o, 4×21/7, Cereghino et al, *Clin Pharmacol Ther* 1975;**18**:733–41).

PHENYTOIN + CARBAMAZEPINE
Phenytoin induces carbamazepine CYP3A4 metabolism, reducing levels, often dramatically (e.g. n=2, Chapron et al, *Drug Intell Clin Pharm* 1993;**27**:708–11), but with some evidence of increased CBZ-E in the CSF. Raised carbamazepine levels may result from withdrawal of phenytoin via removal of enzyme induction (n=2, Chapron et al, *Ann Pharmacother* 1993;**27**:708–11), so carbamazepine levels must be monitored during the de-induction stage to prevent toxicity developing. Raised phenytoin concentrations may occur due to CYP2C19 inhibition (Lakehal et al, *Epilepsy Res* 2002;**52**:79–83) and mean serum levels increase by 35% (some studies by up to 100%), producing neurotoxicity (Browne et al, *Neurology* 1988;**38**:1146–50). The overall clinical effect may be limited but best to monitor the levels of both drugs.

Piperine + carbamazepine
Piperine (used as a spice and adjuvant in traditional Indian medicines) can significantly raise carbamazepine levels (n=20, Pattanaik et al, *Phytother Res* 2009;**23**:1281–6).

Pregabalin + carbamazepine
See pregabalin (*4.5.11*).

Primidone + carbamazepine
The UK SmPC notes that primidone can increase the levels of CBZ-E.

Probenecid + carbamazepine
Probenecid has a minimal effect on carbamazepine kinetics, but can increase the proportion of CBZ-E via enzyme induction (n=10, RCT, open, Kim et al, *Eur J Clin Pharmacol* 2005;**61**:275–80).

Progabide + carbamazepine
Progabide has no effect on carbamazepine (n=24, open, Bianchett et al, *Epilepsia* 1987;**28**:68–73), but may slightly increase CBZ-E levels.

PROTON-PUMP INHIBITORS + CARBAMAZEPINE
Carbamazepine induces the CYP3A4 metabolism of **omeprazole**, but has little or no effect on hydroxylation via CYP2C19 (n=5, open, Bertilsson et al, *Br J Clin Pharmacol* 1997; **44**:186–9). Multiple dose omeprazole may decrease carbamazepine clearance by 40% and thus increase levels (Naidu et al, *Drug Invest* 1994;**7**:8–12). **Pantoprazole** appears to have no effect on carbamazepine (n=20, RCT, Huber et al, *Int J Clin Pharmacol Ther* 1998; **36**:521–4).

Reboxetine + carbamazepine
See reboxetine (*4.3.3.6*).

RIFAMPICIN + CARBAMAZEPINE
Rapid CYP3A4 induction may lower carbamazepine levels (n=1, Zolezzi, *Am J Psychiatry* 2002;**159**:874).

Rosuvastatin + carbamazepine
See statins + carbamazepine.

Rufinamide + carbamazepine
See rufinamide (*4.5.12*).

Saquinavir + carbamazepine
See protease inhibitors + phenytoin.

Sertindole + carbamazepine *
See sertindole (4.2.8).

Sertraline + carbamazepine
See sertraline (*4.3.2.5*).

Simethicone + carbamazepine
There is a report of carbamazepine toxicity after simethicone was started (n=1, Guneysel et al, *J Med Case Reports* 2008;**24**:242).

Smoking + carbamazepine
See carbamazepine + smoking (*4.7.4*).

St John's wort + carbamazepine
See St John's wort (*4.3.3.10*).

Statins + carbamazepine
Transient carbamazepine toxicity has been reported after combination with **atorvastatin** and roxithromycin (n=1, Corbin et al, *Therapie* 2004;**59**:267–9). Carbamazepine reduces the AUC for **simvastatin** by 75% and the peak by 68%, so increased simvastatin doses would be needed (n=12, RCT, c/o, Ucar et al, *Eur J Clin Pharmacol* 2004;**59**:879–82).

Stiripentol + carbamazepine
Stiripentol appears to be a potent inhibitor of CBZ–E formation (n=14, Tran et al, *Clin Pharmacol Ther* 2002;**71**:33; Cazali et al, *Br J Clin Pharmacol* 2003;**56**:526–36).

Tacrolimus + carbamazepine

Tacrolimus levels have been reduced by 50% (after 11 days) and 70% (after 3/12) by carbamazepine (n=1, Wada et al, J Heart Lung Transplant 2009;**28**:409–11).

Terfenadine + carbamazepine

There is a case of raised CBZ levels leading to toxicity after starting terfenadine (n=1, Naranjo=6, Baath et al, Can J Clin Pharmacol 2006;**13**:228–31).

Theophylline/aminophylline+carbamazepine

Theophylline metabolism is accelerated by carbamazepine to give a reduced effect (Mitchell et al, N Z Med J 1986;**99**:69–70).

Thiazides + carbamazepine

Hyponatremia has been reported with the combination (n=1, Ranta and Wooten, Epilepsia 2004;**45**:879).

Tiagabine + carbamazepine

See tiagabine (4.5.13).

Tibolone + carbamazepine

The carbamazepine SmPC states that CBZ may reduce the activity of tibolone.

Topiramate + carbamazepine

See topiramate (4.5.14).

Tramadol + carbamazepine

Carbamazepine may reduce the effectiveness of tramadol.

Trazodone + carbamazepine

Raised carbamazepine levels have been reported with 100mg/d trazodone (n=1, Romero et al, Ann Pharmacother 1999;**33**:1370).

TRICYCLICS + CARBAMAZEPINE

CBZ may induce the CYP3A4 metabolism of imipramine, doxepin and amitriptyline to give plasma levels reduced by 42–50% (e.g. n=51, Leinonen et al, J Clin Psychopharmacol 1991;**11**:313–8), clinically significant, although the free fraction may remain unchanged, so dose increases may not be necessary (n=13, Szymura-Oleksiak et al, Psychopharmacology [Berl] 2001;**154**:38–42).

VALPROATE + CARBAMAZEPINE

Valproate seems to inhibit several carbamazepine metabolic pathways, resulting in raised CBZ-E concentrations (which has led to CBZ-E-induced psychosis, n=1, McKee et al, Lancet 1989;**i**:167, and so watch closely for toxicity), but sometimes with unchanged carbamazepine levels (n=27, Bernus et al, Br J Clin Pharmacol 1997;**44**:21). In one study, carbamazepine levels

fell by about 25% when valproate was added (n=7, open, Levy et al, Epilepsia 1984;**25**:338–45). Valproate may also displace carbamazepine from binding sites on plasma proteins (n=8, open, Macphee, Br J Clin Pharmacol 1988;**25**:59–66). Conversely, carbamazepine induces valproate metabolism, reducing plasma levels by about 20% (n=8, RCT, d/b, c/o, Larkin et al, Br J Clin Pharmacol 1989;**27**:313–22). This is probably minor but a mean 59% increase in valproate levels can occur on carbamazepine withdrawal (n=6, open, Jann et al, Epilepsia 1988;**29**:578–81). Overall, no adjustments in carbamazepine doses are generally necessary, but be aware of the altered metabolite ratio and monitor if clinical symptoms change.

Venlafaxine + carbamazepine

See venlafaxine (4.3.3.9).

Vigabatrin + carbamazepine

See vigabatrin (4.5.16).

Vincristine + carbamazepine

Carbamazepine significantly increases the clearance of vincristine, probably by CYP3A4 induction (n=15, open, Villikka et al, Clin Pharmacol Therapeut 1999;**66**:589–93).

WARFARIN + CARBAMAZEPINE

The metabolism of warfarin is accelerated by carbamazepine, reducing efficacy. Warfarin doses may need to be doubled (n=5+54, Herman et al, Eur J Clin Pharmacol 2006;**62**:291–6), monitored frequently and reduced carefully if carbamazepine is discontinued (n=1, Denbow and Fraser, South Med J 1990;**83**:981).

Zaleplon + carbamazepine

See zaleplon (4.1.5).

Ziprasidone + carbamazepine

See ziprasidone (4.2.9).

Zonisamide + carbamazepine

See zonisamide (4.5.17).

4.5.2 ETHOSUXIMIDE

Carbamazepine + ethosuximide

Carbamazepine induces ethosuximide's metabolism, reducing plasma levels by about 17% (n=6, open, 55/7, Warren et al, Clin Pharmacol Ther 1980;**28**:646–51), probably of minor significance.

Phenytoin + ethosuximide

Phenytoin may reduce ethosuximide plasma levels (n=198, retrospective, Battion et al, Clin Pharmacokinet 1982;**7**:176–80).

Sodium oxybate + ethosuximide
See sodium oxybate (4.6.13).

Valproate + ethosuximide
Valproate may increase ethosuximide plasma levels by up to 50% via enzyme inhibition, although this may only be a transient effect (n = 6, Pisani et al, Epilepsia 1984;**25**:229–33), and standard regular monitoring will probably suffice. Adding ethosuximide to valproate may reduce valproate levels by 28% (n = 4) and stopping ethosuximide from an ethosuximide/valproate combination has led to valproate levels rising by 36% (n = 9). The mechanism is unknown (open, Salke–Kellermann et al, Epilepsy Res 1997;**26**:345–9).

4.5.3 GABAPENTIN

Gabapentin is not metabolised and not protein-bound so there is little chance of an interaction via this mechanism. Excretion is almost completely renal.

Antacids + gabapentin
The antacid 'Maalox' reduces gabapentin levels by 20% when given concurrently. Separating the doses by two hours resulted in only a 5% reduction in levels (Busch et al, Epilepsia 1993;**34**[Suppl 2]:158), although nothing has been reported with other antacids.

Benzodiazepines + gabapentin
No significant interaction has been noted with clonazepam (n = 127, d/b, p/c, UKGSG, Lancet 1990;**335**:1114–7).

Carbamazepine + gabapentin
No significant interaction has been noted (e.g. n = 26, open, Radulovic et al, Epilepsia 1994; **35**:155–61).

Cimetidine + gabapentin
Cimetidine 1200 mg/d reduces gabapentin clearance by about 10%, which requires no dosage adjustment (Busch et al, Epilepsia 1993; **34**[Suppl 2]:158).

Levetiracetam + gabapentin
See levetiracetam (4.5.6).

Lithium + gabapentin
See lithium (4.4).

Oral contraceptives + gabapentin
No change in the kinetics of norethisterone and ethinylestradiol were seen with gabapentin (Busch et al, Epilepsia 1993;**34**[Suppl 2]:158).

Phenobarbital + gabapentin
One study showed no significant interaction

(n = 12, open, 52/7, Hooper et al, Br J Clin Pharmacol 1991;**31**:171–4).

Phenytoin + gabapentin
Only a slight trend towards an increase in phenytoin levels has been observed (e.g. Graves et al, Pharmacotherapy 1989;**9**:196), although toxic phenytoin levels have occurred with gabapentin 600 mg/d (e.g. n = 1, Sanchez-Romero et al, Rev Neurol 2002;**34**:52–3).

Pregabalin + gabapentin
See pregabalin (4.5.11).

Valproate + gabapentin
No significant interaction has been noted (n = 127, d/b, p/c, UKGSG, Lancet 1990; **335**:1114–7).

4.5.4 LACOSAMIDE

Lacosamide has a low protein binding (< 15%).

Alcohol + lacosamide
There is no data on the interaction (SmPC).

Carbamazepine + lacosamide *
Caution is necessary with this combination as enhanced PR prolongation could occur (SmPC), and lacosamide levels may be reduced by 25% (n = 37, Cawello et al, J Clin Pharmacol 2010; **50**:459–71).

Class I antiarrhythmics + lacosamide
Caution is necessary with this combination as enhanced PR prolongation can occur (SmPC).

Digoxin + lacosamide
There is no apparent clinically relevant interaction (SmPC).

Lamotrigine + lacosamide
Caution is necessary with this combination as enhanced PR prolongation could occur (SmPC).

Metformin + lacosamide
There is no apparent clinically relevant interaction (SmPC).

Omeprazole + lacosamide
There is no apparent clinically relevant interaction, although lacosamide levels may increase by 19% (SmPC).

Oral contraceptives + lacosamide
There is no apparent clinically relevant interaction (SmPC).

Phenobarbital + lacosamide
There is no significant pharmacokinetic inter-action, although lacosamide levels may be reduced by 25%.

Phenytoin + lacosamide
There is no significant pharmacokinetic

interaction, although lacosamide levels may be reduced by 25%.

Pregabalin + lacosamide

Caution is necessary with this combination as enhanced PR prolongation can occur (SmPC).

Rifampicin + lacosamide

Rifampicin may induce the metabolism of lacosamide (SmPC).

St John's wort + lacosamide

St John's wort may induce the metabolism of lacosamide (SmPC).

Valproate + lacosamide

There is no significant pharmacokinetic interaction although lacosamide levels may be reduced by 25%.

4.5.5 LAMOTRIGINE

A large naturalistic study showed that lamotrigine levels are lower with co-medication with carbamazepine, ethinylestradiol, fluoxetine, lithium, phenytoin, phenobarbital and topiramate. No other antidepressants or any antipsychotics lowered levels (n = 829, Reimers et al, J Clin Psychopharmacol 2005;**25**:342–8). Lamotrigine seems to have no effect on P450 enzymes.

Aripiprazole + lamotrigine

Aripiprazole has no significant effect on lamotrigine (n = 18, open, 2/52, Schieber et al, Hum Psychopharmacol 2009;**24**:145–52).

Barbiturates + lamotrigine *

Lamotrigine has no significant effect on primidone and phenobarbital (Epilepsia 1991;**32** [Suppl 1]:96), although a blood dyscrasia has been reported with phenobarbital and lamotrigine (n = 1, Siniscalchi et al, Ann Pharmacother 2010; **44**:2031–4).

Benzodiazepines + lamotrigine

Lamotrigine has no significant effect on clonazepam (Epilepsia 1991;**32**[Suppl 1]:96).

Bupropion + lamotrigine

In a small study, steady–state bupropion 300mg/d had no effect on a single 10mg dose of lamotrigine (n = 12, RCT, Odishaw and Chen, Pharmacotherapy 2000;**20**:1448–53).

Carbamazepine + lamotrigine

Toxicity appears more likely to occur when lamotrigine is added to CBZ if the initial CBZ level is high, e.g. greater than 8mg/L, probably via a pharmacodynamic interaction (n = 47, open, Besag et al, Epilepsia 1998;**39**:183–7).

However, lamotrigine does not seem to raise the levels of CBZ-E and, in fact, may reduce the levels of this active but toxic metabolite (n = 14, open, Eriksson and Boreus, Ther Drug Monit 1997;**19**:499–501). Carbamazepine reduces the half-life of lamotrigine from 29 hours to about 15 hours via enzyme induction (n = 23, open, 4/52, Jawad et al, Epilepsia Res 1987;**1**:194–201), with clinically important reductions in lamotrigine plasma concentrations reported (Koch et al, Eur Psychiatry 2003;**18**:42). A case of serious lamotrigine rash has been reported after carbamazepine was stopped, presumably as lamotrigine levels increased (n = 1, Surja et al, J Clin Psychiatry 2005;**66**:400–1), and there is a case of toxic epidermal necrolysis associated with concomitant use of these two drugs (n = 1, Mansouri et al, Arch Dermatol 2005;**141**:788–9).

Citalopram/escitalopram + lamotrigine

See citalopram/escitalopram (4.3.2.1).

Clozapine + lamotrigine

See clozapine (4.2.4).

Eslicarbazepine + lamotrigine *

Lack of interaction has been reported (n = 16, open, 27/7, Almeida et al, Acta Neurol Scand 2010; **121**:257–64).

Fosphenytoin + lamotrigine

See phenytoin + lamotrigine.

Imatinib + lamotrigine

Plasma levels of imatinib do not appear to be affected by lamotrigine (n < 224, p/c, Pursche et al, Curr Clin Pharmacol 2008;**3**:198–203).

Lacosamide + lamotrigine

See lamotrigine + lacosamide (4.5.4).

Levetiracetam + lamotrigine

See levetiracetam (4.5.6).

Lithium + lamotrigine

See lithium (4.4).

LOPINAVIR/RITONAVIR (Kaletra®, Abbott) **+ LAMOTRIGINE**

Kaletra® (Abbott) reduced lamotrigine levels by 55%, with a doubling of lamotrigine dose needed to compensate (n = 24, 31/7, van der Lee et al, Clin Pharmacol Ther 2006;**80**:159–68).

Olanzapine + lamotrigine

See lamotrigine + olanzapine (4.2.5).

ORAL CONTRACEPTIVES + LAMOTRIGINE *

The UK SmPC was changed in June 2005 to include advice that lamotrigine reduces the effectiveness of hormonal contraceptives, and OCs may reduce lamotrigine serum levels

4

(52% in AUC and 39% decrease in Cmax with Microgynon 30® [Schering Health]; n = 7, Sabers et al, Epilepsy Res 2001;**47**:151–4; see also 33% reduction, n = 24, open, Herzog et al, Neurology 2009;**72**:911–4; 50% (range 29–129%) higher during pill-free weeks and on discontinuation; n = 21, Wegner et al, Neurology 2009;**73**:1388–93). The advice is:

- In women starting lamotrigine while on OCs, the normal dose titration should be used.
- In women starting OCs while on lamotrigine, the dose of lamotrigine may need to be increased two-fold (unless also taking any drug that induces lamotrigine glucuronidation).
- In women stopping OCs, lamotrigine levels may double, mostly during the first week, a rapid and significant effect (RCT, 2/12, d/b, p/c, c/o, Christensen et al, Epilepsia 2007;**48**:484–9), so lamotrigine doses may need to be halved (unless also taking any drug-inducing lamotrigine glucuronidation).

In a controlled study, only the ethinylestradiol component of OCs reduced lamotrigine serum levels, but progestogens did not alter the levels (n = 45, Reimers et al, Epilepsia 2005;**46**:1414–7), so advice may need to be considered carefully.

Oxcarbazepine + lamotrigine
See oxcarbazepine (4.5.7).

Phenytoin + lamotrigine
Lamotrigine has no effect on phenytoin but phenytoin reduces the half-life of lamotrigine from 29 hours to about 15 hours via enzyme induction (n = 23, open, 4/52, Jawad et al, Epilepsia Res 1987;**1**:194–201) by increasing lamotrigine's clearance by 125% (n = 570, chart analysis, Weintraub et al, Arch Neurol 2005;**62**:1432–6).

Pregabalin + lamotrigine
See pregabalin (4.5.11).

Risperidone + lamotrigine
See risperidone (4.2.7).

Rufinamide + lamotrigine
See rufinamide (4.5.12).

Sertraline + lamotrigine
Sertraline may increase lamotrigine levels, e.g. sertraline 25 mg/d doubled lamotrigine levels in one case and, in another, a 25 mg/d dose reduction halved lamotrigine levels, despite a 33% lamotrigine dose increase (n = 2, Kaufman and Gerner, Seizure 1998;**7**:163–5).

Smoking + lamotrigine
See lamotrigine + smoking (4.7.4).

Topiramate + lamotrigine
Topiramate does not cause a significant change in lamotrigine levels (n = 24, Berry et al, Epilepsia 2002;**43**:818–23) at standard doses (n = 13, open, 22/52, Doose et al, Epilepsia 2003;**44**:917–22).

VALPROATE + LAMOTRIGINE
Lamotrigine generally has no significant effect on valproate levels (n = 372, open, Mataringa et al, Ther Drug Monit 2002;**24**:631–6) but can potentiate valproate-induced hyperammonemic encephalopathy (Fan et al, Prog Neuropsychopharmacol Biol Psychiatry 2008; **32**: 1747–8). Valproate inhibits lamotrigine glucuronidation, doubling plasma levels (n = 38, RCT, Lalic et al, Eur J Drug Metab Pharmacokinet 2009;**34**:92–9), reducing clearance (by 21%), and lengthening half-life from 29 hours to about 59 hours (e.g. n = 570, chart analysis, Weintraub et al, Arch Neurol 2005;**62**:1432–6), probably a dose-dependent (n = 28, open, Kanner and Frey, Neurology 2000;**55**:588–91), rather than concentration-dependent effect (n = 62, open, Gidal et al, Epilepsy Res 2000;**42**:23–31). Lamotrigine should thus start at half the usual dose when used with valproate. The interaction has been used to enhance the effect of both drugs with striking responses in adults and children with intractable epilepsy (Pisani et al, Lancet 1993;**341**:1224). Enhanced ADRs have been reported, e.g. rash (n = 112, open, Faught et al, Epilepsia 1999;**40**:1135–40), disabling postural and action tremor (n = 3, Reutens et al, Lancet 1993;**342**:185–6), lupus (n = 1, Echaniz–Laguna et al, Epilepsia 1999;**40**:1661–3), delirium (n = 1, Mueller and Beeber, Am J Psychiatry 2004; **161**:1128–9) and toxic epidermal necrolysis (n = 1, Chang et al, Prog Neuropsychopharmacol Biol Psychiatry 2006;**30**:147–50).

Zonisamide + lamotrigine
See zonisamide (4.5.17).

4.5.6 LEVETIRACETAM

Levetiracetam has, as yet, no demonstrable drug interactions. It is not bound to plasma proteins, is not extensively metabolised and does not inhibit or induce CYP1A2, 2A6, 2C8/9/10, 2C19, 2D6, 2E1 and 3A4, nor UGT enzymes.

A review concluded that there was no need to adjust levetiracetam doses if prescribed with any other AED (n = 590, Perucca et al, Epilepsy Res 2003;**53**:47–56).

Review: Levetiracetam, serum levels and influence of dose and other drugs (n = 297, May et al, Ther Drug Monit 2003;**25**:690–9).

Alcohol + levetiracetam
No data is available (UK SmPC).

Carbamazepine + levetiracetam
Lack of pharmacokinetic interaction has been shown, although disabling symptoms consistent with carbamazepine toxicity (but with unchanged levels) have been reported (n = 4, Sisodiya et al, Epilepsy Res 2002;**48**:217–9).

Ciclosporin + levetiracetam
Lack of interaction has been shown in one case (n = 1, Franzoni et al, J Child Neurol 2007; **22**:440–2).

Digoxin + levetiracetam
Lack of pharmacokinetic interaction has been demonstrated (n = 11, RCT, Levy et al, Epilepsy Res 2001;**46**:93–9).

Food + levetiracetam
Levetiracetam absorption is slightly slowed by food, but total absorption remains unchanged.

Gabapentin + levetiracetam
Lack of pharmacokinetic interaction has been demonstrated.

Imatinib + levetiracetam
Plasma levels of imatinib do not appear to be affected by levetiracetam (n < 224, p/c, Pursche et al, Curr Clin Pharmacol 2008;**3**:198–203).

Lamotrigine + levetiracetam
Lack of pharmacokinetic interaction has been demonstrated.

Oral contraceptives + levetiracetam
Lack of pharmacokinetic interaction has been demonstrated (n = 18, RCT, d/b, c/o, Ragueneau et al, Epilepsia 2002;**43**:697–702).

Phenobarbital + levetiracetam
Lack of pharmacokinetic interaction has been demonstrated.

Phenytoin + levetiracetam
Levetiracetam has no effect on the kinetics of phenytoin (n = 6, open, Browne et al, J Clin Pharmacol 2000;**40**:590–5).

Probenecid + levetiracetam
Probenecid may inhibit the clearance of the primary (inactive) metabolite of levetiracetam, but not of the parent drug.

Valproate + levetiracetam
Lack of pharmacokinetic interaction has been demonstrated (n = 16, open, c/o, Coupez et al, Epilepsia 2003;**44**:171–8).

Warfarin + levetiracetam
Lack of pharmacokinetic interaction has been demonstrated (n = 42, RCT, Ragueneau–Majlessi et al, Epilepsy Res 2001;**47**:55–63).

4.5.7 OXCARBAZEPINE

Oxcarbazepine and its metabolite MHD inhibit 2C19 and induce 3A4 and 3A5 at higher (n = 4, open, Patsalos et al, Eur J Clin Pharmacol 1990;**39**:187–8), but probably not at lower doses (n = 8, Larkin et al, Br J Clin Pharmacol 1991;**31**:65–71).

Alcohol + oxcarbazepine
Caution should be exercised if alcohol is taken, as additive sedation can occur.

Antipsychotics + oxcarbazepine
It should be well known that carbamazepine reduces the plasma levels of many antipsychotics. However, as oxcarbazepine seems to have less enzyme-inducing activity when substituted for carbamazepine, it can lead to plasma levels of some antipsychotics (e.g. **haloperidol**, **chlorpromazine** and **clozapine**) increasing by 50–200% over 2–4 weeks (n = 6, Raitasuo et al, Psychopharmacology [Berl] 1994;**16**:115–6). Oxcarbazepine (up to 1200 mg/d), however, may have no effect on **olanzapine** (n = 13) or **risperidone** (n = 12) levels (5/52, Rosaria Muscatello et al, Epilepsia 2005;**46**:771–4). Addition of oxcarbazepine to **amisulpride** has been reported to cause NMS (n = 1, Angelopoulos et al, Gen Hosp Psychiatry 2008;**30**:482–4).

Carbamazepine + oxcarbazepine
Addition of oxcarbazepine to carbamazepine has resulted in a 0–22% decrease in carbamazepine levels and a 40% reduction in MHD levels (UK SmPC), important perhaps during a switch.

Ciclosporin + oxcarbazepine
Trough ciclosporin levels may fall slightly with oxcarbazepine (n = 1, Rosche et al, Clin Neuropharmacol 2001;**24**:113–6).

Cimetidine + oxcarbazepine
Cimetidine has no effect on the kinetics of oxcarbazepine (n = 8, c/o, Keranen et al, Acta Neurol Scand 1992;**85**:239–42).

4

Citalopram + oxcarbazepine

Carbamazepine may induce the metabolism and hence reduce plasma levels of citalopram, and when oxcarbazepine is substituted, citalopram plasma levels may rise (n = 2, Leinonen et al, Pharmacopsychiatry 1996;**29**:156–8).

Corticosteroids + oxcarbazepine *

Oxcarbazepine induces 3A4, reducing hydrocortisone levels, which might be relevant at higher doses or in critical cases (n = 12, p/c, Högler et al, Arch Dis Child 2010;**95**:1065).

Erythromycin + oxcarbazepine

Erythromycin has no effect on the kinetics of oxcarbazepine (n = 8, c/o, Keranen et al, Acta Neurol Scand 1992;**86**:120–3).

Escitalopram + oxcarbazepine

See citalopram + oxcarbazepine.

Felodipine + oxcarbazepine

Repeated doses of oxcarbazepine reduce felodipine AUC and plasma levels by 28% and 34% respectively, which might slightly reduce its clinical effect (n = 8, open, Zaccara et al, Ther Drug Monit 1993;**15**:39–42).

Fosphenytoin + oxcarbazepine

See phenytoin + oxcarbazepine.

Furosemide + oxcarbazepine

There is a case of acute encephalopathy with this combination (n = 1, Siniscalchi et al, Ann Pharmacother 2004;**38**:509–10).

Imatinib + oxcarbazepine

Mean trough levels of imatinib are reduced up to 2.9-fold by oxcarbazepine (n < 224, p/c, Pursche et al, Curr Clin Pharmacol 2008;**3**:198–203).

Lamotrigine + oxcarbazepine

There appears to be no significant interaction (n = 47, RCT, s/b, Theis et al, Neuropsychopharmacol 2005;**30**:2269–74), although ADRs may be more common and a retrospective review suggested that lamotrigine plasma levels may fall by 29% and that reduced lamotrigine doses may be necessary if oxcarbazepine is discontinued (n = 222, May et al, Therap Drug Monit 1999;**21**:175–81).

Lithium + oxcarbazepine

The combination of lithium and oxcarbazepine might theoretically cause enhanced neurotoxicity.

MAOIs + oxcarbazepine

A theoretical risk of interaction exists.

ORAL CONTRACEPTIVES + OXCARBAZEPINE

Oxcarbazepine can produce significant reductions in some OC plasma levels, with some breakthrough bleeding (n = 13, Klosterskov-Jensen et al, Epilepsia 1992;**33**:1149–52; n = 16, RCT, Fattore et al, Epilepsia 1999;**40**:783–7). See oral contraceptives + carbamazepine for advice.

Phenobarbital + oxcarbazepine

Phenobarbital levels raised by 14% and reduced oxcarbazepine/MHD levels by 30% have been observed with the combination. The clinical significance has not been quantified.

Phenytoin + oxcarbazepine *

Doses of oxcarbazepine above 1200 mg/d have been reported to increase phenytoin levels by up to 40% (less than 10% for doses below 1200 mg/d), probably due to CYP2C19 inhibition (e.g. n = 1, Soskin et al, Psychosomatics 2010;**51**:532–5; Lakehal et al, Epilepsy Res 2002;**52**:79–83), and so close monitoring of phenytoin is essential, especially at higher doses.

Propoxyphene + oxcarbazepine

Unlike carbamazepine, propoxyphene has no significant effect on oxcarbazepine kinetics (n = 8, open, Mogensen et al, Acta Neurol Scand 1992;**85**:14–7).

Smoking + oxcarbazepine *

See smoking (4.7.4).

Temozolomide + oxcarbazepine

Temozolomide does not seem to affect oxcarbazepine pharmacokinetics, although the sample size was small (n = 8, Maschio et al, J Neurooncol 2008;**90**:217–21).

Valproate + oxcarbazepine

Valproate levels may rise if oxcarbazepine replaces carbamazepine (n = 4, Patsalos et al, Eur J Clin Pharmacol 1990;**39**:187–8), and may need free-valproate levels to detect (n = 1, Xiong et al, J Clin Psychopharmacol 2008;**28**:472–3). There is also a theoretical increase in the risk of teratogenicity, due to the presence of increased levels of metabolites.

Verapamil + oxcarbazepine

Verapamil can produce a 20% reduction in MHD levels, which could be clinically significant (UK SmPC).

Warfarin + oxcarbazepine

Oxcarbazepine does not appear to affect the anticoagulant activity of warfarin (n = 10, 1/52, Kramer et al, Epilepsia 1992;**33**:1145–8).

4.5.8 PHENOBARBITAL AND PRIMIDONE

Alcohol + barbiturates

See alcohol (4.7.1).

ANTICOAGULANTS + BARBITURATES

A well-documented and clinically significant reduction in anticoagulant levels and effects occur with concurrent barbiturates. Doses of the anticoagulant may need to be raised by up to 60% if a barbiturate is started.

ANTIPSYCHOTICS + BARBITURATES

See antipsychotics (4.2.1) and quetiapine (4.2.6).

Benzodiazepines + barbiturates

See benzodiazepines (4.1.1).

Beta-blockers + barbiturates

Plasma levels of **metoprolol** and **propranolol** are reduced by barbiturates (open, Seideman et al, Br J Clin Pharmacol 1987;**23**:267–71), but **timolol** (n = 12, RCT, c/o, Mantyla et al, Eur J Clin Pharmacol 1983;**24**:227–30), **atenolol** and **nadolol** do not appear to be affected.

Bupropion + phenobarbital

See bupropion (4.6.6).

CALCIUM-CHANNEL BLOCKERS + BARBITURATES

Phenobarbital may induce the CYP3A4 metabolism of verapamil (open, Rutledge et al, J Pharmacol Exp Therap 1988;**246**:7–13), diltiazem, isradipine, nicardipine and nifedipine, reducing efficacy and so some care may be needed.

Carbamazepine + phenobarbital

See carbamazepine (4.5.1).

Charcoal, activated + barbiturates

If given within five minutes, activated charcoal can almost completely prevent barbiturate absorption and can be an effective adjunct in overdose treatment (Neuvonen and Elonen, Eur J Clin Pharmacol 1980;**17**:51–7).

Chloramphenicol + barbiturates

Chloramphenicol's metabolism is accelerated by barbiturates to reduce OC efficacy (n = 1, Koup et al, Clin Pharmacol Ther 1978;**24**:571–5).

CICLOSPORIN + PHENOBARBITAL

Even low dose phenobarbital induces the CYP3A4 metabolism of ciclosporin (Carstensen, et al, Br J Clin Pharmacol 1986;**21**:550–1).

Cimetidine + phenobarbital

Reduced actions of both can occur but this is of very limited significance (n = 8, open, 6/52, Somogyi et al, Eur J Clin Pharmacol 1981; **19**:343).

Clozapine + phenobarbital

See clozapine (4.2.4).

CORTICOSTEROIDS + PHENOBARBITAL

CYP3A4 induction reduces the effect of some corticosteroids (Brooks et al, NEJM 1972;**286**: 1125–8).

Digoxin + phenobarbital

Digitoxin (but not digoxin) levels can be reduced by up to 50% by phenobarbital, probably of little significance (Kaldor et al, Int J Clin Pharmacol Biopharm 1975; **12**:403–7).

Disopyramide + phenobarbital

Barbiturates induce the CYP3A4 metabolism of disopyramide, reducing plasma levels (n = 14, open, Kapil et al, Br J Clin Pharmacol 1987;**24**: 781–91).

Doxorubicin + phenobarbital

Doxorubicin clearance may be increased by barbiturates and so doses may need to be increased (Riggs et al, Clin Pharmacol Ther 1982;**31**:263).

Doxycycline + phenobarbital

Doxycycline levels are reduced via CYP3A4 induction, reducing its effect, with a halved half–life (Neuvonen and Penttila, Br Med J 1974;**2**:535–6). Other tetracyclines appear not to interact.

Ethosuximide + phenobarbital

Reduced phenobarbital and ethosuximide effectiveness has been reported (n = 198, Battino et al, Clin Pharmacokinet 1982;**7**:176–80).

Fenoprofen + phenobarbital

Phenobarbital may slightly increase fenoprofen metabolism and reduce its efficacy (Helleberg et al, Br J Clin Pharmacol 1974;**1**:371).

Furosemide + phenobarbital

One study showed no effect of barbiturates on furosemide's diuretic effect (n = 10, open, Lambert et al, Clin Pharmacol Ther 1983;**34**:170–5).

Gabapentin + phenobarbital

See gabapentin (4.5.3).

Glyceryl trinitrate + phenobarbital

A reduced nitrate effect via enzyme induction may occur.

Griseofulvin + phenobarbital

Cases have been reported of griseofulvin levels reduced by up to 45% by phenobarbital, either by enzyme induction (e.g. Am J Hosp Pharm 1986; **16**:52) or reduced absorption.

Indinavir + barbiturates

The plasma levels of indinavir may be reduced by barbiturates via CYP3A4 induction.

Influenza vaccine + phenobarbital

A transient 20% rise in barbiturate levels has been reported (n = 35, open, Jann and Fidone, Clin Pharm 1986;**5**:817–20).

Isoniazid + primidone

Primidone levels rose by 80% in a patient given

4

isoniazid 300 mg/d (n = 1, Sutton and Kupferberg, *Neurology* 1975;**25**:1179–81). Blood levels should be monitored.

Ketoconazole + phenobarbital
A case exists of reduced ketoconazole levels in a man taking phenobarbital (n = 1, *Antimicrob Ag Chemother* 1982;**21**:151–8).

Lacosamide + phenobarbital
See phenobarbital + lacosamide (*4.5.4*).

Lamotrigine + phenobarbital
See lamotrigine (*4.5.5*).

Levetiracetam + phenobarbital
See levetiracetam (*4.5.6*).

Levonorgestrel + phenobarbital
There is a case of a levonorgestrel implant (Norplant) failing twice in a woman also taking phenobarbital (n = 1, Shane–McWhorter et al, *Pharmacotherapy* 1998;**18**:1360–4).

Levothyroxine (thyroxine) + barbiturates
Levothyroxine metabolism is accelerated by barbiturates to give a reduced effect and this may increase requirements in hypothyroidism.

Lidocaine + barbiturates
Serum lidocaine levels may be lower in people taking barbiturates (LeLorier, *Toxicol Appl Pharmacol* 1978;**44**:657), via CYP3A4 induction.

MAOIs + phenobarbital
See MAOIs (*4.3.4*).

Memantine + phenobarbital
See memantine (*4.6.9*).

Methadone + phenobarbital
See methadone (*4.6.10*).

Metronidazole + phenobarbital
One study showed metronidazole metabolism to be accelerated by barbiturates, reducing levels by a third (*Clin Pharmacol Ther* 1987;**41**:235).

Modafinil + phenobarbital
See modafinil (*4.6.12*).

Nicotinamide + primidone
There are reports of reduced conversion from primidone to phenobarbital (n = 1, Bourgeois et al, *Neurology* 1982;**32**:1122).

NICOUMALONE + BARBITURATES
Nicoumalone metabolism is accelerated by barbiturates, giving a reduced anticoagulant effect.

ORAL CONTRACEPTIVES + PHENOBARBITAL *
See oral contraceptives + carbamazepine.

Oxcarbazepine + phenobarbital
See oxcarbazepine (*4.5.7*).

Paracetamol + phenobarbital
An isolated case of enhanced hepatotoxicity exists (Pirotte, *Ann Int Med* 1984;**101**:403).

Paroxetine + phenobarbital
See paroxetine (*4.3.2.4*).

Pethidine + phenobarbital
Severe CNS sedation with the combination has been reported (n = 12, open, c/o, Stambaugh et al, *J Clin Pharmacol* 1978;**18**:482–90).

Phenylbutazone + phenobarbital
Reduced levels of phenylbutazone may occur (Levi et al, *Lancet* 1968;**i**:1275).

Phenytoin + phenobarbital
See barbiturates + phenytoin (*4.5.9*).

Pregabalin + phenobarbital
See pregabalin (*4.5.11*).

Pyridoxine + phenobarbital
Large doses of pyridoxine (e.g. 200 mg/d) can reduce phenobarbital levels by up to 40–50% (Hansson and Sillanpaa, *Lancet* 1976;**i**:256).

Quetiapine + phenobarbital
See quetiapine (*4.2.6*).

Quinidine + phenobarbital
CYP3A4 induction may reduce quinidine levels by up to 50% (Rogers and Blackman, *Drug Intell Clin Pharm* 1983;**17**:819–20).

Reboxetine + phenobarbital
See reboxetine (*4.3.3.6*).

Rifampicin + barbiturates
Rifampicin can induce barbiturate metabolism, so a decreased efficacy might be predicted (for effect on hexobarbital: n = 40, open, See Richter et al, *Eur J Clin Pharmacol* 1980;**17**:197–202).

Rufinamide + phenobarbital
See rufinamide (*4.5.12*)

Smoking + phenobarbital
See smoking (*4.7.4*).

St John's wort + phenobarbital
See St John's wort (*4.3.3.10*).

Testosterone + phenobarbital
A reduced steroid effect can occur via CYP3A4 induction.

THEOPHYLLINE + BARBITURATES
Theophylline metabolism is accelerated by barbiturates in premature neonates, giving a reduced effect (n = 24, Kandrokas et al, *Ther Drug Monit* 1990;**12**:139–43).

Tiagabine + phenobarbital
See tiagabine (*4.5.13*).

Topiramate + phenobarbital
See topiramate (*4.5.14*).

TRICYCLICS + BARBITURATES
See tricyclics (*4.3.1*).

Tropisetron + phenobarbital

Phenobarbital reduces the plasma levels of tropisetron (BNF).

VALPROATE + PHENOBARBITAL

Valproate may reduce glucuronidation and increase phenobarbital plasma concentrations by up to 25% (mean of 5.87 mg/L, n = 20, Bernus et al, Br J Clin Pharmacol 1994;**38**:411–6), increasing sedation and other side-effects (e.g. Kapetanovic et al, Clin Pharmacol Ther 1981;**99**:314), although this may only be transient (review by Keys, Drug Intell Clin Pharm 1982;**16**:737–9). Reduce phenobarbital dosage if sedation occurs, and monitor blood levels regularly.

Vigabatrin + phenobarbital

See vigabatrin (4.5.16).

WARFARIN + PHENOBARBITAL

See anticoagulants + barbiturates in this section.

Zaleplon + phenobarbital

See zaleplon (4.1.5).

4.5.9 PHENYTOIN

Phenytoin has a narrow therapeutic index and is prone to drug–drug interactions via several mechanisms. It is primarily metabolised by 2C9, secondary is 2C19, with genetic polymorphism affecting levels. It is extensively bound to plasma proteins, induces CYP3A4 and has a saturable metabolism. It can be displaced, giving an increased proportion of free active phenytoin, significant where TDM just measures total phenytoin rather than the proportion of free (hence active) phenytoin. Measuring free phenytoin levels may thus be more appropriate in certain circumstances. Decreased protein binding produces a decline in total concentration, but no change in free levels (Wilkinson, Pharmacol Rev 1987;**39**:1–47).

Thus, low concentrations may appear below the normal therapeutic range, but free (active) levels are appropriate, prompting inappropriately increased doses or discontinuation (see Toler, Ann Pharmacother 1994;**28**:808–9).

Review: pharmacokinetic interactions (Nation et al, Clin Pharmacokinet 1990;**18**:37–60).

Acetazolamide + phenytoin

Acetazolamide may enhance the osteomalacia secondary to phenytoin use in a few patients (n = 2, Mallette, Arch Intern Med 1977;**137**:1013).

ALCOHOL + PHENYTOIN

See alcohol (4.7.1).

Allopurinol + phenytoin

Phenytoin toxicity may occur with repeated high-dose allopurinol (Ogiso et al, J Pharmacobiodyn 1990;**13**:36–43).

AMIODARONE + PHENYTOIN

Amiodarone reduces phenytoin metabolism, toxicity developing over two weeks (n = 7, open, 8/52, Nolan et al, Am J Cardiol 1990;**65**:1252–7), so reduce the phenytoin dose by at least 25%.

Anaesthetics + phenytoin

Case reports exist of phenytoin toxicity following halothane (Karlin and Kutt, J Pediatr 1970;**76**:941–4) and so caution is needed.

Antacids + phenytoin

Antacids probably reduce phenytoin levels, shown in several studies (e.g. n = 6, McElnay et al, Br J Clin Pharmacol 1982;**13**:501) and seizure control could be impaired. It is thus best to separate doses by about three hours or use ranitidine (see also cimetidine).

ANTIPSYCHOTICS + PHENYTOIN

See antipsychotics (4.2.1), clozapine (4.2.4), quetiapine (4.2.6) and risperidone/paliperidone (4.2.7).

ANTIRETROVIRALS + PHENYTOIN

Phenytoin increases lopinavir clearance, and lopinavir and ritonavir reduce phenytoin levels through 2C9 induction (n = 24, Lim et al, J Acquir Immune Defic Syndr 2004;**36**:1034–40). A similar effect on reducing levels occurs with efavirenz (Spak et al, AIDS 2008;**22**:164–5), indinavir (BNF) and nevirapine (n = 36, open, L'homme et al, J Acquir Immune Defic Syndr 2006;**43**:193–6).

Atomoxetine + phenytoin

See atomoxetine (4.6.4).

Ayurvedic herbal mixtures + phenytoin

See shankhapushpi + phenytoin.

Barbiturates + phenytoin

At normal doses phenobarbital probably induces the metabolism of phenytoin, reducing plasma levels, probably of minimal significance (n = 6, open, Browne et al, Neurology 1988;**38**:639–42). Phenytoin serum levels are increased by very high dose barbiturates and the effect may be dose-dependent with a curvilinear relationship (n = 1, Kuranari et al, Ann Pharma-cother 1995;**29**:83–4). Care is also needed if phenobarbital is stopped, as phenytoin levels may change. Phenytoin may raise phenobarbital levels by up to 100%, resulting in increased sedation, probably of minor clinical significance (n = 1, Porro et al, Br

4

J Clin Pharmacol 1982;**14**:294–7) but regular monitoring should still be done, especially as a case of fatal agranulocytosis has been reported with the combination (n = 1, Laurenson *et al*, *Lancet* 1994;**344**:32–3).

Benzodiazepines + phenytoin

Diazepam, clonazepam and chlordiazepoxide have been reported to potentiate phenytoin leading to possible intoxication (e.g. n = 1, Murphy and Wilbur, *Ann Pharmacother* 2003;**37**:659–63), although some studies have not shown this effect. It is best to monitor phenytoin plasma levels regularly. Conversely, phenytoin induces the metabolism of clonazepam, reducing levels by up to 50% (n = 27, open, Sjo *et al*, *Eur J Clin Pharmacol* 1975;**8**:249–54).

Bupropion + phenytoin

See bupropion (*4.6.6*).

Buspirone + phenytoin

See buspirone (*4.1.2*).

Calcium-channel blockers + phenytoin

High dose **diltiazem** (720 mg/d) increases phenytoin levels, and a 40% reduction in phenytoin dose has been needed to stabilise levels (n = 2, Clarke *et al*, *Pharmacotherapy* 1993;**13**:402–5; n = 43, Bahls *et al*, *Neurology* 1991;**41**:740–2). **Isradipine** can raise phenytoin levels, producing toxicity probably by P450 inhibition (n = 1, Cachat and Tufro, *Ann Pharmacother* 2002;**36**:1399–402). Lack of interaction between **nifedipine** and phenytoin has been noted in several studies (e.g. n = 8, open, Schellens *et al*, *Br J Clin Pharmacol* 1991;**31**:175–8), although tremor, headache and restlessness with phenytoin levels tripled has been reported, falling to normal after nifedipine was discontinued (n = 1, Ahmad *et al*, *J Am Coll Cardiol* 1984;**3**:1581). **Verapamil** may inhibit phenytoin metabolism (*Neurology* 1991;**41**:740–2). Almost complete lack of verapamil absorption (at up to 400 mg/d) has been reported (n = 1, Woodcock *et al*, *N Engl J Med* 1991;**325**:1179). The effects of **isradipine** and **nicardipine** may be reduced by phenytoin.

CARBAMAZEPINE + PHENYTOIN

See carbamazepine (*4.5.1*).

Charcoal, activated + phenytoin

Phenytoin absorption is almost completely (98%) prevented if activated charcoal is taken within five minutes and reduced by about 80% if given after one hour (n = 6, open, c/o, Neuvonen *et al, Eur*

J Clin Pharmacol 1978;**13**:213–8). Multiple-dose activated charcoal has been used successfully over several days for phenytoin toxicity secondary to hepatitis and, extraordinarily, may have some use even up to a week after phenytoin ingestion (n = 1, Howard *et al, Ann Pharmacother* 1994;**28**:201–3).

Chinese medicines + phenytoin

Phenytoin poisoning after using Chinese proprietary medicines has been reported (n = 1, Lau *et al, Hum Experimental Toxicol* 2000;**19**:385–6).

Chloral + phenytoin

Dichloralphenazone has been shown to decrease phenytoin levels (n = 5, Riddell *et al, Br J Clin Pharmacol* 1980;**9**:118P), although whether the chloral part of the molecule was responsible for this is not known.

CHLORAMPHENICOL + PHENYTOIN

Phenytoin toxicity may occur with oral chloramphenicol via enzyme inhibition (*Aust J Hosp Pharm* 1987;**17**:51–3). This is an uncommon combination but a well-documented and serious interaction. Monitor very carefully if the combination has to be used.

Chlorphenamine + phenytoin

Two isolated cases exist of phenytoin intoxication (Pugh *et al, Br J Clin Pharmacol* 1975;**2**:173–5) and so care may be needed.

CICLOSPORIN + PHENYTOIN

Ciclosporin levels can be reduced by 80% by phenytoin, by enzyme induction (n = 6, Freeman *et al, Br J Clin Pharmacol* 1984; **18**: 887–93).

Ciprofloxacin + phenytoin

Raised phenytoin levels have been predicted. Raised phenytoin levels from oral ciprofloxacin have been reported (n = 1, Hull, *Ann Pharmacother* 1993;**27**:1283). However, IV ciprofloxacin has led to halved phenytoin levels (n = 1, *Int Pharm J* 1992;**6**:109), and resulted in sub-therapeutic levels, seizures and increased phenytoin dose requirements (Dillard *et al, Ann Pharmacother* 1992;**26**:263; n = 1, Brouwers and de Boer, *Ann Pharmacother* 1997;**31**:498). There is a case of a phenytoin dose increased during ciprofloxacin therapy, only for toxic levels to appear when the antibiotic course was completed (n = 1, Pollak and Slayter, *Ann Pharmacother* 1997;**31**:61–4). More frequent phenytoin plasma level monitoring would be wise.

Clinafloxacin + phenytoin

Higher steady state phenytoin levels have been

reported with clinafloxacin (Randinitis *et al*, *Drugs* 1999;**58**[Suppl 2]:254–5).

CLOZAPINE + PHENYTOIN

See clozapine (4.2.4).

CORTICOSTEROIDS + PHENYTOIN

Steroid metabolism is accelerated by phenytoin to give a reduced effect (McLelland and Jack, *Lancet* 1978;**i**:1096–7) and so higher doses may be needed. Hydrocortisone may be less affected than other steroids. Phenytoin levels may also be changed.

Co-trimoxazole + phenytoin

Raised phenytoin levels have been reported with co-trimoxazole (n = 1, Gillman and Sandyk, *Arch Intern Med* 1985;**102**:559).

DEXAMETHASONE + PHENYTOIN

Phenytoin levels may be halved by dexamethasone (e.g. n = 1, Lackner, *Pharmacother* 1991;**11**:344–7; n = 1, Griffiths and Taylor, *Can J Hosp Pharm* 1999;**52**:96–8), and very high doses of phenytoin may be necessary (e.g. 900mg/d) to maintain levels (case and review by Recueno *et al*, *Ann Pharmacother* 1995;**29**:935). Regular and frequent monitoring of phenytoin levels is thus essential.

Dexibuprofen + phenytoin

Phenytoin acute neurological toxicity has been reported with the combination (n = 1, Llinares–Tello *et al*, *Med Clin* [Barc] 2007;**128**:239).

Dextropropoxyphene + phenytoin

See propoxyphene + phenytoin.

DIAZOXIDE + PHENYTOIN

Reduced phenytoin levels occur via increased metabolism (Turck *et al*, *Presse Med* 1986;**15**:31), so monitor carefully.

DICOUMAROL + PHENYTOIN

Phenytoin levels may rise rapidly by over 100% (Hansen *et al*, *Acta Med Scand* 1971;**189**:15–9) via enzyme inhibition. Avoid the combination if at all possible or monitor very carefully.

Digoxin + phenytoin

Phenytoin reduces digoxin half-life by 30% (n = 6, RCT, open, c/o, Rameis *et al*, *Eur J Clin Pharmacol* 1985;**29**:49–53), so monitor carefully.

DISOPYRAMIDE + PHENYTOIN

Phenytoin reduces the plasma levels of diso-pyramide, possibly to below therapeutic levels (Kessler *et al*, *Clin Pharm* 1982;**1**:263–4).

Disulfiram + phenytoin

Phenytoin toxicity and delirium may occur via enzyme inhibition (e.g. n = 1, Brown *et al*, *Ann Emerg Med* 1983;**12**:310–3).

Dopamine + phenytoin

Hypotension may occur in patients on dopamine if phenytoin is added (n = 5, Bivins *et al*, *Arch Surg* 1978;**113**:245–9), although lack of interaction has been reported in a well studied case (n = 1, Torres *et al*, *Ann Pharmacother* 1995;**29**:1300–1).

Doxifluridine + phenytoin

Elevated phenytoin levels have been reported (n = 1, Konishi *et al*, *Ann Pharmacother* 2002;**36**: 831–4).

DOXYCYCLINE + PHENYTOIN

Doxycycline metabolism is accelerated by phenytoin to give a reduced effect, with a halved half-life (Penttila *et al*, *Br Med J* 1974;**ii**:470). Other tetracyclines appear not to interact, so make dosage adjustments or use an alternative.

Enteral feeds + phenytoin

See nasogastric feeds + phenytoin.

Ethosuximide + phenytoin

See ethosuximide (4.5.2).

FLUCONAZOLE + PHENYTOIN *

Oral fluconazole inhibits phenytoin metabolism producing rapid and severe toxicity (e.g. n = 1, Helldén *et al*, *Eur J Clin Pharmacol* 2010;**66**:791–5; review by Cadle *et al*, *Ann Pharmacother* 1994; **28**:191–5). Continuous phenytoin plasma monitoring is recommended with fluconazole doses of 200mg/d or above (n = 20, RCT, p/c, Blum *et al*, *Clin Pharmacol Ther* 1991;**49**:420–5).

Fluorouracil + phenytoin

Cases exist of elevated phenytoin levels 11 weeks after starting fluorouracil and leucovorin, possibly via CYP2C9 inhibition (n = 1, Gilbar and Brodribb, *Ann Pharmacother* 2001;**35**:1367–70; n = 1, Rosemergy and Findlay, *N Z Med J* 2002; **115**:U124).

FLUOXETINE + PHENYTOIN

Phenytoin levels raised by 66% have been reported two weeks after fluoxetine was added, with levels falling back to nearly normal within a week of stopping fluoxetine (n = 1, Woods *et al*, *N Z Med J* 1994;**107**:19). Conversely, loss of phenytoin efficacy as a result of fluoxetine discontinuation has been reported (n = 1, Shad and Preskorn, *J Clin Psychopharmacol* 1999;**19**:471).

FLUVOXAMINE + PHENYTOIN

Fluvoxamine may toxically triple phenytoin levels, probably by 2C9/19 inhibition (n = 1, Mamiya *et al*, *Ther Drug Monit* 2001;**23**:75–7).

Folic acid + phenytoin

Serum folate decreases when phenytoin is started.

4

Folic acid supplementation should be started with phenytoin as folic acid supplementation in folate-deficient patients changes the kinetics of phenytoin and plasma phenytoin levels are then reduced (n = 4, open, Berg et al, *Ther Drug Monit* 1983;**5**:389–99). If started later, phenytoin levels should be monitored and changes in seizure activity monitored (extensive review by Lewis et al, *Ann Pharmacother* 1995;**29**:726–35).

Furosemide + phenytoin

The diuretic effect may be reduced by up to 50% by phenytoin (e.g. Bissoli et al, *Recenti Prog Med* 1996;**87**:227–8), so larger doses may be needed.

Gabapentin + phenytoin

See gabapentin (*4.5.3*).

Gingko biloba + phenytoin

A fatal seizure has occurred, probably due to reduced phenytoin levels via CYP2C19 induction by GB (n = 1, Kupiec and Raj, *J Anal Toxicol* 2005;**29**:755–8).

Glucagon + phenytoin

Patients on phenytoin may get false negatives with glucagon stimulation tests.

Glucocorticoids + phenytoin

A reduced steroid effect via enzyme induction is possible.

Griseofulvin + phenytoin

It is postulated that reduced griseofulvin levels may occur via enzyme induction (*Am J Hosp Pharm* 1986;**16**:52).

H2-blockers + phenytoin

Phenytoin toxicity has occurred with **cimetidine** (n = 1, Phillips and Hansky, *Med J Aus* 1984; **141**:602), with a 30% increase in phenytoin levels in other reports (n = 9, open, Salem et al, *Epilepsia* 1983;**24**:284–8) and so toxicity may occur, even with OTC cimetidine (n = 9, Rafi et al, *Ann Pharmacother* 1999;**33**:769–74). The effect is rapid and can occur within two days. An alternative is **ranitidine**, where lack of interaction has been shown (e.g. Watts et al, *Br J Clin Pharmacol* 1983;**15**:499–500), although there have been reports of elevated phenytoin levels (e.g. Tse et al, *Ann Pharmacother* 1993;**27**:1448–51), including one case where oral ranitidine produced toxic phenytoin levels, which remained high for a week even though the phenytoin was stopped, and only dropped when the ranitidine was also stopped (Tse and Jagmin, *Ann Intern Med* 1994;**120**:892–3). It is best to monitor phenytoin levels or use an alternative, e.g. **famotidine** (n = 10,

RCT, open, c/o, Sambol et al, *Br J Clin Pharmacol* 1989;**27**:83–7) or **nizatidine** (Bachmann et al, *Br J Clin Pharmacol* 1993;**36**:380–2).

Influenza vaccine + phenytoin

This is reported to reduce total and free phenytoin levels (Smith et al, *Clin Pharm* 1988;**7**:828–32), although one study showed only a transient 60% increase in levels (Jann and Fidone, *Clin Pharm* 1986;**5**:817–20).

Irinotecan + phenytoin

Phenytoin appears to decrease plasma levels of irinotecan (Murry et al, *J Pediatr Hematol Oncol* 2002;**24**:130–3).

ISONIAZID + PHENYTOIN

Phenytoin toxicity may occur via enzyme inhibition (n = 1, Witmer and Ritschel, *Drug Intell Clin Pharm* 1984;**18**:483–6), so observe for toxicity and reduce phenytoin doses if necessary.

KETOCONAZOLE + PHENYTOIN

Phenytoin toxicity may occur via enzyme inhibition. Ketoconazole may also have a reduced effect.

Lacosamide + phenytoin

See phenytoin + lacosamide (*4.5.4*).

Lamotrigine + phenytoin

See lamotrigine (*4.5.5*).

Levetiracetam + phenytoin

See levetiracetam (*4.5.6*).

Levodopa + phenytoin

Levodopa can be completely antagonised by phenytoin (Mendez et al, *Arch Neurol* 1975; **32**:44–6), and so increased levodopa doses may be necessary.

Levothyroxine (thyroxine) + phenytoin

Levothyroxine metabolism is accelerated by phenytoin, increasing requirements (Blackshear et al, *Ann Int Med* 1983;**99**:341–2).

Lidocaine + phenytoin

Phenytoin's central effects may be enhanced if used with lidocaine (Karlsson et al, *Eur J Clin Pharmacol* 1974;**7**:455–9). Sinoatrial arrest has been reported (Wood, *Br Med J* 1971;i:645) which was reversed by isoproterenol.

Lithium + phenytoin

See lithium (*4.4*).

Losartan + phenytoin

Losartan has no effect on phenytoin, but losartan levels may rise via 2C9 inhibition (n = 16, RCT, c/o, Fischer et al, *Clin Pharmacol Ther* 2002; **72**:238–46).

Memantine + phenytoin

See memantine (*4.6.9*).

Methadone + phenytoin

See methadone (4.6.10).

Methotrexate + phenytoin

An increased antifolate effect with phenytoin may occur.

Methylphenidate + phenytoin

See methylphenidate (4.6.11).

METRONIDAZOLE + PHENYTOIN

Phenytoin toxicity via enzyme inhibition is possible (Blyden et al, J Clin Pharmacol Ther 1988; **28**:240–5).

MEXILITINE + PHENYTOIN

Mexilitine levels are reduced by up to 50% via enzyme induction so adjust dosage as necessary (n = 6, open, Begg et al, Br J Clin Pharmacol 1982;**14**:219–23).

MICONAZOLE + PHENYTOIN

Phenytoin toxicity via enzyme inhibition has been reported (n = 2, Rolan et al, Br Med J 1983; **287**:1760).

Mirtazapine + phenytoin

See mirtazapine (4.3.3.4).

Modafinil + phenytoin

See modafinil (4.6.12).

Nasogastric feeds + phenytoin

Reduced phenytoin levels have been reported with nasogastric feeds (e.g. Osmolite®, Ensure® [Abbott]) and other enteral feeds (Pharm J 1989;**243**:181). One study showed that the AUC of phenytoin was unaffected by enteral feeds but that the absorption patterns were significantly different, with phenytoin sodium more rapidly absorbed (n = 10, RCT, Doak et al, Pharmacother 1998;**18**:637–45). Phenytoin dosage should be spaced to one hour before feeding or two hours after feeding (tube may need to be clamped). Monitor plasma levels frequently (comment by Au Yeung and Ensom, Ann Pharmacother 2000;**34**:896–905).

Neuromuscular blocking agents + phenytoin

Phenytoin reduces the effects of most NMBAs, e.g. pancuronium (n = 1, Hickey et al, Anesthesia 1988;**43**:757–9; n = 1, Liberman et al, Int J Clin Pharmacol Ther Toxicol 1988;**26**:371–4) and vecuronium (n = 22, Wright et al, Anesthesiology 2004;**100**:626–33), although atracurium appears unaffected.

NICOUMALONE + PHENYTOIN

Nicoumalone metabolism is induced by phenytoin, reducing its effect, although enhancement has also been reported.

Nitrofurantoin + phenytoin

There is a report of a stable epileptic developing seizures when nitrofurantoin was added, requiring increased phenytoin dosage (n = 1, Heipertz and Pilz, J Neurol 1978;**218**:297–301).

NSAIDs + phenytoin

One study shows no interaction with **ibuprofen** (n = 10, open, Bachmann, Br J Clin Pharmacol 1986;**21**:165–9), but toxicity has been reported (n = 1, Sandyk, S Afr Med J 1982;**62**:592). Phenytoin levels may be increased by **aspirin** via binding displacement (n = 10, open, 11/7, Leonard et al, Clin Pharmacol Ther 1981;**29**:56–60), free levels seeming to remain constant. Transient toxicity may be the only effect and then only at high (900 mg, four-hourly) aspirin doses. Plasma phenytoin levels may be increased by **azapropazone** via enzyme inhibition (n = 5, open, Geaney et al, Br J Clin Pharmacol 1983;**15**:727–34). Phenytoin toxicity may occur with **phenylbutazone** via enzyme inhibition and plasma protein displacement (n = 6, open, Neuvonen et al, Eur J Clin Pharmacol 1979;**15**:263–8). Dosage adjustment may be necessary.

ORAL CONTRACEPTIVES + PHENYTOIN

Contraceptive failure via enzyme induction is well established. See oral contraceptives + carbamazepine for advice (see 4.5.1).

Oxcarbazepine + phenytoin

See oxcarbazepine (4.5.7).

Paroxetine + phenytoin

See paroxetine (4.3.2.4).

Pethidine + phenytoin

Attenuation of pethidine's effect via enzyme induction is possible, with increased metabolite levels (n = 4, open, Pond and Kretschzmar, Clin Pharmacol Ther 1981;**29**:273).

Phenindione + phenytoin

No interaction is thought to occur (n = 54, open, Skovsted et al, Acta Med Scand 1976;**199**:513).

Pregabalin + phenytoin

See pregabalin (4.5.11).

PROGABIDE + PHENYTOIN

Phenytoin levels may rise by up to 40% (n = 6, open, Bianchetti, Epilepsia 1987;**28**:68–73).

Propoxyphene + phenytoin

Large doses of propoxyphene may raise phenytoin levels (Kutt et al, Ann N Y Acad Sci 1971;**179**:704), but normal doses have little or no effect (n = 16, open, Hansen et al, Acta Neurol Scand 1980;**61**:357).

4

Protein kinase inhibitors + phenytoin

Phenytoin decreases **gefitinib**'s levels by about 26% (n = 18, RCT, open, c/o, Chhun *et al*, *Br J Clin Pharmacol* 2009;**68**:226–37) and **imatinib**'s by up to 2.9-fold by phenytoin (n < 224, p/c, Pursche *et al*, *Curr Clin Pharmacol* 2008;**3**:198–203).

Proton pump inhibitors + phenytoin

A lack of effect of **omeprazole** on phenytoin kinetics has been reported, as has a mild rise in phenytoin levels (n = 10, RCT, d/b, c/o, 9/7, Prichard *et al*, *Br J Clin Pharmacol* 1987;**24**:543–5). The SmPC for omeprazole states that there are no significant changes in plasma levels, but patients should be monitored and doses adjusted if necessary. Lack of interaction has been reported with **pantoprazole** (n = 23, RCT, d/b, p/c, c/o, Middle *et al*, *Int J Clin Pharmacol Ther* 1996;**34**:S72–S75).

Pyridoxine + phenytoin

Large doses of pyridoxine (e.g. 200 mg/d) can reduce phenytoin levels by up to 40–50% (Hansson and Sillanpaa, *Lancet* 1976;i:256). Monitoring levels would thus be wise.

Quetiapine + phenytoin

See quetiapine (*4.2.6*).

QUINIDINE + PHENYTOIN

A reduced quinidine effect may occur via enzyme induction (Anon, *N Engl J Med* 1983;**308**:724–5), so monitoring of quinidine levels or effect may be necessary.

RIFAMPICIN + PHENYTOIN

Significant reductions in phenytoin levels may occur via enzyme induction (Abajo, *Br Med J* 1988;**297**:1048).

Rufinamide + phenytoin

See rufinamide (*4.5.12*).

SERTINDOLE + PHENYTOIN *

See sertindole (*4.2.8*).

Sertraline + phenytoin

See sertraline (*4.3.2.5*).

Shankhapushpi + phenytoin

It has been recommended to avoid the Ayurvedic herbal mixture shankhapushpi, as decreased plasma phenytoin levels may occur (mentioned by Fugh-Berman, *Lancet* 2000;**355**:134–8).

Sodium oxybate + phenytoin

See sodium oxybate (*4.6.13*).

Statins + phenytoin

Phenytoin can significantly reduce the therapeutic effect of **simvastatin** and **atorvastatin**, probably via CYP3A4 induction

(n = 1, Murphy and Dominiczak, *Postgrad Med J* 1999;**75**:359–60; n = 1, Khandwala, *South Med J* 2006;**99**:1385–7).

St John's wort + phenytoin

See St John's wort (*4.3.3.10*).

SUCRALFATE + PHENYTOIN

One study showed a small reduction in phenytoin bioavailability (n = 9, open, Hall *et al*, *Drug Intell Clin Pharm* 1986;**20**:607–11) by decreased absorption. This can be avoided by giving phenytoin two hours or more after sucralfate.

Sulphonamides + phenytoin

Phenytoin toxicity is known to be possible via P450 inhibition by co-trimoxazole (Gillman and Sandyk, *Ann Intern Med* 1985;**102**:559) and other sulphonamides, so monitor plasma levels and reduce phenytoin doses if necessary.

Temozolomide + phenytoin

There is a case of delirium probably caused by this combination (n = 1, Levy, *Psychosomatics* 2007;**48**:359–60).

Theophylline + phenytoin

Phenytoin increases theophylline's clearance by 45%, so higher doses may be needed (n = 8, open, Adebayo, *Clin Exp Pharmacol Physiol* 1988;**15**:883–7). Phenytoin absorption may also be reduced (*Int Pharm J* 1989;**3**:98–101). Separating the doses by 1–2 hours may reduce the effect.

Tiagabine + phenytoin

See tiagabine (*4.5.13*).

Ticlopidine + phenytoin

Ticlopidine 500 mg/d inhibits phenytoin clearance so dose adjustment and careful monitoring should be considered (n = 6, Donahue *et al*, *Clin Pharmacol Therapeut* 1999;**66**:563–8; n = 1, Privitera and Welty, *Arch Neurology* 1996; **53**: 1191–2), especially since the onset of phenytoin toxicity may be delayed by several weeks (n = 1, Dahm and Brors, *Tidsskr Nor Laegeforen* 2002;**122**:278–80).

Tolbutamide + phenytoin

Mild phenytoin toxicity may occur via increased free levels (n = 18, Tassaneeyakul *et al*, *Br J Clin Pharmacol* 1992;**34**:494–8).

Topiramate + phenytoin

See topiramate (*4.5.14*).

Trazodone + phenytoin

There is a report of phenytoin toxicity developing when relatively high dose trazodone was added (n = 1, Dorn, *J Clin Psychiatry* 1986;**47**:89).

TRIMETHOPRIM + PHENYTOIN

Plasma phenytoin levels and the antifolate effect may be increased by trimethoprim.

TRICYCLICS + PHENYTOIN

Phenytoin levels may be raised by **imipramine** (Perucca and Richens, *Br J Clin Pharmacol* 1977; **4**:485–6), but not **nortriptyline** (Houghton and Richens, *Int J Clin Pharmacol* 1975;**12**:210–6) or **amitriptyline** (*Clin PharmacolTher* 1975;**18**:191–9), probably due to CYP2C19 inhibition (Shin *et al*, *Drug Metab Dispos* 2002;**30**:1102–7). Phenytoin levels may need to be monitored frequently. Tricyclics may lower the seizure threshold.

VALPROATE + PHENYTOIN

Valproate inhibits phenytoin metabolism and competes for its binding sites. If enzyme saturation has not occurred then this displacement of phenytoin leads to decreased bound, but increased free, phenytoin (n = 12, Lai and Huang, *Biopharm Drug Dispos* 1993;**14**:365–70). More phenytoin is then metabolised so the net result is reduced total and bound concentrations. The free concentration will remain about the same and lower plasma levels will still contain about the same amount of active/free drug. Thus, beware of raising the dose of phenytoin to bring the total plasma concentration into the 'therapeutic range' as it would then be toxic (Keys, *Drug Intell Clin Pharm* 1982;**16**:737–9). If the enzyme is saturated, displacement may lead to a stable total concentration but decreased bound and increased free phenytoin (n = 6, open, Johnson *et al*, *Br J Clin Pharmacol* 1989;**27**:843–9). This could lead to toxic effects within the therapeutic range. In practice, phenytoin levels tend to fall initially by up to 50%, then return to normal over about five weeks. Toxicity is possible if levels were higher at the start so monitoring is essential.

VIGABATRIN + PHENYTOIN

Vigabatrin produces a mean 20–30% reduction in phenytoin levels (n = 8, open, Rimmer and Richens, *Br J Clin Pharmacol* 1989;**27**:27S–33S) and may compromise seizure control (e.g. n = 89, s/b, Browne *et al*, *Neurology* 1987;**37**:184–9).

Vincristine + phenytoin

Phenytoin significantly increases the clearance of vincristine, probably by CYP3A4 induction (n = 15, open, Villikka *et al*, *Clin Pharmacol Therapeut* 1999;**66**:589–93).

Voriconazole + phenytoin

Voriconazole may decrease phenytoin levels

dramatically, where even doubling phenytoin dose is insufficient (Alffenaar *et al*, *Br J Clin Pharmacol* 2009;**68**:462–3).

WARFARIN + PHENYTOIN

Warfarin metabolism is accelerated by phenytoin reducing its effect, although enhanced levels of both and deaths have been reported (n = 1, Panegyres and Rischbieth, *Postgrad Med J* 1991;**67**:98; Meisheri, *J Ass Physicians India* 1996; **44**:661–2).

Zinc + phenytoin

Zinc may reduce phenytoin levels (n=1, *Am J Hosp Pharm* 1988; **18**:297–8).

Zonisamide + phenytoin

See zonisamide (*4.5.17*).

4.5.10 PIRACETAM

Warfarin + piracetam

Significantly prolonged prothrombin time has been reported with piracetam and warfarin (n = 1, Pan and Ng, *Eur J Clin Pharmacol* 1983;**24**:711).

4.5.11 PREGABALIN

Pregabalin is excreted by the kidneys, undergoes little metabolism, has no effect on P450 enzymes, and is not bound to plasma proteins so interactions are unlikely. Lack of interaction has also been shown with antidiabetics, diuretics and insulin.

Alcohol + pregabalin

Pregabalin may potentiate the sedative effects of alcohol (SmPC).

Benzodiazepines + pregabalin

Pregabalin may potentiate the sedative effects of lorazepam (SmPC).

Carbamazepine+ pregabalin

Lack of interaction has been shown (UK SmPC).

Gabapentin + pregabalin

Lack of interaction has been shown (UK SmPC), but pregabalin displaces gabapentin from receptors.

Lacosamide + pregabalin

See pregabalin + lacosamide (*4.5.4*).

Lamotrigine + pregabalin

Lack of interaction has been shown (UK SmPC).

Oral contraceptives + pregabalin

Lack of interaction has been shown (UK SmPC).

Oxycodone + pregabalin

Pregabalin may enhance the cognitive and motor effects of oxycodone (SmPC).

4

Phenobarbital + pregabalin
Lack of interaction has been shown (UK SmPC).
Phenytoin + pregabalin
Lack of interaction has been shown (UK SmPC).
Tiagabine + pregabalin
Lack of interaction has been shown (UK SmPC).
Topiramate + pregabalin
Lack of interaction has been shown (UK SmPC).
Valproate + pregabalin
Lack of interaction has been shown (UK SmPC).

4.5.12 RUFINAMIDE

Rufinamide is almost entirely metabolised by hydrolysis to an inactive metabolite but not by any P450 enzyme. It has no effect on 1A2, 2A6, 2C9, 2C19, 2D6, 2E1 but induces 3A4. It is 34% bound to plasma proteins.
Alcohol + rufinamide
No information is available (UK SmPC).
Benzodiazepines + rufinamide
No changes in the plasma levels of rufinamide are seen with benzodiazepines but rufinamide induces CYP3A4 and reduces levels of, e.g. triazolam (UK SmPC).
Carbamazepine + rufinamide
The plasma levels of rufinamide are reduced by carbamazepine, but carbamazepine is unaffected by rufinamide (UK SmPC).
Lamotrigine + rufinamide
No significant interaction has been seen with this combination (UK SmPC).
Olanzapine + rufinamide
Rufinamide has no effect on olanzapine kinetics (UK SmPC).
Oral contraceptives + rufinamide
Rufinamide can reduce plasma levels of OCs by 14–22%, so adequate additional contraceptive measures are recommended (UK SmPC).
Phenobarbital + rufinamide
The plasma levels of rufinamide are reduced by phenobarbital but rufinamide has no effect on barbiturates (UK SmPC).
Phenytoin + rufinamide
The plasma levels of rufinamide are reduced by phenytoin (UK SmPC) and phenytoin clearance is reduced by rufinamide so phenytoin dose reduction may be necessary.
Topiramate + rufinamide
No significant interaction has been seen with this combination (UK SmPC).

Valproate + rufinamide
Rifinamide plasma levels are increased by valproate (UK SmPC), especially in people with body weight < 30 kg, so start at 200 mg/d but with a maximum of only 400 mg/d. Rufinamide has no effect on valproate (UK SmPC).
Vigabatrin + rufinamide
The plasma levels of rufinamide are reduced by vigabatrin (UK SmPC).

4.5.13 TIAGABINE

Tiagabine appears to be metabolised by CYP3A4.
Alcohol + tiagabine
Lack of interaction has been shown (n = 20, RCT, d/b, p/c, c/o, Kastberg et al, Drug Metabol Drug Interact 1998;**14**:259–73), although some caution is still advised.
Benzodiazepines + tiagabine
No interaction with triazolam has been detected (n = 12, RCT, Richens et al, Drug Metabol Drug Interact 1998;**14**:159–77).
Carbamazepine + tiagabine
Tiagabine clearance is 60% greater with carbamazepine, with plasma levels reduced by a factor of 1.5–3, probably by CYP3A4 induction. Tiagabine has no effect on carbamazepine.
Cimetidine + tiagabine
No interaction has been detected.
Digoxin + tiagabine
Lack of interaction has been shown (n = 13, open, Snel et al, Eur J Clin Pharmacol 1998;**54**:355–7).
Erythromycin + tiagabine
Lack of significant interaction has been shown (n = 13, open, c/o, Thomsen et al, J Clin Pharmacol 1998;**38**:1051–6).
Fosphenytoin + tiagabine
See phenytoin + tiagabine.
Gemfibrozil + tiagabine
Gemfibrozil increased tiagabine levels by 60–75% in one patient (n = 1, Burstein et al, Ann Pharmacother 2009;**43**:379–82).
Oral contraceptives + tiagabine
No interaction has been detected.
Phenobarbital + tiagabine
Tiagabine clearance is 60% greater in people also taking phenobarbital, with plasma levels reduced by a factor of 1.5–3, probably by CYP3A4 induction. There is no effect on phenobarbital.

Phenytoin + tiagabine

Tiagabine clearance is 60% greater in people also taking phenytoin and plasma levels are reduced by a factor of 1.5–3, probably by CYP3A4 induction. There is no effect on phenytoin.

Pregabalin + tiagabine

See pregabalin (4.5.11).

Theophylline + tiagabine

No interaction has been detected.

Valproate + tiagabine

Tiagabine causes a 10–12% reduction in steady-state valproate levels, while valproate increases free tiagabine levels by about 40% (n = 12, open, Gustavson et al, Am J Ther 1998;**5**:73–9).

Warfarin + tiagabine

No interaction has been detected.

4.5.14 TOPIRAMATE

Topiramate is 13–17% bound to plasma proteins (and thus unlikely to interact with highly bound drugs) and not extensively metabolised. Excretion is mainly via the kidneys and it has no major effect on P450 enzymes. Concomitant use with drugs predisposing to nephrolithiasis (renal stone formation) is not recommended, e.g. allopurinol, megadose ascorbic acid, furosemide, methyldopa, phenolphthalein abuse, steroids and Worcester sauce overdose.

Review: Bailer et al, Clin Pharmacokinet 2004; **43**:63–80.

Acetazolamide + topiramate

There may be an increased risk of renal stone formation in susceptible patients.

Antipsychotics + topiramate

Topiramate up to 200mg/d had no significant effect on the plasma levels of **clozapine** and norclozapine (n = 10), olanzapine (n = 12), **ris-peridone** and **paliperidone** (n = 9), or **quetiapine** (n = 7) and was well tolerated (n = 38, 6/52, Migliardi et al, Clin Neuropharmacol 2007;**30**:107–13).

Barbiturates + topiramate

Topiramate has no effect on plasma levels of phenobarbital or primidone (Floren et al, Epilepsia 1989;**30**:646). The effect of the barbiturates on topiramate has not been studied.

Carbamazepine + topiramate

Topiramate has been shown to have no major effect on the plasma levels of CBZ or CBZ–E, although there is a suggestion that it may increase CBZ levels (n = 2 + 23, Mack et al, Seizure 2002;**11**:464–7). However, topiramate clearance is increased two-fold by CBZ and half-life reduced (n = 12 open, Britzi et al, Epilepsia 2005;**46**:378–84), and so topiramate doses may need to be lowered if CBZ is reduced or discontinued (n = 12, open, Sachdeo et al, Epilepsia 1996;**37**:774–80).

Citalopram + topiramate

A case of acute glaucoma has been reported after topiramate was added to stable citalopram (n = 1, Spaccapelo et al, Cases J 2009;**2**:87).

Digoxin + topiramate

Topiramate may decrease digoxin plasma levels, with peak levels reduced by 16%, possibly by reduced bioavailability. Dose reduction or routine digoxin blood levels might be considered.

Eslicarbazepine + topiramate *

Lack of significant interaction has been reported (n = 16, open, 27/7, Almeida et al, Acta Neurol Scand 2010;**121**:257–64).

Fluvoxamine + topiramate

See topiramate + fluvoxamine (4.3.2.3).

Lamotrigine + topiramate

See lamotrigine (4.5.5).

Lithium + topiramate

See lithium (4.4).

ORAL CONTRACEPTIVES + TOPIRAMATE

Serum estrogen levels are reduced by topiramate in patients taking combined oestrogen/ proges-terone oral contraceptives (see SmPC). See oral contraceptives + carbamazepine for additional advice (see 4.5.1).

Phenytoin + topiramate

Decreases in phenytoin clearance may occur in a few patients with topiramate, probably via CYP2C19 inhibition (n = 12, Sachdeo et al, Epilepsia 2002;**43**:691–6). Conversely, topira-mate plasma levels are reduced by about 40% by phenytoin, which could be important if phenytoin is withdrawn.

Posaconazole + topiramate

Posaconazole has been implicated in inducing topiramate toxicity (n = 1, Marriott et al, Ann Intern Med 2009;**151**:143).

Pregabalin + topiramate

See pregabalin (4.5.11).

Rufinamide + topiramate

See rufinamide (4.5.12).

Temozolomide + topiramate

Temozolomide does not seem to affect

topiramate pharmacokinetics (n = 14, Maschio *et al*, *J Neurooncol* 2008;**90**:217–21).

Triamterene + topiramate

There may be an increased risk of renal stone formation in susceptible patients.

Valproate + topiramate

Topiramate has been shown to produce a small but significant increase in valproate clearance, reducing plasma levels, although enhanced valproate side-effects, e.g. apathy, hypothermia and raised LFTs have also been reported (n = 3, Longin *et al*, *Epilepsia* 2002;**43**:451–4), as has reversible hepatic failure (n = 1, Bumb *et al*, *Epileptic Disord* 2003;**5**:157–9) and hyperammonemic encephalopathy (n = 1, Cheung *et al*, *J Child Neurol* 2005;**20**:157–60). Topiramate may enhance the risk and severity of hypothermia from valproate (n = 19, Knudsen *et al*, *J Clin Pharm Ther* 2008;**33**:513–9). Topiramate plasma levels are increased by about 15% by valproate, which could be important if valproate is withdrawn.

Zonisamide + topiramate

See zonisamide (*4.5.17*).

4.5.15 VALPROATE (SODIUM VALPROATE, VALPROIC ACID, DIVALPROEX SODIUM, ETC)

Valproate has a complex metabolism; 50% is metabolised by glucuronidation, 40% by mitochondrial beta-oxidation and 10% by P450 (CYP2C9 and 2C19) enzymes (Sheehan *et al*, *Ann Pharmacother* 2006;**40**:147–50).

Review: DeVane, *Psychopharmacol Bull* 2003; **37**(Suppl 2):25–42.

Antacids + valproate

A slight decrease in valproate absorption with antacids has been noted (n = 7, open, May *et al*, *Clin Pharm* 1982;**1**:244–7).

TRICYCLICS + VALPROATE

Tricyclic levels may be raised by 19% by valproate (n = 15, open, amitriptyline and nortriptyline, Wong *et al*, *Clin Pharmacol Ther* 1996;**60**:48–53) and status epilepticus has been reported, with valproate possibly elevating clomipramine to toxic levels (n = 1, DeToledo *et al*, *Ther Drug Monit* 1997;**19**:71–3; see also Fehr *et al*, *J Clin Psychopharmacol* 2000;**20**:493–4).

Antiretrovirals + valproate

Valproate levels decreased by 48% (resulting in manic relapse) have been reported with lopinavir/ritonavir (Kaletra®, Abbott) probably via glucuronidation-induction (n = 1, Sheehan *et al*, *Ann Pharmacother* 2006;**40**:147–50). Valproate produces a dose-dependent inhibition of zidovudine glucuronidation, leading to raised zidovudine levels (Trapnell *et al*, *Antimicrob Agents Chemother* 1998;**42**:1592–6), possibly by up to three-fold (n = 1, Akula *et al*, *Am J Med Sci* 1997;**31**:244–6), a UK SmPC warning, with severe anaemia reported (n = 1, Antoniou *et al*, *Clin Infect Dis* 2004;**38**:38–40).

Asenapine + valproate

See valproate + asenapine (*4.2.3*).

Aspirin + valproate

Valproate's effect and toxicity may be enhanced by repeated high-dose aspirin (n = 3, Goulden *et al*, *Neurology* 1987;**37**:1392–4), and levels may rise by 12–43% (n = 6, open, Orr *et al*, *Clin Pharmacol Ther* 1982;**31**:642–9).

Benzodiazepines + valproate

See benzodiazepines (*4.1.1*).

BETA-LACTAM and CARBAPENEM ANTIBIOTICS + VALPROATE *

Carbapenems (e.g. doripenem, ertapenem, imipenem, meropenem) can induce a rapid and significant drop in valproate levels and should not be used together (*Drug Safety Update* 2010;**3**:4). Ertapenem (n = 2, Liao *et al*, *Am J Health Syst Pharm* 2010;**67**:1260–4) can reduce valproate levels to almost undetectable levels, a serious interaction and despite increasing the valproate dose, plasma levels may not return to normal, with deaths reported (n = 2, Spriet *et al*, *Am J Health Syst Pharm* 2007;**64**:54–8). A retrospective analysis shows that meropenem reduces valproate levels by about 82% and remain low for a week after meropenem is stopped, gradually returning to normal over the next week (n = 36, Haroutiunian et al, *J Clin Pharmacol* 2009;**49**:1363–9). The decline can be unpredictable and rapid (Naranjo = 7, n = 1, Gu and Huang, *Am J Geriatr Pharmacother* 2009;**7**:26–33).

Bupropion + valproate

See bupropion (*4.6.6*).

CARBAMAZEPINE + VALPROATE

See carbamazepine (*4.5.1*).

Charcoal, activated + valproate

Activated charcoal reduces the absorption of sodium valproate by 65% (n = 6, Neuvonen *et al*, *Eur J Clin Pharmacol* 1983;**24**:243–6) but has no effect on valproate elimination (n = 8, Al-Shareef *et al*, *Br J Clin Pharmacol* 1997;**43**:109–11).

Chitosan + valproate

Chitosan (a weight-loss product) has caused valproate to drop to almost undetectable levels, with resultant seizures (n = 2, *Br Med J* 2009; **339**:b3751).

Clozapine + valproate

See clozapine (*4.2.4*).

Erythromycin + valproate

Valproate levels may rise three-fold when erythromycin is started, resulting in CNS toxicity (n = 1, Redington *et al*, *Ann Intern Med* 1992;**116**:877–8).

Ethosuximide + valproate

See ethosuximide (*4.5.2*).

Fluoxetine + valproate

See fluoxetine (*4.3.2.2*).

Fluvoxamine + valproate

See fluvoxamine (*4.3.2.3*).

Gabapentin + valproate

See gabapentin (*4.5.3*).

Gingko biloba + valproate

There is a case of a fatal seizure with the combination, probably due to reduced valproate levels via CYP2C19 induction (n = 1, Kupiec and Raj, *J Anal Toxicol* 2005;**29**:755–8).

H2-blockers + valproate

One study showed that **cimetidine** reduces the clearance and prolongs the half-life of valproate but **ranitidine** does not interact (n = 12, RCT, Webster *et al*, *Eur J Clin Pharmacol* 1984;**27**:341–3).

Imatinib + valproate

Plasma levels of imatinib do not appear to be affected by valproate (n < 224, p/c, Pursche *et al*, *Curr Clin Pharmacol* 2008;**3**:198–203).

Isoniazid + valproate

Enhanced hepatotoxicity has been reported (n = 1, Dockweiler, *Lancet* 1987;**2**:152).

Lacosamide + valproate

See valproate + lacosamide (*4.5.4*).

LAMOTRIGINE + VALPROATE

See lamotrigine (*4.5.5*).

Levetiracetam + valproate

See levetiracetam (*4.5.6*).

Methylphenidate + valproate

See methylphenidate (*4.6.11*).

Moclobemide + valproate

See valproate + moclobemide (*4.3.3.5*).

Olanzapine + valproate

See valproate + olanzapine (*4.2.5*).

Oral contraceptives + valproate

A reduced contraceptive effect has not been reported with valproate (Mattson *et al*, *JAMA* 1986;**256**:238–40; n = 6, Crawford *et al*, *Contraception* 1986;**33**:23–9), but valproate plasma levels may be higher during drug-free weeks of combined hormonal oral contraceptives than during the 3/52 on it. Indeed, a 23% reduction in valproate levels has been reported when co-prescribed with a combined OC (n = 24, open, Herzog *et al*, *Neurology* 2009; **72**:911–4). There is a wide inter-individual variation and monitoring valproate may be prudent if adding or discontinuing OCs or steroids (n = 9, RCT, c/o, Galimberti *et al*, *Epilepsia* 2006;**47**:1569–72).

Oxcarbazepine + valproate

See oxcarbazepine (*4.5.7*).

Paroxetine + valproate

See paroxetine (*4.3.2.4*).

PHENOBARBITAL + VALPROATE

See phenobarbital (*4.5.8*).

PHENYTOIN + VALPROATE

See phenytoin (*4.5.9*).

Pregabalin + valproate

See pregabalin (*4.5.11*).

Quetiapine + valproate

See quetiapine (*4.2.6*).

Riluzole + valproate *

Increased valproate levels have been reported (n = 1, Veenstra-VanderWeele, *J Child Adolesc Psychopharmacol* 2010:**20**:163–5).

Risperidone + valproate

See valproate + antipsychotics (*4.2.1*).

Rufinamide + valproate

See rufinamide (*4.5.12*).

Smoking + valproate *

See smoking (*4.7.4*).

Sodium oxybate + valproate

See sodium oxybate (*4.6.13*).

Tiagabine + valproate

See tiagabine (*4.5.13*).

Topiramate + valproate

See topiramate (*4.5.14*).

Tricyclics + valproate

See antidepressants + valproate.

Vigabatrin + valproate

See vigabatrin (*4.5.16*).

Warfarin + valproate

Rapidly raised INR (to 3.9) has been reported after a single dose of valproate (Guthrie *et al*, *J Clin Psychopharmacol* 1995;**15**:138–9). Care is needed.

4

Zolpidem + valproate
See zolpidem (*4.1.6*).

Zonisamide + valproate
See zonisamide (*4.5.17*).

4.5.16 VIGABATRIN

Vigabatrin is not metabolised, does not induce enzymes and is not protein bound. It is renally excreted.

Carbamazepine + vigabatrin
A 10% rise in carbamazepine levels has been reported (n = 66, Jedrzejczak *et al*, *Epilepsy Res* 2000;**39**:115–20), as has an 18% reduction in steady-state carbamazepine levels (n = 15, Sanchez-Alcaraz *et al*, *J Clin Pharm Ther* 2002;**27**:427–30).

Oral contraceptives + vigabatrin
Vigabatrin is unlikely to affect consistently the efficacy of oral contraceptives, although in one study two women showed reduced ethinyloestradiol levels (n = 113, Bartoli *et al*, *Epilepsia* 1997;**38**:702–7).

Phenobarbital + vigabatrin
One study reported non-clinically significant 7–11% reductions in barbiturate levels (n=89, s/b, 12/52, Browne *et al*, *Neurology* 1987; **37**:184–9).

PHENYTOIN + VIGABATRIN
See phenytoin (*4.5.9*).

Rufinamide + vigabatrin
See rufinamide (*4.5.12*).

Valproate + vigabatrin
Lack of interaction has been shown (e.g. McKee *et al*, *Epilepsia* 1993;**34**:937–43; see also Mumford, *Eur Hosp Pharm* 1996;**2**:190–1).

4.5.17 ZONISAMIDE

Zonisamide does not inhibit 1A2 or 2D6, and only weakly inhibits 2A6, 2C9, 2C19 and 2E1. It is partly metabolised by 3A4 and partly by N-acetyltransferases and glucuronidation.

Carbamazepine + zonisamide
Zonisamide does not significantly effect carbamazepine, but 3A4 induction by CBZ reduces zonisamide half-life from 65 to 36 hours (n = 18, Ragueneau-Majlessi *et al*, *Epilepsy Res* 2004;**62**:1–11), and an NMS-like state has been reported with the combination (n = 1, Azuma *et al*, *Epilepsia* 2007;**48**:1999–2001).

Cimetidine + zonisamide
Lack of interaction has been shown (SmPC).

Ketoconazole + zonisamide
Lack of interaction has been shown (SmPC).

Lamotrigine + zonisamide
Lack of clinically significant interaction has been shown (n = 20 [c = 18], open, Levy *et al*, *Ther Drug Monit* 2005;**27**:93–8).

Oral contraceptives + zonisamide
There is apparently no interaction (SmPC).

Phenytoin + zonisamide
Lack of clinically relevant interaction has been shown (SmPC).

Rifampicin + zonisamide
An interaction is theoretically possible via 3A4 induction (SmPC).

Topiramate + zonisamide
The UK SmPC recommends caution with the use of zonisamide with carbonic anhydrase inhibitors such as topiramate.

Valproate + zonisamide
Lack of significant interaction has been shown (n = 22 [c = 17], open, Ragueneau-Majlessi *et al*, *Clin Pharmacokinet* 2005;**44**:17–23).

4.6 OTHER DRUGS

4.6.1 ACAMPROSATE

Acamprosate is not protein bound, is renally excreted and is not significantly metabolised and so has a low liability for drug–drug interactions by these mechanisms.

Alcohol + acamprosate
See alcohol (*4.7.1*).

Benzodiazepines + acamprosate
Lack of interaction with diazepam has been shown.

Disulfiram + acamprosate
Lack of interaction has been shown (n = 118, RCT, p/c, 2 years, Besson *et al*, *Alcohol Clin Exp Res* 1998;**22**:573–9).

Food + acamprosate
Food reduces acamprosate's oral absorption.

Naltrexone + acamprosate
Naltrexone significantly increases plasma acam-prosate levels, with some increase in ADRs (n = 23, RCT, d/b, p/c, c/o, 23/7, Johnson *et al*, *J Clin Psychopharmacol* 2003; **23**:281–93).

Tricyclics + acamprosate
There is a lack of interaction with imipramine.

4.6.2 ANTICHOLINERGIC OR ANTIMUSCARINIC AGENTS

The UK SmPC now notes that the antimuscarinic effects of orphenadrine can be enhanced by other drugs with antimuscarinic effects, e.g. antihistamines, antispasmodics, tricyclics, phenothiazines, dopaminergic antiparkinsonian agents (e.g. amantadine), and antiarrhythmics (e.g. disopyramide).

Anticholinesterases + anticholinergics
Some antagonism would be expected.

Antipsychotics + anticholinergics
See antipsychotics (4.2.1).

Benzodiazepines + anticholinergics
See benzodiazepines (4.1.1).

Beta-blockers + anticholinergics
Propantheline increases atenolol bioavailability by 36%, increasing its effect (open, Regardh et al, Biopharm Drug Dispos 1981;2:79–87) but not that of metoprolol (n = 15, open, Briant et al, Eur J Clin Pharmacol 1983;25:353).

Betel nut + anticholinergics
Heavy betel nut consumption has resulted in severe EPSE, possibly by antagonising procyclidine's effect (n = 1, Deahl, Mov Disord 1989;4:330–2).

H2-blockers + anticholinergics
A single–dose study showed possible reduced cimetidine absorption (Kanto et al, Br J Clin Pharmacol 1981;11:629–31), but not with ranitidine (n = 12, open, Donn et al, Pharmacother 1984;4:89–92) or nizatidine (Knadler et al, Clin Pharmac Ther 1987;42:514–20).

Levodopa + anticholinergics
Anticholinergics may reduce the peak blood levels of levodopa and reduce total absorption (Algeri et al, Eur J Pharmacol 1976;35:293–9), possibly by slowed gut motility and increased gut metabolism.

MAOIs + anticholinergics
See MAOIs (4.3.4).

Memantine + anticholinergics
See memantine (4.6.9).

Nitrofurantoin + anticholinergics
Nitrofurantoin bioavailability may be increased by anticholinergics (n = 10, Mannisto, Int J Clin Pharmacol Biopharm 1978;16:223–8).

Paracetamol + anticholinergics
Propantheline delays the absorption of paracetamol (Nimmo et al, Br Med J 1973;i:587–9).

Procarbazine + anticholinergics
Increased sedation could occur.

SSRIs + anticholinergics
There are several cases of the combination probably causing delirium, e.g. **sertraline** and benzatropine (n = 1, Byerly et al, Am J Psychiatry 1996;153:965–6), paroxetine and benzatropine (Armstrong and Schweitzer, Am J Psychiatry 1997;154:581–2) and a variety of adverse effects (n = 5, Roth et al, J Clin Psychiatry 1994;55:491–5). CYP2D6 inhibition seems the likely mechanism.

Thiazide diuretics + anticholinergics
Thiazide bioavailability may be enhanced (open, Beermann et al, Eur J Clin Pharmacol 1978;13:385–7).

Tricyclics + anticholinergics
See tricyclics (4.3.1).

Venlafaxine + anticholinergics
An acute adverse cutaneous reaction has been reported with venlafaxine and orphenadrine (n = 1, Papadimitriou et al, J Eur Acad Dermatol Venereol 2006;20:1019).

Ziprasidone + anticholinergics
See ziprasidone (4.2.9).

4.6.3 ANTICHOLINESTERASES

Review: anticholinesterase interactions (Bentue-Ferrer et al, CNS Drugs 2003;17:947–63).

4.6.3.1 DONEPEZIL

Donepezil is metabolised slowly by CYP2D6 and 3A4 to multiple metabolites, only one of which appears to be pharmacologically active.

Anticholinergics + donepezil
See anticholinesterases + anticholinergics (4.6.2).

Antipsychotics + donepezil
Donepezil 5 mg/d had no effect on **risperidone** pharmacokinetics in schizophrenia and was well tolerated (n = 31, open, 7/7, Reyes et al, Br J Clin Pharmacol 2004;58[Suppl 1]:50–7), although NMS with **bromperidol** (n = 1, Ueki et al, Nippon Ronen Igakkai Zasshi 2001;38:822–4) and severe EPSE with risperidone (n = 1, Magnuson et al, Am J Psychiatry 1998;155:1459) have been reported.

Cimetidine + donepezil
Lack of significant pharmacokinetic interaction has been reported (n = 19, open, Tiseo et al, Br J Clin Pharmacol 1998;46[Suppl 1]:25–9).

Digoxin + donepezil
Lack of significant pharmacokinetic interaction

4

has been reported (n = 12, open, Tiseo et al, Br J Clin Pharmacol 1998;**46**[Suppl 1]:40–4).

Ketoconazole + donepezil

Donepezil levels may rise by around 25% over a week (n = 21, open, Tiseo et al, Br J Clin Pharmacol 1998;**46**[Suppl 1]:30–4).

Memantine + donepezil

See anticholinesterases + memantine (4.6.9).

NMBAs + donepezil

A synergistic effect could be predicted.

NSAIDs + donepezil

The donepezil SmPC recommends additional monitoring of patients at risk of develop-ing ulcers, e.g. if taking concomitant NSAIDs.

SSRIs + donepezil

Lack of interaction has been shown between donepezil 5 mg/d and **sertraline** 100 mg/d (n = 19 [c = 16], RCT, open, c/o, Nagy et al, Br J Clin Pharmacol 2004;**58**(Suppl 1):25–33), although case reports exist with **paroxetine** (Carrier, J Am Geriatr Soc 1999;**47**:1037).

Suxamethonium + donepezil

Donepezil is a cholinesterase inhibitor and would be likely to enhance the effect of suxamethonium-type muscle relaxants (n = 1, Crowe and Collins, Anesthiology 2003;**98**:574–5), e.g. during ECT (Walker and Perks, Anesthesia 2002;**57**:1041).

Theophylline + donepezil

Lack of significant pharmacokinetic interaction has been reported (n = 12, open, Tiseo et al, Br J Clin Pharmacol 1998;**46**[Suppl 1]:35–9).

Warfarin + donepezil

Lack of significant pharmacokinetic interaction has been reported (n = 12, open, Tiseo et al, Br J Clin Pharmacol 1998;**46**[Suppl 1]:45–50).

4.6.3.2 GALANTAMINE

Galantamine is 90% bioavailable, has a large VD, low protein binding, and is metabolised by CYP2D6 and 3A4. Galantamine has a minimal effect on P450 enzymes (review by Farlow, Clin Pharmacokinet 2003;**42**:1383–92).

Anticholinergics + galantamine

See anticholinesterases + anticholinergics (4.6.2).

Antipsychotics + galantamine

Lack of interaction has been reported with risperidone (n = 16, RCT, open, c/o, Huang et al, J Clin Pharmacol 2002;**42**:1341–51).

Beta-blockers + galantamine

As galantamine may cause bradycardia, the SmPC recommends care with drugs that significantly reduce heart rate, e.g. beta-blockers.

Digoxin + galantamine

As galantamine may cause bradycardia, the SmPC recommends care with drugs that significantly reduce heart rate, e.g. digoxin. Galantamine has no effect on the kinetics of digoxin.

Erythromycin + galantamine

A 12% increase in galantamine plasma levels has been reported, probably by CYP3A4 inhibition.

Ketoconazole + galantamine

A 30% increase in galantamine plasma levels has been reported, probably by CYP3A4 inhibition, and so a reduced maintenance dosage might be appropriate.

Memantine + galantamine

See memantine (4.6.9).

Paroxetine + galantamine

A 40% increase in galantamine plasma levels has been reported, probably by CYP2D6 inhibition, and so a reduced maintenance dosage might be appropriate.

Suxamethonium + galantamine

Galantamine is likely to enhance the effect of suxamethonium-type muscle relaxants.

Warfarin + galantamine

Galantamine has been shown to have no effect on the kinetics of warfarin.

4.6.3.3 RIVASTIGMINE

Rivastigmine has minimal protein binding, a short half-life, is metabolised by esterases (but with little effect on P450 enzymes) and lack of significant interaction has been shown with 22 different therapeutic classes (Grossberg et al, Int J Geriatr Psychiatry 2000;**15**:242–7).

Anticholinergics + rivastigmine

See anticholinesterases + anticholinergics (4.6.2).

Atenolol + rivastigmine *

There is a case of true syncope with the combination (n = 1, Paulison and Léos, Cardiovasc Toxicol 2010;**10**:306–10).

Benzodiazepines + rivastigmine

No interaction has been seen in healthy volunteers.

Digoxin + rivastigmine

No interaction in healthy volunteers has been seen.

Fluoxetine + rivastigmine

No interaction in healthy volunteers has been seen.

Memantine + rivastigmine
See anticholinesterases + memantine (4.6.9).

Suxamethonium + rivastigmine
Rivastigmine may enhance the effect of suxamethonium-type muscle relaxants during anaesthesia.

Warfarin + rivastigmine
No interaction in healthy volunteers has been seen.

4.6.4 ATOMOXETINE

Atomoxetine is metabolised by CYP2D6 its half-life may be longer (five hours vs 21 hours) and peak levels five times higher in poor metabolisers and accumulation can occur (Sauer et al, Clin Pharmacokinet 2005;**44**:571–90). It has no clinically significant effect on CYP1A2, 3A4, 2D6 or 2C9. The UK SmPC recommends caution with the potential for potentiation with other noradrenergic drugs, e.g. **tricyclics**, **venlafaxine**, **reboxetine**, **mirtazapine**, **pseudoephedrine** or **phenylephrine**.

Antacids + atomoxetine
Antacids and omeprazole have no effect on atomoxetine bioavailability (UK SmPC).

Aspirin + atomoxetine
Lack of interaction has been shown (UK SmPC).

Benzodiazepines + atomoxetine
Lack of interaction has been shown with diazepam (UK SmPC).

MAOIs + ATOMOXETINE
These should not be used together and a two-week gap is needed after stopping an MAOI before starting atomoxetine (UK SmPC).

Methylphenidate + atomoxetine
Lack of additive cardiovascular effects has been shown (UK SmPC).

Mirtazapine + atomoxetine
See introduction to 4.6.4.

Phenytoin + atomoxetine
Lack of interaction has been shown (UK SmPC).

PPIs + atomoxetine
See antacids + atomoxetine above.

Salbutamol + atomoxetine
Caution is needed with high-dose salbutamol (any route) or other beta-blockers, as the cardiovascular effects of salbutamol can be potentiated (UK SmPC).

SSRIs + atomoxetine
Fluoxetine and paroxetine may increase ato-moxetine levels via 2D6 inhibition (UK SmPC).

Tricyclics + atomoxetine
See introduction to 4.6.4.

Venlafaxine + atomoxetine
There is a case of tic, tremor and speech disturbance, resolving when atomoxetine was discontinued (n = 1, Bond et al, Clin Toxicol [Phila] 2007;**45**:182–5). See also introduction to 4.6.4.

Warfarin + atomoxetine
Lack of interaction has been shown (UK SmPC).

4.6.5 BUPRENORPHINE

Buprenorphine has an extensive first-pass metabolism, but sub-lingual bioavailability is sufficient to allow administration by this route. Half-life can vary widely (3–44 hours), is highly protein bound (96%), and metabolised by CYP2D6 and 3A4. It is a major inhibitor of 2D6 and 3A4, and probably a weak inhibitor of 1A2, 2B6, 2C9, 2C19 and 2E1 (review by Elkader and Sproule, Clin Pharmacokinet 2005;**44**:661–80).

Antiretrovirals + buprenorphine *
Ritonavir can produce a significant increase, albeit asymptomatic, in the AUC for buprenorphine, but this does not happen with **nelfinavir** (n = 7, 15/7, McCance et al, Am J Addict 2010;**19**:30–7), **lopinavir/ritonavir** (e.g. n = 12, open, Bruce et al, J Acquir Immune Defic Syndr 2010;**54**:511–4), **efavirenz, maraviroc** nor **delavirdine** (n = 10, McCance-Katz et al, Clin Infect Dis 2006;**43**[Suppl 4]:S224–34), although there are cases of pharmacokinetic interaction with **atazanavir/ritonavir** (n = 3, Bruce and Altice, AIDS 2006;**20**:783–4), so choose your drugs with care (review by Bruce et al, Clin Infect Dis 2006;**43**[Suppl 4]:S216–23; n = 3, Bruce and Altice, AIDS 2006;**20**:783–4). **Tipranavir/ritonavir** have no significant effect on buprenorphine/naloxone levels but tipranavir levels may be substantially reduced, leading to potential loss of efficacy (n = 12 [c = 10], Bruce et al, Drug Alcohol Depend 2009;**105**:234–9).
Review: * Gruber and McCance-Katz, Curr HIV/AIDS Rep 2010;**7**:152–60.

Benzodiazepines + buprenorphine
See benzodiazepines (4.1.1).

Cocaine + buprenorphine *
Regular cocaine users have lower buprenorphine AUC and Cmax (s = 90, McCance-Katz et al, Am J Addict 2010;**19**:38–46).

Ketoconazole + buprenorphine
Start with half doses of buprenorphine due to ketoconazole's CYP3A4 inhibition (SmPC).

Methadone + buprenorphine
See methadone (4.6.10).

Tricyclics + buprenorphine
See tricyclics (4.3.1).

4.6.6 BUPROPION

Bupropion is 84% protein bound and primarily metabolised by CYP2B6, with a significant first-pass metabolism, although poor metabolisers may accumulate hydroxybupropion, leading to reduced efficacy (n = 12, Pollock et al, Ther Drug Monit 1996;**18**:581–5).

Review: interactions with anticonvulsants (Popli et al, Ann Clin Psychiatry 1995;**7**:99–101).

Alcohol + bupropion
There is an increased risk of seizures, so alcohol should be avoided or minimised. Extreme care is needed in overdose, chronic use and in alcohol withdrawal states.

Antipsychotics + bupropion
The CSM recommends caution due to the possible increased risk of seizures.

Antiretrovirals + bupropion *
Single doses of bupropion have no effect on **lopinavir/ritonavir** but **lopinavir/ritonavir** reduce bupropion levels probably via 2B6 and UGT induction (n = 12, 4/52, Hogeland et al, Clin Pharmacol Ther 2007;**81**:69–75). Ritonavir HD (1200mg/d) and LD (200mg/d) decreases bupropion AUC and Cmax by about 65% and 22% respectively, and so increased bupropion dose (by up to 100%) may be needed, but not above the BNF maximum (Park et al, J Clin Pharmacol 2010;**50**:1180–7).

Baicalin + bupropion
Baicalin (a Chinese herbal medicine) significantly reduces the plasma levels of bupropion via 2B6 induction (n = 17, Fan et al, Eur J Clin Pharmacol 2009;**65**:403–9).

Carbamazepine + bupropion
Carbamazepine induces bupropion metabolism, markedly decreasing bupropion plasma levels (n = 17, RCT, Ketter et al, J Clin Psychopharmacol 1995;**15**:327–33).

Ciclosporin + bupropion
A life-threatening decrease in ciclosporin levels has been reported with bupropion (n = 1, Lewis et al, J Child Adolesc Psychopharmacol 2001; 11:193–8).

Cimetidine + bupropion
Cimetidine may inhibit the metabolism of bupropion, and increase adverse effects, although no effect on bupropion SR was seen in one study (n = 24, RCT, open, Kustra et al, J Clin Pharmacol 1999;**39**:1184–8).

Clonidine + bupropion
Lack of interaction has been reported (n = 8, RCT, d/b, c/o, Cubeddu et al, Clin Pharmacol Ther 1984;**35**:576–84).

Clopidogrel + bupropion
A single-dose study showed clopidogrel to significantly inhibit bupropion's 2B6 metabolism, increasing AUC by 60% (n = 12, Turpeinen et al, Clin Pharmacol Ther 2005;**77**:553–9).

Fluoxetine + bupropion
Bupropion produces no significant changes in fluoxetine levels (n = 24, open, 8/52, Kennedy et al, J Clin Psychiatry 2002;**63**:181–6) but panic disorder (n = 1, Young, J Clin Psychiatry 1996;**57**:177–8) and delirium (n = 1, Chan et al, J Clin Psychopharmacol 2006;**26**:677–9) have been reported.

Fosphenytoin + bupropion
See phenytoin + bupropion.

Ginkgo biloba + bupropion
There is no significant interaction, although hydroxybupropion levels may be reduced (n = 14, 2/52, Lei et al, Br J Clin Pharmacol 2009; **68**:201–6).

Guanfacine + bupropion
There is a report of a grand mal seizure with the combination (n = 1, Tilton, J Am Acad Child Adolesc Psychiatry 1998;**37**:682–3).

MAOIs + bupropion
Animal studies have indicated that acute bupropion toxicity might occur, and the combination is contraindicated.

Lamotrigine + bupropion
See lamotrigine (4.5.5).

Levodopa + bupropion
An increased incidence of side-effects has been reported with the combination.

Moclobemide + bupropion
See MAOIs + bupropion.

Paroxetine + bupropion
Bupropion produces no significant changes in paroxetine levels (open, 8/52, Kennedy et al, J Clin Psychiatry 2002;**63**:181–6), but the CSM recommends caution.

Phenobarbital + bupropion

Phenobarbital may induce the metabolism of bupropion, which would reduce its efficacy.

Phenytoin + bupropion

Phenytoin may induce the metabolism of bupropion, which would reduce its efficacy.

Pseudoephedrine + bupropion

There is a report of acute myocardial ischaemia with the combination (n = 1, Pederson et al, Can J Cardiol 2001;**17**:599–601).

Rifampicin + bupropion

Rifampicin may reduce bupropion's half-life by 50%, reducing plasma levels, probably by CYP2B6 induction (n = 18, Loboz et al, Clin Pharmacol Ther 2006;**80**:75–84).

Selegiline + bupropion

See MAOIs + bupropion.

Sertraline + bupropion

A marked adverse reaction has been reported with the combination, where mood appeared to deteriorate and venlafaxine was added, but was later recognised as serotonin syndrome (n = 1, Munhoz, Clin Neuropharmacol 2004;**27**:219–22).

Smoking + bupropion

In a single-dose study, cigarettes had no detectable effect on bupropion kinetics (open, Hsyu et al, J Clin Pharmacol 1997;**37**:737–43).

St John's wort + bupropion *

See bupropion + St. John's wort (4.3.3.10).

Tamoxifen + bupropion *

See tamoxifen + paroxetine (4.3.2.4).

Ticlopidine + bupropion

A single-dose study showed that ticlopidine significantly inhibited the metabolism of bupropion, increasing AUC by 85% (n = 12, Turpeinen et al, Clin Pharmacol Ther 2005;**77**:553–9).

Tricyclics + bupropion

Bupropion has been reported to increase **imipramine** and **desipramine** levels, through decreased clearance (n = 1, Shad and Preskorn, J Clin Psychopharmacol 1997;**17**:118–9). Also reported with bupropion are seizures with **trimipramine** (n = 1, Enns, J Clin Psychiatry 2001;**62**:476–7), **clomipramine** (n = 1, Shin et al, Clin Neuropharmacol 2004;**27**:192–4) and **nortriptyline** (n = 1, Weintraub, Depress Anxiety 2001;**13**:50–2).

Valproate + bupropion

Valproate does not seem to induce bupropion metabolism, but raised metabolite levels are possible (n = 17, RCT, Ketter et al, J Clin Psychopharmacol 1995;**15**:327–33).

Venlafaxine + bupropion *

Bupropion can significantly increase venlafaxine levels, sometimes dramatically and requiring dose reduction (n = 3, Paslakis et al, J Clin Psychopharmacol 2010;**30**:473–4), but decrease O-desmethylvenlafaxine levels (open, 8/52, Kennedy et al, J Clin Psychiatry 2002;**63**:181–6). See also sertraline + bupropion.

Zolpidem + bupropion

There are some reported cases of antidepressants and zolpidem causing short-lived hallucinations (e.g. Elko et al, Clin Toxicol 1998; **36**:195–203).

4.6.7 CLOMETHIAZOLE

Clomethiazole inhibits CYP2E1.

Alcohol + clomethiazole

See alcohol (4.7.1).

Cimetidine + clomethiazole

Cimetidine inhibits the metabolism of clomethiazole, raising plasma levels.

Methadone + clomethiazole

See methadone (4.6.10).

4.6.8 DISULFIRAM

Disulfiram is a potent inhibitor of CYP1A2, 2B6 and 2E1 (the enzyme that metabolises ethanol), but chronic use could affect other enzymes too (n = 7, Frye and Branch, Br J Clin Pharmacol 2002;**53**:155–62).

Review: disulfiram interactions (Acta Psychiatr Scand 1992;**86**[Suppl 369]:59–66).

Acamprosate + disulfiram

See acamprosate (4.6.1).

ALCOHOL + DISULFIRAM

See disulfiram under 'Alcohol abuse and dependence' (1.4) and alcohol (4.7.1).

Antipsychotics + disulfiram

There is a report of psychotic symptoms reappearing when disulfiram was started and an increased first-pass metabolism of perphenazine has been noted (n = 1, Hansen et al, Lancet 1982;**2**:1472).

Benzodiazepines + disulfiram

Disulfiram may inhibit the metabolism of **diazepam, chlordiazepoxide** and **temazepam** (n = 1, Hardman et al, Lancet 1994;**344**:1231–2), leading to lengthened half-lives, but not with **oxazepam** (open, MacLeod, *Clin Pharmacol Ther* 1978;**24**: 583–9) or **alprazolam** (n = 11, 2/52, Diquet *et al*, *Eur J Clin Pharmacol* 1990; **38**:157–60).

Caffeine + disulfiram
Disulfiram may reduce caffeine clearance by 50% (n = 21, open, Beach *et al*, *Clin Pharmacol Ther* 1986;**39**:265–70).

Cannabis + disulfiram
See cannabis (*4.7.2*).

Carbamazepine + disulfiram
Lack of significant interaction has been shown (n = 7, open, Krag *et al*, *Acta Neurol* 1981;**63**: 395–8).

Cocaine + disulfiram
There is a case of pronounced paranoia with the combination (n = 1, Mutschler *et al*, *J Clin Psychopharmacol* 2009;**29**:99–101).

Colchicine + disulfiram
A potentially fatal interaction between colchicine and disulfiram has been reported (Chen *et al*, *Prog Neuropsychopharmacol Biol Psychiatry* 2009;**33**:1281).

Isoniazid + disulfiram
CNS toxicity has been reported in patients taking isoniazid who then took disulfiram (Rothstein, *JAMA* 1972;**219**:1216).

Lithium + disulfiram
There is no theoretical or clinical reasons why an interaction should occur.

MAOIs + disulfiram
Delirium has been reported with the combination (e.g. n = 1, Blansjaar and Egberts, *Am J Psychiatry* 1995;**152**:296).

Methadone + disulfiram
See methadone (*4.6.10*).

Methylphenidate + disulfiram
See methylphenidate (*4.6.11*).

Metronidazole + disulfiram
Psychotic reactions have been reported (n = 2, Hotson and Langston, *Arch Neurol* 1976;**33**: 41–2).

NICOUMALONE + DISULFIRAM
An enhanced anticoagulant effect is possible.

Omeprazole + disulfiram
There is a report of confusion, disorientation and catatonia with the combination (n = 1, Hajela *et al*, *Can Med Assoc J* 1990;**143**:1207).

Paraldehyde + disulfiram
An enhanced disulfiram reaction is possible

(mentioned in Hadden and Metzner, *Am J Med* 1969;**47**:642).

Phenytoin + disulfiram
See phenytoin (*4.5.9*).

Theophylline + disulfiram
Theophylline levels may be increased via enzyme inhibition. Monitor and reduce the theophylline dose if necessary (n = 20, RCT, Loi *et al*, *Clin Pharmacol Ther* 1989;**45**:476–86).

Tricyclics + disulfiram
See tricyclics (*4.3.1*).

WARFARIN + DISULFIRAM
Prothrombin time can fall by about 10% (Rothstein, *JAMA* 1972;**221**:1051–2), with one study showing a marked effect with reduced warfarin doses sometimes necessary (n = 7, open, O'Reilly, *Clin Pharmacol Ther* 1981;**29**:332). The literature notes this to be a significant effect.

4.6.9 MEMANTINE

Memantine is only minimally metabolised, does not inhibit CYP1A2, 2A6, 2C9, 2D6, 2E1 or 3A, or the FMO system, or epoxide hydrolase or sulphation, and so metabolic interactions are unlikely. Raised urinary pH (e.g. infections, diet change, excessive alkalising gastric buffers, etc) may significantly reduce excretion. Plasma protein binding is 45%.

Alcohol + memantine
See alcohol (*4.7.1*).

Amantadine + memantine
Both are NMDA-antagonists and the combination should be avoided as CNS ADRs may be more frequent. The same may be true with ketamine and dextromethorphan.

Anticholinergics + memantine
The anticholinergic's effects may be enhanced by memantine.

Anticholinesterases + memantine
Lack of interaction has been shown between memantine and **donepezil** (n = 19, open, Periclou *et al*, *Ann Pharmacother* 2004;**38**:1389–94) or **rivastigmine** (n = 16, open, c/o, 7/52, Shua-Haim *et al*, *Clin Drug Investig* 2008;**8**:361–74). A post-marketing survey of patients taking memantine with AChEs suggested that the combination was safe and well-tolerated (n = 158, open, mean 4/52, Hartmann and Mobius, *Int Clin Psychopharmacol* 2003;**18**:81–5).

Antipsychotics + memantine

The antipsychotic effects may be reduced by memantine.

Antispasmodic agents + memantine

The effects may be modified by memantine and dose adjustment may be necessary.

Baclofen + memantine

The effects may be modified by memantine and dose adjustment may be necessary.

Dantrolene + memantine

Dantrolene's effects may be modified by memantine and dose adjustment necessary.

Dextromethorphan + memantine

See amantadine + memantine

Dopamine agonists + memantine

Dopamine antagonists such as bromocriptine may be enhanced by memantine.

H2-blockers + memantine

A theoretical interaction via competition for cationic transport system exists and there is the potential for increased plasma levels.

Hydrochlorthiazide + memantine

There is a theoretical possibility of reduced diuretic effect.

Ketamine + memantine

See amantadine + memantine.

Levodopa + memantine

The effects of levodopa may be enhanced by memantine.

Phenobarbital + memantine

The barbiturate's effects may be reduced by memantine.

Phenytoin + memantine

There is one case report of interaction.

Procainamide + memantine

A theoretical interaction via competition for cationic transport system exists and there is the potential for increased plasma levels.

Quinidine/quinine + memantine

A theoretical interaction via competition for cationic transport systems exists, as is the potential for raised memantine plasma levels.

Smoking + memantine

A theoretical interaction via competition for cationic transport system exists and there is the potential for increased memantine plasma levels.

4.6.10 METHADONE

Methadone is probably metabolised mainly by CYP3A4 (or not, as the case may be; Kharasch

et al, Clin Pharmacol Ther 2008;**84**:506–12) and partly by 2D6 (but genotype has no apparent effect on clearance; Coller *et al, Int J Clin Pharmacol Ther* 2007;**45**:410–7) and 1A2 (and possibly 2B6), and inhibits CYP2D6 and 3A4. Absorption is also variable according to P-glycoprotein status. The (R)-methadone is the active moiety, (S)-methadone being inactive.

Reviews: general (DeMaria, *J Maint Addictions* 2003;**2**:41–57), TDM (Moolchan *et al, J Addict Dis* 2001;**20**:55–73).

Alcohol + methadone

See alcohol (4.7.1).

Antipsychotics + methadone

See methadone + antipsychotics (4.2.1).

Antiretrovirals + methadone *

Antiretrovirals and methadone are not an uncommon combination, and some (but not all) retrovirals can reduce methadone levels significantly, by 3A4 induction.

Atazanavir is a potent CYP3A4 inhibitor, but one study showed no clinically relevant interaction with methadone and no dose adjustment needed (n = 16, 2/52, Friedland *et al, AIDS* 2005; **19**:1635–41), although in another methadone reduced atazanavir plasma levels and AUC by around 40%, which may well be clinically significant (n = 24, Haberl *et al, Eur J Clin Pharmacol* 2010;**66**:375–81).

Didanosine levels can be reduced by about 40% (n = 27, open, Rainer *et al, J AIDS* 2000; **24**:241–8).

Efavirenz can induce (and inhibit) CYP3A4 and produce withdrawal symptoms from reduced methadone levels (n = 1, Pinzani *et al, Ann Pharmacother* 2000;**34**:405–7; n = 1, Marzolini *et al, AIDS* 2000; **14**:1291–2; n = 9 + 52 controls, Esteban *et al, Drug Metab Lett* 2008;**2**:269–79). Indinivir can rasie methadone levels slightly.

Fosamprenavir-ritonavir can reduce methadone AUC by 18%, considered insignificant (n = 26, 18/7, Cao *et al, Pharmacotherapy* 2008;**28**:863–74).

Maraviroc's SmPC says no interaction is expected albeit not formally studied.

Nelfinavir can induce methadone metabolism and clearance, with levels reduced by 40–50%, probably by increasing renal clearance and by altering the S- and R-methadone ratio and despite significant 3A4 inhibition (n = 12, Kharasch *et al, Drug Alcohol Depend* 2009;**101**:158–68).

4

Nevirapine can reduced methadone levels and AUC by 47% (UK SmPC) through CYP3A4 induction, precipitating withdrawal (n = 5 + 52 controls, Esteban et al, Drug Metab Lett 2008;**2**:269–79; n = 7, Altice et al, AIDS 1999;**13**:957–62).

Raltegravir and methadone appear not to interact (n = 12, Anderson et al, J Clin Pharmacol 2010;**50**:1461–6).

Ritonavir may cause a reduction of 40–50% of methadone levvels (Kharasch et al, Clin Pharmacol Ther 2008;**84**:497–505; n = 1, Geletko and Erickson, Pharmacother 2000;**20**:93–4), although **ritonavir/saquinavir** has been used without dose adjustment in AIDS patients (n = 12, Gerber et al, J AIDS 2001;**27**:153–60).

Review: * interactions with antiretrovirals (Gruber and McCance-Katz, Curr HIV/AIDS Rep 2010;**7**:152–60).

Ascorbic acid + methadone
Vitamin C and other urine acidifiers (e.g. ammonium chloride) can decrease methadone plasma levels via increased renal excretion if the pH is less than 6. Methadone's half-life can be halved to around 19–20 hours.

Benzodiazepines + methadone
There is no proven pharmacokinetic interaction but additive sedation can occur (e.g. n = 5, RCT, Preston et al, Drug Alc Dep 1986;**18**:195–202).

Buprenorphine + methadone
An antagonistic effect would be predicted and buprenorphine might displace methadone from Mu-opioid receptors, precipitating withdrawal. Enhanced sedation and respiratory depression may occur.

Cannabis + methadone
An interaction would be possible through CYP3A4 induction.

Carbamazepine + methadone
Reduced methadone levels can occur through CYP3A4 induction (Ketter et al, J Clin Psychopharmacol 1991;**11**:198–203; n = 43, Bell et al, Clin Pharmacol Ther 1988;**43**:623–9), and methadone-induced respiratory depression has been reported after withdrawal of carbamazepine (n = 1, Benitez–Rosario et al, J Pain Symptom Manage 2006;**32**:99–100).

Chloral + methadone
Additive sedation can occur.

Cimetidine + methadone
Raised methadone levels can occur.

Ciprofloxacin + methadone
A course of ciprofloxacin has caused sudden and profound methadone toxicity (n = 1, Herrlin et al, Lancet 2000;**356**:2069–70) and QTc prolongation leading to Torsades de pointes (n = 1, Nair et al, Addiction 2008;**103**:2062–4).

Clomethiazole + methadone
Additive sedation can occur.

Cocaine + methadone *
Regular cocaine users show lower methadone Cmax and AUC (n = 39, retrospective, McCance-Katz et al, Am J Addict 2010;**19**:47–52) possibly by accelerated methadone elimination (Moolchan et al, J Addict Dis 2001;**20**:55–73).

Cyclizine + methadone
There are rare reports of hallucinations with the combination.

Dextromethorphan + methadone
Delirium, hypersomnia and confusion has been reported (n = 1, Lotrich et al, Am J Geriatr Pharmacother 2005;**3**:17–20).

Diphenhydramine + methadone
There are rare reports of additional CNS effects with the combination.

Disulfiram + methadone
Lack of kinetic interaction has been shown (n = 7, Tong et al, J Clin Pharmacol 1980;**20**:506–13).

Domperidone + methadone
Increased absorption has been reported.

Erythromycin + methadone
Raised methadone levels could occur through CYP3A4 inhibition.

Fluconazole/ketoconazole/itraconazole + methadone
Methadone levels can rise by a mean of 27% through CYP3A4 inhibition, although one study did not detect any signs of toxicity with fluconazole (n = 25, RCT, d/b, p/c, 14/7, Cobb et al, Clin Pharmacol Ther 1998;**63**:655–62). Torsade de pointes has been reported after two doses of itraconazole in someone taking methadone (n = 1, NoorZurani et al, Drug Alcohol Rev 2009;**2 8**:688–90).

Fluoxetine + methadone
Lack of significant interaction has been shown (n = 16, open, 9/52, Batki et al, J Clin Psychopharmacol 1993;**13**:243–50).

Fluvoxamine + methadone
Fluvoxamine may inhibit methadone metabolism leading to raised levels (n = 1, DeMaria and Serota, J Addict Dis 1999;**18**:5–12) and severe

hypoventilation has been reported (n = 1, Alderman and Frith, *Aust N Z J Psychiatry* 1999; **33**:99–101).

Fosphenytoin + methadone
See phenytoin.

Grapefruit juice + methadone
Raised methadone levels through CYP3A4 inhibition could theoretically occur.

Hypnotics + methadone
Enhanced sedation can occur.

Lofexidine + methadone
Lofexidine decreases sitting systolic and diastolic bp by 27 and 15 mmHg respectively, and reduced cognitive efficiency compared to placebo when given with methadone, so monitor for cardiovascular and cognitive changes if using the combination (n = 14, d/b, p/c, 11/52, Schroeder *et al, Pharmacotherapy* 2007;**27**:1111–9).

MAOIs + methadone
See MAOIs (*4.3.4*).

Metapyrone + methadone
Metapyrone can cause a withdrawal-like syndrome with methadone (n = 15, open, Kennedy *et al, Br J Addict* 1990;**85**:1133–40).

Naloxone + methadone
This opiate antagonist would block the effect of methadone: this can occur within 5–10 minutes (Tornabene, *Ann Intern Med* 1974;**81**:349–51).

Naltrexone + methadone
This opiate antagonist would block the effect of methadone.

Paroxetine + methadone
See paroxetine (*4.3.2.4*).

Phenobarbital + methadone
Enhanced sedation and respiratory depression may occur. Reduced methadone levels have been reported with phenobarbital (e.g. n = 43, Bell *et al, Clin Pharmacol Ther* 1988;**43**:623–9).

PHENYTOIN + METHADONE
Reduced methadone levels can occur through CYP3A4 induction, with withdrawal symptoms occurring within four days (n = 43, Bell *et al, Clin Pharmacol Ther* 1988;**43**:623–9). Dosage adjustment may be needed.

Quetiapine + methadone
Quetiapine increases the plasma levels of the active R-methadone enantiomer by about 20%, possibly by CYP2D6 inhibition but this is highly variable and probably not clinically significant, (n = 14, Uehlinger *et al, J Clin Psychopharmacol* 2007;**27**:273–8).

Reboxetine + methadone
See reboxetine (*4.3.3.6*).

Rifampicin + methadone
Methadone levels reduce by 30–65% within 4–5 days in 70% patients given rifampicin, through CYP3A4 induction (n = 30, Kreek *et al, N Engl J Med* 1976;**294**:1104–6).

Risperidone + methadone
There is a report of possible interaction, resulting in irritability and aches (n = 1, Wines and Weiss, *J Clin Psychopharmacol* 1999;**19**:65–7).

Sodium bicarbonate + methadone
Sodium bicarbonate and other urinary alkalinisers can increase plasma levels via decreased renal excretion.

St John's wort + methadone
See St John's wort (*4.3.3.10*).

Tricyclics + methadone
Additive sedation might occur and methadone can double desipramine blood levels (n = 5, Maany *et al, Am J Psychiatry* 1989;**146**:1611–3).

Zidovudine + methadone
Raised zidovudine levels have been reported (AUC increased by 41%) (n = 8, McCance-Katz *et al, J Acquir Immune Defic Synd Hum Retrivirol* 1998;**18**:435–43).

4.6.11 METHYLPHENIDATE

Atomoxetine + methylphenidate
See atomoxetine (*4.6.4*).

Carbamazepine + methylphenidate
Carbamazepine has been reported to cause an extreme reduction of methylphenidate levels (n = 1, Behar *et al, J Am Acad Child Adolesc Psychiatry* 1998;**37**:1128–9).

Ciclosporin + methylphenidate
A rise in ciclosporin levels has been reported with methylphenidate (n = 1, Lewis *et al, J Child Adolesc Psychopharmacol* 2001;**11**:193–8).

Cocaine + methylphenidate
No pharmacokinetic or physiological interaction seems to occur (n = 7, p/c, Winhusen *et al, Pharmacol Biochem Behav* 2006;**85**:29–38).

Disulfiram + methylphenidate
There is a case of an acute-onset psychotic episode after a single dose of methylphenidate in a patient taking disulfiram 400 mg/d (n = 1, Caci and Baylé, *Am J Psychiatry* 2007;**164**:1759).

Fluoxetine + methylphenidate
Hallucinations have been reported with the

4

combination (n = 1, Coskun and Zoroglu, *J Clin Psychopharmacol* 2008;**28**:723–5).

Glipizide + methylphenidate

Addition of methylphenidate in a woman also taking glipizide resulted in a 26% reduction in plasma glucose levels, and so an interaction is a possible explanation (n = 1, Gontkovsky et al, *Clin Drug Investig* 2007;**27**:719–25).

MAOIs + methylphenidate

See MAOIs (*4.3.4*).

Modafinil + methylphenidate

See modafinil (*4.6.12*).

Paroxetine + methylphenidate *

Manic switch and serotonin syndrome has been reported with paroxetine added to methylphenidate (n=1, Park and Jung, *Prog Neuropsychopharmacol Biol Psychiatry* 2010;**34**:719-20).

Phenytoin + methylphenidate

Phenytoin toxicity has been reported (n = 3, Ghofrani, *Dev Med Child Neurol* 1988;**30**:267–8).

Sertraline + methylphenidate

Seizures (n = 1, Schertz and Steinberg, *J Child Adolesc Psychopharmacol* 2008;**18**:301–3) and serotonin syndrome (n = 1, Ishii et al, *Psychiatry Clin Neurosci* 2008;**62**:246) have been reported.

St John's wort + methylphenidate

It has been suggested that SJW may reduce the efficacy of methylphenidate in ADHD (Niederhofer, *Med Hypotheses* 2007;**68**:1189).

Tricyclics + methylphenidate

Methylphenidate may inhibit the metabolism of tricyclics producing up to a four-fold increase in levels (e.g. n = 2, Grob and Coyle, *J Dev Behav Pediatrics* 1986;**7**:265–7). Mood and cognitive deterioration has been reported with imipramine and methylphenidate (n = 2, Grob and Coyle, *J Dev Behav Pediatr* 1986;**7**:265–7).

Valproate + methylphenidate

Rapid onset and severe dyskinesia and bruxism has been reported with the combination (n = 2, Gara and Roberts, *J Child Adolesc Psychopharmacol* 2000;**10**:39–43).

4.6.12 MODAFINIL

Modafinil is moderately bound to plasma proteins (62%), essentially to albumin. Renal excretion is the main route of elimination, but it is also metabolised by CYP3A4. It inhibits 2C19, 2D6 and a small and concentration-dependent induction of 1A2, 2B6 and 3A4 (Robertson and Hellriegel, *Clin Pharmacokinet* 2003;**42**:123–37). It has two inactive metabolites.

Amfetamines + modafinil

Low dose amfetamines appear to have no significant effects on steady state modafinil (n = 32, RCT, open, Hellriegel et al, *J Clin Pharmacol* 2002;**42**:450–60).

Benzodiazepines + modafinil

Triazolam levels may be significantly reduced by modafinil, probably via 3A4 induction (n = 41, RCT, 4/52, Robertson, *Clin Pharmacol Ther* 2002; **71**:46–56).

Carbamazepine + modafinil

Carbamazepine might reduce plasma modafinil levels (SmPC).

Ciclosporin + modafinil

The UK SmPC reports a case of a 50% reduction in ciclosporin levels with modafinil.

Cocaine + modafinil

Single doses of IV cocaine have no apparent medical or cardiac interaction with modafinil, although the cocaine euphoria may be significantly blunted (e.g. n = 12, Malcolm et al, *Am J Drug Alcohol Abuse* 2006; **32**:577–87).

Dexamfetamine + modafinil

Dexamfetamine has no apparent effect on steady state modafinil levels (n = 32, RCT, open, Hellriegel et al, *J Clin Pharmacol* 2002;**42**:450–60).

Ethinylestradiol + modafinil

Ethinylestradiol levels may be reduced by modafinil, probably via 3A4 induction (n = 41, RCT, 4/52, Robertson, *Clin Pharmacol Ther* 2002;**71**:46–56).

MAOI + modafinil

See MAOIs (*4.3.4*).

Methylphenidate + modafinil

Low-dose methylphenidate does not appear to interact with modafinil (n = 32, RCT, open, Hellriegel et al, *J Clin Pharmacol* 2002;**41**:895–904), although methylphenidate may slightly slow the absorption of modafinil (RCT, Wong et al, *J Clin Pharmacol* 1998;**38**:276–82).

Oral contraceptives + modafinil *

Modafinil can reduce OC efficacy by 3A4 induction (and for up to two months after stopping). Alternative contraceptive methods or higher dose oral contraceptives containing 50 mcg ethinylestradiol should be used.

Phenobarbital + modafinil

Phenobarbital might reduce plasma modafinil levels (SmPC).

Phenytoin + modafinil
Phenytoin's clearance might be reduced by modafinil (SmPC).

Sodium oxybate + modafinil
See sodium oxybate (4.6.13).

Tricyclics + modafinil
A single dose study showed a clinically important interaction with clomipramine 50mg/d (n=1, Grozinger et al, Clin Neuropharmacol 1998;**21**: 127–9).

Warfarin + modafinil
A single-dose study suggested no interaction (n=28, Robertson et al, J Clin Pharmacol 2002; **42**:205–14), but the UK SmPC recommends caution and additional monitoring as warfarin clearance may be reduced.

4.6.13 SODIUM OXYBATE (GHB)

Sodium oxybate is metabolised by GHB dehydrogenase, eventually to carbon dioxide and water, with no active metabolites. It does not appear to significantly inhibit P450 enzymes 1A2, 2C9, 2C19, 2D6, 2E1, and 3A4 at therapeutic doses.

Alcohol + sodium oxybate
Enhanced CNS depression can occur (SmPC).

Benzodiazepines + sodium oxybate
Respiratory depression might be increased and so the combination should be avoided (SmPC).

Ethosuximide + sodium oxybate
Ethosuximide inhibits GHB dehydrogenase, and so an interaction is theoretically possible but there are no human studies or reports (SmPC).

Modafinil + sodium oxybate *
Lack of interaction has been reported (SmPC), although there is a case of rapid onset depression (n=1, Rossetti et al, Sleep Med 2010; 11:500–1).

Phenytoin + sodium oxybate
Phenytoin inhibits GHB dehydrogenase, and so an interaction is theoretically possible but there are no human studies or reports (SmPC).

Proton-pump inhibitors + sodium oxybate
Lack of interaction has been reported with omeprazole (SmPC).

Tricyclics + sodium oxybate
Lack of interaction has been reported with protriptyline, but adverse effects may be increased with this combination (SmPC).

Valproate + sodium oxybate
Valproate inhibits GHB dehydrogenase, and so

an interaction is theoretically possible but there are no human studies or reports (SmPC).

Zolpidem + sodium oxybate
Lack of interaction has been reported (SmPC).

4.7 NON-PRESCRIBED DRUGS AND 'VICES'

4.7.1 ALCOHOL

Alcohol/ethanol-psychotropic drug interactions can occur frequently and with varied outcome, depending upon:

- alcohol usage (e.g. chronic and/or acute, leading to altered enzymes)
- consumption (amount, time span)
- type of interaction (e.g. additive sedation, antagonism or cross-tolerance)
- what the individual then tries to do (e.g. sleep, drive)
- comorbidity (e.g. asthma).

These variables need to be considered when assessing the effect, or potential effect, of the interaction. Alcohol distribution is wide, with the direct central depressant effect impairing all central functions (e.g. cognition and respiration) which contribute to many of the drug–drug interactions. Alcohol also promotes the action of GABA and may release other amines such as dopamine and endorphins.

Reviews: general (Jang and Harris, Expert Opin Drug Metab Toxicol 2007;**3**:719–31), in older adults (Moore et al, Am J Geriatr Pharmacother 2007;**5**:64–74).

Acamprosate + alcohol
Continued alcohol consumption may negate the therapeutic effect of acamprosate. There is no detectable pharmacokinetic interaction (review by Nalpas et al, Encephale 1990;**16**:175–9).

Agomelatine + alcohol
See agomelatine (4.3.3.1).

ANTIPSYCHOTICS + ALCOHOL
There is no clear evidence that alcohol reduces antipsychotic efficacy (n=31, open, Chetty et al, Eur J Clin Pharmacol 1994;**46**:523–6). However, enhanced CNS depression is well-documented, resulting in impaired concentration, coordination, judgement, drowsiness and lethargy, as well as hypotension and respiratory depression. Alcohol-related drowsiness is significant with **phenothiazines** and **flupentixol**. EPSE may also be

enhanced (Freed, *Med J Aust* 1981;**2**:44–5), as can hepatotoxicity with, eg. **chlorpromazine** (Strubelt, *Biochem Pharmacol* 1980;**29**:1445–9). Single oral doses of **amisulpride** do not seem to enhance the effects of alcohol on the performance and memory of healthy subjects (n = 18, RCT, Mattila *et al, Eur J Clin Pharmacol* 1996;**51**:161). No significant difference in performance or gross motor skills has been shown with **aripiprazole**, although 2.5–10 mg/d increases sedation from alcohol (n = 18, p/c, Kranzler *et al, Alcohol Clin Exp Res* 2008;**32**:573–9). Enhanced CNS sedation would be expected with **olanzapine**, and raised heart rate and increased postural hypotension have been reported. Overall, this is a potentially important interaction, especially in the community. Accidental alcohol over-dosage, especially in people with asthma, respiratory depression or chest infections, could prove fatal if combined with antipsychotics.

BARBITURATES + ALCOHOL

Enhanced or prolonged CNS and respiratory depression can occur, seriously impairing con-centration and performance. Acute alcohol ingestion may increase barbiturate levels but chronic alcohol use may decrease barbiturate levels (Mezey and Robles, *Gastroenterology* 1974; **66**:248–53). The lethal dose of barbiturates is reported to be up to 50% lower when alcohol is also present (Bogan and Smith, *J Forensic Sci* 1967; **7**:37–45). This is mainly due to additive respiratory depression.

BENZODIAZEPINES + ALCOHOL

Alcohol can enhance the sedation caused by benzodiazepines by 20–30%, a well-established, documented and predictable interaction. Synergistic sedation has been reported with **lorazepam** (d/b, c/o, Lister and File, *J Clin Psycho-pharmacol* 1983;**3**:66–71), **clorazepate** and **diazepam**. Larger quantities of alcohol may inhibit benzodiazepine metabolism, especially in those with impaired or borderline hepatic function (review by Guthrie and Lane, *Alcoholism* 1986;**10**:686–90). Acute ethanol consumption decreases diazepam clearance by up to 50%, (Laisi *et al, Eur J Clin Pharmacol* 1979;**16**:263–70). At low dose, alcohol and **temazepam** appear not to interact adversely (n = 24, p/c, c/o, Martin and Siddle, *Brain Cogn* 2003;**53**:58–65).

Beta-blockers + alcohol

Alcohol may slightly reduce propranolol absorption and increase clearance (n = 5, open, Grabowski *et al, Int J Clin Pharmacol Ther Toxicol* 1980;**18**:317–9; Sotaniemi *et al, Clin Pharmacol Ther* 1981;**29**:705–10).

Bupropion + alcohol

See bupropion (*4.6.6*).

Buspirone + alcohol

A minimal interaction and slightly increased sedation has been reported (n = 24, RCT, Erwin *et al, J Clin Psychopharmacol* 1986;**6**:199–209).

BZP (benzylpiperazine) and TFMPP (trifluor-omethylphenylpiperazine) + alcohol *

Severe adverse reactions (agitation, anxiety, hallucinations, vomiting, insomnia, migraine) have been reported with BZP+TFMPP, with or without alcohol, and none with alcohol or placebo comparator groups, and so this appears to hold a significant risk (n = 35, RCT, d/b, p/c, Thompson *et al, J Psychopharmacol* 2010;**24**:1299–308).

Cannabis + alcohol

See cannabis (*4.7.2*).

Carbamazepine + alcohol *

There is virtually nothing published but additive sedation would be expected. In acute carbamazepine intoxication, alcohol does not seem to affect CBZ kinetics (n = 158, Piekoszewski *et al, Pharmacol Rep* 2010;**62**:398–404).

CHLORAL HYDRATE + ALCOHOL

Additive CNS depressant effects occur when alcohol is taken with chloral hydrate. Tachycardia, impaired concentration, disulfiram-like effects and profound vasodilation may also occur (Owen and Taberner, *Br J Pharmacol* 1978; **64**:400).

Clomethiazole + alcohol

Alcohol increases the bioavailability of oral clomethiazole, probably via inhibition of first-pass metabolism (Neuvonen *et al, Int J Clin Pharmacol Ther Toxicol* 1981;**19**:552–60).

Citalopram + alcohol

There is little published at present on this. The UK SmPC notes that citalopram should not enhance the sedation caused by alcohol.

Cocaine + alcohol

See cocaine (*4.7.3*).

DISULFIRAM + ALCOHOL *

Disulfiram inhibits the aldehyde dehydrogenase enzyme, leading to accumulation of acetaldehyde from incomplete alcohol metabolism. The main symptoms of the 'Antabuse reaction' are flushing, sweating, palpitations, hyperventilation, increased pulse, hypotension, nausea and vomiting (often in that order). Arrhythmias and shock can follow. The reaction occurs within 5–15 minutes and can be fatal. Factors affecting the severity of the reaction include the dose of disulfiram, rate and dose of alcohol ingestion, sensitivity, individual aldehyde dehydrogenase activity, concurrent medication (see disulfiram, 4.6.4) and co-existing pulmonary or cardiac disease. Patients should be warned that reactions can occur with disguised sources of alcohol, e.g. Listerine® mouthwashes (which can contain up to 21–27% alcohol), sauces, pharmaceuticals (e.g. cough mixtures) and topical preparations (e.g. shampoo, Stoll and King, *JAMA* 1980;**244**:2045). Delirium has been reported with the combination (Park and Riggio, *Ann Pharmacother* 2001;**35**:32–5).

Escitalopram + alcohol

See citalopram + alcohol.

Fluoxetine + alcohol

Alcohol has no additional significant effect on drowsiness, sedation or task performance tests with fluoxetine 40 mg/d, compared with fluoxetine alone (e.g. Shaw et al, *Hum Psychopharmacol* 1989;**4**:113–20).

Fluvoxamine + alcohol

No significant potentiation of the cognitive effects of 40 g IV alcohol by single and multiple doses of 50 mg fluvoxamine occurred in one study (n = 24, van Harten et al, *Clin Pharmacol Ther* 1992;**52**:427–35).

Lacosamide + alcohol

See alcohol + lacosamide (4.5.4).

Levetiracetam + alcohol

See levetiracetam (4.5.6).

Lithium + alcohol

Impaired driving skills have been suggested and alcohol may produce a slight (12%) increase in peak lithium levels (n = 10, RCT, d/b, p/c, c/o, Anton et al, *Clin Pharmacol Ther* 1985;**38**:52–5).

MAOIs + ALCOHOL

As well as an interaction occurring with alcoholic and low alcoholic drinks (see MAOIs, 4.3.4), alcohol may increase central catecholamine synthesis and release, and MAOIs may inhibit alcohol dehydrogenase, potentiating alcohol (comprehensive review by Weller et al, *Psychosomatics* 1984;**25**:301–9).

MDMA/ecstasy + alcohol *

People aged 18–29 taking both substances become more aroused when intoxicated but psychomotor accuracy is significantly impaired

compared to placebo or either substance alone (n = 16, RCT, d/b, p/c, c/o, Dumont et al, *J Psychopharmacol* 2010;**24**:155–64).

Melatonin + alcohol

See melatonin (4.1.4).

Memantine + alcohol

Memantine has no effect on alcohol-induced performance impairment, but may increase some subjective symptoms (n = 18, 3×3/7, d/b, Bisaga and Evans, *Psychopharmacol [Berl]* 2003; **172**:16–24).

Methadone + alcohol

Predictably, increased sedation and respiratory depression may occur with the combination (Bellville et al, *Clin Pharmacol Ther* 1971;**12**:607–12), especially in overdose, as could hepatotoxicity. Chronic high use of alcohol may induce enzymes requiring higher methadone doses and binge drinking may increase methadone excretion via an enhanced diuretic effect.

MIANSERIN + ALCOHOL

Mianserin causes drowsiness, which is enhanced considerably by alcohol (n = 13, RCT, Seppala et al, *Eur J Clin Pharmacol* 1984;**27**:181–9).

Mirtazapine + alcohol

Lack of pharmacokinetic interaction has been shown, but additive sedation noted (see Timmer et al, *Clin Pharmacokinet* 2000;**38**:461–74).

Moclobemide + alcohol

Some degree of potentiation of the effects of alcohol has been noted (Zimmer et al, *Acta Psychiatr Scand* 1990;**360**[Suppl]:84–6). There has also been a case of a fatality with a moclobemide overdose, plus half a bottle of whisky (n = 1, Bleumink et al, *Neth J Med* 2003; **61**:88–90).

Oxcarbazepine + alcohol

See oxcarbazepine (4.5.7).

Paraldehyde + alcohol

An enhanced sedative effect can be expected.

Paroxetine + alcohol

Lack of interaction has been shown (review by Boyer and Blumhardt, *J Clin Psychiatry* 1992;**53**[Suppl 2]:132–4).

PHENYTOIN + ALCOHOL

Alcohol has a variable effect on phenytoin so monitor plasma levels regularly. The half-life of phenytoin can be up to 50% shorter in an abstaining alcoholic than in a non-drinker (see also n = 1, Bellibas and Tuglular, *Therapie* 1995; **50**:487–8).

4

Pregabalin + alcohol
See pregabalin (4.5.11).

Quetiapine + alcohol
Additive sedation would be expected.

Reboxetine + alcohol
No potentiation of alcohol's cognitive effects has been reported (UK SmPC), and up to 4 mg/d showed no interaction with alcohol in one trial (n = 10, d/b, Kerr et al, Br J Clin Pharmacol 1996; **42**:239–41).

Rufinamide + alcohol
See rufinamide (4.5.12).

Sertraline + alcohol
There is evidence for a lack of interaction (review, Warrington, Int Clin Psychopharmacol 1991;**6**[Suppl 2]:11–21).

Sodium oxybate + alcohol
See sodium oxybate (4.6.13).

Tiagabine + alcohol
See tiagabine (4.5.13).

TRAZODONE + ALCOHOL
Additive sedation has been reported (n = 26, d/b, c/o, Warrington et al, Neuropsychobiology 1986; 15[Suppl 1]:31–7).

TRICYCLICS + ALCOHOL
Enhanced sedation with most tricyclics is known, but surprisingly little has actually been published and most studies refer to the effect on driving performance. Sedation caused by amitriptyline and doxepin is enhanced by alcohol, but less, or minimally so, with nortriptyline and clomipramine. Both alcohol and tricyclics lower the seizure threshold and care is needed in patients susceptible to seizures. Concurrent alcohol may also increase the oral bioavailability of tricyclics by reducing first-pass metabolism (n = 5, open, Dorian et al, Eur J Clin Pharmacol 1983;**25**:325–31).

Venlafaxine + alcohol
There appears to be no significant additive effect between alcohol and venlafaxine (n = 16, RCT, d/b, p/c, c/o, Troy et al, J Clin Pharmacol 1997; **37**: 1073–81).

Zaleplon + alcohol
While zaleplon enhances alcohol performance impairment, the effect appears short-lived and less than triazolam (n = 18, c/o, Roehrs et al, Sleep Med 2001;**2**:323–32) and zolpidem, although less potent on a mg for mg basis (n = 10, RCT, c/o, Drover et al, Clin Ther 2000;**22**:1443–61).

Zolpidem + alcohol
There is no published information available indicating an interaction.

Zopiclone + alcohol
There appears to be no significant interaction (n = 9, RCT, Hindmarch, Int Clin Psychopharmacol 1990;**5**[Suppl 2]:105–13).

4.7.2 CANNABIS (TETRAHYDRO-CANNABINOL, SEE ALSO SMOKING)

Cannabis/marijuana is a frequently (and usually secretively) used drug but, with the exception of perhaps tricyclics, has few known important adverse drug interactions.

Alcohol + cannabis
Decreased ethanol metabolism may occur, with enhanced CNS depression (n = 10, RCT, p/c, d/b, c/o, Consroe et al, Psychopharmacol 1979;**66**:45–50). Cannabis may also reduce peak alcohol levels in modest doses (n = 15, RCT, p/c, Lukas et al, Neuropsychopharmacology 1992;**7**:77–81).

Antidepressants + cannabis
Mental status changes consistent with delirium and tachycardia and other clinically significant adverse events have been reported following use of marijuana and **tricyclics** (n = 4, Wilens et al, J Am Acad Child Adolesc Psychiatry 1997; **36**:45–8). Increased heart rate has been reported, e.g. marked sinus tachycardia, possibly via a combined beta–adrenergic effect (e.g. n = 2, Hillard and Vieweg, Am J Psychiatr 1983;**140**:626–7). Mania has been reported with **fluoxetine** and cannabis (n = 1, Stoll et al, J Clin Psychiatry 1991;**52**:280–1).

Antipsychotics + cannabis
Chlorpromazine clearance has been shown to be increased by cannabis smoking, although the clinical significance is not known (n = 31, Chetty et al, Eur J Clin Pharmacol 1994;**46**:523–6). Cessation of cannabis smoking can lead to **clozapine** intoxication through removal of CYP1A2 induction (n = 1, Zullino et al, Int Clin Psychopharmacol 2002;**17**:141–3). Additive drowsiness has been reported (review by Benowitz and Jones, Clin Pharmacol Ther 1977;**22**:259–68).

Antiretrovirals + cannabis *
Although strong CYP3A4 inhibitors might increase cannabis levels, two studies suggest there is no significant interaction (n = 67, RCT, p/c, Abrams et al, Ann Intern Med 2003;**139**:258–

66; review by Gruber and McCance-Katz, *Curr HIV/AIDS Rep* 2010;**7**:152–60).

Benzodiazepines + cannabis

Additive drowsiness with benzodiazepines and cannabis has been reported (review by Benowitz and Jones, *Clin Pharmacol Ther* 1977;**22**:259–68).

Cocaine + cannabis

See cocaine (4.7.3).

CNS depressants + cannabis

The combination has resulted in additive drowsiness (review by Benowitz and Jones, *Clin Pharmacol Ther* 1977;**22**:259–68), e.g. anticholinergics and barbiturates.

Disulfiram + cannabis

There have been two reported reactions; a hypomanic episode in an alcoholic on disulfiram taking marijuana (n = 1, Lacoursiere and Swatek, *Am J Psychiatry* 1983;**140**:242–4) and an acute confusional state (n = 1, Mackie and Clark, *Br J Psychiatry* 1994;**164**:421).

Lithium + cannabis

There is a case of lithium levels raised into the toxic range by secretive use of cannabis (n = 1, Ratey et al, *J Clin Psychopharmacol* 1981;**1**:32) and additive drowsiness has been reported (review by Benowitz and Jones, *Clin Pharmacol Ther* 1977;**22**:259–68).

Methadone + cannabis

See methadone (4.6.10).

4.7.3 COCAINE *

Cocaine is metabolised by plasma and hepatic esterases, and 10% by CYP3A4 (Gruber and McCance-Katz, *Curr HIV/AIDS Rep* 2010;**7**:152–60).

Alcohol + cocaine

Simultaneous cocaine and alcohol may produce changes in heart rate and blood pressure, increasing the risk of cardiovascular toxicity (Farre et al, *J Pharmacol Exp Ther* 1993;**166**:1364–73). Combined use has led to enhanced cocaine-induced hepatotoxicity.

Antidepressants + cocaine

In combination with cocaine, desipramine may reduce the effect, fluoxetine has no significant effect (n = 5, Walsh et al, *J Clin Psychopharmacol* 1994;**14**:396–407), trazodone has minor physiological effects and MAOIs probably augment the pressor effect.

Antipsychotics + cocaine

Flupentixol may reduce cocaine craving and

haloperidol may moderate the stimulant effects. **Clozapine** increases cocaine levels but reduces the cocaine 'high', and some cardiac events (near–syncopal episode) have been reported, so caution is necessary (n = 8, Farren et al, *Drug Alcohol Depend* 2000;**59**:153–63).

Antiretrovirals + cocaine *

For a review see (Gruber and McCance-Katz, *Curr HIV/AIDS Rep* 2010;**7**:152–60).

Buprenorphine + cocaine

See buprenorphine (4.6.5).

Cannabis + cocaine

Enhanced cardiotoxicity (e.g. increased heart rate) may occur.

Carbamazepine + cocaine

Cocaine may enhance the cardiac effects of carbamazepine.

Disulfiram + cocaine

See cocaine + disulfiram (4.6.8).

Lithium + cocaine

Lithium probably has little effect on cocaine.

Methadone + cocaine

See methadone (4.6.10).

Methylphenidate + cocaine

See methylphenidate (4.6.11).

Modafinil + cocaine

See modafinil (4.6.12).

4.7.4 SMOKING

Many people with mental health problems smoke. There are over 3000 different known chemicals in cigarette smoke, but which ones are significant is not fully known. Only a few smoking drug interactions are significant, and only brief details of the more significant psychotropic ones are included here (review by Schein, *Ann Pharmacother* 1995;**29**:1139–48). The major enzyme metabolising nicotine is probably CYP2A6, with 2B6 and 2D6 playing lesser, but still substantial, roles. Cigarette smoke contains polycyclic aromatic hydrocarbons, which are potent inducers of CYP1A2.

Reviews: general (Zevin and Benowitz, *Clin Pharmacokinet* 1999;**36**:425–38, 128 refs; Desai et al, *CNS Drugs* 2001;**15**:469–94, 100 refs).

Agomelatine + smoking

See agomelatine (4.3.3.1).

Antipsychotics + smoking *

Schizophrenics who smoke tend to receive higher doses of antipsychotics than non-smokers

4

(n = 78, open, Goff et al, Am J Psychiatry 1992; **149**:1189–94), possibly via increased hepatic metabolism and renal excretion (n = 90, RCT, d/b, p/c, Salokangas et al, Schizophren Res 1997;**23**:55–60). Plasma levels of **haloperidol** are around 23% lower in smoking than in non-smoking schizophrenic patients (n = 66, open, Shimoda et al, Ther Drug Monit 1999;**21**:293–6; confirmed by another study, n = 63, Pan et al, Ther Drug Monit 1999;**21**:489). **Chlorpromazine** clearance may be increased by cigarette smoking, but the clinical significance is unclear (n = 31, Chetty et al, Eur J Clin Pharmacol 1994;**46**:523–6) and smoking increases perphenazine clearance, reducing levels (n = 156, Jin et al, J Clin Pharmacol 2010;**50**:73–80).

Olanzapine clearance may be higher and half-life 21% shorter in smokers compared to non-smokers, probably via CYP1A2 induction (review by Lowe and Ackman, Ann Pharmacother 2010;**44**:727–32). Smoking cessation can lead to olanzapine intoxication through removal of CYP1A2 induction (n = 1, Zullino et al, Int Clin Psychopharmacol 2002; **17**:141–3). Lack of interaction has been shown with **amisulpride** levels (n = 85, Bergemann et al, Eur Neuropsychopharmacol 2004;**14**:245–50), **ziprasidone** and **aripiprazole**. There is nothing reported with **risperidone**. Many schizophrenics may smoke to relieve subjective distress from the illness and treatment (review, McEvoy, Curr Opin Psychiatry 2000;**113**:115–9).

Clozapine levels are lowered by smoking (n = 148, open, Haring et al, Am J Psychiatry 1990;**147**:1471–5), the 1A2 induction leading to clozapine non-response, but this usually takes two to four weeks to manifest itself (Zullion et al, Int Clin Psychopharmacol 2002;**17**:141–3). Stopping smoking can be dangerous for someone taking clozapine, e.g. one study showed a mean 72% **increase** in stable clozapine levels on smoking cessation, with one case so extreme it caused a significant ADR (n = 11, open, Meyer, J Clin Psychopharmacol 2001;**21**:569–74). The change in plasma clozapine levels can, in 80% of cases, be predicted by using the formula:

$$\text{Non-smoking level} = 45.3 + (1.474 \times \text{smoking level})$$

Nomograms exist to help predict doses in people on clozapine who smoke, but you will need a colour copy of the best paper (Rostami–Hodjegan et al, J Clin Psychopharmacol 2004;**24**:1–9) to make sense of it (reviews by Lowe and Ackman, Ann Pharmacother 2010;**44**:727–32; and for our Norwegian readers; Molden and Spigset, Tidsskr Nor Laegeforen 2009;**129**:623–3).

Valproate has a variable effect on smoking and clozapine (n = 255, Diaz et al, Pharmacopsychiatry 2008;**41**:81–91):

• Valproate inhibits clozapine metabolism in non-smokers (+16%)
• Valproate induces clozapine metabolism in smokers (–22%)
• Smoking induces clozapine and reduces plasma levels by 20% if not also taking valproate
• Smoking induces clozapine and reduces plasma levels by 46% if taking valproate.

Smoking thus induces clozapine metabolism and this induction may be stronger when the patient is taking valproate, and so the effect may be even more marked when stopping smoking.

Benzodiazepines + smoking

Early studies suggested an increased clearance of benzodiazepines in smokers (review by Schein, Ann Pharmacother 1995;**29**:1139–48). One review noted increased clearance by smoking of alprazolam, lorazepam, oxazepam and diazepam but not chlordiazepoxide (mentioned in Desai et al, CNS Drugs 2001;**15**:469–94).

Beta-blockers + smoking *

Effects of nicotine on heart rate and blood pressure may negate the effects of beta-blockers. Steady-state propranolol levels may be reduced in smokers, via 1A2 induction.

Bupropion + smoking

See bupropion (4.6.6).

Carbamazepine + smoking *

Carbamazepine seems likely to induce 2A6 and lowers nicotine levels, which may lead to increased smoking and exposure to tobacco toxins (n = 8, open, Williams et al, Cancer Epidemiol Biomarkers Prev 2010;**19**:2582–9).

DULOXETINE + SMOKING

See duloxetine (4.3.3.2).

Fluvoxamine + smoking *

Fluvoxamine levels are significantly lower in smokers, probably due to induction of CYP1A2 (n = 30, open, Yoshimura et al, Neuropsychobiology 2002;**45**:32–5), and/or CYP2D6 (n = 32, >4/52, Katoh et al, Biol Pharm Bull 2010;**33**:285–8).

Lamotrigine + smoking
Lamotrigine levels are about 16% lower in smokers compared to non-smokers, probably via UDPGT2B7 induction (n=44, Reinsberger et al, Seizure 2008;**17**:651–3).

Lithium + smoking
Smoking induces CYP1A2 and caffeine is metabolised by CYP1A2. Theoretically, ceasing smoking could raise xanthine levels, which could increase lithium excretion (as with theophylline), lowering levels.

Melatonin + smoking
See melatonin (4.1.4).

Memantine + smoking
See memantine (4.6.9).

Mirtazapine + smoking
Smokers have mirtazapine levels significantly (25%) lower than non-smokers (n=95, Lind et al, Clin Pharmacokinet 2009;**48**:63–70).

Oxcarbazepine + smoking *
Oxcarbazepine seems likely to induce 2A6 and lowers nicotine levels, which may lead to increased smoking and exposure to tobacco toxins (n=6, open, Williams et al, Cancer Epidemiol Biomarkers Prev 2010;**19**:2582–9).

Phenobarbital + smoking
Smoking has been shown not to affect the drowsiness caused by phenobarbital (n=12, d/b, Mirfazaelian et al, Biopharm Drug Dispos 2001;**22**:403–6).

Tricyclics + smoking
Although serum levels of tricyclics fall in smokers, free levels rise, minimising the clinical significance (n=24, open, Perry et al, Ther Drug Monit 1986;**8**:279–84).

Valproate + smoking *
Valproate does not to seem to induce CYP2A6 and does not alter nicotine levels (n=40, open, Williams et al, Cancer Epidemiol Biomarkers Prev 2010;**19**:2582–9). See antipsychotics + smoking.

Zolpidem + smoking
See zolpidem (4.1.6).

4.8 CYTOCHROME P450 DRUG METABOLISM

There are currently at least 58 known P450 enzymes, with 388 isoforms described, regulated by 684 genes (Tomaszewski et al, Acta Pol Pharm 2008;**65**:319–29). The main recognised P450s are 1A1, 1A2, 2A6, 2B6, 2C8, 2C9, 2C18, 2C19, 2D6, 2E1, 3A3, 3A4, 3A5, 3A6, 3A7, 3A43, 21A2.

All have up to 1–70 variations each. These tables (pp. 396–404) may be of use in determining actual or potential interactions. There are many discrepancies in the published literature and these tables may inadvertently perpetuate some inaccuracies or incomplete knowledge. The author would be happy to receive any advice on this.

Some points about P450/CYP interactions:

1. Most have ultrarapid (UM), extensive (EM), intermediate (IM) and poor (PM) metaboliser metabolic variations.
2. Some drugs are metabolised by several enzymes, so if one enzyme is inhibited, another may compensate.
3. A drug may inhibit or induce one enzyme, but be metabolised by another.
4. Onset and offset of inhibition is dependent on the half-life and time to steady state of the inhibitory drug (may be 24 hours to several months) and the drug to be metabolised, but onset is frequently rapid.
5. Onset and offset of induction may take days or several weeks to become apparent, dependent on the inducing drugs half-life, enzyme turnover, age (induction reduces with age) and concurrent liver disease (reduced induction ability).
6. Other enzyme systems are also important. The **UGT** (uridine diphosphate glucuronosyltransferase) enzymes are induced by phenytoin, valproate, phenobarbital and carbamazepine, and lamotrigine is a weak UGT inducer. The Flavin Monoxygenase (**FMO**) system is also important. Humans have FMO1, FMO3, FM04 and FM05 enzymes in the liver, intestine and kidney. Imipramine, chlorpromazine and orphenadrine are known to be metabolised by this enzyme system.

The general rules for avoiding metabolic interactions are:

1. Avoid reported and predictable interactions.
2. With potential interactions, use reduced doses where possible (start low, go slow).
3. Measure plasma levels of drugs with narrow therapeutic indices.

4

CYP1A2

Substrates (drugs metabolised by this enzyme) *

Agomelatine (90%)
Amiodarone
Anagrelide
Asenapine
Caffeine
Carbamazepine (minor)
Chlordiazepoxide
Ciprofloxacin
Clarithromycin
Clopidogrel (minor)
Clozapine (most)
Dextropropoxyphene
Diazepam
Duloxetine
Erlotinib (minor)
Erythromycin
Estradiol
Flecainide
Flutamine
Fluvoxamine (partly)

Haloperidol (partly)
Lefunomide
Lidocaine
Melatonin (partly)
Methadone (minor)
Mexiletine (minor)
Mirtazapine (partly)
Naproxen
Norfloxacin
Olanzapine (partly)
Omeprazole
Ondansetron
Oxfloxacin
Palonosetron (minor)
Paracetamol
Perphenazine
Pimozide (possibly)
Promazine
Propafenone
Propranolol

Ramelteon (95% first-
   pass effect)
Rasagiline (major)
Retinols
Ritonavir
Rofecoxib
Ropinirole
Sibutramine (partly)
Tacrine
Tamoxifen
Theophylline
Tizanidine (main)
Tricyclics (tertiary, e.g.
   amitriptyline, clomipramine,
   desipramine, trimipramine
   imipramine)
Verapamil
Warfarin-R (major)
Zotepine
Ziprasidone (minor)

Significant enzyme inducers (decrease levels of substrates) *

Cabbage
Caffeine (weak, animal studies)
Carbamazepine?
Charcoal-broiled food
Modafinil (small and

dose-dependent)
Omeprazole
Phenobarbital (weak)
Phenytoin (weak)
Rifampin

Ritonavir
Tipranavir (potent)
Tobacco smoke (polycyclic a
   romatic hydrocarbons are
   potent inducers of 1A2)

Significant enzyme inhibitors (increase levels of substrates)

Celery
Cimetidine
Clarithromycin
Diet (low protein/
   high carbohydrates)
Disulfiram (strong)
Erythromycin
Fluoroquinolones, e.g.
   ciprofloxacin and

norfloxacin (strong)
Fluvoxamine (potent
   — other SSRIs only very
   weak inhibitors)
Grapefruit juice
Griseofulvin?
Isoniazid
Ketoconazole
Mirtazapine (very weak)

Moclobemide
Omeprazole
Parsley
Parsnip
Propafenone (major)
Quercetin (weak)
Sertraline (weak)
Ticlopidone

No effect

Anidulafungin
Asenapine
Bevacizumab
Benzodiazepines

Capecitibane
Cranberry juice
Duloxetine
Emtricitabine

Galantamine
Isotretinoin
Lacosamide
Lanthanum

No effect (continued)

Lenalidomide	Palonosetron	Telbivudine
Levetiracetam	Posaconazole	Varenicline
Lithium	Pregabalin	Venlafaxine
Memantine	Rasagiline	Zoledronic acid
Methylnaltrexone	Rufinamide	Zonisamide
Mirtazapine	Sitagliptin	Ziprasidone
Nelarabine	Sulpiride	
Olanzapine	Sunitinib	

CYP1A2 *

1A2 accounts for about 13% of the total liver CYPs, and metabolises 20% of clinically used drugs (Wang and Zhou, *Curr Med Chem* 2009;**16**:4066–218), but may also bioactivate a number of biocarcinogens. Thus, 1A2 induction can increase carcinogenicity (Zhou *et al*, *Curr Drug Metab* 2009;**10**:713–29).

CYP2B6

Substrates (drugs metabolised by this enzyme)

Alfentanil	Ifosfamide	Promethazine
Bupropion	Ketamine	Propofol (main)
Carbamazepine	Lidocaine	Rifampicin
Carteolol	S-methadone (major)	Ropivacaine
Clopidogrel	R-methadone (minor)	Selegiline
Cyclophosphamide	Midazolam	Sevoflurane
Dexamethasone	Nevirapine	Tamoxifen
Diazepam	Nicotine	Testosterone
Ecstasy (MDMA)	Orphenadrine	Thiotepa
Efavirenz	Pethidine	Valproic acid
Estrone	Phenobarbital	
Ethinylestradiol	Procainamide	

Significant enzyme inducers (decrease levels of substrates)

Baicalin, (significant)	Modafinil (minor and	Rifampin
Efavirenz	dose-dependent)	

Significant enzyme inhibitors (increase levels of substrates)

Clopidogrel (potent)	Ketoconazole	fluoxetine, fluvoxamine)
Clotrimazole	Memantine	Thiotepa (potent),
Glabridin (a liquorice	OCs (weak)	Ticopidine
extract)	Orphenadine	Tranylcypromine (modest)
HRT (potent)	Raloxifene	Zolpidem (very weak)
Itraconazole	SSRIs (paroxetine,	

No effect

Anidulafungin	Emtricitabine	Lamotrigine
Benzodiazepines	Isotretinoin	Levetiracetam
Bevacizumab	Lacosamide	Lithium

4

No effect (continued)

Methylnaltrexone	Rufinamide	Venlafaxine
Nelarabine	Sertraline	Zoledronic acid
Palonosetron	Sulpiride	Zonisamide
Posaconazole	Sunitinib	Ziprasidone
Rasagiline	Telbivudine	

CYP2B6 *

2B6 accounts for about 2–10% of the total hepatic CYP content and metabolises about 8% clinically used drugs. It is linked to 3A4 and UGT1A1. There are at least 28 known allelic variants, can be 20–250-fold interindividual variation in 2B6 expression and may be some ethnic variations as well (Mo *et al, Curr Drug Metab* 2009;**10**:730–53; Wang and Tompkins, *Curr Drug Metab* 2008;**9**:598–610). Probes for 2B6 include bupropion (general reviews by Walsky *et al, J Clin Pharmacol* 2006;**46**:1426–38, Turpeinen *et al, Curr Drug Metab* 2006;**7**:705–14) and thioTEPA (Turpeinen *et al, Drug Metab Dispos* 2004;**32**:626–31).

CYP2C9

Substrates (drugs metabolised by this enzyme) *

Agomelatine (10%)	Flurbiprofen	Retinoids
Alosetron	Fluvastatin	Rifampicin
Amiodarone	Glipizide	Rosiglitazone
Amitriptyline	Glyburide	Sibutramine (part)
Arachidonic acid	Irbesartan	Sildenafil (partly)
Atorvastatin	Losartan	Tolbutamide (8/9)
Bupropion (8/9)	Melatonin	Torasemide
Carbamazepine (minor)	Miconazole	Trimethoprim
Celecoxib	NSAIDs (e.g. diclofenac,	Valproate
Cimetidine	naproxen, piroxicam,	Valsartan
Etravirine	tenoxicam 8/9)	S-warfarin (major)
Fluconazole	Phenobarbital	
Fluoxetine	Phenytoin (major)	

Significant enzyme inducers (decrease levels of substrates)

Carbamazepine (weak)	Phenytoin (weak)	Tipranavir (minor)
Dexamethasone	Rifampin	
Phenobarbital (weak)	St John's wort (weak?)	

Significant enzyme inhibitors (increase levels of substrates)

Amiodarone	Fluoxetine	Nilotinib (strong)
Capecitibane	Fluvastatin	Omeprazole
Cimetidine	Fluvoxamine	Paroxetine (weak)
Cyclizine	Gingko biloba (weak)	Phenylbutazone
Disulfiram	Ginseng (weak)	Promethazine
Fluconazole	Miconazole	Sertraline (moderate)
Fluorouracil	Modafinil	Suprofen

Significant enzyme inhibitors (increase levels of substrates) *(continued)*

Tamoxifen	Topiramate	Valproate
Tolcapone (minor)	Tranylcypromine (part)	Zafirlukast

No effect

Anidulafungin	Lenalidomide	Rufinamide
Aripiprazole	Lithium	Sitagliptin
Benzodiazepines	Memantine	Sulpiride
Bevacizumab	Methylnaltrexone	Sunitinib
Cranberry juice	Mirtazapine	Telbivudine
Emtricitabine	Nelarabine	Venlafaxine
Galantamine	Olanzapine	Varenicline
Isotretinoin	Palonosetron	Ziprasidone
Lacosamide	Posaconazole	Zoledronic acid
Lamotrigine	Pregabalin	Zonisamide
Lanthanum	Rasagiline	

CYP2C19

Substrates (drugs metabolised by this enzyme) *

Barbiturates	Flunitrazepam	Proguanil
Cannabis (minor)	Fluoxetine	Promazine
Carisoprodol	Fluvoxamine	Propranolol (part)
Cimetidine	Indomethacin	Quazepam
Citalopram (major 60%)	Lansoprazole	Rabeprazole
Clobazam	Melatonin (partly)	Ramelteon (minor)
Clopidogrel (needs 2C19	Mephenytoin	Rifabutin
to be metabolised	Midazolam (minor)	Rifampicin
from pro-drug)	Moclobemide (major)	Topiramate
Desmethylclobazam	Nelfinavir	Tranylcypromine
Desvenlafaxine	Omeprazole (major)	Tricyclics (tertiary, e.g.
Diazepam (genotype	Perphenazine	amitriptyline, clomipramine,
important)	Pethidine	imipramine, trimipramine)
Etravirine	Phenytoin (minor)	Venlafaxine
Etizolam	Piroxicam	R-warfarin (minor)

Significant enzyme inducers (decrease levels of substrates)

Carbamazepine (weak)	Gingko biloba (low dose,	Rifampin
Common sage (dose-	weak)	St John's wort (low dose)
dependent)	Phenobarbital (weak)	Valerian (weak)

Significant enzyme inhibitors (increase levels of substrates)

Cimetidine	Ginkgo biloba (higher dose,	Modafinil
Felbamate	weak)	Nilotinib (strong)
Fluconazole	Isoniazid (potent)	Omeprazole
Fluoxetine (moderate)	Ketoconazole	Oxcarbazepine
Fluvoxamine	Moclobemide	Paroxetine (weak)

Significant enzyme inhibitors (increase levels of substrates) (continued)

Phenytoin	Ticlopidine	Tranylcypromine (weak)
Sertraline (weak)	Tipranavir (potent)	Tricyclics (e.g. imipramine)
St John's wort (high dose)	Topiramate	Valproate

No effect

Anidulafungin	Levetiracetam	Rufinamide
Aripiprazole	Lithium	Sitagliptin
Benzodiazepines	Memantine	Sulpiride
Bevacizumab	Methylnaltrexone	Sunitinib
Cone flower	Mirtazapine	Telbivudine
Emtricitabine	Nelarabine	Varenicline
Horse chestnut	Olanzapine	Venlafaxine
Isotretinoin	Palonosetron	Ziprasidone
Lacosamide	Posaconazole	Zoledronic acid
Lanthanum	Pregabalin	Zonisamide
Lenalidomide	Rasagiline	

2C is a sub-family, containing many closely related enzymes, e.g. 2C9, 2C10, 2C19, etc. About 20% Asians and 3–5% Caucasians are poor CYP2C19 metabolisers. Around 8% population are 2C19 PM (Carlsson *et al, J Anal Toxicol* 2009;**33**:65–76). 2C9 accounts for around 20% total CYP in the liver, and metabolises about 15% of clinical drugs. It has at least 33 variants (Zhou *et al, Toxicology* 2010; **278**:165–88).

CYP2D6

Substrates (drugs metabolised by this enzyme) *

Amfetamines	Codeine (to morphine)	Haloperidol
Amprenavir	Darifenacin (saturable)	Hydrocodone
Antiarrhythmics type 1c (encainide, flecainide, etc)	Debrisoquine	Indoramin
	Desvenlafaxine	Loratadine
Aripiprazole	Dexfenfluramine	Methadone (part)
Asenapine (minor)	Dextromethorphan	Methamfetamine
Atomoxetine	Diazepam	Mexiletine (main)
Beta-blockers (especially lipophilic, metoprolol, nebivolol, propranolol, timolol)	Donepezil (partly)	Mianserin
	Duloxetine (partly)	Mirtazapine (minor)
	Ecstasy	Morphine derivatives
	Fenfluramine	Imatinib (minor but can be major)
Buprenorphine	Fesoterodine (minor)	
Carvedilol	Flecainide	Nefazodone
Chloroquine	Fluphenazine	Nicotine (partly)
Chlorphenamine	Fluoxetine (partly)	Olanzapine (partly)
Cinnarizine	Fluvoxamine (partly)	Ondansetron
Ciprofloxacin	Gamma-hydroxybutyrate	Oxycodone (partly, to active oxymorphone)
Citalopram (minor)	Galantamine	
Clozapine (minor, unproven)	Gefitinib	Palonosetron (main)

Substrates (drugs metabolised by this enzyme) (continued) *

Paroxetine
Phenothiazines
(e.g. perphenazine,
chlorpromazine,
fluphenazine, thioridazine)
Propafenone
Quinidine
Risperidone (major)

Sertindole (partly)
Tamoxifen (pro-drug,
metabolised to active drug)
Tolcapone (minor)
Tolterodine
Tramadol
Trazodone
Tricyclics — secondary and

tertiary tricyclics (e.g.
nortriptyline, imipramine,
maprotiline, trimipramine,
amitriptyline, clomipramine
and desipramine [weak])
Venlafaxine (major)
Zuclopenthixol

Significant enzyme inducers (decrease levels of substrates)

Carbamazepine (weak)
Ginseng (weak)

Phenobarbital (weak)
Phenytoin (weak)

Rifampin (weak)
Ritonavir (weak)

Significant enzyme inhibitors (increase levels of substrates)

Amidarone
Asenapine (weak)
Buprenorphine (very weak)
Bupropion
Celecoxib
Chloroquine
Chlorphenamine
Chlorpromazine
Cimetidine
Citalopram (very weak/nil)
Clomipramine (moderate)
Cocaine
Cyclizine
Dextromethorphan
Dextropropoxyphene
Diltiazem (weak)
Diphenhydramine
Duloxetine
Escitalopram (weak)
Fenfluramine?
Flecainide

Fluoxetine (strong)
Fluphenazine
Fluvoxamine (very weak)
Haloperidol (dose-
dependent)
Indinavir
Levomepromazine
Methadone (weak?)
Metoclopramide
Metoprolol
Methylnaltrexone (weak)
Mexiletine
Mibefradil
Mirtazapine (very weak/nil)
Moclobemide
Modafinil (small and
dose-dependent)
Nefazodone (very weak/nil)
Nicardipine
Nilotinib (strong)
Norfluoxetine (strong)

Oxycodone
Paroxetine (strong,
dose-related)
Perphenazine
Pindolol
Primaquine
Promethazine
Propafenone
Propanolol
Quinidine
Quinine
Quetiapine
Ritonavir
Sertraline (weak, dose-related,
moderate at 150mg/d)
Terbinafine (potent)
Thioridazine
Timolol
Tipranavir (potent)
Tricyclics (all, strong)
Yohimbine

No effect

Anidulafungin
Aripiprazole
Benzodiazepines
Bevacizumab
Emtricitabine
Galantamine
Isotretinoin
Lacosamide
Lamotrigine
Lanthanum

Lenalidomide
Levetiracetam
Memantine
Mirtazapine
Olanzapine
Palonosetron
Posaconazole
Pregabalin
Rasagiline
Rufinamide

Sitagliptin
Sulpiride
Sunitinib
Telbivudine
Varenicline
Venlafaxine (very weak, nil)
Ziprasidone
Zoledronic acid
Zonisamide

4

CYP2D6 *

2D6 accounts for only about 2–4% of total liver CYPs but metabolises about 25% of current drugs (Zhou, *Clin Pharmacokinet* 2009;**48**:689–723). Metabolism occurs both in the liver and in the brain. An individual's CYP2D6 status (Zhou, *Clin Pharmacokinet* 2009;**48**:761–804) can be determined by giving the probes debrisoquine or dextromethorphan and measuring the ratios of drug and metabolite. Around 5–8% Caucasians, 8.5% African-Americans and 2–10% Asians are slow metabolisers. Up to 29% North Africans and Middle East people (de Leon *et al*, *Psychosomatics* 2006;**47**:75–85) are ultra-rapid metabolisers (three or more 2D6 alleles). All CYP2D6 inhibition is probably concentration-dependent and so inclusion in this list only predicts that an interaction could occur, not that it will.

CYP3A3/4

Substrates (drugs metabolised by this enzyme) *

Alfentanil	Clopidrogel	Fluvoxamine
Alitretinoin	Clotrimazole	Fosaprepitant
Alosetron	Clozapine (partly)	Galantamine
Amiodarone (major)	Cocaine (10%)	Gefitinib
Amprenavir	Codeine	Glibenclamide
Androgens	Colchicine	Glyburide?
Antihistamines, e.g. astemizole	Cortisol	Granisetron
Aripiprazole	Cyclophosphamide	Haloperidol
Asenapine (minor)	Dapsone	Ifosfamide
Benzodiazepines (e.g.	Darifenacin	Imatinib (major)
alprazolam, clonazepam,	Dasatinib	Indinavir
diazepam, flunitrazepam,	Dexamethasone	Irinotecan
midazolam, temazepam and	Dextromethorphan	Isoniazid
triazolam, but not	Digoxin	Isotretinoin
lorazepam)	Disopyramide	Itraconazole
Bromocriptine	Docetaxol	Ivabradine
Budesonide	Donepezil (part)	Ivermectin
Buprenorphine	Doxorubicin	Ketamine
Buspirone	Doxycycline	Ketoconazole
Busulfan	Dutasteride	Lapatinib
Calcium-channel blockers	Efavirez	Levonorgestrel
(e.g. amlodipine,	Ergotamine	Lidocaine
diltiazem, felodipine,	Erlotinib (major)	Lisuride
isradipine, nicardipine,	Estradiol and estrogens	Lopinavir
nifedipine, verapamil)	Ethosuximide	Loratadine
Cannabinoids (main)	Ethinylestradiol	Losartan
Carbamazepine	Etoposide	Macrolides (e.g. erythromycin,
Chloramphenicol	Etravirine	clarithromycin)
Chloroquine	Everolimus	Maravoric
Ciclosporin	Fentanyl	Meloxicam
Cimetidine	Fesoterodine (main)	Methadone (main)
Ciprofloxacin	Fexofenadine	Methylprednisolone
Cisapride (restricted in UK)	Fluconazole	Mianserin
Citalopram (minor, 30%)	Fluoxetine	Mibefradil
Clindamycin	Flutamine	Miconazole

Substrates (drugs metabolised by this enzyme) (continued) *

Mifepristone
Mirtazapine (partly)
Modafinil
Nefazodone
Nelfinavir
Nilotinib
Ondansetron
Orphenadrine
Oxycodone (inactivation)
Paclitaxel
Paracetamol
Paricalcitol (?)
Perphenazine
Pethidine
Phencyclidine
Phenobarbital
Phenytoin
Pimozide (mostly)
Prednisone
Progesterone
Proguanil
Propafenone
Promazine
Protein-pump inhibitors
  (lansoprazole [weak],
  omeprazole, rabeprazole)
Quetiapine (mostly)
Quinidine
Quinine
Ramelteon (minor)

Reboxetine
Rifampin
Rimonabant
Risperidone (partly)
Ritonavir
Saquinavir
Sertindole (partly)
Sertraline
Sibutramine (main)
Sildenafil (partly)
Sirolimus
Sitagliptin (limited except in
  renal failure)
Risperidone (partly)
Ritonavir
Saquinavir
Sertindole (partly)
Sertraline
Sibutramine (main)
Sildenafil (partly)
Sirolimus
Sitagliptin (limited except in
  renal failure)
Sodium fusidate
Sorafenib
Statins (e.g. atorvastatin,
  cerivastatin, lovastatin,
  pravastin, simvastatin)
Steroids (e.g. dexamethasone)
St John's wort

Sunitinib
Tacrolimus
Tamoxifen
Temsirolimus
Testosterone
Theophylline
Tiagabine
Tipranavir
Tolcapone (minor)
Tolterodine
Tolvaptan
Topiramate (possibly)
Trabectedin
Tricyclics — tertiary (e.g.
  imipramine, amitriptyline,
  clomipramine)
Valproate
Vardenafil
Venlafaxine
Vinblastine
Vincristine
Vinorelbine (major)
R-warfarin (minor)
Zaleplon (secondary route)
Ziprasidone (most)
Zolpidem (mainly)
Zonisamide (part)
Zopiclone (mostly)
Zotepine
Zuclopenthixol

4

Significant enzyme inducers (decrease levels of substrates)

Barbiturates (all)
Carbamazepine (induces
  3A4 about 46% more
  than oxcarbazepine)
Cortisol
Dexamethasone
Efavirez
Ethosuximide
Flucloxacillin

Modafinil (small and
  dose-dependent)
Nevirapine (?)
Omeprazole
Oxcarbazepine
Phenobarbital
Phenytoin
Pioglitazone
Prednisone

Primidone
Rifampin (rapid)
Rufinamide (moderate
  effect)
St John's wort (moderate)
Topiramate (dose-
  dependent, especially
  at high doses)
Troglitazone

Significant enzyme inhibitors (increase levels of substrates)

Acetazolamide
Amiodarone
Atazaivir (moderate)
Buprenorphine (weak/

  moderate)
Cannabinoids
Cimetidine (moderate)
Citalopram (weak)

Clotrimazole
Danazol
Dextropropoxyphene
Diltiazem (weaker)

Echinacea purpurea (weak)
Erlotinib
Fluconazole (strong)
Fluoxetine (weak)
Fluvoxamine (moderate)
Fosaprepitant (minor)
Gestodene
Gingko biloba
Grapefruit juice (weak)
Imatinib
Indinavir (moderate)
Isoniazid (potent)
Itraconazole (strong)
Ivabradine (very weak)
Ketoconazole (strong)
Lopinavir

Macrolides (some, e.g.
  clarithromycin,
  erythromycin, strong)
Methadone (weak?)
Metronidazole
Mibefradil
Miconazole (strong)
Mifepristone
Nefazodone (strong)
Nelfinavir
Nilotinib (strong)
Norfluoxetine (moderate)
Orange juice (weak)
Oxycodone
Paroxetine (weak)
Posaconazole (potent)

Quinine
Ritonavir (moderate)
Saquinavir
Sertindole (weak)
Sertraline (minor)
Statins (atorvastatin,
  fluvastatin)
Stiripentol (variable)
Terbinafine
Trazodone
Tricyclics (moderate)
Troleandomycin (strong)
Venlafaxine (very weak)
Verapamil (weak)
Zafirlukast

No effect

Aliskiren
Anidulafungin
Aripiprazole
Asenapine
Benzodiazepines
Bevacizumab
Capecitibane
Cranberry juice
Duloxetine
Emtricitabine
Galantamine
Honey

Isotretinoin
Ivabradine
Lamotrigine
Lanthanum
Lenalidomide
Levetiracetam
Lithium
Memantine
Methylnaltrexone
Mirtazapine
Nelarabine
Olanzapine

Palonosetron
Pioglitazone
Pregabalin
Rasagiline
Rosaconazole
Sitagliptin
Sunitinib
Telbivudine
Varenicline
Zoledronic acid
Zonisamide
Ziprasidone

CYP3A3/4 (very similar structures, and are often grouped together). CYP3A4 is an important P450 enzyme, metabolising at least 50% of all marketed medications (Zhou, *Curr Drug Metab* 2008;**9**:310-22), and may account for up to 50–60% of the total liver P450. There is little generic polymorphism so little inter-individual variation exits. CYP3A4 occurs in the liver, gut, and possibly the brain. Ultra-rapid metabolisers have not yet been identified. Debrisoquine is a probe. Midazolam is more reliable, although simvastatin, lovastatin and buspirone are alternatives (s = 113, Ohno *et al, Clin Pharmacokinet* 2007;**46**:681–96).

Contents

The drugs listed in each section have been reported to cause that condition in some context (e.g. standard dose, high dose, prolonged courses, etc). The main references next to the drug should be consulted to ascertain the circumstances of reports. The references are offered without qualification and no indication of frequency or status of reports can be given, as this information is not really available, except where a side–effect is well recognised, BNF, listed. For completeness, some drugs not available in every country are also listed.

Sub–divisions are based on the UK BNF, chapters: (although many drugs appear in several sections)

- CNS: anxiolytics and hypnotics (including BDZs)
- CNS: antipsychotics (including lithium)
- CNS: antidepressants (including bupropion)
- CNS: analgesics
- CNS: anticonvulsants
- CNS: antiparkinsonian drugs
- CNS: others

- Gastrointestinal drugs
- Cardiovascular drugs
- Respiratory drugs
- Anti-infection drugs
- Endocrine system drugs
- Malignancy and immunosuppressant drugs
- Musculoskeletal and analgesics
- Others

The BNF side-effect categories generally mean:
- Very common = more than one in 10 people get this side–effect
- Common one in 10 to one in 100 (1–10%)
- Uncommon or less common = one in 100 to one in 1000 (0.1–1%)
- Rare = one in 1000 to one in 10000 (0.01–0.1%)
- Very rare = less than one in 10000 ($\leq$0.01%). Each side-effect may be dose-related (the higher the dose, the more likely you are to get it, especially a higher starting dose) and may abate with time.

5.1 ANXIETY, AGITATION AND NERVOUSNESS

- CNS — anxiolytics and hypnotics *
Benzodiazepine withdrawal (n = 43, d/b,
    p/c, 7/52, abrupt is much worse than
    gradual withdrawal, e.g. *Am J Psychiatry*
    1984;**141**:848–52)
Buspirone (n = 3, *J Clin Psychiatry* 1988;**49**:
    165–6)
Clomethiazole
Sodium oxybate (BNF common)
Temazepam
Zopiclone (n = 1, *Ir Med J* 2007;**100**:511; n = 1,
    Prog Neurol Psychiatry 2009;**13**:20–4)

- CNS — antipsychotics
Aripiprazole initiation (n = 2, *J Clin Psychiatry*
    2004;**65**:132–3; n = 3, *Pharmacother* 2007;
    27:1339–42)
 ~ high–dose (n = 1, *J Neuropsychiatry Clin
    Neurosci* 2007;**19**: 481–2)
 ~ after clozapine discontinuation (n = 1, *J Clin
    Psychiatry* 2009;**70**:141–3)
Olanzapine (*Can J Psychiatry* 1998;**43**:1054)
Risperidone (n = 1, *Am J Psychiatry*
    1995;**152**:1096–7; n=1, *Psychiatry Clin
    Neurosci* 1999;**53**:682)
Zotepine (BNF, common)

- CNS — antidepressants
Early worsening of anxiety and agitation with
antidepressants is well–known but very poorly
researched (*Br J Psychiatry* 2009;**194**:483–90).
Bupropion (incidence 9.7%; BNF, common)
Mianserin abrupt withdrawal (n = 1,
    panic anxiety, *Jpn J Psychiatry Neurol*
    1989;**43**:155–9)
Moclobemide (incidence 5–10%, *J Neural
    Transm* 1989;**28** [Suppl]:S77–S89)
Reboxetine (BNF, rare)
SSRIs (BNF, common)
    → citalopram (cases in *Eur J Clin Pharmacol*
        1986;**31**:18–22)
    → fluoxetine (incidence 9%? e.g. *J Clin
        Psychiatry* 1985;**46**(3 Pt 2):32–7)
    → paroxetine (incidence 11%? *Acta Psychiatr
        Scand* 1989;**80**[Suppl 350]:117–37)
    → paroxetine withdrawal (rebound anxiety,
        review, *Can J Clin Pharmacol* 2006;**13**:
        69–74)
    → SSRI withdrawal (BNF)

Tricyclics (e.g. amitriptyline, lofepramine at < 2%,
    review in *Drugs* 1989;**37**:123–40)

- CNS — analgesics
Buprenorphine (BNF, common)
Fentanyl (BNF, common)
Frovatriptan (BNF, less common)
Morphine
Nefopam
Oxycodone (BNF, common)
Pentazocine (e.g. *Br Med J* 1974;**2**:224)
Pizotifen (BNF, rare)
Sumatriptan in people with panic
    disorder (n = 15, RCT, d/b, p/c, *Eur
    Neuropsychopharmacol* 2005;**15**:279–82)

- CNS — anticonvulsants *
Carbamazepine (*J Am Acad Child Adolesc
    Psychiatry* 1988;**27**:500–3)
Clonazepam
Ethosuximide
Gabapentin (BNF, common)
Gabapentin withdrawal (e.g. n = 1, *Am J Health
    Syst Pharm* 2010;**67**:910–2)
Lamotrigine
Levetiracetam (BNF, common)
Phenobarbital and other barbiturates
Piracetam (BNF, uncommon)
Rufinamide (BNF, common; 1–10% incidence,
    UK SmPC)
Topiramate (BNF, common)
Valproate (n = 1, *J Neuropsychiatry Clin Neurosci*
    2001;**13**:528–30)
Vigabatrin
Zonisamide (SmPC)

- CNS — antiparkinsonian drugs
Amantadine
Anticholinergics (BNF, common)
Baclofen (used in Parkinson's Disease, UK SmPC
    change 2009)
Bromocriptine
Levodopa (BNF, common)
Rotigotine (BNF, less common)

- CNS — others *
Alcohol (review, n = 285, *Aggress Behav*
    2007;**33**:327–38)
Anticholinesterases (n = 4, *J Neuropsychiatry
    Clin Neurosci* 1992;**4**:189–94) e.g.:
    → donepezil (n = 1, *Int J Geriatr Psychiatry*

2003;**18**:657–8)
→ rivastigmine (incidence <5%, inc transdermal patches; UK SmPC, common)
Aprepitant (BNF, less common)
Atomoxetine (BNF, common)
Botulinum toxin A injection (BNF, less common; e.g. *South Med J* 1999;**92**:738)
Caffeine (n = 22 children, d/b, p/c, c/o, *J Am Acad Child Adolesc Psychiatry* 1994;**33**:407–15)
Cannabis (n = 79, no association, *Psychiatry Res* 2003;**118**:1–8)
Dexamfetamine
Flumazenil (BNF, common)
Gamma–Hydroxybutyrate (GHB) intoxication (n = 66 with toxicity, 60% incidence, *Am J Emerg Med* 2005;**23**:316–20)
Ginseng (reported, inc. abuse, see *Arch Gen Psychiatry* 1998;**55**:1033–44)
Granisetron (unconfirmed, e.g. *Eur J Cancer* 1990;**26**[Supp 1]:S19–23)
Heroin withdrawal (*Int J Addict* 1992;**27**:25–35)
LSD (n = 16, responds to clonazepam, *Int Clin Psychopharmacol* 2003;**18**:101–5)
Memantine (n = 3, *J Neurol Neurosurg Psychiatry* 2007;**78**:546)
Memantine abrupt discontinuation (n = 2, *Geriatr Gerontol Int* 2009;**9**:202–5)
Metoclopramide (n = 1, *Psychiatry Clin Neurosci* 2007;**61**:193–5)
Modafinil (BNF, common, n = 2, *J Clin Psychopharmacol* 2005;**25**:628–9)
Naltrexone (BNF, common)
Orlistat (BNF, common)
Palonosetron (BNF, less common)
Rimonabant (BNF, common; see SmPC and *Lancet* 2007;**370**:1671–2)
Sibutramine (BNF, common)
Sodium oxybate (BNF, common)
Varenicline (links with agitation but not substantiated, s = 14, n = 4443, *Cochrane Database Syst Rev* 2010;**12**:CD006103)

• Gastrointestinal drugs
Bismuth intoxication (*Postgrad Med J* 1988;**64**:308–10)
H2 blockers (BNF, rare) e.g.:
→ cimetidine (*Adv Psychiatric Treat* 2005;**11**:68)
→ famotidine (mentioned in *Digestion* 1985;**32** [Suppl 1]:24–31)
Misoprostol

Omeprazole

• Cardiovascular drugs
Adrenaline/epinephrine (BNF, common)
Atenolol withdrawal (n = 1, *Am J Psychiatry* 1994;**151**:1840)
Cilostazol (BNF, less common)
Doxazosin (incidence 2.4%)
Epoprostenol (BNF, common)
Fondaparinux sodium (BNF, rare)
Hydralazine (BNF, rare)
Methoxamine
Methyldopa (rare)
Moexipril (BNF, common)
Nicardipine (rare)
Nifedipine (*An Med Interna* 1992;**9**:362)
Ramipril (BNF, less common)
Sodium nitroprusside (BNF, common)
Streptokinase (see *Drugs* 1973;**5**:357)
Telmisartan (BNF, less common)

• Respiratory drugs *
Aminophylline
Dextromethorphan + hydrocodone + propoxyphene (n = 1, *J Psychopharmacol* 2009;**23**:989–91)
Ephedrine (BNF, common)
Mizolastine (BNF, common)
Montelukast (SmPC, FDA warning 2009)
Phenylpropanolamine OD (*Lancet* 1979;**314**:1367–8)
Pseudoephedrine (n = 1, *Eur J Clin Pharmacol* 1978;**14**:253–9)
Salbutamol
Theophylline (*Med Clin (Barc)* 1987;**88**:549–50)

• Anti–infection drugs
Atazanavir (BNF, less common)
Azithromycin (BNF, rare)
Chloroquine (*Adv Psychiatr Treat* 2005;**11**:66)
Clarithromycin (BNF, very rare)
Co–trimoxazole (n = 1, *J Clin Psychopharmacol* 1991;**11**:144–5)
Daptomycin (BNF, less common)
Darunavir (BNF, common)
Efavirenz (BNF, common)
Enfuvirtide (BNF, common)
Ertapenem (BNF, rare)
Ganciclovir (BNF, common; *N Engl J Med* 1990;**322**:933–4; *Adv Psychiatr Treat* 2005;**11**:66)

5

Isoniazid (*Lancet* 1989;**334**:735–6)
Levamisole (rare, *N Engl J Med* 1990;**322**: 352–8)
Lopinavir with ritonavir (BNF, less common)
Mefloquine (BNF, less common; *Pharm J* 1989;**243**:561)
Penicillins (*Adv Psychiatr Treat* 2005;**11**:66)
Piperazine (see *Trans R Soc Trop Med Hyg* 1976;**70**: 358)
Quinine (*Adv Psychiatr Treat* 2005;**11**:66)
Quinupristin with dalfopristin (BNF, less common)
Ribavirin (BNF, common)
Ritonavir (BNF, common)
Stavudine (BNF, less common)
Voriconazole (BNF, common)
Zidovudine (BNF, common)

* Endocrine system drugs
Corticosteroids (BNF, less common; *Adv Psychiatr Treat* 2005;**11**:68; incidence may be as high as 5–6% in adults, usually emerges within a few days or weeks, risk may be higher with higher doses, *MHRA Drug Safety Update* 2007;1–9)
→ dexamethasone — overall risks:
  * dose–related (but not time, duration or severity)
  * female gender
  * PMH (but only weak association, see *Arch Gen Psychiatry* 1981;**38**: 471–7)
→ methyltestosterone
→ prednisone (especially in children, cases in *Clin Paediatr* 1990;**29**: 382–8)
Danazol (BNF, common)
Levothyroxine
Testosterone and esters (BNF, common)
Zoledronic acid (BNF, less common)

* Malignancy and immunosuppressant drugs
Buserelin (BNF, less common)
Ciclosporin (*Adv Psychiatr Treat* 2005;**11**:68)
Clofarabine (BNF, common)
Glatiramer acetate (BNF, common)
Imatinib (BNF, less common)
Interferons, e.g.:
→ interferon alfa (responds to BDZs, n = 2, *J Psychopharmacol* 2004;**18**:41–6)
→ peginterferon alfa 2a + ribavirin (n = 176, incidence < 36%, *Aliment Pharmacol Ther* 2008;**27**:257–65)

Letrozole (BNF, less common)
Octreotide
Trastuzumab (BNF, less common)
Tretinoin (BNF, common)

* Musculoskeletal and analgesics
Abatacept (BNF, less common)
Baclofen (BNF, common)
Etoricoxib (BNF, less common)
Leflunomide (BNF, common)
Methocarbamol (BNF, less common)
NSAIDs (*Adv Psychiatric Treat* 2005;**11**:68), e.g.:
→ ibuprofen (overdose, *Am J Emerg Med* 1998;**16**:549–50)
→ indometacin (n = 1, *South Med J* 1983;**76**:679–80)
→ mefenamic acid
→ naproxen
→ naproxen + chloroquine (*Ann Pharmacother* 1993;**27**: 1058–9)

* Others *
Atropine eye drops (n = 1, *J Ped Ophthalmol Strabis* 1985;**22**: 38–9)
Cyclopentolate eye drops (n = 1, *Nervenarzt* 2009;**80**:967–9)
Deferasirox (BNF, less common)
Flunisolide
Isotretinoin (BNF, rare; n = 45 [c = 23], no association with anxiety, *J Dermatolog Treat* 2004;**15**: 153–7)
Ketamine (BNF, common)
Lead (higher levels, n=1987, *Arch Gen Psychiatry* 2009;**66**:1313-9)
Lidocaine (n = 15, incidence 73%, *Am J Psychiatry* 1987;**144**:159–63)
Neostigmine (cases in *Dtsch Med Wochenschr* 1966;**91**:699)
Organic solvents (n = 77, up to 36% can develop anxiety clusters, *Psychosom Med* 2000;**62**:746–50)
Phenylephrine (rare)
Pyridostigmine (rare)
Ropivacaine (BNF, less common; n = 3 after nerve block, *Reg Anesth Pain Med* 1999;**24**:175–8)
Sevoflurane (n = 169, common, reduced by clonidine, *Anesth Analg* 2005;**101**:1619–22)
Sildenafil (BNF common)
Tacrolimus (BNF, rare; *Adv Psychiatr Treat* 2005;**11**:68)

Vardenafil (BNF, rare)
Yohimbine (mentioned in *Arch Gen Psychiatry* 1998;**55**: 1033–44)
Zafirlukast (FDA warning 2009)

5.2 AGGRESSION, INCLUDING HOSTILITY AND VIOLENCE

Review: Shaw and Fletcher, *Adv Drug React Toxicolog Rev* 2000;**19**: 35–45, 64 refs.

- CNS *

Alcohol (review, n = 285, *Aggress Behav* 2007;**33**:327–38)
Alcohol withdrawal
Amantadine (cases in *Br Med J* 1972;**3**:50)
Amfetamine withdrawal
Anticholinesterases (n = 4, *J Neuropsychiatry Clin Neurosci* 1992;**4**:189–94)
→ donepezil (many e.g. n=1, *Int J Geriatr Psychiatry* 2003;**18**:657–8)
Atomoxetine (*Pediatrics* 2004;**114**:895–6)
Barbiturate withdrawal
Benzodiazepines (incidence < 1%, *J Clin Psychiatry* 1988;**49**:184–8; during prolonged BDZ use: *Can J Psychiatry* 2000; **45**:89–90; aggressogenic effect from diazepam, n = 60 male, *Addict Behav* 2002;**27**: 167–77), e.g.:
→ alprazolam (greater response to provocation, n = 23, RCT, p/c, 8/52, *J Affect Disord* 1995;**35**:117–23)
Carbamazepine
Gabapentin (n = 1, *J Neuropsychiatry Clin Neurosci* 2001;**13**:424; n = 2, *Epilepsia* 1996;**37**:501–2)
Lamotrigine (survey, n = 19, *Epilepsia* 1998;**39**:280–2)
Levetiracetam (SmPC)
Methamphetamine dependence (n = 76, *Arch Gen Psychiatry* 2011;**68**:271–82)
Modafinil (n = 2, *J Clin Psychopharmacol* 2005; **25**:628–9)
Naloxone IV (n = 2, *Ann Pharmacother* 1992; **26**:196–8)
Olanzapine (*Can J Psychiatry* 1998;**43**: 1054)
Paroxetine withdrawal (*Lancet* 1995;**346**:57)
Tricyclics (rare)
Varenicline (n=78 and review, clear association, *Ann Pharmacother* 2010;**44**:1389-94)
Venlafaxine (n = 1, *J Am Acad Child Adolesc Psychiatry* 2003;**42**: 383–4)
Vigabatrin (e.g. *Drugs* 1991;**41**:889–926)

- Others

Anabolic steroids, e.g. oxandrolone
Anabolic steroid withdrawal
Cyproheptadine (n = 1, *J Am Acad Child Adolesc Psychiatry* 1998;**37**:668–70)
Omeprazole
Sildenafil (review, n = 274, *Ann Pharmacother* 2002;**36**:1129–34)
Steroids high dose (*Lancet* 1987;**2**:750–1)
Testosterone (highly variable, n = 56 men, RCT, p/c, c/o, 3x6/52, *Arch Gen Psychiatry* 2000;**57**:133–40)

5.3 BEHAVIOURAL CHANGES

- CNS

Barbiturates
Benzodiazepines:
→ clonazepam (*Dev Med Child Neurol* 1991; **33**: 362–5)
Carbamazepine (*J Paediatrics* 1982;**101**:785–7)
Donepezil (e.g. n = 7, *Am J Psychiatry* 1998;**155**: 1632–3)
Gamma–Hydroxybutyrate (GHB) intoxication (n = 66 with toxicity, 60% incidence, *Am J Emerg Med* 2005;**23**:316–20)
Levetiracetam (n = 553, incidence 7%, *Neurology* 2003; **61**: 1218–21)

- Others

Anabolic steroids (n = 1, bizarre after brief exposure, *Am J Psychiatry* 1992;**149**:271–2)
Bismuth (*Acta Neurologica Belgica* 1979;**79**: 73)
Prazosin (n = 1, bizarre behaviour, *Am J Psychiatry* 2008;**165**:744–5)
Prednisone withdrawal (*JAMA* 1989;**261**:1731)
Theophylline (disputed — not in children, *JAMA* 1992;**267**:2621–4)

5.4 DELIRIUM (ACUTE ORGANIC PSYCHOSIS) AND CONFUSION *

Drug-induced delirium is usually an acute reaction and always with fluctuating levels of awareness of self and environment. It is most frequent in frail or dementing elderly, drug abusers and with pre-existing organic brain disease, and is strongly associated with anticholinergic activity:

- high risk drug groups are tricyclics and typical antipsychotics

5

- medium risk drugs include benzodiazepines, sedatives, dopamine-activating drugs, anticonvulsants, histamine H2 receptor blockers, digoxin, beta-blockers and analgesics. Most of these do not have direct anticholinergic effects but *in vitro* have been shown to bind to muscarinic receptors.

Reviews: * general (Hufschmidt et al, *Acta Neurol Scand* 2009;**120**:436–8; for our German readers, Meyer et al, *Ther Umsch* 2010;**67**:79–83), systematic review (s = 14, Clegg and Young, *Age Ageing* 2011;**40**:23–9), drugs with anticholinergic properties (Cancelli et al, *Neurol Sci* 2009;**30**:87–92).

- CNS — anxiolytics and hypnotics
Benzodiazepine withdrawal
Benzodiazepines, e.g.:
    → alprazolam (n = 1, *Clin Neuropharmacol* 1998;**21**:201–3)
    → diazepam as pre-med (n = 1, *Indian J Ophthalmol* 1989;**37**:35–6)
Chloral and derivatives
Clomethiazole
Clomethiazole withdrawal
Zolpidem (many cases, e.g. n = 1, *Ann Pharmacother* 2001;**35**:1562–4; n = 1, elderly, *Psychosomatics* 2004;**45**:88–9)
Zopiclone withdrawal (n = 1, *Age Ageing* 2005; **34**:526–7)

- CNS — antipsychotics *
Aripiprazole high-dose (n = 1, *J Neuropsychiatry Clin Neurosci* 2007;**19**:481–2)
Butyrophenones
Clozapine (may occur in 10%, especially in older people also taking other anticholinergics; n = 139, *Pharmacopsychiatry* 2003;**36**:156–60)
Clozapine withdrawal (n = 3, *J Clin Psychiatry* 1997;**58**:252–5)
Lithium (many e.g. n = 1, *Psychiatr Prax* 2000; **27**:296–7; n = 1, *Practitioner* 2009; **253**:28–30)
Lithium withdrawal (n=1, complicated by mania, *Gen Hosp Psychiatry* 2010;**32**:102-4)
Olanzapine (n=1, *Psychiatry Investig* 2010;**7**:153-4; n = 1, *Ann Pharmacother* 2006;**40**:135–8)
Olanzapine + opioid (n = 2, *J Pain Symptom Manage* 2005;**29**:330–2)
Phenothiazines (esp. sedative ones)
Quetiapine + lithium (n = 1, *Clin Neuro-*

pharmacol 2008;**31**:176–9)
Quetiapine overdose (n = 1, *Pediatr Emerg Care* 2010;**26**:754–6) and toxicity (n = 1, *Aust N Z J Psychiatry* 2009;**43**:781)
Quetiapine + valproate (n = 2, *Gen Hosp Psychiatry* 2010;**32**:46)
Risperidone (n = 1, *Can J Psychiatry* 1998;**43**:194; n = 1, *J Child Adolesc Psychopharmacol* 2005; **15**:520–5)

- CNS — antidepressants *
Bupropion (cases, e.g. *J Clin Psychiatry* 1990;**51**: 307–8)
Bupropion + fluoxetine (n = 1, *J Clin Psychopharmacol* 2006;**26**:677–9)
MAOIs, e.g.:
    → phenelzine (*J Clin Psychiatry* 1987;**48**: 340–1)
    → tranylcypromine (*J Clin Psychopharmacol* 1997;**17**:430–2)
    → tranylcypromine abuse (*J Clin Psychopharmacol* 2000;**20**:270–1)
Mianserin (n = 5, *Eur Neuropsychopharmacol* 1995;**5**:147–9; in dementia, *J Clin Psychopharmacol* 2010;**30**:467–8)
Mirtazapine (n = 3, *Int Clin Psychopharmacol* 2000;**15**:239–43)
SSRIs, e.g.:
    → fluoxetine (n = 1, *Am J Psychiatry* 1995; **152**:295–6)
    → paroxetine (n = 1, *Pharmacopsychiatry* 2007;**40**:199–200)
    → paroxetine withdrawal (n = 1, *J Neuropsych Clin Neurosci* 2004;**16**:119–20)
    → paroxetine and benzatropine (n = 1, *Am J Psychiatry* 1997;**154**:581–2)
Trazodone (n = 3, *Int Clin Psychopharmacol* 1998;**13**:225–8)
Tricyclics (*J Clin Psychiatry* 1983;**44**:173–6), e.g.:
    → imipramine (n = 1, *Am J Psychiatry* 1983;**140**:1517–8)
Tricyclic withdrawal (n=1, *Aust N Z J Psychiatry* 2010;**44**:863)
Venlafaxine (n = 1, *Can J Psychiatry* 2003;**48**:129)

- CNS — analgesics
Dextropropoxyphene withdrawal
Ergotamine + caffeine (n = 1, *Pharmacother* 2002;**22**:126–9)
Fentanyl (*Anesthesiology* 1995;**83**:869–71)
Methadone (during switch from fentanyl, *J Pain*

Symptom Manage 2001;**21**:177–8)
Nalbuphine
Narcotics
Opioids (n = 1, *J Pain Symptom Manage* 2004;
27:268–73)
Papaveretum
Tramadol (n = 11, *Curr Problems* 1995;**21**:2; n = 1,
Pharmacopsychiatry 2006;**39**:194–9)

- CNS — anticonvulsants *
Barbiturate withdrawal
Barbiturates (dose-related)
Benzodiazepines (common cause, see
anxiolytics)
   → clonazepam (*Mil Med* 1997;**162**:3)
   → midazolam (alone and with propofol, n = 1,
Anesth Prog 2006;**53**:95–7)
Carbamazepine (especially early in therapy; as
part of SIADH, *Psychiatr Prax* 2001;**28**:48–9)
Ethosuximide
Gabapentin abuse (n = 1, *J Psychiatr Pract*
2009;**15**:314–9)
Gabapentin discontinuation (n = 1, *Am J Health
Syst Pharm* 2010;**67**:910–2)
Lacosamide (common, SmPC)
Levetiracetam (n = 1, *Am J Geriatr Pharmacother*
2010;**8**:170–4)
Phenytoin (dose-related)
Pregabalin (SmPC; *Clin Neuropharmacol* 2009;
32:236–7; n = 1, *IMAJ* 2009;**11**:699–700)
Primidone
Phenytoin + temozolomide (n = 1,
Psychosomatics 2007;**48**:359–60)
Topiramate (e.g. reversible dementia, n = 1, *Clin
Neuropharmacol* 2008;**31**:62; n = 1, *Gen Hosp
Psychiatry* 2010;**32**:647)
Valproate (n = 272, usually in first 2/52, can
be serious, more common in elderly,
Pharmacopsychiatry 2009;**42**:61–5;
n = 1, rapidly reversible, *J Am Geriatr Soc*
2010;**58**:799–801)
Valproic acid loading dose (n = 1, *J Clin Psychiatry*
2005;**66**:801–2)
Valproate + lamotrigine (n = 1, *Am J Psychiatry*
2004;**161**:1128–9)
Zonisamide (*J Clin Psychopharmacol* 2004;
4:110–1; SmPC)

- CNS — antiparkinsonian drugs *
Amantadine (n = 1, *Am J Psychiatry*
1980;**137**:240–2)

Amantadine withdrawal (n = 3, *Neurology* 1998;
50:1456–8)
Anticholinergic drugs (e.g. n = 278, *Arch Internal
Med* 2001;**161**:1099–105)
Biperiden IM (*J Neuropsychiatry Clin Neurosci*
2010;**22**:E15)
Bromocriptine
Levodopa (*Lancet* 1973;**ii**:929)
Lisuride
Pergolide withdrawal (*Clin Neuropharmacology*
1988;**11**:545–8)
Ropinirole (common, SmPC)
Selegiline

- CNS — others *
Alcohol + disulfiram (n = 1, *Ann Pharmacother*
2001;**35**:32–5)
Alcohol withdrawal (n = 1, persistent after heavy
use, *Am J Psychiatry* 1997;**154**:846–51)
Amfetamines
Anticholinesterases, e.g.:
   → donepezil (n = 1, *J Clin Psychiatry* 2002;**63**:
250–1)
   → rivastigmine (incidence < 5%)
   → rivastigmine transdermal patches (UK
SmPC, common)
Baclofen (used in Parkinson's Disease, UK SmPC
change 2009)
Betahistine (n = 1, *Ned Tijdschr Geneeskd*
2004;**148**:2338–41)
Caffeine (n = 1, overdose and physical stress, *Am
J Psychiatry* 1978;**135**:855–6)
Cannabis (in cookies, n = 1, *CNS Spectr*
2006;**11**:262)
Cocaine (e.g. n = 333, *Am J Forensic Med Pathol*
1999;**20**:120–7; n = 3 deaths, *Ned Tijdschr
Geneeskd* 2009;**153**:1014–7)
Disulfiram (n = 5, *Am J Psychiatry* 1974;**131**:1281;
n = 1, *Nihon Arukoru Yakubutsu Igakkai Zasshi*
2006;**41**:535–40)
Disulfiram + alcohol (n = 1, *Ann Pharmacother*
2001;**35**:32–5)
Disulfiram + tranylcypromine (n = 1, *Am J
Psychiatry* 1995;**152**:296)
Ergotamine–caffeine (n = 1, *Pharmacother*
2002;**22**:126–9)
Gamma-butyrolactone (GBL) withdrawal (n = 1,
Pharmacopsychiatry 2009;**42**:202–3)
Gamma-hydroxy butyrate (GHB) (n = 1, *Gen
Hosp Psychiatry* 2000;**22**:213–5)
Gamma-hydroxy butyrate (GHB) withdrawal

5

(n = 1, *Ned Tijdschr Geneeskd* 2010;**154**: A1086)

Hyoscine, transdermal (n = 1, *JAMA* 1988;**260**: 478)

MDMA/ecstasy (n = 3, *J Psychoactive Drugs* 1999;**31**:167–70)

Metoclopramide (*J Clin Psychopharmacol* 1987;**7**:281–2; overdose SmPC)

Nabilone

Naltrexone (*Presse Med* 1999;**28**:1361–2)

Nicotine (*J Pain Symptom Manage* 1998;**16**:76–7)

Nicotine withdrawal (e.g. n = 5, *Neurology* 2001;**57**:551–3)

Psilocybin in wild mushrooms (n = 1, *Lakartidningen* 1995;**92**:3779–80)

Sodium oxybate (SmPC)

Solvent intoxication

Varenicline withdrawal (n = 1, *Am J Psychiatry* 2010;**167**:720–1)

- Gastrointestinal drugs

H2 receptor antagonists (*Adv Psychiatr Treat* 2005;**11**:68), e.g.:
  → cimetidine (e.g. *Ann Intern Med* 1992; **115**:658–9)
  → famotidine (n = 1, after switch from cimetidine; *Ann Pharmacother* 2001;**35**:1045–8; n = 6, *Psychosomatics* 1996;**37**:349–55)
  → nizatidine (n = 1, *J Clin Psychiatry* 1997;**58**:327)
  → ranitidine (*Ann Intern Med* 1992;**115**:658–9; n = 1, IV, *Br Med J* 1987; **294**:1616)

Loperamide (*J Pediatr* 1990;**117**:467–71; ibid 1991;**118**:656–7)

Methixene

Misoprostol (n = 1, *Drug Intell Clin Pharm* 1991;**25**:133–4)

Omeprazole (several e.g. n = 1, *Am J Emerg Med* 2008;**26**:519)

Sulfasalazine (*Adv Psychiatr Treat* 2005;**11**:68)

- Cardiovascular drugs *

Alpha–adrenoceptor blockers, e.g. doxazosin, prazosin (*Adv Psychiatr Treat* 2005;**11**:66)

Amiloride

Amiodarone (several e.g. n = 1, *Am J Geriatr Pharmacother* 2010;**8**:170–4)

Beta-blockers (e.g. *Postgrad Med J* 1990;**66**:1050–2)

→ atenolol (n = 1, *Br Med J* 1988;**297**:1048)

→ metoprolol (n = 24, *Cardiovasc Drugs Ther* 2002;**16**:161–5; n = 1, *Ned Tijdschr Geneeskd* 2005;**149**:2183–6)

→ propranolol (*Can J Psychiatry* 2004;**49**:645; n = 3, *Gaoxiong Yi Xue Ke Xue Za Zhi* 1994;**10**:40–7)

Calcium-channel blockers (*Adv Psychiatr Treat* 2005;**11**:66), e.g.:
  → diltiazem + fentanyl (n = 1, *Gen Hosp Psychiatry* 2010;**32**:648)
  → verapamil (n = 1, *Am J Psychiatry* 1987; **144**:248)

Clonidine (n = 7, *Int J Cardiol* 2006;**113**:276–8)

Digitalis (n = 1, *Clin Cardiol* 1995;**18**:351–2)

Digoxin (*Am Heart J* 1983;**106**:419; *J Clin Pharmacol* 1979;**19**:747)

Disopyramide (*Adv Psychiatr Treat* 2005;**11**:66)

Diuretics (via severe K + loss)

Flecainide toxicity (n = 1, *Ann Pharmacother* 2009;**43**:1366–9)

Hydralazine

Lidocaine

Mexilitine

Nitrates (*Adv Psychiatr Treat* 2005;**11**:66)

Procainamide

Sodium nitroprusside (*Psychosomatics* 1995; **36**:83–5)

Spironolactone

Statins (MHRA warning, *Drug Safety Update* 2008;**1**:10)

Sulphonamide diuretics (*Adv Psychiatr Treat* 2005; **11**:66)

- Respiratory drugs *

Aminophylline

Antihistamines, sedating (*Adv Psychiatr Treat* 2005;**11**:68)

Dextromethorphan (n = 1, *Am J Geriatr Pharmacother* 2005;**3**:17–20)

Diphenhydramine (*Psychosomatics* 1994;**35**: 399–402)

Diphenhydramine + linezolid (n = 1, *Ann Pharmacother* 2004;**38**:62–5)

Diphenhydramine + nefopam withdrawal (n = 1, *Prog Neuropsychopharmacol Biol Psychiatry* 2010;**30**:705–6)

Doxapram

Mentholatum (n = 1, *Am J Psychiatry* 2000;**157**: 483–4)

Phenylpropanolamine O/D (*Br Heart J* 1982;

47:51–4)

Promethazine + cyproheptadine overdose
(n = 1, *Australas Psychiatry* 2007;**99**:242–4)

- **Anti-infection drugs** *

These may indirectly cause delirium if inducing diarrhoea and dehydration.

Aciclovir (e.g. n = 1, *Nervenarzt* 1998;**69**:1015–8; n = 1, *Clin Infect Dis* 1995;**21**:435–6)

Amphotericin B (mentioned in *Adv Psych Treat* 2005;**11**:66; *Psychosomatics* 1984;**25**:706)

Azithromycin (several e.g. n = 1, *Med Clin (Barc)* 2006;**126**:439; n = 2, *Surg Neurol* 2003;**59**:509–11)

Cefazolin (n = 1, *Br Med J* 1989;**299**:393)

Cephalexin (n = 1, *J Adolesc Health* 2006; **39**:782–3)

Chloramphenicol (*Clin Pharmacol Ther* 1970; **11**:194)

Chloroquine

Ciprofloxacin (e.g. n = 1, *Age Ageing* 2010;**39**:762; n = 1, *Ann Pharmacother* 1997;**31**:252)

Clarithromycin (n = 1, *Ned Tijdschr Geneeskd* 2001;**145**:225–8; n = 1, *Eur Respir J* 2006;**28**: 671–2; *J Antimicrob Chemother* 2007;**59**:331)

Co-trimoxazole (n = 1, *Hum Exp Toxicol* 2000; **19**:149–51)

Cycloserine

Fluconazole (*Gen Hosp Psychiatry* 2003;**25**:297–8)

Foscarnet sodium (*Adv Psych Treat* 2005;**11**:66)

Gancyclovir (*N Engl J Med* 1990;**322**:933–4)

Gatifloxacin (*Psychosomatics* 2003;**44**:85–6; n = 1, *J Am Geriatr Soc* 2006;**54**:871)

Isoniazid (*Br Med J* 1969;**i**:461)

Itraconazole (*Psychosomatics* 2003;**44**:260–1)

Levofloxacin (*Clin Neurol Neurosurg* 2005; **107**:998–9; n = 1, *Gen Hosp Psychiatry* 2008;**30**:381–3)

Mefloquine (e.g. *Lancet* 1993; **341**:632)

Ofloxacin (*J Clin Psychiatry* 1992;**53**:137–8)

Oseltamivir (n = 1, *Int J Geriatr Psychiatry* 2007; **22**:935–6)

Penicillin

Piperacillin + tazobactam (n = 1, *Nephrol Dial Transplant* 2004;**19**:1341)

Piperazine

Quinine (*Adv Psych Treat* 2005;**11**:66)

Rifampicin

Streptomycin

Sulfadiazine

Sulphonamides

Tobramycin (*JAMA* 1982;**248**:1971–2)

- **Endocrine system drugs** *

Adrenocorticotropin

Clomifene (n = 1, *Psychosomatics* 2007;**48**:65–6)

Corticosteroids (n = 1, *Gen Hosp Psychiatry* 1996;**18**:196–202)

Hypoglycaemics (oral)

Levothyroxine (n = 1, *Sao Paulo Med J* 2009;**127**: 317–8)

Methylprednisolone

Triamcinolone

- **Malignancy and immunosuppressant drugs**

Acytokine

Ciclosporin (*Adv Psychiatr Treat* 2005;**11**:68)

Interferon alfa (several e.g. n = 1, *Am J Psychiatry* 2000;**157**:1705–7)

Interleukin–2 + interferon alfa (n = 1, *Anticancer Res* 2001;**21**:3699–700)

Nelarabine (common, SmPC)

Tamoxifen (n = 273, no adverse effect on cognition, *J Clin Oncol* 2009;**27**:5144–52)

- **Musculoskeletal and analgesics** *

Baclofen

Baclofen withdrawal (n = 1, *Aust N Z J Psychiatry* 2011;**45**:86–7; n = 23, review, *Psychosomatics* 2005;**46**:503–7)

Corticosteroids (incidence may be as high as 5–6% in adults, usually emerges within a few days or weeks, and the risk may be higher with higher doses, *MHRA Drug Safety Update* 2007;1–9)

COX–2 inhibitors:
  → celecoxib (*J Neuropsychiatry Clin Neurosci* 2001;**13**:305–6)
  → rofecoxib (*J Neuropsychiatry Clin Neurosci* 2001;**13**:305–6; *Psychosomatics* 2004;**45**:361–3)

Etodolac (SmPC)

Hydroxychloroquine

Methotrexate (*Adv Psychiatr Treat* 2005;**11**:68)

NSAIDs (*Adv Psychiatr Treat* 2005;**11**:68), e.g.:
  → Aspirin toxicity (n = 1, *Ther Drug Monit* 2010;**32**:700–3)
  → fenoprofen
  → ibuprofen (*Arthritis Rheum* 1982;**25**:1013)
  → ibuprofen + tacrine (n = 1, *Am J Psychiatry* 1996;**153**:842)
  → indometacin, inc. OD (*Drugs*

5

1980;**19**:220–42)
→ ketoprofen (*J Clin Psychopharmacol* 1999;**19**:95–6)
→ naproxen (cases)
→ salicylates? (*Psychosomatics* 1987;**28**:344)
→ sulindac (*JAMA* 1980;**243**:1630)
→ tiaprofenic acid (*CMAJ* 1987;**137**:1022–3)

- Others *

Anesthetic agents (incidence 56%, *Br J Psychiatry* 2001;**178**:360–6)
Atropine and homatropine eye drops
Cyclopentolate eye drops (n = 1, *Nervenarzt* 2009;**80**:967–9)
Herbal medicines (*Psychiatr Serv* 1999;**50**:969–70)
Homatropin eye drops (n = 1, *Clin Neurol Neurosurg* 1987;**89**:53–4)
Iodoform gauze (n = 1, *Lancet* 1997;**350**:1294)
Mercury intoxication (n = 1, *Appl Neuropsychol* 2008;**15**:79–91)
Mouthwash containing alcohol (n = 1, *Mil Med* 2009;**174**:828–31)
Nitrous oxide abuse (n = 1, *Arch Neurol* 1983; **40**:446–7)
Propofol (n = 1, *Can J Anaesth* 1996;**43**:877)
Sevoflurane (*Anesth Analg* 1999;**88**:1308–10; *Minerva Anestesiol* 2002;**68**:402–5)
Strontium (*Prescrire Int* 2009;**18**:216)
Tacrolimus (*Adv Psychiatr Treat* 2005;**11**:68)
Tolterodine + anticholinesterases (*J Am Geriatr Soc* 2002;**50**:1165–6)
Typewriter correction fluid (n = 1, *Psychosomatics* 1986;**27**:665–6)
Valerian root withdrawal (*JAMA* 1998;**280**: 9966–7)

5.5 DEPRESSION (SEE ALSO SUICIDAL IDEATION)

Occurs mainly in patients with a history of depression.
Review: general (Patten and Barbui, *Psychother Psychosom* 2004;**73**:207–99).

- CNS — anxiolytics and hypnotics

Benzodiazepines (BNF, common, especially resistant depression):
→ alprazolam (n = 15, incidence 33% at 3–10mg/d, *Am J Psychiatry* 1987;**144**:664–5; n = 2, *J Clin Psychiatry*

1993;**54**(Suppl):78–84)
→ clobazam (n = 1, *Br Med J* 1983;**286**: 1246–7)
→ clonazepam
→ clorazepate
→ lorazepam (n = 8, incidence 27%, *Am J Psychiatry* 1989;**146**:1230–1)
Benzodiazepine withdrawal (several e.g. n = 3, *Can J Psychiatry* 1988;**33**:626–7; diazepam abuse discontinuation, n = 1, *DICP* 1989;**23**:989–90)
Buspirone (incidence 3%? *J Clin Psychiatry* 1982; **43** [sect 2]:100–2)
Hypnotics (n = 5535 + 2318, increased incidence with hypnotic use, 2% vs 0.9%, *BMC Psychiatry* 2007;**21**:42)
Sodium oxybate (BNF, less common)
Zaleplon (BNF, less common)
Zopiclone (BNF, rare)

- CNS — antipsychotics

Aripiprazole (BNF, less common)
Clozapine (n = 1, managed successfully by SSRIs, *Eur Neuropsychopharmacol* 1998;**8**:239–40)
Fluphenazine depot (n = 1, *Br Med J* 1969;**3**:564–7)
Pimozide (n = 4, *J Clin Psychiatry* 1997;**58**:433–6)
Quetiapine (n = 1, *Clin Neuropharmacol* 2005; **28**:133–5)
Risperidone (BNF, common; n = 17, incidence 29%, *J Clin Psychiatry* 2002;**63**:1040–4)
Ziprasidone (n = 3, *Clin Neuropharmacol* 2007;**30**:357–61)
Zotepine (BNF, common)
Zuclopenthixol

- CNS — antidepressants

Bupropion (BNF, less common)
Duloxetine (induction of ultra-rapid cycling, n = 1, *J Clin Psychopharmacol* 2007;**27**:115–6; n = 2, *Clin Pract Epidemol Ment Health* 2008; **4**:18)
Tricyclics e.g.
→ nortriptyline (n = 2, *Br Med J* 1964;**2**:1593)

- CNS — analgesics

Codeine — long-term use (n = 339, community survey, *J Clin Psychopharmacol* 1999;**19**:373–6)
Eletriptan (BNF, less common)
Fentanyl (transdermal)

Frovatriptan (BNF, less common)

Pentazocine (*South Med J* 1975;**68**:808)

Sumatriptan (n = 1, *J Clin Psychopharmacol* 1995; **15**:81–2)

Tramadol (n = 1, *Am J Psychiatry* 1996;**153**: 843–4)

- CNS — anticonvulsants *

Barbiturates (BNF, less common)

Carbamazepine (BNF, less common)

Ethosuximide (BNF, less common)

Felbamate (FDA warning 2008)

Gabapentin (BNF, uncommon; FDA warning 2008; SmPC update 2010)

Lacosamide (common, SmPC)

Lamotrigine (rare, e.g. n = 1, *J Clin Psychiatry* 2006; **67**:1159–60)

Levetiracetam (BNF, common; n = 2, *Am J Geriatr Pharmacother* 2009;**7**:281–4; n = 1, *J Clin Psychiatry* 2006;**67**:1159–60)

Oxcarbazepine (BNF, uncommon)

Phenobarbital (*Pediatrics* 1990;**85**:1086–91)

Phenytoin (n = 2, *Arch Phys Med Rehab* 1990; **71**:422–3; n = 1, *Harefuah* 1993;**124**:762–4)

Piracetam (BNF, less common)

Pregabalin (BNF, uncommon)

Primidone (n = 241, incidence 42%, *Epilepsy Behav* 2005;**6**:413–6)

Tiagabine (BNF, rare)

Topiramate (BNF, common; n = 70, risk factors, *Epilepsia* 2003;**44**:1573–7; n = 1, *Am J Psychiatry* 2001;**158**:1736)

Vigabatrin (BNF, common; incidence < 10%, *Neurology* 1991;**41**:363–4; n = 10, *J Neurol Neurosurg Psychiatry* 1993;**56**:925–8)

Zonisamide (BNF, common; *J Clin Psychopharmacol* 2004;**24**:110–1)

- CNS — antiparkinsonian drugs

Amantadine (*JAMA* 1972; **222**:792–5)

Anticholinergics, e.g.:
→ benzatropine (BNF, less common)

Botulinum toxin A (n = 1, *South Med J* 1999; **92**:738)

Levodopa (BNF, common, review in *N Engl J Med* 1976;**295**:814–8)

Rasagiline (BNF, common)

Tetrabenazine (BNF, common; n = 1, *J Neurol Neurosurg Psychiatry* 1999;**67**:550)

- CNS — others *

Amfetamine withdrawal (*Br J Hosp Med* 1993; **49**:361–3)

Anticholinesterases, e.g.:
→ galantamine (BNF, common)
→ rivastigmine (BNF, less common)

Atomoxetine (BNF, common)

Botulinum toxin A injection (*South Med J* 1999; **92**:738)

Bupropion (during smoking cessation, rare, *J Clin Psychiatry* 1999;**60**:436–41)

Caffeine withdrawal (review in *N Engl J Med* 1992;**327**:1160–1)

Dexamfetamine withdrawal (BNF, uncommon)

Disulfiram (BNF, rare; case in *Arch Neurol* 1976;**33**:141)

Ergotamine (BNF, very rare)

Flumazenil (incidence < 1%)

Heroin withdrawal (*Int J Addict* 1992;**27**:25–35)

LSD (n = 1, responded to reboxetine, *Isr J Psychiatry Relat Sci* 2002;**39**:100–3)

MDMA/Ecstasy (former chronic users report higher levels of depression than matched controls — n = 29, *J Psychopharmacol* 2001;**15**:181–6; review, *J Psychoactive Drugs* 2007;**39**:31–9; n = 402, suggestion it does not lead to long–term depression, *J Psychopharmacol* 2008;**22**:47–54)

Memantine (BNF, very rare)

Methylphenidate (BNF, common)

Modafinil (BNF, common)

Modafinil + sodium oxybate (n = 1, *Sleep Med* 2010;**11**:500–1)

Nabilone (BNF, less common)

Nalbuphine

Naltrexone (probably not a cause, n = 80, *J Psychiatry Neurosci* 2006;**31**:38–45)

Nicotine dependence and withdrawal (incidence 4%, *Addict Behav* 2003;**28**:461–70)

Ondansetron (n = 1, *Am J Psychiatry* 1995;**152**: 1101; n = 1, *S Afr Med J* 1997;**87**:1013–4)

Orlistat (n = 1, *Can J Psychiatry* 2000;**45**:87)

Oxetorone (n = 1, *Cephalalgia* 1996;**16**:560–1)

Pizotifen (BNF, rare)

Rimonabant (BNF, common; *Lancet* 2007;**370**: 1671–2)

Sibutramine (BNF, common)

Smoking (roughly doubles chance of risk of depression in women; n = 971, *Br J Psychiatry* 2008;**193**:322–6)

Smoking cessation, especially if previous MDD (n = 304, *Am J Psychiatry* 2000;**157**:368–74;

5

n = 100 with history of MDD, *Lancet* 2001;**357**: 1929–32)

Sodium oxybate (SmPC)

Tetrabenazine

Varenicline (links but not substantiated, s = 14, n = 4443, *Cochrane Database Syst Rev* 2010; **12**:CD006103)

- Gastrointestinal drugs

Diphenoxylate

H2-blockers: (BNF, rare), e.g.:
  → cimetidine (several cases, e.g. *Can J Psychiatry* 1981;**26**: 260–1)
  → famotidine (rare reports)
  → ranitidine (several e.g. n = 3, *Aust NZ J Psychiatry* 1991;**25**:4199–8)

Metoclopramide (BNF, less common; e.g. n = 1, *Psychopharmacol Bull* 2002;**36**:82–93)

Proton pump inhibitors (BNF, rare), e.g.:
  → omeprazole (unproven reports)

Sulfasalazine (BNF, less common)

- Cardiovascular drugs *

See also suicidal ideation.

ACE inhibitors, e.g.:
  → enalapril (BNF, less common; n = 1, *South Med J* 1989;**82**: 402–3)
  → imidapril (BNF, less common)
  → lisinopril (rare)
  → quinapril (BNF, less common; n = 1, *Am J Psychiatry* 1999;**156**: 1114–5)
  → ramipril (BNF, less common)

Alpha-blockers (BNF, common; case–control study concluding no association, *Pharmacoepidemiol Drug Saf* 2002;**11**:55–61)

Amiodarone (n = 1, *Br J Psychiatry* 1999;**174**: 366–7)

Beta-blockers (n = 381, concludes no increase in depression in first year, *J Am Coll Cardiol* 2006;**48**:2209–14; but a cohort study showed propranolol is associated with depression in first 3/12, but not with other beta-blockers, n = 5104, *J Clin Psychopharmacol* 2011;**31**:45–50), e.g.:
  → acebutol (mentioned in *Am J Med* 1987; **83**:223–6)
  → atenolol (*J Hum Hypertens* 1987;**1**: 87–93; n = 1, *Actas Esp Psiquiatr* 2006;**34**:352–4)
  → celiprolol (BNF, less common)
  → metoprolol (incidence 5%? review in *Drugs* 1977;**14**: 321–48)

  → nadolol (no difference to placebo, d/b, p/c, *J Neuropsychiatry* 1992;**4**:187–9)
  → nebivolol (BNF, less common)
  → propranolol (n = 1, resolved with switch to atenolol, *Am J Psychiatry* 1982; **139**:1187–8)
  → sotalol (*Ann Pharmacother* 2004;**38**: 1321–2)
  → timolol

Calcium-channel blockers, e.g.:
  → diltiazem (BNF, less common; *Br Med J* 1989;**299**:796)
  → felodipine (*Br Heart J* 1987;**58**:122–8)
  → isradipine (BNF, rare)
  → nicardipine (BNF, uncommon; several cases e.g. n = 2, *J Assoc Physicians India* 2002;**50**:1432–4)
  → nifedipine (n = 1, *Br J Psychiatry* 1991;**159**:447–8; n = 1, *Br J Psychiatry* 1990;**158**;889)

Clonidine (BNF, common; 1% incidence, case study in *Postgrad Med J* 1993;**69**: 327–8; when used for ADHD; *J Clin Psychopharmacol* 2008;**28**:725–6)

Cyclopenthiazide (BNF, rare)

Digoxin (BNF, less common)

Digoxin intoxication (*Psychosomatics* 2001; **42**:369–70)

Doxazosin (BNF, common)

Flecainide (BNF, rare)

Furosemide (BNF, caution in depression)

Hydralazine

Indoramin (BNF, less common)

Losartan (*Ugeskr Laeger* 1997;**159**:2106–8)

Methyldopa (BNF, common; review in *Am J Psychiatry* 1983;**140**: 534–8)

Moxonidine (BNF, C/I)

Prazosin (BNF, uncommon)

Procainamide (BNF, common)

Statins (BNF, less common; n = 2813, no association with depression or suicide and probably lowers incidence [*Arch Intern Med* 2003;**163**:1926–32]. See also suicidal ideation C5.15)

Streptokinase (cases, e.g. *Drugs* 1973;**5**: 357–445)

Telmisartan (BNF, rare)

Valsartan + hydrochlorothiazide overdose (n = 1, *Dtsch Med Wochenschr* 2003;**128**;2534–6)

Verapamil (*Can J Psychiatry* 1993;**38**:299–300)

- Respiratory drugs

Alimemazine

Antihistamines (BNF, rare)

Astemizole (debatable, *Drugs* 1984;**28**:38–61)

Cinnarizine (*Br Med J* 1988;**297**:722; n = 1, *Rev Neurol* 1999;**28**:876–8)

Doxapram (BNF, C/I in depression)

Ephedrine (as part of a psychosis, *Br Med J* 1968;**2**:60)

Hydroxyzine (some reports)

Montelukast (BNF, rare)

Phenylpropanolamine (n = 1, persistent, *Am J Psychiatry* 1990;**147**:367–8; n = 1, *Milit Med* 1986;**151**:387–8)

Pulmicort Turbohaler (n = 1, *Lakartidningen* 1996;**93**:2083)

Theophylline (n = 2, *Br Med J* 1980;**281**:1322)

Zafirlukast (FDA warning 2009)

- Anti-infection drugs *

Amprenavir (BNF, less common)

Antituberculous drugs (*Lancet* 1989;ii:735–6)

Atazanavir (BNF, less common)

Cefradine (n = 1, *Med J Aus* 1973;**2**:742)

Chloramphenicol (BNF, less common; rare mild cases)

Chloroquine (*Adv Psychiatr Treat* 2005;**11**:66)

Clofazimine (*Adv Psychiatr Treat* 2005;**11**:66)

Clotrimazole — oral (review in *Drugs* 1975; **9**:424)

Co-trimoxazole (BNF, very rare but severe cases, e.g. *Drug Intell Clin Pharm* 1988; **22**:267)

Cycloserine (BNF, less common; *Adv Psychiatr Treat* 2005;**11**:66)

Dapsone (n = 1, *Br Med J* 1989;**298**:1524)

Efavirenz (BNF, common; n = 355, not higher risk than placebo, *Clin Infect Dis* 2006;**42**:1790–9)

Ertapenem (BNF, rare)

Ethionamide (*Adv Psychiatr Treat* 2005;**11**:66)

Ganciclovir (BNF, common)

Griseofulvin (as part of psychosis, n = 1, *JAMA* 1974;**229**:1420)

Interferon alfa-2a (concurrent escitalopram for 12/52 does not seem to prevent any induced-depression, n = 133, RCT, d/b, p/c, 12/52, *J Clin Psychiatry* 2011;**72**:522–8)

Linezolid (BNF, common)

Lopinavir with ritonavir (BNF, less common)

Mefloquine (BNF, less common; n = 1, *Pharmacopsychiatry* 2002;**5**:200–2; n = 1, *J Clin Psychopharmacol* 2005;**25**:399–400; CSM

warning, *Curr Prob Pharmacovig* 1999;**25**:15)

Metronidazole (n = 1, *Am J Psychiatry* 1977;**134**:329–30)

Oseltamivir (n = 1, *Psychiatry Investig* 2010; **7**:302–4)

Peginterferon alfa and ribavirin (n = 162, moderate to severe depression seems to be common, especially with higher doses of ribavirin; *J Clin Psychiatry* 2005;**66**:41–8)

Piperazine (cases, e.g. *J Indian Med Assoc* 1976; **66**:33)

Posaconazole (BNF, rare)

Primaquine (n = 1, *Ann Int Med* 1980;**92**:435)

Quinolones (BNF, less common)
  - → ciprofloxacin (very rare)

Ribavirin (BNF, less common)

Stavudine (BNF, less common)

Sulphonamides

Trimethoprim (*Adv Psychiatr Treat* 2005;**11**:66)

Voriconazole (BNF, common)

Zidovudine (BNF, uncommon)

- Endocrine system drugs *

Buserelin (BNF, uncommon)

Cabergoline (BNF, less common)

Choriogonadotropin alfa (BNF, less common)

Clomifene (BNF, common)

Corticosteroids (BNF, rare but incidence may be as high as 5–6% in adults, usually emerges within a few days or weeks, the risk may be higher with higher doses, MHRA *Drug Safety Update* 2007;1–9; *Adv Psychiatr Treat* 2005;**11**:68)
  - → deflazacort (SmPC)
  - → dexamethasone (up to 40% incidence, *Arch Gen Psychiatry* 1981;**38**:471–7)
  - → methyltestosterone (rare)
  - → prednisolone (*J Assoc Physicians India* 1973; **21**:909)
  - → prednisone (review in *Clin Paediatr* 1990; **29**:382–8)

Cyproterone acetate (BNF, C/I in depression)

Danazol (rare cases, *Am J Obstet* 1977;**27**:130)

Depo-Provera (unlikely to cause, n = 495, *Contraception* 1998;**57**:237–40)

Diethylstilbestrol (in utero exposure in females, n = 1612, *Am J Epidemiol* 2010;**171**:876–82)

Estrogens for HRT (BNF, less common)

Finasteride (review, *J Cosmet Dermatol* 2010; **9**:331–2; n = 128, *BMC Clin Pharmacol* 2006;**7**:7)

5

Gestrinone (BNF, common)

Iodine long–term (BNF, common)

Mecasermin (rare, UK SmPC)

Norplant implant (unlikely to cause or exacerbate, n = 910, *Contraception* 1998;**57**:241–5)

Oestrogens for HRT (BNF, uncommon)

Oral contraceptives, combined (BNF, rare; concludes that synthetic estrogen and progestogens may have lower depressive symptoms than placebo, n = 1238, *Psychoneuroendocrinology* 2007;**32**:843–53; opposite conclusion from pilot study in *Expert Opin Drug Saf* 2007;**6**:371–4)

Progestogens (BNF, caution in depression; *Drug Treatment Psychiatry* 1982;**12**:234–5)

Progestogen-only oral contraceptives (BNF, common)

Teriparatide (BNF, common)

Testosterone and esters (BNF, common)

Testosterone abuse cessation (n = 1, *Can J Psychiatry* 1994;**39**:317–8)

Tibolone (BNF, rare)

- Malignancy and immunosuppressant drugs *
Reviews: cytokine-induced (Schiepers *et al,* *Prog Neuropsychopharmacol Biol Psychiatry* 2005; **29**:201–17).

Bicalutamide (BNF, less common)

Bortezomib (BNF, common)

Ciclosporin (n = 1, *Lijec Vjesn* 2007;**129**:74–6; *Adv Psychiatric Treat* 2005;**11**:68)

Cyproterone (BNF, caution in depression)

Dasatinib (BNF, common)

Erlotinib (BNF, less common)

Exemestane (BNF, common)

Glatiramer (BNF, less common)

Gonadorelin agonist therapy for ovarian suppression (treated with sertraline, d/b, p/c, *Fertil Steril* 2000;**74**:984–6)

Gonadorelin analogues (BNF, rare)

Goserelin (n = 1, *Psychosomatics* 2006;**47**:360–1)

Imatinib (BNF, less common)

Interferons (prevalence and management, n = 185 and review, Scalori *et al, Dig Liver Dis* 2005;**37**:102–7; Asnis *et al, Prog Neuropsychopharmacol Biol Psychiatry* 2005; **29**:808–18; *ibid* 201–17), e.g.:

→ aldesleukin

→ interferon + ribavirin (*Psychosomatics* 2006;**47**:254–6)

→ interferon alfa (BNF, uncommon; less likely in people with 5-HTTLPR gene; n = 86, often preceded by insomnia, *Psychiatry Res* 2010;**177**:240–5; n = 1015, 20/52, *Psychosomatics* 2010;**51**:137–48; n = 17 and review, *Int J Neuropsychopharmacol* 2011;**14**:247–53; can be treated with paroxetine [*N Engl J Med* 2001;**344**:961–6], sertraline [*Med J Aus* 2000;**173**:359–61] or methylphenidate [n = 1, *J Psychopharmacol* 2006; **20**:687–9]; review of mechanisms and management, *Br J Hosp Med (Lond)* 2007;**68**:307–10)

→ interferon beta (BNF, caution in depression)

→ peginterferon 2-alpha-2 (prolonged low-dose maintenance is not associated with an increase in depression; n = 129, 3.5 years, *J Affect Disord* 2011;**129**:205–12)

Letrozole (BNF, common; n = 1, *Bipolar Disord* 2006;**8**:516–8)

Leuprolide/leuprorelin (n = 1, *J Clin Psychiatry* 2003;**64**:341–3)

→ leuprolide acetate (BNF, common)

Mesna (BNF, common)

Mithramycin

Mycophenolate mofetil (n = 1, *Pharmacother* 2008;**28**:136–9)

Nilotinib (BNF, less common)

Nilutamide (n = 1, *Therapie* 1997;**52**:79–81)

Octreotide (rare)

Sorafenib (BNF, common)

Tacrolimus (BNF, common)

Tamoxifen (two large studies show no increased risk [n = 2943, *Psychosomatics* 2007;**48**:205–10; n = 11 064, *J Natl Cancer Inst* 2001;**93**:1615–23], n = 1, prevented by venlafaxine, *Psychosomatics* 2009;**50**:162–5)

Toremifene (BNF, less common)

Trastuzumab (BNF, common)

Tretinoin (BNF, common)

Triamcinolone (incidence up to 8%, see *Br Med J* 1969;i:682)

- Musculoskeletal and analgesics
Baclofen (BNF, less common; rare cases, e.g. *Arch Intern Med* 1985;**145**:1717–8; psychotic, n = 1, *J Clin Psychiatry* 1992;**53**:211–2)

Cytokine modulators

→ abatacept (BNF, uncommon)

→ adalimumab (BNF, uncommon)

→ etanercept (BNF, uncommon)

→ infliximab (BNF, uncommon)

→ rituximab (BNF, uncommon)

Dantrolene (BNF, common)

Etodolac (SmPC, rare)

Nabilone

NSAIDs (BNF, uncommon)

→ diflunisal (< 1% incidence)

→ flurbiprofen (> 1% incidence?)

→ ibuprofen (uncommon, *Arthritis Rheum* 1982;**25**:1013)

→ indometacin (BNF, rare; incidence 4%? *Br Med J* 1972;**4**:398)

→ indometacin withdrawal (*Br J Rheumatol* 1992;**31**:211)

→ naproxen (rare)

→ sulindac

- Others *

Acetazolamide (BNF, common)

Acitretin (*J Drugs Dermatol* 2005;**4**:690–6)

Allopurinol

Anagrelide (BNF, less common)

Anesthetic agents (in elderly, n = 140, *Br J Psychiatry* 2001;**178**:360–6)

Apraclonidine (BNF, common)

Betaine (BNF, less common)

Betaxolol eye drops (n = 2, *Aust NZ J Psychiatry* 2001;**35**:569–71)

Brimonidine (BNF, common)

Brinzolamide (BNF, common)

Carbaryl (psychotic, n = 1, *Am J Psychiatry* 1995;**152**:646–7)

Dianette (SmPC)

Dorzolamide eye–drops (*Can J Ophthalmol* 1999;**34**:93–4)

Etretinate (*Br Med J* 1989;**298**:964)

Flunisolide (inhaled, incidence 1–3%)

Isotretinoin (BNF, rare; one review noted an incidence of 1–11%, *Semin Cutan Med Surg* 2007;**26**:210–20; and a larger one showed a statistically significant association, n = 30496, *J Clin Psychiatry* 2008;**69**:526–32; although it may abate over 6/12, n = 100, *Psychol Rep* 2006;**99**:897–906; n = 10, incidence 90% in bipolar patients, *J Affect Disord* 2010;**122**:306–8)

Inositol (n = 3, *Am J Psychiatry* 1996;**153**:839)

Lead (higher levels, n = 1987, *Arch Gen Psychiatry* 2009;**66**:1313–9)

Medroxyprogesterone acetate (Depo-

Provera®; n = 457, 3 years, 12% increase cf non-users, *Contraception* 2000;**61**:385–90)

Mercaptamine (BNF, common)

Mothballs – see paradichlorobenzene

Nitrous oxide (risk factor? *J Clin Psychopharmacol* 2007;**27**:238–9)

Oral contraceptives combined (incidence 16–56%, review in *J Adolescent Health Care* 1981;**2**:53–64)

Organophosphate pesticides (related to cumulative lifetime exposure, n = 29074, *J Occup Environ Med* 2006;**48**:1005–13; n = 761, *Ann Epidemiol* 2002;**12**:389–94)

Paradichlorobenzene (n = 1, *Gen Hosp Psychiatry* 2010;**32**:7–9)

Pegaptanib (BNF, less common)

Sodium phenylbutyrate (BNF, less common)

Tacrolimus (*Adv Psychiatric Treat* 2005;**11**:68)

Vitamin A intoxication (*Psychosomatics* 1992;**33**:117–8)

Xylometazoline (n = 1, child, *JAMA* 1970;**211**:123–4)

5.6 HALLUCINATIONS (INCLUDING VISUAL DISTURBANCES, SEE ALSO PSYCHOSIS)

Where known the type of hallucination is mentioned.

- CNS — anxiolytics and hypnotics *

Benzodiazepines (n = 1, musical, *Can J Psychiatry* 1991;**36**:609–11), e.g.:

→ lorazepam overdose (n = 65, *Ann Pediatr (Paris)* 1984;**31**:286–9)

→ midazolam IV (*Drug Intell Clin Pharm* 1989; **23**:671–2)

→ temazepam (n = 1, visual, *J Am Geriatr Soc* 2006;**54**:1627–8)

→ triazolam (n = 1 in dental surgery, *Anesth Prog* 2005;**52**:17–20)

Benzodiazepine withdrawal (n = 1, visual, *Psychiatr Prax* 1997;**24**:309–10)

Zaleplon (BNF, uncommon; n = 1, dose-related, *Clin Toxicol (Phila)* 2008;**46**:344–5)

Zolpidem (n = 5, *J Toxicol Clin Toxicol* 1998;**36**:195–203; distorted perception, n = 1, *Ann Pharmacother* 2003;**37**:683–6)

Zolpidem overdose (n = 1, command, *J Clin Psychiatry* 2010;**71**:92–3)

Zolpidem + fluvoxamine (n = 1, *Int Psychogeriatr* 2006;**18**:749–51)

5

Zopiclone (BNF, rare; *Pharm J* 1990;**245**:210)

- CNS — antipsychotics

Lithium (n = 1, visual and auditory, *Nervenartz* 1993;**64**:747–9)

Olanzapine (BNF, common; n = 1, hypnopompic hallucinations, *Can J Psychiatry* 2004;**49**:496–7)

- CNS — antidepressants *

Review: factors associated with visual hallucinations with antidepressants (*Hum Psychopharmacol* 2004;**19**:577–84).

Bupropion (BNF, very rare; tactile, n = 2, *J Clin Psychiatry* 2006;**67**:1820–1)

Bupropion + valproate (n = 1, visual and auditory, *Can J Psychiatry* 2000;**45**:198–9)

Duloxetine (BNF, v rare)

MAOIs, e.g.:

- → phenelzine (BNF, rare; n = 1, *Am J Psychiatry* 1994;**151**:450)
- → tranylcypromine (n = 1, *Psychiatr Prax* 1993;**20**:116)

Mirtazapine (n = 3, multimedia, *Int Psychogeriatr* 2010;**22**:837–9)

Moclobemide (pseudohallucinations, n = 1, *Pharmacopsychiatry* 2005;**38**:179–81)

Reboxetine (BNF, very rare)

SSRIs (BNF, uncommon), e.g.

- → citalopram (n = 1, complex visual, *Prog Neuropsychopharmacol Biol Psychiatry* 2009;**33**:575–6)
- → fluoxetine (n = 1, *Am J Psychiatry* 1993; **150**:1750)
- → fluoxetine + zolpidem (n = 1, *J Forensic Sci* 2004;**49**:392–3)
- → fluoxetine + dextromethorphan (n = 1, *Am J Psychiatry* 1992;**149**:1406)
- → paroxetine (n = 1, *Psychiatry Clin Neurosci* 2010;**64**:666–7)
- → paroxetine, excessive use/OD (n = 1, *Psychiatry Clin Neurosci* 2003;**57**:548–9)
- → sertraline (n = 1, *J Clin Psychiatry* 2004;**65**:446–7)

Tricyclics (musical, *Biol Psychiatry* 1996;**40**: 309–10), e.g.:

- → amitriptyline low dose (visual, *J Clin Psychopharmacol* 1988;**8**:75–6)
- → clomipramine (n = 1, visual, *Acta Psychiatr Scand* 1999;**99**:388–90; n = 1, musical, *Br J Psychiatry* 1991;**159**:888–9)

- → doxepin (n = 1, visual, *Aust NZ J Psychiatry* 1982;**16**:295–6)
- → imipramine

Venlafaxine (BNF, uncommon, n = 1, *J Clin Psychiatry* 2009;**70**:601–3)

- CNS — analgesics *

Buprenorphine (rare, incidence < 1%, *Br Med J* 1988;**296**:214)

Buprenorphine-epidural (n = 5, *Br Med J* 1989; **298**:928–9)

Methadone (*J Am Acad Child Adolesc Psychiatry* 1999;**38**:355–6)

Morphine (n = 1, resolved when switched to oxycodone, *Cases J* 2009;**23**:9391)

Morphine SR and methadone (*Lancet* 1987;**2**: 392)

Nefopam (BNF, uncommon; *Curr Probl* 1989; **1**:89)

Oxycodone (n = 1, musical, *Am J Geriatr Psychiatry* 2003;**11**:470)

Oxycodone + sertraline (n = 1, *J Clin Pharmacol* 2001;**41**:224)

Pentazocine

Tramadol (n = 6, *Curr Probl* 1995;**21**:2; n = 1, visual and auditory, *Ann Med Interna* 2003; **20**:493; n = 1, visual, *Acta Clin Belg* 1996;**51**:184–6)

Tramadol + clarithromycin (n = 1, visual-auditory, *Neuropsychopharmacol Hung* 2010;**12**:309–12)

- CNS — anticonvulsants *

Carbamazepine hypersensitivity (n = 1, *Pharmacopsychiatry* 2006;**39**:192–3)

Gabapentin (BNF, rare; n = 1, parasitosis, *South Med J* 2010;**103**:711-2)

Lamotrigine (BNF, common; n = 1, *Am J Psychiatry* 2006;**163**:749–50)

Levetiracetam (BNF, uncommon)

Midazolam (BNF, common; n = 1, visual, *Ann Pharmacother* 1989;**23**:671–2; oral n = 1, visual, *Rev Esp Anestesiol Reanim* 1995; **42**:76–7)

Phenobarbital (BNF, common)

Phenytoin (n = 1, *Epilepsy Behav* 1990;**71**:422–3; IV, n = 1, *Eur J Paediatr Neurol* 2010;**14**:460-3)

Pregabalin (BNF, uncommon)

Primidone (n = 241, incidence 43%; *Epilepsy Behav* 2005;**6**:413–6)

Sodium valproate (BNF, rare)

Topiramate (n = 1, auditory, *J Clin Psychiatry* 2001;**62**:653; *Epileptic Disord* 2008;**10**:240)

Vigabatrin (BNF, visual disturbance common)

Zonisamide (BNF, very rare; e.g. n = 3, *Pharmacotherapy* 2003;**23**:93–6)

● CNS — antiparkinsonian drugs *

Amantadine (BNF, common; e.g. n = 1, musical in PD, *Mov Disord* 2010;**25**:1505–6)

Amantadine overdose (n = 1, *Pediatr Emerg Care* 1991;**7**:89–92)

Anticholinergics, e.g.:

→ trihexyphenidyl (n = 1, tactile, *Rinsho Shinkeigaku* 2005;**45**:125–7; abuse, *Med Clin (Barc)* 1991;**97**:239)

Dopamine agonists:

→ apomorphine (BNF, common)

→ bromocriptine (BNF, common; incidence < 1%, *Ann Int Med* 1984;**101**:149)

→ pergolide (BNF, common; in up to 13%, e.g. *Neurology* 1982;**32**:1181–4)

→ pergolide withdrawal (*Clin Neuro-pharmacology* 1988;**11**:545–8)

→ pramipexole (BNF, common)

→ ropinirole (BNF, common; n = 1, transient, *Prog Neuropharmacol Biol Psychiatry* 2008; **32**:1087–8)

→ rotigotine (BNF, common)

Entacapone (BNF, common)

Levodopa (BNF, common; incidence < 26% in elderly, e.g. *Postgrad Med J* 1989;**65**:358–61)

Levodopa-carbidopa + paroxetine (n = 1, *Ned Tijdschr Geneeskd* 2002;**146**:1056–7)

Rasagaline (BNF, common)

Riluzole added to memantine/bupropion (n = 1, *J Clin Psychopharmacol* 2006;**26**:218–20)

Selegiline (BNF, common; esp. combined with levodopa and/or dopamine agonists, n = 94, *Parkinsonism Relat Disord* 2004;**10**:235–42)

Tolcapone (BNF, common)

● CNS — others *

Alcohol

Amfetamines (*Biol Psychiatry* 1980;**15**:749)

Anticholinesterases, e.g.:

→ donepezil (BNF, common; n = 1, hypnopompic, *J Psychopharmacol* 2000; **14**:303–4)

→ galantamine (BNF, rare)

→ rivastigmine (BNF, very rare)

Atomoxetine (MHRA warning 2009)

Ginseng (n = 1, *Acta Psychiatr Scand* 2002; **105**:76–8)

Guanfacine (n = 1, *J Am Acad Child Adolesc Psychiatry* 2003;**42**:1387)

Hyoscine patch (n = 1, *Lakartidningen* 1995;**92**:638)

Khat (n = 3, hypnagogic, *Acta Psychiatr Scand* 1988;**78**:458–61; n = 4, *Br J Hosp Med* 1995; **54**:322–6)

LSD (*J Nerv Mental Dis* 1991;**179**:173–4)

Meclizine + metaxalone (n=1, *Ann Pharmacother* 2004;**38**:1968–9)

Memantine (BNF, uncommon; n = 3, *J Neurol Neurosurg Psychiatry* 2007;**78**:546; exacer-bation, n = 3, *Neurology* 2005;**65**: 481–2)

Methylphenidate (*Neurology* 2004;**63**:753–4; US FDA warning in children; low-dose n = 1, *J Child Neurol* 2009;**24**:1005–7; visual, n=1, *An Pediatr (Barc)* 2010;**72**:229-30)

Methylphenidate + fluoxetine (n = 1, *J Clin Psychopharmacol* 2008;**28**:723–5)

Metoclopramide OD (SmPC)

Modafinil (n = 1, *J Clin Psychopharmacol* 2009; **29**:408; visual, n = 1, *J Clin Psychopharmacol* 2010;**30**:347–50)

Nabilone (BNF, uncommon)

Naltrexone (BNF, very rare)

Prolintane + diphenhydramine (n = 1, visual, *Pharmacopsychiatry* 2002;**35**:24–5)

Sodium oxybate (SmPC)

Varenicline (UK SmPC; n = 1, *J Med Case Reports* 2009;**3**:7560)

Varenicline withdrawal (n = 1, Am J Psychiatry 2009;**166**:619–20)

● Gastrointestinal drugs

Bismuth toxicity (n = 1, *Actas Luso Esp Neurol Psiquiatr Cienc Afines* 1984;**12**:427–33)

H2-antagonists (BNF, rare)

→ cimetidine (several e.g. *Arch Intern Med* 1983; **98**: 677)

→ famotidine (n = 1, *Pharmacother* 1998;**18**:404–7)

→ ranitidine (n = 1, *Eur J Clin Pharmacol* 1985;**29**:375–6)

Proton-pump inhibitors (omeprazole, lansoprazole etc; BNF, very rare)

Sulfasalazine (BNF, uncommon)

● Cardiovascular drugs *

ACE inhibitors (*Postgrad Med J* 1993;**69**:240), e.g.

5

→ quinapril (*NZ Med J* 1999;**112**:83)

Beta-blockers, e.g.:

→ metoprolol (visual, *Psychosomatics* 2006;**47**:537–8; n = 1, *Tijdschr Psychiatr* 2010;**52**:117–21)

→ pindolol (n = 1, visual, *Harefuah* 1983; **104**:226–7)

→ propranolol (n = 1, musical, *J Nerv Ment Dis* 1998;**186**:192–4; n = 1, *Intensive Care Med* 1999;**25**:336–7)

→ timolol (*JAMA* 1980;**244**:768)

Calcium-channel blockers, e.g.:

→ diltiazem (n = 1, *Psychiatr Prax* 1998; **25**:91–2)

Clonidine (n = 3, *Ann Int Med* 1980;**93**:456–7; n = 1, *Clin Ter* 2000;**991**:45–7)

Clopidogrel (BNF, very rare)

Digoxin (eg. *Arch Neurol* 1983;**40**:386)

Disopyramide

Flecainide (BNF, rare; n = 1, visual, *Postgrad Med J* 1986;**62**:61–2)

Flunarizine (n = 1, *Rev Neurol* 2006;**42**:399–7)

Isosorbide dinitrate (n = 1, visual, *Psychosomatics* 1987;**28**:555–6)

Pentoxifylline (musical, *Neurology* 1993;**43**: 1621–2)

Prazosin (auditory, *J Clin Psychopharmacol* 1988; **8**:228)

Procainamide

Streptokinase (*Drugs* 1973;**5**:357–445)

- Respiratory drugs

Decongestants (containing pseudoephedrine and triprolidine; n = 4, *Br Med J* 1984; **288**:1688; n = 3, *Br Med J* 1984;**288**:1369)

Desloratidine (BNF, very rare)

Dextromethorphan (n = 1, *Psychosomatics* 1996; **37**:71–4)

Doxapram (BNF, common post-op)

Montelukast (BNF, very rare; FDA warning 2009)

Phenylpropanolamine (*JAMA* 1981;**245**:601–2)

Promethazine (*Acta Paediatrica Scand* 1989; **78**: 131–2)

Pseudoephedrine (BNF, rare)

Salbutamol (nebulised) (*Br Med J* 1986; **292**:1430; n = 1, probably due to fluorocarbon propellant, *Pediatr Emerg Care* 1994;**10**:87–8)

Zafirlukast (FDA warning 2009)

- Anti-infection drugs

Aciclovir (BNF, very rare)

Amoxicillin (e.g. n = 1, *Br J Clin Pract* 1996;**50**:279)

Cefalosporins and other beta-lactams (*Adv Psychiatr Treat* 2005;**11**:66)

→ cefaclor (BNF, rare)

→ ceftazidime (*Br Med J* 1998;**297**:858)

→ ertapenem (BNF, very rare)

Chloroquine (*Adv Psychiatr Treat* 2005;**11**:66)

Ciclosporin (visual, *Neurology* 1991;**41**:1996; *Transplantation* 1987;**43**:768–9)

Clarithromycin (n = 1, *Farm Hosp* 2007;**31**: 321–3; n = 1, visual, *Int J Clin Pharmacol Ther* 2002;**40**:20–2; n = 1, visual, *Am J Kidney Dis* 1996;**27**:143–6)

Co-trimoxazole (BNF, rare)

Efavirenz (significantly reduced with stepped dose increase, n = 114, RCT, d/b, *Ann Intern Med* 2009;**151**:149–56)

Erythromycin + nitrazepam/triazolam (n = 1, *Psychiatry Clin Neurosci* 1996;**50**:337–9)

Famciclovir (BNF, very rare)

Flucytosine (BNF, common)

Gatifloxacin (n = 1, *Psychosomatics* 2006;**47**:360)

Gentamicin (*JAMA* 1977;**238**:53)

Isoniazid (n = 1, *Presse Med* 2006;**35**:425–6; *Psychosomatics* 1993;**34**:537–9)

Itraconazole, oral (n = 1, *Clin Infect Dis* 1995; **21**:456)

Maraviroc (uncommon, UK SmPC)

Mefloquine (BNF, uncommon; n = 1, psychotic, *Psychiatr Prax* 1999;**26**:252–4; *Adv Psychiatr Treat* 2005;**11**:66)

Osteltamivir (SmPC, < 1% incidence)

Quinolones (BNF, uncommon; review, esp in elderly, *Prescrire Int* 2008;**17**:20), e.g.:

→ ciprofloxacin (*Arch Intern Med* 1989;**110**:170–1; n = 1, visual, *Arch Soc Esp Oftalmol* 2007;**82**:299–301)

→ levofloxacin (n = 2, visual, *Nippon Ronen Igakkai Zasshi* 1999;**36**:213–7)

→ nalidixic acid (*Nouv Presse Med* 1980;**9**:455)

→ norfloxacin (n = 1, *J Assoc Physicians India* 1996;**44**:504)

Voriconazole (BNF, common; n = 1, *Rev Clin Esp* 2005;**205**:632–3; n = 1, musical, *Infection* 2004;**32**:293–5; n = 12, *Clin Infect Dis* 2008; **47**:7–10)

- Endocrine system drugs

Alendronic acid (n = 1, auditory and visual,

Pharmacotherapy 2004;**24**:799–802)

Cabergoline (BNF, common)

Corticosteroids (incidence may be as high as 5–6% in adults, usually emerges within a few days or weeks, risk may be higher with higher doses, *MHRA Drug Safety Update* 2007;1–9)

Disodium pamidronate (BNF, rare, *Ann Rheum Dis* 1992;**51**:927–8)

Estrogen (n = 1, visual, *Am J Ophthalmol* 2000; **129**:407)

- Malignancy and immunosuppressant drugs*

Bevacizumab (n = 1, visual, *Am J Ophthalmol* 2007; **143**:169–70)

Chlorambucil (n = 1, *Ir Med J* 1984;**77**:288–9)

Hydroxycarbamide

Ifosfamide (n = 6, visual, *Cancer* 1994;**73**:1509–14; n = 5, *Drugs Aging* 2007;**24**:967–73)

Interferon-alfa + ribavirin (n = 1, *Psychosomatics* 2010;**51**:1–7)

Vincristine (n = 2, visual, *Clin Lab Haematol* 1994; **16**:355–7)

- Musculoskeletal and analgesics

Baclofen (BNF, common; used in Parkinson's Disease, UK SmPC change 2009)

COX-2 inhibitors:
→ celecoxib (auditory n = 1, *Am J Psychiatry* 2000;**157**:1022–3)
→ etoricoxib (BNF, very rare)

Hydrochloroquine (n = 1, *Ann Dermatol Venereol* 2004;**131**:471–3)

NSAIDs, e.g.:
→ fenbufen (*Br Med J* 1985;**290**:822)
→ flurbiprofen (BNF, uncommon)
→ indometacin (rare, e.g. n = 1, visual, *Int Clin Psychopharmacol* 1986;**1**:263–6; n = 32, *Can J Anaesth* 2003;**50**:586–8)
→ piroxicam (visual, *Presse Med* 1995; **24**:504)
→ salicylates
→ sulindac (auditory and visual, *Psychosomatics* 1990;**31**:461–2)

Tizanidine (BNF, common)

- Others *

Anagrelide (n = 1, visual, *Eur J Haematol* 2004; **73**:223–4)

Atropine toxicity (n = 1, visual, *Can J Neurol Sci* 1991;**18**:18–27)

Benzydamine (as in Difflam, n = 78, 50%

incidence, *Rev Bras Psiquiatr* 2009;**31**:208–12)

Erythropoietin (e.g. visual, *Psychosomatics* 1998; **39**:83–5; n = 5, *N Engl J Med* 1991;**325**:285)

Isoflurane withdrawal (n = 1, *Acta Paediatr* 1993; **82**:885–6)

Ketamine (BNF, very common; *Minerva Anestesiol* 1983;**49**:299–8; *Anaesthesia* 1990;**45**:422)

Mercaptamine (BNF, rare)

Nitrous oxide (*J Am Dent Assoc* 1980;**101**: 595–7)

Phenylephrine (*JAMA* 1982;**247**:1859)

Propofol (n = 1, *Acta Anaesthesiol Scand* 1998: **42**:739–41; n = 1, erotic, *Rev Esp Anestesiol Reanim* 2000;**47**:90–2)

Radiographic contrast media (n = 2, review, *Br J Clin Pharmacol* 1999;**47**:226–7)

Strontium (*Prescrire Int* 2009;**18**:216)

Tolterodine (n = 1, *BJU Int* 1999;**84**:1109)

5.7 MANIA, HYPOMANIA OR EUPHORIA

- CNS — anxiolytics and hypnotics

Benzodiazepines:
→ alprazolam (*J Clin Psychiatry* 1987;**48**:117–8)
→ clorazepate (n = 5, *Ann Med Psychol (Paris)* 1987;**145**:855–60)
→ midazolam (euphoria possible)

Benzodiazepine withdrawal (n = 1, abrupt, *Acta Psychiatr Scand* 1989;**79**:406–7)

Buspirone (n = 1, *Br J Psychiatry* 1991;**158**: 136–7)

Lorazepam withdrawal (n = 2, *J Affect Disord* 1989;**17**:93–5)

- CNS — antipsychotics *

Review: mania has been reported to be induced by olanzapine, risperidone, quetiapine and ziprasidone, but not (or only very rarely) with clozapine or typicals, including amisulpride (Rachid et al, *J Clin Psychiatry* 2004;**11**:1537–45).

Amisulpride (n = 1, *Prog Neuropsychopharmacol Biol Psychiatry* 2009;**13**:1572–3; n = 1, *Indian J Pharmacol* 2010;**42**:112–3)

Aripiprazole (n = 1, first episode at 55 years, *Psychiatry (Edgmont)* 2010;**7**:37–9; n = 1, *Am J Psychiatry* 2007;**164**:172–3; n = 1, *Pharmacopsychiatry* 2007;**40**:37–8)

Lithium toxicity (n = 3, *Drug Intell Clin Pharm* 1987;**21**:979–81)

5

Lithium + imipramine (n = 1, *Br J Psychiatry* 1988; **153**:828–30)

Lithium withdrawal (n = 1, complicated by delirium, *Gen Hosp Psychiatry* 2010;**32**:102–4)

Olanzapine (review, concludes half of reports are poorly documented but, in the others, mood-elevating effects were prominent, n = 26, *J Clin Psychiatry* 2000;**61**:649–55; Lilly post-hoc analysis of two RCTs failed to show evidence of olanzapine–induced mania; n = 254, Baker *et al, J Affect Disord* 2003;**73**:147–53)

Olanzapine/fluoxetine combination (no greater risk than olanzapine or placebo over 8/52, n = 833, *J Clin Psychiatry* 2005;**66**:611–6)

Quetiapine (many e.g. n = 1, *Can J Psychiatry* 2003;**48**:349–50; n = 1, *Rev Bras Psiquitr* 2009: **31**:286–7)

Paliperidone (n = 1, *J Clin Psychopharmacol* 2010; **30**:202–4; n = 1, *Prog Neuropsychopharmacol Biol Psychiatry* 2010;**34**:1351–2)

Risperidone (review concludes that half of the reports are poorly documented but, in the others, mood-elevating effects were prominent, n = 26, *J Clin Psychiatry* 2000;**61**:649–55)

Risperidone withdrawal (n = 1, *J Clin Psychiatry* 1998;**59**:620–1)

Ziprasidone (n = 14 worldwide, reviewed in *Clin Neuropharmacol* 2005;**28**:83–6; n = 1, *CNS Spectr* 2007;**12**:578–9; n = 1, *J Clin Psychopharmacol* 2008;**28**:711–3)

Ziprasidone + SSRI (n = 1, *J Clin Psychiatry* 2003; **64**:1393–4)

- CNS — antidepressants *

Antidepressant-induced mania is well known (especially in bipolar III), as is the spontaneous swing from depression to hypomania in bipolars. Depressed bipolar II patients may be less vulnerable than in bipolar I to switch to mania/hypomania when treated with an antidepressant and an adjunctive mood stabiliser (n = 184, 10/52, Altshuler *et al, Am J Psychiatry* 2006;**163**:313–5). Risk factors include:

- increased number of antidepressant trials
- history of substance misuse (n = 98, *J Clin Psychiatry* 2006;**67**:1341–5)
- in bipolar depression, during acute and maintenance. Venlafaxine appears worst, sertraline medium and bupropion lowest risk (n = 159, RCT, 10/52, Leverich *et al, Am J Psychiatry* 2006;**163**:232–9)

- Higher doses — SSRI-induced hypomania may be dose-related (n = 2, Ramasubbu, *Acta Psychiatr Scand* 2001;**104**:236–9)

Switching can be reduced by using adjunctive lithium (n = 44, review by Henry *et al, J Clin Psychiatry* 2001;**62**:249–55).

Reviews: * extensive (meta-analysis, s = 73, n = 114,521, Tondo et al, *Acta Psychiatr Scand* 2010;**121**:404–14; Chen *et al, Curr Psychiatry Rep* 2010;**12**:512–21).

Bupropion (rare, e.g. n = 1, within 1/52, *Bipolar Disord* 2001;**3**:159–60; n = 1, *Aust N Z J Psychiatry* 2008; **42**:746)

Bupropion discontinuation (n = 1, *J Clin Psychiatry* 2004;**65**:277)

Desvenlafaxine (n = 1, not bipolar, *J Psychiatr Pract* 2010;**16**:58–62)

Duloxetine (rare in unipolar depression; *J Affect Disord* 2005;**87**:115–9; n = 1, *J Psychopharmacol* 2009;**23**:592–6)

Flupentixol (n = 6, *Eur Psychiatry* 2002;**17**: 349–52)

MAOIs, e.g:
- → isocarboxazid (n = 3, *J Clin Psychiatry* 1986; **47**:40–1)
- → isocarboxazid withdrawal (n = 2, *J Clin Psychopharmacol* 1985;**5**:340–2)
- → phenelzine (e.g. *Biol Psychiatry* 1985;**20**: 1009–14)

Mianserin

Mirtazapine (n=1, *Pharmacopsychiatry* 2010; **43**:37–8; n = 1 after switch from fluoxetine, *J Psychopharmacol* 2009;**23**:220–2; n = 1, *Aust N Z J Psychiatry* 2008;**42**:1070–1)

Mirtazapine withdrawal (n = 1, *Br J Psychiatry* 1999;**175**:390)

Mirtazapine + fluoxetine (n = 1, *Depress Anxiety* 2002;**15**:46–7)

Mirtazapine + sertraline (n = 1, *J Clin Psychiatry* 1998;**59**:320)

Reboxetine (n = 3, *J Clin Psychiatry* 2001;**62**:655–6)

SSRIs, e.g.:
- → citalopram (n = 1, *Gen Hosp Psychiatry* 2007;**29**:374–6; n = 1, *Psychosomatics* 2008; **49**:362–3)
- → citalopram + silbutramine (n = 1, *J Clin Psychiatry* 2002;**63**:165)
- → escitalopram (n = 1, *Eur Psychiatry* 2004; **19**:455–6; n = 2, *Psychopharmacol Bull*

2009;**42**:89–91)
- → fluoxetine (e.g. n = 3, *J Child Adolesc Psychopharmacol* 1998;**8**:73–80)
- → fluvoxamine (n = 1, *World J Biol Psychiatry* 2001;**2**:201–4; n = 1, *J Psychiatry Neurosci* 2003;**28**:134–5)
- → paroxetine (n = 1, psychotic mania, *Am J Psychiatry* 1995;**152**:1399–440; n = 79, incidence 8.9%; *Hum Psychopharmacol* 2003;**18**:565–8)
- → paroxetine + methylphenidate (n = 1, *Prog Neuropsychopharmacol Biol Psychiatry* 2010;**34**:719–20)
- → sertraline (n = 1, *Acta Psychiatr Scand* 2003;**108**:70–4)
- → sertraline withdrawal (*Can J Psychiatry* 2002;**47**:584–5)

St John's wort (n = 12, review in *Int J Clin Pharmacol Ther* 2004;**2**:473–80)

Trazodone (several e.g. n = 3, *Br J Psychiatry* 1991;**158**:275–8)

Tricyclics, e.g.:
- → amitriptyline (*Br Med J* 1991;**303**:331–2, 720, 1200; *Neurology* 1989;**39**:305)
- → amitriptyline withdrawal (n = 1, *J Clin Psychiatry* 1980;**41**:33–4)
- → clomipramine (n = 25, RCT, incidence 24%, *Arch Gen Psychiatry* 1979; **36**:560–5; inc. abuse n = 3, *Addiction* 2007;**102**:1166–7)
- → dosulepin abuse (n = 3, *Addiction* 2007; **102**:1166–7)
- → imipramine (n = 25, RCT, incidence 4%, *Arch Gen Psychiatry* 1979;**36**:560–5)
- → imipramine withdrawal (n = 1, *Am J Psychiatry* 1986;**143**:260)

Tryptophan + MAOI (n = 2, *Am J Psychiatry* 1985;**142**:1487–8)

Venlafaxine (n = 1, *Can J Psychiatry* 2004;**49**:496; n = 1, *Can J Psychiatry* 2004;**49**:786–7)

Venlafaxine withdrawal (n = 1, *Int J Neuropsychopharmacol* 2003;**6**:89–90; n = 1, *Ann Pharmacother* 2007;**41**:359–60)

Venlafaxine + lithium + valproate (n = 1, *Therapie* 2006;**61**:531–3)

Venlafaxine + TMS (n = 1, *J Neuropsychiatry Clin Neurosci* 2010;**22**:E18–9)

- • CNS — analgesics

Buprenorphine (incidence up to 1%, *Br J Clin Pract* 1980; **34**:144–6; n = 1, *Aust N Z J Psychiatry* 2004;**38**:560–1)

Codeine + paracetamol (n = 1, *Aust N Z J Psychiatry* 1998;**32**:586–8)

Frovatriptan (n = 1, *J Neuropsychiatry Clin Neurosci* 2005;**17**:430–1)

Nefopam IM (euphoria, *Br J Anaesth* 1979; **51**:691–5)

Pentazocine (*South Med J* 1975;**68**:808)

Tramadol (n = 1, *Am J Psychiatry* 1997; **154**:1624)

- • CNS — anticonvulsants

Carbamazepine (*J Clin Psychiatry* 1984;**45**:272–4)

Carbamazepine withdrawal (n = 1, *Br J Psychiatry* 1995;**167**:698)

Clonazepam (*Drug Intell Clin Pharm* 1991;**25**: 938–9)

Ethosuximide

Gabapentin (eg n = 1, *Br J Psychiatry* 1995;**166**: 679–80; n = 1, *Br J Psychiatry* 1999;**175**:291)

Lamotrigine (e.g. n = 3, *Am J Psychiatry* 2006; **163**:159–60; n = 1, *Aust N Z J Psychiatry* 2006; **40**:718; no increase in switch to mania in Bipolar I, n = 1258, 6/12, open, p/c, *J Clin Psychiatry* 2009;**70**:1273–80)

Phenobarbital (*Pediatrics* 1984;**74**:1133)

Pregabalin (SmPC)

Topiramate (n = 1, *J Neurol Neurosurg Psychiatry* 2002;**73**:208–9; *J Clin Psychopharmacol* 2005; **25**:196–7)

Vigabatrin (n = 1, *Lancet* 1994;**343**:606–7)

Zonisamide (*J Clin Psychopharmacol* 2004;**24**: 110–1; n = 1, *J Clin Psychopharmacol* 2006;**26**: 439–40)

- • CNS — antiparkinsonian drugs

Amantadine (n = 1, *J Clin Psychiatry* 1989; **50**:143–4)

Bromocriptine (n = 600, incidence 1.3%, *Br Med J* 1984;**289**:1101–3; postpartum mania, n = 1, *J Gynecol Obstet Biol Reprod* [Paris] 2006;**35**:79–81)

Levodopa (e.g. *N Engl J Med* 1971;**285**:1326)

Levodopa + carbidopa (*J Clin Psychopharmacol* 1985;**5**:338–9)

Pramipexole (n = 1, *Am J Psychiatry* 2007;**164**: 351)

Procyclidine abuse (e.g. n = 1 and review, *Br J Psychiatry* 1982;**141**:81–4)

- • CNS — others *

Amfetamine withdrawal (*J Clin Psychiatry* 1980;**41**:33–4)

5

Atomoxetine (MHRA warning 2009; n = 1, *J Clin Psychopharmacol* 2004;**24**:567–8; n = 1, *Pediatrics* 2004;**114**:895–6)

Bromide (n = 1, *Am J Psychiatry* 1976;**133**:228–9)

Caffeine (*Gen Hosp Psychiatry* 2003;**25**:138–9)

Cannabis (n = 4815, dose–related increased risk, *J Affect Disord* 2006;**95**:103–10; comment by Skosnik, *EBMH* 2007;**10**:61; regular use increases illness severity, n = 3459, *J Nerv Ment Dis* 2009;**197**:35–40; n = 1, *Fortschr Neurol Psychiatr* 2010;**78**:223–5; n = 1 and review, *Tijdschr Psychiatr* 2009;**51**:859–63)

Cyclizine

Dexamfetamine (n = 1 and review, *Am J Psychiatry* 1976;**133**:1177–80)

Disulfiram (*J Am Acad Child Adolesc Psychiatry* 1988;**27**:500–3; high dose n = 1, *J Clin Psychopharmacol* 2007;**27**:224–5)

Donepezil (n = 1, *Int Psychogeriatr* 2011; **23**:503–4)

Fenfluramine (e.g. *Am J Psychiatry* 1997;**154**:711)

Ginseng (n = 1, *Acta Psychiatr Scand* 2002;**105**: 76–8)

LSD (n = 1, *Am J Psychiatry* 1981;**138**:1508–9)

Methylphenidate (n = 1, *J Clin Psychiatry* 1986;**47**:566–7; see also n = 137, *Psychopharmacol Bull* 2008;**41**:37–47)

Modafinil (n = 1, *Am J Psychiatry* 2005;**162**:813–4; n = 1, *J Clin Psychiatry* 2006;**67**:1817 see also n = 137, *Psychopharmacol Bull* 2008;**41**:37–47)

Nicotine withdrawal (n = 1, *Am J Psychiatry* 1992;**149**:708; n = 1, *Am J Psychiatry* 1990; **147**:1254–5)

Sibutramine (n = 1, *Int J Neuropsychopharmacol* 2002;**5**:283–4; in OTC diet aid, n=1, *Turk Psikiyatri Derg* 2010;**21**:335-7)

Silbutramine + citalopram (n = 1, *J Clin Psychiatry* 2002;**63**:165)

Varenicline (n=1, *Ir Med J* 2010;**103**:286; n = 1, relapse of pre–existing bipolar, *J Clin Psychiatry* 2007;**68**:1269–70; n = 1, bipolar patient, *Clin Neuropharmacol* 2009; **32**:117–8)

- **Gastrointestinal drugs**

H2 blockers, e.g.:

→ cimetidine (n = 2, *J Clin Psychiatry* 1983; **44**:267–8)

→ famotidine (n = 1, *Pharmacopsychiatry* 2002;**35**:992–4)

→ ranitidine oral (n = 1, after 2/7, *Am J Psychiatry* 1988;**145**:271)

→ ranitidine IV (case in *South Med J* 1987; **80**:1467)

Metoclopramide (n = 1, *J Clin Psychiatry* 1984; **45**:180–1)

- **Cardiovascular drugs**

ACE inhibitors e.g.:

→ captopril (several e.g. n = 1, *Am J Psychiatry* 1993;**150**:1429–30)

→ lisinopril (n = 1, *Psychosomatics* 1995; **36**:508–9)

Beta-blockers, e.g.:

→ propranolol (*South Med J* 1984;**77**:1603)

→ propranolol withdrawal (n = 1, *Am J Psychiatry* 1986;**143**:1633)

Calcium-channel blockers, e.g.:

→ diltiazem (*Clin Cardiology* 1984;**7**:611–2; n = 1, *Clin Cardiol* 1986;**9**:39)

Clonidine (n = 1, *Am J Psychiatry* 1982;**139**:1083)

Clonidine withdrawal (*J Clin Psychopharmacol* 1981;**1**: 93–5; n = 1, *Am J Psychiatry* 1984; **141**:993)

Digoxin (*Med J Rec* 1929;**130**:381–2)

Hydralazine

Isosorbides (*Adv Psych Treat* 2005;**11**:66)

Methyldopa withdrawal (n = 1, *Am J Psychiatry* 1989;**146**:1075–6)

Omega-3 fatty acids (n = 1, *Arch Gen Psychiatry* 2000;**57**:715–6)

Procainamide (n = 1, *Am J Psychiatry* 1988;**145**: 129–30)

- **Respiratory drugs**

Alimemazine (rare cases)

Aminophylline

Beclomethasone aerosol (n = 1, in stable bipolar person, *Am J Psychiatry* 1989;**146**:1076–7)

Beclomethasone nasal spray (n = 1, *Br J Psychiatry* 1989;**155**:871–2)

Cyproheptadine (rare, e.g. *Am J Psychiatry* 1980; **137**:378–9)

Dextromethorphan (*Psychosomatics* 1996;**37**: 71–4; *Psychosomatics* 1996;**37**:571–3)

Dextromethorphan abuse (cases in *Br Med J* 1986;**293**:597; *Br Med J* 1993;**306**:896)

Ephedrine (*J Clin Psychopharmacol* 1983;**3**:97–100; and in a herbal diet supplement, n = 1, *Am J Psychiatry* 1995;**152**:647)

Phenylephrine (*Am J Psychiatry* 1981;**138**:837–8)

Phenylpropanolamine (n = 3, *Am J Psychiatry* 1981;**138**:392)

Pseudoephedrine (several e.g. n = 1, *Tijdschr Psychiatr* 2007;**49**:125–9; n = 1, *NZ Med J* 2002;**199**:86)

Salbutamol

- **Anti-infection drugs** *
Generally low risk, most commonly with (in decreasing order) clarithromycin, ciprofloxacin, ofloxacin, then co-trimoxazole, metronidazole and erythromycin. It can be enduring in a very few people.

Reviews: short review, *Prescrire Int* 2003;**12**:183; n = 103, Abouesh *et al*, *J Clin Psychopharmacol* 2002;**22**:71–81.

Antituberculous drugs (*Lancet* 1989;**ii**:735–6)

Chloroquine (several e.g. n = 6, *Int J Psychiatry Med* 1993;**23**:349–56)

Ciprofloxacin (*Psychosomatics* 2007;**48**:363)

Clarithromycin (n = 1, *Acta Psychiatr Scand* 2010;**122**:267–8; n = 1, *Int J Neuropsychopharmacol* 2004;**7**:99–100)

Dapsone (n = 1, *Br Med J* 1989;**298**:1524)

Efavirenz overdose (n = 1, *Clin Infect Dis* 2001; **33**:270–1)

Ethambutol (n = 1, *Med J Aust* 1996;**164**:445–6)

Foscarnet sodium (*Adv Psychiatr Treat* 2005; **11**:66)

Isoniazid (n = 5, *Br Med J* 1957;**ii**:743–6)

Isoniazid (aka isonicotinic acid hydrazine) and pyridoxine (*Can J Psychiatry* 1988;**33**:675–6)

Ketoconazole (*Adv Psychiatr Treat* 2005;**11**:66)

Mefloquine (n = 1, *South Med J* 2008;**101**:550–1; n = 1, child, *J Child Neurol* 2009;**24**:1008–9; n = 1, *J Clin Psychopharmacol* 2010;**30**:339–41)

Mepacrine (*Mayo Clin Proc* 1989;**64**:129)

Oseltamivir (n = 1, *Am J Psychiatry* 2010; **167**:350)

Quinacrine (n = 1, *Mayo Clin Proc* 1989;**64**: 129–30)

Tetracyclines (*Adv Psychiatr Treat* 2005;**11**:66)

Valaciclovir (n = 1, *Psychosomatics* 2009;**50**:293–6)

Zidovudine (*JAMA* 1988;**259**:3406; n = 2, *Med J Aust* 1989;**150**:339–41)

- **Endocrine system drugs** *
Review: steroid-induced mania (risk factors; *Can J Clin Pharmacol* 2001;**8**:109–12)

Adrenocorticotropin (*Psychosomatic Med* 1953;**15**:280–91)

Androgens (*J Clin Psychiatry* 1985;**46**:354–5)

Clomifene (n = 1, *Psychosomatics* 2007;**48**:65–6)

Corticosteroids (incidence may be as high as 5–6% in adults, usually emerges within a few days or weeks, risk may be higher with higher doses, *MHRA Drug Safety Update* 2007;1–9; may respond to quetiapine, *Can J Psychiatry* 2005;**50**:77–8):

- → cortisone (*Psychosomat Med* 1953;**15**: 589–97)
- → deflazacort (SmPC)
- → dexamethasone (incidence up to 31%, *Arch Gen Psychiatry* 1981;**38**:471–7; n = 1, *Psychopharmacol Bull* 2010;**43**:82–5)
- → hydrocortisone (*J Nerv Ment Dis* 1979; **167**:229–36; n = 1, *Postgrad Med J* 1992; **68**:41–3)
- → prednisolone + clarithromycin (n = 1, *Can J Psychiatry* 1997;**42**:778)
- → prednisone (*J Affect Disord* 1983;**5**:319–24)
- → prednisone + bromocriptine (n = 1, *Gen Hosp Psychiatry* 1991;**13**:345–6)
- → triamcinolone (rare cases)

Dehydroepiandrosterone DHEA (dehydroepiandrosterone, prasterone) (e.g. n = 1, *Encephale* 2002;**28**:563–6; n = 1, *Ann Pharmacother* 2000;**34**:1419–22)

HRT (n = 1, *Am J Geriatr Psychiatry* 1997;**5**: 179–81)

Levothyroxine (n = 1, *J Am Acad Child Adolesc Psychiatry* 2005;**44**:211)

Quinagolide (n = 1, *Gen Hosp Psychiatry* 2007; **29**:464)

Testosterone patches (n = 1, *Am J Psychiatry* 1999;**156**:969)

Triiodothyronine (*J Clin Psychiatry* 1986;**47**:521–32)

- **Malignancy and immunosuppressant drugs** *
Anastrozole (n = 1, *Bipolar Disord* 2006;**8**:516–8)

Ciclosporin (*Biol Psychiatry* 1984;**19**:1161–2)

Interferons (*J Postgrad Med* 2007;**53**:990; *Can J Psychiatry* 2004;**49**:867–8), e.g.:

- → interferon alfa (n = 93, incidence 16%, *J Clin Psychiatry* 2005;**66**:1050–7; n = 1, *J Postgrad Med* 2006; **52**:207–9; n = 4, *Cancer* 2000;**89**:356–62; n = 1, *Ir J Med Sci* 2007;**176**:137–9)
- → interferon alfa withdrawal (n = 44, incidence 5%, *Arch Gen Psychiatry* 1998;**55**:88–9; n = 1, *Psychiatry Clin Neurosci* 2002;**56**:647–8)
- → interferon-alfa-2b (n = 1, *Afr J Psychiatry (Johannesbg)* 2009;**12**:227–8)

→ peginterferon + ribavirin (n = 1, *Am J Psychiatry* 2004;**161**:429)

Letrozole (n = 1, *Bipolar Disord* 2006;**8**:516–8)

Leuprolide (e.g. n = 1, *J Clin Psychiatry* 2010;**71**:1696–8)

Procarbazine (*Br Med J* 1982;**284**:82)

Triptorelin (n = 1, *Br J Psychiatry* 1999;**175**;290–1)

- Musculoskeletal and analgesics *

Baclofen (e.g. *Biol Psychiatry* 1982;**17**:757–9; inc high-dose, e.g. n = 1, *J Clin Psychopharmacol* 1992;**12**:299–7)

Baclofen withdrawal (n = 1, *Am J Psychiatry* 1980; **137**:1466–7)

Indometacin (*J Clin Psychopharmacol* 1987;**7**: 203–4)

Infliximab (n = 1, *Psychiatry Clin Neurosci* 2010; **64**:442–3)

- Others

Aspartame high–dose (n = 1, *Psychosomatics* 1986;**27**:218–20)

Calcium IV (*J Nerv Ment Dis* 1980;**168**: 562–3)

Decongestants

Energy drink containing caffeine, taurine and inositol (*Can J Psychiatry* 2001;**46**:454–5)

Herbal remedies (n = 1, *Am J Psychiatry*1998; **155**:1627)

Horny Goat weed (n = 1, *Psychosomatics* 2004;**45**:536–7)

Inositol (n = 3, *Am J Psychiatry* 1996;**153**:839)

Ma–hung (a herb in weight–loss supplements n = 1, *Pharmacotherapy* 2003;**23**:380–3)

Metrizamide (*N C Med J* 1984;**45**:759)

Sildenafil (relapse, n = 1, *Int J Neuro-psychopharmacol* 2004;**7**:525)

Yohimbine? (see *Arch Gen Psychiatry* 1998; **55**:1033–44)

5.8 MOVEMENT DISORDERS, EXTRA-PYRAMIDAL DISORDERS

Four distinct types of drug-induced extra-pyramidal or movement disorders are common, especially with antipsychotics. These are dystonias, akathisias, pseudoparkinsonism and dyskinesias. All can occur acutely or be delayed (tardive). Acute reactions are usually at the start of treatment or after a dose increase and are usually reversible. The tardive forms are not invariably reversible on discontinuation

of the drug or on dose reduction and can be aggravated by anticholinergics.

Reviews: causes (Thanvi and Treadwell, *Postgrad Med J* 2009;**85**:322–6; Susatia and Fernandez, *Curr Treat Options Neurol* 2009;**11**:162–9).

5.8.1 PSEUDOPARKINSONISM

Pseudoparkinsonism is characterised by akinesia, tremor and rigidity, and generally occurs within a month of the start of treatment.

Reviews: postural induced-tremor in psychiatry (Arbaizar *et al*, *Psychiatry Clin Neurosci* 2008; **62**:638–45), extensive (Mena and de Yébenes, *Expert Opin Drug Saf* 2006;**5**:759–71), in the elderly (Esper and Factor, *Mov Disord* 2008; **23**: 401–4).

- CNS — antipsychotics *

Review: * meta-analysis of SGA head-to-head studies (s = 54, Rummel-Kluge *et al*, *Schizophr Bull* 2011; in press)

Aripiprazole (many cases, e.g. n = 1, *Encephale* 2009;**35**:496–8; *J Psychopharmacol* 2008; **28**:352–3; n = 2, *J Med Case Reports* 2009; **3**:6448)

Chlorpromazine (n = 1, *Psychiatr Pol* 2007;**41**: 495–501)

Clozapine (n = 1, *Ann Pharmacother* 2000;**34**: 615–8)

Lithium

→ short-term (*J Neurol Sci* 2000;**176**: 78–9)

→ long-term (several e.g. n = 2, *Tijdschr Psychiatr* 2009; **51**:123–7)

→ toxicity (n = 1, *Acta Neurol Taiwan* 2007; **16**;231–3)

Olanzapine overdose (n = 1, *Am J Psychiatry* 1998;**155**:1630–1)

Risperidone (may be plasma level/CYP2D6 phenotype dependent, n = 50, *Eur J Pharm Sci* 2010;**41**:289–98)

Ziprasidone IM (n = 1, *Am J Psychiatry* 2005; **23**:92–3)

- CNS — antidepressants *

Review: * (n = 89, *Ann Clin Psychiatry* 2010;**22**:148–56; of which 66% were for duloxetine).

Bupropion (*J Clin Psychopharmacol* 2009;**29**:616–8; *Mov Disord* 2007;**22**:1830–1)

Duloxetine (see above)

MAOIs

Mirtazapine (*J Pain Symptom Manage* 2008;**36**: 5–6)

SSRIs (annual incidence may be around 0.1– 0.2%; Gerber and Lynd, *Ann Pharmacother* 1998;**32**:692–8):

→ fluoxetine (n = 21, *Parkinsonism Relat Disord* 2002;**8**:325–7; mean latency for tremor 54 days, mild and remitted in 50% over a mean of 35 days after discontinuation; n = 1, *Ann Gen Psychiatry* 2010;**9**:5)

→ fluoxetine withdrawal (n = 1, *Am J Psychiatry* 1991;**148**:1263)

→ paroxetine (cases reported in *Current Problems* 1993;**19**:1; incidence as with other SSRIs, *Lancet* 1993;**341**:624)

→ sertraline (n = 1, *Am J Psychiatry* 1994; **151**:288)

→ sertraline and oxycodone (n = 1, *J Clin Pharmacol* 2001;**41**:224)

Trazodone (e.g. n = 1, *Nephron* 2002;**90**:222–3)

Tricyclics

● CNS — analgesics

Nabilone

Pethidine and other opioids

● CNS — anticonvulsants *

Carbamazepine (incidence of tremor may be 22%, *NEJM* 1992;**327**:765–71; CBZ + lithium, n = 1, *Clin Neuropharmacol* 2010;**33**:102–3)

Lacosamide (common, SmPC)

Lamotrigine (n = 1, *Mov Disord* 2006;**21**:2269–70)

Levetiracetam (n = 1, *Clin Neuropharmacol* 2005;**28**:188–90; n = 1, *Clin Neuropharmacol* 2006;**29**:303–4)

Oxcarbazepine (n = 1, *Parkinsonism Relat Disord* 2009;**15**:787–8)

Phenytoin (n = 1, *Singapore Med J* 2006;**47**:981–3)

Pregabalin (n = 1, *Clin Neuropharmacol* 2009; **32**:353–4)

Rufinamide (incidence 1–10%, UK SmPC)

Topiramate + fluvoxamine (n = 1, *Clin Neuro-pharmacol* 2008;**31**:366–7)

Valproate (incidence 5–10%, especially if for > 3 years, *Mov Disord* 2007;**22**:130–3; mechanism unclear as usually unresponsive to levodopa; *Parkinsonism Relat Disord* 1999;**5**:67–8; n = 10, *Pharmacopsychiatry* 2006;**39**:9–12; n = 1, *Ned Tijdschr Geneeskd* 2009;**153**:336)

Zonisamide (SmPC)

● CNS — antiparkinsonian drugs

Bromocriptine

Levodopa

● CNS — others

Anticholinesterases:

→ donepezil (n = 1, *Ann Pharmacother* 1998; **32**:610–1)

→ rivastigmine

Atomoxetine + venlafaxine (n = 1, *Clin Toxicol [Phila]* 2007;**45**:182–5)

Cocaine abuse (*Arch Internal Med* 1997; **157**:241; as a risk factor, review, n = 106, *Psychopharmacol Bull* 2008;**41**:5–10)

Cyclizine

Dexamfetamine

Metoclopramide (n = 1, *J Perianesth Nurs* 2008; **23**:292–9)

Ondansetron (*Ann Pharmacother* 1994; **28**:280; *Ann Pharmacother* 1996;**30**:196)

Tetrabenazine

● Gastrointestinal drugs

Cimetidine (n = 1, possible, *Postgrad Med J* 1982;**58**:527–8)

Domperidone (rare, case in *Helv Paediatr Acta* 1984;**39**:285–8)

Metoclopramide (incidence 2–30%, cases in, e.g. *Ann Int Med* 1989;**149**:2486–92)

Prochlorperazine (common, e.g. *Lancet* 1984; **2**:1082–3)

● Cardiovascular drugs

Review: calcium-channel blockers as cause of EPS (*Ann Pharmacother* 1995;**29**:73–5)

Amiodarone (*Ann Neurol* 1989;**25**:630–2)

Diazoxide (n = 6, *Br Med J* 1973;**3**:474–5)

Diltiazem (*Am J Med* 1989;**87**:95–6)

Flunarizine (*Arq Neuropsiquiatr* 2004;**62**:784–8)

Methyldopa (*Can Med Assoc J* 1966; **95**:928)

Metirosine

Mexilitine

Nifedipine (*Br Med J* 1978;**i**:1619)

Tocainide

Trimetazidine (8% incidence, n = 258, *Therapie* 2005;**60**:419–22)

● Respiratory drugs

Antihistamines:

→ brompheniramine (*NEJM* 1975;**293**:486)

→ cinnarizine (*Arq Neuropsiquiatr*

5

2004;**62**:784–8; *Lancet* 1987;**i**:1324; n = 1, *Rev Neurol* 1999;**28**:876–8)

→ diphenhydramine (*NEJM* 1977;**296**:111)

Montelukast (FDA warning 2009)

Orciprenaline

Promethazine (*Clin Pharm* 1984;**3**:83)

Salbutamol

Terbutaline

Zafirlukast (FDA warning 2009)

- Anti-infection drugs *

Aciclovir

Cephaloridine

Chloroquine

Itraconazole (n = 216, incidence 2%, 20/12, *J Neurol Neurosurg Psychiatry* 2010;**81**:327–9)

- Endocrine system drugs

Mecasermin (rare, UK SmPC)

Medroxyprogesterone

Prednisolone (increases incidence with neuroleptics, review in *JAMA* 1973;**224**:889)

- Malignancy and immunosuppressant drugs

Ciclosporin (n = 1, *Transplant Proc* 2008; **40**:2823–4; 13% point prevalence, n = 60, *Arq Neuropsiquiatr* 2005;**63**:592–6)

Interferons

→ peginterferon-IFN-a 2a (n = 1, *Arq Neuro Psiquiatr* 2009;**67**:715–6)

Nelarabine (very common, SmPC)

Octreotide high-dose (n = 1, *Neurology* 2008; **70**:2345–6)

- Musculoskeletal and analgesics

Etodolac (SmPC)

Fenoprofen

Flurbiprofen (*Br Med J* 1990;**300**:549)

Ibuprofen (n=1, *Postgrad Med J* 1987;**63**:593–4)

Indometacin

Mefenamic acid (n = 1, *J Roy Soc Med* 1983;**76**:35)

Sulindac (n=1, *Ann Neurol* 1985;**17**:104–5)

- Others *

Distigmine bromide (n = 1, *Rinsho Shinkeigaku* 2005;**45**:600–2)

Ethylene glycol + methanol (n = 2, *Clin Pharmacol Ther* 2007;**81**:114–21)

Manganese intoxication (*Chang Gung Med J* 2007;**30**:385–95; review *Neurotoxicology*

2006;**27**:340–6)

Organophosphates (chlorpyrifos overdose; n = 1, *Clin Toxicol (Phila)* 2005;**43**:877–9; incl. Pesticides; n=781, some association between PD and professional pesticide exposure, *Ann Neurol* 2009;**66**:494–504)

5.8.2 AKATHISIA

Characterised by motor restlessness, with an inability to stay still. Onset is around 6–60 days and has been implicated with all antipsychotics, but especially with the high potency ones.

Reviews: * (Kumar and Sachdev, *Curr Opin Psychiatry* 2009;**22**:293–99; Poyurovsky, *Br J Psychiatry* 2010;**96**:89–91).

- CNS — anxiolytics and hypnotics

Alprazolam

Buspirone (several e.g. n = 1, *J Clin Psychopharmacol* 1988;**8**:296–7)

Lorazepam (n = 1, *Oncology* 1990;**47**:415–7)

Melatonin withdrawal (*Mov Disord* 1999; **14**:381–2)

- CNS — antipsychotics *

Review: akathisia is observed with all antipsychotics, but is more common in bipolar than schizophrenia (s = 77, Kane *et al, J Clin Psychiatry* 2009;**70**:627–43).

Aripiprazole (occurs early, is mild-to-moderate severity, leads to few discontinuations and does not compromise efficacy; e.g. n = 4967, *J Psychopharmacol* 2010;**24**:1019–29; n = 1, *J Clin Psychopharmacol* 2011;**31**:134–5)

Clozapine (incidence 6% claimed: *Psychopharmacology* 1995;**118**:52–6; acute nocturnal, n = 1, *J Clin Psychopharmacol* 2007;**27**:205)

Haloperidol (review in *Psychopharmacol* 1985; **21**:69–72)

Lithium (n = 1, *J Neurol Sci* 2000;**176**:78–9)

Olanzapine (incidence 6%)

Pipotiazine (study in *Curr Ther Res* 1981;**29**: 903–14)

Prochlorperazine (n = 140, incidence 44% with IV, *Ann Emerg Med* 1999;**34**:469–75)

Promazine

Quetiapine (e.g. n=1, *Indian J Pharmacol* 2010;**42**:416-7; n = 1, *Aust N Z J Psychiatry* 2006;**40**:607–8)

Risperidone (*Neurology* 1995;**45**:14–9)

Risperidone withdrawal (n = 1, *Am J Psychiatry* 1997;**154**:437–8; n = 2, *Actas Esp Psiquiatr* 2002;**30**:195–7)

Risperidone + levomepromazine (n = 1, *Eur Psychiatry* 2002;**17**:294–5)

Sulpiride (n = 1, *Clin Neuropharmacol* 1994; **17**:481–3)

Ziprasidone dose reduction (n = 5, *Am J Psychiatry* 2006;**163**:546)

Zuclopenthixol (study in *Pharmatherapeutica* 1989;**5**:380–6)

● CNS — antidepressants *

Review: SSRI–induced akathisia (Koliscak and Makela, *J Am Pharm Assoc (2003)* 2009;**49**:e28–36).

Mianserin (n = 1, *J Clin Psychopharmacol* 2010; **30**:338–9; n = 1 after 20 years continuous treatment, *Clin Neuropharmacol* 2010;**33**:50–1)

Mirtazapine (*Med J Aust* 2002;**176**:242; n = 1, *J Clin Psychopharmacol* 2008;**28**:467; after 20 years, n = 1, *Clin Neuropharmacol* 2010; **33**:50–1)

SSRIs, e.g.:
→ citalopram (n = 1, *J Clin Psychiatry* 1988; **49**[Suppl]:18–22; n = 1, *PMR* 2010;**2**:973-5)
→ fluoxetine (e.g. *J Clin Psychiatry* 1991; **52**:491–3; n = 1, dose dependent, *J Psychopharmacol* 2003;**17**:451–2)
→ paroxetine (n = 3, *Compr Psychiatry* 1996; **37**:122–4; *Can J Psychiatry* 2000; **45**:398)
→ sertraline (n = 1, *Am J Psychiatry* 1993;**150**:986–7; mistaken for panic attack, n = 1, *Psychiatr Serv* 2002;**53**:1477–8)

Tricyclics (*Br Med J* 1986;**292**:1529), e.g.:
→ imipramine (n = 1, *J Clin Psychopharmacol* 1987;**7**:254–7)
→ nortriptyline (*Am Fam Physician* 1993; **48**:1024–6)
→ tricyclics and conjugated estrogens (n = 3, *Am J Psychiatry* 1984;**141**:696–7)

Venlafaxine withdrawal (n = 1, *Am Fam Physician* 1997;**56**:455–62)

Venlafaxine + methimazole (n = 1, *Gen Hosp Psychiatry* 2009;**31**:388–90)

● CNS — analgesics

Sumatriptan (n = 1, *J Neurol* 1997;**244**:131–2)

● CNS — anticonvulsants

Carbamazepine (n = 1, *Am J Psychiatry* 1986; **143**:1190–1; *NZ Med J* 1992;**105**:182)

Ethosuximide (n = 1, *Am J Dis Child* 1978; **132**:527–8)

● CNS — antiparkinsonian drugs

Levodopa (review in *Neurology* 1990;**40**:340–5)

● CNS — others *

Alcohol (as trigger factor, *JAMA* 1976; **236**:2422–3)

Antiemetics, e.g. metoclopramide and prochlorperazine (many cases, e.g. n = 3, *Gan To Kagaku Ryoho* 2006;**33**:267–9; n = 56, *Acad Emerg Med* 2007;**14**:799–21)

Cocaine (recent use is a risk factor for antipsychotic-induced, n = 106, *Psychopharmacol Bull* 2008;**41**:5–10)

Methysergide (n = 1, *Clin Neuropharmacol* 1988;**11**:87–9)

Metoclopramide (e.g. n = 1, *Pharm World Sci* 2010;**32**:704–6)

Ondansetron (n = 1, *Cancer* 1992;**69**:1275)

● Cardiovascular drugs

Atenolol (n = 1, *J Clin Psychopharmacol* 1986; **6**:390)

Diltiazem (n = 1, *Ann Intern Med* 1983;**99**:794)

Flunarizine (n = 1, *Rev Clin Esp* 1991;**188**:384)

Midodrine + promethazine (n = 1, *JAMA* 2006;**295**:2000–1)

Trimetazidine (n = 1, *Therapie* 2005;**60**:603–5)

Verapamil (*Lancet* 1991;**338**:893)

● Respiratory drugs

Alimemazine

Cinnarizine (n = 1, *Rev Neurol* 1999;**28**:876–8)

Promethazine + midodrine (n = 1, *JAMA* 2006; **295**:2000–1)

● Malignancy and immunosuppressant drugs

Interferon alfa (*Gen Hosp Psychiatry* 1999; **21**:134–5)

5.8.3 DYSTONIAS

Dystonias includes oculogyric crisis, trismus and torticollis. They may occur within 72 hours of start of therapy and occur more frequently with high-potency antipsychotics.

5

Review: general (van Harten *et al*, *Br Med J* 1999;**319**:623–6, 34 refs).

- CNS — anxiolytics and hypnotics
Benzodiazepines, e.g.:
  → bromazepam (n = 1, *Biomed Pharmacother* 1992;**46**:375–6)
  → diazepam (n = 2, *J Emerg Med* 1988;**6**: 491–3)
  → midazolam (*Br Med J* 1990;**300**:614)
Buspirone (n = 1, *Neurology* 1990;**40**:1904; discussion in *Neurology* 1991;**41**:1850)

- CNS — antipsychotics *
Review: n = 43, *Int J Neuropsychopharmacol* 2001; **4**:393–7.

Amisulpride (e.g. n=1, *Prog Neuropsycho-pharmacol Biol Psychiatry* 2010;**34**:412–3; low dose n = 1, *J Clin Psychopharmacol* 2008;**28**:573–4)

Aripiprazole (many cases, e.g. n=1, *J Clin Psychiatry* 2010;**71**:652–3; n = 1, *J Am Acad Child Adolesc Psychiatry* 2007;**46**:306–7; n = 1, after single dose, *Am J Addict* 2007;**16**:244; n = 1, *Tijdschr Psychiatr* 2009;**51**:761–5)

Clozapine (rare, n = 1, *Am J Psychiatry* 1995;**152**:647–8; n = 1, *Am J Psychiatry* 1994;**151**:1096; occulygyric crisis, n = 3, *Clin Drug Investig* 2007;**27**:861–4)

Clozapine withdrawal, abrupt (cases, *J Clin Psychiatry* 1998;**59**:472–7)

Flupentixol decanoate (n = 1, *Br Med J* 1981; **282**:1756)

Fluspirilene (n = 1, *Nervenarzt* 1994;**65**:647)

Haloperidol (n = 62, incidence 37%, in first episode, *Am J Psychiatry* 1994;**151**:1819–21; *Rev Esp Anaetesiol Reanim* 2004;**51**:229–31)

Lithium (n = 1, *Neurol India* 2002;**50**:473–5)

Loxapine

Olanzapine (n = 1, *Am J Psychiatry* 1999; **156**:1662; tardive n = 1, *Neurol Sci* 2001; **22**:331–2; n = 1, *J Clin Psychopharmacol* 2006;**26**:431; *J Clin Psychiatry* 1998;**59**:384)

Olanzapine overdose (n = 1, *J Emerg Med* 2006; **30**:311–7)

Paliperidone (dystonic dysphagia, n = 1, *J Neuropsychiatry Clin Neurosci* 2010;**22**:451)

Pimozide (low-dose n = 1, *J Am Acad Child Adolesc Psychiatry* 1993;**32**:640–2; n = 1, delayed by 12 hours in child, *J Toxicol Clin Toxicol* 2004;**42**:977–81)

Prochlorperazine

Quetiapine (several, e.g. n = 1, *Aust N Z J Psychiatry* 2006;**40**:607–8; n = 1, *J Am Geriatr Soc* 2009;**57**:918–9)

Risperidone (e.g. may be plasma level/CYP2D6 phenotype dependent, n=50, *Eur J Pharm Sci* 2010;**41**:289-98; persistent, n = 1, *Psychiatr Danub* 2008; **20**:329–31)

Sulpiride (n = 1, *Clin Neuropharmacol* 1991; **14**:463–4)

Ziprasidone (several e.g. 240mg/d, n = 1, *Prog Neuropsychopharmacol Biol Psychiatry* 2007;**31**:546–7; n = 2, *J Clin Psychiatry* 2006;**67**:326–7)

Zuclopenthixol (study in *Acta Psychiatr Scand* 1991;**84**:14–6)

Zuclopenthixol acetate + fluoxetine (laryngeal, n = 1, *Australas Psychiatry* 2010;**18**:174–6)

- CNS — antidepressants *
Amoxapine (n=1, *Indian J Psychiatry* 2009; **51**:327)

Bupropion (BNF, rare; cases e.g. n = 1, *Ann Pharmacother* 2002; **36**:251–4; *J Clin Psychopharmacol* 2009;**29**:616–8)

Bupropion abrupt withdrawal (n = 1, *Prog Neuropsychopharmacol Biol Psychiatry* 2007; **31**:766–8)

Duloxetine (n = 1, *Gen Hosp Psychiatry* 2010;**32**: 646)

MAOIs, e.g.:
  → phenelzine (n = 1, *J Clin Psychopharmacol* 1990;**10**:144–5)
  → tranylcypromine (n = 1, *J Clin Psychopharmacol* 1989;**9**:229–30)

Mirtazapine (n = 1, *J Clin Psychiatry* 2002; **63**:452–3; n=1, *Tijdschr Psychiatr* 2006: **48**:153–7; *Tijdschr Psychiatr* 2006;**48**:993–7)

SSRIs, e.g.:
  → citalopram (dystonic rabbit syndrome; n = 2, *Clin Neuropharmacol* 2005;**28**:289–91)
  → escitalopram (*Clin Neuropharmacol* 2007; **30**:124–6; n = 1, *Int Arch Allergy Immunol* 2006;**140**:27–9)
  → fluoxetine (e.g. n = 1, *Mov Disorder* 2001;**16**:767–9; n = 1, *Rev Neurol* 2004; **38**:99; n = 1, persistent, *Intern Med J* 2008; **38**:672–4)
  → fluvoxamine (*J Clin Psychopharmacol* 1993; **13**:220–1)

→ paroxetine (cases reviewed in *Curr Prob* 1993;**19**:1; n = 1, *J Psychopharmacol* 2002; **16**:395–7)

→ paroxetine withdrawal (n = 1, *Rev Neurol* 2008;**46**:253–4)

→ sertraline (n = 1, *J Clin Psychopharmacol* 1999;**19**:98–100; mistaken for panic attack, n = 1, *Psychiatr Serv* 2002;**53**:1477–8)

Tricyclics, e.g.:

→ amitriptyline (*J Neurol Neurosurg Psychiatry* 1992;**55**:414)

→ amitriptyline and doxepin (n = 1, *Am J Psychiatry* 1988;**145**:649)

→ clomipramine withdrawal (*Aust NZ J Psychiatry* 2001;**35**:696)

Venlafaxine (n = 1, *Mov Disord* 2010;**25**:506–7)

- CNS — analgesics *

Ergotamine (*Mov Disord* 1991;**6**:263–4; *Mov Disord* 1992;**7**:188–9)

Opioid withdrawal (n = 1, *Prog Neuropsychopharmacol Biol Psychiatry* 2011;**35**:640)

Sumatriptan (BNF, very rare; e.g. n = 1, *Ann Pharmacother* 1994;**28**:1199; n = 1, *Cephalagia* 1998;**18**:360–1)

- CNS — anticonvulsants

Carbamazepine (several e.g. n = 1, *Gen Hosp Psychiatry* 2002; **24**:114–5; n = 1, oculogyric crisis, *J Neurosurg* 2008;**109**:944–5)

Gabapentin (n = 1, *Ann Pharmacother* 2005; **39**:380–2; n = 1, possible case, *Br J Anaesth* 2007;**99**:218–20)

Midazolam (n = 1, *Br Med J* 1990;**300**:614)

Phenobarbital (n = 1, *Clin Pediatr (Phila)* 1992;**31**:252)

Phenytoin (n = 1, *Dev Med Child Neurol* 1984; **26**:677–8)

Tiagabine (n = 3, *Epilepsia* 2001;**42**:944–6)

- CNS — antiparkinsonian drugs

Benzatropine (n = 1, child, *Ann Emerg Med* 1986;**15**:594–6)

Bromocriptine (n = 5, *Neurology* 1993;**43**: 2319–22)

Entacapone (BNF, common)

Levodopa (BNF, common)

Rotigotine (BNF, less common)

Tetrabenazine (n = 4, *Ann Neurol* 1985;**17**: 200–2)

Tolcapone (BNF, common)

Trihexyphenidyl withdrawal (n = 1, *Mov Disord* 1989;**4**:349–53)

- CNS — others *

Amfetamine (risk factor with aripiprazole, *Prog Neuropsychopharmacol* 2008;**32**:1756–7)

Amfetamine + haloperidol (n = 2, *Br J Psychiatry* 1994;**165**:276)

Betahistine (n = 1, *Neurologia* 2000;**99**:417; n = 1, oromandibular dystonia after long-term use, *J Clin Neurosci* 2010;**17**:1330–1)

Clebopride (*Rev Neurol* 1997;**25**:2060)

Cocaine (including crack) in its own right or as a risk factor with dopamine-blocking drugs (n = 2, *Am J Emerg Med* 1997;**99**:513–5; n = 1, *South Med J* 1997;**90**:1050–2; n = 29, two years, *J Clin Psychiatry* 1998;**59**:128–30)

Cocaine withdrawal (*Neurology* 1989;**39**:996–7; *Neurology* 1990;**40**:863–4)

Cyclizine (e.g. *Anaesthesia* 2004;**59**:413–4; n = 1, *Anaesthesia* 2003;**58**:257–60)

Disulfiram (n = 1, *Mov Disord* 1991;**6**:166–70)

Domperidone (n = 1, *Mov Disord* 1991;**6**:79–81)

Donepezil (n = 1, cervical, *Rinsho Shinkeigaku* 2010;**50**:147–50)

MDMA/ecstasy (*Mov Disord* 2004;**19**:1386–7; n = 1, *Mov Disord* 1995;**10**:353)

Methamphetamine (n = 1, *Psychiatry Clin Neurosci* 2007;**61**:691–4)

Methylphenidate (n = 1, *J Child Neurol* 1994;**9**: 45–6)

Metoclopramide (BNF, less common; n = 2, *Tidsskr Nor Laegeforen* 2001;**121**:2162–3; incidence 3%, see *NEJM* 1983;**309**:433; cases in, e.g. *Ann Intern Med* 1989;**149**:2486–92)

Ondansetron (n = 1, *Ann Pharmacother* 2011; **45**:e7)

Prochlorperazine (e.g. controlled by hyoscine patch n = 1, *J Emerg Med* 2006;**30**:299–301; n = 1, *Ir J Med Sci* 2007;**176**:53–4)

Rivastigmine (n = 1, *Am J Health Syst Pharm* 2007;**64**:2468–70)

- Gastrointestinal drugs

Cimetidine (n = 1, *Ann Emerg Med* 1987; **16**: 1162–4; n = 1, *J Emerg Med* 2001; **21**:27–9)

Ranitidine (e.g. n = 1, *J La State Med Soc* 1997; **149**:36–8; n = 1, *Am J Emerg* 1999;**17**:258–60)

- Cardiovascular drugs

Amiodarone (isolated case in *Lancet* 1979; 1:81–2)

Flecainide (n = 1, *Mov Disord* 1992;**7**:62–3)

Midodrine + perphenazine (n = 1, *J Neurol* 2008; **255**:767–8)

Midodrine + risperidone (n = 1, *J Neuro- psychiatry Clin Neurosci* 2000;**12**:285–6)

Nifedipine (*Ann Intern Med* 1985;**104**:125)

Propranolol (n = 1, *Arch Neurol* 2000;**57**:570–1)

Verapamil (n = 1, *J Clin Pharmacy Ther* 1998;**23**: 79–80)

- Respiratory drugs

Alimemazine

Cetirizine (*Neurology* 2006;**66**:143–4; n = 1, *Pediatr Emerg Care* 2008;**24**:627–8)

Cinnarizine (n = 101, *Mov Disord* 1989;**4**:139–46)

Dextromethorphan (*J Toxicol Clin Toxicol* 1996; **34**:351–2)

Diphenhydramine:
- → oral (e.g. *Ann Intern Med* 1989;**111**:92–3; n = 1, *Pharmacotherapy* 1994;**14**:491–6)
- → IV (*Ann Intern Med* 1989;**111**:92–3)

Flunarizine (n = 101, *Mov Disord* 1989;**4**:139–46)

Phenylpropanolamine (*Clin Pediatr (Phila)* 1997; **36**:57–8)

Promethazine (n = 1, *Clin Pharm* 1984;**3**:83–5; n = 1, *Pediatr Emerg Care* 1987;**3**:91–2)

- Anti-infection drugs *

Chloroquine (with metronidazole; n = 1, *Drug Intell Clin Pharm* 1988;**22**:308–10)

Erythromycin (n = 1, *Am J Emerg Med* 1992; **10**:616)

Foscarnet (n = 1, *Am J Ther* 2008;**15**:184–6)

Gemifloxacin (n = 1, *Indian J Med Sci* 2009; **63**:557–60)

Lamivudine (n = 2, *Clin Neuropharmacol* 2005; **28**:193–4)

Quinine (*An Med Interna* 2003;**20**:650–1)

Spiramycin (n = 1, *Can J Psychiatry* 1997;**42**:665–6)

- Malignancy and immunosuppressant drugs

Capecitabine (n = 1, *Acta Oncol* 2008:**47**:1161–5)

Etoposide (n = 1, *Drug Intell Clin Pharm* 1988; **22**:41–2)

Peginterferon alfa (*Mov Disord* 2007;**22**:747–8)

- Musculoskeletal and analgesics

Azapropazone (n = 1, *J Neurol Neurosurg Psychiatry* 1988;**51**:731–2)

Indometacin (n = 1, *J Neurol Neurosurg Psychiatry* 1988;**51**:731–2)

Penicillamine (review, *Arch Neurol* 1987;**44**:490–3)

- Others

Acetazolamide (n = 1, *Eur J Neurol* 2000;**7**: 237–40)

Alfentanil (n = 1, *Anesth Analg* 1991;**72**:557–8)

Contrast Media (n = 1, *J Emerg Med* 2001; **21**:499–7)

Copper (n = 1, *Lancet* 1990;**335**:410)

Cyanide (n = 1, *J Neurol Neurosurg Psychiatry* 1992;**55**:198–9)

Insecticides (cholinesterase inhibitors, n = 1, *Drug Intell Clin Pharm* 1988;**22**:311–2)

Ketamine abuse (*Ann Emerg Med* 1982; **11**:673–5)

Permethrin (n = 1, *Pharmacotherapy* 2005;**25**: 448–50)

Propofol (BNF, very rare; n = 45, *Anesth Analg* 2002;**94**:1237–40; n = 1, *Paediatr Anaesth* 2005;**99**:597–601)

Propofol + fentanyl (n = 1, *Br J Anaesth* 2000;**84**: 828–9)

Sevoflurane (*Anaesthesiology* 1999;**90**:1299–6)

5.8.4 DYSKINESIAS

If (tardive) dyskinesia (TD) is of late onset, it can be a potentially irreversible movement disorder with possible relationship to drug, dose and duration (see 6.7).

Review: non-therapeutic risk factors (s = 8, Tenback *et al, Mov Disord* 2009;**24**:2304–15).

- CNS — anxiolytics and hypnotics

Buspirone (n = 1, *J Clin Psychopharmacol* 1988;**8**:296–7; n = 1, *J Clin Psychiatry* 1988; **49**:322–3; n = 2, *Mov Disord* 1993;**8**:331–4)

Midazolam (*Palliat Med* 2000;**14**:435–6)

- CNS — antipsychotics *

In a longitudinal study, the use of first or second generation antipsychotics gave a broadly similar incidence of tardive dyskinesia (n = 352, 4 years, Woods *et al, J Clin Psychiatry* 2010;**71**:463–74).

Amisulpride (e.g. n = 1, *Prog Neuropsychopharmacol Biol Psychiatry* 2010; **34**:728-9; n = 1, *J Neuropsychiatry Clin Neurosci* 2009;**21**:104–5)

Aripiprazole (n = 1, after 18/12 for refractory depression, *CNS Spect* 2006;**11**:435–9; n = 1, *Brain Inj* 2008;**22**:99–102; n = 2, *Prog Neuropsychopharmacol Biol Psychiatry* 2009;**33**:743–4; n=8, wasn't usually reversible on discontinuation, *Mov Disord* 2011;**26**:147-52)

Aripiprazole + tamoxifen (n = 1, *Am J Psychiatry* 2007;**164**:1436–7)

Clozapine (e.g. very low incidence, n=101, *World J Biol Psychiatry* 2009;**10**:919-24; n = 3, *Eur Psychiatry* 2003;**18**:260–1; n = 1, after 10 years, *Am J Psychiatry* 2003;**160**:588)

Clozapine withdrawal, abrupt (n = 4, *J Clin Psychiatry* 1998;**59**:472–7)

Flupentixol decanoate (*Psychopharmacol* 1983; **81**:359–62)

Haloperidol (many cases)

Lithium (n = 130, incidence 9%, *J Clin Psychiatry* 1996;**57**:22–8; n = 1, *J Neurol Sci* 2000;**176**:78–9)

Lithium + carbamazepine (n = 1, *J Clin Psychopharmacol* 1994;**14**:146–7)

Lithium + neuroleptics (n = 1, persistent, *Pharmacopsychiatry* 1998;**31**:201–4)

Loxapine

Olanzapine (e.g. n = 1, *J Clin Psychiatry* 1999; **60**:870; *J Neuropsychiatry Clin Neurosci* 2006;**18**:132; n = 1, *Psychiatry Clin Neurosci* 2003;**57**:605–6)

Pimozide (incidence 35% reported, probably rarer, *Neurology* 1982;**32**:335–6)

Quetiapine (several e.g. n = 1, oropharyngeal and facial dyskinesia, *J Clin Psychopharmacol* 2008;**28**:705–6; n = 1, *World J Biol Psychiatry* 2009;**10**:54–7)

Risperidone (many cases, e.g. n = 1, *Ann Pharmacother* 2000;**34**:1487–8; although a lower incidence has been reported in the elderly with low–dose, n = 330, RCT, open, 12/52, *Am J Psychiatry* 2000;**157**:1150–5; n = 1, *Neurol India* 2009;**57**:94–5)

Risperidone/citalopram abrupt withdrawal (n = 1, *Ann Pharmacother* 2000;**34**:269)

Sulpiride (*Clin Neuropharmacol* 1990;**13**:248–52)

Ziprasidone (e.g. n=1, *Natl Med J India* 2007;**20**: 271–2; n = 1, *Am J Psychiatry* 2004; **161**:175–6; *Can J Psychiatry* 2005;**50**:567–8)

• CNS — antidepressants *
Bupropion (*J Clin Psychiatry* 1997;**58**:218)

Duloxetine (n = 1, *Pharmacopsychiatry* 2006;**39**:237–8; n = 1, *Gen Hosp Psychiatry* 2010;**32**:646)

Mirtazapine (n = 1, *Mov Disord* 2005;**20**:771; n = 1, *Neurol India* 2010;**58**:672–3)

SSRIs (review of movement disorders caused by SSRIs; Leo, *J Clin Psychiatry* 1996;**57**:449–54):
  → citalopram (n = 1, *J Clin Psychiatry* 2007; **68**:803; n = 1, *PMR* 2010;**2**:973–5)
  → escitalopram + itopride (n = 1, *Prog Neuropsychopharmacol Biol Psychiatry* 2009;**33**:380–1)
  → fluoxetine (e.g. n = 5555, incidence 0.2%, *Am J Psychiatry* 1991;**148**:1403; n = 1, *Mov Disord* 1996;**11**:324–6; n = 3, *Psychiatr Serv* 1996;**47**:991–3)
  → fluoxetine + low dose haloperidol (n = 1, *Am J Psychiatry* 1991;**148**:683)
  → fluvoxamine (n = 1, *J Clin Psychopharmacol* 1993;**13**:365–6)
  → paroxetine (*J Clin Psychopharmacol* 1996; **16**:258–9)
  → paroxetine + sumatriptan (n = 1, persistent, *Biol Psychiatry* 1997;**42**:144–6)
  → sertraline (n = 1, *J Clin Psychopharmacol* 1997;**17**:138–9)

Tricyclics, e.g.:
  → clomipramine (n = 9, *Am J Psychiatry* 1993;**150**:165–6)
  → doxepin (10% incidence in study in *J Clin Psychopharmacol* 1987;**7**:243–6)

Venlafaxine

• CNS — analgesics
Fentanyl (*Mov Disorder* 1995;**10**:679–80)

• CNS — anticonvulsants *
Review: Zaatreh, *Expert Opin Drug Saf* 2003;**2**: 385–93.

Carbamazepine (n = 2, *Cleve Clin J Med* 1990; **57**:367–72)

Gabapentin (n = 1, *J Clin Psychopharmacol* 2001; **21**:623–4; n = 1, *Mov Disorder* 2007; **22**:288–9)

Lamotrigine (n = 1, *Eur J Neurol* 2010;**17**:e37)

Lamotrigine overdose (n = 1, *J Child Neurol* 2008; **23**:243)

Midazolam (*Palliat Med* 2000;**14**:435–6)

Oxcarbazepine (n = 1, *J Pediatr Neurosci* 2010; **5**:85–6)

Phenytoin (n = 1, *Arq Neuropsiquiatr* 1999;**57**: 356–60; *Indian Pediatr* 1998;**35**:274–6)

5

- CNS – antiparkinsonian drugs

Apomorphine abuse (n = 1, *Mov Disord* 2005; **20**:105–8)

Bromocriptine (n = 1, low–dose, *Acta Med Port* 1992;**5**:347)

Levodopa (common)

Trihexyphenidyl (n = 1, *Mov Disord* 1993;**8**:512–4)

- CNS — others *

Atomoxetine (n = 2, with other drugs, *Clin Toxicol (Phila)* 2007;**45**:182–5)

Benzatropine (study showed worsening TD — *Neuropsychobiology* 1980;**6**:109)

Cannabis (n = 51, *Schizophr Res* 1993;**11**:3–8)

Cocaine (recent use is a risk factor for antipsychotic-induced, n = 106, *Psychopharmacol Bull* 2008;**41**:5–10; n = 1, *Neurology* 2001;**56**:964–5; 1525)

Donepezil (*Ann Pharmacother* 2000;**34**:1347)

Diphenhydramine (n = 1, *Can J Psychiatry* 1985; **30**:370–1)

Methylphenidate (n = 1, *Prim Care Companion J Clin Psychiatry* 2002;**4**:158–9; n = 1, seven-year-old boy, *Pediatr Neurol* 2007;**37**:287–8; n = 1, short-lived in six-year-old boy, *J Child Adolesc Psychopharmacol* 2007;**17**:378–81)

Metoclopramide (BNF, FDA warning, directly related to total doses taken; <1% incidence, review, *Aliment Pharmacol Ther* 2010;**31**:11–9)

Modafinil (orofacial, n = 1, *J Neurol Neurosurg Psychiatry* 2010;**22**:451)

Norpseudoephedrine (n = 2, *J Neurol* 1994;**241**: 167–9)

Prochlorperazine long-term (n = 1, *South Med J* 1996;**89**:989–91)

Stimulants in ADHD (n = 127, incidence 9% , *Arch Pediatr Adolesc Med* 1994;**148**: 859–61)

- Gastrointestinal drugs

Tiemonium (n = 1, *Fundam Clin Pharmacol* 2007; **21**:657–8)

- Respiratory drugs

Aminophylline (*Pediatr Neurol* 1992;**8**:997)

- Anti-infection drugs

Ciprofloxacin (n = 1, *Hosp Med* 2000;**61**:142–3; n = 1, *J Neurol* 1996;**243**:616–7)

Ofloxacin (n = 1, *Mov Disord* 2004;**19**:731–2)

- Musculoskeletal and analgesics

Baclofen (n = 1, *Arch Phys Med Rehabil* 1993; **74**:766–7)

- Others *

Phenylalanine (exacerbates TD, n = 18, d/b, p/c, *Neuropsychopharmacology* 1997;**16**:136–46)

Propofol (*Anesth Analg* 1996;**83**:420–2)

Sildenafil (n=1, with Parkinson's Disease, *Int J Clin Pharmacol Ther* 2010;**48**:76–8)

5.8.5 OTHER MOVEMENT DISORDERS

5.8.5.1 CATATONIA

Reviews: * in young people (*J Am Acad Child Adolesc Psychiatry* 1999;**38**:1040–6), general (Duggal and Singh, *Drugs Today [Barc]* 2005;**41**:599–607), antipsychotics (n = 127, *J Clin Psychopharmacol* 2010;**30**:3–10).

- CNS — general *

Alcohol withdrawal (n = 1, *Med Sci Monit* 2009;**15**:129–31)

Amfetamine (pseudocatatonia, *Postgrad Med* 1977;**61**:275–7)

Aripiprazole (possible case, *J Clin Psychopharmacol* 2009;**29**:503–4)

Benzodiazepine withdrawal (n = 5, *J Clin Psychopharmacol* 1996;**16**:315–9; *Pharma-copsychiatry* 2001;**34**:41–2)

Bupropion (n = 1, *J Clin Psychiatry* 1992;**53**:210)

Clonazepam withdrawal (n = 1, *Psychosomatics* 2009;**50**:289–92)

Clozapine (*Can J Psychiatry* 2001;**46**:458)

Clozapine withdrawal (e.g. abrupt, n = 1, *Psychosomatics* 2010;**51**:355; *Aust N Z J Psychiatry* 2009;**43**:283–4)

Cocaine (n = 1, *Am J Psychiatry* 1998;**155**:1629)

Disulfiram (e.g. n = 1, dose dependent, *J Clin Pharmacol* 2011;**51**:285-6; n = 1, *Am J Psychiatry* 1992;**149**:1279–80)

Donepezil (n = 1, *No To Shinkei* 2004; **56**:881–4)

Fluphenazine (n = 1, *Br J Psychiatry* 1973;**122**: 240)

Gabapentin (n = 1, *Am J Ger Pharmacother* 2009; **7**:220–4)

Hydroxyzine (n = 1, *No To Shinkei* 2005;**57**: 45–9)

Levetiracetam (n = 1, *Epilepsy Behav* 2006;**8**: 303–7)

Lithium (n = 1, *J Clin Psychopharmacol* 2007;**27**: 410–2)

Loxapine (n = 1, *J Clin Psychiatry* 1983;**44**:10–2)

LSD (n = 1, *Aust N Z J Psychiatry* 1995;**29**:324–7; *Aust N Z J Psychiatry* 1995;**29**:696–7)

MDMA/ecstasy (several e.g. n = 1, *J Am Acad Child Adolesc Psychiatry* 2002;**41**:892)

Methadone overdose (delayed, n = 1, *Neurotoxicity* 2010;**31**:762–4; n = 1, *Prim Care Companion J Clin Psychiatry* 2009;**11**:275–6)

Morphine epidural (n = 1, *Lancet* 1980;**2**: 984; n = 1, *Acta Anaesthesiol Scand* 1981; **25**:445–6)

Paliperidone (n = 1, *West J Emerg Med* 2010; **11**:186–8)

Phenelzine + haloperidol (n = 1, *Can J Psychiatry* 1988;**33**:633–4)

Pipotiazine (n = 1, *Br J Psychiatry* 1988;**152**: 865–6)

Prochlorperazine (n = 1, *Postgrad Med* 1976; **60**:171–3)

Risperidone (n = 1, *Acta Psychiatr Scand* 1999; **99**:223–6)

Tramadol + pethidine (n = 1, *J Formos Med Assoc* 2007;**106**:323–6)

Valproate + risperidone (n = 1, *Neuropsychiatry Neuropsychol Behav Neurol* 1998;**11**:997–63)

Zotepine (n = 1, *Pharmacotherapy* 2005;**25**: 1156–9)

- Others *

Allopurinol (n = 1, *Br Med J* 1991;**302**:970)

Azithromycin (n = 1, *J Clin Psychiatry* 2006;**67**: 492–3)

Baclofen (*J Clin Psychopharmacol* 1986;**6**: 387–8; cases, *Clin Neuropharmacol* 1992;**15**:56–62)

Ciprofloxacin (*J Clin Psychiatry* 1993;**54**:199–6)

Cycloserine

Efavirenz (*AIDS* 2002;**16**:1841–2)

Lead intoxication (n=1, *Cases J* 2009;**2**:8722)

Omeprazole + disulfiram (n = 1, *CMAJ* 1990; **143**:1207–8)

Oral contraceptive (n = 1, *Mov Disord* 2009; **24**:2166–7)

Paracetamol overdose (n = 1, *Prim Care Companion J Clin Psychiatry* 2010; **12**:PCC.09100790)

Phenylpropanolamine overdose (n = 1, *J Clin Psychiatry* 1985;**46**:288–9)

Piperazine (mentioned in *Trans Roy Soc Trop Med Hyg* 1976;**70**:358)

Prednisone (n = 1, *J Geriatr Psychiatry Neurol* 1989;**2**:41–4)

Sibutramine (n = 1, *J Psychosom Res* 2008; **64**:107–9)

Steroids (n = 1, *Br J Psychiatry* 1991;**158**:125–7; *Br J Psychiatry* 1991;**159**:445)

5.8.5.2 CATAPLEXY

Cataplexy is a rare transient sudden loss of muscle tone, often triggered by emotions.

Clomipramine withdrawal (n = 3, *Neurologia* 2002;**17**:113–6)

Clozapine (e.g. *J Neuropsychiatry Clin Neurosci* 2007;**19**:87–8)

Fluoxetine withdrawal (n = 1, *Neurology* 2005; **65**:967–8)

Prazosin (n = 1, *Sleep* 1989;**12**:254–6)

Venlafaxine withdrawal (n = 1, *J Sleep Res* 2005;**14**:207–8)

5.8.5.3 CHOREAS

- CNS — antipsychotics

Chlorpromazine (n = 1, *Postgrad Med J* 1970; **540**:633–4)

Haloperidol (many cases)

Lithium toxicity (n = 1, *Eur J Neurol* 2003;**10**: 743–4; n = 1, *Seishin Shinkeigaku Zasshi* 2003; **105**:1206–12; n = 1, *Mov Disord* 1996;**11**:733–7)

Quetiapine withdrawal (n = 1, *Rev Neurol* 2004; **38**:1094)

Risperidone (n = 1, *J Clin Psychiatry* 1999;**60**:85–7)

Sulpiride (n = 1, *J Psychopharmacol* 1993;**7**:290–2; n = 6, *Clin Neuropharmacol* 1990;**13**:248–52)

- CNS — antidepressants

Fluoxetine (n = 1, *J Clin Psychiatry* 1999;**60**: 868–9; n = 1, *Neurology* 1996;**46**:853)

Mianserin (n = 1, *Br J Psychiatry* 1989;**154**:13–4)

Paroxetine (n = 1, after a single dose, *Br J Psychiatry* 1997;**170**:193–4)

Trazodone low dose (n = 1, *Eur Neurol* 2006; **55**:101–2)

- CNS — anticonvulsants

Review: choreas and anticonvulsants; Zaatreh *et al*, *Seizure* 2001;**10**:596–9).

Carbamazepine (*J Neurol Neurosurg Psychiatry* 1982;**45**:560)

5

Carbamazepine overdose (n = 4, *Neurology* 1988;**38**:755–9)

Gabapentin (several e.g. n = 1, *Clin Rheumatol* 2008;**27**:389–90; *Neurology* 1996;**46**: 851–2)

Lamotrigine (n = 1, *J Child Neurol* 2003;**18**:479–80; *J Child Neurol* 2006;**21**:357–8)

Lamotrigine + phenytoin (n = 3, *Seizure* 2001;**10**: 596–9)

Lamotrigine overdose (n = 1, *J Child Neurol* 2008; **23**:243)

Phenytoin (e.g. n = 3, *Neuropediatrics* 2001; **32**:231–5; *Postgrad Med J* 1990;**66**:1089)

Valproate (n = 1, *Pediatr Neurol* 2006;**35**:356–8; n = 3, *Arch Neurol* 1994;**51**:702–4; n = 1, *Seizure* 2002;**11**:205–6)

- CNS — antiparkinsonian drugs
Anticholinergics (n = 1, *Med J Aust* 1979;**1**:465):
  → trihexyphenidyl (n = 1, *Nippon Ronen Igakkai Zasshi* 1992;**29**:686–9)
Levodopa (BNF)

- CNS — others *
Amfetamines (review, *Emerg Med Australas* 2005;**17**:277–80; n = 1, *Mov Disord* 2004;**19**;840–2)

Cocaine (cases in *Am J Emerg Med* 1991;**9**: 618–20; including crack; *Med Clin (Barc)* 2006;**126**:555; n = 9, *Biol Psychiatry* 1999; **45**:1630–5)

Donepezil (n = 1, *Ann Pharmacother* 2000;**34**: 1347; *J Neurol* 2007;**254**:1752–3)

Methadone (e.g. n = 1, *J Pain Symptom Manage* 2003; **26**:688–91; n = 1, *Clin J Pain* 2001;**17**:375–7)

Methamphetamine (*Ann Intern Med* 1994;**121**: 986)

Methylphenidate (e.g. n = 1, *J Neuropsychiatry Clin Neurosci* 2010;**22**:e352)

Modafinil + tranylcypromine (n= 1, *Am J Psychiatry* 2007;**164**:684)

- Gastrointestinal drugs
H2-blockers, e.g.:
  → cimetidine (n = 1, *Ann Intern Med* 1982; **96**:126; n = 1, *Ann Intern Med* 1982;**96**:531)
  → ranitidine (n = 1, *Lancet* 1988;**2**:158)
Metoclopramide (n = 1, *Am J Ther* 2006;**13**: 543–4; *South Med J* 1986;**79**:1465)
Sulfasalazine (n = 1, *Br Med J* 1991;**302**:1025)

- Anti-infection drugs
Ciprofloxacin (*Mov Disord* 2005;**20**:513–4)
Trimethoprim-sulfamethoxazole (n = 1, *Paediatr Infect Dis J* 2005;**24**:934–5)
Valacyclovir + famciclovir (n = 1, *South Med J* 2001;**94**:655)

- Others *
Anabolic steroids (*Br Med J (Clin Res Ed)* 1981; **283**:349–50)

Baclofen (n = 1, *Mov Disord* 2010;**25**:959–60; *Ann Neurol* 1990;**28**;839)

Ciclosporin (n = 1, *Ann Neurol* 1993;**33**:108–9)

Cyclizine (n = 1, *J Neurol Sci* 1977;**31**:237–44)

Cyproheptadine (n = 1, *Mov Disord* 1989;**4**:81–4)

Dienoestrol/dienestrol

Digoxin toxicity (n = 1, *J Neurol Neurosurg Psychiatry* 1984;**47**:419; n =1, *Mov Disord* 1999;**14**:877–9)

Diphenhydramine (n = 2, *Chudoku Kenkyu* 2007; **20**:125–9)

Estrogen as topical vaginal cream (n = 1, *Mov Disord* 1991;**6**:355–7)

HRT (n = 1, *Br Med J* 1991;**302**:762)

Interferons:
  → interferon alfa (*Neurology* 2002;**58**:328–30; n = 1, *Nippon Naika Gakkai Zasshi* 1997; **86**:1036–8)

Levofloxacin (n = 1, *Nippon Ronen Igakkai Zasshi* 1999;**36**:213–7)

Luteinizing hormone–releasing hormone analog (n = 1, *J Neurol* 2008;**255**:1264–5)

Oral contraceptives (BNF, rare; n = 1, *J Neurol Neurosurg Psychiatry* 2004;**75**:327–8; n = 2, *Rev Med Chil* 1999;**127**:468–71)

Propofol (n = 1, *Anesth Analg* 1996;**82**:670)

Sildenafil (n = 1, with Parkinson's Disease, *Int J Clin Pharmacol Ther* 2010;**48**:76–8)

Trimetazidine (*Rev Med Intern* 2008;**29**:512–5)

5.8.5.4 TICS (including exacerbation of Tourette's syndrome)
- CNS — general *
Amisulpride (n = 1, *Clin Neuropharmacol* 2006; **29**:163–4)

Atomoxetine (many e.g. n = 1, *CNS Spectr* 2008;**13**:301–3; n = 2, *Int J Psychiatry Med* 2007;**37**:499–24)

Atomoxetine + venlafaxine (n = 1, *Clin Toxicol [Phila]* 2007;**45**:182–5)

Caffeine (n = 2, *Pediatrics* 1998;**101**:E4)

Carbamazepine (e.g. n = 1, *Epileptic Disord* 2000;**2**:39–40; n = 3, *Epilepsia* 1993;**34**: 965–8)

Clozapine (n = 1, *Am J Psychiatry* 1995;**152**:649; n = 1, *Aust NZ J Psychiatry* 2005;**39**:202; n = 1, exacerbation, *Aust N Z J Psychiatry* 2008; **42**:1068–70)

Cocaine (several e.g. *NEJM* 1986;**315**:398; n = 1, *Am J Psychiatry* 1996;**153**:965)

Escitalopram (n = 1, *Int Clin Psychopharmacol* 2005;**20**:177–8)

Fluoxetine (cases in *Ann Pharmacother* 1993; **27**:725–6; n = 1, Tourette's, *Am J Psychiatry* 1994;**151**:946–7)

Haloperidol (n = 2, tics, *Am J Psychiatry* 1986; **143**:1176–7)

Lamotrigine (several e.g. n = 5, *Epilepsia* 2000;**41**:862–7; n = 1, vocal and motor tics, *Am J Psychiatry* 2006; **163**:159)

Quetiapine (n = 1, *J Clin Psychiatry* 2002;**63**: 1184–5)

Risperidone withdrawal (n = 1, *J Am Acad Child Adolesc Psychiatry* 1997;**36**:162–3)

Sertraline (e.g. n = 1, *Int Clin Psychopharmacol* 2005;**20**:177–8; n = 1, *Pharmacopsychiatry* 2007;**40**:289–90)

Stimulants (frequent cause, especially in children treated for ADHD, incidence may be about 8% with methylphenidate, 6% with dexamfetamine; n = 555, chart review, Varley et al, *Compr Psychiatry* 2001;**42**:228–33):
- → amfetamines (*JAMA* 1982;**247**:1729–31, n = 1, *Mov Disord* 2004;**19**:840–2)
- → dexamfetamine (see amfetamines)
- → methylphenidate (*JAMA* 1982;**247**:1729–31)

Sulpiride (review of n = 17, *Seishin Shinkeigaku Zasshi* 2006;**108**:459–65)

Ziprasidone (n = 1, vocal, *J Clin Psychopharmacol* 2009;**29**:611–2)

- Others

Anabolic steroids (e.g. methandrostenolone, testosterone; *NEJM* 1990;**322**:1674)

Clonidine (n = 1, *J Child Neurol* 2001;**16**:380–1; n = 1, *J Am Acad Child Adolesc Psychiatry* 1989; **28**:583–6)

Growth hormone (human, n = 1, *Eur Neurol* 2007;**57**:116–7)

Mercury poisoning (n = 1, *Arch Dis Child* 2000; **83**:174–5)

Ofloxacin (n = 1, *Ann Pharmacother* 1996;**30**: 138–41)

Sibutramine (BNF, may exacerbate)

Prednisolone (n = 2, *Nervenarzt* 1998;**69**:1111–4)

5.9 NEUROLEPTIC MALIGNANT SYNDROME

NMS is mostly related to the use of therapeutic or high doses of neuroleptics, particularly phenothiazines and high potency drugs. It frequently occurs within 4–11 days of initiation, or alteration of dosages of neuroleptic therapy. NMS may be due to a sudden and profound reduction in dopaminergic function, caused by dopamine blocking drugs. See 6.8.

Reviews: atypicals as causes (*Expert Opin Drug Saf* 2003;**2**:21–35; Trollor et al, *CNS Drugs* 2009; **23**:477–92).

- CNS — antipsychotics *

Be aware that NMS with atypicals might actually be serotonin toxicity via 5HT1A partial agonism (Odagaki, *Curr Drug Saf* 2009;**4**:84–93).

Amisulpride (n = 1, *Clin Neuropharmacol* 2007; **30**:245–6; n = 1, *J Neuropsychiatry Clin Neurosci* 2007;**19**:488–9)

Amisulpride + oxcarbazepine (n = 1, *Gen Hosp Psychiatry* 2008;**30**:482–4)

Amisulpride withdrawal (n = 1, Ball et al, *Med Sci Law* 2009;**49**:298–300)

Aripiprazole (e.g. n = 1 without fever, *J Okla State Med Assoc* 2006;**99**:435–8; n = 1, Naranjo high probability, *Clin Neuropharmacol* 2007;**30**:47–51; low dose, *J Psychiatr Pract* 2007;**13**:117–9; n = 1, *Mov Disord* 2010;**25**:2475–6; n = 1 in clozapine-intolerant patient, *Am J Health Syst Pharm* 2010; **67**:1254–9)

Aripiprazole + clozapine (n = 1, *Prog Neuropsychopharmacol Biol Psychiatry* 2010; **34**:427–8)

Aripiprazole + fluoxetine (n = 1, possible, *Am J Psychiatry* 2005;**162**:397–8)

Aripiprazole + lithium (n = 1, *J Clin Psychopharmacol* 2006;**26**:434–6)

Bromperidol + donepezil (n = 1, *Nippon Ronen Igakkai Zasshi* 2001;**38**:822–4)

Chlorpromazine (e.g. n = 2, *Biol Psychiatry* 1983; **18**:1441–6; n = 1, *Trop Doct* 1992;**22**:92–3)

Clozapine (rare, but cases exist, e.g. n = 2 and

5

review, *Ann Pharmacother* 1999;**33**:623–30;
long-term n = 1, *Chang Gung Med J* 2001;**24**:
522–5; n = 1, *Ann Intern Med* 2002;**137**:374;
after 30 years uneventful treatment;
n = 1, *Anasthesiol Intensivmed Notfallmed
Schmerzther* 2006;**41**:125–7; after 10 years,
n = 1, *Crit Care Resusc* 2007; **9**:338–40)

Clozapine + paroxetine (n = 1, *Aging Clin Exp
Res* 2006;**18**:266–70)

Clozapine + risperidone (n = 1, *Prog
Neuropsychopharmacol Biol Psychiatry*
2002;**26**:407–9)

Clozapine + venlafaxine (n = 1, *Can J Psychiatry*
2004;**49**:497–8)

Flupentixol (SmPC, n = 1, possible, *Br J Psychiatry*
1988;**152**:558–9)

Fluphenazine (reviewed in *Compr Psychiatry*
1985;**26**:63–70)

Fluphenazine decanoate (n = 1, *Ann
Pharmacother* 2005;**39**:1131–5)

Haloperidol (many cases, e.g. in pregnancy, n = 1,
Obstet Gynecol 2001;**98**:906–8; following
clozapine discontinuation, n = 1, *Aust NZ J
Psychiatry* 2005;**39**:947–8)

Haloperidol + olanzapine (n = 1, *Am J Psychiatry*
2001;**158**:650–1)

Levomepromazine discontinuation (n=1, *J
Neuropsychiatry Clin Neurosci* 2010;**22**:E16)

Lithium (possible cases in *J Clin Psychopharmacol*
1987;**7**:339–41)

Lithium + amitriptyline (n = 1, *J Psychiatry
Neurosci* 1995;**20**:305–6)

Lithium + risperidone (possible case in *Am J
Psychiatry* 1995;**152**:1096)

Lithium + ziprasidone (n = 1, *Ann Pharmacother*
2006;**40**:139–42)

Loxapine (n=1, *Br J Psychiatry* 1991;**159**:572–3)

Olanzapine (many e.g. atypical syndrome,
n = 1, *Pharmacotherapy* 2002;**22**:641–4;
n = 1, with severe hypernatraemia, *Hum
Psychopharmacol* 2001;**16**:279–81; 2.5 mg/d,
n = 1, *Am J Psychiatry* 2003;**160**:796; n = 1,
atypical with normal CK, *Acta Psychiatr Scand*
2005;**112**:238–40)

Olanzapine + chlorpromazine overdose (n = 1, *J
Med Toxicol* 2009;**5**:27–31)

Olanzapine + fluphenazine (n = 1, *J Clin Psychopharmacol* 2003;**23**:672–4)

Olanzapine + levomepromazine (n = 1, *Acta
Psychiatr Scand* 2000;**102**:231–3)

Olanzapine + lithium (n = 1, *Pharmacother* 2003;
23:255–9)

Olanzapine + rivastigmine (n = 1,
Pharmacotherapy 2008;**28**:403–5)

Paliperidone (several, e.g. n = 1, *J Clin
Psychopharmacol* 2010;**30**:89–91; atypical,
n = 1, *Prog Neuropsychopharmacol Biol
Psychiatry* 2011;**35**:650–1)

Paroxetine + alprazolam (n = 1, Naranjo = 6,
Neuropsychopharmacol Biol Psychiatry
2006;**30**:1176–8)

Perphenazine (n = 1, *Otolaryngol Head Neck
Surg* 1992;**106**:206–8; n = 1, *Pharmacol Toxicol*
1987;**60**:221–3)

Promazine

Quetiapine (atypical n = 1, *J Clin Psychopharmacol*
2009;**29**:497–9; n = 1 after no dose changes
and review of n = 13, *Ann Pharmacother*
2009;**43**:785–91; n = 1, Stanley and Hunter,
Br J Psychiatry 2000;**176**:497; n = 1, in XYY
syndrome, *Am J Health Syst Pharm* 2010;
67:459–61)

Quetiapine + fluvoxamine (n = 1, *Am J Psychiatry*
2005;**162**:812)

Risperidone (many cases, e.g. n = 1, *J Child
Adolesc Psychopharmacol* 2005;**15**:844–5;
n = 1, *Curr Drug Saf* 2009;**4**:119–20; n = 1, *J
Natl Med Assoc* 2009;**101**:273–5)

Risperidone + haloperidol (during switch, n = 1,
Ann Pharmacother 2001;**35**:698–701)

Risperidone + lithium (*J Clin Psychopharmacol*
2003;**23**:315–7; n = 1, *J Clin Psychiatry* 2004;
65:724)

Risperidone + ritonavir + indinavir (n = 1,
Psychosomatics 2000;**41**:453–4)

Ziprasidone (*J Clin Psychopharmacol* 2002;**22**:
624–6; n = 1, adolescent, *Clin Ther* 2004;**26**:
1105–8; n = 1, on second day, *World J Biol
Psychiatry* 2007;**8**:42–4)

Zotepine + valproate + benzodiazepine (n = 2,
Psychiatr Clin Neurosci 2003;**57**:369–71)

Zuclopenthixol (n = 1, *Br J Psychiatry* 1989;**154**:
562–3)

- CNS — antidepressants

Amoxapine + lithium (n = 1, *Ann Clin Psychiatry*
2000;**12**:107–9)

SSRIs:

→ citalopram overdose (n = 1, *Can J
Psychiatry* 2000;**45**:941–2)

→ fluoxetine monotherapy (n = 1, *Biol
Psychiatry* 1990;**28**:518–21)

→ paroxetine monotherapy (n = 1, *Rinsho Shinkeigaku* 2006;**46**:575–8; n = 1, *Seishin Shinkeigaku Zasshi* 2004;**106**:723–6)

→ paroxetine + olanzapine (n = 1, *J Clin Psychopharmacol* 2003;**23**:671–2)

→ paroxetine + promethazine (n = 1, *Nervenartz* 1997;**68**:664–6)

→ sertraline withdrawal (n = 1, *J Clin Psycho-pharmacol* 2009;**29**:300–1)

Tricyclics:

→ clomipramine (n = 1, *Br Med J* 2004; **329**:1333–5)

→ desipramine (n = 1, *Neurology* 1990; **40**:1797–8)

→ imipramine withdrawal (n = 1, *J Clin Psychopharmacol* 1987;**7**:53–4)

→ nortriptyline (n = 1, *Am J Emerg Med* 1999; **17**:736–7)

→ trimipramine (n = 1, *J Clin Psychiatry* 1989;**50**:144–5)

→ overdose (*J Assoc Physicians India* 2002; **50**:614)

Phenelzine (many cases, e.g. *Can Med Assoc J* 1991;**145**:817–9)

Venlafaxine (n = 1, *J Formos Med Assoc* 2006;**105**: 90–3; n = 1, *Lancet* 2000;**355**:2164–5)

Venlafaxine + trifluoperazine (n = 1, *Lancet* 2000;**354**:289–90)

- CNS — anticonvulsants

Carbamazepine (may also complicate symptoms, n = 1, *Br J Psychiatry* 1994;**164**:270; n = 1, *South Med J* 1991;**84**:1378–80)

Carbamazepine withdrawal (n = 1, *Am J Psychiatry* 1990;**147**:1687)

Oxcarbazepine + amisulpride (n = 1, *Gen Hosp Psychiatry* 2008;**30**:482–4)

Phenytoin toxicity (*S Afr Med J* 1988;**73**:620–1)

Tiapride (n = 1, *Clin Neuropharmacol* 1996;**19**: 539–40; n = 1, *Rev Rhum Ed Fr* 1994;**61**:362)

Zonisamide + carbamazepine (n=1, *Epilepsia* 2007;**48**:1999–2001)

- CNS — antiparkinsonian drugs

Amantadine (SmPC)

Amantadine withdrawal (e.g. n = 1, *Am J Psychiatry* 1994;**151**:451–2; n = 1, *Eur J Pediatr* 2001; **160**:401)

Anticholinergic withdrawal (n = 1, *Int Clin Psychopharmacol* 1996;**11**:207–9)

Bromocriptine to pergolide (rapid switch, n = 1,

Parkinsonism Relat Disord 2002;**9**:116)

Fava bean abrupt withdrawal (n = 1, *Mov Disord* 2005;**20**:630–1; NB Fava beans contain appreciable amounts of levodopa)

Levodopa (n = 1, *Intern Med* 1992;**31**:1298–302)

Levodopa withdrawal (several e.g. n = 1, *Med J Aust* 1991;**155**:53–4; n = 1, *J Clin Anesth* 1995;**7**:652–6)

Levodopa and bromocriptine withdrawal (n = 1, *Singapore Med J* 2001;**42**:85–8)

Tetrabenazine long–term (n=1, *Mov Disord* 1997;**12**:246–8; *Mov Disord* 1996;**11**:95)

Tolcapone withdrawal (n = 1, *Am J Med* 2000; **108**:517–8)

- CNS — others

Anticholinesterases (n = 1, *Int J Geriatr Psychiatry* 2006;**21**:193–4), e.g.:

→ donepezil (n = 1, *Int J Neuro-psychopharmacol* 2004;**7**:101–3)

→ donepezil + maprotiline (n = 1, *Neurology* 2003;**60**:1050–1)

→ donepezil + olanzapine (n = 1, *Nat Clin Pract Neurol* 2008;**4**:170–4)

Cocaine (review, *Am J Emerg Med* 1996;**14**: 425–8; n = 1, *Tijdschr Psychiatr* 2006;**48**; 399–404)

Cocaine + amfetamine overdose (fatal, n = 1, *Med Clin (Barc)* 1996;**106**:717–8)

Domperidone (n = 1, *Dig Dis Sci* 1992;**37**:946–8)

LSD (n = 1, fatal, *J Neurol Neurosurg Psychiatry* 1991;**54**:741–3)

LSD + alcohol (n = 1, *Br J Addict* 1990;**85**:990–1)

Methylphenidate (n = 1, *Pediatr Neurol* 1998;**19**: 299–301; n = 1, *Prim Care Companion J Clin Psychiatry* 2006;**8**:47)

Metoclopramide (e.g. *Ann Pharmacother* 1999;**33**:644–5; n = 1, *J Burn Care Res* 2006; **27**:237–41)

Metoclopramide withdrawal (n = 1, *Aust N Z J Med* 1995;**25**:261)

Prochlorperazine (n = 1, *J Emerg Med* 1996;**14**: 727–9)

- Others *

Alimemazine (n = 1, *Eur J Pediatr* 2002;**161**:259–61)

Baclofen abrupt withdrawal (n = 1, *J Psycho-pharmacol* 2001;**99**:61–3; n = 1, *Med Clin (Barc)* 2006;**127**:79)

Compulsive water drinking (*Med J Aust* 1989; **150**:457–8)

5

Diphenhydramine (n = 1, *Vet Hum Toxicol* 1988; **30**:58–9)

Diphenhydramine + diprophyllin overdose (n = 1, *J Neurol Sci* 1999;**162**:108–9)

Ganciclovir (n = 1, *Pharmacother* 2000;**20**: 479–83)

Iron (low levels? *Lancet* 1987;i:1234–6)

Oral contraceptives (n = 1, *Drug Intell Clin Pharm* 1989;**23**:811)

Organophosphate poisoning (n = 1, *Can J Anesth* 1995;**42**:1027–30)

Promethazine (n = 1, *Aust N Z J Psychiatry* 2005; **39**:113–4)

Promethazine + lorazepam (n = 1, *Aust N Z J Psychiatry* 2001;**35**:250–1)

Rifampicin + chlorpromazine (n = 1, *J Korean Med Sci* 2008;**23**:734–6)

Simvastatin (complicated n = 1, *Clin Neuro-pharmacol* 2009;**32**:348–9)

5.10 OBSESSIVE-COMPULSIVE SYMPTOMS

- CNS — anxiolytics and hypnotics

Benzodiazepine withdrawal (n = 1, *Br J Psychiatry* 1987;**150**:272; n = 1, *J Nerv Ment Dis* 1988; **176**:688–91)

- CNS — antipsychotics *

Reviews: FGA–induced OCD (*Prog Neuropsycho-pharmacol Biol Psychiatry* 2003;**27**;333–46). There is a 3% incidence with clozapine, olanzapine and risperidone in Asians, although in this study no cases were reported with quetiapine (Mahendran et al, *J Clin Psychiatry* 2007;**68**:542–5). Severity is associated with longer duration of olanzapine treatment (e.g. n = 113, *J Clin Psychiatry* 2002;**63**: 104–7; n = 6, *J Clin Psychopharmacol* 2002;**22**: 461–7; n = 2, *J Child Adolesc Psychopharmacol* 2003;**13** Suppl 1:S89–92).

Clozapine (e.g. n = 40, 20% incidence, *Compr Psychiatry* 2009;**50**:437–42; n = 59 on clozapine, 24% had OCD; Mukhopadhaya et al, *J Psychopharmacol* 2009;**23**:6–13; although one study showed it might be of some use for OCD symptoms in people with schizophrenia; n = 15, Reznik et al, *Pharmacopsychiatry* 2004;**37**:52–6; n = 7, *Clin Neuropharmacol* 2009;**32**:227–9)

Haloperidol (n = 20, 10% incidence, *Compr Psychiatry* 2009;**50**:437–42)

Olanzapine (e.g. severity associated with duration of treatment: n = 113, *J Clin Psychiatry* 2002; **63**:104–7; review, n = 9, *Int Clin Neuropsychopharmacol* 2004;**7**:375–7)

Quetiapine (a few cases e.g. n = 1, *Aust N Z J Psychiatry* 2009;**43**:1185; n = 5, *J Clin Psychopharmacol* 2006;**26**:396–400)

Risperidone (e.g. dose dependent case, *Aust N Z J Psychiatry* 1998;**32**:299–301; n = 2, children, *J Child Adolesc Psychopharmacol* 2003;**13**[Suppl 1]:S89–92)

- CNS — antidepressants

Fluoxetine (n = 3, *Am J Psychiatry* 1991;**148**: 1262–3)

- CNS — analgesics

Codeine abuse (n = 2, *Acta Psychiatr Scand* 1989; **79**:619–20)

- CNS — anticonvulsants *

Gabapentin withdrawal (n = 1, *J Clin Psychiatry* 1998;**59**:131)

Lamotrigine (n = 1, *J Psychopharmacol* 2010;**24**:1001–3)

Topiramate (n = 1, *Psychiatry Clin Neurosci* 2006; **60**:394)

- CNS — others

Methamphetamine (*J Clin Psychiatry* 1999;**60**: 337–8; n = 1, *J Am Acad Child Adolesc Psychiatry* 1998;**37**:135)

Methylphenidate (several e.g. n = 1, *Can J Psychiatry* 2001;**46**:89; n = 1, *CNS Spectr* 2003;**8**:612–3)

Modafinil (n = 2, exacerbation of symptoms, *Prim Care Companion J Clin Psychiatry* 2008; **10**:164–5)

Stimulants (n = 1, *Biol Psychiatry* 1985;**20**:1332–7)

- Anti-infection drugs

Isoniazid (*J Clin Psychiatry* 1990;**51**:387)

- Endocrine system drugs

Corticosteroids (may respond to fluvoxamine, *Clin Neuropharmacol* 2009;**32**:176–7):
  → cortisone (n = 1, *Pharmacopsychiatry* 2002; **35**:72–4)

- Malignancy and immunosuppressant drugs

Interferons (*Gen Hosp Psychiatry* 2006;**28**: 357–8)

- Others *

Isotretinoin (n = 1 after 7 years, *Neuropsychiatr Dis Treat* 2010;**6** :719–22)

5.11 PANIC ATTACKS

- CNS — anxiolytics and hypnotics

Benzodiazepines:
  - → alprazolam (*J Am Board Fam Pract* 2002;**15**: 69–72)
  - → clobazam withdrawal (n = 2, *Br Med J* 1981; **282**:1931–2)
  - → diazepam discontinuation after long-term abuse (n = 1, *Drug Intell Clin Pharmacy* 1989; **23**:989–90)

Buspirone (case + correspondence in *Lancet* 1989;**2**:46–7, 615, 682–3)

- CNS — antipsychotics

Review: long-term (n = 45, incidence 20%, *Psychiatry Clin Neurosci* 1999; **53**: 91–4).

Clozapine (n = 1, *Am J Psychiatry* 2000;**157**:2056)

Olanzapine (e.g. hyperventilation, n = 1, *J Psych Neurosci* 2002;**27**:360–3)

Risperidone (in people with post-LSD visual disorder, n = 3, *J Clin Psychopharmacol* 1996; **16**:238–41)

- CNS — antidepressants *

Amitriptyline abrupt discontinuation (n = 1, *Am J Psychiatry* 1981;**138**:117–8)

Mianserin discontinuation (n = 1, *Jpn J Psychiatry Neurol* 1989;**43**:995–9)

Mirtazapine discontinuation (*Can J Psychiatry* 2000;**45**:570–1)

SSRIs:
  - → citalopram (n = 1, *South Med J* 2002;**95**; 1088–9)
  - → fluoxetine (unless initial doses kept very low, e.g. *J Clin Psychopharmacol* 1987; **7**:329–32; n = 1, *J Neuropsychiatry Clin Neurosci* 1989;**1**: 219–20)
  - → fluoxetine + bupropion (*J Clin Psychiatry* 1996;**57**:177–8)
  - → sertraline (n = 1, *Clin Neuropharmacol* 2000;**23**:164–8; n = 1, *Bol Asoc Med P R* 2009;**101**:59–60)

Trazodone

- CNS — analgesics

Opiate blockade (*J Clin Psychopharmacol* 1987;**7**:361–2)

Sumatriptan (n = 125, incidence 7.2%, *Am J Psychiatry* 1996;**153**:1505; single dose n = 15, RCT, d/b, p/c, *Eur Neuropsychopharmacol* 2005;**15**:279–82)

- CNS — anticonvulsants

Pregabalin (BNF, less common)

Topiramate (n = 1, *J Clin Psychopharmacol* 2001;**21**:461–2; n = 1, *J Clin Psychiatry* 2006; **67**:326–7; *Pharmacopsychiatry* 2008;**41**:79)

- CNS — antiparkinsonian drugs

Amantadine (n = 1, *J Clin Psychiatry* 1996;**57**:374)

Levodopa (n = 31, *Acta Neurol Scand* 1993;**87**: 14–8)

Pramipexole (*Eur J Neurol* 2007;**14**:e1)

- CNS — others *

Amfetamines (n = 3, *Biol Psychiatry* 1992;**32**:91–5; n = 1, *J Clin Psychopharmacol* 1998;**18**:95–6; methamphetamine n = 1, *J Anxiety Disord* 1997;**11**:113–6)

Caffeine hyperreactivity (e.g. n = 98, RCT, d/b, 1/52, *Psychiatry Res* 2009;**169**:149–53)

Cannabis (n = 1, *Acta Psychiatr Scand* 1998;**98**: 254–5; *J Am Acad Child Adolesc Psychiatry* 2000;**39**:1467)

Cocaine (e.g. reviews: *Am J Drug Alcohol Abuse* 1992;**18**:57–62; *Biol Psychiatry* 1996;**40**:938–40; *J Addict Dis* 1992;**11**:47–58)

Fenfluramine (n = 1, *Braz J Med Biol Res* 1997; **30**:887–90)

MDMA/Ecstasy (n = 3, *Biol Psychiatry* 1992;**32**: 91–5)

Metoclopramide (n = 1, *Psychopharmacol Bull* 2002;**36**:82–93)

Naltrexone (n = 1, *Am J Psychiatry* 1998;**155**: 447)

Sibutramine (n = 1, *Am J Psychiatry* 2002;**159**: 1793–4; n = 1, *Riv Psichiatr* 2009;**44**:64–7)

Smoking cessation (n = 2, *J Clin Psychiatry* 2002; **63**:594–5)

Sumatriptan (n = 125, incidence 7%, panic being interpretation of side-effects such as chest pain, palpitations, etc, *Am J Psychiatry* 1996;**153**:1505)

Varenicline (BNF, less common)

- Gastrointestinal drugs

Pentagastrin (laboratory probe, n = 14,

incidence 86% in people with OCD, p/c, *Psychopharmacology (Berl)* 1996;**126**: 339–44; n = 25, RCT, p/c, d/b, c/o, *Psycho-neuroendocrinology* 2002;**27**:417–29)

- Cardiovascular drugs

Carvedilol (n = 1, *Ann Pharmacother* 2002;**36**: 1736–40)

Isoproterenol (n = 131, incidence 66%, p/c, d/b, *Biol Psychiatry* 1988;**24**:891–902)

Pentoxifylline (n = 1, *Am J Psychiatry* 1994;**151**: 290)

- Respiratory drugs

Doxapram (*Biol Psychiatry* 1993;**33**:295–7; n = 10, s/b, *Psychiatry Res* 2005;**133**:253–61)

Epinephrine/adrenaline (n = 25, incidence 67%, d/b, p/c, *J Affect Disord* 1996;**39**:133–40; n = 50, incidence 68%, RCT, d/b, *Biol Psychiatry* 1998;**44**:1017–26)

Salbutamol (n = 1, *Eur Neuropsychopharmacol* 1997;**7**:241–2)

Theophylline (n = 1, *An Med Interna* 1990;**7**:53; n = 1, *Rev Clin Esp* 1988;**183**:280)

- Anti-infection drugs

Chloroquine and mefloquine (*Adv Psychiatr Treat* 2005;**11**:66)

Co-trimoxazole (n = 1, *J Clin Psychopharmacol* 1991;**11**:144–5)

Mefloquine (BNF, less common; incidence 0.3%, n = 35,370, *Drug Saf* 2004;**27**:203–13)

Metronidazole (*South Med J* 1985;**78**:627)

Rifampicin (n = 1, *Pharmacotherapy* 2005;**25**: 435–7)

- Endocrine system drugs

Dexamethasone (e.g. *J Adolesc Health* 1994;**99**: 345–7; *J Psychiatry Neurosci* 1997;**22**:346–7)

Estrogen (n = 1, *Am J Psychiatry* 1994;**151**:1246; *Psychosomatics* 1988;**29**:433–5)

Levonorgestrel implant (n = 2, *J Clin Psychiatry* 1994;**55**:478–80)

Oral contraceptive, combined (n = 2, *J Clin Psychiatry* 1992;**53**:163–5; n = 1, *Acta Obstet Gynecol Scand* 1992;**71**:87–90)

TRH (thyrotropin releasing hormone) (n = 99, *Depress Anxiety* 2003;**17**:78–87)

- Malignancy and immunosuppressant drugs

Interferons (n = 1, *Gen Hosp Psychiatry* 2005;**27**: 329–37)

- Musculoskeletal and analgesics

Infliximab (n = 1, *Dig Dis Sci* 2006;**51**:1056)

Oxaprozin (n = 1, *Am J Psychiatry* 1995;**152**:149)

- Others *

Aspartame (n = 1, unproven, high dose, *Lancet* 1986;**12**:631)

Carbon dioxide (mentioned in *Am J Psychiatry* 1994;**151**:292–3)

Flumazenil (n = 36, incidence 9%, d/b, *J Psychopharmacol* 1998;**12**:146–50; n = 1, given as part of ECT, *J ECT* 2009;**25**:145)

Isotretinoin (n = 1, *Rev Med Chil* 2006;**134**: 1565–7)

Lactate oral (e.g. in calcium lactate tablets, case in *Ann Pharmacother* 1995;**29**:539–40)

Lead (higher levels, n = 1987, *Arch Gen Psychiatry* 2009;**66**:1313-9)

Organic solvents (n = 3, *Am J Psychiatry* 1987; **144**:1056–8)

Oxymetazoline withdrawal (n = 1, *J Clin Psychiatry* 1987;**48**:293)

Phenylephrine (n = 1, *Br J Psychiatry* 1980;**136**: 297–9)

Procaine (in Penicillin G, n = 3, *Am J Psychiatry* 1988;**145**:1317)

Sodium lactate (study in *Arch Gen Psychiatry* 1989;**46**:135–40)

Tyramine (*J S C Med Assoc* 2002;**98**:187–92)

Yohimbine (see *Arch Gen Psychiatry* 1998;**55**: 1033–44; n = 16, p/c, *Psychiatry Res* 1993;**48**: 119–33)

5.12 PARANOID OR SCHIZOPHRENIC-LIKE PSYCHOSES (SEE ALSO HALLUCINATIONS 5.6)

This is characterised by paranoid delusions and hallucinations in a person with little clouding of consciousness. The literature on drug-induced psychosis is extensive but mainly case reports and short uncontrolled studies. A classification has been proposed:

- Intoxication mimicking functional: (e.g. drug-induced), eg. stimulants and cannabis. Persists for several days until the drug has cleared.

- Psychoactive drugs altering the clinical presentation of an existing psychosis: e.g. cannabis or amfetamines, etc. creating a more aggressive and disturbed schizophrenic patient (Davison and Roth, *Br J Psychiatry* 1996;**168**:651).

- Chronic hallucinations induced by substance abuse: insight usually present, no clouding of consciousness, continue despite long-term abstinence, e.g. alcoholic hallucinosis, LSD or cannabis flashbacks.
- Drug-induced relapse of functional psychosis: e.g. schizophrenia.
- Withdrawal states: e.g. delirium tremens, benzodiazepine or barbiturate withdrawal.
- Others: acute intoxication/confusion with clouding of consciousness, post-intoxication depression, e.g. post-amfetamine crash, panic/anxiety attacks, e.g. from hallucinogens such as LSD.
- True drug-induced psychosis: any psychotic symptoms which occur with drug intoxication and then persist after elimination of the causing drug, e.g. one to two drug-free weeks.

Review: substance-induced psychosis (Mathias et al, J Clin Psychiatry 2008;**69**:358–67).

- CNS — hallucinogens, etc (major cause)

Cannabis — see CNS Others

Dimethoxy-methylamfetamine (DOM)

LSD

Khat chewing (n = 4, Br J Hosp Med 1995;**54**: 322–6)

Mescaline

MDE/Eve (n = 1, Arch Gen Psychiatry 1993;**50**:75)

MDMA/Ecstasy (n = 1, Br J Psychiatry 1991;**159**: 713–5)

Petrol (n = 2, Am J Psychiatry 1964;**120**:757–61)

Phencyclidine (angel dust)

Psilocybin (magic mushrooms) (n = 3, Br J Psychiatry 1978;**132**:602)

- CNS — stimulants (major cause)

Review: systematic (s = 54, Curran et al, Br J Psychiatry 2004;**185**:196–204).

Adderall® (n = 1, J Am Board Fam Pract 2002; **99**:498–500)

Amfetamines (e.g. treatment/review in Topic Emerg Med 1985;**7**:18–32; Gen Hosp Psychiatry 1996;**18**:117–20)

Cocaine (n = 50, incidence 68%, Am J Psychiatry, 1991;**148**:495–8)

Diethylpropion (e.g. n = 1, Int Clin Psychopharmacol 1993;**8**:67–70)

Ephedrine (review in Br J Psychiatry 1987;**150**: 252–5)

Methamfetamine (n = 1, Am J Psychiatry 1999;**4**:662; Australas Psychiatry 2006;**14**:86–9)

Phencyclidine (n = 10, South Med J 1988;**81**:565–7)

Phentermine (n = 1, Zhonghua Yi Xue Za Zhi [Taipei] 1998;**61**:44–7)

Phenylephrine (e.g. JAMA 1982;**247**:1859–60)

Phenylpropanolamine (e.g. n = 1, Am J Psychiatry 2000; **157**:1021–2)

Pseudoephedrine (many cases, e.g. South Med J 1990;**83**:64–5)

Solvents (e.g. review, Nihon Arukoru Yakubutsu Igakkai Zasshi 2005;**40**:471–84)

- CNS — anxiolytics and hypnotics

Benzodiazepines: (see also anticonvulsants)
  - → alprazolam
  - → lorazepam (e.g. Br J Psychiatry 1986;**148**:344; pre-operative, n = 1, Anaesthesia 2003;**58**:1036)
  - → lormetazepam (n = 1, Pharmacopsychiatry 1993;**26**:102–3)
  - → midazolam (possible case in Drug Intell Clin Pharm 1989;**23**:671–2)
  - → nitrazepam (BNF, C/I in psychosis)
  - → nitrazepam normal-dose withdrawal (n = 2, J UOEH 1988;**10**:337–40)
  - → triazolam (e.g. Pharmaco-psychiatry 1989;**22**:115–9)
  - → triazolam withdrawal (J Clin Psychiatry 1987;**48**:168–9)

Benzodiazepine withdrawal (Int J Geriatr Psychiatry 1995:**10**:901–2; Psychosomatics 1997;**38**:160–1)

Buspirone (e.g. J Psychopharmacol 1993;**7**:295–300; n = 1, Psychosomatics 1992;**33**:332–5)

Chloral

Melatonin (n = 1, Ann Pharmacother 1997;**31**:1408)

Oxybate (BNF, less common)

Zolpidem (e.g. n = 2, Ann Clin Psychiatry 1996; **8**: 89–91; n = 1, J Am Geriatr Soc 1997;**45**:533–4)

Zolpidem withdrawal (n = 2, Ugeskr Laeger 1993;**155**:2711–3)

Zopiclone (some cases reported — WHO Drug Information 1990;**4**:179)

- CNS — antipsychotics *

Antipsychotic withdrawal (rebound psychosis as opposed to relapse; n = 1, Can J Psychiatry

5

1989;**34**:227–9; in Tourette's; *Biol Psychiatry* 1993;**34**:341–2)

Aripiprazole (n = 1, *J Clin Psychiatry* 2005;**66**: 1339; n = 4, *Int Clin Psychopharmacol* 2004; **19**:45–8; as both add-on and during tapered crossover; and as adjunct to risperidone, n = 1, *J Clin Psychiatry* 2007;**68**:1445–6; added to clozapine, n = 1, *Prog Neuropsychopharmacol Biol Psychiatry* 2011;**35**:291–2)

Chlorpromazine (n = 1, *Can Med Assoc J* 1970: **102**:642; n = 1, *Brain Inj* 1993;**7**:77–83)

Clozapine withdrawal (e.g. rebound psychosis, study in *Psychopharmacol* 1988;**24**:260–3; n = 3, *J Clin Psychiatry* 1997;**58**:252–5)

Haloperidol (*Drug Intell Clin Pharm* 1981;**15**:209)

Olanzapine (psychotic mania, *Eur Psychiatry* 1999;**14**:410–1)

Risperidone (n = 1, *J Child Adolesc Psycho-pharmacol* 2005;**15**:520–5)

- CNS — antidepressants *

Antidepressants may account for 8% admissions due to drug-induced psychosis or mania (n = 533, *J Clin Psychiatry* 2001;**62**:30–3)

Bupropion (many cases, e.g. *J Psychiatr Pract* 2007;**13**:336–8; n = 1, *J Am Board Fam Med* 2008;**21**:244–5; overdose n = 1, *Prog Neuropsychopharmacol Biol Psychiatry* 2005; **29**:149–51)

Mirtazapine (BNF, may aggravate psychotic states; caused by dissociated sleep-wakefulness, n = 1, *Pharmacotherapy* 2010;**30**: 145–50)

Phenelzine (BNF, rare; e.g. n = 1, *Br J Psychiatry* 1991;**159**:716–7)

SSRIs, e.g.:
- → citalopram (n = 1, *Prog Neurol Psychiatry* 2009;**13**:40–1)
- → fluoxetine (e.g. n = 1, *J Am Acad Child Adolesc Psychiatry* 2007;**46**:944–5)
- → fluvoxamine (e.g. n = 1, *Can J Psychiatry* 2000; **45**:762; n = 1, *Hum Psychopharmacol* 2003;**18**:477–8)
- → paroxetine (case of psychotic mania, *Am J Psychiatry* 1995;**152**:1399–440)
- → sertraline (n = 4, *Ann Clin Psychiatry* 1997; **9**:99–7)

St John's wort (n = 1, *Hum Psychopharmacol* 2004;**19**:275–6; review, n = 17, possible association, *Int J Clin Pharmacol Ther* 2004;

42:473–80)

Trazodone (n = 1, *J Neuropsych Clin Neurosci* 2005;**17**:253–4)

Tricyclics (BNF, may aggravate psychosis; review, concludes any psychosis is temporary and rare, s = 20, n = 177, *J Affect Disord* 2008; **106**:279–84)

Venlafaxine (n = 1, also occurred on rechallenge, *Indian J Psychiatry* 2009;**51**:308–9)

Venlafaxine + propafenone (*Int J Psychiatr Med* 2001;**31**:427–32)

- CNS — analgesics

Buprenorphine (BNF, less common)

Buprenorphine withdrawal (n = 1, *Am J Psychiatry* 2008;**165**:399–400)

Butorphanol (*J Neuropsychiatry Clin Neurosci* 1998;**10**:236–7)

Codeine OD (n = 1, *Neurobehavioral Toxicol Teratol* 1985;**7**:93–4)

Diamorphine (BNF, caution in psychosis)

Dipipanone (BNF, uncommon)

Fentanyl (BNF, v rare)

Methadone withdrawal (e.g. n = 2, *J Clin Psychiatry* 1995;**56**:73–6)

Morphine intrathecal (*Anesth Analg* 1993;**77**: 1298–9)

Naltrexone (after heroin detox, n = 1, *Am J Addict* 2005;**14**:486–7)

Oxycodone (BNF, caution in psychosis)

Paracetamol overdose (*Gen Hosp Psychiatry* 1997;**19**; 149–50)

Pentazocine (esp. hallucinations, e.g. *Br Med J* 1974;**2**:224)

- CNS — anticonvulsants *

Psychosis induced by anticonvulsants may be the result of 'forced normalisation'. Risk factors include temporal lobe epilepsy (TLE), treatment resistance, past history of psychosis or affective disorder, and becoming suddenly seizure-free (best to do this gradually). Drug regimens should be changed gradually and compliance should be maintained to prevent epileptic psychoses (n = 44, Matsuura, *J Neurol Neurosurg Psychiatry* 1999;**67**:231–3).

Carbamazepine (BNF, rare)

Carbamazepine toxicity (*Lancet* 1989;**i**:167)

Carbamazepine withdrawal (n = 1, *Br J Clin Pract* 1996;**50**:350–1)

Clonazepam (n = 1, *J Nerv Ment Dis* 1982;**170**: 117)

Clonazepam withdrawal (*J Clin Psychopharmacol* 1986;**6**:193)

Ethosuximide (BNF, rare)

Gabapentin (exacerbation of psychosis in schizophrenic, n = 1, *Can J Psychiatry* 2002;**47**:975–6)

Lamotrigine (*Epilepsy Behav* 2007;**11**:476; n = 4, incidence 0.2%, *Epilepsy Behav* 2007;**11**:133–9)

Levetiracetam (BNF, less common; cases within n = 517, *Neurology* 2003;**61**:704–6; n = 1, long-term, *Can J Psychiatry* 2004;**49**:868; n = 1, *Med Clin [Barc]* 2007;**129**:278)

Oxcarbazepine (n = 1, *Epilepsy Behav* 2008; **12**:492–3)

Phenytoin toxicity (e.g. n = 1 for trigeminal neuralgia, *Epilepsy Behav* 2003;**4**:771–2; *Clin Pediatr [Phila]* 1993;**32**:107–10)

Pregabalin (n = 1, *Seizure* 2006;**15**:208–10)

Tiagabine (BNF, rare; RCT shows no significant risk; n = 554, *Epilepsia* 2002;**43**:394–8; n = 1, *Neuropsychiatr* 2007;**21**:59–61; n = 596, 1.5% incidence, esp. with previous episodes, *Epilepsy Behav* 2003;**4**:548–52)

Topiramate (n = 596, 1.5% incidence, esp. with previous episodes, *Epilepsy Behav* 2003; **4**:548–52; n = 1, migraine prophylaxis, *Am J Health Syst Pharm* 2010;**67**:1178–80; n = 2, *Clin Neuropharmacol* 2006;**29**:168–9)

Valproate (isolated cases, e.g. *Clin Electroencephalography* 1982;**13**:50–3)

Vigabatrin (BNF, less common; e.g. n = 1, *Acta Med Port* 2000;**13**:111–4; review, *Acta Neurol Scand* 1996;**93**:1–8)

Vigabatrin withdrawal (*Med J Aust* 1992;**156**: 291; letter in *Lancet* 1990;**335**:1279)

Zonisamide (BNF, less common; n = 74, incidence 13–18%, *Seizure* 2000;**9**:65–70; n = 1, *Am J Psychiatry* 2007;**164**:682)

- CNS — antiparkinsonian drugs

The incidence with Parkinsonian treatments may be as high as 20–30%.

Review: Kuzuhara, *J Neurol* 2001;**248**(Suppl 3): 28–31.

Amantadine (n = 2, exacerbation of schizophrenia, *Am J Psychiatry* 1986;**143**: 1170–1; overdose, n = 1, *Ann Emerg Med* 1990;**19**:668–70)

Anticholinergics (in people with Alzheimer's disease, n = 230, *Clin Pharmacol Ther* 2008; **84**:63–8):
- → biperidin (*Med Clin (Barc)* 1992;**99**:79)
- → trihexyphenidyl

Barbiturates

Cabergoline (BNF, caution in psychosis; n = 2, exacerbation of schizophrenia when used as adjunct, *Gen Hosp Psychiatry* 2008;**30**:378–80)

Dopamine agonists:
- → bromocriptine (BNF, rare; cases inc. *An Med Interna* 2003;**20**:50–1; low-dose n = 1, *Acta Obstet Gynecol Scand* 1991;**70**:375–6; n = 2, *Harefuah* 1990;**118**:203–4)
- → bromocriptine + pseudoephedrine (n = 1, *J Fam Pract* 1997;**45**:164–6)
- → pergolide (BNF, caution in psychosis; esp. hallucinations, incidence ≤ 13%, e.g. *Neurology* 1982;**32**:1181–4)
- → pramipexole (BNF, *Psychiatry Clin Neurosci* 2008;**62**:245)
- → ropinirole (BNF, less common; n = 95, 14% incidence, *Ann Pharmacother* 2009;**43**:1426–32; n = 1, *Prog Neuropsychopharmacol Biol Psychiatry* 2008;**32**:1087–8; n = 1, *Am J Psychiatry* 2006;**163**:457–8)
- → rotigotine (BNF, less common)

Levodopa (esp. hallucinations — *Arch Neurol* 1970;**23**:193–200)

Lisuride (a few cases, e.g. *Lancet* 1986;**2**:510)

Selegiline (a few cases, e.g. *Neurology* 1981;**31**: 19–23)

- CNS — others *

Review: drug-induced symptoms in Parkinson's disease (Kuzuhara, *J Neurol* 2001;**248**(Suppl 3): 28–31).

Adderall® (n = 1, *J Am Board Fam Pract* 2002; **99**:498–500)

Alcohol

Alcohol, caffeine and 'vigueur fit' (n = 1, *Med Sci Law* 2001;**41**:331–6)

Amfetamine (*Gen Hosp Psychiatry* 1996;**18**:117–20; treatment for this, review *Cochrane Database Syst Rev* 2009;**1**:CD003026)

Atomoxetine (n = 1, transient, *J Child Adolesc Psychopharmacol* 2009;**19**:319–20)

Bupropion (n = 1, *Indian J Psychiatry* 2009;**51**: 53–4; n = 2, *Pharm World Sci* 2009;**31**:238–40)

Caffeine (n = 1, *CNS Spectr* 2009;**14**:127–9)

5

Cannabis:

Cannabis (acute onset, usually resolves in 2–7 days. See box below)

Cocaine (review of risk factors, e.g. low BMI, n = 69, Isr J Psychiatry Relat Sci 2005;**42**:45–50; review, Rev Med Leige 2010;**65**:623-7)

Cocaine + OTC cold cure (J Clin Psychiatry 1989;**50**:147)

Dexamfetamine (BNF, less common; Pediatrics 2004;**113**:1466)

Dexfenfluramine (Am J Psychiatry 1997;**154**: 1624–5)

Diethylpropion (n = 1, Int Clin Psychopharmacol

The case for cannabis causing psychosis and/or schizophrenia *

- Earlier use is associated with a greater risk of developing psychosis (n = 472, Acta Psychiatr Scand 2008;**118**:209–13; n = 3801, Arch Gen Psychiatry 2010;**67**:440–7; n = 116, Eur Psychiatry 2009;**24**:282–6) and at an earlier age (n = 68, Dragt et al, Can J Psychiatry 2010;**55**:165–71).
- Patients in the prodromal phase and at ultra-high risk for psychosis seem more vulnerable to the negative effects of cannabis (n = 121, Aust NZ J Psychiatry 2009;**43**:1155–62).
- Regular use may increase illness severity (n = 3459, J Nerv Ment Dis 2009;**197**:35–40).
- Cannabis may also reduce brain volume over five years (n = 82, Am J Psychiatry 2008;**165**: 490–6).
- The risk appears to be higher with skunk, use for over five years (n = 280 [c = 174], Di Forti et al, Br J Psychiatry 2009;**195**:488––91) and over 10 years (Foti et al, Am J Psychiatry 2010;**167**:987–93).
- There is a significant interindividual sensitivity (n = 190, Goldberger et al, Int J Neuropsycho-pharmacol 2010;**13**:1145–54), e.g. having the COMT Val(158)Met polymorphism (n = 157, Estrada et al, Acta Psychiatr Scand 2011;**123**:485–92), or at ultra high risk (n = 284, Psychol Med 2009;**39**:951–6; n = 121, Aust NZ J Psychiatry 2010;**44**:230–6).
- In someone with schizophrenia, stopping cannabis can lead to a clear improvement (n = 92, Gonzalez-Pinto et al, Schizophr Bull 2011;**37**:631–9).

The case against cannabis causing psychosis and/or schizophrenia *

- Cannabis use has risen steadily since the mid-1990s, and there is no evidence of increasing schizophrenia or psychosis in people aged 16–44 (n = 600 000 a year, or 2.3% UK population aged 16–44, Frisher et al, Schizophr Res 2009;**113**:123–8), although it could of course hasten the onset (n = 116, Sugranyes et al, Eur Psychiatry 2009;**24**:282–6; Int J Drug Policy 2010;**21**:10–9).
- Cannabis is neither a sufficient nor necessary cause for psychosis (Arseneault et al, Br J Psychiatry 2004;**184**:110–7; systematic review, s = 35, Lancet 2007;**370**:319–28).

Conclusion: *
- Cannabis use brings forward the onset of psychosis which might otherwise have had good prognostic indicators, and continued use makes the psychosis more difficult to treat (n = 99, Leeson et al, Schiphr Bull 2011; in press).
- At higher doses, cannabis is a risk factor for the development or relapse of schizophrenia.
- Use in vulnerable adolescents carries a high risk (Casadio et al, Neurosci Biobehav Rev 2011;**35**:1779–87.
- You would have to stop 5000 people smoking cannabis to prevent one case of schizophrenia.
- Cannabis should be avoided if it makes psychotic symptoms worse. If antipsychotic compliance is good, positive symptoms unchanged on consumption, occasional modest use may carry a relatively lower risk.

Review: meta-analysis (s = 35, Koskinen et al, Schizophr Bull 2010;**36**:1115–30).

1993;**8**:67–70; n = 5, *Clin Neuropharmacol* 1988;**11**:183–8)

Disulfiram (BNF, rare; C/I in psychosis; e.g. n = 1, *Ned Tijdschr Geneeskd* 2002;**146**:965):

→ low-dose (n = 1, *Prog Neuropsychopharmacol Biol Psychiatry* 2008; **32**;311–2)

→ high-dose (n = 1, *J Clin Psychopharmacol* 2007;**27**:224–5)

Ephedra alkaloids (in 'vigueur fit' tablets; n = 1, *Med Sci Law* 2001;**41**:331–6; n = 7, *South Med J* 2003;**96**:718–20)

Gamma-hydroxybutyrate (GHB) withdrawal (n = 8, *Ann Emerg Med* 2001;**37**:147–53)

Hyoscine (n = 4 plus review, *Fortschr Neurol Psychiatr* 1998;**66**:289–95)

Hyoscine transdermal patches (e.g. Transderm®, *Neurology* 2000; **54**:1877; n = 3, *Can J Hosp Pharm* 1994;**47**:67–9)

Khat (n = 1, *Tijdschr Psychiatr* 2007;**49**:763–7; review of association in Somalia, n = 4854, *BMC Med* 2005;**3**:5; n = 1, *Ethiop Med J* 1997; **35**:137–9)

Khat + mushrooms (n = 4, *World J Biol Psychiatry* 2004;**5**:49–53)

MDMA/ecstasy (n = 1, *Lijec Vjesn* 2000;**122**:27–30; n = 1, persistent after single dose, *Psychosomatics* 2001;**42**:525–7; n = 1, very persistent, *Psychol Rep* 2004;**95**:192–6; n = 32, *Eur Addict Res* 2002;**8**:133–40)

Memantine (BNF, less common; n = 1, in bipolar, *J Clin Psychiatry* 2010;**71**:957; n = 1, *J Clin Psychiatry* 2005; **66**:658–9; n = 3, *Neurology* 2005;**65**:481–2)

Methamphetamine (n = 21, 6/12 follow-up, *Zhonghua Yi Xue Za Zhi [Taipei]* 2001; **64**:388–94; n = 309, incidence 13%, *Addiction* 2006;**101**:1473–8; n = 39, *Psychiatry Res* 2008;**157**:273–7)

Methylphenidate (BNF, v rare; n = 3 in adults, *Clin Neuropharmacol* 2010;**33**:204–6)

Methysergide (n = 1, *Neuropsychobiology* 1989; **22**:125–7)

Metoclopramide (n = 2, *Ann Pharmacother* 2002; **36**:1387–90)

Modafinil (may exacerbate: n = 1, *Arch Gen Psychiatry* 2002;**59**:292–3; n = 1, *Am J Psychiatry* 2005;**162**:1983; n = 1, *Intern Med J* 2008;**38**:677–8)

Nabilone (BNF, common)

Naltrexone (after heroin detox, n = 1, *Am J Addict* 2005;**14**:486–7)

Nandrolone (n = 1, *Psychiatr Prax* 2003;**30**(Suppl 3):S73–4)

Nicotine, abrupt withdrawal (n = 1, *Am J Psychiatry* 1994;**151**:452)

Promethazine (rare but possible, e.g. *NEJM* 1960;**263**:747)

Silbutramine (e.g. n = 1, *Prog Neuropsychopharmacol Biol Psychiatry* 2010;**34**:1359–60; in OTC diet aid n = 1, *Turk Psikiyatri Derg* 2010;**21**:335–7; n = 1, *J Psychosom Res* 2008;**64**:107–9)

Sodium oxybate (SmPC)

Varenicline (n = 1, relapse of pre-existing schizophrenia, *J Clin Psychiatry* 2007;**68**:1269; n = 1, *CNS Spectr* 2010;**15**:470–2; n = 1, *Pharmacotherapy* 2009;**29**:852–7)

Varenicline withdrawal (n = 1, *Am J Psychiatry* 2010;**167**:720–1)

- Gastrointestinal drugs

Antidiarrheals (OTC) (n = 1, *Br J Psychiatry* 1990; **157**:758–9)

Bismuth toxicity (*Am Fam Physician* 1988;**38**: 244–6)

Cimetidine (*Indian Pediatr* 1989;**26**:1061–2; n = 1, *Am J Psychiatry* 1980;**137**:1112–3)

Dicycloverine

- Cardiovascular drugs

ACE inhibitors, e.g.:

→ lisinopril (*Psychiatr Prax* 1998;**25**:204)

Amyl nitrate (Martindale, 1993)

Beta–blockers (see under depression for differentials), e.g.:

→ atenolol (rare, n = 1, *Am J Psychiatry* 1983; **140**:1382)

→ propranolol (well known, e.g. n = 1, *Am J Emerg Med* 1995;**13**:536–7)

→ propranolol withdrawal (*Biol Psychiatry* 1989;**25**:351–4)

Calcium–channel blockers, e.g.:

→ diltiazem (n = 1, *Arch Intern Med* 1991; **151**:373–4; *J R Soc Med* 1988;**81**:296–7)

→ enalapril (n = 1, *Drug Intell Clin Pharm* 1991; **25**:558–9)

→ nifedipine (e.g. *Am J Med* 1987;**83**:389; n = 1, *Am J Med* 1986;**81**:705–6)

→ quinapril (n = 1, *J Am Geriatr Soc* 2000;**48**: 1533)

Clonidine (n = 1, *Prog Neuropsychopharmacol* 1980;**4**:21)

5

Clonidine withdrawal (n = 3, *Am J Psychiatry* 1982;**139**:110–2)

Digoxin toxicity (BNF, v rare; *J Nerv Mental Dis* 1978;**166**:817; *Lijec Vjesn* 1991;**113**:417–9)

Disopyramide (BNF, very rare; e.g. *Lancet* 1978;**1**: 858 + 1152)

Dopamine infusion (*Biol Psychiatry* 1992;**31**: 1225–7)

Doxazosin (n = 1, *Br Med J* 1997;**314**:1869)

Hydralazine

Lidocaine IV (n = 6, *Ann Intern Med* 1982;**97**: 149–50)

Losartan (*Cardiology* 1996;**87**:569–70)

Methyldopa (BNF, mild psychosis is common; *Adv Psych Treat* 2005;**11**:66)

Mexilitine (n = 1, *Am Heart J* 1984;**107**:1091–8)

Nitrates, e.g. isosorbides (*Adv Psychiatr Treat* 2005;**11**:66)

Pentoxifylline (*J Assoc Physicians India* 1992;**40**: 479)

Procainamide (BNF, uncommon; *Crit Care Nurse* 1993;**13**:70–2)

Quinidine (n = 1, *Med J Aust* 1990;**153**:47–9)

Simvastatin (n = 3, *Ned Tijdschr Geneeskd* 1993; **137**:1312–5)

Tocainide (*Br Med J* 1984;**288**:606–7)

- **Respiratory drugs** *

Betamethasone (n = 1, *No To Shinkei* 1992;**44**: 913–6)

Chlorphenamine OD (n = 1, *Med J Aust* 1973; **1**:382–6)

Coricidin cold medicine (*Ann Pharmacother* 2005;**39**:9977–8)

Cyproheptadine (*Indian J Pediatr* 1989;**56**:521–3; n = 1, *Pediatr Emerg Care* 1986;**2**:183–5)

Dextromethorphan (review, *Addict Biol* 2005;**10**:325–7; n = 1, *Am J Psychiatry* 2000; **157**:304)

Dextromethorphan + hydrocodone + propoxyphene (n = 1, *J Psychopharmacol* 2009;**23**:989–91)

Diphenhydramine (e.g. *Am J Emerg Med* 1997;**99**: 548–9; n = 2, *Chudoku Kenkyu* 2007;**20**:125–9)

Diphenhydramine overdose (n = 1, *Dtsch Med Wochenschr* 1988;**113**:180–3)

Ephedrine (n = 1, *Harefuah* 1994;**127**:166–8;299)

Phenylpropanolamine (e.g. with caffeine, *Biol Psychiatry* 1991;**30**:401–4; n = 1, *Am J Psychiatry* 2000;**157**:1021–2)

Phenylpropanolamine + amantadine (n = 1, *Gen Hosp Psychiatry* 1995;**17**:457–8)

Promethazine (n = 1, *Psychosomatics* 2004;**45**: 89–90)

Salbutamol (*Biol Psychiatry* 1989;**26**:631–3)

Salbutamol inhaler (n = 1, *J Clin Psychopharmacol* 1995;**99**:446–7)

Theophylline (n = 1, *J Clin Psychopharmacol* 1989; **9**:65–6)

- **Anti-infection drugs** *

Aciclovir (BNF, rare; *Adv Psych Treat* 2005;**11**:66)

Amoxicillin + clarithromycin (n = 1, *Paediatr Anaesth* 2005;**99**:703–5)

Amoxicillin (co-amoxiclav; n = 1, *Praxis (Bern 1994)* 2009;**98**:765–6)

Amoxicillin + clarithromycin + pantoprazole (n = 1, *Neuropsychiatr* 2010;**24**:144–50)

Antifungals, e.g.:

   → amphotericin B IV (n = 1, *Ariz Med* 1972; **29**:322)

   → griseofulvin (*Adv Psychiatr Treat* 2005;**11**: 66)

   → posaconazole (BNF, common)

Antimalarials, e.g.:

   → chloroquine (n = 1, *Am J Ther* 2007;**14**: 406–7; n = 1, recurrent, *Indian J Med Sci* 1996;**50**:302–4; n = 1, *Presse Med* 2003; **32**:117; *Lancet* 1985;**2**:37)

   → lariam (severe is extremely low, e.g. one in 6000, *Pharm J* 1996;**256**:184)

   → mefloquine (BNF, less common; n = 179, more common in females and first-time users; *Eur J Clin Pharmacol* 2002;**58**:441–5; n = 1, after a single dose, responded to quetiapine, *Malar J* 2006;**5**:74)

   → quinine (*Br J Psychiatry* 1988;**153**:575–6)

Antiretrovirals, e.g.:

   → efavirenz (BNF, less common; e.g. n = 1, *Clin Infect Dis* 2007;**45**:128–30; n = 1, *Clin Infect Dis* 2005;**40**:22–3)

Antituberculous drugs (*Lancet* 1989;**ii**:105; 735–6):

   → cycloserine (BNF, common; *Adv Psychiatr Treat* 2005;**11**:66)

   → ethambutol toxicity (n = 1, *Int J STD AIDS* 2007;**18**:287–8)

   → isoniazid (BNF, common; caution in psychosis; *Gen Hosp Psychiatry* 2007;**29**:85–6; n = 1, *Pediatr Emerg Care* 2002;**18**:25–7)

   → rifampicin (*Indian J Lepr* 1992;**64**:537–9)

Carbaryl (n = 1, *Am J Psychiatry* 1995;**152**:466–7)

Cephalosporins (*Aust NZ J Psychiatry* 2003;**37**: 627–8), e.g.:
→ cefuroxime (*Lancet* 1984;i:965)
→ cephalexin (n = 1, *Med J Aust* 1973;i:497)
→ cephalothin (*Drug Intell Clin Pharm* 1974;**8**: 71)

Ciclosporin (n = 1, *Lijec Vjesn* 2007;**129**:75–6)

Colistin (BNF, rare)

Co-trimoxazole (several e.g. n = 1, *Pharmacopsychiatry* 2006;**39**:236–7)

Dapsone (BNF, uncommon at low doses; e.g. *J Indian Med Assoc* 1989;**87**:120–1; n = 1, *J Trop Med Hyg* 1993;**96**:274–6; *Br Med J* 1989;**299**:324)

Ethambutol (n = 1, *Ann Thoracic Med* 2008;**3**: 149–51)

Ethionamide (*Adv Psychiatr Treat* 2005;**11**:66)

Foscarnet (BNF, common; *Adv Psychiatr Treat* 2005;**11**:66)

Ganciclovir (BNF, less common; n = 1, *Pharmacother* 2000;**20**:479–83; *N Eng J Med* 1996;**335**:1397)

Gatifloxacin (*Am J Geriatr Psychiatry* 2003; **11**:470–1; n = 1, *J Am Geriatr Soc* 2006;**54**: 871; *Psychosomatics* 2007;**48**:87)

Isoniazid (n = 1, *Ann Thoracic Med* 2008;**3**:149–51; n = 1, *Psychosomatics* 2009;**50**:640–1)

Ketoconazole (n = 1, idiosyncratic and v rare, *Am J Psychiatry* 1990;**147**:677)

Levamisole (*Ann Pharmacother* 1998;**32**:134–5)

Macrolides, e.g.:
→ clarithromycin (BNF, v rare; e.g. *Med J Malaysia* 2006;**61**:263; n = 1, *Psychiatr Bull* 2004;**28**:98–9)
→ erythromycin (n = 2, *Arch Internal Med* 1986;**146**:897–9)
→ erythromycin + bromocriptine (n = 1, *Neurologia* 1997;**12**:429)
→ nalidixic acid (a few cases, e.g. *Br Med J* 1965;**2**:590)

Mefloquine (n = 1, child, *J Child Neurol* 2009;**24**: 1008–9)

Mepacrine (BNF, rare, transient)

Metronidazole (BNF, v rare; *J Fam Pract* 1988;**27**: 323–5; n = 1, *Am J Psychiatry* 1997;**154**:1170–1)

Nitrofurantoin (*Adv Psychiatr Treat* 2005;**11**:66)

Oseltamivir (no evidence for increased risk of neuropsychiatric ADRs in people aged 1–21; *Int J Adolesc Med Health* 2009;**21**:79–89)

Penicillin (several cases, e.g. *Br J Psychiatry* 1990; **156**:554)

Primaquine (n = 1, *Ann Intern Med* 1980;**92**:435)

Quinacrine (e.g. n = 1, *Hum Psychopharmacol* 2002;**17**:357–9)

Quinolones (*Adv Psychiatr Treat* 2005;**11**:66), e.g.:
→ ciprofloxacin (many e.g. n = 1, *Eur Psychiatry* 2003;**18**:262–3; n = 1, *Psychosomatics* 2007;**48**:269; n = 1, *Arch Ophthalmol* 2002; **120**:665–6)
→ levofloxacin (rare but can be serious, SmPC, n = 1, *Gen Hosp Psychiatry* 2008;**30**:381–3)
→ nalidixic acid (BNF, less common; injection n = 1, *J Forensic Sci* 1986;**31**:1145–9)
→ norfloxacin (*J Assoc Physicians India* 1994;**42**: 844)
→ ofloxacin (*Psychiatr Prax* 1996;**23**:251; n = 2, *Int J STD AIDS* 2003;**14**:636–7)
→ pefloxacin (n = 1, *Prog Neuropsycho-pharmacol Biol Psychiatry* 1996;**20**:343–7)

Sulfadiazine (n = 2, *Clin Infect Dis* 1992;**99**:556–7)

Tobramycin (a few cases, e.g. *Pediatr Pulmonol* 1988;**4**:201–4)

Trimethoprim (*Adv Psychiatr Treat* 2005;**11**:66)

Triple therapy for H Pylori (*J Am Board Fam Pract* 2002;**99**:66–8)

Valaciclovir (n = 1, *Psychosomatics* 2009;**50**: 293–6)

- **Endocrine system drugs**

Adrenocorticotropin

Carbimazole

Clomifene (n = 1, *Hum Reprod* 1997;**12**:706–7; n = 2, *Am J Psychiatry* 1997; **154**:1169–70)

Corticosteroids (aggravation of schizophrenia, incidence may be as high as 5–6% in adults, usually emerges within a few days or weeks, risk may be higher with higher doses, *MHRA Drug Safety Update* 2007;1–9; review, *Gen Hosp Psychiatry* 2003;**25**:27–33):
→ corticosteroid withdrawal (*J Pain Symptom Manage* 2007;**34**:118–9)
→ deflazacort (aggravation of symptoms, SmPC)
→ dexamethasone withdrawal (*Lijec Vjesn* 1988;**110**:94–6)
→ prednisone (usually > 40 mg/d, e.g. case and discussion in *Br J Psychiatry* 1993;**162**:549–53; low dose n = 1, *Endocr J* 2006;**53**:255–8)
→ prednisolone + clarithromycin (n = 1, *Gen Hosp Psychiatry* 1998;**20**:325–6)
→ triamcinolone (SmPC, dose–related;

5

nasal spray n = 1, *Prog Neurol Psychiatry* 2007;**11**:31–2)

Desmopressin (n = 1, *Lancet* 1981;**2**:808)

Estrogen withdrawal (review, n = 26, *J Acta Psychiatr Scand* 2001;**104**:323)

Iodine, radioactive (n = 1, *Am J Psychiatry* 2009; **166**:1067–8)

Insulin abuse (*Br Med J* 1971;**4**:792–3)

Methyltestosterone (*Lancet* 1987;**i**:863)

Quinagolide (BNF, v rare)

- Malignancy and immunosuppressant drugs *

Ciclosporin (*Psychosomatics* 1993;**34**:101–2)

5-fluorouracil (n=1, *Clin Colorectal Cancer* 2009;**8**:166-8)

Gonadorelin (*Br J Psychiatry* 1999;**175**:290–1)

Ifosfamide (BNF, common; e.g. n = 1, *Farm Hosp* 2006;**30**:399–6; n = 1, *Psychooncology* 2007;**16**:956–60)

Interferons e.g.:

  → interferon-alfa (e.g. n = 1, psychotic depression, *J Psychopharmacol* 2005;**19**: 102–5; n = 1, *Pharmacopsychiatry* 2007;**40**:146–8; n = 1, persistent, *J Clin Psychopharmacol* 2006;**26**:446–7)

  → peginterferon alfa 2b + ribavirin (n = 1, *Int Clin Psychopharmacol* 2005;**20**:289–90; n = 1, *Braz J Infect Dis* 2006;**10**:406–7)

  → interferon-alfa + ribavirin (n=1, *Psychosomatics* 2009;**50**:538-42)

  → interferon-beta-1b (n=1, *Psychiatry Clin Neurosci* 2010;**64**:584-6)

Leuprolide (n=1, *J Clin Psychiatry* 2010;**71**:1696-8)

Leuprorelin acetate (n = 1, *Nervenarzt* 2007;**78**: 691–5)

Tacrolimus (BNF, rare; n = 1, *Int J Neuro-psychopharmacol* 2006;**9**:493–4)

- Musculoskeletal and analgesics *

Allopurinol (n = 1, causing relapse, *Schizophr Res* 2007;**93**:409)

Aspirin (*JAMA* 1965;**193**:555–8)

Baclofen (many e.g. n=1, *Ann Pharmacother* 2006; **40**:2071–3; intoxication, n = 18, *Przegl Lek* 2004;**61**:389–91)

Baclofen withdrawal (n=1, *J Neuropsychiatry Clin Neurosci* 2009;**21**:476)

Carisoprodol withdrawal (n = 1, *Ann Clin Psychiatry* 2008;**20**:173–4)

Chloroquine (BNF, rare)

Hydroxychloroquine (BNF, rare)

Indometacin (rare, e.g. cases within n = 32, *Can J Anaesth* 2003;**50**:586–8; n = 1, *Postgrad Med J* 2000;**76**:736–7)

Indometacin + ciprofloxacin (n =1, *Rev Clin Esp* 1992;**191**:401)

Pyridostigmine (n = 1, *Deutsch Med Wschr* 1966; **9**:699)

Sulindac (*JAMA* 1980;**243**:1420)

- Others *

Atropine (oral, IV, eye drops, e.g. *DICP Ann Pharmacother* 1990;**24**:708–9; n = 4 plus review, *Fortschr Neurol Psychiatr* 1998;**66**:289–95; *J Assoc Physicians India* 1990; **38**:444–5)

Brimonidine eye drops (*Arch Ophthalmol* 2000; **118**:1132–3)

Butane (n = 1, *Psychiatry Clin Neurosci* 2001;**55**:163)

Colubrina — see Mabi bark

Cyanide (*Arch Environ Health* 1997;**52**:245–6)

Cyclobenzaprine (n = 1, *Can J Psychiatry* 2000;**45**: 763–4)

Cyclopentolate eye drops (several e.g. n = 1, *J Cataract Refract Surg* 2003;**29**:1026–30)

Distigmine bromide (n = 1, *Eur Psychiatry* 2003; **18**:318–9)

Energy drinks (n = 1, *Am J Psychiatry* 2010; **167**:353)

Flumazenil (*Lancet* 1992;**339**:488–9)

Herbal preparations and supplements (n = 1, *Int J Psychiatry Med* 2007;**37**:279–82; n = 1, *S D Med* 2008;**61**:173–7)

Inhalants (n = 40, responds to carbamazepine, *Psychiatr Serv* 1998;**49**:812–5)

Insect repellant (*Psychosomatics* 2001;**42**:78–80; n = 1, after 2/52 topical application of DEET, *Am J Psychiatry* 1987;**144**:1103–4)

Iohexol (n = 1, *Neuroradiology* 1994;**36**:141)

Isotretinoin (no evidence for causing psychosis or any other psychiatric disorder, n = 21911, *Arch Dermatol* 2000;**136**:1231–6; n = 5, *Int Clin Psychopharmacol* 2005;**20**:39–41)

Ketamine (discussion, *Am J Psychiatry* 1997;**154**: 805–11)

Ketorolac (BNF, less common)

Lactate oral (e.g. in calcium lactate tablets, case in *Ann Pharmacother* 1995;**29**:539–40)

Mabi bark tea (n = 1, *Br J Psychiatry* 1992;**161**: 404–7; hotly disputed, *Br J Psychiatry* 1993; **162**:275)

Methazolamide (n = 1, *Pharmacotherapy* 1997;
17:387–9)

Metrizamide (n = 1, prolonged, *Psychosomatics*
1986;**27**:373–5)

Mouthwash containing alcohol (n = 1, *Mil Med*
2009;**174**:828–31)

Nitrous oxide abuse (n = 1, *J Med Toxicol* 2006;
2:71–4)

Nutmeg (*J R Soc Med* 1993;**86**:179–80; *Br J
Psychiatry* 1993;**162**:131)

Oral contraceptive, combined (n = 1, *Gynecol
Endocrinol* 2007;**23**:361–2)

Organic solvents (n = 2, *Nihon Arukoru Yakubutsu
Igakkai Zasshi* 2007;**42**:76–81)

Oxybutynin (n = 2, *Clin Drug Investig* 2006;**26**:
603–6)

Oxymetazoline nasal spray (several e.g. *CMAJ*
1994;**150**: 375–6)

Peyote plant (n = 1, *J Clin Psychiatry* 2004;**65**:
1433–4)

Phenylephrine (*JAMA* 1982;**247**:1859)

Pilocarpine (*Psychosomatics* 2005;**46**:88)

Procaine penicillin (n = 1, *Int J Dermatol* 1995;
34:627–9)

Salvia divinorum (n = 1, *Am J Psychiatry* 2009;
166:832)

Styrene exposure (n = 1, *J Clin Exp Neuropsychol*
1990;**12**:798–806)

Thallium poisoning (n = 1, *J Assoc Physicians India*
2006;**54**:53–5)

Timolol eye drops (n = 163 from National
Registry reports, *J Clin Psychopharmacol* 1987;
7:264–7)

Toluene (*Br J Psychiatry* 1991;**158**:578)

Trichloroethylene abuse (n = 1, *Arch Neurobiol
(Madr)* 1989;**52**:198–202)

Yohimbine (unproven, see *Arch Gen Psychiatry*
1998;**55**:1033–44)

5.13 SEROTONIN SYNDROME (SS)

Serotonin syndrome (SS) has been reported
with a variety of antidepressants, buspirone,
carbamazepine, pethidine, dextromethorphan
and levodopa, usually in combination but can
be monotherapy or in overdose. There was an
FDA alert on SS with SSRIs/SNRIs and triptans,
but other data suggests SS is rare and the
combination should not be prohibited (n = 29,
MedGenMed 2007;**9**:48). There were 7349
reported cases of SS and 93 deaths in USA in
2002 (Bush et al, *J Palliat Med* 2006;**9**:1257–9).
Few SS reports have been fully documented
or peer reviewed and so are not confirmed.
It is not idiopathic, but a predictable adverse
consequence of excess serotonergic agonism.

Reviews: * prevention, recognition, management
(Ables and Nagubilli, *Am Fam Physician* 2010;
81:1139–42), misdiagnosis (n = 7, Attar–Herzberg
et al, *Isr Med Assoc J* 2009;**11**:367–70).

* Monotherapy *

Amantadine (n = 1, *Am J Emerg Med* 2008;
26:5–6)

Bupropion OD (n = 1, *J Med Toxicol*
2010;**6**:168–71)

Chlorphenamine? (*Singapore Med J* 2006;**47**:
1014)

Dexfenfluramine (n = 1, *JAMA* 1996;**276**:1220–1)

Dextromethorphan (n = 1, *Geriatr Gerentol Int*
2011;**11**:121–2)

Duloxetine (n = 1, *Aust N Z J Psychiatry* 2009;
43:581–2)

MDMA/ecstasy (review of risks; *Aust N Z J
Psychiatry* 2007; **41**:649–55; *Pharmacol
Biochem Behav* 2002;**71**:837–44)

Methadone (n = 1, *J Palliat Med* 2006;**9**:
1257–9)

Milnacipran (n = 1, *Neurology* 2010;**74**:699–
700)

Mirtazapine (n = 1, *Rev Esp Anestesiol Reanim*
2009;**56**:515-6; n = 1, *Clin Neuropharmacol*
2003;**26**: 54–7)

Pethidine (n = 1, *Br J Anaesth* 2009;**103**:369–70)

SSRIs, e.g.:

→ citalopram (n = 1, *Kaohsiung J Med Sci*
2005;**21**:326–8; n = 1, after a first–time
low dose, *Neurotoxicology* 2007;**28**:1272–4;
n = 1, misdiagnosed as fibromyalgia, *Phys
Ther* 2008;**88**:757–65)

→ fluoxetine (several, e.g. n= 1,
Psychopharmacol Bull 2008;**41**:76–9)

→ fluvoxamine (e.g. after single dose
n = 1, *Ann Emerg Med* 1999; **34**:806–7;
mild syndrome may occur in 43% on
fluvoxamine alone, n = 37, *Int J Neurosci*
2001;**109**:165–72)

→ paroxetine (at standard dose in 80-
year-old, n = 1, *Am J Ther* 2006;**13**:550–2;
delayed effect, n = 1, *Consult Pharm* 2009;
24:64–8; OD n = 1, fatal, *Psychosomatics*
2010;**51**:437–42)

5

→ sertraline low dose (*J Clin Psycho-pharmacol* 2000;**20**:713–4; single 50 mg dose in nine-year-old, *Clin Toxicol (Phila)* 2008;**46**:845–9; 25 mg, n = 1, *Seishin Shinkeigaku Zasshi* 2009;**111**:1041–6)

→ sertraline overdose (n = 1, *Arch Pediatr Adolesc Med* 1997;**151**:1064–7)

Sibutramine overdose (n = 1, child, *Clin Toxicol [Phila]* 2009;**47**:598–601)

Suanzaorentang (*J Clin Psychopharmacol* 2008; **28**:113–4)

Tandospirone (n = 1, *Rinsho Shinkeigaku* 2002; **42**:892–4)

Trazodone (*Int J Geriatr Psychiatry* 1997; **12**:129–30)

Tricyclics e.g.:

→ amitriptyline (n = 1, *Postgrad Med J* 2000;**76**: 254–6)

→ clomipramine (*J Clin Psychopharmacol* 1999;**19**:285–7; possible case after withdrawal of clozapine: *Ann Pharmacother* 2001;**35**:180–2)

→ dosulepin overdose (n = 1, *J Child Adolesc Psychopharmacol* 1998;**8**:201–4)

Venlafaxine (several e.g. n = 1, *Psychiatry Clin Neurosci* 2006;**60**:121–2; 37.5 mg/d, n = 1, *Ann Pharmacother* 2003;**37**:209–11)

Ziprasidone (n = 1, *Psychiatry Clin Neurosci* 2010;**64**:338–9)

- Combinations, including SSRIs *

A self-confessed expert in SS concludes that there is no evidence for serious SS with SSRIs and triptans, and that patients will be denied effective treatment if this combination is banned (Gillman, *Headache* 2010;**50**:264–72).

Citalopram + buspirone (n = 1, *Int Clin Psychopharmacol* 1997;**12**:61–3)

Citalopram + fluconazole (n = 2, Levin *et al*, *Gen Hosp Psychiatry* 2008;**30**:372–7)

Citalopram/trazodone + linezolid (n = 1, *Ann Pharmacother* 2005;**39**:956–61)

Citalopram + linezolid (n = 1, *J Am Med Dir Assoc* 2004;**5**:111–3; n=1, *Ir J Med Sci* 2011;**180**:285-6)

Citalopram + linezolid + mirtazapine (n = 1, *J Intensive Care Med* 2005;**20**:351–3)

Citalopram + methylene blue + (n = 1, *Med J Aust* 2008;**189**:534–5)

Citalopram + moclobemide (*Med Clin [Barc]* 1999;**113**:677–8)

Citalopram overdose + moclobemide (many fatal e.g. n = 1, *Anaesthetist* 2006;**55**:1189–96; n = 1, *J Anal Toxicol* 2001;**25**:147–51)

Citalopram + pethidine (n = 1, *Psychosomatics* 2007;**48**:361–3)

Citalopram + quetiapine (n = 1, *N Z Med J* 2006;**119**:2058)

Citalopram + St John's wort (*Pharm J* 2007; **278**:487)

Citalopram + tramadol (n = 1, *Am J Psychiatry* 2004;**161**:1129)

Citalopram + trazodone + linezolid (n = 1, *Ann Pharmacother* 2005;**39**:956–61)

Escitalopram + cyclobenzaprine (a tricyclic muscle-relaxant, n = 1, *Am J Emerg Med* 2008; **26**:1069)

Fluoxetine + moclobemide + clomipramine overdose (fatal case in *Anaesth Intensive Care* 1995;**23**:499–502)

Fluoxetine + buspirone (*Ann Pharmacother* 2000;**34**:871–4)

Fluoxetine + carbamazepine (n = 1, *Lancet* 1993; **42**:442–3)

Fluoxetine + dextromethorphan (n = 1, *Gen Hosp Psychiatry* 2006;**28**:78–80)

Fluoxetine + hydromorphone (n = 1, *Prescrire Int* 2004;**13**:57)

Fluoxetine + olanzapine (n = 1, *World J Biol Psychiatry* 2004;**5**:114–5)

Fluoxetine + lithium (n = 1, *Ugeskrift for Laeger* 1995;**157**:1204–5)

Fluoxetine + mirtazapine (*Int J Geriatr Psychiatry* 1998;**13**:495–6; n = 1, *Ann Pharmacother* 2001;**35**:1217–20)

Fluoxetine + moclobemide (e.g. *Pharmaco-psychiatry* 1996;**29**:162; n = 1, *Can J Anaesth* 2000;**47**:246–50)

Fluoxetine + nefazodone (n = 1, *J Clin Psychiatry* 2000;**61**:146)

Fluoxetine + paroxetine (n = 1, *Am Fam Physician* 1995;**52**:1475–82)

Fluoxetine + pethidine (n = 1, *Anesthesiology* 2003;**98**:9911–2)

Fluoxetine + sertraline (n = 1, *Clin Pharmacol Ther* 1993;**1**:84–8)

Fluoxetine + tramadol (n = 1, *J Royal Soc Med* 1999;**92**:474–5)

Fluoxetine + tranylcypromine/trifluoperazine (n = 1, *Anaesthesia* 1991; **46**:507–8)

Fluoxetine + trazodone (*Biol Psychiatry* 1996; **39**:384–5)

Fluoxetine + venlafaxine (*Ann Pharmacother* 1998;**32**:432–6)

Fluvoxamine + oxycodone (n = 1, *Ann Pharmacother* 2006;**40**:155–7)

Paroxetine + lithium (n = 1, *Pharmacopsychiatry* 1997;**30**:106–7)

Paroxetine + methylene blue (n = 1, *Can J Anaesth* 2008;**55**:36–41)

Paroxetine + methylphenidate (n = 1, *Prog Neuropsychopharmacol Biol Psychiatry* 2010; **34**:719–20)

Paroxetine + moclobemide (n = 1, fatal, *J Anal Toxicol* 1997;**21**:518–20; *J Accid Emerg Med* 1999;**16**:293–5)

Paroxetine + moclobemide + selegiline (all low dose, n = 1, *J Chin Med Assoc* 2009;**72**:446–9)

Paroxetine + nefazodone (n = 1, *Ann Emerg Med* 1997;**29**:113–9)

Paroxetine + OTC cold remedy (*Am J Emerg Med* 1994;**12**:642–4)

Paroxetine + risperidone (*J Clin Psychopharmacol* 2000;**20**:103–5)

Paroxetine + tramadol (n = 11, *Int Clin Psychopharmacol* 1997;**12**:181–2)

Paroxetine + trazodone (*Psychosomatics* 1995; **36**:159–60)

Sertraline + amitriptyline (*Ann Pharmacother* 1996;**30**:1499–500)

Sertraline + bupropion + venlafaxine (n = 1, *Clin Neuropharmacol* 2004; **27**:219–22)

Sertraline + buspirone + loxapine (n = 1, *Therapie* 1999;**54**:269–71)

Sertraline + clomipramine (n = 1, *J Med Assoc Thai* 2005;**88**:993–6)

Sertraline + dolasetron (n = 1, *J Psychopharmacol* 2002;**16**:191)

Sertraline + erythromycin (n = 1, *Pharmacotherapy* 1999;**19**:894–6)

Sertraline + indometacin (n = 1, *J Clin Psychopharmacol* 2010;**30**:468–70)

Sertraline + linezolid (n = 1, *Clin Infect Dis* 2002;**34**:1651–2; n = 1, *Pharmacotherapy* 2006;**26**:269–76)

Sertraline + metoclopramide (n = 1, *Ann Pharmacother* 2002;**36**:67–71)

Sertraline + phenelzine (n = 1, *Ann Pharmacother* 1994;**28**:732–5)

Sertraline + risperidone + trazodone (n = 1, *CNS Spectr* 2007;**12**:396–8)

Sertraline + tramadol (several e.g. n = 1, *Aust Pres* 2002;**25**:19; n = 1, *Clin Neuropharmacol* 2004;**27**:150–1)

Sertraline + tranylcypromine (n = 1, *Clin Pharm* 1993;**12**:222–5)

SSRIs + risperidone (n = 2 [one fatal], *Ann Pharmacother* 2003;**37**:388–91)

SSRIs + dextromethorphan (supra-therapeutic dextromethorphan doses may be needed with an SSRI to create SS [n = 2, *Clin Toxicol (Phila)* 2008;**46**:771–3])

- Combinations, including MAOIs/ moclobemide (see also above) *

Moclobemide + clomipramine overdose (*Intensive Care Med* 1997;**23**:122–4; *J Toxicol Clin Toxicol* 1998;**36**:31–2)

Moclobemide + clomipramine (n = 1, *Br Med J* 1993;**306**:248)

Moclobemide + pethidine (possible case, *Med J Aust* 1995;**162**:554)

Moclobemide + venlafaxine overdose (n = 1, *Forensic Sci Int* 2009;**184**:16-20)

Phenelzine + clomipramine (n = 1, *Clin Pharmacol Therap* 1993;**53**:84–8)

Phenelzine + cyclobenzaprine (n = 1, *Anesth Analg* 2006;**103**:1466–8)

Phenelzine + dextromethorphan (n = 1, *Clin Pharmacol Therap* 1993;**53**:84–8)

Phenelzine + quetiapine (n = 1, *CNS Spectr* 2007;**12**:396–8)

Tranylcypromine + modafinil? (n = 1, *Am J Psychiatry* 2007;**164**:684),

Tranylcypromine + SSRIs + tyramine (n=1, fatal, *Pharmacopsychiatry* 2010;**43**:284-5)

Tranylcypromine + venlafaxine (cases in *Vet Hum Toxicol* 1996;**38**:358–61; *Hum Exp Toxicol* 1997;**16**:14–7)

- Other combinations (see also above) *

Buprenorphine + naloxone (Suboxone single dose, n = 1, *Am J Emerg Med* 2008;**26**:840)

Clomipramine + olanzapine (n = 1, *Minerva Anestesiol* 2008;**74**:41–5)

Dextromethorphan + chlorphenamine (n = 1, *Pediatr Emerg Care* 2007;**23**:829–31)

Duloxetine + cyclobenzaprine (n = 1, *Anesth Analg* 2006;**103**:1466–8)

Duloxetine + olanzapine, but only when olanzapine was discontinued (n=1, *Pharmacopsychiatry* 2011;**44**:75-7)

Fentanyl + 5HT3 antagonist (n = 1, *Psychosomatics* 2001;**42**:258–60)

5

Herbal detox cocktail (*Am J Emerg Med* 2004; **22**:625–6)

Linezolid + duloxetine (n = 1, *J Clin Psychopharmacol* 2006;**26**:681–3)

Linezolid (shortly after stopping paroxetine, n = 1, *Clin Infect Dis* 2002;**34**:1651–2; review of cases, *Pharmacotherapy* 2006;**26**:1784–93)

Linezolid + pethidine (n = 1, *Clin Infect Dis* 2008; **46**:264–5)

Linezolid + tryptophan + metoclopramide (n = 1, *Med Intensiva* 2009;**33**:360–1)

Methylene blue (review, n = 25, *Psychosomatics* 2010;**51**:194–200)

Mirtazapine + tramadol + olanzapine (n = 1, *Am J Psychiatry* 2002;**159**:672–3)

Nortriptyline + selegiline (n = 1, *J Neurol* 2000; **247**:811)

St John's wort + buspirone (n = 1, *J Psychopharmacol* 2002;**16**:401)

Tramadol + venlafaxine + mirtazapine (n = 1, *Ann Pharmacother* 2004;**38**:411–3)

Tramadol abuse added to sertraline + trazodone (n = 1, *Indian J Psychiatry* 2009; **51**:68)

Tramadol OD (n = 1, *Pediatr Neurol* 2011; **44**:72–4; n = 158, 5% incidence, *Clin Toxicol (Phila)* 2010;**48**:337–41)

Trazodone + amitriptyline (n = 1, *Int Clin Psychopharmacol* 1996;**11**:289–90)

Trazodone + nefazodone (n = 1, *Am J Psychiatry* 2000;**157**:1022)

Venlafaxine + amitriptyline (n = 1, *Postgrad Med J* 2000;**76**:254–6)

Venlafaxine + Antiparkinsonian drugs (n = 1, *J Clin Psychopharmacol* 2010;**30**:620–2)

Venlafaxine + co-amoxiclav (n = 1, *J R Soc Med* 2003;**96**:233–4)

Venlafaxine + dexamfetamine (n = 1, *Med J Aust* 2002;**176**:240–1)

Venlafaxine + linezolid (n = 1, *J Antimicrob Chemother* 2004;**54**:289–90; n = 1, *Ann Pharmacother* 2005;**39**:956–61)

Venlafaxine + lithium + valproate (n = 1, *Therapie* 2006;**61**:531–3)

Venlafaxine + maprotiline + reboxetine (n = 1, *Eur Psychiatry* 2004;**19**:456–7)

Venlafaxine + methadone + ciprofloxacin (n=1, *Psychosomatics* 2009;**50**:639–9)

Venlafaxine + metoclopramide (n = 1, *Ann Pharmacother* 2002;**36**:67–71)

Venlafaxine + mirtazapine (n = 1, *World J Biol Psychiatry* 2002;**3**:167)

Venlafaxine + selegiline (n = 1, *J Clin Psychopharmacol* 1997;**17**:66–7)

Venlafaxine + sour date nut (n = 1, *Am J Psychiatry* 2004;**161**:1129–30)

Venlafaxine + St John's wort? (*Presse Med* 2000; **29**:1285–6)

Venlafaxine + trazodone (n = 1, *Am J Psychiatry* 2001;**158**:2088–9)

5.14 SLEEP PROBLEMS

5.14.1 SLEEP DISTURBANCES

Review of non-psychotropic causes: Novak and Shapiro, *Drug Safety* 1997;**16**:133–49.

- CNS — anxiolytics and hypnotics

Lorazepam

Zolpidem (hypnagogic, on temporary withdrawal, n = 1, *J Toxicol Clin Toxicol* 2003; **41**:869–72)

- CNS — antipsychotics

Benperidol

Chlorpromazine

Clozapine abrupt withdrawal (n = 1, *Eur Arch Psychiatry Clin Neurosci* 1996;**246**:79–82)

Fluspirilene

Olanzapine (somnambulism, n = 2, *Am J Psychiatry* 2001;**158**:1158)

Risperidone (sleep-related eating disorder, n = 1, *J Clin Psychiatry* 2004;**65**:273–4)

Sulpiride

- CNS — antidepressants

Bupropion (incidence 11%)

Duloxetine (insomnia, BNF common)

MAOIs (hypersomnia, mainly tranylcypromine and phenelzine, *Am J Psychiatry* 1989; **146**:1078; n = 8, dose-related, *Am J Psychiatry* 1988;**145**:1552–6)

Mirtazapine (n = 1, *Br J Clin Pharmacol* 2009;**67**: 135–6)

SSRIs (all SSRIs can disrupt sleep architecture so are best taken in the morning, RCT, n = 14, *J Clin Psychiatry* 2001;**62**:642–52; somnambulism, n = 1, *J Pharm Tech* 1999; **15**:204–7):
  - → fluoxetine
  - → paroxetine (somnambulism, n = 1, *J Clin Psychiatry* 2003;**64**:483)

Trazodone

Tricyclics

- CNS — analgesics

Nefopam

- CNS — anticonvulsants

Lamotrigine (n = 109, incidence 6%, dose-related, *Epilepsia* 1999;**40**:322–5)

Levetiracetam (hypersomnia, n = 1, *Epilepsia* 2005;**46**:588–9)

Phenytoin

Rufinamide (insomnia, incidence 1–10%, UK SmPC)

- CNS — antiparkinsonian drugs

Amantadine (4% incidence, *J Clin Psychiatry* 1981;**42**:9; *Rev Neurol* 1997;**25**:2062)

Biperiden withdrawal (n = 2, *Int Clin Psychopharmacol* 2000;**15**:357–9)

Bromocriptine

Pramipexole (n = 6, *Mov Disord* 2000;**15**:658–63; n = 40, 52% incidence of somnolence, *Mov Disord* 2000;**99**:658–63)

Ropinirole and/or pramipexole (n = 2, *Pharmacother* 2000;**20**:724–6)

- CNS — others

Anticholinesterases:
→ donepezil (n = 2, *J Am Geriatr Soc* 1998; **46**:119–20)
→ rivastigmine (incidence < 5%)

Ginseng (common, *Drugs Exp Clin Res* 1996; **22**:65–72)

Methylphenidate

Methysergide

Modafinil (UK SmPC)

Nicotine (n = 252, *J Clin Psychiatry* 2001;**62**: 319–24)

Raltegravir (n = 2, *AIDS Patient Care STDS* 2009; **23**:689–90)

Sibutramine

Sodium oxybate (SmPC)

- Gastrointestinal drugs

Bismuth toxicity (*Postgrad Med J* 1988;**64**: 308–10)

Propantheline

Ranitidine (see *Adv Psychiatr Treat* 1999;**5**:30–8)

Sulfasalazine

- Cardiovascular drugs

Amiodarone (frequent, e.g. *Am J Cardiol* 1983; **52**:975–9)

Beta-blockers:
→ atenolol (very common, *Adv Psychiatr Treat* 1999;**5**:30–8)
→ carvedilol (n = 1, *Ann Pharmacother* 2002; **36**:1736–40)
→ propranolol (very common, *Adv Psychiatr Treat* 1999;**5**:30–8)

Calcium-channel blockers:
→ diltiazem (see *Adv Psychiatr Treat* 1999; **5**:30–8)
→ isradipine (up to 3%, *Am J Med* 1989; **86**[Suppl 4A]:98–102)
→ nifedipine (see *Adv Psychiatr Treat* 1999; **5**:30–8)

Clonidine for ADHD (*J Clin Psychopharmacol* 2008;**28**:725–6)

Digoxin (see *Adv Psychiatr Treat* 1999;**5**:30–8)

Statins (MHRA warning, *Drug Safety Update* 2008;**1**:10; *Drug Saf* 2008;**31**:1115–23), e.g.:
→ lovastatin (*Lancet* 1994;**343**:973)

- Respiratory drugs

Aminophylline

Brompheniramine

Montelukast (FDA warning 2009)

Pseudoephedrine

Theophylline

Zafirlukast (FDA warning 2009)

- Anti-infection drugs *

Cefalosporins (*Adv Psychiatr Treat* 2005;**11**:66)

Chloroquine (*Presse Med* 1991;**20**:659)

Cinoxacin

Ciprofloxacin (n = 1, *Lancet* 1986;**1**:819–22)

Efavirenz (dose-related, *J Acquir Immune Defic Syndr* 2001;**28**:399–400)

Fleroxacin (n = 2, *Int Clin Psychopharmacol* 1994; **9**:295–6)

Ganciclovir (*Adv Psychiatr Treat* 2005;**11**:66)

Griseofulvin (*Adv Psychiatr Treat* 2005;**11**:66)

Interferon-alfa (n = 86, insomnia often precedes depression, *Psychiatry Res* 2010; **177**:240–5)

Maraviroc (insomnia, common, UK SmPC)

Nitrofurantoin (*Adv Psychiatr Treat* 2005; **11**:66)

Quinolones (*Adv Psychiatr Treat* 2005;**11**:66)

- Endocrine system drugs

Clomifene

Corticosteroids (incidence may be as high as 5–6% in adults, usually emerges within a few days or weeks, risk may be higher with

5

higher doses, *MHRA Drug Safety Update* 2007;1–9)
→ deflazacort (SmPC)
→ triamcinolone
Tolazamide

- Malignancy and immunosuppressant drugs
Thalidomide cessation (n = 1, *Gastroenterology* 2001;**120**:1567–8)
Trabectedin (insomnia, common, UK SmPC)

- Musculoskeletal and analgesics
Diclofenac
Diflunisal
Etodolac (insomnia, SmPC)
Fenoprofen
Indometacin
Naproxen (*Eur J Rheumatol Inflamm* 1981;**4**: 87–92)
Sulindac

- Others
Eculizumab (insomnia, uncommon, SmPC)
Mercury poisoning (n = 99, *Arq Neuropsiquiatr* 2000;**58**:32–8)
Sarin toxicity (n = 161, *Percept Mot Skills* 2005; **100**:1121–6)

5.14.2 VIVID DREAMS AND NIGHTMARES *

Nightmares — a review noted that drugs affecting serotonin, noradrenaline and dopamine are clearly associated with reports of nightmares, and that immunological drugs and those affecting GABA, histamine and acetylcholine are also possible causative agents (Pagel and Helfter, *Hum Psychopharmacol* 2003;**18**:59–67).

Baclofen
Beta-blockers:
→ atenolol (*Clin Pharm Ther* 1979;**25**:8)
→ propranolol (*Adv Drug React Bull* 1983; **99**:364)
Ciprofloxacin (n = 1, *Indian J Psychiatry* 2008; **50**:305–6)
Clonidine (*Adv Drug React Bull* 1983;**99**:364)
Digoxin toxicity (*Ann Intern Med* 1980; **93**:639)
Duloxetine (insomnia, SPC common)
Famotidine (n = 1, *Pharmacother* 1998;**18**:404–7)

Galantamine (n = 1, nightmares, *J Am Geriatr Soc* 2009;**57**:565)
Indometacin (rare, n = 202, 2.5 years, incidence 0.5%, *Br Med J* 1965;**2**:1281–4)
Mirtazapine (SmPC at < 1 in 10,000; causing psychosis, n = 1, *Pharmacotherapy* 2010;**30**:145–50)
Nalbumetone (*Pharm J* 1990;**244**:764)
Nicotine patches (*Pharm J* 1992;**249**:384)
Pergolide (e.g. *Clin Neuropharmacol* 1986;**9**: 160–4)
Rivastigmine (REM sleep behaviour disorder, n = 1, *J Clin Sleep Med* 2010;**6**:192–5)
SSRI withdrawal
Verapamil (*NEJM* 1988;**318**:929–30)
Withdrawal from barbiturates, benzodiazepines, narcotics, etc

5.15 SUICIDAL IDEATION (SEE ALSO DEPRESSION)

Although suicidal ideation is not the same as actual suicide, more suicidal ideation is associated with more suicide attempts and completions (1,404,470 reports on 832 drugs, Robertson and Allison, *PloS One* 2009;**4**:e7312). In men, suicide risk is strongly inversely related to BMI, but not height or physical activity (n = 1829, Mukamal *et al, Arch Intern Med* 2007;**167**:468–75), except in extreme obesity where attempted suicide increases (Dong *et al, Int J Obes (Lond)* 2006;**30**:388–90). For example, up to 8.8% of 10–24-year-olds considered or attempted suicide in 2002, whereas the actual suicide rate was 0.0028% (Seemüller *et al, Acta Psychiatr Scand* 2009;**119**:166–7, reply by Castelpietra).

- CNS — anxiolytics and hypnotics *
Insomnia is an independent predictor of suicidal ideation in depression, so needs treating (n = 60, RCT, d/b, 9/52, McCall *et al, Sleep Med* 2010;**11**:822–7). Anxiety disorders are also associated with increased suicide attempts, e.g. PTSD (AOR = 1.81), panic (AOR = 1.3) increase the risk by 50%, and comorbid panic and personality disorder increased risk to AOR = 5.76 (n = 34653, Nepon *et al, Depress Anxiety* 2010;**27**:791–8).
Benzodiazepines (n = 1, *Br J Gen Pract* 2007;**57**: 407–9):
→ alprazolam (caution in SmPC)

→ chlordiazepoxide (SmPC)
Sodium oxybate (SmPC; BNF less common)
Zaleplon (BNF caution)
Zolpidem (SmPC)

- CNS — antipsychotics (including lithium)*
Antipsychotics can cause akathisia, with the associated risk of suicide (review, *CNS Spectr* 2007;**12**(9 Suppl 14):1–13).

Aripiprazole (BNF very rare, SmPC now says that there is no increased risk of suicidality in bipolar disorder; n = 20489, in schizophrenia or bipolar, no increase in events, *Pharmacoepidemiol Drug Saf* 2010;**19**:1124–30; actually reduced suicide rate as adjunct in MDD, s = 2, n = 737, RCT, d/b, p/c, *J Clin Psychiatry* 2011;**72**:548–55)
Flupentixol (SmPC; BNF)

CNS antidepressants, including bupropion

The stats:

- **Depression is a risk factor for suicide:** Suicide practically does not occur without the presence of mental health problems, most commonly depression, then alcoholism.
- **Suicidal ideation is not necessarily the same as actual suicide or suicide attempt.**
- **The absolute risk of suicide during acute antidepressant treatment is about one in 3000**, and serious suicide attempts is one in 1000, with no evidence of a statistically significant increase in suicide or ideation in the first four weeks with newer antidepressants (n = 65103, Simon *et al, Am J Psychiatry* 2006;**163**:41–7).
- **Any suicidal ideation with antidepressants may have several causes:** e.g. increasing motivation, short-term akathisia and misdiagnosis of bipolar depression. Risk factors include drug abuse, severe MDD, melancholic features and younger age (n = 1090, Zisook *et al, J Affect Disord* 2009;**117**:63–73).
- **The risk with SSRIs is increased in adolescents,** reduced in adults and much reduced in older adults (s = 8, n > 200,000, WHO systematic review, Barbui *et al, CMAJ* 2009;**180**:291–7; s = 372, n = 99231, Stone *et al, Br Med J* 2009;**339**:b2880):

Age	Suicidal behaviour	Suicidal ideation
<25	Increased (OR 2.3)	Increased (OR 1.6)
25–64	No significant change (OR 0.87)	Possibly reduced (OR 0.79)
>64	Decreased (OR 0.06)	Decreased (OR 0.37)

- **The risk is in the first few weeks in children and adolescents**: (meta-analysis, s = 16, n = 2741, RCTs, Dubicka *et al, Br J Psychiatry* 2006;**189**:393–8), peaking at 3/52 and predicted by high baseline suicidal ideation, family conflict, and drug and alcohol use; the median time to non-suicidal event was 2/52, predicted by previous history of non-suicidal self-injury and venlafaxine (n = 334, Brent *et al, Am J Psychiatry* 2009;**166**:418–26).
- **Antidepressants can cause akathisia** (see 5.8.2) and anxiety/jitteriness, but this is poorly defined and unproven (s = 107, Sinclair *et al, B J Psychiatry* 2009;**194**:483–90).

The case against antidepressants causing suicide:

- An analysis of all FDA trials for nine antidepressants was unable to find any link with increased suicide from any antidepressants compared to placebo (n = 49277; 77 suicides, Khan *et al, Am J Psychiatry* 2003;**160**:790–2)
- A meta-analysis of SSRIs showed no increased the risk of suicide in adults (s=477, n=>40000, RCTs, p/c, Gunnell *et al, Br Med J* 2005;**330**:385; see also n=146095, Martinez *et al, Br Med J* 2005;**330**:389–93).

CNS antidepressants, including bupropion (*continued*)

- In Denmark, the suicide rate (1995–1999) dropped, particularly in people treated with SSRIs or older antidepressants (n = 438625), compared to those not treated with antidepressants (n = 1199057) (four years, Søndergård et al, Acta Psychiatr Scand 2006;**114**:168–76).
- Improving diagnosis and treatment of MDD in Sweden (1995–2002) led to increased antidepressant use and decreased suicides (Henriksson and Isacsson, Acta Psychiatr Scand 2006;**114**:159–67).
- For every extra DDD of antidepressant used per 1000 population in Japan, the suicide rate reduced by 6% (Nakagawa et al, J Clin Psychiatry 2007;**68**:908–16).
- A Swedish study of suicides concluded the only explanation for the findings is that antidepressants reduce suicide (n = 18922 suicides, Isacsson et al, Acta Psychiatr Scand 2010; **122**:454–60).
- Reduced antidepressant use (2003–6) in younger people led to a reduction in SSRI use in <19s in 22% reduction of SSRI use in <19s in the Netherlands (22%) and USA (30%). This resulted in an increase in suicides in the Netherlands (49%, from 0.86 to 1.28 per 100000 population) and USA (14%, from 2.83 to 3.23 per 100000 population), an abrupt reversal of 20-year trends (Gibbons et al, Am J Psychiatry 2007;**164**:1356–63; see also n = 943,313, Libby et al, Arch Gen Psychiatry 2009;**66**:633–9; disputed by Wheeler et al, Br Med J 2008;**336**:542–5).
- Of n = 142,090 people in Germany prescribed antidepressants, there were only 33 (0.02%, 1 in 4300) cases of suicide (14 probably antidepressant-related, 19 possibly) with 23 associated with akathisia (Stübner et al, J Clin Psychiatry 2010;**71**:1293–307).

Minimising the potential for antidepressants to cause suicidal ideation:

- **Be alert for bipolar depression presenting as unipolar depression, especially in the under-25s:** The increase in younger people may be because bipolar disorder is often (as yet) undiagnosed in younger people, and antidepressants without mood stabilisers may promote mixed states and hence suicidal ideation, although the actual antidepressant used seems to make no difference (n = 20906 on antidepressants, nine years, Schneeweiss et al, Pediatrics 2010;**125**:876–88), except venlafaxine (n = 334, Brent et al, Am J Psychiatry 2009;**166**:418–26)
- **Avoid antidepressants toxic in overdose:** SSRIs and other newer agents have low toxicity in overdose but tricyclics and MAOIs can be toxic in overdose (seven years, Hawton et al, Br J Psychiatry 2010;**196**:354–8; n = 287543 adults on antidepressants, nine years, Schneeweiss et al, Arch Gen Psychiatry 2010;**67**:497–506).
- **Start antidepressants slowly,** especially in adolescents: there is a higher risk on initiation (OR = 3.42) and dose titration (up OR = 2.62; down OR = 2.19) (n = 52261, Valuck et al, J Clin Psychiatry 2009;**70**:1069–77).
- **Take care early in treatment** and monitor for akathisia, agitation.
- **Avoid polypharmacy:** Three or more psychotropics from different classes may increase the risks (n = 318, Fontanella et al, Ann Pharmacother 2009;**43**:1939–47).
- **Treat any insomnia:** see CNS — anxiolytics and hypnotics. SSRIs can disrupt sleep architecture so must be taken with breakfast.
- **Ensure antidepressants are not stopped prematurely or too abruptly:** Discontinuation (esp. within first 56 days) shows an increased risk (OR = 1.61) (n = 52261, Valuck et al, J Clin Psychiatry 2009;**70**:1069–77).
- **Not using antidepressants has its own risk:** People with MDD who have committed suicide have seldom been treated with antidepressants. If depression improves, suicidal ideation reduces (n = 1693, Olfson and Marcus, J Clin Psychiatry 2008;**69**:425–32).

Duloxetine (SmPC; BNF rare; case series, *J Clin Psychopharmacol* 2008;**28**:101–2; n = 2, *Clin Pract Epidemol Ment Health* 2008;**4**:18)

MAOIs:
→ isocarboxazid (SmPC; BNF in susceptible persons)
→ phenelzine (SmPC; BNF in susceptible persons)

Mirtazapine (SmPC; BNF rare; associated with statistically significantly lower suicide risk cf. placebo: s = 15, RCT, d/b, p/c, Kasper *et al, World J Biol Psychiatry* 2010;**11**:36–44)

Moclobemide (SmPC)

SSRIs:
→ citalopram (SmPC: may be genetic linkage; n = 1447, incidence 8.6%, *Arch Gen Psychiatry* 2007;**64**:689–97; n = 1915, incidence 6%, 14/12, *Am J Psychiatry* 2007; **164**:1530–8)
→ escitalopram (SmPC; lower than with nortriptyline, n = 811, RCT, open, 12/52, *BMC Med* 2009;**7**:60)
→ fluoxetine (SmPC; two Lilly analyses of the FDA databases on suicide show no increase in the risk of treatment-emergent suicide with use of fluoxetine for MDD [s = 18, n = 3751, Beasley *et al, J Clin Psychopharmacol* 2007;**27**:682–6], nor for non-MDD conditions [s = 53, n = 11448, d/b, p/c, *Psychol Med* 2007;**37**:1585–93], although older data suggested a possible problem [*Am J Psychiatry* 1990;**147**:1570–2; disproven in s = 17, n = 3065, d/b, *Br Med J* 1991;**303**:685–92])
→ fluvoxamine
→ paroxetine (SmPC, may be higher than formally reported, *BMC Psychiatry* 2006; **6**:55)
→ paroxetine withdrawal (n = 4, *J Psychopharmacol* 2008;**22**:330–2; overall incidence of suicidal behaviour with paroxetine is the same as placebo but higher in adults < 30 years old (s = 57, n = 14911, p/c, *J Affect Disord* 2010;**120**:40–7)
→ sertraline (SmPC, but a meta-analysis showed that the 0.04% incidence of suicides with sertraline [n = 4 from n = 10917] was similar to 0.03% with placebo [n = 3 from n = 9006], s = 126, n = 19923, d/b, p/c, *J Clin Psychiatry* 2009; **70**:674–83)

Reboxetine (SmPC; BNF rare)

Trazodone (SmPC)

Tricyclics:
→ clomipramine (SmPC)
→ lofepramine (SmPC)
→ nortriptyline (SmPC)
→ trimipramine (SmPC)

Tryptophan (SmPC; BNF)

Venlafaxine (SmPC; BNF very rare; has higher suicide rate than citalopram, fluoxetine and dosulepin but there may be confounding factors, e.g. use in more severe MDD might explain this; n = 219,088, *BMJ* 2007;**334**:242)

- CNS — analgesics *

Dihydrocodeine (SmPC)

Paracetamol

Tramadol (FDA warning 2010)

Ziconotide (SmPC, uncommon; IT, n = 1, *Pain* 2011;**152**:235–7)

- CNS — anticonvulsants *

A meta-analysis showed that 32.5% of all deaths of people with epilepsy are from suicide and 13.5% of all registered suicides are committed by epileptics so suicide in epilepsy is disturbingly frequent (s = 30, n = 51216, Pompili *et al, Epilepsy Behav* 2006;**9**:641–8). The BNF states that AEDs are associated with a small increase in risk of suicidal thoughts and behaviour, sometimes as soon as one week after starting. The data is contradictory:

- Levetiracetam, tiagabine and topiramate may lead to a 3-fold increase in suicidal behaviour, but not older AEDs (n = 9415, *Neurology* 2010;**75**:335–40)

- Clonazepam, valproate, lamotrigine, phenobarbital seem to double the suicide risk, but only for relatively shortly after initiation (n = 6780, Olesen *et al, Pharmacoepidemiol Drug Saf* 2010;**19**:518–24).

- Compared to topiramate and carbamazepine, increased suicidal acts may occur with gabapentin (HR = 1.42), lamotrigine (HR = 1.84), oxcarbazepine (HR = 2.07), tiagabine (HR = 2.41) and possibly valproate (HR = 1.65) (n = 29620, < 180/7, Patorno *et al, JAMA* 2010;**303**:1401–9; comment by Procopio, *EBMH* 2010;**13**:102), but:

5

- There was no increase in suicide-related events in people with epilepsy or bipolar taking AEDs, but was increased in people with depression taking AEDs and those taking AEDs but not having epilepsy, depression or bipolar (n = 5,130,795, Arana et al, N Engl J Med 2010;**363**:542–51).
- Consistent taking of AEDs is associated with a substantial reduction in risk of SI (cf lithium (n = 16645, Smith et al, J Affect Disord 2009;**117**:162–7).
- The increase with AEDs in epilepsy may be disease-related rather than AED-related (appear to actually be protective in bipolars; n = 47918, Gibbons et al, Arch Gen Psychiatry 2009;**66**:1354–60).

Review: * Mula et al, Curr Neurol Neurosci Rep 2010;**10**:327–32.

Barbiturates (BNF uncommon)
Benzodiazepines, e.g.:
→ clobazam (SmPC, especially in elderly or children)
→ clonazepam, diazepam, flurazepam, loprazolam, lorazepam, midazolam, nitrazepam, temazepam (SmPC; BNF rare)
Carbamazepine (suicidality, FDA warning 2008)
Ethosuximide (SmPC)
Felbamate (suicidality, FDA warning 2008)
Gabapentin (BNF, uncommon; suicidality, FDA warning 2008; pharmacoepidemiological study concluded that gabapentin reduced the risk of suicide attempt in people with psychiatric disorders [n = 131,178, Gibbons et al, Pharmacoepidemiol Drug Saf 2010;**19**:1241–7], but another guarded appraisal came to the opposite conclusion [Ziemba et al, Neurologist 2010;**16**:325–8])
Lacosamide (SmPC)
Lamotrigine (suicidality, FDA warning 2008)
Levetiracetam (suicidality, FDA warning 2008; SmPC; BNF rare)
Oxcarbazepine (SmPC, FDA warning 2008)
Phenytoin (SmPC)
Pregabalin (suicidality, FDA warning 2008; reports, SmPC addition)
Rufinamide as adjunct in bipolar (n = 2, Epilepsy Behav 2011;**20**:386–9)
Tiagabine (suicidality, FDA warning 2008; SmPC)
Topiramate (SmPC; BNF less common, FDA warning 2008)

Valproate (reports, SmPC addition, FDA warning 2008, but no increased risk of suicide in a range of indications, s = 13, n = 1327, p/c, Ann Gen Psychiatry 2011;**10**:1)
Vigabatrin (BNF rare)
Zonisamide (SmPC; BNF less common, FDA warning 2008)

- CNS — antiparkinsonian drugs
Levodopa (SmPC; BNF very rare)

- CNS — others *
Acamprosate (mentioned SmPC)
Alcohol (risk of suicide is primarily associated with the quantity of alcohol consumed per drinking day, but not with drinking frequency or overall alcohol consumption; n = 47,654, Soc Psychiatry Psychiatr Epidemiol 2007;**42**:153–60)
Atomoxetine (SmPC; BNF less common, n = 1, J Paediatr Child Health 2008;**44**:596–8)
Bupropion (SmPC, rare)
Caffeine (in bipolars, high coffee consumption is significantly associated [OR 1.79] with suicidal acts; n = 352, Bipolar Disorder 2009; **11**:494–503)
Cannabis (young users may possibly be more at risk, n = 2033, Acta Psychiatr Scand 2008; **118**:395–403; n = 1, Case Report Med 2009;**2009**:321456)
Disulfiram (SmPC)
Galantamine (SmPC, very rare)
Memantine (association, SmPC; BNF very rare)
Methylphenidate (SmPC; BNF less common)
Modafinil (SmPC; BNF rare)
Naltrexone (BNF rare)
Nicotine (high nicotine consumption is significantly associated [OR 2.42] with suicidal acts in bipolar people [n = 352, Bipolar Disorder 2009;**11**:494–503] and in adolescent females [OR 4.7, n = 508, Compr Psychiatry 2009;**50**:293–8])
Oxybate (n = 1, J Neuropsychiatry Clin Neurosci 2010;**22**:352)
Sibutramine (SmPC)
Varenicline (SmPC; BNF less common, links but not substantiated, s = 14, n = 4443, Cochrane Database Syst Rev 2010;**12**:CD006103; no association, n = 80,660, BMJ 2009; **339**:b3805; n = 1, J Anal Toxicol 2009;**33**: 118–20)

- Cardiovascular drugs

ACE inhibitors (a review has shown that there is no greater risk of suicidal ideation with ACE inhibitors, n = 58 529, *Br J Clin Pharmacol* 2001;**52**: 313–8; n = 743, *Eur J Clin Pharmacol* 2007;**63**:591–6)

Beta-blockers (one review has shown that users of medium and high lipid-soluble beta-blockers may be associated with an increased risk of suicide, n = 58 529, *Br J Clin Pharmacol* 2001;**52**: 313–8; but another study showed no increased risk; n = 743, *Eur J Clin Pharmacol* 2007;**63**:591–6)

Calcium-channel blockers (reviews have shown no greater risk of suicidal ideation with calcium-channel blockers, n = 58 529, *Br J Clin Pharmacol* 2001;**52**: 313–8; n = 743, *Eur J Clin Pharmacol* 2007;**63**:591–6; n = 153 458, *Br Med J* 2000;**320**: 1251)

Omega-3 fatty acids (low plasma levels may be a risk factor for suicide or depression: *Am J Psychiatry* 2006;**163**:1100–2)

Statins — there is insufficient evidence that low cholesterol is associated with increased risk of suicidal ideation and might actually be lower (n = 2813, *Arch Intern Med* 2003;**163**:1926–32; see also n = 930, *J Clin Psychiatry* 2008;**69**:1920–7), but increased dietary intake may reduce impulsive and aggressive behaviours (*Pharmacopsychiatry* 2002;**35**:1–5). Other data had suggested a higher incidence of low cholesterol in parasuicide [n = 100, *Br J Psychiatry* 2000;**177**:77–83] and suicide [n = 783, *Acta Psych Scand* 2001;**104**:37–41]; but high risk of violent suicide with high cholesterol, n = 37 635, *Am J Psychiatry* 2000;**157**: 648–50). Statins are implicated (MHRA warning, *Drug Safety Update* 2008;**1**:10), e.g.

  → atorvastatin (very low-density lipoprotein cholesterol levels are not associated with increased suicide, n = 10001, *Am J Cardiol* 2007;**100**:747–52)
  → simvastatin (*Curr Problems* 1992;33: n = 4, *Lancet* 1993;**341**:14)

- Respiratory drugs *

Montelukast (FDA change 2009; SmPC, rare; BNF very rare; s = 116, n = 20131 on montelukast, 17633 controls, no completed suicides, only one suicidal ideation, no

evidence of a problem, *J Allergy Clin Immunol* 2009;**124**:691–6)

- Anti-infection drugs *

Antiretrovirals — multiple switching of agents is associated with higher distress and suicide than single or non-switchers in ART therapy (n = 779, *Int J STD AIDS* 2007;**18**:700–4):

  → disoproxil (SmPC; BNF less common)
  → emtricitabine (SmPC; BNF less common)
  → efavirenz (SmPC; BNF less common; not associated with increased suicide risk, n = 355, 48/52, *Clin Infect Dis* 2006; **42**: 1790–9)
  → tenofovir (SmPC; BNF less common)

Cycloserine (SmPC, psychosis with suicidal tendencies)

Fluoroquinolone (n = 1, *Gen Hosp Psychiatry* 2010;**32**:108–10)

Levofloxacin (SmPC, very rare)

Ofloxacin (SmPC, very rare)

Mefloquine (SmPC, rare; BNF rare; n = 1, *Presse Med* 2006;**35**:789–92)

Ribavirin (SmPC; BNF oral, more common in children)

- Endocrine system drugs *

Levothyroxine (n = 1, *Sao Paulo Med J* 2009; **127**:317–8)

Systemic corticosteroids (SmPC; BNF especially high doses and during withdrawal):

  → beclomethasone (SmPC, BNF as above)
  → cortisone (SmPC, BNF as above)
  → deflazacort (SmPC, BNF as above)
  → dexamethasone (SmPC, BNF as above)
  → fludrocortisone (SmPC, BNF as above)
  → hydrocortisone (SmPC, BNF as above)
  → methylprednisolone (SmPC, BNF as above)
  → prednisolone (SmPC, BNF as above)
  → testosterone (lack of clear association between high levels and suicide attempts, but more data needed, n = 149, *Neuropsychobiology* 2011;**63**:125–30)
  → triamcinolone (SmPC, BNF as above)

- Malignancy and immunosuppressant drugs *

Aldesleukin (suicide, n = 1, *J Am Osteopath Assoc* 1993;**93**:799–800)

Interferons:

5

→ interferon alfa
→ interferon-alfa + ribavirin (n = 1, *Psychosomatics* 2009;**50**:538–42)
→ interferon beta-1a and 1b (n = 11, *Clin Neuropharmacol* 2010;**33**:312–6)
→ peginterferon alfa (SmPC; BNF uncommon, contraindication for some in severe depression or suicidal ideation)

• Musculoskeletal and analgesics *
Infliximab (n = 1, *J Crohns Colitis* 2010;**4**:591–3)

• Others *
Alitretinoin (SmPC, very rare)
Baclofen (SmPC)
Isotretinoin (SmPC; BNF rare; n = 5756, mean 15-year follow-up; 1.57x increased risk for all attempts inc repeat attempts, 1.36x risk of 1st attempts occurring during treatment, and for 6/12 after treatment finishes, Sundström *et al, Br Med J* 2010;**341**:c5812; prospective study in Finnish male military conscripts showed that in fact depressive symptoms declined with isotretinoin and was not associated with treatment-emergent depression or suicidal ideation among young men, although idiosyncratis reactions could not be excluded, n = 135 [c = 126], 12/52, Rehn *et al, J Eur Acad Dermatol Venereol* 2009;**23**:1294–7; retrospective chart review, no cases reported, n = 1743, *Australas J Dermatol* 2010;**51**:248–53; n = 30496, statistically significant association, *J Clin Psychiatry* 2008;**69**:526–32; n = 300, incidence 30% in bipolar patients, *J Affect Disord* 2010; **122**:306–8)
Zafirlukast (FDA warning 2009)

MANAGEMENT OF SIDE-EFFECTS

Contents

Without wishing to state the blindingly obvious, we know that all drugs have side-effects. These may range from being mild and transient to being intolerable or life-threatening. If switching or discontinuing the causative agent is not clinically possible (e.g. patient preference, clinical response), managing undesirable adverse effects may allow continued treatment, improve compliance and lead to better outcomes.

STANDARD STRATEGIES TO TRY FIRST INCLUDE:

- Drug — alter formulation (i.e. SR/MR, liquid, injection).
- Dose — adjust total daily dose (increasing rarely works, but a systematic and gradual decrease should be tried to determine the minimum effective dose).
- Dose — manipulate frequency and timings (e.g. split, or load to one particular time).
- Dose — consider drug holiday (e.g. omitting doses on particular days, although this is likely only to be helpful for some specific ADRs).
- Dose — consider slower dose escalation (including stopping and restarting more gently), particularly with buspirone, many tricyclics and SSRIs.
- Monitor plasma levels to optimise the dose if possible, e.g. tricyclic ADRs are clearly correlated with plasma levels (review for our Polish readers by Grzesiak et al, Psychiatr Pol 2003;**37**:825–37).
- Switch to a drug from a different chemical group.
- Discontinue completely.
- Discontinue any concurrent drugs that might be interacting.
- Wait for the side-effect to wear off, or at least to get more tolerable.
- Initiate adjunctive therapies (additional drugs, physical management strategies).

All of these routine strategies may be of some importance and relevance for each side-effect. This chapter comments on some of the above, along with additional strategies. Data in this area of therapy is notably sparse, and the author would be grateful for any additional ideas.

Disclaimers:
- Some drug doses are quoted as total daily doses but many will need to be given as divided doses.
- Drugs and strategies are not in any particular order within each section, and are in alphabetical order where possible.

6

6.1 Anticholinergic and related side-effects

Anticholinergic, blurred vision

Antidepressants	**Switch** to an antidepressant with less anticholinergic side-effects (see *2.1.2*). Beware of glaucoma developing (see *3.6*).
	Bethanechol 30–90 mg/d may be effective but often poorly tolerated.
	Pilocarpine 1% drops QDS may restore pupilary responsiveness and have been used if desipramine-induced (Salah and Cameron, *Am J Psychiatry* 1996;**153**:579).

Anticholinergic, constipation

Antidepressants	Ensure adequate fluid intake.
(usually tricyclics)	Usually requires bran or a bulking or lubricating laxative, e.g. lactulose, docusate.
	Bethanechol 30–90 mg/d may be effective but often poorly tolerated.

Clozapine	As for tricyclics, but it is important to take this seriously as it may lead on to potentially fatal paralytic ileus, with or without previous abdominal symptoms (there are over 30 cases of fatal clozapine-induced constipation, e.g. n = 2, Hibbard *et al, Psychosomatics* 2009;**50**:416–9; review, n = 102, Palmer *et al, J Clin Psychiatry* 2008;**69**:759–68).

Risk factors for clozapine-induced constipation:
* Recently starting clozapine
* High clozapine dose or plasma level
* Use of concomitant anticholinergics
* Intercurrent illness

Additional actions:
* Regular physical monitoring, especially during higher risk times
* Appropriate and timely use of laxatives
* Ensure adequate fluid intake
* Early referral before life-threatening pathological changes start

Once resolved, preventative measures (high-fibre diet, adequate fluid intake, stool softeners and exercise) must be used to allow clozapine to continue safely (n = 1, Pelizza *et al, Acta Biomed* 2007;**78**:144–8).

Anticholinergic, dry mouth (xerostomia)
General advice
* **Stimulate salivary flow** — sugarless gum and other confectionary (e.g. wine gums) stimulate salivary flow (avoid those with sugar as this can promote dental caries and weight gain).
* Artificial **saliva sprays** (most contain methylcellulose or glycerin, e.g. Glandosane® [Fresenius Kabi]).
* Ensure adequate **hydration**.
* **Distigmine** bromide, but this has its own notable adverse effects, e.g. digestive, urinary and dermatological (n = 25, open, Wolpert *et al, Fortschr Neurol Psychiatr Grenzgeb* 1980;**48**:224–33).
* **Pilocarpine** 10–30 mg/d, as 2–3 times a day, may resolve the problem within a day if caused by clozapine, olanzapine, benzatropine, tricyclics or mirtazapine, with no significant side-effects (naturalistic overview, Masters, *Am J Psychiatry* 2005;**162**:1023).

Review: dietary and dental advice to avoid dental consequences (Boyd *et al, Nutr Rev* 1997;**55**:362–8).

SSRIs	**Switching** to fluvoxamine may be effective if paroxetine-induced (n = 1, Arima *et al, Ann Pharmacother* 2005;**39**:567–71). **Stop any olanzapine**, which may enhance the effect (n = 1, Hori *et al, Prog Neuropsychopharmacol Biol Psychiatry* 2006;**30**:758–60).
Tricyclics	**Coffee** — chewing 15 g cappuccino coffee for five minutes may help (n = 10, open, Chodorowski, *Przegl Lek* 2002;**59**:392–3). **Pilocarpine** (peripheral cholinergic) may not be effective but **bethanechol** has been used at 5–10 mg at night, or up to 60 mg/d sublingually to promote salivation (titrate dose slowly upwards, may be poorly tolerated). **Yohimbine** 4 mg/d may be effective for 3–4 hours (Bagheri *et al, Br J Clin Pharmacol* 1994;**37**:93–6).

Anticholinergic, urinary retention
Tricyclics	Once other physical causes have been excluded, the best course of action is probably to discontinue and/or switch. It can be a medical emergency (Tueth, *Am J Emerg Med* 1994;**12**:212–6) so must be taken seriously. **Bethanechol** 30–90 mg/d may be effective, albeit poorly tolerated (Hermesh *et al, Drug Intell Clin Pharm* 1987;**21**:877–9).
Antipsychotics	**Aripiprazole** 10 mg/d has been successful as an alternative antipsychotic

for urinary retention caused by haloperidol, olanzapine and risperidone (n = 1, Sahoo, *Isr J Psychiatry Relat Sci* 2007;**44**:74–5).

Urinary hesitancy (see also anticholinergic effects)

Reboxetine — **Doxazosin** 1 mg/d (n = 1, Szabadi, *Br J Psychiatry* 1998;**173**:441–2).
Tamsulosin 0.4 mg/d may be rapidly successful (within 20 minutes) and well tolerated (n = 8 males, Kasper and Wolf, *Eur Neuropsychopharmacol* 2002;**12**:119–22; n = 1, Kasper, *Psychopharmacol* 2002;**159**:445–6).

Urinary incontinence

Venlafaxine — **Sertraline**, switch to (n = 1, Polimeni et al, *Clin Neuropharmacol* 2005;**28**:247–8).
Duloxetine might be an alternative if stress-related.

6.2 Blood disorders

Review: Haematological toxicity from psychotropics and how to treat (Flanagan and Dunk, *Hum Psychopharmacol* 2008;**23**:27–41).

Bleeding

SSRIs — **Discontinue**, or **switch** to a non-SSRI may be the best option.
Stop any NSAIDs (inc. aspirin), prescribe a less gastrotoxic NSAID or co-prescribe gastroprotective drugs (Dalton et al, *CNS Drugs* 2006;**20**:143–51; Mort et al, *Pharmacotherapy* 2006;**26**:1307–13).
Vitamin C 500 mg/d has been used (n = 1, Tielens, *Am J Psychiatry* 1997;**153**:883; Rasker, *Ned Tijdschr Genneesk* 1993;**137**:618).

Blood dyscrasias

Neutropenia, agranulocytosis

Clozapine — **'Red result' — immediate cessation mandatory**
Even a major **dose reduction** is unlikely to help in the short-term.
GCSF/filgrastim may be effective and logical (e.g. n = 1, Schuld et al, *Acta Psychiatr Scand* 2000;**102**:153–5), and may shorten the duration of hospitalisation (n = 11, Chengappa et al, *Psychopharmacol Bull* 1996;**32**:111–21). It can also be used long term (11–48/12, n = 3, Hagg et al, *Int Clin Psychopharmacol* 2003;**18**:173–4). Doses above 0.3 mg/wk may be more successful, although any rechallenge still needs extreme care (n = 5, Joffe et al, *Am J Psychiatry* 2009;**166**:236).
'Amber result' — advice on management
Exclude any interacting or contributing drugs, e.g. carbamazepine (e.g. Imbarlina et al, *Eur Psychiatry* 2004;**19**:506–9; see *Chapter 4.2.3*), antibiotics, etc.
Take the blood sample in the afternoon: neutrophil levels have a diurnal variation and a transient and harmless neutropenia (not requiring discontinuation) may occur in the morning (morning pseudoneutropenia, n = 1, Esposito et al, *World J Biol Psychiatry* 2003;**4**:192–4).
Exercising before a sample, **B12** and oral **folate** have also been used.
*****Lithium** (e.g. n = 1, Pinninti et al, *J Clin Psychopharmacol* 2010;**30**:219–21; n = 1, Brunoni et al, *Prog Neuropsychopharmacol Biol Psychiatry* 2008;**32**:2006–7) has been used to prevent transition to 'red' by reversing a low wbc, e.g. during an 'amber' phase or raising baseline wbc where a low count exists, allowing clozapine to start. Although lithium protects against neutropenia, it does not protect against it progressing to agranulocytosis (Paton and Esop, *Psychiatr Bull* 2005;**29**:186–8). Plasma levels of 0.4 mmol/l have been used.
After care and re-exposure:
After clozapine rechallenge post-leucopenia or neutropenia, 38% had

6

a further dyscrasia and in most it was more severe, longer-lasting and occurred more quickly (incidence peaks at 5.5 weeks), but 55% of these 53 were rechallenged successfully and remained in treatment (n = 53, Dunk *et al, Br J Psychiatry* 2006;**188**:255–63).

Reviews: * management (Esposito *et al, Eur J Clin Pharmacol* 2005;**60**:759–64), rechallenge (Ghaznavi *et al, Am J Psychiatry* 2008;**165**:813–8), general (Herceg *et al, Psychiatr Danub* 2010;**22**:85–9).

Eosinophilia

Clozapine

Clozapine-induced eosinophilia has an incidence of 13%, and resolves in nearly all without intervention (n = 160, Chatterton, *Aust N Z J Psychiatry* 1997;**31**:874–6) and probably is not a predictor of neutropenia (n = 70, Ames *et al, J Clin Psychiatry* 1996;**57**:579–81), but monitor carefully anyway, especially in women (n = 118, > 3/52, Banov *et al, J Clin Psychiatry* 1993;**54**:466–9).

Switching to quetiapine can be a successful alternative (n = 1, Zipris *et al, Isr J Psychiatry Relat Sci* 2007;**44**:54–6).

6.3 Cardiac effects

Hypertension

Antipsychotics

Beta-blockers and other general strategies are often adequate, e.g. **propranolol** has been used if the hypertension is aripiprazole-induced (n = 1, Borras *et al, Am J Psychiatry* 2005;**162**:2392).

Clozapine

Hypertension is usually transient over the first month, so reduce the dose or rate of upward titration.

Antihypertensives may be necessary if persistent or severe (**Pindolol** 5 mg BD has been used when clozapine-induced (e.g. review of 82 cases with clozapine; Henderson *et al, J Clin Psychiatry* 2004;**65**:686–9).

Review: management (Shiwach, *Clin Neuropharmacol* 1998;**21**:139–40).

MAOIs

For hypertensive crisis, refer to a specialist unit immediately for specialist care, e.g. using British Hypertension Society guidelines for malignant hypertension (see also Elliot, *J Clin Hypertens* [*Greenwich*] 2004;**6**:587–92).

Hypotension

MAOIs

Hypotension occurs in about 10% people on MAOIs (n = 61, Remnick *et al, Prog Neuropsychopharmacol Biol Psychiatry* 1989;**13**:497–504) and usually needs specialist medical care.

Metoclopramide (Patterson, *J Clin Psychopharmacol* 1987;**7**:112–3).

Plasma expansion, e.g. salt tablets or fludrocortisone (review by Cockhill and Remick, *Can J Psychiatry* 1987;**32**:803–8).

Postural (orthostatic) hypotension

General strategies: (review by Freeman, *Semin Neurol* 2003;**23**:435–42)

- Self-care (e.g. if lying down, dangle legs for a minute before rising slowly and attempting to stand).
- Use support stockings.
- Slower dose titration.
- Plasma volume expansion, e.g. fluid and increased sodium chloride intake.
- Desmopressin, indomethacin and erythropoietin can be used in extreme cases.
- Midodrine, an alpha-adrenergic agonist, is licensed and available in some countries (review by McClellan *et al, Drugs Aging* 1998;**12**:76–86), e.g. for tricyclics (n = 1, Maskall and Lam, *J Psychiatry Neurosci* 1993;**18**:276–7).

Additional strategies:

Tricyclics

Fludrocortisone has been used but obviously has long-term side-effects

	(Chobanian *et al*, *N Engl J Med* 1979;**301**:68–73).
	Yohimbine 12 mg/d (n = 12, d/b, c/o, p/c, Lacomblez *et al*, *Clin Pharmacol Ther* 1989;**45**:241–51).
MAOIs	**Brewed coffee** (Pollack and Rosenbaum, *J Clin Psychiatry* 1987;**48**:3–8).
	Fludrocortisone (Simonson, *Am J Psychiatry* 1964;**120**:1118–9).
	Levothyroxine or liothyronine has been suggested (see review, Whybrow and Prange, *Arch Gen Psychiatry* 1981;**38**:106–13).
	Methylphenidate 10–15 mg (case series, Feighner *et al*, *J Clin Psychiatry* 1985;**46**:206–9), but beware of ADRs.
	Salt tablets 600–1800 mg BD (n = 1, Munjack, *J Clin Psychiatry* 1984;**45**:89–90; mentioned in Pollack and Rosenbaum, *J Clin Psychiatry* 1987;**48**:3–8).
	Review: general (Cockhill and Remick, *Can J Psychiatry* 1987;**32**:803–8).
Antipsychotics	The effect is probably alpha-adrenergic-related so slower dose titration and lower doses are logical. Tolerance usually develops.
Clozapine	**Bovril and moclobemide** has been used for severe clozapine-induced postural hypotension (n = 1, Taylor *et al*, *Br J Psychiatry* 1995;**167**:409–10).
	Fludrocortisone (n = 1, Testani, *J Clin Psychiatry* 1994;**55**:497–8).

QTc prolongation

General strategies (see *Chapter 3.2* for risk factors and short review)

- **Switching** drugs is usually essential. If not possible, use the lowest doses in simple drug regimens.
- Avoiding metabolic interactions minimises the impact.
- **Magnesium** ion (Mg^{++}) orally at a mean dose of magnesium oxide 15 mg/kg/d shortens QTc, and can be given long term with appropriate monitoring. Magnesium sulphate by IV injection has been recommended by the American Heart Association (n = 24, Bachman, *J Clin Psychiatry* 2003;**64**:733–4).
- **Beta-blockers** are often ineffective (mentioned by Bachman, *J Clin Psychiatry* 2003;**64**:733–4).

Reviews: antipsychotics and QTc prolongation (Vieweg, *Prim Care Companion J Clin Psychiatry* 2003;**5**:205–15; Taylor, *Acta Psychiatr Scand* 2003;**107**:85–95; Zareba and Lin, *Psychiatr Q* 2003;**74**:291–306).

Tachycardia

Antipsychotics	Amisulpride may be slightly safer than olanzapine for tachycardia (n = 33, Wang *et al*, *Neuropsychobiology* 2008;**57**:200–5).
Clozapine	Tachycardia is common (up to 67%) early in treatment, but usually resolves over 4–6 weeks (n = 100, Marinkovic *et al*, *Prog Neuropsychopharmacol Biol Psychiatry* 1994;**18**:537–44). However, it may be the first, or only, presenting symptom of (often fatal) cardiomyopathy and so this must be fully excluded first. If the tachycardia is persistent and/or associated with chest pain, this may also indicate myocarditis (review of n = 26 where it was fatal in 46% of cases, Hagg *et al*, *J Clin Psychopharmacol* 2001;**21**:382–8). Myocarditis is most common (80%) in the first month (n = 25, Hill and Harrison-Woolrych, *N Z Med J* 2008;**121**:68–75), but can occur at any time, e.g. even after six years therapy (n = 1, Tanner and Culling, *Postgrad Med J* 2003;**79**:312–3) where discontinuation would be essential.
	Slower dose escalation may help.
	Manage nicotine and caffeine intake.
	Discontinuation usually results in rapid resolution (e.g. n = 1, Stampfer and Swanepoel, *Australas Psychiatry* 2005;**13**:80–2).
	Beta-blockers may help if the tachycardia is anticholinergic/noradrenergic-related, although the literature on this is minimal. Metoprolol is often used first-line as it has a short half-life, and can be converted to atenolol, which may be effective over five years with carvedilol and captopril (n = 1, Rostagno *et al*, *Gen Hosp Psychiatry* 2008;**30**:280–3).

6

6.4 Central adverse effects

Abnormal dreams and nightmares *

Antidepressants	**Take in the morning**, especially if serotonergic.

* Discontinue or switch drugs may be the only option. For mirtazapine-induced dissociated sleep-wakefulness switch to, e.g. bupropion (n = 1, Felthous et al, *Pharmacotherapy* 2010;**30**:145–50)

Discontinue any tramadol (n = 1, Devulder et al, *Acta Clin Belg* 1996;**51**: 184–6) and possibly other similar drugs that may exacerbate the effect.

Anorexia

Valproate Anorexia could be a sign of impending hepatic failure. Investigate immediately and discontinue if necessary.

Ataxia

Lithium This is usually a sign of lithium toxicity and neurotoxicity, and requires immediate action, e.g. discontinuation or dose reduction. If acute, dialysis may be needed. Consider also the global clinical picture, as ataxia may occur with 'normal' therapeutic lithium plasma levels.

Discontinue any exacerbating drugs, e.g. clozapine (Lee and Yang, *Zhonghua Yi Xue Za Zhi [Taipei]* 1999;**62**:184–7).

Buspirone (high-dose) has been used for ataxia due to lithium toxicity (n = 1, Megna and O'Dell, *Arch Phys Med Rehabil* 2001;**82**:1145–8).

Delirium

- Discontinue any causative agent (see 5.4).
- There is very limited evidence (no p/c studies) for the use of antipsychotics to treat delirium (s = 14, Seitz et al, *J Clin Psychiatry* 2007;**68**:11–21; atypicals for delirium, Peritogiannis et al, *Psychiatry Clin Neurosci* 2009;**63**:623–31).

Review: systematic review (Campbell et al, *J Gen Intern Med* 2009;**24**:848–53).

Antidepressants **Donepezil** may help if tricyclic overdose-induced (rapidly effective in n = 1, Noyan et al, *Prog Neuropsychopharmacol Biol Psychiatry* 2003;**27**:885–7).

Antipsychotics **Reduce** any concurrent anticholinergics.

Switch to an antipsychotic with low anticholinergic effects (*Table 2.1.4*) or discontinue if no clear indication. **Quetiapine** has been used if risperidone-induced (n = 1, Kato et al, *Psychosomatics* 2005;**46**:374–5) and **haloperidol** used if clozapine-induced (Spisla and Bunter, *Psychiatr Prax* 1997;**24**:308).

Reduce dose, e.g. clozapine-induced delirium appears to be dose-related (n = 139, Centorrino et al, *Pharmacopsychiatry* 2003;**36**:156–60).

Propofol has been used successfully for post-ictal delirium with clozapine-ECT therapy (n = 1, Sienaert et al, *J ECT* 2004;**20**:254–7).

Depression

Tetrabenazine **Discontinue**, or use antidepressants.

Reboxetine (n = 1, Schreiber et al, *J Neurol Neurosurg Psychiatry* 1999;**67**:550)

Drowsiness or sedation (see also fatigue)

Antipsychotics Wait, as tolerance often partly develops.

Adjust dose, e.g. lower dose, bias full dose to night or early evening or spread out throughout the day.

Avoid any other concurrent CNS depressants.

Methylphenidate 20–40 mg/d has been used if clozapine-induced (with great care; Miller, *Am J Psychiatry* 1996;**153**:1231–2).

Modafinil 200 mg/d has been used if sedation is induced by clozapine (n = 3, Makela et al, *J Clin Psychiatry* 2003;**64**:485–6), risperidone or olanzapine, with no exacerbation of psychosis. However, a pilot study was unable to show a significant effect from modafinil for clozapine-induced sedation (n = 35, d/b, p/c, 8/52, Freudenreich *et al, J Clin Psychiatry* 2009;**70**:1674–80) and a critical review concludes that the evidence is fairly poor but it may work (s = 6, Saavedra-Velez *et al, J Clin Psychiatry* 2009;**70**:104–12).

Levetiracetam	Can be minimised by starting at a lower dose.
MAOIs	For phenelzine-induced daytime somnolence, triazolam (or presumably another short-acting hypnotic) can help sleep and reduced daytime somnolence (n = 3, Gray, *Am J Psychiatry* 1989;**146**:1078).
Mirtazapine	**Start at higher dose**: 30 mg/d may produce less drowsiness than 15 mg/d (mirtazapine is a highly potent H1 receptor blocker, and at 30 mg/d the noradrenergic enhancement may counteract some of the histamine blockade).
SSRIs	**Modafinil**, used adjunctively to SSRIs at the start of treatment, may enhance the onset of action in people with MDD and fatigue (n = 29, open, 6/52, Ninan *et al, J Clin Psychiatry* 2004;**65**:414–20, MS; n = 16, 3/52, open, Schwartz *et al, J Clin Psychiatry* 2004;**65**:1223–7).
Topiramate	**Modafinil** (Berigan, *Prim Care Companion J Clin Psychiatry* 2002;**4**:249–50).
Valproate	**Investigate immediately** and discontinue if necessary. May be indicative of impending hepatic failure or encephalopathy.
	Modafinil (Berigan, *Can J Psychiatry* 2004;**49**:72–3).

Dysphoria

Antipsychotics	**Procyclidine** can help (n = 51, King *et al, Br J Psychiatry* 1995;**167**:480–2).
	Review: Voruganti and Awad, *Can J Psychiatry* 2004;**49**:285–9.

Fatigue (see also drowsiness or sedation)

Antipsychotics	**Adjust dose** or spread the doses out throughout the day.
	Modafinil has limited efficacy. A small study failed to show any differences vs placebo on fatigue, attention, working memory and executive functioning (n = 24 [c = 20], 8/52, d/b, p/c, Sevy *et al, J Clin Psychiatry* 2005;**66**:839–43), although a smaller study showed it may be effective in some people (n = 11, open, 4/52, Rosenthal and Bryant, *Clin Neuropharmacol* 2004;**27**:38–43).
Topiramate	**Modafinil** (Berigan, *Prim Care Companion J Clin Psychiatry* 2002;**4**:249–50).

Hypomania

Antidepressants	Mania from antidepressants is restricted to people with bipolar disorder (previously diagnosed or not). It may be aprt of the natural course but **discontinuation** is the absolute priority, with short-term management of the manic episode.
	Switch antidepressants if needed once resolved; venlafaxine appears to have the highest risk of inducing mania, sertraline has an intermediate risk and bupropion the lowest (n = 159, RCT, 10/52, Leverich *et al, Am J Psychiatry* 2006;**163**:232–9). **Adjunctive mood stabilisers**, e.g. lithium, should be used.

Insomnia

Antidepressants (SSRIs, bupropion, venlafaxine)	**Standard hypnotic therapy** (time-limited) may be adequate, e.g. zolpidem 5–10 mg/d if SSRI-induced (n = 190, RCT, d/b, 5/52, Asnis *et al, J Clin Psychiatry* 1999;**60**:668–76).
	Adjust time of doses, e.g. prefer morning doses, as all serotonergic antidepressants can disrupt sleep architecture.
	Quetiapine 50 mg/d was effective for phenelzine-induced insomnia non-responsive to BDZs, Zs and antihistamines (n = 1, Sokolski and Brown, *Ann Pharmacother* 2006;**40**:567–70).
	Trazodone 50–75 mg may be effective in patients on MAOIs, SSRIs (n = 12, d/b, p/c, c/o, 2 × 7/7, Kaynak *et al, Sleep Med* 2004;**5**:15–20), bupropion (67% improved, n = 17, RCT, p/c, d/b, c/o, Nierenberg *et al, Am J Psychiatry*

6

	1994;**151**:1069–72) and venlafaxine (especially in people with increased inner tension; n = 50[c = 42], open, 4/52, Bertschy *et al*, *Pharmacol Res* 2005;**51**:79–84).
Antidepressants (MAOIs)	**Adjust time of doses**, e.g. last dose of the day should be before 3.00 PM **Switch** to isocarboxazid. **Hypnotics** may help sleep but have no effect on daytime somnolence (n = 8, Teicher *et al*, *Am J Psychiatry* 1988;**145**:1552–6).
Aripiprazole	Add a hypnotic agent during the first days of treatment, administer in the morning or divide the dose of aripiprazole into two daily doses (AM and PM — Aitchison *et al*, *J Psychopharmacol* 2009;**23**:231–40).
Lamotrigine	Insomnia is probably dose-related so reduce dose, switch (n = 109, Sadler, *Epilepsia* 1999;**40**:322–5) or use hypnotics.
Methylphenidate	**Mirtazapine** can be used (chart review, Adler *et al*, *Curr Psychiatry Rep* 2006;**8**:409–15).

Irritability, jitteriness or agitation

SSRIs	**Slower dose titration** (or restarting more slowly) usually helps. **Valproate** has been used for fluoxetine-induced irritability in autism (Anagnostou *et al*, *J Clin Psychopharmacol* 2006;**26**:444–6).
Tricyclics	**Slower dose titration** (or restarting more slowly) usually helps. **Iron supplements** to resolve any low serum iron (Yeragani *et al*, *Neuropsychobiology* 1992;**25**:8–10). **Perphenazine** has been used (n = 2, Pohl *et al*, *J Clin Psychiatry* 1986;**47**:427).
Aripiprazole	Agitation is common when switching to aripiprazole and must be managed. **Benzodiazepines** (esp. lorazepam) can be used during switch-over period (Aitchison *et al*, *J Psychopharmacol* 2009;**23**:231–40). **Anticholinergic** drugs. **Antihistaminic** drugs (e.g. diphenhydramine; Aitchison *et al*, *J Psychopharmacol* 2009;**23**:231–40). **Valproic acid** as an adjunct. **Gabapentin** as an adjunct. **Review:** Cassano *et al*, *Clin Drug Invest* 2007;**27**:1–13.

Nausea

Antidepressants	**Slower dose increases** help initially. See *Table 2.1.2* for comparative incidence of nausea with antidepressants. **Cisapride** has been used so presumably similar short-term antiemetics may be effective. **Slow-release** tablets/capsules reduce the peak plasma level effect, as would splitting doses throughout the day. **Gorei-san** (TJ-17), a Japanese herbal medicine may help if SSRI-induced (n = 3, open, Yamada *et al*, *Psychiatr Clin Neurosci* 1999;**53**:681). **Mirtazapine** may help if the nausea is SSRI-induced (Pedersen and Klysner, *Int Clin Psychopharmacol* 1997;**12**:59–60) and 15 mg at night may be effective within four days (n = 1, Caldis and Gair, *Can J Psychiatry* 2004;**49**:707). **Milnacipran and olanzapine** have been used for severe antidepressant-induced nausea (n = 1, Yoshida *et al*, *Pharmacopsychiatry* 2007;**40**:84–5).
Antipsychotics	**Antiemetics**, e.g. ondansetron may be effective but **avoid** metoclopramide or prochlorperazine for the first 1–2 months, or if there is a history of EPSE. **Prochlorperazine** has been effective for quetiapine-withdrawal nausea, where ondansetron had failed (n = 1, Kim and Staab, *Am J Psychiatry* 2005;**162**:1020), but see warning above.
Aripiprazole	Nausea is usually transient so administer aripiprazole with or after food, reduce the dose or add an antiemetic if other measures fail (review, Cassano

	et al, Clin Drug Invest 2007;**27**:1–13), e.g. domperidone (Aitchison *et al, J Psychopharmacol* 2009;**23**:231–40).
Galantamine	**Switching** to the XL preparation has a disappointingly low impact on reducing nausea (n = 965, RCT, d/b, p/c, 6/12, Dunbar *et al, Clin Ther* 2006;**28**:365–72, MS). Rivastigmine patches might be an alternative.

Nocturnal enuresis (see also urinary incontinence) *

Clozapine	**Avoid or reduce fluids** at night or after 6.00 PM, have planned night awakenings, enuresis alarms, and voiding before going to bed.
	Adjust dose and bias towards morning if possible.
	Desmopressin can be used intranasally at 10 mcg in each nostril at bedtime (e.g. n = 1, Aronowitz *et al, Am J Psychiatry* 1995;**152**:472), although it risks hyponatraemia (n = 1, Sarma *et al, Aust N Z J Psychiatry* 2005;**39**:949).
	Oxybutinin (mentioned in Lurie and Hosmer, *J Clin Psychiatry* 1997;**58**:404).
	Tolterodine (there is one case where it did **not** work, whereas desmopressin did: n = 1, English *et al, Ann Pharmacother* 2001;**35**:867–9).
	Trihexyphenidyl 5 mg/d at bedtime (n = 2, Poyurovsky *et al, Int Clin Psychopharmacol* 1996;**11**:61–3).
Sertraline	* **Switch** to fluoxetine (n = 1, Maalouf and Gilbert, *J Child Adolesc Psychopharmacol* 2010;**20**:161–2)

Obsessive-compulsive symptoms

Antipsychotics	**Standard treatments** may be adequate, e.g. **fluoxetine** if quetiapine-induced (n = 1, Ozer *et al, Prog Neuropsychopharmacol Biol Psychiatry* 2006;**30**:724–7).
	Valproate has been used for augmentation in clozapine-induced OCD (n = 1, Zink *et al, Pharmacopsychiatry* 2007;**40**:202–3).
	Aripiprazole 20 mg/d adjunctively has been effective for clozapine-induced OCD (n = 7, Englisch *et al, Clin Neuropharmacol* 2009;**32**:227–9)
	Reduced dose — clozapine-induced OCD symptoms may be related to high clozapine/norclozapine plasma levels, so try reducing the dose or measuring plasma levels (n = 39, Lin *et al, Ther Drug Monit* 2006;**28**:303–7).
Benzodiazepines	Pregabalin has been successful if BDZ-induced (Oulis *et al, Prog Neuropsychopharmacol Biol Psychiatry* 2008;**32**:2000–1).

Panic

SSRIs	Discontinue if panic symptoms are citalopram-induced (n = 1, Brauer *et al, South Med J* 2002;**95**:1088–9).

Sedation (see drowsiness)
Seizures *

Clozapine	Clozapine-induced seizures are usually dose-related, so reduce the dose or rate of increase, or stop and restart if seizures occur. The incidence rises markedly above 600 mg/d.
	Discontinue any other drugs likely to reduce the seizure threshold. Carry out an **EEG** to test for ictal activity, as abnormal EEGs are not uncommon with clozapine or olanzapine (n = 323, Centorrino *et al, Am J Psychiatry* 2002;**159**:109–15).
	Valproate is standard management (case of successful concurrent valproate at low-dose clozapine 125 mg/d; n = 1, Foster and Olajide, *J Psychopharmacol* 2005;**19**:93–6), but the literature is remarkably sparce on this. It may be underused as only 24% patients on clozapine at risk of seizures may receive prophylactic valproate (n = 81, Sparshatt *et al, Psychiatric Bull* 2008;**32**:262–5).
	* **Other anticonvulsants** include gabapentin ($\leq$2100 mg/d, n = 1, Usiskin *et al, Am J Psychiatry* 2000;**157**:482–3), lamotrigine (n=1, Muzyk *et al, J*

6

Psychiatr Pract 2010;**16**:125–8) and **topiramate** (Navarro *et al*, *Am J Psychiatry* 2001;**158**:968–9).

Review: * management (Wong *et al*, *Can J Psychiatry* 2007;**52**:457–63; Herceg *et al*, *Psychiatr Danub* 2010;**22**:85–9).

6.5 Dermatological effects

Lithium is a major cause of cutaneous reactions, often characterised by pathological findings of neutrophilic infiltration (can cause or make worse). The general advice with lithium is:

- Check personal and family history of skin diseases before prescribing; the incidence is also higher in males (n = 108, Chan *et al*, *J Affect Disord* 2000;**57**:107–13; review by Yeung and Chan, *Am J Clin Dermatol* 2004;**5**:3–8).
- For mild or moderate dermatoses — use specific or systemic therapy.
- For severe or persistent dermatoses — use specific or systemic therapy; try dose reduction or discontinuation or rechallenge at lower dose.
- Most reactions seem to be dose-related, usually not too serious and may resolve despite continuation. Dose reduction and discontinuation are obvious options.
- Exclude other factors, e.g. infections, other medication changes.

Review: cutaneous reactions from lithium (Yeung and Chan, *Am J Clin Dermatol* 2004;**5**:3–8)

Acne

Lithium	**Systemic antibiotics** (avoid tetracycline because of interaction, see Malt, *Br Med J* 1978;**2**:502)
	Topical retinoids (tretinoin; Remmer and Falk, *J Clin Psychiatry* 1986;**47**:48). **Reduce dose or discontinue.**
	Wait (may spontaneously resolve even with continued treatment, n = 2, Kusumi, *Dis Nerv Sys* 1971;**32**:853–4).

Alopecia

- Check trace minerals, as low plasma levels of copper and zinc may predispose to hair loss, so oral supplementation may be effective (Ftemi and Calabrese, *Ann Pharmacother* 1995;**29**:1302).
- Other standard management includes hair care techniques and minoxidil.

Review: McKinney *et al*, *Ann Clin Psychiatry* 1996;**8**:183–5.

Carbamazepine	May occur in 6% and resolve after withdrawal, but can take several months.
Lithium	May occur in 12–19% patients (Mercke *et al*, *Ann Clin Psychiatry* 2000;**12**:35-42), either *de novo* or exacerbated. It may occur in the first 6/12 of treatment, and is more common in women.
	Alopecia may resolve with continued treatment (Ghadirian *et al*, *J Clin Psychiatry* 1986;**47**:212–3) or withdrawal (but might take several months).
	Exclude hypothyroidism as a causative factor (9%, Mortimer and Dawber, *Int J Dermatol* 1984;**23**:603–4) and other causes, e.g. stress, co-medication.
SSRIs	Occurs more in women and there may be an association with sertraline so switch if appropriate, e.g. to paroxetine or trazodone (may help if sertraline-induced; n = 1, Gautam, *Ann Pharmacother* 1999;**33**:631–7).
	Review: Hedenmalm *et al*, *Pharmacoepidemiol Drug Safety* 2006;**15**:719–25.
Valproate	The incidence is 5–6% (range 2.6–15%). It is usually transient and slight and often resolves without alteration of dose, although may take 6/12 to regrow.
	Dose reduction may help as alopecia is considered to be dose-dependent (28% incidence at high dose, 5% at low dose) so dose reduction may help (Mercke *et al*, *Ann Clin Psychiatry* 2000;**12**:35–42).
	Check copper and zinc levels as low levels may predispose to hair loss with valproate (Ftemi and Calabrese, *Ann Pharmacother* 1995;**29**:1302; Tasaki *et al*, *J Dermatol* 1993;**20**:21–4).

Darier's disease
Lithium   Topical retinoids.

Exfoliative dermatitis
Lithium   **Discontinue** — although rare (e.g. Sarantidis and Waters, *Br J Psychiatry*
                           1983;**143**:42–50) it is serious and discontinuation is usually the only option.

Folliculitis
Lithium   **Observation** (as it is often transient, starting several months after
                           commencing lithium and resolving spontaneously), keep lithium levels stable.
                           Topical antibiotics and corticosteroids.

Hair loss
Venlafaxine   **Discontinue or switch**, and it may resolve within a month (Pitchot and
                           Ansseau, *Am J Psychiatry* 2001;**158**:1159–60).

Maculopapular eruption
Lithium   Usually occurs within three weeks of starting treatment.
                           Topical corticosteroids.
                           Oral antihistamines.
                           Reduce dose or discontinue (can recur on rechallenge).

Photosensitivity
Antipsychotics   **Exclude other causes**, e.g. SLE and porphyria.
                           Avoid direct sunlight or sun-lamps.
                           Use a high factor sun-block cream.
                           Reduce doses or **switch** drugs (there is no reliable comparative information
                           but chlorpromazine is almost certainly the worst).
                           Reviews: antipsychotics (Warnock and Morris, *Am J Clin Dermatol* 2002;
                           3:629–36), antipsychotics, antidepressants and anxiolytics (Harth and
                           Rapoport, *Drug Saf* 1996;**14**:252–9).

Phenytoin   Can be the presenting symptom of serious reactions (review by Scheinfeld,
                           Expert Opin Drug Saf 2004;**3**:655–65).
                           If mild, can reintroduce cautiously but discontinue immediately if it recurs.

Pigmentation
Imipramine   Blue-grey pigmentation, often facial, is probably due to melanin deposits.
                           Laser (Q-switched alexandrite and ruby) treatment may be effective,
                           better with higher doses (n = 1, Atkin and Fitzpatrick, *J Am Acad Dermatol*
                           2000;**43**:77–80).
                           Switch to an SSRI (e.g. sertraline, n = 1, Metelitsa *et al, J Cutan Med Surg*
                           2005;**9**:341–5).

Chlorpromazine   **Withdrawal** — chlorpromazine-pigmentation is almost completely
                           reversible on withdrawal. CPZ lenticular pigmentation may persist whereas
                           corneal changes may resolve slowly over several years on discontinuation.
                           Switch drugs, e.g. levomepromazine (n = 4), trifluoperazine (n = 1),
                           combination (n = 5) (Bloom *et al, Acta Psychiatr Scand* 1993;**87**:223–4) can
                           help. Other data supports a switch to haloperidol (n = 4, Thompson *et al,
                           Acta Psychiatr Scand* 1988;**78**:763–5).

Psoriasis
Lithium   Lithium takes about a month to exacerbate psoriasis (but this is not
                           inevitable: Skoven and Thormann, *Arch Dermatol* 1979;**115**:1185–7) and 10
                           months to induce it *de novo*.
                           Conventional topical therapy (e.g. topical corticosteroids and calcipotriol).
                           Oral retinoids.
                           Reduce dose (as it is apparently dose-dependent) or discontinue (rarely
                           necessary and takes many weeks to resolve on discontinuation).

6

Rash

Review: ACHSS (anticonvulsant hypersensitivity syndrome; n = 32, Newell *et al, Pediatr Dermatol* 2009;**26**:536–46).

| Anticonvulsants (general) | **Switch AED:** Skin rash with one AED seems to increase risk of rash with another, especially combinations involving carbamazepine or phenytoin. Specific cross-sensitivity rates may be useful for AED selection and counselling of patients (n = 1875, Hirsch *et al, Neurology* 2008;**71**:1527–34). |

Rash with first AED	Second AED	Chance of rash with second AED
Carbamazepine	Lamotrigine	20% (n = 50)
Carbamazepine	Oxcarbazepine	33% (n = 15)
Carbamazepine	Phenobarbital	26.7% (n = 30)
Carbamazepine	Phenytoin	57.6% (n = 59)
Lamotrigine	Carbamazepine	26.3% (n = 38)
Lamotrigine	Oxcarbazepine	20% (n = 15)
Lamotrigine	Phenytoin	38.9% (n = 36)
Oxcarbazepine	Carbamazepine	71.4% (n = 7)
Oxcarbazepine	Lamotrigine	37.5% (n = 8)
Phenobarbital	Carbamazepine	66.7% (n = 12)
Phenobarbital	Phenytoin	53.3% (n = 15)
Phenytoin	Carbamazepine	42% (n = 81)
Phenytoin	Lamotrigine	18.9% (n = 74)
Phenytoin	Phenobarbital	19.5% (n = 41)

Oral corticosteroids (n = 1, Verrotti *et al, Int J Immunopathol Pharmacol* 2000;**13**:49–53).

Antihistamines, topical corticosteroids and H2-blockers have also been used.

Avoid paracetamol — adverse cutaneous reactions with carbamazepine and valproate (e.g. EM, SJS and TEN) can be enhanced by paracetamol (n = 72, Gau *et al, J Clin Psychopharmacol* 2008;**28**:509–17).

| Carbamazepine | Occurs in about 10–13% of people and there may be a genetic susceptibility (Hung *et al, Pharmacogenet Genomics* 2006;**16**:297–306), e.g. in Chinese (n = 24, Miller, *Epilepsy Curr* 2008;**8**:120–1). |

If treating the rash rather than discontinuing, full laboratory test monitoring (including LFTs, FBC, U&E) must be carried out frequently to exclude agranulocytosis, aplastic anaemia (n = 10, Cates and Powers, *Ann Pharmacother* 1998;**32**:884–7) or internal organ involvement, which may occur in rare cases and be potentially fatal.

Slow increments (syrup 0.1 mg/d, doubling on alternate days over 4/52) has been successful in preventing recurrence of rash (n = 1, Boyle and Lawlor, *Am J Psychiatry* 1996;**153**:1234).

Oral corticosteroids, e.g. prednisone (n = 20, only four had to discontinue carbamazepine, Murphy *et al, Neurology* 1991;**41**:144–5).

| Lamotrigine | **Take very seriously**: although relatively rare, rash may be the first sign of a potentially fatal Stevens-Johnson syndrome (n = 1175, RCT, Ketter *et al, J Clin Psychiatry* 2006;**67**:400–6) or toxic epidermal necrolysis (review: Antai-Otong, *Perspect Psychiatr Care* 2005;**41**:193–6). |

Prevention:

Risk factors: It is more common in females (relative risk of 1.8; Wong *et al,*

Ann Pharmacother 1999;**33**:1037–42), people with a previous anticonvulsant rash and in the under 13s (n = 988, Hirsch *et al*, *Epilepsia* 2006;**47**:318–22).

Slow dose titration — the risk of rash is almost abolished by following the manufacturer's recommended titration schedule (n = 254, Huang *et al*, *Kaohsiung J Med Sci* 2002;**18**:66–72), especially the initial dose (n = 1955, Calabrese *et al*, *J Clin Psychiatry* 2002;**63**:1012–9). The starting dose in adults should be 25 mg/d for two weeks, then 50 mg/d for two weeks, then increasing every 1–2 weeks, halved if added to valproate (where rash is also more likely to occur) or if allergic to trimethoprim, and doubled if combined with concurrent enzyme-inducing drugs, e.g. phenytoin, carbamazepine, etc.

Preventative dermatological advice should be given, e.g. avoid other new medicines, foods, cosmetics, deodorants, detergents and fabric softeners, and avoid sunburn or exposure to poison ivy/oak (n = 100, Ketter *et al*, *J Clin Psychiatry* 2005;**66**:642–5). This may be effective in minimising the danger of this serious adverse reaction.

Valproate is currently not contraindicated but lamotrigine must be added to valproate only if started at very low initial doses (n = 108, Faught *et al*, *Epilepsia* 1999;**40**:1135–40), as the risk is 3–4 times more common with the combination (n = 103, Li *et al*, *Arq Neuropsiquiatr* 1996;**54**:47–9).

Management:

Corticosteroids for mild non-progressive types.

IV immunoglobulins and corticosteroids are essential in specialist care settings for more severe reactions. **Toxic epidermal necrolysis** caused by lamotrigine has responded to intravenous immunoglobulin and amniotic membranes (n = 1, Schwartz *et al*, *Arch Dermatol* 2008;**144**:724–6).

Switching may be the best option in epilepsy (long-term follow up, n = 2, Feliciani *et al*, *Int J Immunopathol Pharmacol* 2003;**16**:89–93).

Aftercare:

Very careful rechallenge may be possible in some patients with a much slower dose escalation. Leave a gap of 1–2 months, then restart at 0.1 mg/d (n = 7, Besag *et al*, *Seizure* 2000;**9**:2820–6), then 2.5–5 mg/d for 2/52, increasing by 5 mg/d every 2/52 to 25 mg/d, then as per SmPC (n = 52, P-Codrea Tigaran *et al*, *Acta Neurol Scand* 2005;**111**:191–4). In one trial, 88% re-exposures were successful, with a very slow titration rate crucial in reducing recurrence (n = 44, Lorberg *et al*, *Int J Neuropsychopharmacol* 2009;**12**:257–65).

Phenytoin
Rash can be the presenting symptom of serious reactions (review by Scheinfeld, *Expert Opin Drug Saf* 2004;**3**:655–65).

If mild, can re-introduce cautiously but discontinue immediately if it recurs.

Antipsychotics
* **Clozapine** — slow introduction, starting at 0.0125 mg/d doubled over four days, reaching 250 mg/d after 105 days (n = 1, Raju, Southern *et al*, *Progress Neurol Psychiatry* 2010;**14**:30–1).

Antidepressants
Fluoxetine — care is needed, as rash can develop into more serious Stevens-Johnson syndrome or toxic epidermal necrolysis (Lyell syndrome).

Switching may not be effective as there can be cross-reactivity with other SSRIs (e.g. n = 1, Sannicandro *et al*, *Pharmacotherapy* 2002;**22**:516–8; paroxetine and sertraline n = 1, Warnock and Azadian, *Ann Pharmacother* 2002;**36**:631–3).

Avoid chocolate, which might be a precipitant (n = 1, Cederberg *et al*, *BMC Psychiatry* 2004;**4**:36), although this could be a tough call for some people.

Antihistamine and topical steroids are widely mentioned in the literature

6

as effective where rash is mild and self-limiting, e.g. fluoxetine and paroxetine rash has responded to oral diphenhydramine and a topical hydrocortisone cream (n = 1, Sannicandro et al, Pharmacotherapy 2002;**22**:516–8).

Rivastigmine Rash and itchiness with rivastigmine patches is a well recognised ADR, is mild in about 20% of patients but is common with all transdermal preps. The two mechanisms are allergic dermatitis (tends to spread out from the patch) and irritant dermatitis (just the patch area itself). Management includes:

Varying the site — the best areas compared to the back are the upper arm and chest, with the lower back better than the upper back. Do not apply to excessively hairy, broken, burned, cut or irritated skin; move the patch application site daily and do not use the exact same site for at least 14 days.

Skin care: If cleaning the skin before patch application, gently wash with water and dab dry with a cloth or towel.

- Avoid shaving, vigorous rubbing or use of alcohol-based cleansers or gels on the area as they may damage the integrity of the stratum corneum, the thin outer layer of skin.
- Gently clean the skin and apply moisturisers after every patch removal to reduce irritation and promote healthy skin.
- Remove the patch carefully to avoid surface damage to frail skin.
- Any irritant dermatitis (localised to the patch) should be left to resolve spontaneously, usually within several days without any intervention.

Treat any allergic dermatitis (hypersensitivity to patch adhesive or rivastigmine, presenting as localised redness that can spread beyond the edge of the patch) should be left to resolve spontaneously, usually within two weeks once the patch is removed. However, once allergic, patients will continue to experience skin reactions with subsequent use.

- **Use moisturising creams** and lotions for skin irritation (dryness, scaling, fissures or cracks).
- **Antihistamines and calamine lotion** can help itchiness but have no effect on irritant or allergic dermatitis.
- **Potent topical corticosteroids** may help severe allergic dermatitis, with referral to a dermatologist and discontinuation considered.

Seborrheic dermatitis

Lithium Ketoconazole shampoo. Topical or systemic antifungal agents.

Sweating

Antidepressants **Discontinuation** or dose-reduction usually improves this rapidly.

Adjunctive therapies

Sweating can be a significantly irritating ADR for patients, especially those on tricyclics. Drugs tried include:

- **Aripiprazole** 10–20 mg/d has been used for SSRI/duloxetine-induced sweating in women (Lu et al, J Clin Psychopharmacol 2008;**28**:710–1).
- **Beta-blockers** (propranolol, atenolol, labetalol) probably make sweating worse and should be excluded before other therapies are tried (n = 1, Butt, J Clin Psychiatry 1989;**50**:146–7).
- **Benzatropine** 0.5–1 mg/d if venlafaxine-induced (Pierre and Guze, J Clin Psychopharmacol 2000;**20**:269).
- **Clonidine** 0.2 mg/d may help dramatically within 24 hours, (n = 1, Feder, J Clin Psychiatry 1995;**56**:35; and for nortriptyline and paroxetine-induced; n = 1, Mago and Monti, J Clin Psychiatry 2007;**68**:639–40), although stopping it sometimes helps (Leeman, J Clin Psychiatry 1990;**51**:258–9).
- **Cyproheptadine** 4 mg either BD or at night (n = 5, open, Ashton and

Weinstein, *Am J Psychiatry* 2002;**159**:874–5).

- **Mirtazapine** has been successful for 'hot flushes' in women (n = 22[c = 16], Perez *et al*, *J Support Oncol* 2004;**2**:50–6), although sedation was a tolerance problem (n = 27[c = 20]), open, 12/52, Biglia *et al*, *Breast J* 2007;**13**:490–5). It may be dose-dependent, perhaps via 5-HT2/3 antagonism and influence on regulation of body temperature and diaphoresis (n = 1, Buecking *et al*, *Eur J Clin Pharmacol* 2005;**61**:543–4).
- **Terazosin** 2 mg/d (e.g. very effective if venlafaxine or sertraline-induced, n = 1, Mago and Monti, *J Clin Psychiatry* 2007;**68**:639–40).

Review: Marcy and Britton, *Ann Pharmacother* 2005; **39**:748–52.

6.6 Endocrine effects

Metabolic syndrome is a term used to describe a series of endocrine disturbances such as weight gain, hypertriglyceridemia and increased insulin, glucose, and low-density lipoprotein cholesterol levels. These are associated with antipsychotic use and raise the risk of diabetes and cardiac problems.

Reviews: Hert *et al*, *World Psychiatry* 2009;**8**:15–22; Meyer and Stahl, *Acta Psychiatr Scand* 2009;**119**: 4–14.

Diabetes:

Diabetes insipidus

Diabetes insipidus (not related to diabetes mellitus) is caused by poor kidney function or inadequate antidiuretic hormone production and is commonly reported with lithium and clozapine. It is becoming more common anyway, and often underdiagnosed. Screening before prescribing psychotropics helps exclude pre-existing diabetes, for which any medication would obviously get the blame.

- Discontinuing or replacing the causative drug if possible is the obvious strategy if possible.
- If urine volumes exceed 4 L/day, use thiazides and/or amiloride.
- NSAIDs (e.g. indometacin) may help in severe cases.

Diabetes mellitus

Type 1: person is unable to produce any insulin (previously known as insulin-dependent diabetes).

Type 2: person is unable to produce enough insulin or the insulin fails to work (insulin resistance, formerly non-insulin dependent diabetes mellitus [NIDDM], mature-onset diabetes).

- May be caused by decreased insulin sensitivity and weight gain.
- Monitor carefully if there is a family history or risk factors exist.

General management includes: *

- The most effective strategies are to adjust lifestyle changes, e.g. weight, smoking, exercise and diet.
- * Sleep loss or deprivation increases the risk of diabetes and weight gain and is a novel independent risk factor, through altered leptin and ghrelin signals, decreased glucose tolerance and insulin sensitivity (n = 12, RCT, 2x2/7, c/o, Spiegel *et al*, *Ann Intern Med* 2004;**141**:846–50), especially if associated with activation of the stress system which leads to consumption of comfort food (n = 21, Pejovic *et al*, *J Sleep Res* 2010;**19**:552–8).
- Oral hypoglycaemics, e.g. metformin (increases utilisation, but not production, of insulin; n = 40, RCT, d/b, 14/52, Baptista *et al*, *Can J Psychiatry* 2006;**1**:192–6) or insulin can be considered.

Review: diabetes and atypicals (Clarke and Burge, *Diabetes Technol Ther* 2003;**5**:669–83).

Clozapine	**Discontinue** (although it may not always resolve, n = 2, Tovey *et al*, *J Psychopharmacol* 2005;**19**:207–10).
	Orlistat has been used (Pavlovic, *Eur Psychiatry* 2005;**20**:520).
	Review: Henderson, *CNS Drugs* 2002;**16**:77–89.
Olanzapine	**Discontinue** drug (may not always resolve, see Koller and Doraiswamy, *Pharmacotherapy* 2002;**22**:841–52).
	Reduced dosage may help (n = 237, Koller and Doraiswamy, *Pharmacotherapy* 2002;**22**:841–52).

6

Switch to an alternative antipsychotic, e.g. quetiapine (n = 6 and review, Ashim et al, J Psychopharmacol 2004;**18**:128–32), risperidone (n = 1, Wu et al, Psychiatry Clin Neurosci 2006;**60**:115–6), aripiprazole (De Hert et al, Diabetes Care 2006;**29**:2329–30) or ziprasidone (Spivak et al, Am J Psychiatry 2002;**159**:1606; mean −14 mg/dL reduction in serum glucose, n = 84, Montes et al, Prog Neuropsychopharmacol Biol Psychiatry 2007;**31**:383–8).

Rosiglitazone — 4–8 mg/d improved glycaemic control in olanzapine metabolic disturbance but not Hb1c or lipids (n = 30, RCT, d/b, p/c, 12/52, Baptista et al, Pharmacopsychiatry 2009;**42**:14–9) and 4 mg/d non-significantly improved glucose utilisation and insulin sensitivity and reduced LDL in clozapine metabolic disturbance (n = 18, RCT, d/b, p/c. 8/52, Henderson et al, Acta Psychiatr Scand 2009;**119**:457–65).

Risperidone *

Telmisartan has been used successfully as an adjunct (n = 1, Yamaguchi and Tsutsumi, Intern Med 2010;**49**:919–23).

Hepatotoxicity

Valproate

Early discontinuation and supportive therapy is usually vital (Konig et al, Epilepsia 1999;**40**:1036–40)

Dose reduction may be possible if monitored with extreme care (n = 1, Lackmann, Pharmacology 2004;**70**:57–8).

L-carnitine can help, especially if given IV and within the first five days (n = 92, Bohan et al, Neurology 2001;**56**:1405–9; n = 1, Romero-Falcon et al, Eur J Intern Med 2003;**14**:338–40), and it can also be given prophylactically (review of evidence by Leheureux et al, Crit Care 2005;**9**:431–40).

Garlic organosulfur and **gingko biloba** use has been postulated (Sabayan et al, Med Hypotheses 2007;**68**:512–4).

Hyperammonaemia *

Valproate

Discontinuation, as this is usually rapidly reversible (e.g. n = 2, Carlson et al, J Am Acad Child Adolesc Psychiatry 2007;**46**:356–61) but can lead to coma.

* **Reduce dose**, as it may be plasma level related (n = 2, Wadzinski et al, J Am Board Fam Med 2007;**20**:499–502), or stop and add lactulose (n = 1) or IV normal saline (n = 1) (n = 2, Shan et al, J Psychopharmacol 2010;**24**:943–5).

* **Stop other drugs that may exacerbate**, e.g. phenobarbital (n = 1, Vivekanandan and Nayak, Ann Indian Acad Neurol 2010;**13**:145–7), topiramate (e.g. n = 1, Deutsch et al, Clin Neuropharmacol 2009;**32**:350–2) or pivmecillinam (n = 1, Lokrantz et al, Acta Neurol Scand 2004;**109**:297–301).

L-carnitine can correct carnitine deficiency (Segura-Bruna et al, Acta Neurol Scand 2006;**114**:1–7) and be well tolerated (n = 19, LoVecchio et al, Am J Emerg Med 2005;**23**:321–2).

Review: * Vivekanandan and Nayak, Ann Indian Acad Neurol 2010;**13**:145–7.

Hypercalcemia (hyperparathyroidism) *

Lithium

Although very rare, hypercalcemia/hyperparathyroidism is a recognised ADR (review, Saunders et al, World J Surg 2009;**33**:2314–23):

* **Surgery** (bilateral or unilateral parathyroidectomy), albeit only effective in less than half patients (n = 71, 6/12, Järhult et al, Br J Surg 2010;**97**:1680–5).

Calcimimetic therapy (a potential alternative to parathyroidectomy).

Hypercholesterolaemia

Antipsychotics

Standard treatments for reducing cholesterol, e.g. statins are effective (n = 28, Ojala et al, J Psychopharmacol 2008;**22**:33–8).

Switch drugs, e.g. aripiprazole (significant decrease, n = 15 olanzapine, n = 9 others, Spurling et al, J Clin Psychiatry 2007;**68**:406–9) or ziprasidone (mean 24.1 mg/dL total cholesterol, n = 84, Montes et al, Prog Neuropsychopharmacol

Biol Psychiatry 2007;**31**:383–8).

Discontinue any beta-blockers, which may enhance clozapine's effect on cholesterol (n = 50, Batmiller *et al*, *Schizophr Res* 2003;**59**:49–57).

Hyperglycaemia

Clozapine

Standard hypoglycaemic therapies

Orlistat has been used (Pavlovic, *Eur Psychiatry* 2005;**20**:520).

Amisulpride has a lower hyperglycaemic effect compared to clozapine (n = 22, 12–16/52, Rettenbacher *et al*, *J Psychopharmacol* 2007;**21**:400–4), although unlikely to be therapeutically equivalent.

Review: Henderson, *CNS Drugs* 2002;**16**:77–89.

Hyperlipidaemia

Antipsychotics

Hyperlipidaemia has been reported with all antipsychotics (decreasing incidence from clozapine, olanzapine, risperidone, quetiapine, ziprasidone to first generation) except aripiprazole.

Manage risk factors, such as weight gain, dietary changes and glucose intolerance (Koro and Meyer, *Essent Psychopharmacol* 2005;**6**:148–57).

Discontinue any beta-blockers which may enhance the effects on lipids (n = 50, Batmiller *et al*, *Schizophr Res* 2003;**59**:49–57).

Lipid-lowering therapy, e.g. rosuvastatin (n = 100, 3/12, De Hert *et al*, *J Clin Psychiatry* 2006;**67**:1889–96).

Switch drugs:

- **Amisulpride or ziprasidone** (Rettenbacher *et al*, *Int Clin Psychopharmacol* 2006;**21**:369–72) and **risperidone** (n = 15, Su *et al*, *Psychopharmacology* [Berl] 2005;**183**:383–6) may be alternatives if olanzapine or clozapine-induced.

- **Aripiprazole** has resolved clozapine (n = 1, Ball *et al*, *Ann Pharmacother* 2005;**39**:1570–2) and olanzapine-induced hyperlipidaemia (s = 3, n=546, RCT, Newcomer *et al*, *Schizophr Res* 2008;**106**:300–7) and may be the best option (n = 13,133 vs 17,240, Olfson *et al*, *Am J Psychiatry* 2006;**163**:1821–5; mean –6.2 mg/dL in triglycerides, n = 84, Montes *et al*, *Prog Neuropsychopharmacol Biol Psychiatry* 2007;**31**:383–8), although raised lipids and triglycerides have been linked with improved PANSS scores (n = 55, RCT, p/c, d/b, 8/52, Procyshyn *et al*, *J Psychiatry Neurosci* 2007;**32**:31–8).

- **Fluvoxamine** 50 mg/d has been used for clozapine-induced hyperlipidaemia, partly by altering the clozapine:norclozapine ratio and possibly partly by facilitating a reduced clozapine dose via CYP1A2 inhibition (n = 68, RCT, 12/52, Lu *et al*, *J Clin Psychiatry* 2004;**65**:766–71).

Hyperprolactinaemia

Hyperprolactinaemia is more common in bipolar disorder and schizophrenia (Bushe and Shaw, *J Psychopharmacol* 2007;**21**:768–73) and is linked to longer-term clinical sequelae, such as osteoporosis, hip fractures and possibly breast cancer.

Reviews: general (Bostwick *et al*, *Pharmacotherapy* 2009;**29**:64–73), drug causes (review, Torre and Falorni, *Ther Clin Risk Manag* 2007;**3**:929–51)

Antidepressants

Switch — occurs in 22% women and 4.5% men with fluoxetine (n = 87, open, 12/52, Papakostas *et al*, *J Clin Psychiatry* 2006;**67**:952–7).

Antipsychotics

Reducing the dose of the causative agent may help.

Check clinical relevance or importance (remembering the potential long-term effects of raised prolactin), especially if it is resulting in amenorrhoea in women or testosterone deficiency in men.

Test for a lesion by stopping the drug temporarily (or switching to a prolactin-sparing antipsychotic) to see if prolactin returns to normal, and/or

6

performing a CT scan (Molitch, *Mayo Clin Proc* 2005;**80**:1050–7).

HRT/combined oral contraceptive in women and **exogenous testosterone** in men (see Molitch, *Mayo Clin Proc* 2005;**80**:1050–7) may help, and avoid the need to switch drugs (Miller, *CNS Spectr* 2004;**9**[8 Suppl 7]:28–32).

Switch drugs:

Switching to a prolactin sparing drug (*Table 2.1.4*) is first-line strategy.
A comparison of the prolactin-raising effect of antipsychotics in children and adolescents concludes that quetiapine, ziprasidone and clozapine are best, amisulpride and risperidone worst, but there is insufficient data on the rest (s = 29, Roke *et al*, *J Child Adolesc Psychopharmacol* 2009:**19**:403–14).

- **Aripiprazole** may be an alternative as it can reduce prolactin in its own right, but is not always successful. In a switching study, augmenting with aripiprazole or switching (either abruptly or cross-over) to aripiprazole significantly reduced prolactin levels within a week, maintained for eight weeks (n = 269, 8/52, Byerly *et al*, *Schizophr Res* 2009;**107**:218–22; see also n = 23 [n = 20], Lu *et al*, *Prog Neuropsychopharmacol Biol Psychiatry* 2008;**32**:1978–81; n = 555, RCT, open, 26/52, Hanssens *et al*, *BMC Psychiatry* 2008;**22**:95; MS).

- **Olanzapine** has been used if risperidone-induced (n = 17, c/o, Lin *et al*, *J Clin Psychiatry* 2006;**67**:1470–1).

- **Quetiapine** has a low incidence of hyperprolactinaemia (20%; n = 70, Stevens *et al*, *J Child Adolesc Psychopharmacol* 2005;**15**:893–900) and switching to quetiapine from typicals may be successful in about 65% of cases (n = 69, Nakajima *et al*, *Pharmacopsychiatry* 2005;**38**:17–9).

- * **Risperidone** — switching patients from oral to RLAI may reduce prolactin levels, possibly by reducing surges in 9-OH-risperidone levels (35% reduction, n = 25, open, 12/52, Bai *et al*, *J Clin Psychopharmacol* 2007;**27**:306–8). Paliperidone and risperidone cause the same amount of prolactin elevation (n = 76, 6/7, RCT, d/b, Berwaerts *et al*, *J Psychopharmacol* 2010;**24**:1011–8).

Adjunctive therapies: *

- * **Aripiprazole** augmentation may be useful:
    - ~ * **Benzamide**: only 10% had normalised prolactin (n = 10, 8/52, open, Chen *et al*, *Prog Neuropsychopharmacol Biol Psychiatry* 2010; **34**:1495–9).
    - ~ **Haloperidol**: aripiprazole 15–30 mg/d can reduce prolactin levels, with 88% normal after 8/52 (cf. 4% with placebo) and reversal of symptoms in most (n = 56, p/c, 8/52, Shim *et al*, *Am J Psychiatry* 2007;**164**:1404–10), albeit with some exacerbation of hallucinations (n = 7, Lee *et al*, *Prog Neuropsychopharmacol Biol Psychiatry* 2006;**30**:714–7).
    - ~ * **Risperidone**: 93% had normalised prolactin with aripiprazole 5–20 mg/d (n = 15, 8/52, open, Chen *et al*, *Prog Neuropsychopharmacol Biol Psychiatry* 2010; **34**:1495–9). In 16 females the effect occurred over four weeks at 3 mg/d, plateaued at 6 mg/d with no advantage above 12 mg/d (n = 16, Yasui-Furukori *et al*, *J Clin Psychopharmacol* 2010;**30**:596–9). 15 mg/d has been used for risperidone depot (Wahl and Ostroff, *Am J Psychiatry* 2005;**162**:1542–3) induced hyperprolactinaemia.
    - ~ **Olanzapine**: aripiprazole 15 mg produced complete resolution (n = 1, Aggarwal *et al*, *Indian J Pharmacol* 2010;**42**:58–9).

~ * **Paliperidone** (n = 1, Rocha et al, Prog Neuropsychopharmacol Biol Psychiatry 2010;**34**:1153–4).

Dopamine agonists should generally be avoided as they may precipitate psychosis, but with careful monitoring and dose adjustment may be successful in selected cases where other strategies have failed (review of bromocriptine and cabergoline; Colao et al, Nat Clin Pract Endocrinol Metab 2006;**2**:200–10). There may be significant differences in tolerability of dopamine agonists, with cabergoline probably the best (review by Chanson et al, Ann Endocrinol [Paris] 2007;**68**:113–7).

* **Amantadine** has been successful in 90% patients (n = 10, open, 7/52, Correa et al, J Clin Psychopharmacol 1987;**7**:91–5).
* **Bromocriptine** 2.5–10 mg/d reduces prolactin over four weeks then plateaus, with no relapses (n = 60 [c = 48], RCT, s/b, p/c, 8/52, Lee et al, Psychiatry Clin Neurosci 2010;**64**:19–27).
* **Cabergoline** is longer-acting, better tolerated and may be superior to bromocriptine in efficacy. Cabergoline 0.125–0.25 mg/d has been used if risperidone-induced (58% had a statistically significant reduction, with no adverse affects and no deterioration in psychosis; n = 19, 8/52, Cavallaro et al, J Clin Psychiatry 2004;**65**:187–90). Use a lower dose as the standard starting dose of 0.5mg/d or higher might cause psychosis (n = 2, Chang et al, Gen Hosp Psychiatry 2008;**30**:378–80).
* **Pergolide** – mentioned in some reviews (see below).
* **Peony-glycyrrhiza decoction** (PGD, a herbal medicine) 45 g/d was as effective as bromocriptine 5 mg/d at reducing risperidone-induced hyperprolactinaemia in women with schizophrenia, and also improved symptoms of raised prolactin (n = 20, RCT, c/o, 3x4/52, Yuan et al, J Clin Psychopharmacol 2008;**28**:264–70).

Reviews: * management (Madhusoodanan et al, Hum Psychopharmacol 2010;**25**:281–97), general (Verhelst and Abs, Treat Endocrin 2003;**2**:23–32).

Hyperthyroidism

Lithium   Lithium can raise TSH levels, which has been linked strongly with an increased risk of depression, so monitor regularly and manage (s = 2, n = 32, RCT, d/b, p/c, 18/12, Frye et al, Acta Psychiatr Scand 2009;**120**:10–3).
Carbimazole (n = 9 and review, Barclay et al, Clin Endocrinol [Oxf] 1994; **40**:759–64).
Radioactive iodine (n = 3, Dwarakanathan, Endocr Pract 1998;**4**:201–3).

Hyponatraemia

Risk factors for hyponatraemia include older age, female gender, low body weight, concurrent drugs (e.g. diuretics, NSAIDs, carbamazepine, cancer chemotherapy), reduced renal function, comorbidity (e.g. hypothyroidism, diabetes, COPD), and hotter weather (review by Jacob and Spinler, Ann Pharmacother 2006;**40**:1618–22), so monitor serum sodium over several weeks in higher risk patients. Rapid correction is extremely hazardous.

* On causative drug withdrawal, sodium usually returns to normal within two weeks.
* Smoking may exacerbate hyponatraemia.
* Rechallenge may be possible without recurrence (review, Kirby and Ames, Int J Geriatr Psychiatry 2001;**16**:484–93). If necessary, restart at low dose, increase slowly and monitor carefully.
* If sodium > 125 mmol/l, monitor daily until above 135 mmol/L. If < 125 mmol/L, refer for urgent specialist medical care.
* Loop diuretics have been used (Jacob and Spinler, Ann Pharmacother 2006;**40**:1618–22).
* Restrict fluid intake.

Review: Management (Munger, Am J Health Syst Pharm 2007;**64**:253–65).

6

Antidepressants	May be due to inappropriate antidiuretic hormone secretion (SIADH). **Use a lower risk antidepressant.** According to CSM data to 2005, the risks are as follows (although there is doubtless under-reporting for all drugs):

- Highest risk (> 1% incidence): citalopram, escitalopram, fluoxetine, sertraline.
- Medium risk (0.5–1% incidence): amitriptyline, clomipramine, dosulepin, doxepin, imipramine, lofepramine, moclobemide, paroxetine, venlafaxine.
- Lowest risk (<0.5% incidence): nortriptyline, trazodone, phenelzine, tranylcypromine, mirtazapine, reboxetine.

Mirtazapine appears, overall, to have the lowest risk based on current evidence and the level of reported problems (cases have been reported, e.g. profound hyponatraemia; n = 2, Cheah et al, Am J Geriatr Pharmacother 2008;**6**:91–5), although all antidepressants have reported associations.
If it recurs on rechallenge and antidepressants are essential, consider water restriction and/or careful use of demeclocycline.
Demeclocycline use is controversial and some texts recommend avoiding it with antidepressants.
Review: Cawley, Ann Pharmacother 2007;**41**:840–50.

Antipsychotics
Can be caused by water intoxication, SIADH or severe hyperlipidaemia and/or hyperglycaemia.
If caused by water intoxication (serum and urine osmolality both low):

- **Fluid restriction** (refer to DGH if sodium < 125 mmol/L).
- **Switch drugs**, e.g. clozapine (may reverse hyponatraemia/hypoosmolemia; n = 8, 18–24/52, open, Canuso and Goldman, J Neuropsychiatry Clin Neurosci 1999;**11**:86–90), olanzapine, risperidone or quetiapine.
- There is no evidence that altering doses is effective.

If caused by SIADH (high urine but low serum osmolality):

- **Fluid restriction** (refer to DGH if sodium < 125 mmol/L).
- **Switch** antipsychotic as soon as possible. A low incidence has been reported with aripiprazole (Bachu et al, Am J Ther 2006;**13**:370–2).
- **Consider** demeclocycline (probably directly blocks the renal tubular effect of antidiuretic hormones; usual dose range is 0.9–1.2 g daily, reduced to 600–900 mg/d for maintenance, see standard texts).
- **Discontinue any concurrent desmopressin** (n = 1, Sarma et al, Aust N Z J Psychiatry 2005;**39**:1726–31).
- **Lithium** has been used (mentioned in Madhusoodanan et al, Adverse Drug React Toxicol Rev 2002;**21**:17–29).

Hypothyroidism
Lithium
Lithium inhibits thyroid release but compensatory mechanisms operate in most patients. It is more common in people with circulating thyroid antibodies (n = 150, Bocchetta et al, J Endocrinol Invest 2007;**30**:363–6). Refer to an endocrinologist if TSH levels are repeatedly abnormal.
Lithium withdrawal tends to resolve euthyroid or hypothyroid goitres.
Supplementary thyroxine therapy is indicated for overt hypothyroidism. Treatment with thyroxine for subclinical hypothyroidism is controversial.
Manage weight, especially during the first year, as this can be highly predictive of hypothyroidism (Henry, J Psychiatry Neurosci 2002;**27**:104–7).
Reviews: general (Fagiolini et al, Epidemiol Psichiatr Soc 2006;**15**:123–7), mechanisms (Bocchetta and Loviselli, Clin Pract Epidemiol Ment Health 2006;**12**:23; Johnson and Eagles, Br J Psychiatry 1999;**175**:336–9).

Polyuria and renal impairment (often a symptom of diabetes insipidus)

Lithium   About 20% of people on lithium develop decreased renal function and polyuria, but this is probably only progressive in a few, with a change in therapy only recommended if serum creatinine concentration rises above 200 micromol/l (van Gerven and Boer, *Ned Tijdschr Geneeskd* 2006;**150**:1715–8). It may be due to lithium's effect on vasopressin at a hypothalamic level and a decrease in GFR. The main strategies are:

- **Reduce dose** to the lowest possible, making it once daily (if not already), although there is little data to support this.
- **Switch** to an alternative drug if possible (e.g. valproate has been used; n = 7, Stoll et al, *J Clin Psychiatry* 1996;**57**:356–9).
- **Discontinue** any other drugs that might be contributing.
- **Stop any serotonergic antidepressants** that may enhance polyuria (n = 75, Movig et al, *Br J Psychiatry* 2003;**182**:319–23).
- **Diuretics** such as amiloride have been used (n = 1, Finch et al, *Pharmacotherapy* 2003;**23**:546–50), but great care is needed with interactions, see *Chapter 4.4* (mentioned in van Gerven and Boer, *Ned Tijdschr Geneeskd* 2006;**150**:1705–9).
- **NSAIDs** such as ketoprofen 100 mg IV have been effective in acute lithium toxicity presenting as severe nephrogenic diabetes mellitus (n = 1, Tran-Van et al, *Presse Med* 2005;**34**:1137–40), as has indomethacin 150 mg (rapidly effective, within 36 hours; e.g. n = 1, Lam and Kjellstrand, *Ren Fail* 1997;**19**:183–8), probably by blocking lithium's prostaglandin-inducing activity. Adequate hydration is essential.
- **Refer** to renal specialists for advice (although they are likely to recommend discontinuation).

Reviews: effect of lithium on renal function (n = 20, Turan et al, *Prog Neuropsychopharmacol Biol Psychiatry* 2002;**26**:561–5), general (van Gerven and Boer, *Ned Tijdschr Geneeskd* 2006;**150**:1705–9), risk factors (n = 75, Movig et al, *Br J Psychiatry* 2003;**182**:319–23).

Weight gain

Numerous mechanisms for drug-induced weight gain have been proposed, including:

- Sedation — leading to decreased activity.
- Thirst — anticholinergic dry mouth may lead to an increased intake of fluids and calories.
- Reduced metabolism — fat and carbohydrate oxidation.
- Increased food intake via neurotransmitter-mediated increase in appetite, e.g. via blockade of receptors such as 5-HT2A, 5-HT2C, H1 or H2 and perhaps D2, and polypeptides such as CCK. 5-HT2C polymorphism appears to determine circulating leptin levels so might explain the mechanism (e.g. n = 30, RCT, d/b, Kluge et al, *J Clin Psychopharmacol* 2007;**27**:662–6).
- Changes in levels of leptin (Baptista and Beaulieu, *Can J Psychiatry* 2002;**47**:742–9; Gorobets, *Bull Exp Biol Med* 2008;**146**:348–50), a multifunctional polypeptide produced by fat cells to reduce appetite (by signalling the size of the adipose tissue to the brain) and to increase energy expenditure. Weight gain induced by clozapine, olanzapine and other antipsychotics may be related to an increase in leptin levels via hypothalamic neurons that mediate the effects of leptin on the control of food intake (Reynolds et al, *J Psychopharmacol* 2006;**20**[4 Suppl]:15–8).
- Other polypeptides may also be implicated, e.g. reductin and cytokines, tumour necrosis factor alpha (TNF-alpha) and ghrelin (a fast-acting hormone which plays a role in meal initiation; clozapine, olanzapine, risperidone, amisulpride all cause raised ghrelin but quetiapine does not; n = 112, Esen-Danaci et al, *Prog Neuropsychopharmacol Biol Psychiatry* 2008;**32**:1434–8).
- Induction of abdominal fat deposition, combined with a dysfunction of the normal leptin control of weight (n = 46, 10/52, Zhang et al, *Br J Psychiatry* 2004;**184**:58–62).

6

- Fluid retention — via peripheral oedema, a minor effect.
- Endocrine effects — increased prolactin levels (which may promote adiposity and is related to weight gain in men; open, p/c, Baptista et al, Pharmacopsychiatry 1997;**30**:250–5), variation in cortisol or altered insulin secretion.
- * Poor sleep quality — there are non-endocrine reasons for weight gain (thanks to Dr Neil Stanley for alerting me to this). Sedation caused by drugs producing sedated sleep is NOT the same as having restorative sleep and short sleep duration is consistently associated with concurrent and future obesity (s = 36, n = 1392345, Patel and Hu, Obesity 2008;**16**:643–53). Poor sleep or sleep deprivation leads to increased hunger and chances to eat (leading to increased calorific intake), and increased fatigue and altered thermoregulation (leading to reduced energy need). This leads to obesity:

  >7 hours sleep per day = category with lowest prevalence of adiposity

  <5.5 hours sleep per day = category with highest prevalence of adiposity

  People with <5.5 hours sleep eat the same meals the next day but increase their calorific intake from snacks, especially between 7.00PM and 7.00AM, but without an increase in energy expenditure (n = 11, 2x14/7, Nedeltcheva et al, Am J Clin Nutr 2009;**89**:126–33). Late night watching of television and computer screens may inhibit or suppress the release of melatonin, which does not trigger normal sleep-wake cycle (wearing yellow glasses helps apparently).

Reviews: * sleep (Knutson And Van Cauter, Ann N Y Acad Sci 2008;**1129**:287–304), general (s = 248, Gentile, Obes Rev 2009;**10**:527–42; Ruetsch et al, Encephale 2005;**31**:507–16), non-pharmacological interventions (Alvarez-Jiménez et al, Br J Psychiatry 2008;**193**:101–7; comment by McIntyre, EBMH 2009;**12**:52), therapeutic options (Cordes et al, Fortschr Neurol Psychiatr 2008;**76**:703–14), in bipolar (Torrent et al, Acta Psychiatr Scand 2008;**118**:4–18).

Antidepressants *	Weight change in depression is well known and weight loss or gain can be part of the presenting symptoms. Although weight gain with antidepressants may be the reversal of a pre-treatment weight loss in some people (although heavier people are more likely to gain weight if they become depressed), the main causes with tricyclics are drug-induced carbohydrate craving (Paykel, Br J Psychiatry 1973; **123**:501–7) and a decreased metabolic rate (Fernstein et al, Biol Psychiatry 1985;**20**:688–92), rather than improved mood. **Switching** to agomelatine, trazodone or reboxetine are options.
SSRIs	There is a tendency for weight loss over the first six weeks (increased metabolic rate, suppressed appetite, and increased basal body temperature; n = 20, RCT, p/c, Bross and Hoffer, Am J Clin Nutrition 1995;**61**:1020–5), gradually to regained over six months, and then many may gain weight over the longer-term (reviewed by Sussman and Ginsberg, Psychiatr Ann 1998;**28**:89–97). **Topiramate** up to 250mg/d has produced a mean 4kg loss of weight (n = 15, open, 10/52, Van Ameringen et al, J Clin Psychiatry 2002;**63**:981–4). **Bupropion** for SSRI-induced weight gain (see review by Demyttenaere and Jaspers, J Psychopharmacol 2008;**22**:792–804). **Review:** * review and meta-analysis (s = 116, Serretti and Mandelli, J Clin Psychiatry 2010;**71**:1259–72).
Mirtazapine *	Weight gain is difficult to manage and so switching may be the only option. Global data (MI) has suggested starting at 30mg/d may reduce weight gain. **Ranitidine** at night is probably of no use.
Antipsychotics *	**Education**; WWW (warn, weigh, watch): Warn: * counsel patients with a higher risk of weight gain, e.g. female, prone to overeating under stress, narcissistic personality traits, family or personal history of obesity and a greater than 6.5kg difference between

adult maximum and minimum weights, e.g. weight gain with olanzapine (mean 13 mg/d) continues to increase but most is in the first 2/12, slows in months 2–4, but still continues to increase over six months in 85% (s = 86, n = 12425, Millen *et al, J Psychopharmacol* 2011;**25**:639–47). Weigh: take a baseline weight, warn of the unpredictable nature of weight gain, that the effect plateaus after several months, and the need to optimise calorie intake.

Watch: most weight is gained in the first few months, so ensure the patient seeks advice from a dietician early, since it is easier to prevent weight gain than lose it once it has happened. Moderate physical exercise may be helpful and intake of high calorie fluids should be avoided. Weight management includes all possible variations on 'eat less, move more', but should also include 'sleep better'.

Manage more carefully where risk factors exist:

- Increased parents' BMI
- Patient's pre-morbid BMI (higher predicts 12.5% of gain with olanzapine)
- Female gender
- Schizophrenia spectrum disorder (trend)
- Age (negative correlation, more common in younger, gain is reduced by 0.6 kg for every extra 10 years of age)
- High cumulative olanzapine dose

(n = 118; 12/52, Smith *et al, Int Clin Psychopharmacol* 2008;**23**:130–7; n = 65, Gebhardt *et al, J Psychiatr Res* 2009;**43**:620–6; n = 164, < 24/52, Ujike *et al, J Clin Psychiatry* 2008;**69**:1416–22).

Cochrane concludes that modest weight loss can be achieved with selected pharmacological and non-drug therapies but that the data is limited by small sample sizes, duration and intervention variety (s = 23, Faulkner *et al, Cochrane Database Syst Rev* 2007:**1**:CD005148).

Behavioural interventions:

Dietary interventions and nutritional education may be effective, e.g:

- Regular dietician visits and self-directed dieting with weight loss as a treatment goal (n = 35 [c = 29], 15/12, Kalarchian *et al, J Clin Psychiatry* 2005;**66**:1058–63).
- Individual nutritional education for 3–6/12 after starting olanzapine may be successful, although studies are small and excluded obese people (Evans *et al, Aust N Z J Psychiatry* 2005;**39**:479–86; critical review by Isaacs, *EBMH* 2006;**9**:11; programme focused on nutrition, exercise and motivation; n = 31 [c = 21], 12/12, Menza *et al, J Clin Psychiatry* 2004;**65**:471–7).
- Weight management programmes may be effective (e.g. n = 48 [c = 36], RCT, 12/52, Kwon *et al, J Clin Psychiatry* 2006;**67**:547–53). Attending group sessions regularly over a year also helps (n = 93, Pendlebury *et al, Acta Psychiatr Scand* 2007;**115**:286–94).

Exercise may help. Those doing light jogging for 30 minutes three times a week plus reducing food intake by 500 kcal/d gained 2 kg less than those just receiving olanzapine 10–20 mg/d for mania (n=28, RCT, 8/52, Milano *et al, Adv Ther* 2007;**24**:123–34).

Lifestyle intervention and metformin were both superior for antipsychotic-induced weight gain on all measures, with the combination being the most effective (n = 128, RCT, p/c, 12/52, Wu *et al, JAMA* 2008;**299**:185–93).

Medication interventions:

Reduce dose, as there is preliminary evidence that weight gain with

6

clozapine and olanzapine is related to **plasma** levels, but not dose. However, there is insufficient evidence on other second generation antipsychotics (Simon et al, J Clin Psychiatry 2009;**70**:1041–50).

Slower introduction has been postulated to lead to a lower final weight gain.

Switch drugs: (see Table 6.6.1 for the relative risks; review s = 4, n = 636, Mukundan et al, Cochrane Database Syst Rev 2010;**12**:CD006629)

Aripiprazole (see also adjunctive) — a meta-analysis in schizophrenia showed a mean 2.55 (+1.5) kg weight loss when switching to aripiprazole from other antipsychotics (s = 9, n = 784, Barak and Aizenberg, J Obes 2011;**2011**:898013), e.g. olanzapine and risperidone (n = 15, Su et al, Psychopharmacology (Berl) 2005;**183**:383–6; n = 121, Meyer et al, Clin Ther 2005;**27**:1930–41), although when switched to aripiprazole in a small study, a third deteriorated mentally, and in the remainder who improved, there was no alteration in weight or metabolic outcomes (n = 15, open, 4/12, Kim et al, J Clin Psychopharmacol 2007;**27**:365–8).

Quetiapine — in olanzapine-induced weight gain, a Lilly study showed that switching to quetiapine led to increased relapses and no significant weight improvements (n = 133, 13/52, Deberdt et al, Ther Clin Risk Manag 2008;**4**:713–20).

Adjunctive therapies: *

Might outperform placebo (in order; s = 32, n = 1482, p/c, Maayan et al, Neuropsychopharmacology 2010;**35**:1520–30):

- * **Metformin** used at the start of treatment with antipsychotics

TABLE 6.6.1: RELATIVE WEIGHT GAIN WITH ANTIPSYCHOTICS

Drug	Long-term change †	Range (95% CI)	Change at 10/52 ‡
Perphenazine	5.8	0.4–11.1	–
Clozapine	5.7	4.3–7	4 (2.7–5.3)
Chlorpromazine	4.2	2.9–5.4	2.1 (0.9–3.4)
Olanzapine	4.2	3.7–4.6	3.5 (3.3–3.7)
Sertindole	2.9	2.7–3.2	3 (1.8–5.2)
Quetiapine	2.5	<1.5–3.5	(0?)
Risperidone	1.7	1.4–2	2 (1.6–2.4)
Fluphenazine	1.1	0.1–2.2	0.4 (-0.7–1.5)
Non-drug controls	0.8	0.1–1.6	1.3 (0.8–1.8)
Polypharmacy	0.5	0.2–0.7	1.2 (0.4–2.1)
Haloperidol	0.5	0.2–0.8	0.5 (0.1–1)
Ziprasidone	0.3	-0.3–0.8	0 (-0.5–0.6)
Trifluoperazine	0.3	-0.9–1.5	–
Placebo	-1	-1.8–0.1	0.4 (-1.3–1.5)
Pimozide	-2.7	-9.3–3.9	–

(Allison et al, Am J Psychiatry 1999;**156**:1686–96, 96 refs, review by Fenton, EBMH 2000;**3**:58; n = 427, Brecher et al, In J Psychiatr Clin Pract 2000;**4**:287–91)

† longer-term weight change in kg (random effects mode)

‡ weight change at 10 weeks (fixed effects mode)

Please bear in mind that this is aggregated data, so is subject to error, weight was often measured at a different time and there may be a dose-relationship and a huge inter-individual variation.

significantly reduces weight gain and waist circumference (s = 6, n = 336, RCT, p/c, Ehret *et al*, *J Clin Psychiatry* 2010;**71**:1286–92), but has no effect on the risk of diabetes or aid loss of olanzapine-induced weight gain (n = 40, RCT, d/b, p/c, 14/52, Baptista *et al*, *Can J Psychiatry* 2006;**51**:192–6). In patients stable on clozapine, addition of metformin 500–1000 mg/d can lead to a mean weight loss of 1.87 kg (n = 61 [c = 56], RCT, d/b, p/c, 14/52, Carrizo *et al*, *Schizophr Res* 2009;**113**:19–26). Metformin only increases utilisation of insulin not the production, so can be safe long-term but not without the risk of, e.g. lactic acidosis.

- **Sibutramine** 15 mg/d significantly reduced olanzapine-induced weight gain (8 lb *vs* 2 lb), but increased bp and disturbed sleep in some patients (n = 37, RCT, d/b, p/c, 12/52, Henderson *et al*, *Am J Psychiatry* 2005;**162**:954–62). However, it was ineffective for clozapine-induced weight gain (n = 21, RCT, d/b, p/c, 12/52, Henderson *et al*, *Acta Psychiatr Scand* 2007;**115**:101–5). Addition of sibutramine (10–20 mg/d) to metformin (850–1700 mg/d) was no more effective than metformin alone for reducing olanzapine-induced weight gain (n = 28, d/b, p/c, 12/52, Baptista *et al*, *Psychiatry Res* 2008;**159**:250–3). It is contraindicated in 'psychiatric illness' so care is needed.

- ***Topiramate** 100 mg/d started with olanzapine can actually result in weight loss and improved metabolic measures (n = 72, RCT, d/b, p/c, 12/52, Narula *et al*, *Schizophr Res* 2010;**118**:218–23). The most effective dose may be 200 mg/d (n = 66, RCT, d/b, p/c, 12/52, Ko *et al*, *Clin Neuropharmacol* 2005;**28**:169–75), with reduced adiposity in women (n = 43, RCT, d/b, p/c, 10/52, Nickel *et al*, *J Clin Psychopharmacol* 2005;**25**:211–7). Adjunctive topiramate (mean 200 mg/d) in overweight schizophrenics can produce continued weight loss over 6/12 (n = 10, Lévy *et al*, *Can J Clin Pharmacol* 2007;**14**:234–9) and improve mood (both depressive and manic) and drop BMI by two points at 12/52 in refractory obese bipolar patients (n = 30, open, 12/52, Gabriel, *Eat Weight Disord* 2007;**12**:48–53).

- **Modafinil** 200 mg/d reduced the weight gained with olanzapine by 50% (from 0.89 to 0.47 kg/m2; n = 50 [c = 40], RCT, d/b, p/c, 3/52, Roerig *et al*, *Biol Psychiatry* 2009;**65**:607–13), the effect being maintained for three years in a patient on clozapine, possibly by reducing clozapine-induced fatigue, reversed on discontinuation (n = 1, Henderson *et al*, *Ann Clin Psychiatry* 2005;**17**:95–7).

- **Reboxetine** co-prescribed when starting olanzapine may help (n = 26 [c = 20], RCT, p/c, d/b, 6/52, Poyurovsky *et al*, *Am J Psychiatry* 2003;**160**:297–302).

Newer options and case reports:

- **Acetazolamide** has been used as an alternative to topiramate (n = 1, Schneiderhan and Marvin, *Am J Ther* 2007;**14**:581–4).

- ***Aripiprazole** 15 mg/d (see also switching) significantly reduced weight and BMI from olanzapine, but had no effect on overall cholesterol, although serum triglycerides, VLDC and VLDL all decreased significantly (d/b, p/c, c/o, 10/52, Henderson *et al*, *J Clin Psychopharmacol* 2009;**29**:165–9). In patients stable on clozapine who had gained > 2.5 kg, addition of aripiprazole 5–15 mg/d resulted in statistically significant weight loss cf placebo (mean -2.5 kg vs -0.4 kg) (n = 207, RCT, d/b, p/c, 16/52, Fleischhacker *et al*, *Int J Neuropsychopharmacol* 2010;**13**:1115–25).

6

- **Bofu-tsusho-san** (an Oriental herbal medicine) can attenuate weight gain from olanzapine (Yamamoto and Inada, *Psychiatry Clin Neurosci* 2008;**62**:747).
- **Bupropion** 150–300 mg/d as an adjunct to olanzapine (mean duration 26/12) produces modest weight loss, with 50% losing > 3% (n = 8 [c = 7], open, 24/52, Gadde *et al*, *J Clin Psychopharmacol* 2006;**6**:409–13; review by Gadde and Xiong, *Expert Rev Neurother* 2007;**7**:17–24).
- **Memantine** augmentation had a significant effect for clozapine-induced weight gain (n = 1, Scharfer *et al*, *Pharmacopsychiatry* 2007;**40**:149–51).
- * **Mifepristone** 600 mg/d can attenuate weight gain from olanzapine (n = 57, RCT, d/b, 2/52, Gross *et al*, *Adv Ther* 2009;**26**:659–69).
- **Quetiapine** has been used as an adjunct to clozapine; after six months' therapy patients had 25% of their dose converted to quetiapine (using ratio 1 mg clozapine:2 mg quetiapine) for 10 months. Average weight loss was 0.22–10.5 kg after one month, and maintained, with 100% user satisfaction reported (review by Werneke *et al*, *Int Clin Psychopharmacol* 2002;**17**:145–60).
- * **Switching to orodispersible olanzapine** — although an RCT failed to show any loss of weight with orodispersible compared to plain tablets (RCT, d/b, p/c, 16/52, Karagianis *et al*, *Schizophr Res* 2009;**113**:41–8; MS), there are continued reports, e.g. a mean weight loss 6.6 kg; (e.g. n = 2, weight loss 15 kg maintained for 12/12, Kozumplik *et al*, *Psychiatr Danub* 2009;**21**:71–4; especially in males and Americans, n = 149, 16/52, Karajans *et al*, *Int J Clin Pract* 2010;**64**:1520–9).
- * **Add ziprasidone** if clozapine-induced (dose-dependent, n = 1, Roy-Desruisseaux and Grignon, *Hum Psychopharmacol* 2010;**25**:428).

Not significantly superior to placebo:

- **Amantadine** 100–300 mg/d may be well-tolerated and attenuate weight gain in some patients who had already gained weight with olanzapine 5–20 mg/d (n = 125, RCT, d/b, p/c, 16/52, Deberdt *et al*, *Eur Neuropsychopharmacol* 2005;**15**:13–21), but not in all studies (n = 25, Bahk *et al*, *Psychiatr Clin Neurosci* 2004;**58**:163–7).
- **Appetite suppressants** may exacerbate psychosis or fail to work.
- * **Orlistat** has a modest effect that may only be seen in men (n = 71 [c = 63], RCT, d/b, p/c, 16/52, Joffe *et al*, *J Clin Psychiatry* 2008;**69**:706–11), with no effect after 16/52 in non-responders (n = 44; RCT, p/c, d/b, 16/52; then open 16/52, Tchoukhine *et al*, *J Clin Psychiatry* 2011;**72**:326–30).
- **Fluoxetine** is ineffective if olanzapine-induced (e.g. n = 31, RCT, d/b, Bustillo *et al*, *Neuropsychopharm* 2003;**28**:527–9).
- **Fluvoxamine** (50 mg/d) may allegedly attenuate weight gain and metabolic disturbances from clozapine, perhaps by allowing lower doses to be used, although the interaction can be dramatic and dangerous (n = 68, RCT, 12/52, Lu *et al*, *J Clin Psychiatry* 2004;**65**:766–71).
- **H2-antagonists** such as famotidine (n = 14, d/b, p/c, 6/52, Poyurovsky *et al*, *Eur Neuropsychopharmacol* 2004;**14**:332–6) and nizatidine are ineffective for olanzapine-induced weight gain (n = 175, d/b, p/c, 16/52, Cavazzoni *et al*, *Eur Neuropsychopharmacol* 2003;**13**:81–5), but may have some effect (n = 59, RCT, d/b, 8/52, Atamaca *et al*, *Hum Psychopharmacol* 2003;**18**:457–61). Ranitidine reduced the weight gain from olanzapine in 60% cases (RCT, open, Lopez-Mato *et al*, *Vertex* 2003;**14**:85–96) and may

stop weight gain with quetiapine, although not reduce any weight already gained (n = 47, RCT, Atmaca et al, *Hum Psychopharmacol* 2004; **19**:37–40).

- **Phenylpropanolamine** is ineffective if clozapine-induced (n = 16, RCT, d/b, 12/52, Borovicka et al, *J Clin Psychiatry* 2002; **63**:345–8).

Reviews: * general (s = 21, n = 3391, RCT, d/b, p/c, Parsons et al, *Schizophr Res* 2009; **110**:103–10: Maayan and Correll, *Expert Rev Neurother* 2010; **10**:1175–200).

Lithium	Weight gain, the second most common reason for non-compliance, is reported to occur in around 33% people (perhaps up to 65%, n = 70, open, Vendsborg et al, *Acta Psychiatr Scand* 1976; **53**:139–47), of which 25% are probably obese (review: Sachs and Guille, *J Clin Psychiatry* 1999; **60** [Suppl 21]:16–9). Weight increase occurs predominantly during the first two years of treatment, more often in people already overweight and may be more common in women than men.

Manage thirst, as increased thirst has been noted in 89% and strongly correlates with weight gain. Increased hunger/food intake has not been directly shown (*J Psychopharmacol* 1990; **4**:303), and so the predominant mechanism may be increased intake of high-calorie drinks.

Thyroid status should also be assessed as a possible contributory cause.

Counselling, e.g. use of plain/low-calorie beverages, along with normal sodium intake, dietary advice and monitoring, particularly during the first year, may be adequate.

Lamotrigine may be an alternative as it is associated with weight loss, there being no significant differences in non-obese patients (n = 554, s = 2, d/b, p/c, 12/12, Bowden et al, *Am J Psychiatry* 2006; **163**:1199–201).

Topiramate can safely be added to lithium or valproate in bipolar I manic or mixed episodes to significantly reduce weight (n = 287, RCT, d/b, p/c, 12/52, Chengappa et al, *J Clin Psychiatry* 2006; **67**:1698–1706; MS).

Anticonvulsants *	There is less likelihood of gaining weight with AEDs if physical activity is included as well as dieting (n = 66, < 8/12, Gaspari and Guerreiro, *Arq Neuropsiquiatr* 2010; **68**:277–81).

Gabapentin is not a good alternative as weight gain can be a significant adverse effect of gabapentin (n = 44, 12/12, DeToledo et al, *Ther Drug Monit* 1997; **19**:394–6).

Levetiracetam at normal doses is usually weight neutral (s = 4, n = 970, RCT, p/c, Gidal et al, *Epilepsy Res* 2003; **56**:121–6)

Topiramate has been reported to produce weight loss, e.g. a dose-related weight loss occurred in 50% patients in a trial in bipolar disorder, with a mean 14.2 lb weight loss (n = 76, open, Ghaemi et al, *Ann Clin Psychiatry* 2001; **13**:185–9) and, compared to lithium and valproate, it produced an average of 1.2 kg weight loss (n = 214, open, chart, Chengappa et al, *Clin Ther* 2002; **24**:1576–84). It has even been abused to try to promote weight loss (n = 1, Colom et al, *J Clin Psychiatry* 2001; **62**:475–6). The effect appears dose-related, with average amounts lost ranging from 1.1 kg/1.5% (up to 200 mg/d) to 5.9 kg/7% (800 mg/d or above). The effect peaks at 12–15 months, is greater in people with higher starting weights, and is at least partially reversible (MI).

Carbamazepine	Weight gain may be due to increased appetite. It is reversed by discontinuation but not by dieting (n = 4, Lampl et al, *Clin Neuropharmacol* 1991; **14**:251–5).
Valproate	* Weight gain with valproate seems more common in people with normal or below normal weight before starting (n = 70, Corman et al, *Can J Neurol*

Sci 1997;**24**:240–4) and so warning people in advance may be advantageous (review of mechanisms, Verrotti *et al, Obes Rev* 2011;**12**:32–43).

Get a new set of genes (n = 5 twin pairs, Klein *et al, Obes Res* 2005;**13**:1330–4). OK, it's not realistic, but may help to explain to some people that weight gain with valproate isn't all their 'fault'.

6.7 Movement disorders

Blepharospasm (see also tardive dystonia)
Blepharospasm is a sustained, forced, involuntary closing of the eyelids, often a presenting symptom of tardive dystonia.

Antipsychotics	Switching antipsychotics is usually the main effective strategy, e.g. to **clozapine**, (n = 4, Levin and Reddy, *J Clin Psychiatry* 2000;**61**:140–3) or **quetiapine** (n = 1, Reeves and Liberto, *Mov Disord* 2003;**18**:1072–3). **ECT** has been used (n = 1, Sienaert and Peuskens, *J ECT* 2005;**21**:132–4).

Bruxism (teeth grinding)
Bruxism is defined as grinding, clenching and forceful teeth or jaw movements, usually during sleep. Almost everyone bruxes, but bruxism is where it is severe enough to cause damage or distress.
Review: general; Lobbezoo *et al, J Oral Rehabil* 2006;**33**:293–300.

Antidepressants	**Dose reduction** usually leads to resolution (n = 4, Ellison and Stanziani, *J Clin Psychiatry* 1993;**54**:432–4) but can take several months to resolve (n = 1, Alonso-Navarro *et al, Clin Neuropharmacol* 2009;**32**:111–2). * **Switching** to duloxetine has alleviated if venlafaxine-induced (n = 1, Chang *et al, Prog Neuropsychopharmacol Biol Psychiatry* 2011;**35**:307). * **Buspirone** has been used if bruxism is induced by venlafaxine (40 mg/d, significantly effective over 4/52: Pavlovic, *Int J Neuropsychopharmacol* 2004;**7**:523–4; n = 1, Kuloglu *et al, J Psychopharmacol* 2010;**24**:627–8), or SSRIs (n = 4, Bostwick and Jaffee, *J Clin Psychiatry* 1999;**60**:857–60), e.g. fluoxetine (n = 1, Sabuncuoglu *et al, Spec Care Dentist* 2009;**29**:215–7). **Gabapentin**, if venlafaxine-induced (n = 1, Brown and Hong, *J Am Dent Assoc* 1999;**130**:1467–9). **ECT**, if fluvoxamine-induced (n = 1, Miyaoka *et al, J ECT* 2003;**19**:170–2).
Antipsychotics	**Dose reduction** usually leads to resolution. **Switch** to low-dose clozapine (n = 1, 16/52, Mendhekar and Andrade, *J Neuropsychiatry Clin Neurosci* 2009;**21**:105–6). **Propranolol** (case where concurrent akathisia also improved; n = 2, Amir *et al, Clin Neuropharmacol* 1997;**20**:86–9). **Lamotrigine** has been used successfully (n = 1, McMeekin, *J S C Med Assoc* 2007;**103**:69–73).

Dysphagia
Difficulty in swallowing or painful swallowing has been reported with many antipsychotics.
Review: drug-induced (O'Neill and Remington, *Ann Pharmacother* 2003;**37**:1675–84)

Antipsychotics	Dysphagia generally responds rapidly to discontinuation (e.g. n = 1, Stewart, *Dysphagia* 2003;**18**:274–5). In life-threatening dysphagia, **benzodiazepines** (clonazepam) or oral **anticholinergics** may be effective (trihexyphenidyl, n = 2, Hayashi *et al, Clin Neuropharmacol* 1997;**20**:77–81; benzatropine, n = 1, Nair *et al, Gen Hosp Psychiatry* 2001;**23**:231–2), although if used regularly, anticholinergics may be a causative or exacerbating factor.

EPSE, akathisia
Neuroleptic-induced akathisia (NIA) is a subjective unpleasant feeling of inner restlessness and the

urge to move, with rocking while standing or sitting, lifting feet as if marching on the spot, and crossing and uncrossing legs while sitting. NIA has been associated with suicidal behaviour (s = 83, Hansen, *Hum Psychopharmacol* 2001;**16**:495–505) and subjective cognitive dysfunction and so needs treating (n = 67, Kim and Byun, *J Clin Pharm Ther* 2007;**32**:461–7). It is probably an imbalance of cortical and nigrostriatal dopaminergic innervation and has been reported with other drugs.

Reviews: effect on clinical outcome (n = 34, Luthra *et al*, *Gen Hosp Psychiatry* 2000;**22**:276–80), use of serotonin-based drugs (Poyurovsky and Weizman, *Br J Psychiatry* 2001;**179**:4–8; including an algorithm), NIA and violence (Leong and Silva, *J Forensic Sci* 2003;**48**:187–9).

Antidepressants	**Reduce** the dose, as it is dose-related at least for fluoxetine (n = 1, Hansen, *J Psychopharmacol* 2003;**17**:451–2).

Switch antidepressants, e.g. **paroxetine** for fluoxetine-induced (n = 1, Bauer *et al*, *J Clin Psychiatry* 1996;**57**:593–4).

Propranolol has also been used if fluoxetine-induced (Fleischhacker, *Biol Psychiatry* 1991;**30**:531–2).

Review: SSRI-induced akathisia (Koliscak and Makela, *J Am Pharm Assoc* 2009;**49**:28–36).

Antipsychotics

* **Reducing the dose or switching** antipsychotics is the main strategy, e.g. switch to risperidone (4 mg/d) and quetiapine (300 mg/d) for olanzapine-induced (n = 1, Peritogiannis and Tsouli, *J Psychopharmacol* 2010;**24**:1121–5). For **aripiprazole**, reduce dose, use benzodiazepines, adrenoceptor antagonists (propranolol), gabapentin or anticholinergic agents (review, Cassano *et al*, *Clin Drug Invest* 2007;**27**:1–13; Aitchison *et al*, *J Psychopharmacol* 2009;**23**:231–4).

Adjunctive therapies:

The following drugs may be useful in the short or long-term if the dose or drug cannot be changed:

- **Anticholinergics** may have some efficacy but are generally considered less useful. Biperiden 5 mg IV may be rapidly effective (< 10 minutes) for severe akathisia (n = 23, open, Hirose and Ashby, *Int J Psychiatry Med* 2000;**30**:185–94). Cochrane concludes that there is no reliable evidence to support or refute the use of anticholinergics for acute NIA (Lima *et al*, *CDSR* 2006;**4**:CD003727).

- **Benzodiazepines**, e.g. clonazepam 0.5–3 mg/d (mean 1.7 mg/d) have been used and 81% patients in one study improved, with the effect prominent in two days (n = 21, open, *Acta Psychiatr Scand* 1989;**80**:106–7). Diazepam 10–17 mg IV (at 5 mg/30 seconds) has also provided rapid relief of acute NIA (n = 18, open, Hirose and Ashby, *J Clin Psychiatry* 2002;**63**:524–7).

- **Beta-blockers**, e.g. propranolol 30–80 mg/d can produce a dramatic and persistent improvement (especially if not part of an EPSE), but may take up to three months to act in chronic cases (d/b, p/c, Kramer *et al*, *Biol Psychiatry* 1988;**24**:823–7). Other lipophilic beta-blockers, e.g. metoprolol (RCT, Adler *et al*, *Biol Psychiatry* 1990;**27**:673–5) may be effective if olanzapine-induced (n = 1, Kurzthaler *et al*, *Am J Psychiatry* 1997;**154**:1316). Nadolol, sotalol and atenolol are probably ineffective.

- **Cyproheptadine** 16 mg/d may be effective, supported by a robust trial (n = 30, RCT, d/b, 7/7, Fischel *et al*, *J Clin Psychopharmacol* 2001;**21**:612–5).

- **Diphenhydramine** IV may rapidly (over 30 minutes) reduce the symptoms of acute NIA from IV prochlorperazine (n = 87, open, Vinson, *J Emerg Med* 2004;**26**:265–70).

- **Gabapentin**, where a dose-related response has been reported (n = 1, Pfeffer *et al*, *Int Clin Psychopharmacol* 2005;**20**:179–81).

6

- **Mianserin** 5 mg/d may produce a significant improvement in NIA and dysphoria (n = 15, RCT, 5/7, Poyurovsky et al, Br J Psychiatry 1999;**174**:238–42; n = 1, Stryjer et al, Eur Psychiatry 2004;**19**:237–8).
- **Mirtazapine** has a 53% response rate (cf placebo 8%) in NIA (s = 5, n=125, Hieber et al, Ann Pharmacother 2008;**42**:841–6), probably via 5HT2A/2C antagonism.
- **Ropinirole** 18 mg/d has helped aripiprazole-induced tardive akathisia (n = 1, Hettema and Ross, J Clin Psychiatry 2007;**68**:1814–5).
- **Thiamine** (vitamin B1) high-dose (1.2 g/d) may be useful for acute NIA (n = 20, RCT, p/c, d/b, 5/7, Lerner et al, J Clin Psychiatry 2004;**65**:1550–4).
- * **Trazodone** 100mg/d showed definite and statistically significant activity against NIA, probably by 5HT2A postsynaptic receptor antagonism, in a small but perfectly-formed study (n = 13, RCT, d/b, p/c, c/o, 6/7, Stryjer et al, Clin Neuropharmacol 2010;**33**:219–22).
- **Zolmitriptan** (a selective 5HT1D inhibitor) 7.5 mg/d can produce a significant and rapid improvement in NIA, even in chronic and resistant cases, warranting further trials (n = 8, open, 3/7, Gross-Isseroff et al, Int Clin Psychopharmacol 2005;**20**:23–5).

Less use:

Other drugs tried, usually without success, include:

- **Amantadine** (n = 4, Zubenko et al, J Clin Psychopharmacol 1984;**4**:218–20).
- **Apomorphine** low dose may reduce objective (movement) effects but not subjective distress (Karstaedt and Pincus, Neurology 1993;**43**:611–3).
- **Buspirone** has only a minor effect, with only 20% showing any effect (n = 10, Poyurovsky and Weizman, Int Clin Psychopharmacol 1997;**12**:263–8).
- * **Fluvoxamine** for aripiprazole-induced (n = 2, Furuse and Hashimoto, Ann Gen Psychiatry 2010;**9**:11).
- **Granisetron** is ineffective (n = 10, 4/7, Poyurovsky and Weizman, Int Clin Psychopharmacol 1999;**14**:357–60).
- **Iron supplements** — although there is no relationship between plasma iron and chronic akathisia (Barnes et al, Br J Psychiatry 1992;**161**:791–6), IV iron has been used successfully in iron-deficient akathisia (n = 1, Cotter and O'Keeffe, J Neurol Neurosurg Psychiatry 2007;**78**:548).
- **Moclobemide** (n = 1, Ebert and Demling, Pharmacopsychiatry 1991;**24**:29–31).
- **Tryptophan** (n = 6, open, Biol Psychiatry 1990;**27**:671–2).

Lithium

- **Lorazepam** (Yassa and Grouix, J Clin Psychopharmacol 1989;**9**:70–1).
- **Mianserin** (n = 1, Poyurovsky et al, Int Clin Psychopharmacol 1995;**10**:261–3).

EPSE, dyskinesias (acute or tardive)

Tardive dyskinesia (TD) is an involuntary hyperkinesia, which increases with anxiety, goes away during sleep and in some cases may be irreversible. Symptoms include choreas, tics, dystonias and orolingual dyskinesias, but not tremor. It is generally seen as repetitive, involuntary and purposeless movements of, e.g. the tongue, neck and jaw. It may be a late symptom of schizophrenia and antipsychotics might in fact just bring such symptoms forward (rather than cause them), e.g. brain structures are similar (n = 93, McCreadie et al, Arch Gen Psychiatry 2002;**59**:332–6) and TD fluctuates with time (n = 37, McCreadie et al, Br J Psychiatry 2002;**181**:135–7).

Risk factors include the length of exposure to antipsychotics in the elderly, alcohol consumption, advancing age, being male, previous head injury, presence of organic brain disease, structural brain damage, earlier drug-induced Parkinsonism, akathisia or dystonias, being left-handed, being diabetic, concurrent affective or negative symptoms and having a parent with schizophrenia who themselves has or had a dyskinesia.

Reviews: general (Correll and Schenk, *Curr Opin Psychiatry* 2008;**21**:151–6; Soares-Weiser and Fernandez, *Semin Neurol* 2007;**27**:159–69), in children (Correll and Kane, *J Child Adolesc Psychopharmacol* 2007;**17**:647–56), 'miscellaneous' treatments (s = 7, Soares-Weiser and Joy, *Cochrane Database Syst Rev* 2003;**2**:CD000208).

Antidepressants	**Mirtazapine** has been used for bupropion-induced TD (n = 1, Kohen and Sarcevic, *Movement Disord* 2006;**21**:584–5).
Antipsychotics	**Withdrawal** or **dose reduction** are the usual strategies, although the risk of relapse may be high.

Drug 'holidays' seem detrimental.

Transient dose increases may help occasionally, but only in the short-term.

Withdraw or reduce any anticholinergic drugs if possible, as these can provoke or exacerbate TD, although are not a risk factor as such (Soares and McGrath, *Cochrane Database Syst Rev* 2000;**2**:CD000204). Indeed, trihexyphenidyl is now contraindicated for use in TD.

Switching antipsychotics: *

Switching to a SGA is usually considered the main strategy, e.g. switching to risperidone or olanzapine can be equally effective (n = 60, RCT, s/b, 24/52, Chan et al, *J Clin Psychiatry* 2010;**71**:1226–33).

- **Aripiprazole** may be effective if induced by quetiapine (n = 1, Rizos et al, *World J Biol Psychiatry* 2009;**10**:54–7), risperidone (Caykoylu et al, *Prog Neuropsychopharmacol Biol Psychiatry* 2009;**33**:571–2) or haloperidol (n = 3, Osorio et al, *Neurotox Res* 2010;**17**:432–4).
- **Clozapine** may improve TD, especially with dystonic features, e.g. > 50% reduction in symptoms has been seen (n = 7, open, Bassitt et al, *Eur Arch Psychiatr Clin Neurosci* 1998;**248**:209–11), and may also be effective over the longer term (n = 7, open, five years, Louza and Bassitt, *J Clin Psychopharmacol* 2005;**25**:180–2).
- **Olanzapine**, with reports of a marked reduction in pre-existing symptoms of TD (e.g. n = 2, Agarwal and Kumar, *J Clin Psychiatry* 2001;**62**:298–9).
- * **Quetiapine** where, in a switch study, it maintained psychotic symptom control but reduced TD compared to haloperidol (n = 45, RCT, 12/12, s/b, Emsley et al, *J Clin Psychiatry* 2004;**65**:696–701). Adjunctive quetiapine has been used for risperidone (n = 1, Nelson et al, *Clin Neuropharmacol* 2003;**26**:297–8) and olanzapine-induced TD (n = 1, Peritogiannis and Tsouli, *J Psychopharmacol* 2010;**24**:1121–5).
- **Risperidone**, where the response may occur in a few weeks and then be maintained (n = 40, 48/52, Bai et al, *Int Clin Psychopharmacol* 2005;**20**:79–85; n = 49, RCT, d/b, p/c, 16/52, Bai et al, *J Clin Psychiatry* 2003;**64**:1342–8; MS; review by Tandon, *EBMH* 2004;**7**:83).

Adjunctive therapies:

Adjunctive therapies are usually considered to be of low efficacy, although tetrabenazine is licensed:

- * **Tetrabenazine** is licensed in the UK, with a starting dose of 12.5 mg, titrated to 25–75 mg/d (maximum 200 mg/d). In refractory TD, tetrabenazine (mean 58 mg/d) has significantly improved AIMS scores (n = 20, 20/52, Ondo et al, *Am J Psychiatry* 1999;**156**:1279–81). It may have long-term efficacy (n = 448, mean 2.3 years, Kenney et al, *Mov Disord* 2007;**22**:193–7; review by Fasano and Bentivoglio, *Expert Opin Pharmacother* 2010;**11**:2883–96).
- **Amantadine** was superior to placebo in one study (d/b, c/o, p/c, 18/52, Angus et al, *J Clin Psychopharmacol* 1997;**17**:88–91).

6

- **Buspirone** at up to 180 mg/d may be useful (n = 8, open, 12/52, Moss *et al, J Clin Psychopharmacol* 1993;**13**:204–9).
- **Cyproheptadine** at 8–24 mg/d has significantly improved haloperidol-induced TD (n = 10, open, Lee *et al, J Serotonin Res* 1994;**1**:91–5).
- **Donepezil**, a pilot study indicated 5–10 mg/d might suppress symptoms of TD (n = 10, open, 8/52, Caroff *et al, J Clin Psychiatry* 2001;**62**:772–5).
- **Gabapentin** has improved long-term TD, with an average improvement of 47.5% (n = 25, open, 12/12, Hardoy *et al, J Affect Disord* 2003;**75**:125–30).
- **Galantamine** 8–24 mg/d as an adjunct to stable antipsychotic doses has reduced AIMS-rated scores, but not statistically significant, although there was a statistically significant deterioration on discontinuation (n = 35, RCT, d/b, p/c, c/o, 2 × 12/52, Caroff *et al, J Clin Psychiatry* 2007;**68**:410–5; MS).
- * **Ginkgo biloba,** in a Chinese population an extract of GB significantly reduced AIMS scores cf placebo with no effect on PANSS scores (n = 157 [c = 152], RCT, d/b, p/c, 12/52, Zhang *et al, J Clin Psychiatry* 2011;**72**:615–21).
- * **Levetiracetam** (500–3000 mg/d) was well tolerated and significantly reduced AIMS scores (43% vs 19%) compared to placebo (n = 50, RCT, d/b, p/c, 12/52, Woods *et al, J Clin Psychiatry* 2008;**69**:546–54; n = 1, Chen and Liu, *J Clin Psychopharmacol* 2010;**30**:205–7).
- **Melatonin** 10 mg/d has been shown to decrease AIMS scores in TD (n = 22, d/b, p/c, c/o, 6/52, Shamir *et al, Arch Gen Psychiatry* 2001;**58**:1049–52).
- **Naltrexone** plus clonazepam have reduced TD scores (n = 23, RCT, d/b, p/c, Wonodi *et al, J Clin Psychopharmacol* 2004;**24**:441–5).
- **Ondansetron** (a 5-HT3 antagonist) 12 mg/d has been used successfully (n = 12, open, 12/52, Sirota *et al, Am J Psychiatry* 2000;**157**:287–9; although this could have been an interaction).
- **Piracetam** (mean 4800 mg/d) appears to be effective (n = 40, RCT, d/b, p/c, c/o, 2 × 4/52, Libov *et al, J Clin Psychiatry* 2007;**68**:1031–7).
- **Pyridoxine** (Vitamin B6) 200 mg/d has produced a rapid and sustained reduction in TD symptoms and 1200 mg/d was clearly superior to placebo for reducing the symptoms of TD (n = 50, RCT, d/b, p/c, c/o, 26/52, Lerner *et al, J Clin Psychiatry* 2007;**68**:1648–54).
- **Sodium oxybate** resolved olanzapine-induced TD, with a 2/52 latency of onset (n = 1, Berner, *J Clin Psychiatry* 2008;**69**:862).
- **Thiamine** was effective in one small but careful study (n = 15, RCT, d/b, p/c, 4/52, Lerner *et al, Am J Psychiatry* 2001;**158**:1511–4).
- **Yi-gan san**, Japanese herbal medicine (n = 22, open, 12/52, Miyaoka *et al, Prog Neuropsychopharmacol Biol Psychiatry* 2008;**32**:761–4).
- **Zopiclone** has been used (n = 1, Sugawara *et al, Prog Neuropsychopharmacol Biol Psychiatry* 2009;**33**:727–8).

Less useful:

Many adjunctive therapies have been tried but few have any real use. The following are not in the useful group:

- **Baclofen**, see GABA agonists.
- **Benzodiazepines** have been used but Cochrane concludes that they have no proven advantage over placebo (s = 3, n = 56, Bhoopathi and Soares-Weiser, *Cochrane Database Syst Rev* 2006;**3**:CD000205).
- **Calcium-channel blockers** are not supported by any robust studies (s = 0, n = 0, Soares-Weiser and Rathbone, *Cochrane Database Syst Rev* 2004;**1**:CD000206).

- **Cholinergic drugs** (e.g. choline, lecithin, ACEIs) are probably ineffective (see systematic review; s = 11, n = 261, RCTs, Tammenmaa *et al*, *Prog Neuropsychopharmacol Biol Psychiatry* 2004;**28**:1099–107).
- **Citalopram** was ineffective in one study (n = 13, Korsgaard *et al*, *Clin Neuropharmacol* 1986;**9**:52–7).
- **GABA agonists/enhancers such as baclofen and valproate**. Cochrane concludes from the eight small, short-term studies that the evidence is inconclusive and unconvincing (s = 8, n = 547, Soares *et al*, *Cochrane Database Syst Rev* 2004;**4**:CD000203).
- **Insulin** (low-dose) has been suggested to be as superior to placebo (see McGrath and Soares, *Cochrane Database Syst Rev* 2000;**2**:CD000208).
- **Lithium** has no consistent positive effect (e.g. Yassa *et al*, *Can J Psychiatry* 1984;**29**:36–7) and may even be detrimental.
- **Valproate**, see GABA agonists.
- **Vitamin E** probably has no significant effect (up to 1600 iu/d; n = 158, RCT, up to two years, Adler *et al*, *Arch Gen Psychiatry* 1999;**56**:836–41; Soares and McGrath, *Cochrane Database Syst Rev* 2000;**2**:CD000209), but may perhaps be effective in a small subgroup of patients (s = 18, Boomershine *et al*, *Ann Pharmacother* 1999;**33**:1195–202).

EPSE, Parkinsonism

Pseudoparkinsonism or Parkinsonian side-effects include akinesia, rigidity, bradykinesia and coarse tremor at rest. They are usually associated with antipsychotics but can occur with many drugs (see *Chapter 5.8*).

Antidepressants, (especially tricyclics)	* **Switch drugs** (e.g. to reboxetine if paroxetine-induced; n = 1, Kuloglu *et al*, *J Psychopharmacol* 2010;**24**:623–4), or treat as per antipsychotics. **Benzodiazepines**, e.g. diazepam (mentioned in Pollack and Rosenbaum, *J Clin Psychiatry* 1987;**48**:3–8). **Propranolol** 40–120 mg/d has been used (mentioned in Pollack and Rosenbaum, *J Clin Psychiatry* 1987;**48**:3–8).
Antipsychotics	**Dose reduction** of any antipsychotic. **Switch** to an antipsychotic with lower EPS, e.g. quetiapine, olanzapine or aripiprazole. **Anticholinergics** (antimuscarinics) are first-line treatments. They include **benzatropine** (also has antihistaminic properties and a long half-life of up to 24 hours), **orphenadrine** (which is probably more toxic: Slørdal and Gjerden, *Br J Psychiatry* 1999;**174**:275–6), **procyclidine** (with a disputed abuse potential) and **trihexyphenidyl** (benzhexol; with a reported abuse and dependence potential; Frauger *et al*, *Therapie* 2003;**58**:541–7). They may improve survival (n = 88, 10-year prospective study, Waddington *et al*, *Br J Psychiatry* 1998;**173**:325–9) and compliance, and may actually only be detrimental to positive symptoms during acute phases (when excess dopaminergic activity is thought to occur) but not during stable phases (Tandon and Dequardo, *Am J Psychiatry* 1995;**152**:814–5). Anticholinergics may adversely effect memory, exacerbate TD, and abrupt withdrawal can produce rebound EPS and cholinergic rebound. They are best prescribed only for overt symptoms and discontinued gradually after three months, reinstated only if symptoms reappear. If, however, they aid long-term compliance that may be a benefit that outweighs the risks.

6

Adjunctive therapies:

- **Diphenhydramine** 25–300 mg (oral or parenteral) may be effective within minutes and maintenance with 25–50 mg TDS has been widely used (n = 5, RCT, Granana *et al, Medicina [B Aires]* 1999;**59**:38–42).

- **Donepezil** may have some use in treating EPSE in the elderly (n = 7, open, Bergman *et al, J Clin Psychiatry* 2005;**66**:107–10).
- **Estrogen** at high plasma levels has been reported to reduce hyperkinetic symptoms of EPSE in women with psychosis (n = 25, RCT, Thompson *et al, Acta Psychiatr Scand* 2000;**101**:130–4).
- **Iron supplementation** may help EPSE if it is associated with iron-deficient anaemia (n = 1, Yoshida *et al, Nihon Shinkei Seishin Yakurigaku Zasshi* 2004;**24**:29–31).
- **Kava special extract** WS1490 has been claimed to be effective (n = 42, open, Boerner and Klement, *Wien Med Wochenschr* 2004; **154**:508–10).
- **Zolpidem** 5mg QDS has been used for persistent and refractory EPSE (n = 1, Farver and Khan, *Ann Pharmacother* 2001; **35**:435–7).

Less use:
Some drugs that have been tried but failed include:

- **Amantadine** is not recommended for EPSE but may be effective (d/b, c/o, Silver *et al, J Clin Psychiatry* 1995;**56**;167–70) and better tolerated than anticholinergics (review by Mamo *et al, Drug Saf* 1999; **20**:269–75).
- **Calcium** orally.
- **Mianserin** is ineffective (Korsgaard and Friis, *Psychopharmacol [Berl]* 1986;**88**:109–11).
- **Quinine**.

EPSE, dystonia (including oculogyric crisis)

Dystonia is a syndrome of sustained or slow involuntary muscular contractions, resulting in twisting of the neck, limbs, trunk or face. Acute dystonia from antipsychotics is more likely to occur in younger and more severely ill people, especially if antipsychotic-naïve. It can present as an oculogyric crisis (review by Abe, *World J Biol Psychiatry* 2006;**7**:70–4).
Review: general (Balash and Giladi, *Eur J Neurol* 2004;**11**:361–70).

Antidepressants	**Switching drugs** is the main strategy.
	Epinephrine 0.3mg has been used for escitalopram-induced oculogyric dystonia (n = 1, Patel and Simon, *Int Arch Allergy Immunol* 2006;**140**:27–9).
	Mianserin has been used at low dose for fluoxetine-induced dystonia (Poyurovsky *et al, Mov Disord* 1997;**12**:1102–5).
Antipsychotics	***Acute dystonia:***

Acute dystonia:
- **Anticholinergics** are usually effective for acute dystonias (e.g. laryngeal dystonia: Christodoulou and Kalaitzi, *J Psychopharmacol* 2005;**19**:307–11) and **procyclidine** is the standard UK treatment.
- **Diphenhydramine** (oral or parenteral) can be used and has been reported to produce rapid reversal of dystonic reactions, e.g. oculogyric crisis (Leigh *et al, Ann Neurol* 1987;**22**:3–17).

Tardive dystonia:
Switching antipsychotic is the first choice strategy:
- **Clozapine** may improve severe and persistent (e.g. Sieche and Giedke, *J Clin Psychiatry* 2000;**61**:949).
- **Olanzapine** may have some role (n = 4, s/b, Lucetti *et al, Clin Neuropharmacol* 2002;**25**:71–4).
- **Quetiapine** has been used if the dystonia is induced by risperidone, olanzapine (n = 2, Gourzis *et al, Clin Neuropharmacol* 2005;**28**:195–6) or amisulpride (n = 1, Fountoulakis *et al, Schizophr Res* 2006;**88**:232–4).

Others:
In resistant cases, other strategies may be worth trying:

- **Benzodiazepines** — a multiple drug-resistant disabling dystonia responded partly to clozapine and virtually completely when clonazepam was added (n = 1, Shapleske *et al*, *Br J Psychiatry* 1996;**168**:516–8).
- **Botulinum toxin** may possibly relieve the pain and symptoms of dystonia (n = 34, open, Tarsy *et al*, *Clin Neuropharmacol* 1997;**20**:90–3).
- **Levodopa** combined with an anticholinergic has been used (n = 1, Looper and Chouinard, *Can J Psychiatry* 1998;**43**:646–7).
- **Levetiracetam** has helped generalised dystonia (n = 1, 20/52, Sullivan *et al*, *Parkinsonism Relat Disord* 2005;**11**:469–71).
- **Tetrabenazine** has been used for olanzapine-induced tardive dystonia (n = 1, Rauchverger *et al*, *J Neuropsychiatry Clin Neurosci* 2007;**19**:484–5).

  Less useful:
- **Anticholinergics** are less effective in tardive dystonia (e.g. n = 32, Wojcik *et al*, *Am J Psychiatry* 1991;**148**:1055–9).
- **Carbamazepine** is ineffective (*Psychopharmacol Bull* 1985;**21**;345–6). Other drugs tried include baclofen and bromocriptine.

Laryngospasm (see also dystonia)

Benzodiazepines	**Flumazenil** may be effective in 25 minutes if laryngospasm is midazolam-induced (n = 1, Davis *et al*, *Ann Emerg Med* 1998;**32**:263–5).

Myoclonus

Myoclonus presents as shock-like, involuntary movements. It can also be caused by CNS infections, systemic metabolic disorders or neurodegenerative disorders. General management includes:

- It can be a symptom of serotonin syndrome and akathisia, so exclude these first.
- **Discontinuation, switching** or **dose reduction** usually resolves myoclonus.
- **Discontinue** any other causative drugs, e.g. levodopa, tricyclics, lamotrigine (n = 1, Rosenhagen *et al*, *J Clin Psychopharmacol* 2006;**26**:346–7) and bismuth salts (including OTC products).

Review: Jimenez-Jimenez, *CNS Drugs* 2004;**18**:93–104.

Other strategies:

Antidepressants	**Valproate**, if sertraline-induced (n = 1, Ghaziuddin *et al*, *J Child Adolesc Psychopharmacol* 2001;**11**:199–202).
Antipsychotics	**Carbamazepine**, if clozapine-induced, but beware of the potential interaction (n = 5, Bak *et al*, *J Clin Psychiatry* 1995;**56**:418–22).
	Haloperidol may be an alternative if olanzapine-induced (n = 1, Camacho *et al*, *Clin Neuropharmacol* 2005;**28**:145–7).
	Valproate, if clozapine-induced (n = 1, Meltzer and Ranjan, *Am J Psychiatry* 1994;**151**:1246–7).

Pisa syndrome (antipsychotic-induced pleurothonus)

Persistent dystonia of the trunk is a rare ADR from long-term antipsychotics.

Review: Suzuki and Matsuzaka, *CNS Drugs* 2002;**16**:165–74.

Antipsychotics	**Switching** to olanzapine has worked if risperidone-induced (n = 1, Nishimura *et al*, *J Neuropsychiatry Clin Neurosci* 2007;**19**:202–3).
	Switching to clozapine has worked if olanzapine-induced, with psychotic symptoms improved and Pisa syndrome declined over six weeks (n = 1, Arora *et al*, *Ann Pharmacother* 2006;**40**:2273–5).
	Anticholinergics help about 40% (n = 1, Bhattacharya *et al*, *Mov Disord* 2000;**15**:1285–7; Suzuki *et al*, *J Clin Psychopharmacol* 1999;**19**:277–80).
Galantamine	**Memantine** has been used as an alternative (Chen *et al*, *Int J Geriatr Psychiatry* 2008;**23**:660–1).

Restless legs (may also be akathisia)

Antidepressants *	Although there are anecdotal reports, there is no clear association between antidepressants and restless legs (n = 200, Brown *et al*, *Sleep Med*

6

2005;**6**:443–50).

* Re-exposure may be possible without recurrence with **mirtazapine** (n = 1, Pae et al, Psychiatr Clin Neurosci 2004;**58**:669–70), or has resolved when switched to bupropion (n = 1, Park et al, Psychiatry Investig 2009;**6**:313–5).
Exclude other drugs, e.g. D2 receptor antagonists such as domperidone (n = 1, Chang et al, Prog Neuropsychopharmacol Biol Psychiatry 2006;**30**:316–8), tramadol and dopamine-blockers, plus possibly antihistamines and non-opioid analgesics (n = 14, Kim et al, Hum Psychopharmacol 2008;**23**:615–20).
Bupropion may be a therapy in its own right (n = 3, Kim et al, Clin Neuropharmacol 2005;**28**:298–301).

Antipsychotics	* **Switch** — olanzapine-induced may resolve if switched to risperidone, quetiapine or aripiprazole (n = 3, Aggarwal et al, Curr Drug Saf 2010;**5**:129–31). **Benzodiazepines**, e.g. clonazepam have been used (n = 1, Horiguchi et al, Int Clin Psychopharmacol 1999;**14**:33–6). **Ropinirole** — has been used if caused by olanzapine (n = 5, Kang et al, J Psychopharmacol 2009;**23**:597–601) or quetiapine (n = 2, Urbano and Ware, J Clin Psychopharmacol 2008;**28**:704–5).
Carbamazepine*	Vitamin D deficiency can be a cause (n = 1, Prakash et al, Gen Hosp Psychiatry 2010;**32**:228).

Tremor (see EPSE, Parkinsonism and under 'others')

6.8 Neuroleptic malignant syndrome (NMS)

NMS is a rare and potentially fatal idiosyncratic dose-independent ADR resulting in a sudden loss in control of body temperature. The main symptoms are hyperthermia or fever and severe muscle rigidity, with two or more of: diaphoresis, dysphagia, tremor, incontinence, altered consciousness, tachycardia, altered blood pressure, leucocytosis and raised creatinine phosphokinase concentration. Body temperature rises rapidly and can be fatal in 1–3 days, although death rates are reducing due to increased awareness, early intervention, and the use of newer antipsychotics. It is probably caused by a sudden over-blockade of dopaminergic function, disrupting the thermoregulatory centre.

Risk factors include:

* **History** (previous NMS, known cerebral compromise, previous ECT).
* **Mental state** (agitation, overactive and/or in need of restraint or seclusion, catatonia, affective disorder [Berardi et al, Hum Psychopharmacol 2002;**17**:99–102], mental retardation).
* **Physical state** (dehydration, postpartum, Parkinson's disease, young and male, high serum creatinine phosphokinase [n = 32, Hermesh et al, J Clin Psychopharmacol 2002;**22**:252–6]).
* **Drugs** (see Chapter 5.9, e.g. high potency antipsychotics, IM therapy, high doses over short periods, abrupt or recent changes, rapid neuroleptisation, and concurrent MAOIs and carbamazepine).
* **Genetic** vulnerability (n = 2 siblings, Ziegenbein et al, Ann Pharmacother 2006;**40**:574–5).
* **Catatonia**, also a prodromal state (n = 17, White and Robins, CNS Spectr 2000;**5**:58–65).

Neuroleptic rechallenge:

Rechallenge with antipsychotics may show a high rate of recurrence, although most people may be able to tolerate antipsychotics again if monitored carefully and a two-week recovery period is allowed (n = 15, Rosebush et al, J Clin Psychiatry 1989;**50**:295–8). Rechallenge with clozapine has been successful (Weller and Kornhuber, Br J Psychiatry 1992;**161**:855–6). Depots are contraindicated.

Reviews: risk factors (Gupta et al, Int J Psychiatry 2003;**45**:30–5; n = 15, controls n = 45, Viejo et al, Acta Psychiatr Scand 2003;**107**:45–9), general (Strawn et al, Am J Psychiatry 2007;**164**:870–6).

Antipsychotics	**Immediate management** is essential. **Withdraw** any antipsychotics, lithium and antidepressants. **Correct** any dehydration and hyperpyrexia, e.g. using ice packs, re-hydration, and sedation with benzodiazepines if necessary.

Measure WCC, U&E, LFT and CPK to assess diagnosis, cause and response.
Manage acute symptoms, initially using a first-line agent below:

First line strategies:

- **Dantrolene** IV (a skeletal muscle relaxant used for malignant hyperthermia) is usually the treatment of choice. It reduces the duration and mortality of NMS (n = 9, Nisijima and Ishiguro, *Biol Psychiatry* 1993;**33**:45–8) and reduces body temperature in 2–24 hours, although it might prolong the course compared to supportive therapy (Rosebush *et al*, *Br J Psychiatry* 1991;**148**:709–12).
- **Bromocriptine** 7.5–60 mg/d reduces the duration and mortality of NMS (Sakkas *et al*, *Psychopharmacol Bull* 1991;**27**:381–4). There are some views that it might sometimes prolong the course of symptoms compared to supportive therapy (Rosebush *et al*, *Br J Psychiatry* 1991;**148**:709–12).
- **Amantadine** 100 mg BD may be the third-line choice (mentioned by Waldorf, *AANA J* 2003;**71**:389–94).

Other strategies:

- **Anaesthetics** have been used for emergency treatment in a person recovering from NMS (Parke and Wheatley, *Anesthesia* 1992;**47**:908–9).
- **Anticoagulants** used to provide complete anticoagulation have been suggested as adjunctive therapy to reduce death as a result of pulmonary embolism (van Harten and van Agtmael, *Am J Psychiatry* 1995;**152**:1103).
- **Apomorphine** s/c 2 mg three-hourly for three days then 2 mg QD for two days can improve NMS significantly (n = 1, Lattanzi *et al*, *Am J Psychiatry* 2006;**163**:1450–1), and as rapidly as monotherapy (e.g. n = 1, Gambassi *et al*, *Aging Clin Exp Res* 2006;**18**:266–70).
- * **Benzodiazepines** (e.g. high-dose lorazepam and diazepam; n = 1, Tsai and Huang, *Chang Gung Med J* 2010;**33**:576–80) can be used if dantrolene and bromocriptine have failed. Predominantly, catatonic symptoms may rapidly respond to diazepam, including via continuous IV administration (Miyaoka *et al*, *Am J Psychiatry* 1997;**153**:882), although its longer half-life may complicate recovery (Velamoor, *Br J Psychiatry* 1992;**160**:135–6).
- **ECT** has been used for low-dose quetiapine-induced NMS (n = 1, Bora *et al*, *Eur Psychiatry* 2003;**18**:323).
- **Levodopa** IV may be an effective alternative to dantrolene (Nisijima *et al*, *Biol Psychiatry* 1997;**41**:913–4), as may carbidopa/levodopa (Shoop and Cernek, *Ann Pharmacother* 1997;**31**:119).
- **Nifedipine** 25 mg s/l has been used (Talley and Taylor, *Psychosomatics* 1994;**35**:168–70).

Aftercare:

1. Review NMS symptoms to confirm diagnosis.
2. Review psychiatric diagnosis and the need for further antipsychotics.
3. Consider alternative management strategies.
4. Leave as long a gap as possible before restarting antipsychotics (e.g. 14 days), considering also the risks of untreated psychosis.
5. Choose an antipsychotic from a different group to the causative agent, particularly of low potency or any previously used without problem. Start low and go slow. Contraindicate depots.
6. Perform alternate day CPK monitoring, interpreted in the context of the global clinical picture.
7. Perform daily temperature, pulse and muscle tone measures, weekly wbcs and ensure adequate hydration and nutrition.

6

8. Obtain an informal or formal second opinion, as informed consent for re-exposure may not be possible. Inform family and carers of the decisions and risks (and document this).
9. Educate patients, carers and care team of the symptoms of early NMS and of the appropriate action to take, i.e. seek urgent medical advice.

Review: guidelines for the re-introduction of antipsychotics following NMS (Williams and MacPherson, *Irish J Psychiatr Med* 1997;**14**:147–8).

6.9 Serotonin syndrome

This potentially dangerous adverse reaction is attributed to a toxic hyperserotonergic state from hyper-stimulation of the brain stem and spinal chord 5HT1A and 5HT2 receptors. Onset is usually within a few hours of drug or dose changes, usually resolves in about 24 hours and can be fatal.

Sternbach's diagnostic criteria

1. At least three of the following: mental state changes (e.g. confusion), agitation/restlessness, sweating, diarrhoea, fever, hyperreflexia, tachycardia, myoclonus, lack of co-ordination, shivering, and tremor. Other symptoms can include nausea, vomiting, tachycardia, myoclonus, hypertension, convulsions and multiple organ failure.
2. Other causes ruled out, e.g. infection, metabolic disturbances, substance abuse or withdrawal.
3. No concurrent antipsychotic dose changes.

The Hunter Serotonin Toxicity Criteria (Dunkley *et al*, *QJM* 2003;**96**:635–42) may be more specific and an alternative to Sternbach's criteria.

Reviews: general (Isbister *et al*, *Med J Aust* 2007;**187**:361–5; Boyer and Shannon, *N Engl J Med* 2005;**352**:1112–20; Gillman, *Biol Psychiatry* 2006;**59**:1046–51), Serotonin Syndrome Rating Scale to aid diagnosis (Hegerl *et al*, *Eur Arch Psych Clin Neurosci* 1998;**248**:96–103).

All drugs	**Discontinue** all serotonergic drugs (see *Chapter 5.13*), including over-the-counter sympathomimetics (usually adequate management in mild cases).

Symptomatic support, e.g. cooling blankets and fans.

Benzodiazepines, e.g. lorazepam (1–2 mg by slow IV injection every 30 minutes until excessive sedation occurs) may be superior to clonazepam, which has a lower affinity for peripheral benzodiazepine receptors (e.g. Nierenberg and Semprebon, *Clin Pharmacol Ther* 1993;**53**:84–8).

Chlorpromazine has been used for its sedative effect (n = 1, Graham, *Med J Aust* 1997;**166**:166–7).

Cyproheptadine (a non-specific 5-HT blocker) at 4–8 mg orally (but perhaps as high as 10–20 mg), repeated every 2–4 hours up to 0.5 mg kg/d maximum (beware of urinary retention) has been claimed to be the best antiserotonergic drug strategy, with case reports of rapid success (n = 3, McDaniel, *Ann Pharmacother* 2001;**35**:870–3; Baigel, *Eur J Anaesthiol* 2003;**20**:586–8; n=2, Levin *et al*, *Gen Hosp Psychiatry* 2008;**30**:372–7).

* **Lipids** (20% lipid emulsion IV bolus) have been used for venlafaxine, lamotrigine and diazepam OD (n=1, *Minerva Anestesiol* 2011;**77**:93–5).

Mirtazapine blocks 5-HT2 and 5-HT3 receptors and may reduce serotonergic toxicity (Hoes, *Pharmacopsychiatry* 1996;**29**:81).

Nitroglycerin (2 mg/kg/min) has been reported to be rapidly successful in severe SS (e.g. n = 1, Brown and Skop, *Ann Pharmacother* 1996;**30**:191; n = 1, Brown, *Am J Emerg Med* 2004;**22**:510).

Propranolol (1–3 mg every five minutes, up to 0.1 mg/kg) may be useful, as it blocks 5-HT1A and 5-HT2 receptors (Guze and Baxter, *J Clin Psychopharmacol* 1986;**6**:119–20).

General
The main stages of sexual activity that can be affected by psychotropics (as well as, of course, the conditions they may be treating) are libido, arousal/lubrication, erectile issues and orgasmic disorders. Many studies do not differentiate between these stages and refer to generic 'sexual dysfunction'. This section includes general advice and then stage-specific strategies to improve sexual problems.
Review: female sexual dysfunction (Clayton, *J Clin Psychiatry* 2006;**67**:991–2).

General sexual dysfunction

Anticonvulsants	**Switching drugs**:

- **Lamotrigine** improves sexual function, testosterone levels and gonadal efficiency compared to carbamazepine and phenytoin (n = 85, Herzog *et al*, *Neurology* 2005;**65**:1016–20). It improves most measures of sexual function, especially in women, including people both starting on lamotrigine as a first anticonvulsant (n = 79) and those switching (n = 62) on to it (n = 141, open, 8/12, Gil-Nagel *et al*, *Seizure* 2006;**15**:142–9).
- **Levetiracetam** has no apparent adverse sexual or endocrine effects in men or women (n = 136, p/c, Svalheim *et al*, *Epilepsy Behav* 2009;**16**:281–7).
- **Oxcarbazepine** — in 228 males with epilepsy and pre-existing sexual dysfunction, 79% improved when switched to oxcarbazepine with the effect more marked if they had previously been on an enzyme-inducing AED (n=673, 12/52, Luef *et al*, *Acta Neurol Scand* 2009;**119**:94–9). Carbamazepine significantly reduces testosterone and androgen levels in men and women, which adversely effects sexual function (n = 160, RCT, d/b, 12/12, Lossius *et al*, *Epilepsia* 2007;**48**:1875–82), so don't switch to it.

Exogenous testosterone and **aromatase inhibitors** (to reduce testosterone's metabolism) have been tried for male sexual dysfunction.
Review: general (Montouris *et al*, *Epilepsy Behav* 2005;**7** Suppl 2:S7–14).

Antidepressants *	**General interventions** include behavioural strategies, psychotherapy,

delaying drug intake until after sexual activity, reduction in dosage, drug holidays, adjuvants and switching. Sexual side-effects from SSRIs do not seem to abate with time (n = 119, Landén *et al*, *J Clin Psychiatry* 2005;**66**:100–6), but untreated depression has a greater impact on global sexual functioning than actual antidepressant ADRs (e.g. n=70, RCT, d/b, 8/52, Lanza di Scalea *et al*, *J Clin Psychiatry* 2009;**70**:423–8; with duloxetine, n = 288, d/b, p/c, 52/52, Montejo *et al*, *J Sex Med* 2011;**8**:773–82).
Switch drugs:
Switching antidepressants is often the main strategy. The adverse effect in decreasing order of impact is sertraline, venlafaxine, citalopram, paroxetine, fluoxetine, imipramine, phenelzine, duloxetine, escitalopram, and fluvoxamine, with no difference from placebo shown with agomelatine, amineptine, bupropion, moclobemide and mirtazapine (meta-analysis by Serretti and Chiesa, *J Clin Psychopharmacol* 2009;**29**:259–66).

- **Agomelatine** has minimal effect compared to paroxetine (n = 92 healthy males, RCT, p/c, d/b, 8/52, Montejo *et al*, *J Psychopharmacol* 2010;**24**:111–20) and venlafaxine (n = 276 [n = 193 sexually active; n = 111 remitted], d/b, 12/52, Kennedy *et al*, *J Clin Psychopharmacol* 2008;**28**:329–33).
- ***Bupropion** has placebo-level sexual ADRs (s = 7, n = 1463, RCT, d/b, Thase *et al*, *J Clin Psychiatry* 2005;**66**:974–81), and has helped on all

6

domains of sexual dysfunction from SSRIs in men using three different scales (n = 234, RCT, d/b, p/c, 12/52, Safarinejad, *BJU Int* 2010;**106**:832–9).

- **Escitalopram** has been claimed to have less sexual ADRs than similar antidepressants (Ashton *et al, J Sex Marital Ther* 2005;**31**:257–62).
- **Mirtazapine** has lower sexual ADRs than other antidepressants, apart from the potentially counter-productive sedation (e.g. n = 78, open, 6/12, Saiz-Ruiz *et al, Hum Psychopharmacol* 2005;**20**:435–40).
- **Moclobemide** may have lower sexual ADRs (n = 5, open, Ramasubbu, *J Psychiatr Neurosci* 1999;**224**:45–50).
- **Pregabalin** has reversed citalopram-induced sexual dysfunction within 3/7 in GAD in males suffering from poor libido, arousal and orgasmic satisfaction (n = 2, Oulis *et al, J Clin Psychopharmacol* 2008;**28**:362–3).
- **Reboxetine** lacks serotonin-related sexual ADRs (n = 450, RCT, d/b, 8/52, Clayton *et al, Int Clin Psychopharmacol* 2003;**18**:151–6; 6% incidence *vs* 39% with citalopram in women; n = 357, RCT, d/b, 24/52, Langworth *et al, J Clin Psychopharmacol* 2006;**26**:121–7).

Adjunctive therapies:

- **Ephedrine** 50mg was shown to be effective for SSRI-induced sexual dysfunction but, then again, so was placebo (n = 19 women, RCT, p/c, c/o, 8/52, Meston, *J Sex Marital Ther* 2004;**30**:57–68).
- **Gingko biloba** has produced some spectacular individual responses but nothing statistically significant different (n = 24 [c = 11], RCT, t/b, p/c, 12/52, Wheatley, *Hum Psychopharmacol* 2004;**19**:545–8).
- **Ropinirole** up to 2–4mg/d was effective in 54% (n = 13 [3F, 10M], open, 4/52, Worthington *et al, Int Clin Psychopharmacol* 2002; **17**:307–10).
- **Sildenafil** 50–100mg may help all domains of sexual function in women (n = 49, RCT, d/b, p/c, 8/52, Nurnberg *et al, JAMA* 2008;**300**:395–404).
- **Trazodone**, a 5HT2A antagonist, may help as an adjunct in SSRI-induced sexual dysfunction in all four domains (n = 20 [c = 15], Stryjer *et al, Clin Neuropharmacol* 2009;**32**:82–4).

No efficacy:

- **Granisetron** does not help (n = 12, RCT, d/b, p/c, 14/7, Jespersen *et al, Int Clin Psychopharmacol* 2004;**19**:161–4).
- **Methylphenidate** OROS was ineffective in improving antidepressant-induced sexual dysfunction but at least it did not exacerbate the problem (Pae *et al, Clin Neuropharmacol* 2009;**32**:85–8).

Reviews: antidepressant-induced sexual dysfunction (Taylor, *Curr Psychiatry Rep* 2006;**8**:431–6; Rudkin *et al, Cochrane Database Syst Rev* 2004;**4**:CD003382; Tayor *et al, J Affect Disord* 2005;**88**:241–54; Balon and Segraves, *J Sex Marital Ther* 2008;**34**:353–65), sexual ADRs of newer antidepressants (Schweitzer *et al, Aust N Z J Psychiatry* 2009;**43**:795–808).

Antipsychotics *   Sexual dysfunction occurs at higher rates in schizophrenia (86–96%) than in the general population (n = 179, MacDonald *et al, Br J Psychiatry* 2003;**182**:50–6) and is high with antipsychotics, especially in men (n = 243, Montejo *et al, J Sex Med* 2010;**7**:3404–13), with only 37% spontaneously reporting it. Sexual dysfunction may occur in 45% people on typicals, with hyperprolactinaemia the predominant cause (n = 101, Smith *et al, Br J Psychiatry* 2002;**181**:49–55). However, raised prolactin may not necessarily be the only cause as in first episodes sexual dysfunction may occur despite normal prolactin levels (n = 74, open, van Bruggen *et al, Psychoneuroendocrinology* 2009;**34**:989–95).

General principles:

Normalise prolactin, e.g. by switching to a prolactin-sparing antipsychotic such as olanzapine or quetiapine (cf risperidone and fluphenazine; n = 27, RCT, d/b, Kelly and Conley, *Psychoneuroendocrinology* 2006;**31**:340–6).

Aripiprazole has helped either as an alternative (45%) or adjunct (55%) to another antipsychotic, with prolactin significantly reduced, improvement in libido, and reduced erectile, ejaculation and menstrual dysfunction, established from 12/52 and maintained for 6/12 (n = 27 [c = 22], 26/52, open, Mir *et al, J Psychopharmacol* 2008;**22**:244–53; see also (n = 555, RCT, open, 26/52, Hanssens *et al, BMC Psychiatry* 2008;**8**:95). However, **olanzapine** might be suitable in the short-term, prolactin levels may be little different to haloperidol at 9/12 (n = 63, RCT, 9/12, Costa *et al, J Psychopharmacol* 2007;**21**:165–70).

Reviews: in men (Khawaja, *J Ayub Med Coll Abbottabad* 2005;**17**:73–5) and in women (Smith, *J Clin Psychopharmacol* 2003;**23**[3 Suppl 1]:S27–32).

Libido (see also general advice section)

Libido and desire is controlled by the mesolimbic dopamine reward pathway and facilitated by NA and 5-HT. Testosterone is essential for male and estrogen and progesterone for female sexual behaviour. It is unclear to what extent psychotropics effect libido specifically.

Antidepressants	**Switch drugs** to, e.g. **moclobemide** (n = 5, open, Ramasubbu, *J Psychiatr Neurosci* 1999;**224**:45–50), **bupropion** or **mirtazapine**.
Antipsychotics	**Raised prolactin** may be the predominant cause, so check and, if raised, see the hyperprolactinaemia section for options, as bromocriptine may be of use (review, Zeitlin and Rajfer, *Rev Urol* 2000;**2**:39–42).

Arousal (lubrication and erection) — (see also general advice section)

Arousal mechanisms involve acetylcholine (facilitates erection/lubrication), adrenergic fibres (cause detumescence), cAMP (smooth muscle relaxation), dopamine (stimulates sexual arousal in females), and nitric oxide (activates the production of cGMP).

Review: options for oral pharmacotherapy in ED (Vitezic and Pelcic, *Int J Clin Pharmacol Ther* 2002; **40**;393–403).

Antidepressants	**Switching drugs** is the main strategy, e.g. to:

- **Bupropion** (n = 18 ethnic minority women, open, 10/52, Dobkin *et al, J Clin Psychopharmacol* 2006;**26**:21–6).
- **Moclobemide** (n = 5, open, Ramasubbu, *J Psychiatr Neurosci* 1999;**224**: 45–50).
- **Mirtazapine**.

Adjunctive therapies:

- **PDE-5 inhibitors**, e.g. sildenafil are effective for drug-induced erectile dysfunction (s = 15, n = 904, Taylor *et al, J Affect Disord* 2005;**88**:241–54), including men with ED at the time of diagnosis of MDD that then persists, despite the resolution of the depressive symptoms (RCT, 12/52, Tignol *et al, Int Clin Psychopharmacol* 2004;**19**:191–9).
- **Yohimbine** given 1–2 hours pre-intercourse has been shown to improve antidepressant-induced ED (review by Labbate *et al, J Clin Psychiatry* 2003; **64**[Suppl 10]:11–9).

Antipsychotics	**Switching drugs** is the main strategy, e.g. to:

- **Olanzapine**, if haloperidol-induced (n = 570, Bitter *et al, Int Clin Psychopharmacol* 2005;**20**:19–21; part of SOHO study).
- **Quetiapine** (n = 28) may improve erectile function and lubrication compared to other antipsychotics (n = 86, 6/12, open, Montejo-Gonzalez *et al, J Clin Psychopharmacol* 2005;**25**:533–8).

Adjunctive therapies:

6

- **Amantadine** 100 mg/d may help (n = 6, open, 6/52, Valevski *et al, Clin Neuropharmacol* 1998;**21**:355–7).
- **PDE-5 inhibitors**, e.g. sildenafil can be effective if ED is induced by olanzapine (n = 10, 4/52, Atmaca *et al, Int J Impot Res* 2002;**14**:547–9) or risperidone (n = 32 [c = 31], RCT, d/b, p/c, c/o, Gopalakrishnan *et al, Am J Psychiatry* 2006;**163**:494–9). Cochrane concludes that sildenafil may be useful but the data is very limited (Berner *et al, Cochrane Database Syst Rev* 2007;**1**:CD003546). Vardenafil 10 mg is also well-tolerated and effective for ED in chronic schizophrenia, and independent of ED severity or prolactin levels (n = 25 [c = 21], open, 12/52, Mitsonis *et al, J Clin Psychiatry* 2008;**69**:206–12).

Carbamazepine	**Oxcarbazepine**, switch to (n = 4, Sachdeo and Sathyan, *Curr Med Res Opin* 2005;**21**:1065–8).

Anorgasmia (see also general advice section)

Noradrenaline exerts an excitatory or facilitatory action on orgasm. Serotonin 5HT2A receptor agonism is inhibitory on orgasm.

Antidepressants	Anorgasmia from antidepressants is a common phenomenon. A minor effect can be advantageous in some men (by delaying ejaculation), but almost invariably considered disadvantageous in women.

Dose adjustment:

- reduce dose
- omit selected doses (e.g. at weekends)
- use a single daily dose, e.g. one taken at night will give trough levels the next evening, useful if that is when sexual activity occurs
- partial drug holiday i.e. missing specific days (although as David Baldwin once said, you'd need a sabbatical for fluoxetine, due to its long half-life).

Wait for spontaneous resolution (occurs in less than a third).

Withdraw drug — anorgasmia is rapidly reversible on drug withdrawal.

Switch drugs:

Switching drugs may often be the main choice, but frequently a major problem if the patient has responded to the causative agent:

- **Bupropion** (probably fairly useful as it has a low serotoninergic effect) SR may be successful for escitalopram-induced anorgasmia (s = 2, n = 830, RCT, d/b, p/c, 8/52, Clayton *et al, J Clin Psychiatry* 2006;**67**:736–46).
- **Duloxetine** is alleged to have a lower anorgasmic effect (s = 4, n = 1466, RCT, d/b, p/c, Delgado *et al, J Clin Psychiatry* 2005;**66**:686–92).
- **Escitalopram** may be better than paroxetine (Bielski *et al, Ann Clin Psychiatry* 2005;**17**:65–9).
- **Mirtazapine** has placebo-level effects on orgasmic capacity. This is probably because although it increases serotonin, it blocks serotonin's anorgasmic effect on 5HT2A receptors.
- **Trazodone** 50–200 mg/d may help men with psychogenic ED, if the person can stay awake long enough (s = 6, n = 396 men, RCTs, > 1/52, Fink *et al, BJU Int* 2003;**92**:441–6).
- **Venlafaxine** 75 mg daily had no effect on premature ejaculation and therefore might be better than an SSRI at not causing it (n = 31, p/c, s/b, c/o, Kilic *et al, Int J Androl* 2005;**28**:47–52).

Adjunctive therapies:

Many adjunctive therapies have been tried and may work for some individuals. These are purely in alphabetical order as there is no robust way of assessing their relative efficacies:

- **Bethanechol** taken 1–2 hours before intercourse has been claimed to relieve tricyclic-induced anorgasmia, but may only occasionally be successful.
- **Bupropion** was effective in 46% of women and 75% of men, most improvement occurring in the first two weeks (open, n = 24, 7/52, Gitlin *et al*, *J Sex Marital Ther* 2002;**28**:131–8), but an RCT failed to show an effect in SSRI-induced anorgasmia (n = 30, RCT, p/c, Masand *et al*, *Am J Psychiatry* 2001;**158**:805–7).
- **Buspirone** 20–60 mg/d has improved 58% people with SSRI-induced sexual problems (cf. 30% on placebo; n = 117, p/c, > 4/52, Landen *et al*, *J Clin Psychopharmacol* 1999;**19**: 268–71).
- **Cyproheptadine** 2–4 mg 30–60 minutes before sex (provided one can then stay awake) may help if SSRI-induced, although relapse of depression has been reported (see *4.3.2.2*). 4 mg (but not 2 mg) the day before intercourse has been used for anorgasmia induced by citalopram (being referred to by the male patient as 'the catapult pills' Lauerma, *Acta Psychiatr Scand* 1996;**93**:69–70).
- **Dronabinol**, a synthetic cannabinol, one hour before sex has increased libido, arousal, lubrication, orgasm and overall quality, but beware of people wandering around with a grin on their faces in case they get tested for illicit drug use (n = 1, Salerian, *J Clin Psychiatry* 2004;**665**:1146–7).
- **Loratadine** 15 mg/d may rapidly reverse SSRI-induced anorgasmia in men and women (n = 10, case series, Brubaker, *J Clin Psychiatry* 2002;**63**:534).
- **Methylphenidate** (Roeloffs *et al*, *J Clin Psychiatry* 1996;**57**:548) and dextroamfetamine (15–20 mg/d) have been used successfully for SSRI-induced anorgasmia (n = 5, Bartlik, *J Sex Marital Ther* 1995;**21**:264–71).
- **Mianserin** 7.5–15 mg/d as add-on for SSRI-induced 'sexual dysfunction' may be successful in 65% within 1–2 weeks, with no adverse effects (n = 17, open, 3/12, Dolberg *et al*, *Psychopharmacol* [Berl] 2002;**161**:404–7), although the only RCT showed no significant difference in women (n = 75, RCT, d/b, p/c, 4/52, Michelson *et al*, *J Psychiatr Res* 2002;**36**:147–52).
- **Mirtazapine** improved function in premenopausal females with SSRI-induced sexual side-effects (n = 148, RCT, p/c, 6/52, Michelson *et al*, *J Psychiatr Res* 2002;**36**:147–52). Stimulation of the 5HT2A receptor inhibits orgasm, but mirtazapine blocks 5HT2A receptors, reversing the anorgasmic effect, and this may happen at relatively low doses, e.g. 7.5–15 mg/d.
- **PDE-5** inhibitors such as **sildenafil** 50–100 mg, taken 30–60 minutes pre-sex, may help SSRI-induced anorgasmia in men (n = 90, RCT, p/c, 6/52, Nurnberg *et al*, *JAMA* 2003;**289**:56–64) and in women (n = 98 [c = 89], RCT, d/b, p/c, 8/52, Nurnberg *et al*, *JAMA* 2008;**300**:395–404), but high doses may be needed (50–200 mg/d) to overcome the problem (n = 21, open Seidman *et al*, *J Clin Psychiatry* 2003;**64**:721–5).
- **Yohimbine** 5.4–10.8 mg has been used if SSRI-induced, although it was no better than placebo in the main RCT (n = 148, RCT, p/c, 6/52, Michelson *et al*, *J Psychiatr Res* 2002;**36**:147–52). Yohimbine can cause insomnia, so rolling over and going to sleep afterwards may be trickier.

Less useful:

- **Amantadine** 200–300 mg/d was ineffective in the main study (n = 57, RCT, p/c, 8/52, Michelson *et al*, *Am J Psychiatry* 2000;**157**:239–43), but there are cases of successful use in SSRI-induced anorgasmia (n = 596, Keller Ashton *et al*, *J Sex Marital Ther* 1997;**23**:165–75).

6

- **Ginkgo biloba** has failed to show any significant reversal of SSRI-induced sexual dysfunction (n = 37, RCT, p/c, 2/12, Kang *et al, Hum Psychopharmacol* 2002;**17**:279–84).
- **Granisitron** (5-HT3 antagonist) has been used to treat fluoxetine-induced anorgasmia, but 1–2 mg was ineffective in one study, although a significant placebo response was noted (n = 20, p/c, c/o, Nelson *et al, J Clin Psychiatry* 2001;**62**:469–73).

Antipsychotics

Switch drugs:
- **Quetiapine** has a lower incidence of problems than risperidone and fluphenazine (n = 27, RCT, d/b, Kelly and Conley, *Psychoneuroendocrinology* 2006;**31**:340–6).

Adjunctive therapies:
- **Amantadine** 100 mg/d did not help in one study (n = 6, open, 6/52, Valevski *et al, Clin Neuropharmacol* 1998;**21**:355–7).

Opiates

Buprenorphine probably has less sexual ADRs than methadone as buprenorphine causes less suppression of plasma testosterone (n = 105, Bliesener *et al, J Clin Endocrinol Metab* 2005;**90**:203–6).

Methadone produces a dose-dependent inhibition of orgasm (n = 92, Brown *et al, J Addict Disord* 2005;**24**:91–106), so dose reduction may help.

Anticonvulsants *

Reduce dose or discontinue as it may be dose-related for topiramate (n = 7, Sun *et al, Headache* 2006;**46**:1450–3) and oxcarbazepine (e.g. n = 1, Calabrò *et al, Epilepsy Behav* 2010;**17**:287–8; n = 1, Boora *et al, Prim Care Companion J Clin Psychiatry* 2009;**11**:173–4).

Ejaculation problems (see also general advice section)

All drugs

Discontinue or reduce dose, e.g. if tricyclic-induced. Retrograde ejaculation from risperidone 8 mg/d promptly responds to dose reduction (n = 1, Loh *et al, Int Clin Psychopharmacol* 2004;**19**:111–2). Discontinuation generally works for clozapine (n = 3, Talmon *et al, Harefuah* 1994;**126**:509–10). Trazodone ejaculatory inhibition resolves within 48 hours of discontinuing (n = 1, Kaufman *et al, J Sex Marital Ther* 2007;**33**:225–30).

Switch drugs, e.g. ED and inappropriate ejaculation with reboxetine resolved when switched to sertraline (n = 1, Sivrioglu *et al, Prog Neuropsychopharmacol Biol Psychiatry* 2007;**31**:548–50).

Tamsulosin has been used for reboxetine-induced painful ejaculation (n = 2, Demyttenaere and Huygens, *Eur Neuropsychopharmacol* 2002;**12**:337–41), and intermittent use may help with other causes (n = 405, Goktas *et al, J Urol* 2006;**175**:650–2).

Priapism

Early treatment (within 4–6 hours, before local hypoxemia) reduces morbidity, the need for invasive procedures and impotence, and may prevent or minimise long-term complications.

- Immediate short-term treatment includes conservative measures, e.g. pain control, vigorous hydration, and cold compress before urology consultation.
- Active treatments include cavernosal penile aspiration, irrigation, instillation of vasoactive agents, intracavernosal injection of phenylephrine (n = 1, Davol and Rukstalis, *Urology* 2005;**66**:880) and, if necessary, shunting procedures.

Terbutaline orally may be effective for about 40% (cf. 15% with placebo), so may be worth a try (n = 68, RCT, p/c, Priyadarshi, *Int J Impot Res* 2004;**16**:424–6; n = 75, RCT, p/c, Lowe and Jarow, *Urology* 1993;**42**:51–4).

Switching — if antipsychotic related, switch to one with a lower propensity to cause priapism (highest with chlorpromazine, and risperidone; see review by Compton and Miller, *J Clin Psychiatry* 2001;**62**:362–6).

Reviews: general (Wang *et al, Int Clin Psychopharmacol* 2006;**21**:245–8; Kalsi *et al, Hosp Med* 2002; **63**:224–5), antipsychotics (Sood *et al, Int Clin Psychopharmacol* 2008;**23**:9–17).

6.11 Others, side-effects

Gastric irritation (see also nausea)

Valproate — Take with or after food.

Slow-release or enteric-coated tablets may help.

Avoid fizzy drinks with the liquid or soluble tablets.

Glaucoma (see also glaucoma section in *Chapter 3*)

Topiramate — **Discontinuation** usually quickly leads to reversal (Anon, *Prescrire Int* 2003;**12**:61).

Methylprednisolone and mannitol may be rapidly effective if acute (n = 1, Rhee *et al, Am J Ophthalmol* 2006;**141**:1133–4).

Laser surgery or peripheral iridectomy may be longer-term options (n = 83, Fraunfelder *et al, Ophthalmology* 2004;**111**:109–11).

Hypersalivation (see also sialorhoea)

Lithium — **Propantheline** may give some symptomatic relief (n = 1, Donaldson, *Am J Psychiatry* 1982;**139**:1350–1).

Incontinence (see also noctural enuresis)

Clozapine — This may be due to alpha-adrenergic antagonism with an incidence of up to 44% (persistent in 25%) (n = 61, >3/12, Lin *et al, Acta Psychiatr Scand* 1999;**100**:158–61) and, in nearly all cases, usually resolves spontaneously within 3/12 (n = 16, Warner *et al, Int Clin Psychopharmacol* 1994;**9**:207–9).

Reducing fluid intake during the evening may help.

* **Aripiprazole** 10–15 mg/d as an adjunct may be useful (n = 2, Lee and Kim, *J Korean Med Sci* 2010;**25**:333–5) .

Alpha-adrenergic agonists; ephedrine was rapidly effective at 150 mg at night in 16 patients with the problem, with response maintained over 12/12 (n = 57, Fuller *et al, J Clin Psychiatry* 1996;**57**:514–8).

DDAVP® (Ferring)/**Desmopressin** intranasally has been used symptomatically (n = 1, English *et al, Ann Pharmacother* 2001;**35**:867–9).

Oxybutinin has been used (Lurie and Hosmer, *J Clin Psychiatry* 1997;**58**:404).

Tolterodine has been used, albeit unsuccessfully (n = 1, English *et al, Ann Pharmacother* 2001;**35**:867–9).

Review and case series: Warner *et al, Int Clin Psychopharmacol* 1994;**9**:207–9.

Jaundice (see also hepatotoxicity)

Valproate — Could be a sign of impending hepatic failure. Investigate immediately and discontinue if necessary.

Mastalgia (see also hyperprolactinaemia)

Venlafaxine — **Check prolactin** and take appropriate action.

Bromocriptine 5 mg/d has been used for mastalgia occurring in weeks 5–13 of therapy, with no recurrence on discontinuation (n = 1, Bhatia *et al, J Clin Psychopharmacol* 2000;**20**:590–1).

Megaloblastic anaemia

Anticonvulsants — Folic acid may be used if caused by, e.g. phenytoin or phenobarbital.

Oedema

Lithium — **Reduce dose**, as this common effect may be dose-related.

Diuretics may be useful but see *Chapter 4.4* for interactions.

Trazodone — **Reduction** in dose or **discontinuation** may be rapidly successful (n = 10, Barnett *et al, J Clin Psychopharmacol* 1985;**5**:161–4).

6

Valproate	**Discontinuation** — oedema can occur after long-term treatment (but can be after short-term use), can fluctuate and rapidly improve if valproate is stopped (n = 2, Lin et al, *Int J Neuropsychopharmacol* 2009;**12**:991–3).

Osteopenia (see also osteoporosis and hyperprolactinaemia)

Antipsychotics	**Correct** any raised prolactin abnormalities. **Standard therapies**, e.g. alendronic acid 5 mg/d has improved spine and hip T-scores by 7% and 9% respectively over a year (n = 1, Howes and Smith, *Am J Psychiatry* 2004;**161**:756).

Osteoporosis (see also osteopenia)

General	**Beer drinking** — I couldn't resist mentioning that quantitative bone ultrasound values for women (pre-, peri- and post-menopausal) are greater in beer drinkers (in moderation of course), compared to non-beer or non-wine drinkers, possibly due to the phytoestrogen content (n = 1697, Pedrera-Zamorano et al, *Nutrition* 2009;**25**:1057–63).

Pain at site of injection

Depots	**Warm baths** and regular exercise can help. **Change site** or systematically alternate injection sides. **Check injection technique**, as Z-tracking technique may not always be meticulously followed (Belanger-Annable, *Canadian Nurse* 1985;**81**:1–3).

Raised LFTs

Valproate	Raised LFTs are not uncommon but usually transient, so monitor LFTs (including prothrombin time) until they return to normal. **Discontinue** if the prothrombin time is abnormally prolonged. **Salicylates** (inc. OTC) may exacerbate so should be discontinued.

Sialorhoea (hypersalivation)

Clozapine	Hypersalivation with clozapine may be a lack of the swallowing reflex (rather than excess saliva production; n = 17, Rabinowitz et al, *Biol Psychiatry* 1996;**40**:1132–4), or due to clozapine's pharmacology, e.g. M4 activation or alpha-2 blockade, so hypersalivation may be an inaccurate term for this side-effect, albeit descriptive. **Review:** Cochrane concludes there is insufficient evidence for any treatment (s = 15, Syed et al, *Cochrane Database Syst Rev* 2008;**3**:CD005579; comment by Sockalingham and Remington, *EBMH* 2009;**12**:12). ***Physical strategies:*** • Propping pillows up at night helps a little in some people. • Reduce caffeine intake (n = 1, Odom-White and de Leon, *J Clin Psychiatry* 1996;**57**:175–6). ***Adjunctive therapies:*** Adjunctive therapies are usually the only realistic option for this unpleasant and common, but not life-threatening ADR. The following are probably in descending order of efficacy: • **Atropine** 1% eye drops, one drop given orally at bedtime may be rapidly effective (n = 3, Antonello and Tessier, *J Psychiatry Neurosci* 1999;**24**:250; Comley et al, *Aust N Z J Psychiatry* 2000;**34**:1033–4). • * **Glycopyrrolate** (glycopyrronium) was superior to biperiden and placebo, and had minimal effect on cognitive function, unlike biperiden (RCT, d/b, c/o, 3 × 4/52, Liang et al, *Schizophr Res* 2010;**119**:138–44). • **Hyoscine** hydrobromide 300 mcg sucked and swallowed up to TDS. Hyoscine is erratically absorbed and so the tablets should be sucked and swallowed to optimise efficacy. • * **Moclobemide** 150–300 mg/d showed a beneficial effect in 66% patients

(n = 53, 6/52, c/o, Kreinin et al, World J Biol Psychiatry 2011; in press).

- **Pirenzepine** (M1/M4 blocker) 25–100 mg/d is frequently used (e.g. n = 29, Schneider et al, Pharmacopsychiatry 2004;**37**:43–5).
- **Quetiapine**, through allowing reduced clozapine dosage.
- **Sulpiride** (150–300 mg/d) may have some efficacy (n = 18, open, 3/52, Kreinin et al, Isr J Psych Relat Sci 2005;**42**:61–3), as may amisulpride ('strong ameliorating effect'; n = 20, RCT, d/b, p/c, c/o, Kreinin et al, Int Clin Psychopharmacol 2006;**21**:99–103).
- **Tricyclics** (e.g. amitriptyline; Praharaj and Arora, Br J Clin Pharmacol 2006;**63**:128–9) can be useful, mainly for their anticholinergic effect.

Less use:

- * **Amisulpride** 150 mg/d has been used (e.g. n = 1, Praharaj et al, Am J Ther 2011;**18**:84–5), with a 74% improvement in one study (n = 53, 6/52, c/o, Kreinin et al, World J Biol Psychiatry 2011; in press).
- * **Anticholinergics** or antimuscarinics are generally ineffective, although trihexyphenidyl 5–15 mg/d at bedtime reduced secretions by 44% in one study (n = 14, open, Spivak et al, Int Clin Psychopharmacol 1997;**12**:213–5; n=1, Aggarwal et al, Indian J Med Sci 2009;**63**:470-1). Trihexyphenidyl plus terazosin 2 mg/d (Reinstein et al, Clin Drug Invest 1999;**17**:97–102) may be better than either drug alone. **Biperiden** was superior to placebo (but not as good as glycopyrrolate) but significantly reduced MMSE scores (RCT, d/b, c/o, 3x4/52, Liang et al, Schizophr Res 2010;**119**:138–44).
- **Botulinum toxin** (injected into the parotid gland) has been used successfully (n = 9, p/c, 16/52, Steinlechner et al, Psychopharmacology (Berl) 2010;**207**:593–7), although the evidence is weak (s = 6, Lim et al, Clin Otolaryngology 2006;**31**:267–72).
- **Bupropion** has helped (n = 1, Stern et al, Prog Neuropsychopharmacol Biol Psychiatry 2009;**33**:1578–80).
- **Chewing gum** has been used to stimulate salivation and swallowing.
- **Clonidine** 50–100 mcg/d increases adrenergic tone and reduces patient-reported hypersalivation (wet area on pillow) without adverse effects (n = 12, open, 4/52, Parharaj et al, J Psychopharmacol 2005;**19**:426–8), although it might exacerbate depression and psychosis. Clonidine patches (0.1 mg/week) have been used.
- **Guanfacine** (Webber et al, J Clin Psychopharmacol 2004;**24**:675–6).
- **Ipratropium** (sublingually or intranasal spray) has limited efficacy (e.g. Freudenreich et al, J Clin Psychopharmacol 2004;**24**:98–100) and the only RCT showed no sublingual efficacy compared to placebo (n = 20, RCT, d/b, p/c, 6/52, Sockalingam et al, J Clin Psychiatry 2009;**70**:1114–9).
- **Lofexidine** 0.2 mg BD has been used as an alpha-2 agonist in the short-term (testing the theory that hypersalivation is due to clozapine's alpha-2 antagonism; n = 1, 1/12, Corrigan et al, Br J Psychiatry 1995;**167**:412; rebuttal of theory by Szabadi, Br J Psychiatry 1996;**169**:380–1).
- **Propantheline** 7.5 mg/d has been used.
- **Scopolamine** patches (Gaftanyuk and Trestman, Psychiatr Serv 2004; **55**:318).
- **Septoplasty** was dramatically successful in one patient with a deviated septum causing him to breathe through his mouth (n = 1, Conry et al, Am J Psychiatry 1996;**153**:444).

Reviews: general (Praharaj et al, Psychopharmacol [Berl] 2006;**185**:265–73; Freudenreich, Drugs Today [Barc] 2005;**41**:411–8).

6

Tremor (see also EPSE, Parkinsonism)

Lithium   **Dose reduction** is appropriate since tremor is dose/plasma level related.
Beta-blockers are standard therapy, e.g. **propranolol** 30–40 mg/d (n = 5, Lapierre, *Can Med Assoc J* 1976; **114**:619–20), **metoprolol** (comparison with propranolol, Zubenko *et al*, *Psychiatry Res* 1984; **11**:163–4), **atenolol** and **nadolol** (for a hepatically-compromised patient; n = 1, Dave and Langbart, *Ann Clin Psychiatry* 1994; **6**:51–2).
Pregabalin (n = 1, Marks *et al*, *Int J Neuropsychopharmacol* 2008; **11**:879–81).
Vitamin B6 900–1200 mg/d was completely effective in 80% patients (open, n = 5, Miodownik *et al*, *Int J Psychiatr Med* 2002; **32**:103–8).
Linoleic acid is ineffective (Schou, *Prostaglandins Med* 1980; **5**:343–4; Anton, *Prostaglandins Med* 1980; **5**:321–2).
Review: Gelenberg and Jefferson, *J Clin Psychiatry* 1995; **56**:283–7.

Vomiting (see also nausea)

Valproate   Could be impending hepatic failure. Investigate immediately and discontinue if necessary.

PSYCHOTROPIC DRUGS

This section details currently and formerly available psychotropic drugs in the UK. The dates are rarely definitive. A drug may be licensed but not launched, it may be different in different countries, may be launched but not promoted, different salts or presentations may exist; medicines may be discontinued but not withdrawn, or there may be much stock left so continues to be used. Patents may exist for the drug, manufacturing process, different salts, presentation/formulation appearance, packaging or license. Patent extension or protection may be gained. The author would be grateful for any clarifications and corrections.

NAME (UK GENERIC, TRADE AND OTHERS)	UK LAUNCH	UK PATENT EXPIRY	UK STATUS	COMMENTS
Acamprosate (Campral EC®)	1996	Expired 2002	Available	
Acetazolamide (Diamox®)	1953	Expired	Available	
Agomelatine (Valdoxan®)	2009	February 2016	Available	
Alprazolam (Xanax®)	1983	Expired 1990	Available	Black list in UK
Amisulpride (Solian®)	1997	Expired 2001	Available	
Amitriptyline (Tryptizol®, Lentizol®)	1961 SR caps 1971	Expired	Available	SR caps discontinued 2000
Amobarbital (amylobarbital, amylobarbitone, Amytal®)	c1923	Expired	Tablets discontinued 2006 Injection 2000	Low use
Amoxapine (Asendis®)	1989	Expired	Discontinued 2006	Low use
Asenapine (Saphris®)	2012	February 2020	License applied	Available USA 2009
Aripiprazole (Abilify®)	2004 IM inj 2008	October 2014	Available	
Atomoxetine (Strattera®)	2004	2019	Available	
Beclamide (Nydrane®)	c1956	Expired	Discontinued 1987	Low use
Benperidol (Anquil®)	1973	Expired	Available	
Benzatropine, benztropine (Cogentin®)	1950s	Expired	Discontinued 2008	Injection available only, as UK import
Benzoctamine (Tacitin®)	1971	Expired	Discontinued 1983	Low use
Biperiden (Akineton®)	c1957	Expired	Discontinued 2003	Low use
Bromazepam (Centrax®)	1984	Expired	Discontinued 2002	Low use
Buprenorphine (Subutex®, Suboxone®, Temgesic®)	1980 (USA 2003) 1999 for SM	Expired 2006	Available	Suboxone 2007 (with naloxone)

Name	UK LAUNCH	UK PATENT EXPIRY	UK STATUS	Comments
Bupropion (Zyban®, Welbutrin®)	2000 (US 1985 for depression)	Expired 2009	Available	
Buspirone (Buspar®)	1987	Expired 2000	Available	
Butobarbitone (Sonergan®)	1931	Expired	Available	
Butriptyline (Evadyne®)	1975	Expired	Discontinued 1993	Low use
Carbamazepine (Tegretol®, Carbatrol®)	1962 (1965 for epilepsy), SR tabs 1989 Suppositories 1994	Expired	Available	
Chloral Hydrate (Noctec®)	1870s	Expired	Available	First synthesis 1832, first medical use 1869. Noctec capsules discontinued 1996
Chlordiazepoxide (Librium®)	1960	Expired	Available	Injection discontinued 1988
Chlormethiazole, clomethiazole (Heminevrin®)	First patent 1938 First used for DTs in 1959 Syrup 1972	Expired	Available	Infusion discontinued 2000 Syrup discontinued 2009
Chlormezanone (Trancopal®)	c1961	Expired	Withdrawn 1996 worldwide	Toxic epidermal necrolysis
Chlorpromazine (Largactil®, Thorazine®)	1954	Expired	Available	
Chlorprothixene (Taractan®)	1959	Expired	Discontinued 1987	Low use
Citalopram (Cipramil®, Celexa®)	1995 Drops 2000	Expired 2002	Available	
Citrated calcium carbimide (Abstem®)	1977	Expired	Discontinued 1984	Low use
Clobazam (Frisium®)	1979	Expired 1997	Available	
Clomipramine (Anafranil®)	1970	Expired	Available	Injection discontinued 2002, syrup 2001
Clonazepam (Rivotril®)	1974	Expired c1995	Available	
Clorazepate Dipotassium (Tranxene®)	1973	Expired c1988	Discontinued 2005	Lack of use
Clozapine (Clozaril®, Zaponex®, Denzapine®, Leponex®, Clopine®, Klozapol®, Faxaclo®)	1990 Suspension	Expired	Available	

Name	UK LAUNCH	UK PATENT EXPIRY	UK STATUS	Comments
Cyclobarbitone (Rapidal®, Phanodorm®)	c1920s	Expired	Discontinued 1988	Lack of use and toxicity
Deprol® (meprobamate and benactyzine)	1965	Expired	Discontinued 1970s	Low use
Desipramine (Pertofran®)	1963	Expired c1988	Discontinued 1997	Low use/toxicity
Dexamphetamine (dexamfetamine, dextroamphetamine) (Dexadrine®)	1937	Expired	Available	First synthesised 1887. Marketed 1932 for nasal congestion, as stimulant 1935 and Dexadrine® launched 1937
Diazepam (Valium®)	1963	Expired	Available	
Dibenzepine (Noveril®)	1970	Expired	Discontinued 1981	Low use
Dichloralphena-zone (Welldorm®)	1940s?	Expired	Discontinued 1992 (converted to chloral betaine)	Production problems
Disulfiram (Antabuse®)	1949 (1951 in USA)	Expired	Available	First synthesised 1881
Donepezil (Aricept®)	1997	Expires 13th Feb 2012	Available	
Dosulepin, dothiepin (Prothiaden®)	1969	Expired	Available	
Doxepin (Sinequan®, Adapin®)	1969	Expired	Available	
Droperidol (Droleptan®)	c1980	Expired	Withdrawn 2001	Due to QTc issues
Duloxetine (Cymbalta®, Yentrene®)	2004 for stress incontinence 2005 (depression)	Expires 2012	Available	Basic US patent expired 2008
Escitalopram (Cipralex®, Lexapro®)	2002	Expires May 2014	Available	
Eslicarbazepine (Zebinix®)	2009	2021	Available	
Ethosuximide (Zarontin®, Emeside®)	1982ish	Expired	Available	
Ethotoin (Peganone®)	1957	Expired	Discontinued 1985	Low use
Fencamfamin (Reactivan®)	c1965	Expired	Withdrawn 1986	Abuse and dependency
Fenfluramine (Ponderax®)	1968	Expired	Withdrawn 1997	Toxicity (deaths) and abuse
Flumazenil (Anexate®)	1988	Expired 2002	Available	

7

Name	UK LAUNCH	UK PATENT EXPIRY	UK STATUS	COMMENTS
Flunitrazepam (Rohypnol®)	1982	Expired	Withdrawn 1986	Abuse
Fluoxetine (Prozac®)	1989, Liquid 1992	Expired 2000	Available	
Flupentixol (Fluanxol®, Depixol®)	1965	Expired	Available	
Flupentixol decanoate (Depixol®)	1972 Low vol 1992	Expired	Available	
Fluphenazine decanoate (Modecate®)	1968	Expired	Available	
Fluphenazine enanthate (Moditen®)	1966	Expired	Discontinued 1991	Low use
Fluphenazine HCl (Moditen®)	c1967	Expired	Discontinued 2008	Low use
Flurazepam (Dalmane®)	1973	Expired	Available	
Fluspirilene (Redeptin®)	1975	Expired	Discontinued 1995	Low use, import in UK
Fluvoxamine (Faverin®, Luvox®)	1987	Expired 1996	Available	
Fosphenytoin (Pro-Epanutin®)	1998	Expired US 2007	Available	
Gabapentin (Neurontin®)	1993	Expired 2000	Available	
Galantamine (Reminyl®, Nivalin®, Razadyne®)	2000 Syrup 2003 XL 2004	Expires 15th January 2012	Available	
Glutethimide (Doriden®)	1954	Expired	Discontinued 1983	Low use
Haloperidol (Haldol®, Serenace®)	1959	Expired	Available	
Haloperidol decanoate (Haldon Decanoate®)	1982	Expired 2000	Available	
Heptabarbitone (Medomin®)	1950s?	Expired	Discontinued 1985	Low use
Hexobarbital (Citopan®)	c1940	Expired	Discontinued1960s	Low use
Hydergine® (codergocrine)	c1975	Expired	Discontinued 2005	Low use
Hydroxyzine (Atarax®, Vistaril®)	c1958	Expired	Available	
Imipramine (Tofranil®)	1959	Expired	Available	
Iprindole (Prondol®)	c1972	Expired	Discontinued 1995	Low use
Iproniazid (Marsilid®)	1958	Expired	Discontinued 1987	Low use
Isocarboxazid (Marplan®)	1959–60	Expired	Available	
Ketazolam (Anxon®)	1980	Expired	Discontinued 1990	Low use

NAME	UK LAUNCH	UK PATENT EXPIRY	UK STATUS	COMMENTS
Lacosamide (Vimpat®)	2008	2023	Available	
Lamotrigine (Lamictal®)	1991 Dispersible tablets 1994	Expired 2005	Available	
Levetiracetam (Keppra®)	2000 syrup 2005	Expired 2010	Available	
Levomepromazine/ methotrimeprazine (Nozinan®)	c1950s	Expired	Available	
Limbitrol® (amitriptyline and chlordiazepoxide)	c1966	Expired	Discontinued 1994	Low use
Lithium carbonate (Camcolit®, Priadel®, Liskonum®, Phasal®)	c1955 (first USA mania license in 1970) Priadel 1968 Liskonum 1980	Expired	Available	
Lithium citrate tablets (Litarex®)	1982	Expired	Discontinued 2001	Low use
Lofepramine (Gamanil®)	1983	Expired	Available	
Lofexidine (Britlofex®)	1992	Expired 2003	Available	
Loprazolam (Dormonoct®)	1983	Expired 1995	Available	
Lorazepam (Ativan®, Temesta®)	1971	1982	Available	
Lormetazepam (Noctamid®)	1980	Expired	Available	
Loxapine (Loxapac®)	1989	Expired 1996	Discontinued 2003	Low use
Maprotiline (Ludiomil®)	1975	Expired c1989	Discontinued 2005	Low use
Mazindol (Teronac®)	1960s (1973 USA)	Expired	Discontinued 1992	Low use
Meclofenoxate (Lucidril®)	1966	Expired	Discontinued 1982	Low use
Medazepam (Nobrium®)	1968	Expired	Discontinued 1994	Lack of use after black-listing
Memantine (Ebixa®, Axura®)	2002	Expires May 2014	Available	
Meprobamate (Equanil®)	1955	Expired	Discontinued 2002	Low use
Methadone (Physeptone®, Methadose®)	c1947 (as analgesic)	Expired	Available	First synthesised 1937
Methixene (Tremonil®)	1970s	Expired	Discontinued 1994	Low use
Methohexitone (Brietal®)	c1957	Expired	Discontinued 1999	Low use

7

Name	UK LAUNCH	UK PATENT EXPIRY	UK STATUS	Comments
Methoin (Mesontoin®)	1940s	Expired	Discontinued 1981	Low use
Methylphenidate (Ritalin®, Concerta®, Medikinet®, Equasym®, Daytrana®)	1954 (for fatigue and depressi on) Equasym 2000 Concerta 2002 Medikinet 2007	Expired	Available	First synthesised 1944, off market in mid-1980s, reintroduced 1995
Methylphenobarbitone (Prominal®)	1935	Expired	Discontinued 2001	Low use
Methyprylon(e) (Noludar®)	c1958	Expired	Discontinued 1989	Adverse effects and low use
Mianserin (Norval®, Bolvidon®)	1976	Expired	Available	
Midazolam (Hypnovel®)	1982	Expired 1995	Available	
Mirtazapine (Zispin®, Remeron®, Avanza®)	1997	Expired 2005	Available	
Moclobemide (Manerix®, Aurorix®)	1993	Expired 2002	Available	
Modafinil (Provigil®, Modavigil®)	1998	Expired 2003	Available	
Motipress® (fluphenazine 1.5mg and nortriptyline 30mg)	1976	Expired	Discontinued 2003	Low use
Motival® (fluphenazine 0.5mg and nortriptyline 10mg)	1973	Expired	Discontinued 2006	Low use
Naltrexone (Nalorex®, Opizone®, Revia®)	1988	Expired 2007	Available	
Nefazodone (Dutonin®)	1995	Expired 2007	Withdrawn 2002	Hepatic ADRs
Nialamide (Niamid®)	1950s	Expired	Discontinued 1970s	Low use
Nitrazepam (Mogadon®, Remnos®, Somnite®)	1965	Expired	Available	
Nomifensine (Merital®)	1977	Expired	Withdrawn worldwide 1986	Haemolytic anaemia
Nortriptyline (Allegron®, Aventyl®, Pamelor®)	1963	Expired c1988	Available	
Olanzapine (Zyprexa®, Zalasta®, Zolafren®)	1996 Velotabs 2001 IM injection 2005 Depot 2010	Expired Sept 2011	Available	

Name	UK LAUNCH	UK PATENT EXPIRY	UK STATUS	Comments
Olanzapine pamoate/embonate (Zypadhera®)	2010	-	Available	
Opipramol (Insidon®)	1970s	Expired	Discontinued 1981	Available in Germany
Orphenadrine (Disipal®, Norflex®, Biorphen®)	c1951	Expired	Available	Injection discontinued 1990
Oxazepam (Serenid®)	c1965	Expired c1987	Available	
Oxcarbazepine (Trileptal®)	2000	Expired 2000	Available	
Oxprenolol (Trasicor®)	c1968 1983 for anxiety	Expired	Available	
Oxypertine (Integrin®)	c1950s	Expired	Discontinued 2002	Low use
Paliperidone (Invega®)	2007	2014	Available	
Paliperidone palmitate (Xeplion®, Invega Sustenna®)	2011	2018	Available	
Paraldehyde	First used as AED in 1882	Expired	Discontinued UK 2009	Available as special only in UK
Paramethadione (Paradione®)	1970s?	Expired	Discontinued UK 1984	Low use
Paroxetine (Seroxat®, Aropax®, Paxil®)	1991 (liquid 1997)	Expired 2006	Available	
Parstelin® (tranylcypromine 10mg, trifluoperazine 1mg)	<1964	Expired	Discontinued 1999	Low use
Pemoline (Volital®, Kethamed®, Ronyl®)	1975 in USA	Expired	Withdrawn 1997	Withdrawn worldwide 2005 due to liver toxicity
Pentobarbital (Nembutal®)	c1919	Expired	Discontinued 1986	Low use
Pericyazine (Neulactil®)	1966	Expired	Available	
Perphenazine (Fentazin®, Triafon®)	1957	Expired 1987	Available	Injection discontinued 1990
Phenelzine (Nardil®)	1959–60	Expired	Available	
Phenobarbitone sodium (Gardenal®)	1912	Expired	Available	
Phenytoin (Epanutin®, Dilantin®)	1938	Expired	Available	
Pimozide (Orap®)	1971	Expired	Available	
Pipothiazine (Piportil®)	1983	Expired	Available	
Piracetam (Nootropil®)	1992	Expired	Available	
Pramindole	1968	Expired	Discontinued 1981	Low use

7

Name	UK LAUNCH	UK PATENT EXPIRY	UK STATUS	COMMENTS
Prazepam (Centrax®)	1982	Expired c1988 in US	Discontinued 1988	Lack of use after black-listing
Pregabalin (Lyrica®)	2004 (epilepsy) 2007 (GAD)	Expires 2018	Available	
Primidone (Mysoline®)	1952	Expired	Available	Suspension discontinued 2000
Prochlorperazine (Stemetil®, Buccastem®)	1950s	Expired	Available	
Procyclidine (Kemadrin®)	1951 UK	Expired	Available	
Promazine (Sparine®)	1955	Expired	Available	
Promethazine (Phenergan®)	c1951 (USA)	Expired	Available	OTC in UK from 1985
Propranolol (Inderal®)	1965 1973 (anxiety)	Expired	Available	
Protriptyline (Concordin®)	1967	Expired	Discontinued 2000	Low use
Quetiapine (Seroquel®)	1997, 2009 (bipolar) 2009 XL Bipolar depression 2010	Expires 2012	Available	
Reboxetine (Edronax®)	1997	Expired 2004	Available	
Remoxipride (Roxiam®)	1990	Expired	Suspended 1993, withdrawn 1994	Aplastic anaemia
Risperidone (Risperdal®, Ridal®, Sizodon®)	1993 Quicklets 2003 Consta 2002	Expired 2007 Consta expires 2014	Available	
Rivastigmine (Exelon®)	1998, liquid 2001 Patches 2007	July 2012	Available	
Secobarbital (Seconal sodium)	1934	Expired	Discontinued 2009	Was quinalbarbitone
Sertindole (Serdolect®, Serlect®)	1996	Expired March 2011	Discontinued UK 2010	Voluntarily withdrawn 1998, reintroduced 2003 on named-patient basis only. Launched Australia 2011
Sertraline (Lustral®, Zoloft®)	1991	Expired 2005	Available	
Sodium oxybate (Xyrem®)	2006	2019 (USA)	Available	

Name	UK LAUNCH	UK PATENT EXPIRY	UK status	Comments
Sodium valproate (Epilim®, Episenta®, Depakene®)	1977 1988 injection 1993 Convulex 1994 Chrono	Expired	Available	
Sulpiride (Dolmatil®, Sulpitil®, Dogmatil®, Modal®)	1983	Expired	Available	
Sulthiame (Ospolot®)	c1965	Expired	Discontinued 1986	Low use
Tacrine (Cognex®)	Licensed 1997 in UK	Expired	Never marketed in UK	
Temazepam (Normison®, Euhypnos®, Restoril®)	1969	Expired	Available	
Tetrabenazine (Nitoman®, Xenazine®)	1950s	Expired	Available	
Thiopropazate (Dartalan®)	c1950s	Expired	Discontinued 1984	Low use
Thioproperazine (Majeptil®)	1950s	Expired	Discontinued 1981	Low use
Thioridazine (Melleril®, Mellaril®, Thoril®)	1958	Expired	Voluntarily withdrawn 2005 (liquids 2004)	Restricted due to QTc prolongation.
Thiothixene (Navane®)	1967	Expired	Discontinued c1980	Low use
Tiagabine (Gabitril®)	1998	Expired June 2011	Available	
Topiramate (Topamax®)	1995	Expired 2009	Available	
Tranylcypromine (Parnate®)	1959–60	Expired	Available	
Trazodone (Molipaxin®, Desyrel®, Trittico®)	1980 SR tabs 1992	Expired	Available	
Triazolam (Halcion®)	1978	Expired	License revoked 1993	Adverse effects
Triclofos sodium	1962	Expired	Discontinued 2010	Lack of availability of ingredient
Trifluoperazine (Stelazine, Eskazine®)	1958 Spansules 1967	Expired	Available	Injection discontinued 1995
Trifluperidol (Triperidol®)	1967	Expired	Discontinued 1981 Reintroduced c1986 Discontinued 1995	Low use
Trihexyphenidyl, benzhexol (Artane®)	c1955	Expired	Available	
Trimipramine (Surmontil®)	1966	Expired c1988	Available	

7

Triptafen® preps (perphenazine + amitriptyline	1970s	Expired	Available	
Troxidone (Triodone®)	1960s	Expired	Withdrawn 1985	Toxicity (especially teratogenicity) and low use
Tryptophan (Optimax®, Pacitron®)	Available as food supplement Licensed for depression Optimax® 1971, Pacitron® 1976	Expired	Available	Discontinued 1990 after reports of Eosinophilia Myalgia Syndrome. Reintroduced 1994
Tybamate (Solacen®)	1966	Expired	Discontinued 1970s	Low use
Valproate semisodium (Depakote®)	2000	Expired 2008	Available	
Valproic acid (Convulex®)	1993	Expired	Available	
Venlafaxine (Efexor®, Effexor®, Foraven®, Polirid®)	1995	Expired 2008 XL expiry 2012	Available	
Vigabatrin (Sabril®)	1989	Expired 2001	Available but restricted	
Viloxazine (Vivalan®)	1974	Expired	Discontinued 2000	Low use and toxicity
Zaleplon (Sonata®)	2000	Expired 2011	Available	
Zimelidine (Zelmid®)	1982	Expired	Withdrawn 1983	Guillaine-Barré syndrome
Ziprasidone (Zeldox®, Geodon®)	Licensed but never launched	N/K	Never launched in UK	SPC restrictions made non-viable
Zolpidem (Stilnoct®, Ambien®)	1994	Expired 2002	Available	
Zonisamide (Zonegran®)	2005	Expired 2008	Available	
Zopiclone (Zimovane, Imovane®)	1999	Expired 1993	Available	
Zotepine (Zoleptil, Nipolept®)	1998	Expired	Discontinued December 2010	Japan since 1982
Zuclopenthixol acetate (Clopixol Acuphase®)	1990	Expired	Available	Clopenthixol until 1985
Zuclopenthixol decanoate (Clopixol®)	1978	Expired	Available	Clopenthixol until 1985
Zuclopenthixol oral (Clopixol®, Cisordinol®)	1982	Expired 1994	Available	Clopenthixol until 1985

NEW DRUGS EXPECTED

Name, trade name and manufacturer	Details
Aripiprazole IM depot injection (Abilify®) *	Aripiprazole IM depot is a lyophilised cake that when reconstituted with water forms an injectable monthly suspension. The major phase III trial as maintenance for schizophrenia was terminated early (in 2010) due to meeting efficacy criteria ahead of schedule. It may thus be launched in Europe and UK earlier than expected.
Armodafinil (Nuvigil®, Cephalon) *	Armodafinil is the r-enantiomer of modafinil, presumably with similar effects but a longer half-life (12–15 hours). For excessive sleepiness in sleep apnea and comorbid depression (n = 249, RCT, d/b, p/c, Krystal et al, J Clin Psychiatry 2010;**71**:32–40). Approved USA 2007. Phase III studies underway in 2011 as an adjunct in bipolar depression.
Bapineuzumab (Pfizer) *	An IV or SC anti-beta-amyloid monoclonal antibody being trialled for a positive effect on removing plaques, although the potential for meningitis and oedema is a current limitation. Phase III planned. Inconclusive phase 2 trial as ability to slow disease progression, and vasogenic oedema appears dose-limiting and potentially severe (n = 234, 78/52, Salloway et al, Neurology 2009;**73**:2061–70). FDA considering application in Q2 2011. Reviews (Panza et al, Immunotherapy 2010;**2**:767–82; Kerchner and Boxer, Expert Opin Biol Ther 2010;**10**:1121–30).
Blonanserin (Lonasen®, Dainippon) *	Blonanserin is a D2 and 5HT antagonist antipsychotic and has been compared successfully to haloperidol (n = 307, d/b, p/c, RCT, 6/52, Garcia et al, CNS Drugs 2009;**23**:615–25). Launched 2010 in Japan and Korea.
Brivaracetam (Rikelta®, UCB) *	In phase III for partial-onset seizures and myoclonic seizures, and is related to levetiracetam. FDA and EMA granted orphan drug status for myoclonus. **Review:** Malawska and Kulig, Expert Opin Investig Drugs 2008;**17**:361–9
Buprenorphine implants	Early US study showing a possible relapse prevention effect, overcoming poor adherence and the diversion potential (n = 163 [c = 88], RCT, d/b, p/c, 24/52, Ling et al, JAMA 2010;**304**:1576–83). No European trials or marketing at moment.
Cariprazine (Forest and Gedeon Richter)	Orally active potent D3/D2 partial agonist, with low potency for other receptors, in Phase III in USA for schizophrenia and mania, although a Phase II for bipolar depression was promising. **Review:** use in schizophrenia, bipolar mania and depression (Gründer, Curr Opin Investig Drugs 2010;**11**:823–32).
Carisbamate (Comfyde®, J&J) *	Novel neuromodulator in phase III for epilepsy (Kulig and Malawska, Idrugs 2007;**10**:720–7; safe in elderly; n = 48, RCT, d/b, p/c, Levy et al, Epilepsy Res 2008;**79**:22–30). Status unclear; license declined by FDA (2009).
Desvenlafaxine (Pristiqs®, Pfizer) *	Metabolite of venlafaxine, for depression, anxiety and non-hormonal vasomotor symptoms associated with menopause. Launched USA in 2008 for depression, see Chapter 1 (depression, unlicensed)
Dimebolin (Dimebon, Pfizer and Medivation) *	Dimebolin (also known as latrepirdine) is a neuroprotective for Alzheimer's and Huntington's diseases. It is also an antihistamine, but seems to work via mitochondria. UK license possible 2012. It is effective for mild-to-moderate Alzheimer's (n = 183, RCT, d/b, p/c, 26/52, Doody et al, Lancet 2008;**372**:207–15; review as novel neuroprotector and cognitive enhancer (n = 14, open, Bachurin et al, Ann N Y Acad Sci 2001;**939**:425–35; also Sachdeva and Burns, CNS Neurosci Ther 2011;**17**:199–205).

7

NAME, TRADE NAME AND MANUFACTURER	DETAILS
Docosahexaenoic acid	An omega-3 fatty acid supplement, in phase III for Alzheimer's (2008).
Guanfacine (Tenex®, Intuniv®, Shire)	An alpha-2-adrenoceptor agonist for ADHD (and hypertension). Closes HCN channels when binding to alpha-2 receptors, which enhances dopamine and other transmitters. This is similar to clonidine but appears more specific to the pre-frontal cortex. It seems effective in combination with methylphenidate, especially in partial responders. Approved in USA 2009, UK trials underway.
Iloperidone (Zomaril®, Fanapt®, Novartis/Vanda) *	Iloperidone is an antagonist of NA-alpha2C, D2, D3, 5HT1A and 5HT6 receptors approved in USA for schizophrenia. Its high alpha(1)-adrenoceptors affinity can lead to haemodynamic adverse effects (Bishara and Taylor, Drugs 2008;**68**:2269–92). A monthly depot being investigated. It is effective for schizophrenia (s = 3, n = 1943, RCT, d/b, p/c, 6/52, J Clin Psychopharmacol 2008;**28**[Suppl 1]:S4–11; Citrome, Int J Clin Pract 2009;**63**:1237–48; s = 3, n = 1644 [c = 1326], RCT, d/b, Kane et al, J Clin Psychopharmacol 2008;**28**[2 Suppl 1]:S29–35; s = 3, n = 1943, RCT, d/b, p/c, 6/52, Potkin et al, J Clin Psychopharmacol 2008;**28**[2 Suppl 1]:S4–1).
Indiplon MR® (Neurocrine Biosciences/Pfizer) *	Quick-acting GABA-A modulator for transient sleep disorders. Approvable in USA subject to more trials (2008), but development appears to have been discontinued. Has been used for post-bedtime dosing in people with difficulty maintaining sleep (n = 264, RCT, d/b, p/c, 4/52, Roth et al, Sleep 2007;**30**:1731–8) and in the elderly (n = 358, RCT, d/b, p/c, 2/52, Walsh et al, Sleep Med 2007;**8**:753–9).
Leuprolide acetate or leuprorelin (Lupron®, Eligard®, Pfizer) *	Licensed for prostate cancer but now in phase III for Alzheimer's disease (2010), although ADRs are a problem. **Review:** Wilson et al, Expert Opin Investig Drugs 2007;**16**:1851–63.
Lisdexamfetamine dimesylate (Vyvance®, Shire) *	Vyvance is lisdexamphetamine, which is dexamfetamine bound to the amino acid, l-lysine and is a long-acting pro-drug of d-amfetamine. It is inactive until metabolised in the GI tract but mostly metabolised in the blood, releasing d-amphetamine, reducing the abuse potential in people with a history of stimulant abuse. It is licensed in USA and Canada since 2009 for ADHD, including adults (n = 36, Jasinski and Krishnan, J Psychopharmacol 2009;**23**:419–27). 2012 launch in UK possible. **Reviews:** Weber and Siddiqui, CNS Drugs 2009;**23**:419–25; Cowles, Ann Pharmacother 2009;**43**:669–76; Najib, Clin Ther 2009;**31**:142–76.
Loxapine nasal spray (Staccato) *	Loxapine nasal spray has undergone phase III trials for acute agitation in mania and schizophrenia. The hand-held single-dose inhalator received a negative opinion from FDA in early 2011.
Lurasidone (Latuda®, Dainippon/Takeda) *	Lurasidone blocks D2, 5HT7, 5HT2A, 5HT1A and alpha2C recptors. It may be useful for memory impairment in schizophrenia. Phase III studies (e.g. PEARL 2) in schizophrenia have been positive. Launched US in February 2011. The dose is 40–120 mg/d and appears weight neutral. **Review:** Meyer et al, Expert Opin Investig Drugs 2009;**18**:1715–26.
Masitinib *	Tyrosine kinase inhibitor for Alzheimer's Disease. Phase II at present. Licensed in 2009 by EMA for cancer in animals.

NAME, TRADE NAME AND MANUFACTURER	DETAILS
Methylphenidate (Daytrana®, Shire)	Daytrana® is a daily patch with a nine-hour duration. Shire are doing an additional study to confirm efficacy. It appears as effective as oral methylphenidate (n = 282, RCT, d/b, p/c, 7/52, Findling et al, J Clin Psychiatry 2008;**69**:149–59).
Mifepristone (Corlux®, Mifegyne®, Exelgym) *	A glucocorticoid type-II receptor (GRII) antagonist and progesterone receptor antagonist for depression and psychosis, approval awaited in USA, and available in many European countries for endogenous hypercortisolism.
Naltrexone depot (Vivitrol®, Alkermes) *	Naltrexone extended-release depot suspension, licensed in USA as long-term relapse prevention in alcohol and opioid dependence. UK license delayed. **Review:** Swainston Harrison et al, CNS Drugs 2007;**21**:83–7.
Nalmefene (Revex®, Lundbeck) *	Nalmefene is an opioid antagonist related to naltrexone, being investigated for alcohol dependence. Targeted use may be viable (n = 403, RCT, d/b, p/c, 28/52, Karhuvaara et al, Alcohol Clin Exp Res 2007;**31**:1179–87). 2012 launch in UK possible.
Nemonapride (Emilace®, Yamanouchi) *	Nemonapride is a D2/D3 receptor antagonist similar in structure to sulpiride, which has been available in Japan since 1991 (Bishara and Taylor, Drugs 2008;**68**:2269–92).
Nicergoline (Sermion®, Farmitalia) *	In phase III studies for Alzheimer's disease, and may help protect cells against beta-amyloid toxicity (Caraci et al, Brain Res 2005;**1047**:30–7). Available in many countries.
Ramelteon (Rozerem®, Takeda) *	Ramelteon is an MT1, MT2 and MT3 receptor agonist marketed for insomnia, with no abuse potential in previous sedative abusers, even at massive doses (n = 14, d/b, p/c, c/o, 18/7, Johnson et al, Arch Gen Psychiatry 2006;**63**:1149–57). It is available in USA, but the European license application has been withdrawn. **Review:** Pandi-Perumal et al, Nat Clin Pract Neurol 2007;**3**:221–8.
Retigabine (Trobalt®, GSK/ Valeant) *	Retigabine is a neuronal KCNQ/Kv7 potassium channel opener, licensed by EMEA in April 2011, as adjunctive therapy (n = 399 [c = 279], RCT, d/b, 16/52, Porter et al, Neurology 2007;**68**:1197–204) to treat adult epilepsy patients with partial-onset seizures (failed neuropathic pain trials).
Rolipram *	This MAOI/PDE-4 inhibitor is licensed in some countries for depression, but as it is also an antiflammatory it is being investigated for Alzheimer's disease.
Rosiglitazone (Avandamet®, GSK) *	This thiazolidinedione is in phase III trials for a potential for delaying cognitive decline (n = 30, RCT, d/b, p/c, 6/12, Watson et al, Am J Geriatr Psychiatry 2005;**13**:950–8), especially in people with diabetes.
Selegiline Transdermal System (Emsam®, BMS) *	Selegiline Transdermal System (6–12 mg/24 hours) is licensed in USA for depression, with insomnia and application-site reactions the main adverse effects (n = 265, RCT, d/b, p/c, 8/52, Feiger et al, J Clin Psychiatry 2006;**67**:1354–61) and relapse prevention over a year in responders (n = 322, d/b, p/c, 52/52, Amsterdam and Bodkin, J Clin Psychopharmacol 2006;**26**:579–86).

7

Name, trade name and manufacturer	Details
Talnetant (GSK) *	Talnetant is an orally active NK3 antagonist, under phase II/III trials for schizophrenia. Development appears to have been discontinued.
Tasimelteon (Vanda) *	Tasimelteon is a melatonin agonist (VEC-162) acting on M1 and M2 receptors. Phase II and III studies have been successful (s = 2, n = 450, RCT, d/b, p/c, Rajaratnam *et al, Lancet* 2009;**373**:482–91). To be researched in MDD (phase III). It has been granted orphan drug status in USA for non-24-hour sleep/wake disorder. **Review:** (Hardeland, *Curr Opin Investig Drugs* 2009;**10**:691–701)
Tramiprosate (Alzhemed®, Neurochem) *	Phase III trials for Alzheimer's as an anti-amyloid protein agent were not successful (Wright, *Drugs Today [Barc]* 2006;**42**:291–8; see Santa-Maria *et al, Mol Neurodegener* 2007;**2**:17).
Vilazodone (Viibryd®) *	An SSRI and 5HT1A partial agonist antidepressant, with negligible affinity for other serotonin receptors and a rate of sexual side-effects and weight gain comparable to placebo. Main side-effects were diarrhoea (28.0% in treatment group versus 9.2% in placebo), nausea (23.4% versus 5.1%) and dizziness (8.5% versus 4.6%). Launched in USA 2011.
Zolpidem CR (Sanofi-Aventis)*	European development appears to have been discontinued.

INDEX

All the main psychotropic drugs are indexed according to their BNF or other main indications in *Chapter 1*, but obviously may appear elsewhere. In order to keep the index down to a manageable size, you are then referred to the index listing for that drugs chemical or therapeutic group. Individual drugs should be looked up under their drug group.

Abbreviations

FOR DETAILS OF STUDIES:
* = new or updated entry
n = number of patients
RCT = randomised controlled trial
d/b = double-blind
c/o = cross-over
o/p = out-patient
s/b = single blind (trial)
p/c = placebo-controlled
MS = manufacturer's study

OTHER ABBREVIATIONS:
AAPCD = American Academy of Pediatrics Committee on Drugs
ACh = acetylcholine
ACEI = ACE inhibitors
AD = Alzheimer's disease
ADHD = attention deficit hyperactivity disorder
ADD = attention deficit disorder
ADL = activities of daily living
ADME = absorption, distribution, metabolism and excretion
ADR = adverse drug reaction
AED = anti-epileptic drug
AFP = alpha-fetoprotein
AIMS = abnormal involuntary movement scale
AN = anorexia nervosa
APE = acute psychiatric emergency
APA = American Psychiatric Association
AWS = alcohol withdrawal syndrome
BAP = British Association for Psychopharmacology
BD = twice a day
BDD = body dysmorphic disorder
BDI = Beck Depression Inventory

BDZ = benzodiazepine(s)
BMA = British Medical Association
BMI = body mass index
BNF = British National Formulary
BPD = borderline psychiatric disorder
BPRS = Brief Psychiatric Rating Scale
BPSD/BPSSD = behavioural and psychological (signs and) symptoms of dementia
bp = blood pressure
BP = British Pharmacopoeia
CBT = cognitive behavioural therapy
CBZ = carbamazepine
CBZ-E = carbamazepine-epoxide
CCK = cholecystokinin
CGI = clinical global impression
ChEIs = cholinesterase inhibitors
CHD = coronary heart disease
CNS = central nervous system
CPK = creatinine phosphokinase
CSE = convulsive status epilepticus
CSM = Committee on the Safety of Medicines
CVAE = cerebrovascular adverse events
D1 = dopamine-1 (receptor)
D2 = dopamine-2 (receptor)
DA = dopamine
DDD = defined daily dose
DSM-IV = Diagnostic Statistical Manual IV
DT = delirium tremens
e/c = enteric-coated
ECG = electrocardiogram
ECT = electroconvulsive therapy

EBMH = Evidence-Based Mental Health (Journal)
EEG = electro-encephalogram
EPO = Evening primrose oil
EPSE = extra-pyramidal side-effects
FBC = full blood count
FDA = Federal Drug Agency
GABA = gamma-aminobutyric acid
GAD = generalised anxiety disorder
GB = Ginkgo Biloba
GFR = glomerular filtration rate
GTC = generalised tonic-clonic (seizure)
HAL-PRO - haloperidol + promethazine
5-HT = 5-hydroxytryptamine
HF = heart failure
IED = intermittent explosive disorder
IV = intravenous
IM = intramuscular
INR = international normalised ratio
IPT = interpersonal therapy
ISE = ion-selective electrode
ITT = intention to treat
L/A = long-acting
LD = low dose
LFT = liver function tests
LTG = lamotrigine
MAOI = mono-amine oxidase inhibitor
MCM = major congenital malformations
MDD = major depressive disorder
MHRA = Medicines and Healthcare products Regulatory Agency (was CSM/MCA)
MI = manufacturers' information
MMSE = Mini-mental state examination

MS = mood stabiliser
NA = noradrenaline
NCSE = non-convulsive status epilepticus
NE = norepinephrine
NICE = National Institute for Clinical Excellence
N/K = not known
NMDA = N-methyl-D-aspartate receptor
NMS = neuroleptic malignant syndrome
NPI = Neuropsychiatric Inventory
NNH = numbers needed to harm
NNT = numbers needed to treat
NPSA = National Patient Safety Agency
NSAIDs = non-steroidal anti-inflammatory drugs
OCD = obsessive-compulsive disorder
O/C = oral contraceptive
OD = overdose
OFC = olanzapine-fluoxetine combination
OTC = over-the-counter (medicine)
PD = personality disorder

Pro-drug
PMH = previous medical history
PMS = pre-menstrual syndrome
PPHN = persistent pulmonary hypertension in the newborn
PT = prothrombin time
PTSD = post-traumtic stress disorder
PUFA = polyunsaturated fatty acid
QoLS = Quality of Life Scale
QTc = corrected QT interval
REM = rapid eye movement
RIMA = reversible inhibitor of monoamine-A
RPSGB = Royal Pharmaceutical Society
RT = rapid tranquillisation Society of Great Britain
RT = rapid tranquillisation
SA = short-acting
SAD = seasonal affective disorder
s/c = subcutaneous
SDS = Severity of Dependence scale
SF = sugar-free
SFQ = sexual functioning questionnaire

SIB = self-injurious behaviour
SIDS = sudden infant death syndrome
SJW = St John's wort
SPC = summary of product characteristics
SSRI = serotonin-selective reuptake inhibitor
STEP-BD = systematic treatment enhancement program for bipolar disorder
SUD = substance use disorders
t½ = half life
TCA = tricyclic antidepressant
TD = tardive dyskinesia
TDM = therapeutic drug monitoring
TEAEs = treatment emergent adverse events
THC = tetrahydrocannabinol
TIA = transient ischaemic attack
TRS = treatment-resistant schizophrenia
U&E = urea and electrolytes
USP = United States Pharmacopoeia
VaD = vascular dementia
YMRS = Young Mania Rating scale